BATES'

Guide to
Physical
Examination
and History Taking

BATES'

Guide to
Physical
Examination
and History Taking

Eleventh Edition

Lynn S. Bickley, MD, FACP
Clinical Professor of Internal Medicine
School of Medicine
University of New Mexico
Albuquerque, New Mexico

Peter G. Szilagyi, MD, MPH
Professor of Pediatrics
Chief, Division of General Pediatrics
University of Rochester School of Medicine and Dentistry
Rochester, New York

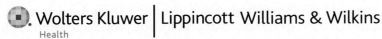
Wolters Kluwer | Lippincott Williams & Wilkins
Health
Philadelphia • Baltimore • New York • London
Buenos Aires • Hong Kong • Sydney • Tokyo

Acquisitions Editor: Elizabeth Nieginski/Susan Rhyner
Product Manager: Annette Ferran
Editorial Assistant: Ashley Fischer
Design Coordinator: Joan Wendt
Art Director, Illustration: Brett MacNaughton
Manufacturing Coordinator: Karin Duffield
Indexer: Angie Allen
Prepress Vendor: Aptara, Inc.

11th Edition

9 8 7 6 5 4 3 2 1

Printed in China

Library of Congress Cataloging-in-Publication Data

Bickley, Lynn S.
  Bates' guide to physical examination and history-taking.—11th ed./Lynn S. Bickley, Peter G. Szilagyi.
    p.; cm.
  Guide to physical examination and history-taking
  Includes bibliographical references and index.
  ISBN 978-1-60913-762-5 (hardback : alk. paper)
  I. Szilagyi, Peter G. II. Bates, Barbara, 1928–2002. Guide to physical examination and history-taking.
III. Title. IV. Title: Guide to physical examination and history-taking.
  [DNLM: 1. Physical Examination—methods. 2. Medical History Taking—methods. WB 205]
  616.07'54—dc23
                                                                2012029587

CCS0912

To

Randolph B. Schiffer,

for his lifelong care and support,
and to our students world-wide committed to clinical excellence.

Acknowledgments

For his ever-thoughtful insights into improving the examination of children and adolescents, we highlight the important contribution of Peter Szilagyi, MD, MPH, our pediatrics author, to *Chapter 18, Assessing Children: Infancy Through Adolescence* in our 11th edition of *Bates' Guide to Physical Examination and History Taking*. He has been a responsive and valued coauthor over the past three editions.

As with each edition, many experts across the nation enriched the 11th edition. We are grateful to two colleagues at the University of New Mexico School of Medicine: George Comerci, MD, Division of Integrative Medicine, an excellent internist and teacher, provided an intensive look at *Chapter 9, The Cardiovascular System;* and Carla Herman, MD, MPH, Chief of Geriatrics, suggested many useful updates for *Chapter 20, The Older Adult.* Andrew Dentino, MD, from Texas Tech University Health Sciences Center School of Medicine also lent enthusiastic comments to the text of *Chapter 20.* We appreciate the helpful revisions proposed by Susan Langer, MD, psychiatrist, which guided changes in *Chapter 3, Interviewing and the Health History,* and *Chapter 5, Mental Status and Behavior.* Ron Rapini, MD, from the University of Texas Health Sciences Center in Houston offered valuable suggestions for *Chapter 6, The Skin, Hair, and Nails,* as did Elaine Dannefer, PhD and Nancy Obuchowski, PhD, at the Cleveland Clinic in their reviews of *Chapter 2, Clinical Reasoning, Assessment, and Recording Your Findings.* Several contributors deserve special mention for enhancing the focus on women's health: Justina Trott, MD, from Women's Health Services in Santa Fe and the Robert Wood Johnson Center for Health Policy at the University of New Mexico, who facilitated a general women's health content review; Julie Craig, MD, MPH, also from Women's Health Services, who thoroughly updated *Chapter 19, The Pregnant Woman;* and Kim Templeton, MD, University of Kansas, who provided detailed scrutiny of *Chapter 16, The Musculoskeletal System.* Valuable contributors to *Chapter 9, The Cardiovascular System; Chapter 10, The Breasts and Axillae;* and *Chapter 14, Female Genitalia* include Annabelle Volgman, MD, Rush Heart Center for Women; Patricia Dawson, MD, PhD, Swedish Cancer Institute and the University of Washington School of Medicine; Janice Werbinski, MD, Borgess Women's Health and Michigan State University; and Dutima Batra, MD, Permanente Medical Group. Jennifer Pierce, MD, PhD, Women's Health Services in Santa Fe, assessed *Chapter 8, The Thorax and Lungs,* and also reviewed *Chapter 16.* Randolph Schiffer, MD displayed his customary excellence clarifying the challenging content in *Chapter 17, The Nervous System.*

We would also like to thank Michael Barone, MD, The Johns Hopkins University School of Medicine; Anne Gadomski, MD, Mary Imogene Bassett Center; Nancy Mogielnicki, Child Health Associate; Mark Craig; and multiple fellows and medical students for their excellent reviews of *Chapter 18, Assessing Children: Infancy Through Adolescence.*

As always, this book reflects the special talents and expertise of the publishing team at Wolters Kluwer/Lippincott Williams & Wilkins. Annette Ferran, Supervising Product Manager, tackled the innumerable details of editing each chapter and aligning content, layout, and illustration with perseverance and unflagging attention to excellence for both the 11th edition and *Bates Pocket Guide to Physical Examination and History Taking,* 7th edition. Chris Miller, Project Manager with Aptara, has brought meticulous care to every aspect of the book's production, ensuring its polished appearance and easy-to-follow format for students and teachers. Brett MacNaughton, Art Director, has overseen the valued integration of both photographs and illustrations with layout and text. Marcelo Oliver and Body Scientific International are responsible for the new, beautifully rendered illustrations in the 11th edition. We remain grateful to these people, as well as to the many staff members of Wolters Kluwer/Lippincott Williams & Wilkins who have contributed so much to the editions of this textbook over the decades.

Finally, for his invaluable and cheerful help answering requests for the hundreds of references reviewed for this new edition, we applaud Arthur Robinson, medical librarian at the Christus St. Vincent Regional Medical Center in Santa Fe.

Contents

List of Tables

Introduction

Bates' Guide to Physical Examination and History Taking is designed for students of health professions who are learning to talk with patients, to perform their physical examinations, and to apply clinical reasoning to understanding and assessing patient concerns. The 11th edition has many new features to facilitate student learning. As with previous editions, these changes spring from three sources: the queries and feedback of students and teachers; the goal of making the book easier to read and more efficient to use; and the abundant new evidence that underpins the techniques of interviewing, examination, and promoting health.

Bates' 11th helps students build on basic knowledge of human anatomy and physiology as they acquire the timeless skills of patient assessment. Throughout the Guide, we emphasize common or important problems rather than the rare and esoteric. Occasionally, physical signs of rare disorders are included if they hold a solid niche in classic physical diagnosis or represent a disorder that is critical to the life of the patient. Each chapter explicitly reflects a strong *evidence-based perspective*, listing key citations that closely align content with new evidence from the health care literature. Color helps readers find chapter sections and tables more easily, and highlights insets of key information and special tips for challenging aspects of examination such as examining the eye or assessing the jugular venous pressure. More than 200 new and revised photographs and drawings have been added to better illustrate key points in the accompanying text. All tables remain vertical so readers can page through the chapters more easily without turning the book to its side.

Bates' 11th: Special Highlights and Changes in Brief

The 11th edition features extensive new content, substantial revisions, and many new photos and illustrations to help students master the important skills of patient assessment. As in the past two editions, the 11th edition comprises three units: *Foundations of Health Assessment, Regional Examinations,* and *Special Populations.*

- *Unit 1, Foundations of Health Assessment. Chapter 1, Overview: Physical Examination and History Taking,* and *Chapter 2, Clinical Reasoning, Assessment, and Recording Your Findings,* follow a logical sequence that introduces students to the overall process of history taking and physical examination. Importantly, these chapters include how to sequence the examination and a case example of the written record for a comprehensive assessment and for an office progress note. Discussion and tables clarify the differences between subjective and objective data and between comprehensive and focused examinations. There are guidelines for ensuring a succinct and well-organized clinical record and how to analyze clinical data, as well as details about needed equipment and standard and universal precautions to minimize infection. *Chapter 2* explores the process of clinical reasoning and methods for assessing clinical data. *Chapter 3, Interviewing and the Health History*, has been reorganized to better lead students through the techniques of skilled interviewing. *Chapter 3* now contains sections on the Fundamentals of Skilled Interviewing; the Sequence and Context of the Interview, including the cultural context of the interview; Advanced Interviewing; and Ethics and Professionalism. Look for new content on motivational interviewing to help patients address health promotion through changing lifestyle and behaviors.

- *Unit 2, Regional Examinations.* This unit, spanning *Chapters 4* through *17*, again begins with the important general survey of the patient and techniques for accurate measurement of the vital signs in *Chapter 4*. This chapter provides evidence-based information on current guidelines for assessing obesity and nutrition and managing acute and chronic pain. Because assessment of mood, affect, and mental health begins at the outset of every patient encounter, *Chapter 5, Behavior and Mental Status* follows, with new information on personality disorders and the major mental health issues affecting our population.

Subsequent chapters are devoted to the techniques of regional examination for each of the body systems, with both updated and classic references documenting the value of physical examination. These chapters are arranged in a "head-to-toe" sequence, just as you would examine the patient. Each of these chapters contains:

- A review of relevant anatomy and physiology
- Key questions for pertinent health history
- Updated information useful for health promotion and counseling
- Well-described and well-illustrated techniques of examination
- Examples of the written record for the physical examination of that system
- Extensive citations from the clinical literature, and
- Tables to help students recognize and compare abnormalities in selected clinical conditions

Key features and revisions in the regional examination chapters are highlighted below.

- In *Chapter 5, Behavior and Mental Status,* readers will again find discussion of the often perplexing *Medically Unexplained Symptoms* and suggestions for recommended clinical approaches.

- In *Chapter 7, The Head and Neck*, the Anatomy and Physiology and Techniques of Examination sections for each of the component examinations for the Head, the Eyes, the Ears, the Nose, the Throat, and the Neck remain combined to facilitate student learning of the complex examination techniques involved.

- *Chapter 9, The Cardiovascular System*, is notable for extensive updates on Health Promotion and Counseling, featuring the challenges of attaining "ideal cardiovascular health," risks for special populations such as women and African Americans, steps for risk factor screening, and how to promote lifestyle and risk factor modification. In this chapter and *Chapter 8, The Thorax and Lungs*, look for new evidence-based guidelines that address tobacco cessation, adult immunizations for influenza and pneumonia, hypertension screening, and risk factor screening for cardiovascular disease, dyslipidemia, and metabolic syndrome.

- Likewise, in *Chapter 10, The Breasts and Axillae*, look for the similar updates on risk assessment for breast cancer, the Gail and Claus screening models, BRCA1 and BRCA2 mutations, and recommendations about mammography and clinical and breast self-examination.

- Other notable features include discussion of new screening guidelines for peripheral vascular disease, Pap smears, prostate cancer, colon cancer, and risk factors for stroke and new information on sexually transmitted infections.

- *Unit 3, Special Populations.* In this unit, *Chapters 18* through *20*, readers will again find chapters relating to special stages in the life cycle: infancy through adolescence, pregnancy, and aging. There is updated content throughout *Chapter 18, Assessing Children: Infancy Through Adolescence*, with a stronger focus on health promotion for children and adolescents. *Chapter 19, The Pregnant Woman*, has been thoroughly revised in this edition, with many new references. In *Chapter 20, Assessing the Older Adult*, there are updated guidelines for functional assessment and minimizing risk of falls and new discussion and tables on the cultural dimensions of aging. In conjunction with *Chapter 17, The Nervous System*, students will find a significant emphasis on differentiating delirium, dementia, and depression.

Suggestions for Students Using the Book

Although the health history and the physical examination are both essential for patient assessment and care, students often learn them separately, sometimes even from different faculty members. Students learning interviewing are advised to return to *Chapter 3, Interviewing and the Health History*, as they gain experience talking with patients of different temperaments and ages. As they develop a smooth sequence of examination, students may wish to review the sequence of examination outlined in *Chapter 1, Overview: Physical Examination and History Taking*. Students learning interviewing and physical examination over several months or even a year are encouraged to refer back to *Bates' 11th* regularly and use the book as a continuing guide to mastery of these time-honored skills of patient assessment.

As students begin integrating the patient's story with the patient's physical findings, we suggest that they study the related portions of the Health History as they learn successive areas of regional physical examination. Often, symptom clusters prompt examination of more than one body system. For example, chest pain prompts evaluation of both the thorax and lungs and the cardiovascular system. The symptoms of the urinary tract are relevant to the chapters on the abdomen, the prostate, and male and female genitalia.

Students may study and review the Anatomy and Physiology sections according to their individual needs. They can study Techniques of Examination to learn how to perform the relevant examination, practice it under faculty guidance, and review the Techniques section again afterward to consolidate their learning. Students and faculty will benefit from identifying common abnormal findings, which appear in two places. The right-hand column of the Techniques of Examination sections presents possible abnormal findings. These are highlighted in red and placed directly adjacent to the relevant text. Distinguishing abnormal from normal findings improves learners' observations and clinical acumen. For further information on abnormalities, readers also can turn to the Tables of Abnormalities at the end of each of the regional examination chapters. These tables display or describe various abnormal conditions in a convenient format that allows students to compare and contrast types of abnormalities in a single table.

As students progress through the body systems and regions, they should study the write-ups of the sample patient, Mrs. N, found in *Chapter 2, Clinical Reasoning, Assessment, and Recording Your Findings.* They should also refer frequently to the sections in each of the regional examination chapters entitled Recording Your Findings that display sample write-ups of the examination. This cross-checking will help students learn how to describe and organize information from the interview and physical examination into standard written format. Furthermore, understanding the precepts of *Chapter 2* will help students to select and analyze the data they are learning to collect.

Close scrutiny of the Tables of Abnormalities deepens student knowledge of important clinical conditions, what they should be looking for, and why they are asking certain questions. However, rather than memorize all the detail that is presented, students should return to the related physical signs and abnormalities whenever a patient, real or described, appears with a problem. Students should use this book to try to analyze the concern or finding, and make use of other clinical texts or journals to pursue the patient's problems in as much depth as necessary. The Citations and Additional References at the end of each chapter provide many additional references for further study.

During clinical rotations, as students deepen their skills of history taking and physical examination they should use the book as a guide to empathic listening and clinical mastery, with particular emphasis on the Examples of Abnormalities columns in red. These columns contain useful information on the clinical conditions pertinent to physical findings and, when available, their statistical significance.

Related Learning Material

As a companion to the 11th edition, we recommend *Bates' Pocket Guide to Physical Examination and History Taking, 7th edition*, by Lynn Bickley and Peter Szilagyi. The Pocket Guide is an updated, abbreviated version of this text, designed for portability, review, and convenience. The pocket guide does not stand alone; readers should refer to the text and illustrations of *Bates' Guide to Physical Examination and History Taking* whenever more comprehensive study and understanding is needed.

Bates' Visual Guide to Physical Examination is a comprehensive, highly informative series of 18 videos keyed to this text. Individual and sets of modules in a variety of formats are available from Lippincott Williams & Wilkins.

Footage from these videos focusing on Head-to-Toe Examination and Approach to the Patient is available on Lippincott's thePoint Web site, along with additional instructor and student resources.

Foundations of Health Assessment

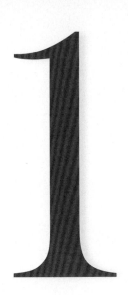

Overview: Physical Examination and History Taking

The techniques of physical examination and history taking that you are about to learn embody time-honored skills of healing and patient care. Gathering a sensitive and nuanced history and performing a thorough and accurate examination deepens your relationships with patients, focuses your assessment, and sets the direction of your clinical reasoning. The quality of your history and physical examination governs your next steps with patient assessment and guides your choices from among the initially bewildering array of secondary testing and technology. As you become an accomplished clinician, you will continually polish these important relational and clinical skills.

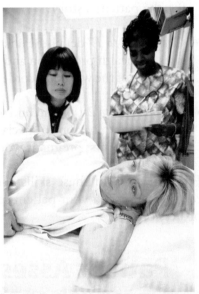

As you enter the realm of patient assessment, you begin integrating the essential elements of clinical care: empathic listening; the ability to interview patients of all ages, moods, and backgrounds; the techniques for examining the different body systems; and, finally, the process of clinical reasoning. Your experience with history taking and physical examination will grow, and will trigger the steps of clinical reasoning from the first moments of the patient encounter: identifying symptoms and abnormal findings; linking findings to underlying pathophysiology or psychopathology; and establishing and testing a set of explanatory hypotheses. Working through these steps will reveal the multifaceted profile of the patient before you. Paradoxically, the skills that allow you to assess all patients also shape the image of the unique human being entrusted to your care.

This chapter provides a guide to clinical proficiency in two critical areas: the *Health History* and the *Physical Examination*. It describes the components of the health history and how to organize the patient's story; it gives an overview of the physical examination with a sequence for ensuring patient comfort; and it provides brief descriptions of techniques of examination for each component of the physical examination, from the General Survey through the Nervous System. Chapter 2, Clinical Reasoning, Assessment, and Recording Your Findings, follows with the third area for proficiency—the written record, or "write-up," which contains the all-important *Assessment and Plan*. By studying the subsequent chapters and perfecting the

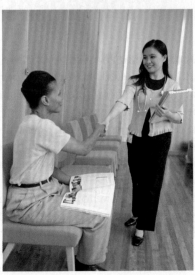

skills of examination and history taking described, you will move to active patient assessment, gradually at first, but then with growing confidence and expertise, and ultimately to clinical competence.

Included in each chapter are citations from the medical literature and pertinent further readings, so that you can continue to expand your knowledge. Beginning with Chapter 4, sections on Health Promotion and Counseling provide updated guidelines to help you promote and protect your patients' health and well-being.

- *Chapter 2, Clinical Reasoning, Assessment, and Recording Your Findings,* explores the steps of clinical reasoning and how to document your evaluations, diagnoses, and plans for patient care clearly and effectively. Your record sets the guideposts for the many members of the health care team.

- *Chapter 3, Interviewing and the Health History,* expands on the essential, varied, and often challenging skills of building patient rapport and eliciting the patient's story.

- *Chapters 4 to 17* detail the anatomy and physiology, health history, guidelines for health promotion and counseling, techniques of examination, and examples of the written record relevant to specific body systems and regions.

- *Chapters 18 to 20* extend and adapt the elements of the adult history and physical examination to special populations: newborns, infants, children, and adolescents; pregnant women; and older adults.

From mastery of these skills and the mutual trust and respect of caring relationships with your patients emerge the timeless rewards of the clinical professions.

Patient Assessment: Comprehensive or Focused

Determining the Scope of Your Assessment.   As you build your skills in taking the health history and performing the physical examination, you will face the question "How much should I do?" and ask "Should my assessment be comprehensive or focused?" For patients you are seeing for the first time in the office or hospital, you will usually choose to conduct a *comprehensive assessment*, which includes all the elements of the health history and the complete physical examination. Nevertheless, in many situations, a more flexible *focused* or *problem-oriented assessment* is appropriate, particularly for patients you know well who are returning for routine office care or for patients with specific "urgent care" concerns like sore throat or knee pain. You will adjust the scope of the history and physical examination to the situation at hand, keeping several factors in mind: the magnitude and severity of the patient's problems; the need for thoroughness; the clinical setting—inpatient or outpatient, primary or subspecialty care; and the time available. Mastery of all the components of a comprehensive assessment allows you to select the elements that are most pertinent to the patient's concerns yet meet clinical standards for best practice and diagnostic accuracy.

The History and Physical Examination: Comprehensive or Focused?

Comprehensive Assessment	Focused Assessment
▶ Is appropriate for new patients in the office or hospital	▶ Is appropriate for established patients, especially during routine or urgent care visits
▶ Provides fundamental and personalized knowledge about the patient	▶ Addresses focused concerns or symptoms
▶ Strengthens the clinician–patient relationship	▶ Assesses symptoms restricted to a specific body system
▶ Helps identify or rule out physical causes related to patient concerns	▶ Applies examination methods relevant to assessing the concern or problem as precisely and carefully as possible
▶ Provides baselines for future assessments	
▶ Creates platform for health promotion through education and counseling	
▶ Develops proficiency in the essential skills of physical examination	

As you can see, the *comprehensive examination* does more than assess body systems. It is a source of fundamental and personalized knowledge about the patient that strengthens the clinician–patient relationship. Most people seeking your care have specific worries or symptoms. The comprehensive examination provides a more complete basis for assessing these concerns and answering patient questions.

For the *focused examination*, you will select the methods relevant to thorough assessment of the targeted problem. The patient's symptoms, age, and health history help determine the scope of the focused examination, as does your knowledge of disease patterns. Of all the patients with sore throat, for example, you will need to decide who may have infectious mononucleosis and warrants careful palpation of the liver and spleen and who, by contrast, has a common cold and does not need this examination. The clinical reasoning that underlies and guides such decisions is discussed in Chapter 2.

What about the *routine clinical check-up*, or *periodic physical examination?* Numerous studies have scrutinized the usefulness of the comprehensive physical examination for the purposes of screening and prevention of illness, in contrast to evaluation of symptoms.[1–7] Findings have validated the importance of physical examination techniques: blood pressure measurement, assessment of central venous pressure from the jugular venous pulse, listening to the heart for evidence of valvular disease, detection of hepatic and splenic enlargement, and the pelvic examination with Papanicolaou smears. Various consensus panels and expert advisory groups have further expanded recommendations for examination and screening. A growing body of evidence documents the utility of many features of clinical assessment and techniques of examination.[8–11]

Subjective vs. Objective Data. As you acquire the techniques of history taking and physical examination, remember the important differences between *subjective information* and *objective information,* as summarized in the table below. Knowing these differences helps you cluster patient information. These distinctions are equally important for organizing written and oral presentations about patients into a logical and understandable format.

Differences Between Subjective and Objective Data

Subjective Data	Objective Data
What the patient tells you	What you detect during the examination
The history, from Chief Complaint through Review of Systems	All physical examination findings
Example: Mrs. G is a 54-year-old hairdresser who reports pressure over her left chest "like an elephant sitting there," which goes into her left neck and arm.	*Example:* Mrs. G is an older, overweight white female, who is pleasant and cooperative. Height 5′4″, weight 150 lbs, BMI 26, BP 160/80, HR 96 and regular, respiratory rate 24, temperature 97.5°F

Comprehensive Assessment of the Adult

THE COMPREHENSIVE ADULT HEALTH HISTORY

Overview. Below are the seven components of the *Comprehensive Adult Health History:*

- Identifying Data and Source of the History; Reliability

- Chief Complaint(s)

- Present Illness

- Past History

- Family History

- Personal and Social History

- Review of Systems

See Chapter 18, Assessing Children: Infancy Through Adolescence, for comprehensive pediatric health histories, pp. 765–891.

As you will learn in Chapter 3, Interviewing and the Health History, when you talk with the patient, the health history rarely emerges in this order. The interview is more fluid; you will closely follow the *patient's* cues to elicit the patient's narrative of illness, provide empathy, and strengthen rapport. You will quickly learn where to fit different aspects of the patient's story into the more formal format of the oral presentation and written record. You will transform the patient's language and story into the components of the health history familiar to all members of the health care team. This restructuring organizes your clinical reasoning and provides a template for your expanding clinical expertise.

As you begin your clinical journey, review the components of the adult health history, then study the more detailed explanations that follow.

Overview: Components of the Adult Health History

Identifying Data	▶ *Identifying data*—such as age, gender, occupation, marital status
	▶ *Source of the history*—usually the patient, but can be a family member or friend, letter of referral, or the medical record
	▶ If appropriate, establish *source of referral*, because a written report may be needed.
Reliability	▶ Varies according to the patient's memory, trust, and mood
Chief Complaint(s)	The one or more symptoms or concerns causing the patient to seek care
Present Illness	▶ Amplifies the *Chief Complaint;* describes how each symptom developed
	▶ Includes patient's thoughts and feelings about the illness
	▶ Pulls in relevant portions of the *Review of Systems,* called "pertinent positives and negatives" (see p. 10)
	▶ May include *medications, allergies,* and habits of *smoking* and *alcohol,* which are frequently pertinent to the present illness
Past History	▶ Lists childhood illnesses
	▶ Lists adult illnesses with dates for at least four categories: medical, surgical, obstetric/gynecologic, and psychiatric
	▶ Includes health maintenance practices such as immunizations, screening tests, lifestyle issues, and home safety
Family History	▶ Outlines or diagrams age and health, or age and cause of death, of siblings, parents, and grandparents
	▶ Documents presence or absence of specific illnesses in family, such as hypertension or coronary artery disease
Personal and Social History	Describes educational level, family of origin, current household, personal interests, and lifestyle
Review of Systems	Documents presence or absence of common symptoms related to each major body system

Initial Information

Date and Time of History. The date is always important. Be sure to document the time you evaluate the patient, especially in urgent, emergent, or hospital settings.

Identifying Data. These include age, gender, marital status, and occupation. The *source of history* or *referral* can be the patient, a family member or friend, an officer, a consultant, or the medical record. Designating the *source of referral* helps you to assess the type of information provided and any possible biases.

Reliability. Document this information if relevant. For example, "The patient is vague when describing symptoms, and the details are confusing." This judgment reflects the quality of the information provided by the patient and is usually made at the end of the interview.

Chief Complaint(s). *Make every attempt to quote the patient's own words.*

For example, "My stomach hurts and I feel awful." Sometimes patients have no specific complaints. Report their goals instead. For example, "I have come for my regular check-up" or "I've been admitted for a thorough evaluation of my heart."

Present Illness. This section of the history is a complete, clear, and chronologic account of the problems prompting the patient to seek care. The narrative should include the onset of the problem, the setting in which it has developed, its manifestations, and any treatments.

- Each principal symptom should be well-characterized, with descriptions of (1) location; (2) quality; (3) quantity or severity; (4) timing, including onset, duration, and frequency; (5) the setting in which it occurs; (6) factors that have aggravated or relieved the symptom; and (7) associated manifestations. These *seven attributes* are invaluable for understanding all patient symptoms. It is important to include "pertinent positives" and "pertinent negatives" from sections of the *Review of Systems* related to the *Chief Complaint(s)*. These indicate the presence or absence of symptoms relevant to the *differential diagnosis,* which identifies the most likely diagnoses explaining the patient's condition.

See Chapter 3, Interviewing and the Health History, pp. 55–102.

- Other information is frequently relevant, such as risk factors for coronary artery disease in patients with chest pain, or current medications in patients with syncope.

- The *Present Illness* should reveal the patient's responses to his or her symptoms and what effect the illness has had on the patient's life. Always remember, *the data flow spontaneously from the patient, but the task of oral and written organization is yours.*

- Patients often have more than one symptom or concern. Each *symptom* merits its own paragraph and a full description.

- *Medications* should be noted, including name, dose, route, and frequency of use. Also list home remedies, nonprescription drugs, vitamins, mineral or herbal supplements, oral contraceptives, and medicines borrowed from family members or friends. Ask patients to bring in all their medications so you can see exactly what they take.

- *Allergies*, including *specific reactions* to each medication, such as rash or nausea, must be recorded, as well as allergies to foods, insects, or environmental factors.

- Note *tobacco use*, including the type. Cigarettes are often reported in pack-years (a person who has smoked 1½ packs a day for 12 years has an 18-pack-year history). If someone has quit, note for how long.

- *Alcohol and drug use* should always be investigated. (Avoid restricting the *Personal and Social History* to these topics if you place them there.)

See Chapter 3, Interviewing and the Health History, for suggested questions, pp. 55–102.

Past History

- *Childhood illnesses*, such as measles, rubella, mumps, whooping cough, chickenpox, rheumatic fever, scarlet fever, and polio, are included in the *Past History*. Also included are any chronic childhood illnesses.

- Provide information relative to *Adult Illnesses* in each of four areas:

  - *Medical:* Illnesses such as diabetes, hypertension, hepatitis, asthma, and HIV; hospitalizations; number and gender of sexual partners; and risky sexual practices

  - *Surgical:* Dates, indications, and types of operations

  - *Obstetric/Gynecologic:* Obstetric history, menstrual history, methods of contraception, and sexual function

  - *Psychiatric:* Illness and time frame, diagnoses, hospitalizations, and treatments

- Cover selected aspects of *Health Maintenance*, especially immunizations and screening tests. For *immunizations,* find out whether the patient has received vaccines for tetanus, pertussis, diphtheria, polio, measles, rubella, mumps, influenza, varicella, hepatitis B, *Haemophilus influenzae* type B, pneumococci, and herpes zoster. For *screening tests,* review tuberculin tests, Pap smears, mammograms, stool tests for occult blood, colonoscopy and cholesterol tests, together with results and when they were last performed. If the patient does not know this information, written permission may be needed to obtain prior medical records.

Family History.
Under *Family History,* outline or diagram the age and health, or age and cause of death, of each immediate relative, including parents,

grandparents, siblings, children, and grandchildren. *Review each of the following conditions and record whether they are present or absent in the family:* hypertension, coronary artery disease, elevated cholesterol levels, stroke, diabetes, thyroid or renal disease, arthritis, tuberculosis, asthma or lung disease, headache, seizure disorder, mental illness, suicide, substance abuse, and allergies, as well as symptoms reported by the patient. Ask about any history of breast, ovarian, colon, or prostate cancer. Ask about any genetically transmitted diseases.

Personal and Social History. The *Personal and Social History* captures the patient's personality and interests, sources of support, coping style, strengths, and fears. It should include occupation and the last year of schooling; home situation and significant others; sources of stress, both recent and long-term; important life experiences, such as military service, job history, financial situation, and retirement; leisure activities; religious affiliation and spiritual beliefs; and activities of daily living (ADLs). Baseline level of function is particularly important in older or disabled patients. The *Personal and Social History* includes lifestyle habits that promote health or create risk, such as *exercise and diet,* including frequency of exercise, usual daily food intake, dietary supplements or restrictions, and use of coffee, tea, and other caffeinated beverages, and *safety measures,* including use of seat belts, bicycle helmets, sunblock, smoke detectors, and other devices related to specific hazards. Include any *alternative health care* practices.

See p. 931 for the ADLs frequently assessed in older patients.

You will learn to intersperse personal and social questions throughout the interview to make the patient feel more at ease.

Review of Systems. Understanding and using *Review of Systems* questions may seem challenging at first. These "yes-no" questions should come at the end of the interview. Think about asking a series of questions going from "head to toe." It is helpful to prepare the patient for the questions by saying, "The next part of the history may feel like a hundred questions, but it is important to make sure we have not missed anything." Most *Review of Systems* questions pertain to symptoms, but on occasion some clinicians include diseases like pneumonia or tuberculosis. Note that you may also draw on *Review of Systems* questions related to the Chief Complaint to establish "positives and negatives" that help clarify the diagnosis.

See Chapter 3, Interviewing and the Health History, for discussion of the role of pertinent positives and negatives in the differential diagnosis, p. 71.

Start with a fairly general question as you address each of the different systems. This focuses the patient's attention and allows you to shift to more specific questions about systems that may be of concern. Examples of starting questions are "How are your ears and hearing?" "How about your lungs and breathing?" "Any trouble with your heart?" "How is your digestion?" "How about your bowels?" Note that you will vary the need for additional questions depending on the patient's age, complaints, and general state of health and your clinical judgment.

The *Review of Systems* questions may uncover problems that the patient has overlooked, particularly in areas unrelated to the *present illness.* Significant health events, such as a major prior illness or a parent's death, require full exploration. Remember that *major health events should be moved to the Present Illness or Past History in your write-up*. Keep your technique flexible. Interviewing the patient yields findings that you organize into formal written format only after the interview and examination are completed.

Some clinicians do the *Review of Systems* during the physical examination, asking about the ears, for example, as they examine them. If the patient has only a few symptoms, this combination can be efficient. If there are multiple symptoms, however, the flow of both the history and the examination can be disrupted, and necessary note taking becomes awkward.

Listed below is a standard series of review-of-system questions. As you gain experience, the "yes or no" questions will take no more than several minutes. For each regional "system" you will ask: "Have you ever had any...?"

General: Usual weight, recent weight change, clothing that fits more tightly or loosely than before; weakness, fatigue, or fever.

Skin: Rashes, lumps, sores, itching, dryness, changes in color; changes in hair or nails; changes in size or color of moles.

Head, Eyes, Ears, Nose, Throat (HEENT): *Head:* Headache, head injury, dizziness, lightheadedness. *Eyes:* Vision, glasses or contact lenses, last examination, pain, redness, excessive tearing, double or blurred vision, spots, specks, flashing lights, glaucoma, cataracts. *Ears:* Hearing, tinnitus, vertigo, earaches, infection, discharge. If hearing is decreased, use or nonuse of hearing aids. *Nose and sinuses:* Frequent colds, nasal stuffiness, discharge, or itching, hay fever, nosebleeds, sinus trouble. *Throat (or mouth and pharynx):* Condition of teeth and gums, bleeding gums, dentures, if any, and how they fit, last dental examination, sore tongue, dry mouth, frequent sore throats, hoarseness.

Neck: "Swollen glands," goiter, lumps, pain, or stiffness in the neck.

Breasts: Lumps, pain, or discomfort, nipple discharge, self-examination practices.

Respiratory: Cough, sputum (color, quantity), hemoptysis, dyspnea, wheezing, pleurisy, last chest x-ray. You may wish to include asthma, bronchitis, emphysema, pneumonia, and tuberculosis.

Cardiovascular: "Heart trouble," high blood pressure, rheumatic fever, heart murmurs, chest pain or discomfort, palpitations, dyspnea, orthopnea, paroxysmal nocturnal dyspnea, edema, results of past electrocardiograms or other cardiovascular tests.

Gastrointestinal: Trouble swallowing, heartburn, appetite, nausea. Bowel movements, stool color and size, change in bowel habits, pain with defecation, rectal bleeding or black or tarry stools, hemorrhoids, constipation, diarrhea. Abdominal pain, food intolerance, excessive belching or passing of gas. Jaundice, liver or gallbladder trouble, hepatitis.

Peripheral vascular: Intermittent claudication; leg cramps; varicose veins; past clots in the veins; swelling in calves, legs, or feet; color change in fingertips or toes during cold weather; swelling with redness or tenderness.

Urinary: Frequency of urination, polyuria, nocturia, urgency, burning or pain during urination, hematuria, urinary infections, kidney or flank pain, kidney stones, ureteral colic, suprapubic pain, incontinence; in males, reduced caliber or force of the urinary stream, hesitancy, dribbling.

Genital: *Male:* Hernias, discharge from or sores on the penis, testicular pain or masses, scrotal pain or swelling, history of sexually transmitted infections and their treatments. Sexual habits, interest, function, satisfaction, birth control methods, condom use, and problems. Concerns about HIV infection. *Female:* Age at menarche, regularity, frequency, and duration of periods, amount of bleeding; bleeding between periods or after intercourse, last menstrual period, dysmenorrhea, premenstrual tension. Age at menopause, menopausal symptoms, postmenopausal bleeding. If the patient was born before 1971, exposure to diethylstilbestrol (DES) from maternal use during pregnancy (linked to cervical carcinoma). Vaginal discharge, itching, sores, lumps, sexually transmitted infections and treatments. Number of pregnancies, number and type of deliveries, number of abortions (spontaneous and induced), complications of pregnancy, birth-control methods. Sexual preference, interest, function, satisfaction, any problems, including dyspareunia. Concerns about HIV infection.

Musculoskeletal: Muscle or joint pain, stiffness, arthritis, gout, backache. If present, describe location of affected joints or muscles, any swelling, redness, pain, tenderness, stiffness, weakness, or limitation of motion or activity; include timing of symptoms (e.g., morning or evening), duration, and any history of trauma. Neck or low back pain. Joint pain with systemic features such as fever, chills, rash, anorexia, weight loss, or weakness.

Psychiatric: Nervousness, tension, mood, including depression, memory change, suicide attempts, if relevant.

Neurologic: Changes in mood, attention, or speech; changes in orientation, memory, insight, or judgment; headache, dizziness, vertigo, fainting, blackouts; weakness, paralysis, numbness or loss of sensation, tingling or "pins and needles," tremors or other involuntary movements, seizures.

Hematologic: Anemia, easy bruising or bleeding, past transfusions, transfusion reactions.

Endocrine: "Thyroid trouble," heat or cold intolerance, excessive sweating, excessive thirst or hunger, polyuria, change in glove or shoe size.

■ THE COMPREHENSIVE ADULT PHYSICAL EXAMINATION

Beginning the Examination: Setting the Stage

Before you begin the physical examination, take time to prepare for the tasks ahead. Think through your approach to the patient, your professional demeanor, and how to make the patient feel comfortable and relaxed. Review the measures that promote the patient's physical comfort and make any adjustments needed in the environment.

See Chapter 18, Assessing Children: Infancy Through Adolescence, for the comprehensive examination of infants, children, and adolescents, pp. 765–891.

Preparing for the Physical Examination

> ▶ Reflect on your approach to the patient.
> ▶ Adjust the lighting and the environment.
> ▶ Check your equipment.
> ▶ Make the patient comfortable.
> ▶ Choose the sequence of examination.

Reflect on Your Approach to the Patient. When first examining patients, feelings of insecurity are inevitable, but these will soon diminish with experience. Be straightforward. Identify yourself as a student. Appear calm, organized, and competent, even when you feel differently. Forgetting part of the examination is common, especially at first. Simply examine that area out of sequence, but smoothly. It is not unusual to go back to the bedside and ask to check one or two items that you might have overlooked.

Beginners need to spend more time than experienced clinicians on selected portions of the examination, such as the ophthalmoscopic examination or cardiac auscultation. To avoid alarming the patient, warn the patient ahead of time by saying, for example, "I would like to spend extra time listening to your heart and the heart sounds, but this doesn't mean I hear anything wrong."

Most patients view the physical examination with some anxiety. They feel vulnerable, physically exposed, apprehensive about possible pain, and uneasy about what the clinician may find. At the same time, they appreciate your concern about their problems and respond to your attention. With this in mind, the skillful clinician is thorough without wasting time, systematic without being rigid, gentle yet not afraid to cause discomfort should this be required. The skillful clinician examines each region of the body, and at the same time senses the whole patient, notes the wince or worried glance, and shares information that calms, explains, and reassures.

As a beginner, *avoid interpreting your findings.* You are not the patient's primary caregiver, and your views may be conflicting or wrong. As you grow in experience and responsibility, sharing findings will become more appropriate. If the patient has specific concerns, discuss them with your teachers before providing reassurance. At times, you may discover abnormalities such as an ominous mass or a deep oozing ulcer. Always avoid showing distaste, alarm, or other negative reactions.

Adjust the Lighting and the Environment.　Several environmental factors affect the caliber and reliability of your physical findings. To achieve superior techniques of examination, it is important to "set the stage" so that both you and the patient are comfortable. You will find that awkward positions impair the quality of your examination. Take the time to adjust the bed to a convenient height (but be sure to lower it when finished), and ask the patient to move toward you if this makes it easier to examine a region of the body more carefully.

Good lighting and a quiet environment make important contributions to what you see and hear but may be hard to arrange. Do the best you can. If a television interferes with listening to heart sounds, politely ask the nearby patient to lower the volume. Most people cooperate readily. Be courteous and remember to thank the patient as you leave.

Tangential lighting is optimal for inspecting structures such as the jugular venous pulse, the thyroid gland, and the apical impulse of the heart. It casts light across body surfaces that throws contours, elevations, and depressions, whether moving or stationary, into sharper relief. When light is perpendicular to the surface or diffuse, shadows are reduced and subtle undulations across the surface are lost. Experiment with focused, tangential lighting across the tendons on the back of your hand; try to see the pulsations of the radial artery at your wrist.

Check Your Equipment.　Equipment necessary for the physical examination includes the following:

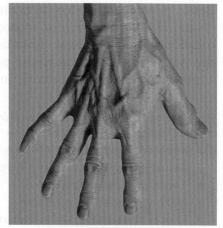

TANGENTIAL LIGHTING

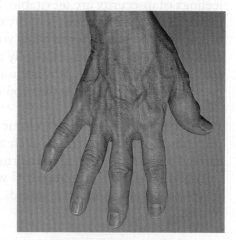

PERPENDICULAR LIGHTING

Equipment for the Physical Examination

▸ An ophthalmoscope and an otoscope. If you are examining children, the otoscope should allow for pneumatic otoscopy.
▸ A flashlight or penlight
▸ Tongue depressors
▸ A ruler and flexible tape measure, preferably marked in centimeters
▸ Often a thermometer
▸ A watch with a second hand
▸ A sphygmomanometer

(continued)

> ### Equipment for the Physical Examination (*continued*)
>
> ▶ A stethoscope with the following characteristics:
>   ▶ Ear tips that fit snugly and painlessly. To get this fit, choose ear tips of the proper size, align the ear pieces with the angle of your ear canals, and adjust the spring of the connecting metal band to a comfortable tightness.
>   ▶ Thick-walled tubing as short as feasible to maximize the transmission of sound: approximately 30 cm (12 inches), if possible, and no longer than 38 cm (15 inches)
>   ▶ A bell and a diaphragm with a good changeover mechanism
> ▶ Gloves and lubricant for oral, vaginal, and rectal examinations
> ▶ Vaginal specula and equipment for cytologic and perhaps bacteriologic study
> ▶ A reflex hammer
> ▶ Tuning forks, ideally one of 128 Hz and one of 512 Hz
> ▶ Q-tips, safety pins, or other disposable objects for testing sensation and two-point discrimination
> ▶ Cotton for testing the sense of light touch
> ▶ Two test tubes (optional) for testing temperature sensation
> ▶ Paper and pen or pencil, or desktop or laptop computer

Make the Patient Comfortable. Your access to the patient's body is a unique and time-honored privilege of your role as a clinician. Showing concern for privacy and patient modesty must be ingrained in your professional behavior. These attributes help the patient feel respected and at ease. Be sure to close nearby doors and draw the curtains in the hospital or examining room before the examination begins. Wash your hands carefully each time you examine a patient.

You will acquire the art of *draping the patient* with the gown or draw sheet as you learn each segment of the examination in the chapters ahead. *Your goal is to visualize one area of the body at a time.* This preserves the patient's modesty and helps you to focus on the area being examined. With the patient sitting, for example, untie the gown in back to better listen to the lungs. For the breast examination, uncover the right breast but keep the left chest draped. Redrape the right chest, then uncover the left chest and proceed to examine the left breast and heart. For the abdominal examination, only the abdomen should be exposed. Adjust the gown to cover the chest and place the sheet or drape at the inguinal level.

To help the patient prepare for potentially awkward segments of the examination, briefly describe your plans before starting. As you proceed with the examination, keep the patient informed, especially when you anticipate embarrassment or discomfort, as when checking for the femoral pulse. Try to gauge whether the patient wants to know about any of your findings. Is the patient curious about the lung findings or your method for assessing the liver or spleen?

Make sure your instructions to the patient at each step in the examination are courteous and clear. For example, "I would like to examine your heart now, so please lie down."

As in the interview, be sensitive to the patient's feelings and physical comfort. Watching the patient's facial expressions and even asking "Is it okay?" as you move through the examination often reveals unexpressed worries or sources of pain. To ease discomfort, it may help to adjust the slant of the patient's bed or examining table. Rearranging the pillows or adding blankets for warmth shows your attentiveness to the patient's well-being.

When you have completed the examination, tell the patient your general impressions and what to expect next. For hospitalized patients, make sure the patient is comfortable and rearrange the immediate environment to the patient's satisfaction. Be sure to lower the bed to avoid risk of falls and raise the bedrails if needed. As you leave, wash your hands, clean your equipment, and dispose of any waste materials.

Choose the Sequence of the Examination. It is important to recognize that *the key to a thorough and accurate physical examination is developing a systematic sequence of examination.* Organize your comprehensive or focused examination around three general goals:

- Maximize the patient's comfort.

- Avoid unnecessary changes in position.

- Enhance clinical efficiency.

In general, move from "head to toe." Avoid examining the patient's feet, for example, before checking the face or mouth. You will quickly see that some segments of the examination are best obtained while the patient is sitting, such as examination of the head and neck and of the thorax and lungs, whereas others are best obtained with the patient supine, such as the cardiovascular and abdominal examinations.

Often you will need to examine a patient *at bedrest,* especially in the hospital, where patients frequently cannot sit up in bed or stand. This often dictates changes in your sequence of examination. You can examine the head, neck, and anterior chest with the patient lying supine. Then roll the patient onto each side to listen to the lungs, examine the back, and inspect the skin. Roll the patient back and finish the rest of the examination with the patient again supine.

With practice, you will develop your own sequence of examination, keeping the need for thoroughness and patient comfort in mind. At first, you may need notes to remind you what to look for as you examine each region of the body, but with practice, you will acquire a routine sequence of your own. This sequence will become habit and remind you to return to a segment of the examination you may have skipped, helping you to be thorough.

For an overview of the physical examination sequence, study the following outline.

The Physical Examination: Suggested Sequence and Positioning

- General survey
- Vital signs
- Skin: upper torso, anterior and posterior
- Head and neck, including thyroid and lymph nodes
- *Optional:* nervous system (mental status, cranial nerves, upper extremity motor strength, bulk, tone, cerebellar function)
- Thorax and lungs
- Breasts
- Musculoskeletal as indicated: upper extremities
- Cardiovascular, including JVP, carotid upstrokes and bruits, PMI, S_1, S_2; murmurs, extra sounds
- Cardiovascular, for S_3 and murmur of mitral stenosis
- Cardiovascular, for murmur of aortic insufficiency
- *Optional:* thorax and lungs—anterior
- Breasts and axillae
- Abdomen
- Peripheral vascular
- *Optional:* skin—lower torso and extremities

- Nervous system: lower extremity motor strength, bulk, tone, sensation; reflexes; Babinski reflex
- Musculoskeletal, as indicated
- *Optional:* skin, anterior and posterior
- *Optional:* nervous system, including gait
- *Optional:* musculoskeletal, comprehensive
- *Women:* pelvic and rectal examination
- *Men:* prostate and rectal examination

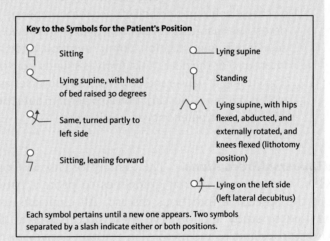

Key to the Symbols for the Patient's Position

- Sitting
- Lying supine, with head of bed raised 30 degrees
- Same, turned partly to left side
- Sitting, leaning forward
- Lying supine
- Standing
- Lying supine, with hips flexed, abducted, and externally rotated, and knees flexed (lithotomy position)
- Lying on the left side (left lateral decubitus)

Each symbol pertains until a new one appears. Two symbols separated by a slash indicate either or both positions.

Techniques of Examination

Focus on the more detailed description of the physical examination in the section following. Review the cardinal techniques of examination, sequencing and positioning for the examination, and the need for universal precautions.

Cardinal Techniques of Examination. Note that the physical examination relies on four classic techniques: inspection, palpation, percussion, and auscultation. You will see in later chapters that several maneuvers are also used to amplify physical findings, such as having the patient lean forward to better detect the murmur of aortic regurgitation or balloting the patella to check for joint effusion.

Cardinal Techniques of Examination

Inspection	Close observation of the details of the patient's appearance, behavior, and movement such as facial expression, mood, body habitus and conditioning, skin conditions such as petechiae or ecchymoses, eye movements, pharyngeal color, symmetry of thorax, height of jugular venous pulsations, abdominal contour, lower extremity edema, and gait.
Palpation	Tactile pressure from the palmar fingers or fingerpads to assess areas of skin elevation, depression, warmth, or tenderness, lymph nodes, pulses, contours and sizes of organs and masses, and crepitus in the joints.
Percussion	Use of the striking or *plexor finger*, usually the third, to deliver a rapid tap or blow against the distal *pleximeter finger*, usually the distal third finger of the left hand laid against the surface of the chest or abdomen, to evoke a sound wave such as resonance or dullness from the underlying tissue or organs. This sound wave also generates a tactile vibration against the pleximeter finger.
Auscultation	Use of the diaphragm and bell of the stethoscope to detect the characteristics of heart, lung, and bowel sounds, including location, timing, duration, pitch, and intensity. For the heart, this involves sounds from closing of the four valves and flow into the ventricles as well as murmurs. Auscultation also permits detection of bruits or turbulence over arterial vessels.

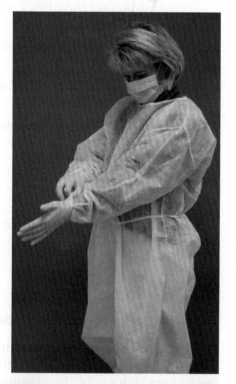

Standard and Universal Precautions.   The Centers for Disease Control and Prevention (CDC) have issued several guidelines to protect patients and examiners from the spread of infectious disease. All clinicians examining patients are advised to study and observe these precautions at the CDC Web sites. Advisories for standard and methicillin-resistant *Staphylococcus aureus* (*MRSA*) precautions and for universal precautions are summarized below.[12–15]

● *Standard and MRSA Precautions:* Standard Precautions are based on the principle that all blood, body fluids, secretions, excretions except sweat, nonintact skin, and mucous membranes may contain transmissible infectious agents. These practices apply to all patients in any setting. They include hand hygiene; when to use gloves, gowns, and mouth, nose, and eye protection; respiratory hygiene and cough etiquette; patient isolation criteria; precautions relating to equipment, toys, solid surfaces, and laundry handling; and safe needle-injection practices.

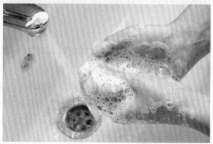

Be sure to wash your hands before and after examining the patient. This will show your concern for the patient's welfare and display your awareness of a critical component of patient safety. Antimicrobial fast-drying soaps are often within easy reach. *Change your white coat frequently,* because cuffs can become damp and smudged and transmit bacteria.

- *Universal precautions:* Universal precautions are a set of guidelines designed to prevent transmission of human immunodeficiency virus (HIV), hepatitis B virus (HBV), and other blood-borne pathogens when providing first aid or health care. The following fluids are considered potentially infectious: all blood and other body fluids containing visible blood, semen, and vaginal secretions; and cerebrospinal, synovial, pleural, peritoneal, pericardial, and amniotic fluids. Protective barriers include gloves, gowns, aprons, masks, and protective eyewear. All health care workers should *observe the important precautions for safe injections and prevention of injury from needlesticks, scalpels, and other sharp instruments and devices.* Report to your health service immediately if such injury occurs.

Scope and Positioning for the Examination. As you review the Techniques of Examination summarized on pp. 17–19, note that clinicians vary in where they place different segments of the examination, especially the examinations of the musculoskeletal system and the nervous system. Some of these options are indicated in red in the right-hand column.

As you develop your own sequence of examination, *an important goal is to minimize how often you ask the patient to change position* from supine to sitting, or from standing to lying supine. Some suggestions for patient positioning during the different segments of the examination are also indicated in the right-hand column in *red* throughout the book.

This book recommends examining the patient from the patient's right side, moving to the opposite side or foot of the bed or examining table as necessary. This is the standard position for the physical examination and has several advantages compared with the left side: estimates of jugular venous pressure are more reliable, the palpating hand rests more comfortably on the apical impulse, the right kidney is more frequently palpable than the left, and examining tables are frequently positioned to accommodate a right-handed approach.

Left-handed students are encouraged to adopt right-sided positioning, even though at first it may seem awkward. It still may be easier to use the left hand for percussing or for holding instruments such as the otoscope or reflex hammer.

Overview—The Physical Examination

Read carefully this "head-to-toe" sequence, the techniques for examining each region of the body, and how to optimize patient comfort and minimize changes in the patient position.

General Survey. Observe the patient's general state of health, height, build, and sexual development. Obtain the patient's weight. Note posture, motor activity, and gait; dress, grooming, and personal hygiene; and any odors of the body or breath. Watch the patient's facial expressions and note manner, affect, and reactions to people and things in the environment. Listen

This general survey continues throughout the history and examination.

to the patient's manner of speaking and note the state of awareness or level of consciousness.

Vital Signs. Measure the blood pressure. Count the pulse and respiratory rate. If indicated, measure the body temperature.

The patient is sitting on the edge of the bed or examining table. Stand in front of the patient, moving to either side as needed.

Skin. Observe the skin of the face and its characteristics. Assess skin moisture or dryness and temperature. Identify any lesions, noting their location, distribution, arrangement, type, and color. Inspect and palpate the hair and nails. Study the patient's hands. Continue your assessment of the skin as you examine the other body regions.

Head, Eyes, Ears, Nose, Throat (HEENT). ***Head:*** Examine the hair, scalp, skull, and face. ***Eyes:*** Check visual acuity and screen the visual fields. Note the position and alignment of the eyes. Observe the eyelids and inspect the sclera and conjunctiva of each eye. With oblique lighting, inspect each cornea, iris, and lens. Compare the pupils, and test their reactions to light. Assess the extraocular movements. With an ophthalmoscope, inspect the ocular fundi. ***Ears:*** Inspect the auricles, canals, and drums. Check auditory acuity. If acuity is diminished, check lateralization (Weber test) and compare air and bone conduction (Rinne test). ***Nose and sinuses:*** Examine the external nose; using a light and a nasal speculum, inspect the nasal mucosa, septum, and turbinates. Palpate for tenderness of the frontal and maxillary sinuses. ***Throat (or mouth and pharynx):*** Inspect the lips, oral mucosa, gums, teeth, tongue, palate, tonsils, and pharynx. *(You may wish to assess the cranial nerves during this portion of the examination.)*

The room should be darkened for the ophthalmoscopic examination. This promotes pupillary dilation and visibility of the fundi.

Neck. Inspect and palpate the cervical lymph nodes. Note any masses or unusual pulsations in the neck. Feel for any deviation of the trachea. Observe the sound and effort of the patient's breathing. Inspect and palpate the thyroid gland.

Move behind the sitting patient to feel the thyroid gland and to examine the back, posterior thorax, and lungs.

Back. Inspect and palpate the spine and muscles of the back. Observe shoulder height for symmetry.

Posterior Thorax and Lungs. Inspect and palpate the spine and muscles of the *upper* back. Inspect, palpate, and percuss the chest. Identify the level of diaphragmatic dullness on each side. Listen to the breath sounds; identify any adventitious (or added) sounds, and, if indicated, listen to the transmitted voice sounds (see p. 314).

Breasts, Axillae, and Epitrochlear Nodes. In a woman, inspect the breasts with her arms relaxed, then elevated, and then with her hands pressed on her hips. In either sex, inspect the axillae and feel for the axillary nodes. Feel for the epitrochlear nodes.

The patient is **still sitting**. Move to the front again.

A Note on the Musculoskeletal System. By this time, you have made some preliminary observations of the musculoskeletal system. You have inspected the hands, surveyed the upper back, and, at least in women, made a fair estimate of the shoulders' range of motion. Use these and subsequent observations to decide whether a full musculoskeletal examination is warranted. If indicated, *with the patient still sitting,* examine the hands, arms, shoulders, neck, and temporomandibular joints. Inspect and palpate the joints and check their range of motion. *(You may choose to examine upper extremity muscle bulk, tone, strength, and reflexes at this time, or you may decide to wait until later.)*

Palpate the breasts, while at the same time continuing your inspection.

The patient position is supine. Ask the patient to lie down. You should stand at the *right side* of the patient's bed.

Anterior Thorax and Lungs. Inspect, palpate, and percuss the chest. Listen to the breath sounds, any adventitious sounds, and, if indicated, transmitted voice sounds.

Cardiovascular System. Observe the jugular venous pulsations and measure the jugular venous pressure in relation to the sternal angle. Inspect and palpate the carotid pulsations. Listen for carotid bruits.

Elevate the head of the bed to approximately 30 degrees for the cardiovascular examination, adjusting as necessary to see the jugular venous pulsations.

Inspect and palpate the precordium. Note the location, diameter, amplitude, and duration of the apical impulse. Listen at each auscultatory area with the diaphragm of the stethoscope. Listen at the apex and the lower sternal border with the bell. Listen for the first and second heart sounds and for physiologic splitting of the second heart sound. Listen for any abnormal heart sounds or murmurs.

Ask the patient to roll partly onto the left side while you listen at the apex for an S_3 or *mitral stenosis.* The patient should sit, lean forward, and exhale while you listen for the murmur of *aortic regurgitation.*

Abdomen. Inspect, auscultate, and percuss the abdomen. Palpate lightly, then deeply. Assess the liver and spleen by percussion and then palpation. Try to feel the kidneys, and palpate the aorta and its pulsations. If you suspect kidney infection, percuss posteriorly over the costovertebral angles.

Lower the head of the bed to the flat position. **The patient should be supine.**

Lower Extremities. Examine the legs, assessing three systems while the patient is still supine. Each of these three systems can be further assessed when the patient stands.

The patient is **supine**.

With the patient supine:

- *Peripheral Vascular System.* Palpate the femoral pulses and, if indicated, the popliteal pulses. Palpate the inguinal lymph nodes. Inspect for lower extremity edema, discoloration, or ulcers. Palpate for pitting edema.

- *Musculoskeletal System.* Note any deformities or enlarged joints. If indicated, palpate the joints, check their range of motion, and perform any necessary maneuvers.

- *Nervous System.* Assess lower extremity muscle bulk, tone, and strength; also assess sensation and reflexes. Observe any abnormal movements.

With the patient standing:

- *Peripheral Vascular System*. Inspect for varicose veins.

- *Musculoskeletal System*. Examine the alignment of the spine and its range of motion, the alignment of the legs, and the feet.

- *Genitalia and Hernias in Men*. Examine the penis and scrotal contents and check for hernias.

- *Nervous System*. Observe the patient's gait and ability to walk heel-to-toe, walk on the toes, walk on the heels, hop in place, and do shallow knee bends. Do a Romberg test and check for pronator drift.

The patient is standing. You can sit on a chair or stool.

Nervous System. The complete examination of the nervous system can also be done at the end of the examination. It consists of the five segments described below: *mental status, cranial nerves* (including funduscopic examination), *motor system, sensory system,* and *reflexes.*

The patient is sitting or supine.

Mental Status. If indicated and not done during the interview, assess the patient's orientation, mood, thought process, thought content, abnormal perceptions, insight and judgment, memory and attention, information and vocabulary, calculating abilities, abstract thinking, and constructional ability.

Cranial Nerves. If not already examined, check sense of smell, strength of the temporal and masseter muscles, corneal reflexes, facial movements, gag reflex, and strength of the trapezia and sternomastoid muscles.

Motor System. Muscle bulk, tone, and strength of major muscle groups. *Cerebellar function:* rapid alternating movements (RAMs), point-to-point movements, such as finger-to-nose (F → N) and heel-to-shin (H → S), gait.

Sensory System. Pain, temperature, light touch, vibration, and discrimination. Compare right with left sides and distal with proximal areas on the limbs.

Reflexes. Including biceps, triceps, brachioradialis, patellar, Achilles deep tendon reflexes; also plantar reflexes or Babinski reflex (see pp. 725–731).

Additional Examinations. The *rectal* and *genital* examinations are often performed at the end of the physical examination. Patient positioning is as indicated.

Rectal Examination in Men. Inspect the sacrococcygeal and perianal areas. Palpate the anal canal, rectum, and prostate. If the patient cannot stand, examine the genitalia before doing the rectal examination.

The patient is lying on his left side for the rectal examination (or standing and bending forward).

Genital and Rectal Examinations in Women. Examine the external genitalia, vagina, and cervix. Obtain a Pap smear. Palpate the uterus and adnexa bimanually.

Learn the principles of clinical reasoning, the skills of interviewing and therapeutic rapport, and the techniques of physical examination in the chapters to follow.

> The patient is **supine in the lithotomy position.** You should be seated during examination with the speculum, then standing during bimanual examination of the uterus, adnexa (and rectum as indicated).

Bibliography

Citations

1. U.S. Preventive Services Task Force. Guide to Clinical Preventive Services 2010-2011. Recommendations of the U.S. Preventive Services Task Force. Available at http://www.ahrq.gov/clinic/pocketgd.htm. See also http://www.uspreventiveservicestaskforce.org/recommendations.htm. Accessed August 27, 2011.
2. Chacko KM, Anderson RJ. The annual physical examination: important or time to abandon? Am J Med 2007;120:581–583.
3. Boulware LE, Marinopoulos S, Phillips KA et al. Systematic review: the value of the periodic health evaluation. Ann Intern Med 2007;146:289–300.
4. Culica D, Rohrer J, Ward M et al. Medical check-ups: who goes not get them. Am J Public Health 2002;92:88–91.
5. Laine C. The annual physical examination: needless ritual or necessary routine? Ann Intern Med 2002;136:701–702.
6. Oboler SK, Prochazka AV, Gonzales R et al. Public expectations and attitudes for annual physical examinations and testing. Ann Intern Med 2002;136:652–659.
7. Hesrud DD. Clinical preventive medicine in primary care: background and practice. Rational and current preventive practice. Mayo Clin Proc 2000;75:1165–1172.
8. Reilly BM. Physical examination in the care of medical inpatients: an observational study. Lancet 2003;362:1100–1105.
9. Simel DL, Rennie D. The clinical examination. An agenda to make it more rational. JAMA 1997;277:572–574.
10. Sackett DL. A primer on the precision and accuracy of the clinical examination. JAMA 1992;267:2638–2644.
11. Evidence-Based Working Group. Evidence-based medicine. A new approach to teaching the practice of medicine. JAMA 1992;268:2420–2425.
12. Centers for Disease Control and Prevention (CDC). Standard precautions. Guidelines for isolation precautions: preventing transmission of infectious agents in healthcare settings 2007. Updated October 2007. Available at http://www.cdc.gov/hicpac/pdf/isolation/Isolation2007.pdf. Accessed August 27, 2011.
13. Centers for Disease Control and Prevention. Guide to infection prevention in outpatient settings. Minimum expectations for safe care. May 2011. Available at http://www.cdc.gov/HAI/pdfs/guidelines/standatds-of-ambulatory-care-7-2011.pdf. Accessed August 27, 2011.
14. Centers for Disease Control and Prevention. Precautions to prevent the spread of MRSA in healthcare settings. Reviewed August 2010. Available at http://www.cdc.gov/mrsa/prevent/healthcare/precautions.html. Accessed August 27, 2011.
15. Centers for Disease Control and Prevention. Bloodborne infectious diseases: HIV/AIDS, Hepatitis B, Hepatitis C. Universal precautions for the prevention for transmission of bloodborne infections, p. 66. Updated October 2007. Available at http://www.cdc.gov/hicpac/pdf/isolation/Isolation2007.pdf. Accessed August 27, 2011.

Additional References

Physical Examination and History Taking

Grady D. Scientists at work: Dr. Abraham Verghese. Physician revives a dying art: the physical. New York Times. October 12, 2010.

Koh HK. A 2020 vision for healthy people. N Engl J Med 2010;362:1653–1658.

McGee S. Evidence-Based Physical Diagnosis, 2nd ed. St. Louis: Saunders, Elsevier, 2007.

Orient JM, Sapira JD (eds). Sapira's Art & Science of Bedside Diagnosis, 3rd ed. Philadelphia: Lippincott Williams & Wilkins, 2005.

Peltier D, Regan-Smith M, Wofford J et al. Teaching focused histories and physical exams in ambulatory care: a multi-institutional randomized trial. Teach Learn Med 2007;19:244–250.

Phoon CK. Must doctors still examine patients. Perspect Biol Med 2000;43:548–561.

Anatomy and Physiology

Agur AMR, Dalley AF. Grant's Atlas of Anatomy, 12th ed. Philadelphia: Wolters Kluwer Health/Lippincott Williams & Wilkins, 2009.

Buja LM, Krueger GRF, Netter FH. Netter's Illustrated Human Pathology. Teterboro, NJ: Icon Learning Systems, 2005.

Koeppen BM, Stanton BA, Berne RM. Berne and Levy Physiology, 6th ed. Philadelphia: Mosby/Elsevier, 2010.

Hall JE, Guyton AC. Guyton and Hall Textbook of Medical Physiology, 12th ed. Philadelphia: Saunders/Elsevier, 2011.

Moore KL, Dalley AF, Agur AMR. Clinically Oriented Anatomy, 6th ed. Philadelphia: Wolters Kluwer Health/Lippincott Williams & Wilkins, 2010.

Standring S, Gray H. Gray's Anatomy: The Anatomical Basis of Clinical Practice, 40th ed. Edinburgh: Churchill Livingstone/Elsevier, 2008.

Medicine, Surgery, and Geriatrics

Barker LR, Burton JR, Zeive PD. Barker, Burton, and Zieve's Principles of Ambulatory Medicine, 7th ed. Philadelphia: Lippincott Williams & Wilkins, 2007.

Becker JB, Berkley KJ, Geary N et al. Sex Differences in the Brain: From Genes to Behavior. New York: Oxford University Press, 2008.

Cassel C, Leipzig RM, Cohen HJ, Larson EB, Meier DE. Geriatric Medicine: An Evidence-based Approach, 4th ed. New York: Springer, 2003.

Cecil RL, Goldman L, Ausiello DA. Cecil Textbook of Medicine, 23rd ed. Philadelphia: Saunders Elsevier, 2008.

Hazzard WR, Halter JB. Hazzard's Geriatric Medicine and Gerontology, 6th ed. New York: McGraw-Hill Medical Publishing Division, 2009.

Jong EC, Stevens DL. Netter's Infectious Diseases. New York: Elsevier, 2012.

Longo D, Harrison TR et al (eds). Harrison's Principles of Internal Medicine, 18th ed. New York: McGraw-Hill, 2011.

Mandell GL. Essential Atlas of Infectious Diseases, 3rd ed. Philadelphia: Current Medicine, 2005.

Mandell GL, Gordon R, Bennett JE, Dolin R (eds). Mandell, Douglas, and Bennett's Principles and Practice of Infectious Diseases, 7th ed. Philadelphia: Elsevier–Churchill Livingstone, 2010.

Sabiston DC, Townsend CM (eds). Sabiston Textbook of Surgery: The Biological Basis of Modern Surgical Practice, 18th ed. Philadelphia: Saunders/Elsevier, 2008.

Schwartz SI, Brunicardi CF. Schwartz's Principles of Surgery, 9th ed. New York: McGraw-Hill, 2010.

Health Promotion and Counseling

American Public Health Association. Public Health Links (for public health professionals). Available at: http://www.apha.org/about/Public+Health+Links. Accessed September 16, 2011.

Boulware LE, Marinopoulos S, Phillips KA et al. Systematic review: the value of the periodic health evaluation. Ann Intern Med 2007;146:289–300.

Centers for Disease Control and Prevention. CDC Health Disparities & Inequalities Report - United States, 2011. Available at http://www.cdc.gov/minorityhealth/CHDIReport.html. Accessed September 18, 2011.

Centers for Disease Control and Prevention. QuickStats: Health status among persons aged ≥ 25 years, by education level – National health Interview Survey, United States 2009. Available at http://www.cdc.gov/mmwr/preview/mmwrhtml/mm5951a7.htm?s_cid=mm5951a7. Accessed September 16, 2011.

Centers for Disease Control and Prevention. Vaccines and Immunizations. Available at http://www.cdc.gov/vaccines. Also Diseases and Conditions. Available at http://www.cdc.gov/diseasesconditions. Accessed September 16, 2011.

Federal Interagency Forum on Aging Statistics. Older Americans 2010 – Key Indicators of Well-Being. Available at http://www.agingstats.gov/agingstatsdotnet/Main_Site/Data/2010_Documents/Docs/OA_2010.pdf. Accessed September 16, 2011.

Hesrud DD. Clinical preventive medicine in primary care: background and practice. Rational and current preventive practice. Mayo Clin Proc 2000;75:1165–1172.

National Quality Measures Clearinghouse. Measures by Topic. Agency for Healthcare Research and Quality (AHRQ). Available at http://www.qualitymeasures.ahrq.gov/browse/by-topic.aspx. Accessed September 16, 2011.

Office of Women's Health. U.S. Department of Health and Human Services. A-Z Health Topics. Available at http://www.womenshealth.gov. Accessed September 16, 2011.

U.S. Preventive Services Task Force. Tools for Using Recommendations in Primary Care Practice. Available at http://www.uspreventiveservicestaskforce.org/tools.htm. Accessed September 16, 2011.

The Bates' suite offers these additional resources to enhance learning and facilitate understanding of this chapter:

- Bates' *Pocket Guide to Physical Examination and History Taking*, 7th edition
- Bates' *Visual Guide to Physical Examination*
- thePoint online resources, for students and instructors: http://thepoint.lww.com

Clinical Reasoning, Assessment, and Recording Your Findings

Once you have gained your patient's trust, gathered a detailed history, and completed the requisite portions of the physical examination, you reach the critical step of formulating your *Assessment* and *Plan*. Using sound clinical reasoning, you must now analyze your findings and identify the patient's problems. You must share your impressions with the patient, eliciting any concerns and making sure that he or she understands and agrees to the steps ahead. Finally, you must document your findings in the patient's record in a succinct and legible format that communicates the patient's story and the rationale for your assessment and plan to other members of the health care team. As you make clinical decisions, you will turn to clinical evidence, calling on your knowledge of sensitivity, specificity, predictive value, and other analytical tools.

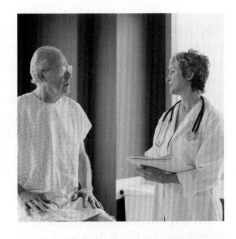

This chapter follows a stepwise approach designed to help you acquire the important skills of clinical reasoning, assessment, and recording your findings; it does not cover decisions about prognosis and therapy.

Chapter Overview

▶ Assessment and Plan: The process of clinical reasoning
▶ Recording your findings: The record of Mrs. N and the challenges of clinical data
▶ Recording your findings: Checklist for a clear and accurate record
▶ Evaluating clinical evidence: sensitivity, specificity, predictive value, likelihood ratio, kappa measurement
▶ Lifelong learning: Integrating clinical reasoning, assessment, and analysis of clinical evidence

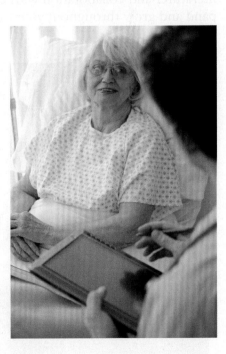

The comprehensive health history and physical examination build the foundation of your clinical *Assessment*. As you learned in Chapter 1, through skilled interviewing, you gather the history from the patient or the family, termed *subjective data*, and conduct the physical examination and testing, known as *objective data*. This information is primarily descriptive and factual. As you move to *Assessment*, you go beyond description and observation to analysis and interpretation. You select and cluster relevant pieces of information, analyze their significance, and try to explain them logically using principles of biopsychosocial and biomedical science. Your clinical reasoning process is pivotal to how you interpret the patient's history and physical examination, single out problems identified in the *Assessment,* and move from each problem to its action plan.

The *Plan* is often wide-ranging and incorporates patient education, changes in medications, needed tests, referrals to other clinicians, and return visits for counseling and support. However, a successful *Plan* does more than just describe the approach to a problem. It must include the patient's responses to the problems identified and to the diagnostic and therapeutic interventions that you recommend. It requires good interpersonal skills and sensitivity to the patient's goals, economic means, competing responsibilities, and family structure and dynamics.

The *patient record* serves a dual purpose—it reflects your analysis of the patient's health status, and it documents the unique features of the patient's history, examination, laboratory and test results, assessment, and plan in a formal written format. In a well-constructed record, each problem in the *Assessment* is listed in order of priority with an explanation of supporting findings and a differential diagnosis, followed by a *Plan* for addressing that problem. The patient record facilitates clinical reasoning, promotes communication and coordination among the professionals who care for your patient, and documents the patient's problems and management for medicolegal purposes.

Study the record of "Mrs. N." later in this chapter on pp. 31–35 to see how clinical findings are assembled and to practice your own clinical reasoning.

With experience, commitment to lifelong learning and pursuit of clinical literature, and collaboration with colleagues, your clinical acumen will expand and grow throughout your career.

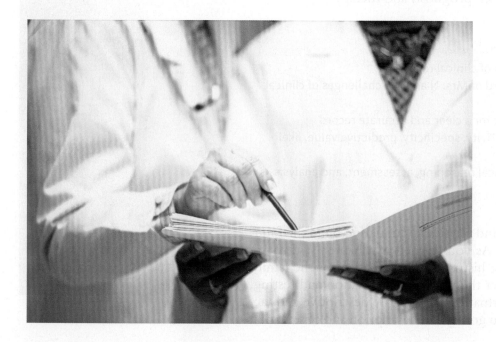

ASSESSMENT AND PLAN: THE PROCESS OF CLINICAL REASONING

Because assessment takes place in the clinician's mind, the process of clinical reasoning may seem inaccessible and even mysterious to beginning students. Experienced clinicians often think quickly, with little overt or conscious effort. They differ widely in personal style, communication skills, clinical training, experience, and interests. Some clinicians may find it difficult to explain the logic behind their clinical thinking. As an active learner, you will be expected to ask teachers and clinicians to elaborate on the fine points of their clinical reasoning and decision making.[1,2]

Cognitive psychologists have shown that clinicians use three types of reasoning for clinical problem solving: pattern recognition, development of schemas, and application of relevant basic and clinical science.[3–6] As you gain experience, your clinical reasoning will begin at the outset of the patient encounter, not at the end. Study the steps described here, then apply them to the *Case of Mrs. N* that follows. Think about these steps as you see your first patients. As with all patients, focus on determining "What explains this patient's concerns?" and "What are the problems and diagnoses?"[7,8]

For clinical examples of excellent and faulty reasoning and strategies to avoid cognitive errors, turn to Kassirer et al, *Learning Clinical Reasoning.*[9]

Identifying Problems and Making Diagnoses: Steps in Clinical Reasoning

> ▶ Identify abnormal findings.
> ▶ Localize findings anatomically.
> ▶ Interpret findings in terms of probable process.
> ▶ Make hypotheses about the nature of the patient's problem.
> ▶ Test the hypotheses and establish a working diagnosis.
> ▶ Develop a plan agreeable to the patient.

- **Identify abnormal findings.** Make a list of the patient's *symptoms,* the *signs* you observed during the physical examination, and any laboratory reports available to you.

- **Localize these findings anatomically.** This step may be easy. The symptom of scratchy throat and the sign of an erythematous inflamed pharynx, for example, clearly localize the problem to the pharynx. A complaint of headache leads you quickly to the structures of the skull and brain. Other symptoms, however, may present greater difficulty. Chest pain, for example, can originate in the coronary arteries, the stomach and esophagus, or the muscles and bones of the chest. If the pain is exertional and relieved by rest, either the heart or the musculoskeletal components of the chest wall may be involved. If the patient notes pain only when carrying groceries with the left arm, the musculoskeletal system becomes the likely culprit.

When localizing findings, be as specific as your data allow, but bear in mind that you may have to settle for a body region, such as the chest, or a body system, such as the musculoskeletal system. On the other hand, you may be able to define the exact structure involved, such as the left pectoral muscle. Some symptoms and signs cannot be localized, such as fatigue or fever, but are useful in the next set of steps.

● **Interpret the findings in terms of the probable process.** Patient problems often stem from a *pathologic process* involving diseases of a body structure. There are several such processes, variably classified, including congenital, inflammatory or infectious, immunologic, neoplastic, metabolic, nutritional, degenerative, vascular, traumatic, and toxic. Possible pathologic causes of headache, for example, include concussion from trauma, subarachnoid hemorrhage, or even compression from a brain tumor. Fever and stiff neck, or nuchal rigidity, are two of the classic signs of headache from meningitis. Even without other signs, such as rash or papilledema, they strongly suggest an infectious process.

Other problems are *pathophysiologic*, reflecting derangements of biologic functions, such as congestive heart failure or migraine headache. Still other problems are *psychopathologic*, such as disorders of mood like depression or headache as an expression of a somatization disorder.

● **Make hypotheses about the nature of the patient's problem.** Here you draw on all the knowledge and experience you can muster, and it is here that reading is most useful for learning about patterns of abnormalities and diseases that help you cluster your patient's findings.

By consulting the clinical literature, you embark on the lifelong goal of **evidence-based decision making.**[10,11]

Until you gain broader knowledge and experience, you may not be able to develop highly specific hypotheses, but proceed as far as you can with the data and knowledge you have. The following steps should help:

Clinical Reasoning: Developing Hypotheses About Patient Problems

1. *Select the most specific and critical findings to support your hypothesis.* If the patient reports "the worst headache of her life," nausea, and vomiting, for example, and you find a change in mental status, papilledema, and meningismus, build your hypothesis around elevated intracranial pressure rather than gastrointestinal disorders. Although other symptoms are useful diagnostically, they are much less specific.

2. Using your inferences about the structures and processes involved, *match your findings against all the conditions you know that can produce them.* For example, you can match your patient's papilledema with a list of conditions affecting intracranial pressure. Or you can compare the symptoms and signs associated with the patient's headache with the various infectious, vascular, metabolic, or neoplastic conditions that might produce this clinical picture.

(continued)

**Clinical Reasoning: Developing Hypotheses
About Patient Problems** (*continued*)

3. *Eliminate the diagnostic possibilities that fail to explain the findings.* You might consider cluster headache as a cause of Mrs. N's headaches (see The Case of Mrs. N, pp. 31–35), but eliminate this hypothesis because it fails to explain the patient's throbbing bifrontal localization with intermittent nausea and vomiting. Also, the pain pattern is atypical for cluster headache—it is not unilateral, boring, or occurring repetitively at the same time over a period of days, nor is it associated with lacrimation or rhinorrhea.

4. *Weigh the competing possibilities and select the most likely diagnosis* from among the conditions that might be responsible for the patient's findings. You are looking for a close match between the patient's clinical presentation and a typical case of a given condition. Other clues help in this selection, too. The *statistical probability* of a given disease in a patient of this age, sex, ethnic group, habits, lifestyle, and locality should greatly influence your selection. You should consider the possibilities of osteoarthritis and metastatic prostate cancer in a 70-year-old man with back pain, for example, but not in a 25-year-old woman with the same complaint. The *timing of the patient's illness* also makes a difference. Headache in the setting of fever, rash, and stiff neck that develops suddenly over 24 hours suggests quite a different problem than recurrent headache over a period of years associated with stress, visual scotoma, and nausea and vomiting relieved by rest.

See section on Evaluating Clinical Evidence, pp. 43–49.

5. Finally, as you develop possible explanations for the patient's problem, *give special attention to potentially life-threatening and treatable conditions* such as meningococcal meningitis, bacterial endocarditis, pulmonary embolus, or subdural hematoma. Here you make every effort to minimize the risk for missing conditions that may occur less frequently or be less probable but that, if present, would be particularly ominous. *One rule of thumb is always to include "the worst case scenario" in your list of differential diagnoses* and make sure you have ruled out that possibility based on your findings and patient assessment.

- **Test your hypotheses.** Now that you have made a hypothesis about the patient's problem, you are ready to *test your hypothesis*. You are likely to need further history, additional maneuvers on physical examination, or laboratory studies or x-rays to confirm or rule out your tentative diagnosis or to clarify which of two or three possible diagnoses are most likely. When the diagnosis seems clear-cut—a simple upper respiratory infection or a case of hives, for example—these steps may not be necessary.

- **Establish a working diagnosis.** You can now establish a working definition of the problem. Make this at the highest level of explicitness and certainty that the data allow. You may be limited to a symptom, such as "tension headache, cause unknown." At other times, you can define a problem explicitly in terms of its structure, process, and cause. Examples include "bacterial meningitis, pneumococcal," "subarachnoid hemorrhage, left temporoparietal lobe," or "hypertensive cardiovascular disease with left ventricular dilatation and congestive heart failure."

Although diagnoses are based primarily on identifying abnormal structures, altered processes, and specific causes, you will frequently see patients whose complaints do not fall neatly into these categories. Some symptoms defy analysis and are medically unexplained. You may never be able to move beyond simple descriptive categories such as "fatigue" or "anorexia." Other problems relate to stressful events in the patient's life. Events such as losing a job or loved one may increase the risk for subsequent illness. Identifying these events and helping the patient develop coping strategies are just as important as managing a headache or a duodenal ulcer.

See Chapter 5, Behavior and Mental Status, section on "Medically Unexplained Symptoms," pp. 142–143.

Another increasingly prominent category on problem lists is *Health Maintenance*. Routinely listing Health Maintenance helps you track several important health concerns more effectively: immunizations, screening measures (e.g., mammograms, prostate examinations), instructions regarding nutrition and breast or testicular self-examinations, recommendations about exercise or use of seat belts, and responses to important life events.

- **Develop a plan agreeable to the patient.** Identify and record a *Plan* for each patient problem. Your *Plan* flows logically from the problems or diagnoses you have identified. Specify which steps are needed next. These steps range from tests to confirm or further evaluate a diagnosis, to consultations for subspecialty evaluation, to additions, deletions, or changes in medication, to arranging a family meeting. You will find that you follow many of the same diagnoses over time; however, your *Plan* is often more fluid, encompassing changes and modifications that emerge from each patient visit. The *Plan* should make reference to diagnosis, therapy, and patient education.

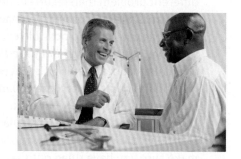

Before finalizing your *Plan*, it is important to share your assessment and clinical thinking with the patient and seek out his or her opinions, concerns, and willingness to proceed with any further testing or evaluation. Remember that patients may need to hear the same information multiple times and ways before they comprehend it. The patient should always be an active participant in the plan of care.

RECORDING YOUR FINDINGS: THE CASE OF MRS. N AND THE CHALLENGES OF CLINICAL DATA

Now turn to the case of Mrs. N and scrutinize the history, physical examination, assessment, and plan. Apply your own clinical reasoning to the findings presented and begin to analyze her concerns. See if you agree with the Assessment and Plan and the priority of the problems listed.

The Case of Mrs. N

8/25/12 11:00 AM

Mrs. N is a pleasant, 54-year-old widowed saleswoman residing in Espanola, New Mexico.

Referral. None

Source and Reliability. Self-referred; seems reliable.

Chief Complaint: "My head aches."

Present Illness: For about 3 months, Mrs. N has had increasing problems with frontal headaches. These are usually bifrontal, throbbing, and mild to moderately severe. She has missed work on several occasions because of associated nausea and vomiting. Headaches now average once a week, usually related to stress, and last 4 to 6 hours. They are relieved by sleep and putting a damp towel over the forehead. There is little relief from aspirin. No associated visual changes, motor-sensory deficits, or paresthesias.

"Sick headaches" with nausea and vomiting began at age 15, recurred throughout her mid-20s, then decreased to one every 2 or 3 months and almost disappeared.

The patient reports increased pressure at work from a new and demanding boss; she is also worried about her daughter (see *Personal and Social History*). She thinks her headaches may be like those in the past, but wants to be sure because her mother died following a stroke. She is concerned that they interfere with her work and make her irritable with her family. She eats three meals a day and drinks three cups of coffee a day and tea at night.

   Medications. Aspirin, 1 to 2 tablets every 4 to 6 hours as needed. "Water pill" in the past for ankle swelling, none recently.

   *Allergies. Ampicillin causes rash.

   Tobacco. About 1 pack of cigarettes per day since age 18 (36 pack-years).

   Alcohol/drugs. Wine on rare occasions. No illicit drugs.

Past History

Childhood Illnesses.   Measles, chickenpox. No scarlet fever or rheumatic fever.

Adult Illnesses.   *Medical:* Pyelonephritis, 1998, with fever and right flank pain; treated with ampicillin; developed generalized rash with itching several days later. Reports x-rays were normal; no recurrence of infection. *Surgical:* Tonsillectomy, age 6; appendectomy, age 13. Sutures for laceration, 2001, after stepping on glass. *Ob/Gyn:* 3-3-0-3, with normal vaginal deliveries. Three living children. Menarche age 12. Last menses 6 months ago. Little interest in sex, and not sexually active. No concerns about HIV infection. *Psychiatric:* None.

Health Maintenance.   *Immunizations:* Oral polio vaccine, year uncertain; tetanus shots × 2, 1991, followed with booster 1 year later; flu vaccine, 2000, no reaction. *Screening tests:* Last Pap smear, 2008, normal. No mammograms to date.

Gravida (G)-Parity, or # deliveries (P)-Miscarriages (M)-Living (L), or G-P-M-L 3-3-0-3

---

*You may wish to add an asterisk or underline important points.

(continued)

The Case of Mrs. N (continued)

Family History

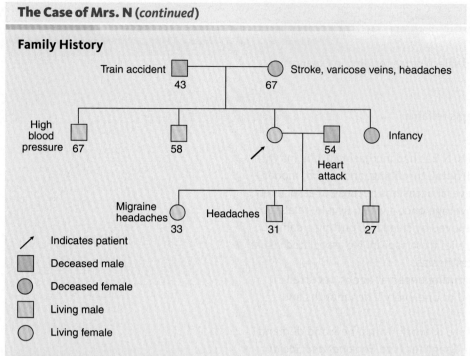

Father died at age 43 in train accident. Mother died at age 67 from stroke; had
varicose veins, headaches

One brother, 61, with hypertension, otherwise well; one brother, 58, well
except for mild arthritis; one sister, died in infancy of unknown cause

Husband died at age 54 of heart attack

Daughter, 33, with migraine headaches, otherwise well; son, 31, with headaches; son, 27, well

No family history of diabetes, tuberculosis, heart or kidney disease, cancer,
anemia, epilepsy, or mental illness.

Personal and Social History: Born and raised in Las Cruces, finished high
school, married at age 19. Worked as sales clerk for 2 years, then moved with
husband to Espanola, had 3 children. Returned to work 15 years ago because of
financial pressures. Children all married. Four years ago Mr. N died suddenly
of a heart attack, leaving little savings. Mrs. N has moved to a small apartment to be near daughter, Isabel. Isabel's husband, John, has an alcohol problem. Mrs. N's apartment now a haven for Isabel and her 2 children, Kevin,
6 years, and Lucia, 3 years. Mrs. N feels responsible for helping them; feels
tense and nervous but denies depression. She has friends but rarely discusses
family problems: "I'd rather keep them to myself. I don't like gossip." No church
or other organizational support. She is typically up at 7:00 A.M., works 9:00 to
5:30, eats dinner alone.

Exercise and diet. Gets little exercise. Diet high in carbohydrates.

Safety measures. Uses seat belt regularly. Uses sunblock. Medications kept
in an unlocked medicine cabinet. Cleaning solutions in unlocked cabinet
below sink. Mr. N's shotgun and box of shells in unlocked closet upstairs.

(continued)

The Family History can be recorded
as a diagram or a narrative. The diagram is more helpful than the narrative for tracing genetic disorders.
The negatives from the family history should follow either format.

The Case of Mrs. N (*continued*)

Review of Systems

General.   *Has *gained* about 10 lbs in the past 4 years.

Skin.   No rashes or other changes.

Head, Eyes, Ears, Nose, Throat (HEENT).   See *Present Illness.* No history of head injury. *Eyes:* Reading glasses for 5 years, last checked 1 year ago. No symptoms. *Ears:* Hearing good. No tinnitus, vertigo, infections. *Nose, sinuses:* Occasional mild cold. No hay fever, sinus trouble. *Throat (or mouth and pharynx):* Some bleeding of gums recently. Last dental visit 2 years ago. Occasional canker sore.

Neck.   No lumps, goiter, pain. No swollen glands.

Breasts.   No lumps, pain, discharge. Does breast self-examination sporadically.

Respiratory.   No cough, wheezing, shortness of breath. Last chest x-ray, 1986, St. Mary's Hospital; unremarkable.

Cardiovascular.   No known heart disease or high blood pressure; last blood pressure taken in 2007. No dyspnea, orthopnea, chest pain, palpitations. Has never had an electrocardiogram (ECG).

Gastrointestinal.   Appetite good; no nausea, vomiting, indigestion. Bowel movement about once daily, *though sometimes has hard stools for 2 to 3 days when especially tense; no diarrhea or bleeding. No pain, jaundice, gallbladder or liver problems.

Urinary.   No frequency, dysuria, hematuria, or recent flank pain; nocturia × 1, large volume. *Occasionally loses some urine when coughs hard.

Genital.   No vaginal or pelvic infections. No dyspareunia.

Peripheral Vascular.   Varicose veins appeared in both legs during first pregnancy. For 10 years, has had swollen ankles after prolonged standing; wears light elastic pantyhose; tried "water pill" 5 months ago, but it didn't help much; no history of phlebitis or leg pain.

Musculoskeletal.   Mild, aching, low back pain, often after a long day's work; no radiation down the legs; used to do back exercises but not now. No other joint pain.

Psychiatric.   No history of depression or treatment for psychiatric disorders. (See also *Present Illness* and *Personal and Social History.*)

Neurologic.   No fainting, seizures, motor or sensory loss. Memory good.

Hematologic.   Except for bleeding gums, no easy bleeding. No anemia.

Endocrine.   No known thyroid trouble, temperature intolerance. Sweating average. No symptoms or history of diabetes.

Physical Examination

Mrs. N is a short, overweight, middle-aged woman, who is animated and responds quickly to questions. She is somewhat tense, with moist, cold hands. Her hair is well-groomed. Her color is good, and she lies flat without discomfort.

(continued)

The Case of Mrs. N (*continued*)

Vital Signs.   Ht (without shoes) 157 cm (5′2″). Wt (dressed) 65 kg (143 lb). BMI 26. BP 164/98 right arm, supine; 160/96 left arm, supine; 152/88 right arm, supine with wide cuff. Heart rate (HR) 88 and regular. Respiratory rate (RR) 18. Temperature (oral) 98.6°F.

Skin.   Palms cold and moist, but color good. Scattered cherry angiomas over upper trunk. Nails without clubbing, cyanosis.

Head, Eyes, Ears, Nose, Throat (HEENT).   **Head:** Hair of average texture. Scalp without lesions, normocephalic/atraumatic (NC/AT). **Eyes:** Vision 20/30 in each eye. Visual fields full by confrontation. Conjunctiva pink; sclera white. Pupils 4 mm constricting to 2 mm, round, regular, equally reactive to light. Extraocular movements intact. Disc margins sharp, without hemorrhages, exudates. No arteriolar narrowing or A-V nicking. **Ears:** Wax partially obscures right tympanic membrane (TM); left canal clear, TM with good cone of light. Acuity good to whispered voice. Weber midline. AC > BC. **Nose:** Mucosa pink, septum midline. No sinus tenderness. **Mouth:** Oral mucosa pink. Several interdental papillae red, slightly swollen. Dentition good. Tongue midline, with 3 × 4 mm shallow white ulcer on red base on undersurface near tip; tender but not indurated. Tonsils absent. Pharynx without exudates.

Neck.   Neck supple. Trachea midline. Thyroid isthmus barely palpable, lobes not felt.

Lymph Nodes.   Small (<1 cm), soft, nontender, and mobile tonsillar and posterior cervical nodes bilaterally. No axillary or epitrochlear nodes. Several small inguinal nodes bilaterally, soft and nontender.

Thorax and Lungs.   Thorax symmetric with good excursion. Lungs resonant. Breath sounds vesicular with no added sounds. Diaphragms descend 4 cm bilaterally.

Cardiovascular.   Jugular venous pressure 1 cm above the sternal angle, with head of examining table raised to 30 degrees. Carotid upstrokes brisk, without bruits. Apical impulse discrete and tapping, barely palpable in the 5th left interspace, 8 cm lateral to the midsternal line. Good S_1, S_2; no S_3 or S_4. A II/VI medium-pitched midsystolic murmur at the 2nd right interspace; does not radiate to the neck. No diastolic murmurs.

Breasts.   Pendulous, symmetric. No masses; nipples without discharge.

Abdomen.   Protuberant. Well-healed scar, right lower quadrant. Bowel sounds active. No tenderness or masses. Liver span 7 cm in right midclavicular line; edge smooth, palpable 1 cm below right costal margin (RCM). Spleen and kidneys not felt. No costovertebral angle tenderness (CVAT).

Genitalia.   External genitalia without lesions. Mild cystocele at introitus on straining. Vaginal mucosa pink. Cervix pink, parous, and without discharge. Uterus anterior, midline, smooth, not enlarged. Adnexa not palpated due to obesity and poor relaxation. No cervical or adnexal tenderness. Pap smear taken. Rectovaginal wall intact.

Rectal.   Rectal vault without masses. Stool brown, negative for occult blood.

Extremities.   Warm and without edema. Calves supple, nontender.

(*continued*)

The Case of Mrs. N (continued)

Peripheral Vascular.   Trace edema at both ankles. Moderate varicosities of saphenous veins both in lower extremities. No stasis pigmentation or ulcers. Pulses (2+ = brisk, or normal):

	Radial	Femoral	Popliteal	Dorsalis Pedis	Posterior Tibial
RT	2+	2+	2+	2+	2+
LT	2+	2+	2+	Absent	2+

Musculoskeletal.   No joint deformities. Good range of motion in hands, wrists, elbows, shoulders, spine, hips, knees, ankles.

Neurologic.   **Mental Status:** Tense but alert and cooperative. Thought coherent. Oriented to person, place, and time. **Cranial Nerves:** II–XII intact. **Motor:** Good muscle bulk and tone. Strength 5/5 throughout. **Cerebellar:** Rapid alternating movements (RAMs), point-to-point movements intact. Gait stable, fluid. **Sensory:** Pinprick, light touch, position sense, vibration, and stereognosis intact. Romberg negative.

Reflexes:

	Biceps	Triceps	Brachio-radialis	Patellar	Achilles	Plantar
RT	2+	2+	2+	2+	1+	↓
LT	2+	2+	2+	2+/2+	1+	↓

OR

Laboratory Data
None currently. See Plan.

> See Muscle Strength Grading, p. 710.

> Two methods for recording reflexes may be used: a tabular form or a stick picture diagram; 2+ = brisk, or normal. See p. 725 for grading system.

Assessment and Plan

1. **Migraine headaches.** A 54-year-old woman with migraine headaches since childhood, with a throbbing vascular pattern and frequent nausea and vomiting. Headaches are associated with stress and relieved by sleep and cold compresses. There is no papilledema, and there are no motor or sensory deficits on the neurologic examination. The differential diagnosis includes tension headache, also associated with stress, but there is no relief with massage, and the pain is more throbbing than aching. There are no fever, stiff neck, or focal findings to suggest meningitis, and the lifelong recurrent pattern makes subarachnoid hemorrhage unlikely (usually described as "the worst headache of my life").

(continued)

Assessment and Plan (continued)

Plan:

- Discuss features of migraine vs. tension headaches.
- Discuss biofeedback and stress management.
- Advise patient to avoid caffeine, including coffee, colas, and other carbonated beverages.
- Start NSAIDs for headache, as needed.
- If needed next visit, begin prophylactic medication because patient is having more than three migraines per month.

2. **Elevated blood pressure.** Systolic hypertension is present. May be related to anxiety from first visit. No evidence of end-organ damage to retina or heart.

Plan:

- Discuss standards for assessing blood pressure.
- Recheck blood pressure in 1 month.
- Check basic metabolic panel; review urinalysis.
- Introduce weight reduction, exercise programs, or both (see #4).
- Reduce salt intake.

3. **Cystocele with occasional stress incontinence.** Cystocele on pelvic examination, probably related to bladder relaxation. Patient is perimenopausal. Incontinence reported with coughing, suggesting alteration in bladder neck anatomy. No dysuria, fever, flank pain. Not taking any contributing medications. Usually involves small amounts of urine, no dribbling, so doubt urge or overflow incontinence.

Plan:

- Explain cause of stress incontinence.
- Review urinalysis.
- Recommend Kegel exercises.
- Consider topical estrogen cream to vagina next visit if no improvement.

4. **Overweight.** Patient 5'2", weighs 143 lbs. BMI is ~26.

Plan:

- Explore diet history, ask patient to keep food intake diary.
- Explore motivation to lose weight, set target for weight loss by next visit.
- Schedule visit with dietitian.
- Discuss exercise program, specifically, walking 30 minutes most days a week.

5. **Family stress.** Son-in-law with alcohol problem; daughter and grandchildren seeking refuge in patient's apartment, leading to tensions in these relationships. Patient also has financial constraints. Stress currently situational. No current evidence of major depression.

Plan:

- Explore patient's views on strategies to cope with stress.
- Explore sources of support, including Al-Anon for daughter and financial counseling for patient.
- Continue to monitor for depression.

(continued)

See Chapter 3, Interviewing and the Health History, section on Motivational Interviewing, p. 72, and Table 3-1, Motivational Interviewing: A Clinical Example, p. 101.

Assessment and Plan (*continued*)

6. **Occasional musculoskeletal low back pain.** Usually with prolonged standing. No history of trauma or motor vehicle accident. Pain does not radiate; no tenderness or motor-sensory deficits on examination. Doubt disc or nerve root compression, trochanteric bursitis, sacroiliitis.

   Plan:
   - Review benefits of weight loss and exercises to strengthen low back muscles.

7. **Tobacco abuse.** 1 pack per day for 36 years.

   Plan:
   - Check peak flow or FEV_1/FVC on office spirometry.
   - Give strong warning to stop smoking.
   - Offer referral to tobacco cessation program.
   - Offer patch, current treatment to enhance abstinence.

8. **Varicose veins, lower extremities.** No complaints currently.

9. **History of right pyelonephritis, 1998.**

10. **Ampicillin allergy.** Developed rash but no other allergic reaction.

11. **Health maintenance.** Last Pap smear 2008; has never had a mammogram.

    Plan:
    - Teach patient breast self-examination; schedule mammogram.
    - Pap smear sent today.
    - Provide three stool guaiac cards; next visit discuss screening colonoscopy.
    - Suggest dental care for mild gingivitis.
    - Advise patient to move medications and caustic cleaning agents to locked cabinet, if possible, above shoulder height. Advise patient to move gun and cartridges to a locked gun cabinet.

Generating the Problem List

Now that you have completed your assessment and written record, you will find it helpful to generate a *Problem List* that summarizes the patient's problems for the front of the office or hospital chart. *List the most active and serious problems first, and record their date of onset.* Some clinicians make separate lists for active or inactive problems; others make one list in order of priority. On follow-up visits, the *Problem List* helps you remember to check the status of problems the patient may not mention. The *Problem List* also allows other members of the health care team to review the patient's health status at a glance.

A sample *Problem List* for Mrs. N is provided on the following page. You may wish to give each problem a number and use the number when referring to specific problems in subsequent notes.

Clinicians organize problem lists differently, even for the same patient. Problems can be symptoms, signs, past health events such as a hospital admission or surgery, or diagnoses. You might choose different entries from those above. Good lists vary in emphasis, length, and detail, depending on the clinician's philosophy, specialty, and role as a provider. Some clinicians would find this list too long. Others would be more explicit about "family stress" or "varicose veins."

Problem List: The Case of Mrs. N

Date Entered	Problem No.	Problem
8/30/12	1	Migraine headaches
	2	Elevated blood pressure
	3	Cystocele with occasional stress incontinence
	4	Overweight
	5	Family stress
	6	Low back pain
	7	Tobacco abuse since age 18
	8	Varicose veins
	9	History of right pyelonephritis 1998
	10	Allergy to ampicillin
	11	Health maintenance

The list illustrated here includes problems that need attention now, like Mrs. N's headaches, as well as problems that need future observation and attention, such as her blood pressure and cystocele. Listing the allergy to ampicillin warns you not to prescribe medications in the penicillin family. Some symptoms such as canker sores and hard stools do not appear on this list because they are minor concerns and do not require attention during this visit. Problem lists with too many relatively insignificant items are distracting. If these symptoms increase in importance, they can be added at a later visit.

The Challenges of Clinical Data. As you can see from the case of Mrs. N, organizing the patient's clinical data poses several challenges. The beginning student must decide whether to cluster the patient's symptoms and signs into one problem or several. The amount of data may appear unmanageable. The quality of the data may be prone to error. Guidelines to help you address these challenges are provided here.

- **Clustering data into single versus multiple problems.** One of the greatest difficulties facing students is how to cluster clinical data. Do selected data fit into one problem or several problems? The patient's *age* may help; young people are more likely to have a single disease, whereas older people tend to have multiple diseases. The *timing* of symptoms is often useful. For example, an episode of pharyngitis 6 weeks ago is probably unrelated to the fever, chills, pleuritic chest pain, and cough that prompt an office visit today. To use timing effectively, you need to know the natural history of various diseases and conditions. A yellow penile discharge followed 3 weeks later by a painless penile ulcer suggests two problems: gonorrhea and primary syphilis. In contrast, a penile ulcer followed in 6 weeks by a maculopapular skin rash and generalized lymphadenopathy suggest two stages of the same problem: primary and secondary syphilis.

Involvement of the *different body systems* may help you to cluster the clinical data. If symptoms and signs occur in a single system, one disease may explain them. Problems in different, apparently unrelated, systems often require more than one explanation. Again, knowledge of disease patterns is necessary. You might decide, for example, to group a patient's high blood pressure and sustained apical impulse together with flame-shaped retinal hemorrhages, place them in the cardiovascular system, and label the constellation "hypertensive cardiovascular disease with hypertensive retinopathy." You would develop another explanation for the patient's mild fever, left lower quadrant tenderness, and diarrhea.

Some diseases involve more than one body system. As you gain knowledge and experience, you will become increasingly adept at recognizing *multisystem conditions* and building plausible explanations that link together their seemingly unrelated manifestations. To explain cough, hemoptysis, and weight loss in a 60-year-old plumber who has smoked cigarettes for 40 years, you probably would rank lung cancer high in your differential diagnosis. You might support your diagnosis with your observation of the patient's cyanotic fingernails. With experience and continued reading, you will recognize that his other symptoms and signs can be linked to the same diagnosis. Dysphagia would reflect extension of the cancer to the esophagus, pupillary asymmetry would suggest pressure on the cervical sympathetic chain, and jaundice could result from metastases to the liver.

In another case of multisystem disease, a young man who presents with odynophagia, fever, weight loss, purplish skin lesions, leukoplakia, generalized lymphadenopathy, and chronic diarrhea is likely to have AIDS. Related risk factors should be explored promptly.

● **Sifting through an extensive array of data.** It is common to confront a relatively long list of symptoms and signs, and an equally long list of potential explanations. One approach is to *tease out separate clusters of observations and analyze one cluster at a time,* as described above. You can also *ask a series of key questions* that may steer your thinking in one direction and allow you to temporarily ignore the others. For example, you may ask what produces and relieves the patient's chest pain. If the answer is exercise and rest, you can focus on the cardiovascular and musculoskeletal systems and set the gastrointestinal system aside. If the pain is substernal, burning, and occurs only after meals, you can logically focus on the gastrointestinal tract. A series of discriminating questions helps you form a decision tree or algorithm that is helpful in collecting and analyzing clinical data and reaching logical conclusions and explanations.

● **Assessing the quality of the data.** Almost all clinical information is subject to error. Patients forget to mention symptoms, confuse the events of their illness, avoid recounting embarrassing facts, and may slant their stories to what the clinician wants to hear. Clinicians misinterpret patient statements, overlook information, fail to ask "the one key question," jump prematurely to conclusions and diagnoses, or forget an important part of the examination, such as the funduscopic examination in a woman with headache. You can avoid some of these errors by acquiring the habits of skilled clinicians, summarized below.

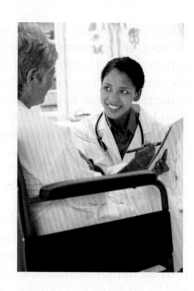

> **Tips for Ensuring the Quality of Patient Data**
>
> ▸ Ask open-ended questions and listen carefully and patiently to the patient's story.
> ▸ Craft a thorough and systematic sequence to history taking and physical examination.
> ▸ Keep an open mind toward both the patient and the data.
> ▸ Always include "the worst-case scenario" in your list of possible explanations of the patient's problem, and make sure it can be safely eliminated.
> ▸ Analyze any mistakes in data collection or interpretation.
> ▸ Confer with colleagues and review the pertinent medical literature to clarify uncertainties.
> ▸ Apply principles of data analysis to patient information and testing.

Compose the record as soon after seeing the patient as possible, before your findings fade from memory. At first you may take notes, but work toward recording each segment of the health history during the interview, leaving spaces for filling in details later. Jot down blood pressure, heart rate, and key abnormal findings to prompt your recall when you complete the record later.

See Table 2-1, p. 53, for a Sample Progress Note for the follow-up visit of Mrs. N.

RECORDING YOUR FINDINGS: CHECKLIST FOR A CLEAR AND ACCURATE RECORD

A clear, well-organized clinical record is one of the most important adjuncts to patient care. Your skill in recording your patient's history and physical examination should evolve in parallel with your growing skills in clinical reasoning and your ability to formulate the patient's *Assessment* and *Plan*. Your goal should be a clear, concise, but comprehensive report that documents the key findings of your patient assessment and communicates the patient's problems in a succinct and *legible* format to other providers and members of the health care team. Even though your institution or agency may have printed or electronic forms for recording patient information, you should always be able to generate your own record.

Regardless of your experience, certain principles will help you to organize a good record. Think especially about the *order and readability* of the record and the *amount of detail* needed. How much detail to include often poses a vexing problem. As a student, you may wish (or be required) to be quite detailed. This helps build your descriptive skills, vocabulary, and speed—admittedly a time-consuming process. Ultimately, however, the pressures of workload and time management will force some compromises. Nonetheless, a good record always provides the supporting evidence from the history, physical examination, and laboratory findings for all the problems or diagnoses identified.

Is the Order Clear?

Order is imperative. Make sure that future readers, including yourself, can easily find specific points of information. Keep the *subjective* items of the history, for example, in the history; do not let them stray into the physical examination. Did you . . .

● Make the headings clear?

● Accent your organization with indentations and spacing?

● Arrange the *Present Illness* in chronologic order, starting with the current episode, then filling in relevant background information?

Do the Data Included Contribute Directly to the Assessment?

You should spell out the supporting evidence, both positive and negative, for every problem or diagnosis that you identify. Be sure there is sufficient detail to support your Assessment and Plan.

Are Pertinent Negatives Specifically Described?

Often portions of the history or examination suggest that an abnormality might exist or develop in that area.

For the patient with notable bruises, record the "pertinent negatives," such as the absence of injury or violence, familial bleeding disorders, or medications or nutritional deficits that might lead to bruising.

For the patient who is depressed but not suicidal, record both facts. In the patient with a transient mood swing, on the other hand, a comment on suicide is unnecessary.

Are There Overgeneralizations or Omissions of Important Data?

Remember that data not recorded are data lost. No matter how vividly you can recall selected details today, you will probably not remember them in a few months. The phrase "neurologic exam negative," even in your own handwriting, may leave you wondering in a few months' time, "Did I really do the sensory exam?"

Is There Too Much Detail?

Is there excess information or redundancy?

Is important information buried in a mass of detail, to be discovered by only the most persistent reader? *Omit most of your negative findings* unless they relate directly to the patient's complaints or to specific exclusions in your diagnostic assessment. *Do not list abnormalities that you did not observe. Instead, concentrate on a few major ones, such as* "no heart murmurs," and try to describe structures in a concise, positive way. You can omit certain body structures even though you examined them, such as normal eyebrows and eyelashes.

"Cervix pink and smooth" indicates you saw no redness, ulcers, nodules, masses, cysts, or other suspicious lesions, but this description is shorter and readable.

Are Phrases and Short Words Used Appropriately? Is There Unnecessary Repetition of Data?

- Omit unnecessary words, such as those in parentheses in the examples below. This saves valuable time and space.

  "Cervix is pink (in color)." "Lungs are resonant (to percussion)." "Liver is tender (to palpation)." "Both (right and left) ears with cerumen." "II/IV systolic ejection murmur (audible)." "Thorax symmetric (bilaterally)."

- Omit repetitive introductory phrases such as "The patient reports no . . . ," because readers assume the patient is the source of the history unless otherwise specified.

- Use short words instead of longer, fancier ones when they mean the same thing, such as "felt" for "palpated" or "heard" for "auscultated."

- *Describe what you observed, not what you did.* "Optic discs seen" is less informative than "disc margins sharp."

Is the Written Style Succinct? Are There Excessive Abbreviations?

Records are scientific and legal documents, so they should be clear and understandable.

- Using words and brief phrases instead of whole sentences is common, but abbreviations and symbols should be used only if they are readily understood.

- Likewise, an overly elegant style is less appealing than a concise summary.

- Be sure your record is legible; otherwise, all that you have recorded is worthless to your readers.

Are Diagrams and Precise Measurements Included Where Appropriate?

Diagrams add greatly to the clarity of the record.

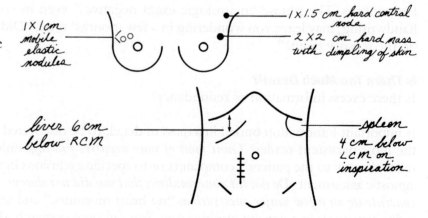

To ensure accurate evaluations and future comparisons, make measurements in centimeters, not in fruits, nuts, or vegetables.

- "1 × 1 cm lymph node" versus a "pea-sized lymph node . . ."

- Or "2 × 2 cm mass on the left lobe of the prostate" versus a "walnut-sized prostate mass."

Is the Tone of the Write-up Neutral and Professional?

It is important to be objective. Hostile, moralizing, or disapproving comments have no place in the patient's record. Never use inflammatory or demeaning words, penmanship, or punctuation.

Comments such as "Patient DRUNK and LATE TO CLINIC AGAIN!!" are unprofessional and set a bad example for other providers reading the chart. They also might prove difficult to defend in a legal setting.

EVALUATING CLINICAL EVIDENCE

Symptoms, physical findings, tests, and x-rays should help reduce uncertainty about whether a patient does or does not have a given condition. Clinical data, including laboratory work, however, are inherently imperfect. Learn to apply the principles of *reliability, validity, sensitivity, specificity,* and *predictive value* to your clinical findings and the tests you order. These test characteristics will help you decide how confident you can be in your findings and test results as you assess the presence or absence of a disease or problem. You should also understand and apply two additional concepts: the *kappa (κ) measurement of agreement* and *likelihood ratios (LRs)*. These seven statistical tools are common measures for assessing evidence that you will find in the clinical literature. Take the time to work through these measures with your teachers, and practice using them. They will enhance lifelong learning, strengthen your clinical reasoning, and improve decision making in your clinical practice.

Principles of Test Selection and Use

Reliability. Indicates how dependably repeated measurements of the same relatively stable phenomenon will give the same result, also known as precision. Reliability may be measured for one observer or for more than one observer.

Example: If on several occasions, one clinician consistently percusses the same span of a patient's liver dullness, *intraobserver reliability* is good. If, on the other hand, several observers find quite different spans of liver dullness on the same patient, *interobserver reliability* is poor.

(continued)

Principles of Test Selection and Use (continued)

Validity. Indicates how closely a given observation agrees with "the true state of affairs," or the best possible measure of reality.

Example: Blood pressure measurements by mercury-based sphygmomanometers are less valid than intra-arterial pressure tracings.

Sensitivity. Identifies the proportion of people who test positive in a group of people known to have the disease or condition, or the proportion of people who are *true positives* compared with the total number of people who actually have the disease. When the observation or test is negative in people with the disease, the result is termed *false negative. Good observations or tests have a sensitivity of more than 90%, and, when negative, help rule out disease because there are few false negatives. Such observations or tests are especially useful for screening.*

Example: The sensitivity of Homan's sign in the diagnosis of deep venous thrombosis (DVT) of the calf is 50%. In other words, compared with a group of patients with deep vein thrombosis confirmed by phlebograms, a much better test, only 50% will have a positive Homan's sign; so this sign, if absent, is not helpful because 50% of patients with DVTs have a negative Homan's sign.

To help remember this, experts state "when the **S**ensitivity of a symptom or sign is high, a **N**egative response rules *out* the target disorder; the acronym for this property is *"SnNout."*[12]

Specificity. Identifies the proportion of people who test negative in a group of people known to be *without* a given disease or condition, or the proportion of people who are "true negatives" compared with the total number of people without the disease. When the observation or test is positive in people without the disease, the result is termed *false positive. Beneficial observations or tests have a specificity of more than 90% and help "rule in" disease because the test is rarely positive when disease is absent, and there are few false positives.*

Example: The specificity of serum amylase in patients with possible acute pancreatitis is 70%. In other words, of 100 patients without pancreatitis, 70 will have a normal serum amylase; in 30, the serum amylase will be falsely elevated.

Likewise, when the **Sp**ecificity is high, a **P**ositive test result rules *in* the target disorder. The acronym is *"SpPin."*[12]

Predictive Value. Indicates how well a given symptom, sign, or test result, either positive or negative, predicts the presence or absence of disease.

(continued)

Principles of Test Selection and Use (*continued*)

Positive predictive value is the probability of disease in a patient with a positive (abnormal) test, or the proportion of "true positives" out of the total population with the disease.

Example: In a group of women with palpable breast nodules in a cancer screening program, the proportion with confirmed breast cancer would constitute the *positive predictive value* of palpable breast nodules for diagnosing breast cancer.

Negative predictive value is the probability of not having the condition or disease when the test is negative, or normal, or the proportion of "true negatives" out of the total population without the disease.

Example: In a group of women without palpable breast nodules in a cancer screening program, the proportion without confirmed breast cancer constitutes the *negative predictive value* of absence of breast nodules.

Displaying Clinical Data

To use these principles, it is important to display the data in the 2 × 2 format diagrammed in the following chart. Using this format will ensure the accuracy of your calculations of sensitivity, specificity, and predictive value. Note that the presence or absence of disease implies use of the *highest standards* to establish whether the disease is truly present or absent. This is usually the best test available, such as a coronary angiogram for assessing coronary artery disease or a tissue biopsy for malignancy.

Note that the numbers related to presence or absence of disease are displayed **down the table** in the left and right columns (*present* = a + c; *absent* = b + d). Numbers related to the observation or test are displayed **across the table** in the upper and lower rows (*test positive* = a + b; *test negative* = c + d).

Be careful when reading the medical literature, as there are many discrepancies in the display of rows and columns.

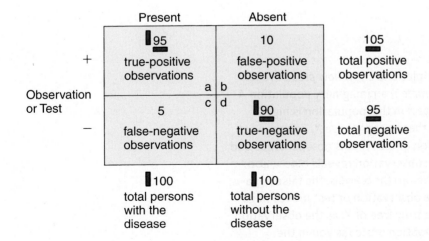

Now you are ready to make your calculations:

$$\text{Sensitivity} = \frac{a}{a+c} = \frac{\text{true-positive observations (95)}}{\text{total persons with disease (95}+5)} \times 100 = 95\%$$

$$\text{Specificity} = \frac{d}{b+d} = \frac{\text{true-negative observations (90)}}{\text{total persons with disease (90}+10)} \times 100 = 90\%$$

$$\text{Positive predictive value} = \frac{a}{a+b} = \frac{\text{true-positive observations (95)}}{\text{total positive observations (95}+10)} \times 100 = 90.5\%$$

$$\text{Negative predictive value} = \frac{d}{c+d} = \frac{\text{true-negative observations (90)}}{\text{total negative observations (90}+5)} \times 100 = 94.7\%$$

Now return to the data chart. *The **vertical red bars** designate sensitivity (a/a + c) and specificity (d/b + d), and the **horizontal red bars** designate positive predictive value (a/a + b) and negative predictive value (d/c + d).* The data displayed indicate that the hypothetical test has excellent test characteristics. The sensitivity and specificity of the test are both more than 90%, as are the positive and negative predictive values. Such a test would be clinically useful for assessing the presence or absence of a disease or condition in your patient.

Prevalence and Predictive Value.   Note that the predictive value of a test or observation depends heavily on the *prevalence* of the condition within the population studied. Prevalence is the proportion of people in a defined population at any given point in time who have the condition in question. When the prevalence of a condition is *low,* the positive predictive value of the test will fall. When the prevalence, sensitivity, and specificity are *high,* the positive predictive value is high, and the negative predictive value approaches zero. To work further on these relationships, turn to the boxes on Prevalence and Predictive Value, and practice making the calculations described.

Prevalence and Predictive Value

Two examples further illustrate these principles and show *how predictive values vary with prevalence.* Consider first (*Example 1*) an imaginary population *A* with 1,000 people. The prevalence of disease *X* in this population is high—40%. You can quickly calculate that 400 of these people have *X.* You then set out to detect these cases with an observation or test that is 90% sensitive and 80% specific. Of the 400 people with *X,* the observation reveals 0.90 × 400, or 360 (the true positives). It misses the other 40 (400 – 360, the false negatives). Out of the 600 people without *X,* the observation or test proves negative in 0.80 × 600, or 480. These people are truly free of *X,* as the observation suggests (the true negatives). But the observation misleads you in the

(continued)

Prevalence and Predictive Value (*continued*)

remaining 120 (600 – 480). These people are falsely labeled as having *X* when they are really free of it (the false positives). These figures are summarized below:

Example 1. Prevalence of Disease X = 40%

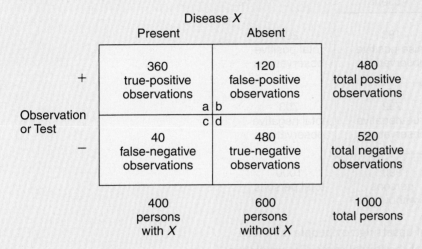

As a clinician who does not have perfect knowledge of who really does or does not have disease *X*, you are faced with a total of 480 people with positive observations. You must try to distinguish between the true and the false positives and will undoubtedly use additional kinds of data to help you in this task. Given only the sensitivity and specificity of your observation, however, you can determine the probability that a positive observation is a true positive, and you may wish to explain it to the concerned patient. This probability is calculated as follows:

$$\text{Positive predictive value} = \frac{a}{a+b} = \frac{\text{true positives (360)}}{\text{total positives (360} + \text{120)}} \times 100 = 75\%$$

Thus, 3 out of 4 of the people with positive observations really have the disease, and 1 out of 4 does not.

By a similar calculation, you can determine the probability that a negative observation is a true negative. The results here are reasonably reassuring to the involved patient:

$$\text{Negative predictive value} = \frac{d}{c+d} = \frac{\text{true negatives (480)}}{\text{total negatives (40} + \text{480)}} \times 100 = 92\%$$

As *prevalence* of the disease in a population diminishes, however, the predictive value of a positive observation diminishes considerably, while the predictive value of a negative observation rises further. In *Example 2,* in a second population (*B*) of 1,000 people, only 1% have disease *X*. Now there are only 10 cases of *X* and 990 people without *X*. If this population is screened with the

(*continued*)

Prevalence and Predictive Value (*continued*)

same test, which has a 90% sensitivity and an 80% specificity, here are the results:

Example 2. Prevalence of Disease X = 1%

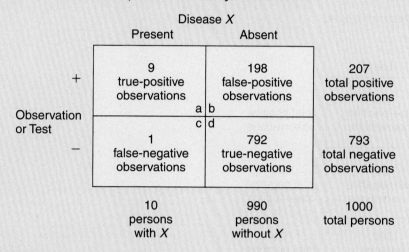

You are now confronted with the possibly of upsetting 207 people (all those with positive observations) to detect 9 out of the 10 real cases. The predictive value of a positive observation is only 4%. Improving the specificity of your observation without diminishing its sensitivity would be helpful, if it were possible. For example, if you could increase the specificity of the observation from 80% to 98% (given the same prevalence of 1% and sensitivity of 90%), the positive predictive value of the observation would improve from 4% to 31%—scarcely ideal but certainly better. Good observations or tests have a sensitivity and specificity of 90% or greater.

Because prevalence strongly affects the predictive value of an observation, prevalence also influences the assessment process. Because coronary artery disease is much more common in middle-aged men than in young women, you should pursue angina as a cause of chest pain more actively in the former group. The effect of prevalence on predictive value explains why your odds of making a correct assessment are better when you hypothesize a common condition rather than a rare one. The combination of fever, headache, myalgias, and cough probably has the same sensitivity and specificity for influenza throughout the year, but your chance of making this diagnosis correctly by using this cluster of symptoms is much greater during a winter flu epidemic than it is during a quiet August.

Prevalence varies significantly with clinical setting as well as with season. Chronic bronchitis is probably the most common cause of hemoptysis among patients seen in a general medical clinic. In the oncology clinic of a tertiary medical center, however, lung cancer might head the list, whereas in a group of postoperative patients on a general surgical service, irritation from an endotracheal tube or pulmonary infarction might be most likely. In certain parts of Asia, by contrast, one should think first of a worm called a lung fluke.

Likelihood Ratios and Kappa Measurement. Two other statistics are also clinically useful: likelihood ratios and the κ statistic for measuring degree of observer agreement. Students are encouraged to pursue these concepts through further reading.[13–15]

Likelihood ratio (LR). Conveys the odds that a finding occurs in a patient with the condition compared to a patient without the condition. When the LR is >1.0, the probability of the condition goes up; when the LR is <1.0, the probability of the condition goes down.

▶ A positive LR $= \dfrac{\text{sensitivity}}{(1-\text{specificity})}$

▶ A negative LR $= \dfrac{(1-\text{sensitivity})}{\text{specificity}}$

Example. The LR of subarachnoid hemorrhage (SAH) is 10 if neck stiffness is present, and 0.4 if neck stiffness is absent.[8] The odds of SAH are 10 times higher if neck stiffness is present compared to patients without SAH. When neck stiffness is absent, the odds that the patient has SAH are reduced to 0.4

For example, suppose the pretest probability of SAH in the patient is 25% or a pretest odds of 1:3. If the patient has neck stiffness, the posttest probability is revised upwards by the LR to 77% (posttest odds of 10:3.) If there is no neck stiffness, the posttest probability is revised downwards by the negative LR to 12% (posttest odds of 4:30.)

Kappa (κ) measurement of interobserver agreement. Measures the degree of observer agreement, or precision, of a clinical finding compared to agreement by chance alone.

Conventional levels of κ are slight agreement = 0.0–0.2; fair = 0.2–0.4; moderate = 0.4–0.8; substantial = 0.8–1.0.[12]

Example. Two clinicians agree 89% of the time that a patient has a migraine headache. Calculations show that their expected agreement is 59% based on chance alone. Their remaining potential agreement beyond chance (100%–59%) is 41%, and their actual agreement beyond chance is 30% (89%–59%). The κ measure of their agreement is 30%/41%, or 0.73. The chance of two clinicians agreeing that migraine is present is moderately high.

LIFELONG LEARNING: INTEGRATING CLINICAL REASONING, ASSESSMENT, AND ANALYSIS OF CLINICAL EVIDENCE

The concepts of sensitivity and specificity help in both the collection and the analysis of data and underlie some of the basic strategies of interviewing. Questions with high sensitivity, if answered in the affirmative, may be particularly useful for screening and for gathering evidence to support a hypothesis. For example, "Have you had any discomfort or pain in your chest?" is a highly sensitive question for diagnosing angina pectoris. For patients with this condition, there would be few false-negative responses and, thus, it is a good first screening question. However, because there are many other causes of chest discomfort, it is not highly specific. Pain that is retrosternal, pressing, and less than 10 minutes in duration—each a reasonably sensitive attribute of angina—would add significantly to the growing evidence for the diagnosis. To confirm your hypothesis, an affirmative answer to a more specific question is needed, such as "Is the pain precipitated by exertion?" or "Is the pain relieved by rest?"

Data for testing hypotheses also come from the physical examination. Heart murmurs are good examples of findings with varying sensitivity and specificity. The vast majority of patients with significant valvular *aortic stenosis* have systolic ejection murmurs audible in the aortic area. Presence of a systolic murmur has a high sensitivity for aortic stenosis. It is present in most cases and the false-negative rate is low. On the other hand, many other conditions produce systolic murmurs, such as increased blood flow across a normal valve, or aortic sclerosis, the sclerotic changes associated with aging, so the finding of a systolic murmur is not very specific. Using such a murmur as your only criterion for diagnosing aortic stenosis would lead to many false positives.

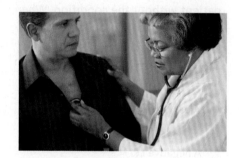

In contrast, a high-pitched, soft blowing decrescendo diastolic murmur best heard along the left sternal border is quite specific for *aortic regurgitation*. This murmur is almost never heard in normal hearts, and it is present in very few other conditions, so there are few false positives.

Combining data from the history and physical examination allows you to test your hypotheses, screen for selected conditions, build your case, and confirm a diagnosis even before obtaining further diagnostic tests. Consider the following list of evidence: cough, fever, a shaking chill, left-sided pleuritic chest pain, dullness throughout the left lower posterior lung field with crackles, bronchial breathing, and egophony. Cough and fever are good screening items for pneumonia, the next items support the hypothesis, and bronchial breathing with egophony in this distribution is specific for lobar pneumonia. A chest x-ray would confirm the diagnosis.

Absence of selected symptoms and signs is also diagnostically useful, especially when they are usually present in a given condition (i.e., their sensitivity is high). For example, if a patient with cough and left-sided pleuritic chest pain does not have fever, bacterial pneumonia becomes much less likely (except possibly in infancy and old age). Likewise, in a patient with severe dyspnea, the absence of orthopnea makes left ventricular failure less probable as an explanation for shortness of breath.

Skilled clinicians use this kind of logic even if they are unaware of its statistical underpinnings. They begin to generate tentative hypotheses as soon as the patient describes the *Chief Complaint,* then build evidence for one or more of these hypotheses and discard others as they continue with the history and examination, avoiding premature conclusions that can lead to diagnostic errors.[16,17] In developing a *Present Illness,* they borrow items from other parts of the history, such as the *Past Medical History,* the *Family History,* and the *Review of Systems.* In a 55-year-old man with chest pain, the skilled clinician does not stop with the attributes of pain, but moves on to probe risk factors for coronary artery disease such as family history, hypertension, diabetes, lipid abnormalities, and smoking. In both the history and physical examination, the clinician searches explicitly for other possible manifestations of cardiovascular disease such as congestive heart failure or the claudication or diminished lower extremity pulses of atherosclerotic peripheral vascular disease. By generating hypotheses early and testing them sequentially, experienced clinicians improve their efficiency and enhance the relevance and value of the data they collect.

A growing body of literature describes the sources of cognitive errors arising from faults in hypothesis generation, context formulation, information gathering, estimations of relevance, test interpretation, verification, and causal models.[9,18–22]

This sequence of collecting data and testing hypotheses is diagrammed here:

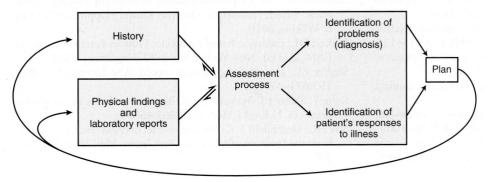

After the plan has been implemented, the process recycles. The clinician gathers more data, assesses the patient's progress, modifies the problem list if indicated, and adjusts the plan accordingly. As you gain experience, the interplay of assessment, data collection, and knowledge from the clinical literature will become increasingly familiar. You will come to value the challenges and rewards of clinical reasoning and assessment that make patient care meaningful.

Bibliography

Citations

1. Peterson MC, Holbrook JH, Von Hales DE et al. Contributions of the history, physical examination, and laboratory investigation in making medical diagnoses. West J Med 1992; 156:163–165.
2. Hampton JR, Harrison MJ, Mitchell JRA et al. Relative contributions of history-taking, physical examination, and laboratory investigation to diagnosis and management of medical outpatients. Br Med J 1975;2(5969):486–489.
3. Bowen J. Educational strategies to promote clinical diagnostic reasoning. New Engl J Med 2006;355:2217–2225.
4. Coderre S, Mandin H, Harasym P et al. Diagnostic reasoning strategies and diagnostic success. Med Educ 2003;37:695–703.
5. Elstein A, Schwarz A. Clinical problem solving and diagnosis decision making: selective review of the cognitive literature. Br Med J 2002;324(7339):729–732.
6. Norman, G. Research in clinical reasoning: past history and current trends. Med Educ 2005;39:418–427.
7. Schneiderman H. Bedside Diagnosis. An Annotated Bibliography of Literature on Physical Examination and Interviewing, 3rd ed. Philadelphia: American College of Physicians, 1997.
8. McGee S. Evidence Based Physical Diagnosis, 2nd ed. St. Louis: Saunders/Elsevier, 2007.
9. Kassirer J, Wong J, Kopelman R. Learning Clinical Reasoning, 2nd ed. Philadelphia: Wolters Kluwer/Lippincott Williams & Wilkins, 2010.
10. Evidence-Based Medicine Working Group. Evidence-based medicine: a new approach to teaching the practice of medicine. JAMA 1992;268:2420–2425. *Launched the Rational Clinical Examination Series.*

11. Guyatt G. Users' Guide to the Medical Literature: A Manual for Evidence-Based Clinical Practice. New York: McGraw-Hill Medical, 2008.

12. Sackett D. A primer on the precision and accuracy of the clinical examination. JAMA 1992;267(19):2638–2644.

13. Fletcher RH, Fletcher SW. Clinical Epidemiology: The Essentials, 4th ed. Philadelphia: Lippincott Williams & Wilkins, 2005.

14. Black E (ed). Diagnostic Strategies in Common Medical Problems, 2nd ed. Philadelphia: American College of Physicians, 1999.

15. Sackett DL. Evidence-based medicine: How to Practice and Teach EBM, 2nd ed. New York: Churchill Livingstone, 2000.

16. Dubeau CE, Voytovich AE, Rippey RM. Premature conclusions in the diagnosis of iron-deficiency anemia: cause and effect. Med Decis Making 1986;6:169–173.

17. Kuhn GJ. Diagnostic errors. Acad Emerg Med 2002;9:740–750.

18. Graber ML, Franklin N Gordon R. Diagnostic error in internal medicine. Arch Intern Med 2005;165:1493–1499.

19. Redelmeier DA. Improving patient care: the cognitive psychology of missed diagnoses. Ann Intern Med 2005;142:115–120.

20. Berner ES, Graber ML. Overconfidence as a cause of diagnostic error in medicine. Am J Med 2008;121:S2–S23.

21. Norman GR, Eva KW. Diagnostic error and clinical reasoning. Med Educ 2010;44:94–100.

22. Newman-Toker DE, Pronovost PJ. Diagnostic errors—the next frontier for patient safety. JAMA 2009;301:1060–1062.

23. Donnelly WJ. Viewpoint: patient-centered medical care requires a patient-centered medical record. Acad Med 2005; 80:33–38.

Additional References

Alfaro-LeFevre R. Critical Thinking and Clinical Judgment: A Practical Approach to Outcome-Focused Thinking, 4th ed. St. Louis; WB Saunders/Elsevier, 2009.

Carpenito-Moyet LJ. Nursing Diagnosis: Application to Clinical Practice, 13th ed. Philadelphia: Wolters Kluwer/Lippincott Williams & Wilkins, 2010.

Cherry B, Jacob SR. Contemporary Nursing: Issues, Trends, and Management, 5th ed. St. Louis: Elsevier/Mosby, 2011.

Fletcher RH, Fletcher, SW. Clinical Epidemiology: The Essentials, 4th ed. Philadelphia: Lippincott Williams & Wilkins, 2005.

Guyatt GH, Oxman AD, Vist GE et al. GRADE: what is "quality of evidence" and why is it important to clinicians? BMJ 2008;336:995–988.

Guyatt GH, Oxman AD, Vist GE et al. GRADE: and emerging consensus on rating quality of evidence and strength of recommendations. BMJ 2008;336:924–926.

Inui TS. Establishing the doctor–patient relationship: science, art, or competence? Schweiz Med Wochenschr 1998;128:225.

Laditka JN, Laditka SB. Race, ethnicity, and hospitalization for ambulatory care sensitive conditions in the USA. Ethn Health 2006;11:247–263.

Luce BR, Kramer JM, Goodman SN et al. Rethinking randomized clinical trials for comparative effectiveness research: the need for transformational change. Ann Intern Med 2009;151:206–209.

Nettina SM. The Lippincott Manual of Nursing Practice Handbook, 9th ed. Philadelphia: Wolters Kluwer/Lippincott Williams & Wilkins, 2010.

Sackett DL. Evidence-based Medicine: How to Practice and Teach EBM, 2nd ed. New York: Churchill Livingstone, 2000.

Siegler EL. The evolving medical record. Ann Intern Med 2010; 153:671–677.

Song Y, Skinner J, Bynurm J et al. Regional variations in diagnostic practices. N Engl J Med 2010;363:45–53.

Sox HC, Greenfield S. Comparative effectiveness research: a report from the Institute of Medicine. Ann Intern Med 2009;151:203–205.

The Bates' suite offers these additional resources to enhance learning and facilitate understanding of this chapter:

- Bates' *Pocket Guide to Physical Examination and History Taking*, 7th edition
- Bates' *Visual Guide to Physical Examination*
- thePoint online resources, for students and instructors: http://thepoint.lww.com

Table	
2-1	**Sample Progress Note**

A month later, Mrs. N returns for a follow-up visit. The format of the office progress note is quite variable, but it should meet the same standards as the initial assessment. The note should be clear, sufficiently detailed, and easy to follow. It should reflect your clinical reasoning and delineate your assessment and plan. Be sure to learn the documentation standards for billing in your institution, because this can affect the detail and type of information needed in your progress notes.

The note below follows the SOAP format: **S**ubjective, **O**bjective, **A**ssessment, and **P**lan. You will see many other styles, some focused on the "patient-centered" record.[23] The terms for SOAP are often not listed, but implied. Frequently clinicians record the history and physical examination, then document the plan by listing of each problem and its assessment.

9/25/12

Mrs. N returns to the clinic for follow-up of her migraine headaches. She states that she has fewer headaches since avoiding caffeinated beverages. She is now drinking decaffeinated coffee and has stopped drinking tea. She has joined a support group and started exercising to reduce stress. She is still having one to two headaches a month with some nausea, but they are less severe and generally relieved with NSAIDs. She denies any fever, stiff neck, associated visual changes, motor-sensory deficits, or paresthesias.

She has been checking her blood pressure at home. It is running about 150/90. She is walking 30 minutes three times a week in her neighborhood and has reduced her daily caloric intake. She has been unable to stop smoking. She has been doing the Kegel exercises but still has some leakage with coughing or laughing.

Medications: Motrin 400 mg up to three times daily as needed for headache
Allergies: Ampicillin causes rash
Tobacco: 1 pack per day since age 18

Physical Examination: Pleasant, overweight, middle-aged woman, who is animated and somewhat tense. Ht 157 cm (5′ 2″). Wt 63 kg (140 lbs). BMI 26. BP 150/90. HR 86 and regular. RR 16. Afebrile.

Skin: No suspicious nevi. *HEENT*: Normocephalic, atraumatic. Pharynx without exudates. *Neck*: Supple, without thyromegaly. *Lymph nodes*: No lymphadenopathy. *Lungs*: Resonant and clear. *CV*: JVP 6 cm above the right atrium; carotid upstrokes brisk, no bruits. Good S_1, S_2. No murmurs heard today. No S_3, S_4. *Abdomen*: Active bowel sounds. Soft, nontender, no hepatosplenomegaly. *Extremities*: Without edema.

Labs: Basic metabolic panel and urinalysis from 8/25/12 unremarkable. Pap smear normal.

Impression and Plan

1. Migraine headaches—now down to one to two per month due to reductions in caffeinated beverages and stress. Headaches are responding to NSAIDs.
   - Will defer daily prophylactic medication for now because patient is having fewer than three headaches per month and feels better
   - Affirm need to stop smoking and to continue exercise program
   - Affirm patient's participation in support group to reduce stress
2. Elevated blood pressure—BP remains elevated at 150/90.
   - Will initiate therapy with a diuretic
   - Patient to take blood pressure three times a week and bring recordings to next office visit
3. Cystocele with occasional stress incontinence—stress incontinence improved with Kegel exercises but still with some urine leakage. Urinalysis from last visit—no infection
   - Initiate vaginal estrogen cream
   - Continue Kegel exercises
4. Overweight—has lost ~4 lbs.
   - Continue exercise
   - Review diet history; affirm weight reduction.
5. Family stress—patient handling this better. See Plans above.
6. Occasional low back pain—no complaints today
7. Tobacco abuse—see Plans above
8. Health maintenance—Pap smear sent last visit. Mammogram scheduled. Colonoscopy recommended.

Interviewing and the Health History

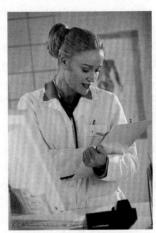

The health history interview is a conversation with a purpose. As you learn to elicit the patient's history, you will draw on many of the interpersonal skills that you use every day, but with unique and important differences. In social conversation, you freely express your own needs and are responsible only for yourself. In contrast, the primary goals of the patient interview are to *listen* and to improve the well-being of the patient through a trusting and supportive relationship.

Relating effectively with patients is among the most valued skills of clinical care. For the patient, "a feeling of connectedness . . . of being deeply heard and understood . . . is the very heart of healing."[1] For the clinician, this deeper relationship enriches the rewards of patient care.[2–4]

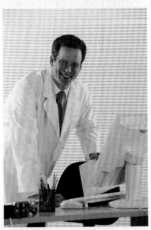

This chapter introduces you to the essentials of interviewing and establishing trust, the foundations of your therapeutic alliance with your patients. At first, you will focus on gathering information, but with experience and empathic listening, you will allow the patient's story to unfold in its most authentic and detailed form.

The process of interviewing is both an art and a skill. It is primarily *patient-centered*. It "encourages patients to express what is most important to them. They express their personal concerns in addition to symptoms," creating a narrative that includes "the personal context of the patient's symptoms and disease."[5] Experts have defined patient-centered interviewing as "following the patient's lead to understand their thoughts, ideas, concerns and requests, without adding additional information from the doctor's perspective." In contrast, in the more symptom-focused, clinician-centered approach, the clinician "takes charge of the interaction to meet her or his own need to acquire the symptoms, their details and other data that will help her or him identify a disease," which can overlook the personal dimensions of the illness.[5,6] Evidence suggests that the patient is best served by integrating these interviewing styles, leading to a more complete depiction of the patient's illness and allowing clinicians to more fully convey the caring attributes of "respect, empathy, humility and sensitivity."[5] Current evidence shows that this approach is not only more satisfying for the patient and the clinician, but it is also more effective in achieving the desired health outcomes.[7–9]

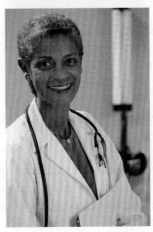

The *interviewing process* is quite different from the format of the health history, presented in Chapter 1. The interview consists of more than just asking a series of questions; it requires a highly refined sensitivity to the patient's feelings and behavioral cues. The *health history format* provides an important framework for organizing the patient's story into various categories pertinent to the patient's present, past, and family health. The purposes of the interview and the health history format are complementary but distinct. Keep these in mind as you learn the techniques of skilled interviewing.

The *interviewing process* that generates the patient's story is fluid and requires empathy, effective communication, and the relational skills to respond to patient cues, feelings, and concerns. As you will see, it is "open-ended," drawing on a range of techniques that affirm and empower the patient—active listening, guided questioning, nonverbal affirmation, empathic responses, validation, reassurance, and partnering. These techniques are especially pertinent to eliciting the patient's chief concerns and the History of the Present Illness.

The *health history format* is a structured framework for organizing patient information in written or verbal form. This format focuses your attention on the specific kinds of information you need to obtain, facilitates clinical reasoning, and clarifies communication of patient concerns, diagnoses, and plans to other health care providers involved in the patient's care. "Clinician-centered," closed-ended "yes-no" questions are more pertinent to the Past Medical History, the Family History, the Personal and Social History, and the Review of Systems.

Above all, the interview involves a commitment to masterful *listening*, easily sacrificed to the time pressures of daily health care. In the words of Sir William Osler, one of our greatest clinicians and co-founder of Johns Hopkins School of Medicine in 1893: "Listen to your patient. He is telling you the diagnosis" and "The good physician treats the disease; the great physician treats the patient who has the disease."

DIFFERENT KINDS OF HEALTH HISTORIES

As you learned in Chapter 1, the scope and detail of the history depends on the patient's needs and concerns, your goals for the encounter, and the clinical setting (inpatient or outpatient, the amount of time available, primary care or subspecialty).

See Chapter 1, Overview: Physical Examination and History Taking, pp. 3–24.

- For new patients, in most settings, you will do a *comprehensive health history.*

- For patients who seek care for specific complaints, for example, cough or painful urination, a more limited interview tailored to that specific problem may be indicated; this is sometimes known as a *focused* or *problem-oriented history.*

- For patients who seek care for ongoing or chronic problems, an interview focusing on the patient's self-management, response to treatment, functional capacity and quality of life, is most appropriate.[10]

- Primary care clinicians frequently schedule visits specifically for health maintenance to address screening and issues, like smoking, weight, or high-risk sexual behaviors.

- A specialist may need a more comprehensive history to evaluate a problem with numerous possible causes.

Knowing the content and relevance of the components of a comprehensive health history enables you to select the elements most pertinent to the patient's concerns and your shared goals for the patient's health.

This chapter, reorganized for this edition to facilitate learning, sets the guideposts for interviewing and the health history: the fundamentals of skilled interviewing; the sequence and social context of the interview; advanced interviewing, including strategies for addressing challenging patients and sensitive topics; and ethics and professionalism.

Chapter Overview

The Fundamentals of Skilled Interviewing
▶ The Techniques of Skilled Interviewing: Active listening. Emphatic responses. Guided questioning. Nonverbal communication. Validation. Reassurance. Partnering. Summarization. Transitions. Empowering the patient.

The Sequence and Context of the Interview
▶ Preparation: Reviewing the medical record. Setting goals for the interview. Reviewing your clinical behavior and appearance. Adjusting the environment.
▶ The Sequence of the Interview: Greeting the patient and establishing rapport. Taking notes. Establishing the agenda for the interview. Inviting the patient's story. Identifying and responding to emotional cues. Expanding and clarifying the patient's story. Generating and testing diagnostic hypotheses. Sharing the treatment plan. Closing the interview and the visit. Taking time for self-reflection.
▶ The Cultural Context of the Interview: Demonstrating cultural humility—a changing paradigm.

Advanced Interviewing
▶ Challenging Patients: The silent patient. The confusing patient. The patient with impaired capacity. The talkative patient. The angry or disruptive patient. The patient with a language barrier. The patient with low literacy or low health literacy. The hearing impaired patient. The blind patient. The patient with limited intelligence. The patient seeking personal advice. The seductive patient.
▶ Sensitive Topics: The sexual history. The mental health history. Alcohol and prescribed and illicit drug use. Intimate partner and family violence. Death and dying.

Ethics and Professionalism

THE FUNDAMENTALS OF SKILLED INTERVIEWING

You may have many reasons for choosing to enter the health care professions, but building effective and healing relationships is undoubtedly paramount. "Those who suffer empower healers to witness, explain, and relieve their suffering."[2] This section describes the fundamental and essential techniques of therapeutic interviewing, the timeless skills you will continually polish in your work with patients. These skills require practice and feedback from your teachers so you can monitor your progress. Over time, you will learn to select the techniques best suited to the ever changing dynamics of human behavior in your patient relationships. Key among these techniques are active listening and empathy, the golden links to a therapeutic alliance.

The Techniques of Skilled Interviewing

▶ Active listening
▶ Empathic responses
▶ Guided questioning
▶ Nonverbal communication
▶ Validation

▶ Reassurance
▶ Partnering
▶ Summarization
▶ Transitions
▶ Empowering the patient

Active Listening. The habit of *active listening* lies at the heart of all interviewing techniques. Active listening is the process of closely attending to what the patient is communicating, being aware of the patient's emotional state, and using verbal and nonverbal skills to encourage the speaker to continue and expand upon important concerns. Active listening allows you to understand the meaning of those concerns at multiple levels of the patient's experience.[11] This takes practice. It is easy to drift into thinking about your next question or possible diagnoses when you and the patient are best served by your concentration on listening.

Empathic Responses. Empathic responses are vital to patient rapport and healing.[12,13] Empathy has been described as the capacity of the clinician to identify with the patient and feel the patient's pain as the clinician's own.[14] Empathy "requires a willingness to suffer some of the patient's pain in the sharing of suffering that is vital to healing."[15] As patients talk with you, they may convey, in words or in facial expression or demeanor, feelings they may or may not have consciously acknowledged. These feelings are crucial to understanding their illnesses. *To express empathy, you must first recognize the patient's feelings.* This requires a willingness on your part to then elicit emotional content. At first this may seem uncomfortable but will deepen mutual trust. When you sense important but unexpressed feelings from the patient's face, voice, behavior or words, gently ask: "How do you feel about that?" or "That seems to trouble you, can you say more?" Do not assume you know the meaning of these feelings. Unless you affirm your concern, important dimensions of the patient's experience may go untapped.

Once the patient has shared these feelings, reply with understanding and acceptance. Your responses may be as simple as: "That sounds upsetting" or "You must be feeling sad." *For a response to be empathic, it must convey that you feel what the patient is feeling.* Empathy may also be nonverbal—placing your hand on the patient's arm or offering tissues when the patient is crying.

If your response to the death of a parent, for example, addresses how upset the patient must have felt when, in fact, the death relieved the patient of long-standing emotional harm, you have acted on your own assumptions in place of supporting the patient's feelings and life experiences. Instead, you can ask: "You have lost your father. What has that been like for you?"

Guided Questioning: Options for Expanding and Clarifying the Patient's Story. There are several ways you can ask for more information from the patient without interfering with the flow of the patient's story. Your goal is to facilitate full communication, in the patient's own words, and without interruption. Guided questions show your sustained interest in the patient's feelings and deepest disclosures. They may help you avoid questions that prestructure or even shut down the flow of the patient's ideas. A series of "yes-no" questions makes the patient feel more passive, leading to a loss of significant detail. Your goal is to absorb the patient's story.

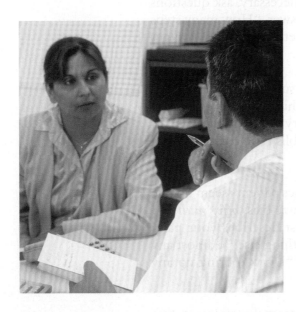

Types of Guided Questioning

- ▶ Moving from open-ended to focused questions
- ▶ Using questioning that elicits a graded response
- ▶ Asking a series of questions, one at a time
- ▶ Offering multiple choices for answers
- ▶ Clarifying what the patient means
- ▶ Encouraging with continuers
- ▶ Using echoing

For further practice see Smith, *Patient-Centered Interviewing.*[5]

Moving From Open-Ended to Focused Questions. Your questioning should proceed from general to specific. Think about a cone, open at the top then tapering to a focal point. Start with the most general questions like, "How can I help?" and move to still open but focused ones like, "Tell me more about your experience with the medicine." Then pose closed questions like, "Did the new medicine cause any problems?" Begin with a truly open-ended question that does not inadvertently include an answer. A possible sequence might be:

"Tell me about your chest discomfort." (Pause)
"What else?" (Pause)
"Where did you feel it?" (Pause) "Show me."
"Anywhere else?" (Pause) "Did it travel anywhere?" (Pause) "To which arm?"

You should avoid *leading questions* that include the answer in the question or suggest your desired response: "Has your pain been improving?" or "You don't have any blood in your stools, do you?" If you ask "Is your pain like a pressure?" and the patient answers yes, your words may turn into the patient's words. Adopt the more neutral "Please describe your pain."

Questioning That Elicits a Graded Response. If necessary, ask questions that require *a graded response* rather than a single answer. "How many steps can you climb before you get short of breath?" is better than "Do you get short of breath climbing stairs?"

Asking a Series of Questions, One at a Time. Be sure to *ask one question at a time*. "Any tuberculosis, pleurisy, asthma, bronchitis, pneumonia?" may lead to a negative answer out of sheer confusion. Try "Do you have any of the following problems?" Be sure to pause and establish eye contact as you list each problem.

Offering Multiple Choices for Answers. Sometimes patients seem unable to describe their symptoms without help. To minimize bias, *offer multiple-choice answers:* "Which of the following words best describes your pain: aching, sharp, pressing, burning, shooting, or something else?" Almost any specific question has at least two possible answers. "Do you bring up any phlegm with your cough, or is it dry?"

Clarifying What the Patient Means. At times, patients make statements that are ambiguous or have unclear associations. To understand their meaning, you need to *request clarification,* as in "Tell me exactly what you meant by 'the flu'" or "You said you were behaving just like your mother. What did you mean?"

Encouraging With Continuers. Without even speaking, you can use posture, gestures, or words to encourage the patient to say more. Pausing with a nod of the head or remaining silent, yet attentive and relaxed, is a *cue for the patient to continue.* Leaning forward, making eye contact, and using phrases like "Mm-hmm," or "Go on," or "I'm listening" all sustain the flow of the patient's story.

Echoing. A simple repetition of the patient's last words, or *echoing*, encourages the patient to expand on factual details and feelings, as shown in the following example:

Patient: "The pain got worse and began to spread." (Pause)
Response: "Spread?" (Pause)
Patient: "Yes, it went to my shoulder and down my left arm to the fingers. It was so bad that I thought I was going to die." (Pause)
Response: "Going to die?"
Patient: "Yes, it was just like the pain my father had when he had his heart attack, and I was afraid the same thing was happening to me."

This reflective technique helped to reveal not only the location and severity of the pain but also its meaning to the patient. It did not bias the story or interrupt the patient's train of thought.

Nonverbal Communication. Communication that does not involve speech occurs continuously and provides important clues to feelings and emotions. Being more sensitive to nonverbal messages allows you to both "read the patient" more effectively and send messages of your own. Pay close attention to eye contact, facial expression, posture, head position and movement such as shaking or nodding, interpersonal distance, and placement of the arms or legs—crossed, neutral, or open. Be aware that some nonverbal language is universal and some is culturally bound.

Just as mirroring your position can signify the patient's increasing sense of connectedness, matching your position to the patient's can signal increased rapport. You can also mirror the patient's *paralanguage,* or qualities of speech, such as pacing, tone, and volume, to increase rapport. Moving closer or physical contact like placing your hand on the patient's arm can convey empathy or help the patient gain control of difficult feelings. Bringing nonverbal communication to the conscious level is the first step to using this crucial form of patient interaction.

Validation. Another way to affirm the patient is to validate or acknowledge the legitimacy of his or her emotional experience. A patient who has been in a car accident but has no physical injury may still be experiencing significant distress. Stating something like, "Being in that accident must have been very scary. Car accidents are always unsettling because they remind us of our vulnerability and mortality. That could explain why you still feel upset," reassures the patient. It helps the patient feel that such emotions are legitimate and understandable.

Reassurance. When you are talking with patients who are anxious or upset, it is tempting to try to reassure them. You may find yourself saying, "Don't worry. Everything is going to be all right." Although this may be appropriate in nonprofessional relationships, as a clinician such comments are usually counterproductive. You may mistakenly reassure the patient about the wrong thing. Moreover, premature reassurance may block further disclosures. Your patient may feel that you are uncomfortable with anxiety or that you have not appreciated the depth of your patient's distress.

The first step to effective reassurance is simply identifying and acknowledging the patient's feelings. This promotes a feeling of connection. More meaningful reassurance comes later after you have completed the interview, the physical examination, and perhaps some laboratory studies. At that point, you can interpret for the patient what you think is happening and deal openly with expressed concerns. Reassurance comes from making the patient feel confident that problems have been fully understood and are being addressed.

Partnering.   When building your relationships with patients, be explicit about your commitment to an ongoing partnership. Make patients feel that regardless of what happens with their illness, you envision continuing their care. Even as a student, especially in a hospital setting, this support can make a big difference.

Summarization.   Giving a capsule summary of the patient's story during the course of the interview serves several functions. It communicates to the patient that you have been listening carefully. It identifies what you know and what you don't know. "Now, let me make sure that I have the full story. You said you've had a cough for 3 days, that it's especially bad at night, and that you have started to bring up yellow phlegm. You have not had a fever or felt short of breath, but you do feel congested, with difficulty breathing through your nose." Following with an attentive pause, or asking "Anything else?" lets the patient add other information and corrects any misunderstandings.

You can use summarization at different points in the interview to structure the visit, especially at times of transition (see below). This technique also allows you, the clinician, to organize your clinical reasoning and to convey your thinking to the patient, making the relationship more collaborative. It is also a useful technique for learners when they draw a blank on what to ask next.

Transitions.   Patients may be apprehensive during a health care visit. To put them more at ease, tell them when you are changing directions during the interview. Just as clear signs along the highway give a sense of confidence, this "signposting" gives patients a greater sense of control. As you move from one part of the history to the next and on to the physical examination, orient the patient with brief transitional phrases like "Now I'd like to ask some questions about your past health." Make clear what the patient should expect or do next. "Before we move on to reviewing all your medications, was there anything else about past health problems?" "Now I would like to examine you. I will step out for a few minutes. Please undress and put on this gown."

Empowering the Patient.   The clinician–patient relationship is inherently unequal. Your feelings of inexperience as a student predictably evolve over time into confidence in your knowledge, skills, and authority in your role as a clinician. But patients have many reasons to feel vulnerable. They may be in pain or worried about a symptom. They may be unfamiliar or overwhelmed by even getting to see you, a situation you may take for granted. Differences of gender, ethnicity, race, or class may also contribute to power differentials. However, ultimately, patients are responsible for their own care.[16] Patients who are self-confident and understand your recommendations are most likely to adopt your advice, make lifestyle changes, or take medications as prescribed.

Listed next are principles that help you share power with your patients. Although many of them have been discussed previously in this chapter, the need to reinforce patients' primary responsibility for their health is so fundamental that it is worth summarizing them here.

Empowering the Patient: Principles of Sharing Power

▶ Evoke the patient's perspective.
▶ Convey interest in the person, not just the problem.
▶ Follow the patient's leads.
▶ Elicit and validate emotional content.
▶ Share information with the patient, especially at transition points during the visit.
▶ Make your clinical reasoning transparent to the patient.
▶ Reveal the limits of your knowledge.

THE SEQUENCE AND CONTEXT OF THE INTERVIEW

Preparation: Reviewing the medical record. Setting goals for the interview. Reviewing your clinical behavior and appearance. Adjusting the environment.

The Sequence of the Interview: Greeting the patient and establishing rapport. Establishing the agenda for the interview. Inviting the patient's story. Exploring the patient's perspective. Identifying and responding to emotional cues. Expanding and clarifying the patient's story. Generating and testing diagnostic hypotheses. Sharing the treatment plan. Closing the interview and the visit. Taking time for self-reflection.

The Cultural Context of the Interview: Demonstrating cultural humility—a changing paradigm.

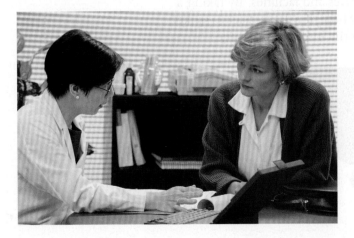

Now that you have learned the fundamental techniques for skilled interviewing, you are ready to turn to the interview itself. First, prepare for the interview by reviewing the record and setting goals for the interview ahead.

Review your appearance and make sure the patient is comfortable and the environment is conducive to the very personal information soon to be shared. You will find that each interview has a rhythm and sequence. Master the components that are described. Finally, the interview has important societal dimensions. As you create a therapeutic alliance, be aware of any biases that may affect your responses to the patient and the patient's need for a therapeutic partnership.

Preparation

Interviewing patients requires planning. As you launch or renew your relationship with the patient, consider several steps that are crucial to success: reviewing the medical record, setting goals for the interview, reviewing your behavior and appearance, and adjusting the environment.

Reviewing the Medical Record.   Before seeing the patient, review the medical records. This helps you gather information and plan the areas you need to explore. Look closely at identifying data such as age, gender, address, and health insurance, and peruse the problem list, the medication list, and details such as documented allergies. The chart often provides valuable information about past diagnoses and treatments, but do not let previous diagnoses deflect you from making your own assessment based on new approaches or ideas. The medical record evolves from many observers and is not designed to depict the unique individual you are about to see. Data may be incomplete or even disagree with what the patient tells you. Recognizing and correcting discrepancies in the record may prove helpful to the patient's care.

Setting Goals for the Interview.   Before you talk with the patient, clarify your goals for the interview. As a student, your primary purpose may be to complete a comprehensive history required for your rotation. As a practicing clinician, your goals can range from assessing a new concern, to treatment follow-up, to completing forms. *The clinician must balance these provider-centered goals with patient-centered goals,* weighing multiple agendas arising from the needs of the patient, the patient's family, and health care agencies and facilities. By taking a few minutes to think through your goals ahead of time, it will be easier to strike a healthy balance among the various purposes of the interview to come.

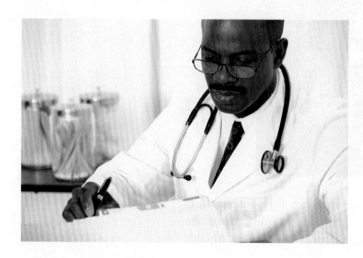

Reviewing Your Clinical Behavior and Appearance.   Just as you carefully observe the patient throughout the interview, the patient will be watching you. Consciously or not, you send messages through both your words and your behavior. Posture, gestures, eye contact, and tone of voice all convey the extent of your interest, attention, acceptance, and understanding. The skilled interviewer seems calm and unhurried, even when time is limited. Reactions that betray disapproval, embarrassment, impatience, or boredom block communication, as do any behaviors that condescend, stereotype, criticize, or belittle the patient. Professionalism requires equanimity and "unconditional positive regard" to nurture healing in relationships with patients.[17] Your personal appearance is also important. Patients find cleanliness, neatness, conservative dress, and a name tag reassuring. Remember to keep *the patient's perspective* in mind if you want to build the patient's trust.

Adjusting the Environment.   Make the interview setting as private and comfortable as possible. You may have to talk with the patient under difficult circumstances, such as a two-bed room or the corridor of a busy emergency department, but a conducive environment improves communication. If there are privacy curtains, ask permission to pull them shut. Suggest moving to an empty room instead of talking in a waiting area. Adjust the room temperature for the patient's comfort when needed. *As the clinician, it is part of your job to make adjustments to the location and seating that make the patient more comfortable.* These efforts are always worth the time.

The Sequence of the Interview

Once you have prepared for the interview, you are ready to listen and elicit the patient's concerns using the techniques you have learned. In general, an interview moves through several stages. *Throughout this sequence, as the clinician, you must always be attuned to the patient's feelings, help the patient express them, respond to their content, and validate their significance.* A typical sequence follows throughout this section.

As a student, you will concentrate primarily on gathering the patient's story and creating a shared understanding of the patient's concerns. When you become a practicing clinician, reaching agreement on a plan for further evaluation and treatment becomes more important. Whether the interview is comprehensive or focused, pay close attention to the patient's feelings and affect, always working on strengthening the relationship as you move through this sequence. When gathering data and forming hypotheses, including the patient's feelings, ideas, and expectations leads to therapeutic interventions best suited to the patient's needs, coping skills, and life circumstances.

Greeting the Patient and Establishing Rapport.   The initial moments of your encounter with the patient lay the foundation for your ongoing relationship. How you greet the patient and other visitors in the room, provide for the patient's comfort, and arrange the physical setting all shape the patient's first impressions.

As you begin, *greet the patient* by name and introduce yourself, giving your own name. If possible, shake hands with the patient. If this is the first contact, explain your role, including your status as a student and how you will be involved in the patient's care. Repeat this part of the introduction on subsequent meetings until you are confident that the patient knows who you are: "Good morning, Mr. Peters. I am Susannah Martinez, a third-year medical student. You may remember me. I was here yesterday talking with you about your heart problems. I am part of the medical team taking care of you."

In general, use a formal title to address the patient, Mr. O'Neil or Ms. Washington for example.[18–20] Except with children or adolescents, avoid first names unless you have specific permission from the patient or family. Calling an unfamiliar adult "granny" or "dear" can depersonalize and demean. If you are unsure how to pronounce the patient's name, don't be afraid to ask. You can say, "I am afraid of mispronouncing your name. Could you say it for me?" Then repeat it to make sure that you heard it correctly.

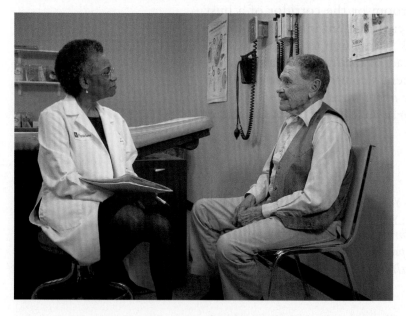

When visitors are in the room, be sure to acknowledge and greet each one in turn, inquiring about each person's name and relationship to the patient. Whenever visitors are present, *you are obligated to maintain the patient's confidentiality.* Let the patient decide if visitors or family members should remain in the room, and ask for the patient's permission before conducting the interview in front of them. For example, "I am comfortable with having your sister stay for the interview, Mrs. Jones, but I want to make sure that this is also what you want" or "Would you prefer if I spoke to you alone or with your sister present?"

Always be attuned to the patient's comfort. In the office or clinic, help the patient find a suitable place for coats and belongings. In the hospital, after greeting the patient, ask how the patient is feeling and if you are coming at a convenient time. Arranging the bed to make the patient more comfortable or allowing a few minutes for the patient to say goodbye to visitors or to finish using the bathroom demonstrates your awareness of the patient's needs. In any setting, look for signs of discomfort, such as shifting position or facial expressions show-

See Chapter 18, Assessing Children, Infancy Through Adolescence, for discussion of visitors present during pediatric visits, pp. 765–891.

ing pain or anxiety. You must attend to pain or anxiety first, both to encourage the patient's trust and to provide enough comfort for the interview to proceed.

Consider the best way to *arrange the room* and how distant you should be from the patient. Remember that cultural background and individual taste influence preferences about interpersonal space. Choose a distance that facilitates conversation and allows good eye contact. You should probably be within several feet, close enough to be intimate but not intrusive. Pull up a chair and, if possible, sit at eye level with the patient. Move any physical barriers, like desks or bedside tables, out of the way. In an outpatient setting, sitting on a rolling stool, for example, allows you to change distances in response to patient cues. Avoid arrangements that convey disrespect or inequality of power, such as interviewing a woman already positioned for a pelvic examination. Lighting also makes a difference. If you sit between a patient and a bright light or window, your view might be good but the patient may have to squint to see you, making the interaction more like an interrogation than a supportive interview.

As you begin the interview, give the patient your undivided attention. Spend enough time on small talk to put the patient at ease, and avoid looking down to take notes, read the chart, or scan a computer screen. Show interest in the patient as a person. For example, you can begin by asking, "So that I can get to know you, tell me about yourself."[21]

Taking Notes. As a novice, you may need to write down much of what you learn during the interview. Even though experienced clinicians recall much of the interview without taking notes, no one can remember all the details of a comprehensive history. Jot down short phrases, specific dates, or words rather than attempting a final format; but do not let note taking or written or electronic forms distract you from the patient. Maintain good eye contact, and whenever the patient is talking about sensitive or disturbing material, put down your pen or move away from the keyboard. Most patients are accustomed to note taking, but for those who find it uncomfortable, explore their concerns and explain your need to make an accurate record. When using an electronic health record, review the patient's record before entering the room; elicit the patient's story while directly facing the patient, maintaining eye contact, and observing all nonverbal behavior; and face the viewing screen only after engaging the patient in the goals for the visit.[22]

Establishing the Agenda. Now that you have established rapport, you are ready to pursue the patient's reason for seeking health care. This reason is traditionally designated the *chief complaint,* but in the ambulatory setting, where there are often three or four reasons for the visit, the phrase *presenting problem(s)* may be preferable. An additional benefit to this phrase is that it does not characterize the patient as a complainer. Begin with **open-ended questions** that allow full freedom of response: "What concerns bring you here today?" or "How can I help you?" Helpful open-ended questions are "Are there specific concerns that prompted you to schedule this appointment?" and "What made you decide to come in to see us today?" These questions encourage the patient to express not just medical problems but any possible concerns. As you elicit the patient's story, note that the first problem the patient mentions may not be the one that is most important.[23] At times the patient may even offer one reason for the visit to the nurse and another to you. For some visits, patients do not have a specific concern and only "want a check-up."

Identifying all the concerns at the outset allows you and the patient to negotiate the concerns that are most pressing and those that can be postponed to a later visit. Questions such as "Is there anything else?", "Have we got everything?", or "Is there anything we missed?" help the patient to express all the reasons for seeking care. The clinician may want to address different issues, like an elevated blood pressure or an abnormal clinical finding or test result. Identifying the full agenda or even "the real reason" for the visit protects time for the most important issues and avoids insufficient attention to late-emerging concerns. However, even negotiating the agenda at the outset does not avert the "oh by the way" concerns that suddenly emerge at the end of the visit.[24]

Inviting the Patient's Story. Once you have elicited, negotiated, and prioritized the agenda, invite the patient's story by asking about the foremost concern, "Tell me more about . . ." Continue to encourage patients to tell their stories in their own words, using an open-ended approach. Avoid biasing the patient's story—*inject no new information* and *do not interrupt*. Instead, use active listening skills: lean forward as you listen; add continuers such as nodding your head and phrases like "uh huh," "go on," or "I see." Train yourself to *follow the patient's leads*. If you intervene too early or ask specific questions prematurely, you risk suppressing the very information you are seeking. Studies show that clinicians interrupt patients during office visits after only 18 seconds.[23] Once interrupted, patients usually do not return to telling their stories. After the patient's initial description of each issue, use a *focusing approach to explore the patient's story in more depth*. Ask *"How would you describe the pain?" "What happened next?" "What else did you notice?"* Using additional guided questioning helps you avoid missing any of the patient's concerns.

See pp. 60–61 for discussions of *continuers*.

See pp. 59–61 for discussions of *guided questioning*.

Exploring the Patient's Perspective. It is critical to explore the deeper meanings patients attach to their symptoms. The ***disease/illness distinction model*** acknowledges the different yet complementary perspectives of the clinician and the patient.[25] ***Disease*** is the explanation that the *clinician* brings to the symptoms. It is the way that the clinician organizes what he or she learns from the patient that leads to a clinical diagnosis. ***Illness*** can be defined as how the *patient* experiences all aspects of the disease, including its effects on relationships, function, and sense of well-being. Many factors may shape this experience, including prior personal or family health, the effect of symptoms on everyday life, individual outlook and style of coping, and expectations about medical care. The melding of these two perspectives forms the basis for planning evaluation and treatment. *The clinical interview needs to incorporate both these views of reality.*

Even a straightforward complaint like sore throat can illustrate these divergent views. The patient may be most concerned about pain and difficulty swallowing, missing time from work, or a cousin who was hospitalized with tonsillitis. The clinician, however, may focus on specific points in the history that differentiate streptococcal pharyngitis from other etiologies, or on a questionable history of allergy to penicillin. To understand the patient's expectations, the clinician needs to go beyond just the attributes of a symptom. Learning about the patient's perception of illness means asking patient-centered questions in the four domains listed below. This information is crucial to patient satisfaction, effective health care, and patient follow-through.[5,26]

Exploring the Patient's Perspective (F-I-F-E)

▶ The patient's **F**eelings, including fears or concerns, about the problem
▶ The patient's **I**deas about the nature and the cause of the problem
▶ The effect of the problem on the patient's life and **F**unction
▶ The patient's **E**xpectations of the disease, of the clinician, or of health care, often based on prior personal or family experiences

---

Exploring the patient's perspective encompasses different types of questions. To uncover the patient's feelings the clinician might ask, "What concerns you most about the pain?" or "How has this been for you?" To explore the patient's thoughts about the cause of the problem you could say, "Why do you think you have this stomachache?" or "What have you tried?" because therapeutic attempts suggest explanatory models. A patient may worry that the pain is a symptom of serious disease and want reassurance. Alternatively, the patient may be less concerned about the cause of the pain and just want relief. To determine the effect of the illness on the patient's lifestyle and function, particularly for patients with chronic illness, ask, "What can't you do now that you could do before? How has your backache (shortness of breath, etc.) affected your ability to work? Your life at home? Your social activities? Your role as a parent? Your function in intimate relationships? The way you feel about yourself as a person?" You need to find out what the patient expects from you, the clinician, or from health care in general ... "I am glad that the pain is almost gone, how specifically can I help you now?" Even if the stomach pain is almost gone, the patient may need a work excuse to take to an employer. A mnemonic for the patient's perspective on the illness is *FIFE—Feelings, Ideas, effect on Function, and Expectations.*

Identifying and Responding to the Patient's Emotional Cues. Emotional distress is frequently associated with illness; 30% to 40% of patients show significant levels of anxiety and depression in primary care practices.[27] Patient visits tend to be longer when clinicians miss opportunities to acknowledge emotional clues.[24] Patients may withhold their true concerns in up to 75% of acute care visits but may offer clues to these concerns, which may be direct or indirect, verbal or nonverbal, and expressed as ideas or emotions.[28,29] Acknowledging and responding to these clues help build rapport, expand the clinician's understanding of the illness, and improve patient satisfaction.

If the patient does not mention the impact of the illness, probe the broader personal context of the illness by asking "How has this affected you?" or "What do you make of this?" Seek the patient's related emotions directly or indirectly by stating "How did you feel about that?" or "Many people would be frustrated by something like this." See the box on the next page for a taxonomy of the clues about the patient's perspective on illness.

Clues to the Patient's Perspective on Illness

▶ Direct statement(s) by the patient of explanations, emotions, expectations, and effects of the illness[17]

▶ Expression of feelings about the illness without naming the illness

▶ Attempts to explain or understand symptoms

▶ Speech clues (e.g., repetition, prolonged reflective pauses)

▶ Sharing a personal story

▶ Behavioral clues indicative of unidentified concerns, dissatisfaction, or unmet needs such as reluctance to accept recommendations, seeking a second opinion, or early return appointment

Source: Lang F, Floyd MR, Beine KL. Clues to patients' explanations and concerns about their illnesses: a call for active listening. Arch Fam Med 9:222–227, 2000.

Learn to respond immediately when you observe an emotional cue. Appropriate response techniques include reflection, synonyms, and feedback indicating support and partnership. A mnemonic for responding to emotional cues is *NURes: N*aming—"That sounds like a scary experience"; *U*nderstanding or legitimization—"It's understandable that you feel that way"; and *Re*specting—"You've done better than most people would with this."

Expanding and Clarifying the Patient's Story. After eliciting the patient's story in a nondirective manner as fully as possible and exploring the patient's lived experience of the illness, guide the patient to elaborate on the areas of the health history that seem most significant. As a clinician, you must clarify the attributes of each symptom, including context, associations, and chronology. For pain and many other symptoms, understanding these essential characteristics, summarized as the seven key attributes of a symptom, is critical.

To pursue the seven attributes, two mnemonics may help:

● **OLD CARTS,** or **O**nset, **L**ocation, **D**uration, **C**haracter, **A**ggravating/ **A**lleviating Factors, **R**adiation, and **T**iming, *and*

● **OPQRST,** or **O**nset, **P**alliating/**P**rovoking Factors, **Q**uality, **R**adiation, **S**ite, and **T**iming

The Seven Attributes of a Symptom

1. *Location.* Where is it? Does it radiate?
2. *Quality.* What is it like?
3. *Quantity or severity.* How bad is it? (For pain, ask for a rating on a scale of 1 to 10.)
4. *Timing.* When did (does) it start? How long does it last? How often does it come?
5. *Setting in which it occurs.* Include environmental factors, personal activities, emotional reactions, or other circumstances that may have contributed to the illness.
6. *Remitting or exacerbating factors.* Is there anything that makes it better or worse?
7. *Associated manifestations.* Have you noticed anything else that accompanies it?

Whenever possible, *use the patient's words*, making sure you clarify their meaning. Although using medical terms is tempting, it confuses and frustrates patients. Be aware of how quickly jargon like "take a history" and "work you up" can creep into your discussions. Choose instead plain expressions such as "I'd like to learn more about your illness" or "Doing these tests can help us understand what's causing your illness."

It is important to establish *the sequence and time course* of each of the patient's symptoms if you are to arrive at accurate assessments. To encourage a chronologic account, ask questions like "What then?" or "What happened next?" or "Please start at the beginning, or the last time you felt well, and go step by step." To fill in specific details, vary the types of questions and interviewing techniques that you use, including focused questions for information that is still missing. *In general, an interview moves back and forth from open-ended questions to increasingly focused questions and then on to another open-ended question, returning the lead in the interview to the patient.*

See the Techniques of Skilled Interviewing and discussion of focused questions, pp. 58–63.

Generating and Testing Diagnostic Hypotheses.   As you gain experience listening to patient concerns, you will acquire the skills of clinical reasoning. You will *generate and test diagnostic hypotheses* about what disease process might be present. Identifying the attributes of each symptom and pursuing related details are fundamental to recognizing patterns of disease and to generating the *differential diagnosis*. As you learn more about epidemiology and clusters of presenting symptoms, knowing what to listen for and seeking further information become more automatic.

Some students visualize the process of evoking a full description of the symptom(s) as "the cone":

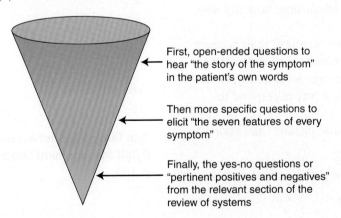

First, open-ended questions to hear "the story of the symptom" in the patient's own words

Then more specific questions to elicit "the seven features of every symptom"

Finally, the yes-no questions or "pertinent positives and negatives" from the relevant section of the review of systems

Each symptom has its own "cone," which becomes a paragraph in the History of Present Illness in the written record.

For example, in a patient with a cough, these questions would come from the Respiratory section of the Review of Systems, on pp. 20–21.

Appropriate questions about symptoms are also suggested in each of the chapters on the regional physical examinations. This is one way that you build evidence for and against various diagnostic possibilities. The challenge is to avoid letting this kind of inquiry dominate the interview, displacing goals like eliciting the patient's perspective or conveying concern for the patient's well-being.

See also Chapter 2, Clinical Reasoning, Assessment, and Recording Your Findings, pp. 49–51.

Sharing the Treatment Plan. Learning about the disease and conceptualizing the illness give you and the patient the opportunity to create a shared picture of the patient's problems. This multifaceted picture then forms the basis for planning further evaluation (e.g., physical examination, laboratory tests, consultations) and negotiating a treatment plan. Shared planning plays an important role in building rapport.

See also Chapter 2, Clinical Reasoning, Assessment, and Recording Your Findings, for more specific techniques for negotiating a plan.

Behavior Change and Motivational Interviewing. Many of your patient visits will close with a discussion of behavior change that "goes beyond the 'big four' lifestyle habits (smoking, excessive drinking, lack of exercise, and unhealthy diet)" to include use of medications, sleep regimens, or steps to improve management of disease.[30] Advanced skills such as motivational interviewing and the therapeutic use of the doctor–patient relationship are beyond the scope of this book. Nonetheless, it is worthwhile to introduce the principles of motivational interviewing, a set of well-documented techniques that improves health outcomes, especially for patients with substance abuse.[31] Motivational interviewing helps patients "to say why and how they might change, and is based on the use of a guiding style" of interviewing rather than direct advice. It engages patients to express the pros and cons of a given behavior. Motivational interviewing makes the assumption that many patients already know what is best for them and helps them confront their ambivalence to change.[32] Using three core skills empowers *the patient* to provide ideas, solutions, and a timetable for change, as shown in the following table.

See Table 3-1, Motivational Interviewing: A Clinical Example, p. 101.

The Guiding Style of Motivational Interviewing

▶ "Ask" open-ended questions—invite the patient to consider how and why they might change

▶ "Listen" to understand your patient's experience—"capture" their account with brief summaries or reflective listening statements such as "quitting smoking feels beyond you at the moment"; these express empathy, encourage the patient to elaborate, and are often the best way to respond to resistance

▶ "Inform"—by asking permission to provide information, and then asking what the implications might be for the patient.

Source: Quoted directly from Rollnick S, Butler CC, Kinnersly P et al. Motivational Interviewing. BMJ 340:1242–1245, 2010.

See Table 3-2, Brief Action Planning: A Self-Management Support Tool, p. 102.

Closing the Interview. You may find that ending the interview is difficult. Patients often have many questions, and if you have done your job well, they are engaged and affirmed as they talk with you. Let the patient know that the end of the interview is approaching to allow time for any final questions. Make sure the patient understands the mutual plans you have developed. For example, before gathering your papers or standing to leave the room, you can say, "We need to stop now. Do you have any questions about what we've covered?" As you close, reviewing future evaluation, treatments, and follow-up is helpful. "So, you will take the medicine as we discussed, get the blood test before you leave today, and make a follow-up appointment for 4 weeks. Do you have any questions about this?" Even better, ask the patient to relate the plan back to you.[33,34]

The patient should have a chance to ask any final questions; however, these few minutes are not the time to bring up new topics. If this happens and the concern is not life threatening, simply assure the patient of your interest and make plans to address the problem at a future time. "That knee pain sounds concerning. Why don't you make an appointment for next week so we can discuss it?" Reaffirming your on-going commitment to the patient's health is always appreciated and transmits caring and esteem.

Taking Time for Self-Reflection. The value of self-reflection as a vital quality of truly empathetic clinicians cannot be overemphasized. As you encounter people of diverse ages, gender identities, social class, race, and ethnicity, being consistently respectful and open to individual differences is an ongoing challenge of clinical care. Because we bring our own values, assumptions, and biases to every encounter, we must look inward to clarify how our own expectations and reactions affect what we hear and how we behave. *Self-reflection is a continual part of professional development in clinical work. It brings a deepening personal awareness to our work with patients. This personal awareness is one of the most rewarding aspects of patient care.*[35]

The Cultural Context of the Interview

Demonstrating Cultural Humility—A Changing Paradigm. Communicating effectively with patients from every background has always been an important professional skill. Nonetheless, the disparities in risks of disease, morbidity, and mortality are marked and broadly documented across different population groups, reflecting inequities in health care access, income level, type of insurance, educational level, language proficiency, and provider decision making.[36,37] To moderate these disparities, clinicians are increasingly urged to prove their own attributes and responsiveness as they experience diversity in their clinical practices.[38,39]

Cultural competence is commonly viewed as "a set of attitudes, skills, behaviors, and policies that enable organizations and staff to work effectively in cross-cultural situations. It reflects the ability to acquire and use knowledge of the health-related beliefs, attitudes, practices, and communication patterns of clients and their families to improve services, strengthen programs, increase community participation, and close the gaps in health status among diverse population groups."[40] Culturally competent care requires "understanding of and respect for the cultures, traditions, and practices of a community."[41] For example, Asians and Pacific Islanders for Reproductive Health have cited environmental toxins as threats to food safety, and the Native American Women's Health Education Resource Center has included sovereignty and the right to parent as Native Americans in their agendas for health.

See Chapters 4–20, sections on Health Promotion and Counseling: Evidence and Recommendations and selected notations in the Examples of Abnormalities columns.

Experts caution that too often cultural competence is reduced to a static decontextualized set of traits and beliefs for particular ethnic groups that objectifies patients as "other," implicitly reinforcing the perspectives of the dominant, often Western, culture.[42,43] Instead, "culture is ever-changing and always being revised within the dynamic context of its enactment." However, "this dynamic is often compromised by various sociocultural mismatches between patients and providers."[44] Such mismatches arise from providers' lack of knowledge about patient beliefs and lived experiences as well as unintentional or intentional enactment of stereotypes and bias during patient encounters.

Instead, move toward the precepts of *cultural humility*. Cultural humility is defined as a "process that requires humility as individuals continually engage in self-reflection and self-critique as lifelong learners and reflective practitioners."[44] It is a process that includes "the difficult work of examining cultural beliefs and cultural systems of both patients and providers to locate the points of cultural dissonance or synergy that contribute to patients' health outcomes."[45] It calls for clinicians to "bring into check the power imbalances that exist in the dynamics of (clinician)–patient communication" and maintain mutually respectful and dynamic partnerships with patients and communities. To attain these attributes, seek out the more effective training models that continue to emerge.[46–51]

Begin your commitment to self-reflective practice by studying the vignettes that follow. These examples illustrate how cultural differences and unconscious bias can unwittingly lead to poor communication and disrupt the quality and outcomes of patient care.

See discussion of self-reflection, p. 73.

Cultural Humility: Scenario 1

A 28-year-old taxi driver from Ghana who had recently moved to the United States complained to a friend about U.S. medical care. He had gone to the clinic because of fever and fatigue. He described being weighed, having his temperature taken, and having a cloth wrapped tightly, to the point of pain, around his arm. The clinician, a 36-year-old woman from Washington, D.C., asked the patient many questions, examined him, and wanted to take blood, which the patient had refused. The patient's final comment was ". . . and she didn't even give me chloroquine!"—his primary reason for seeking care. The man from Ghana was expecting few questions, no examination, and treatment for malaria, which is what fever usually means in Ghana.

In this example, cross-cultural miscommunication is understandable and thus less threatening to explore. Unconscious bias leading to miscommunication, however, occurs in many clinical interactions. Consider the scenario on the next page that is closer to daily practice.

Cultural Humility: Scenario 2

A 16-year-old high school student came to the local teen health center because of painful menstrual cramps that interfered with her concentration at school. She was dressed in a tight top and short skirt and had multiple piercings, including in her eyebrow. The 30-year-old male clinician asked the following questions: "Are you passing all of your classes? What kind of job do you want after high school? What kind of birth control do you want?" The teenager felt pressured into accepting birth control pills, even though she had clearly stated that she had never had intercourse and planned to postpone it until she got married. She was an honor student and planning to go to college, but the clinician did not elicit these goals. The clinician glossed over her cramps by saying, "Oh, you can just take some ibuprofen. Cramps usually get better as you get older." The patient will not take the birth control pills that were prescribed, nor will she seek health care soon again. She experienced the encounter as an interrogation, so failed to gain trust in her clinician. In addition, the clinician's questions made assumptions about her life and did not show respect for her health concerns. Even though the provider pursued important psychosocial domains, she received ineffective health care because of conflicting cultural values and clinician bias.

In both of these cases, the failure stems from mistaken assumptions or biases. In the first case, the clinician did not consider the many variables affecting patient beliefs about health and expectations for care. In the second case, the clinician allowed stereotypes to dictate the agenda instead of listening to the patient and respecting her as an individual. Each of us has our own cultural background and our own biases. These do not simply fade away as we become clinicians.

As you provide care for an ever-expanding and diverse group of patients, you must recognize how culture shapes not only the patient's beliefs, but also your own. *Culture* is the system of shared ideas, rules, and meanings that influences how we view the world, experience it emotionally, and behave in relation to other people. It can be understood as the "lens" through which we perceive and make sense out of the world we inhabit. The meaning of culture is much broader than the term "ethnicity." Cultural influences are not limited to minority groups; they are relevant to everyone.

Avoid allowing knowledge about specific cultural groups to turn into stereotyping. For example, you may have learned that Hispanic patients convey their pain in a more dramatic fashion. Recognize that this is a stereotype. You must evaluate each patient with pain as an individual, not decreasing the amount of analgesic you would typically use, but being aware of your reactions to the patient's style. Work on an appropriate and informed clinical approach to all patients by becoming aware of your own values and biases, developing communication skills that transcend cultural differences, and building therapeutic partnerships based on respect for each patient's life experience. This type of framework, described in the next section, will allow you to approach each patient as a unique individual.

The Three Dimensions of Cultural Humility

▸ *Self-awareness.* Learn about your own biases; we all have them.
▸ *Respectful communication.* Work to eliminate assumptions about what is "normal." Learn directly from your patients; they are the experts on their culture and illness.
▸ *Collaborative partnerships.* Build your patient relationships on respect and mutually acceptable plans.

Self-Awareness. Start by exploring your own cultural identity. How do you describe yourself in terms of ethnicity, class, region or country of origin, religion, and political affiliation? Don't forget the characteristics that we often take for granted—gender, life roles, sexual orientation, physical ability, and race—especially if we belong to majority groups. What aspects of your family of origin do you identify with, and how are you different from your family of origin? How do these identities influence your beliefs and behaviors?

A more challenging task in learning about ourselves is to bring our own values and biases to a conscious level. *Values* are the standards we use to measure our own and others' beliefs and behaviors. These may appear to be absolutes. *Biases* are the attitudes or feelings that we attach to perceived differences. Being attuned to difference is normal; in fact, in the distant past, detecting differences may have preserved life. Intuitively knowing members of one's own group is a survival skill that we may have outgrown as a society, but that is still actively at work.

Feeling guilty about our biases makes it hard to recognize and acknowledge them. Start with less threatening constructs, like the way an individual relates to time, a culturally determined phenomenon. Are you always on time—a positive value in the dominant Western culture? Or do you tend to run a little late? How do you feel about people whose habits are opposite to yours? Next time you attend a meeting or class, notice who is early, on time, or late. Is it predictable? Think about the role of physical appearance. Do you consider yourself thin, mid-size, or heavy? How do you feel about your weight? What does prevailing U.S. culture teach us to value in physique? How do you feel about people who have different weights?

Respectful Communication. Given the complexity of culture, no one can possibly know the health beliefs and practices of every culture and subculture. Let your patients be the experts on their own unique cultural perspectives. Even if patients have trouble describing their values or beliefs in the abstract, they should be able to respond to specific questions. Find out about the patient's cultural background. Maintain an open, respectful, and inquiring attitude. "What did you hope to get from this visit?" If you have established rapport and trust, patients will be willing to teach you. Be aware of questions that contain assumptions. And always be ready to acknowledge your areas of ignorance or bias. "I know very little about Ghana. What would have happened at a clinic there if you had these concerns?" Or, with the second patient and with much more difficulty, "I mistakenly made

Use some of the same questions discussed earlier in the section, Sharing the Treatment Plan, p. 72.

assumptions about you that are not right. I apologize. Would you be willing to tell me more about yourself and your future goals?"

Learning about specific cultures is valuable because it broadens what areas you, as a clinician, need to explore. Do some reading about the life experiences of individuals in ethnic or racial groups that live in your area. There may be historic reasons for loss of trust in clinicians and health care.[51] Go to movies that are filmed in foreign countries and present the perspectives of different cultures. Learn about the concerns of different consumer groups with explicit health agendas. Get to know healers of different disciplines and learn about their practices. Most importantly, be open to learning from your patients. Do not assume that what you have learned about a cultural group applies to the individual before you.

Collaborative Partnerships. Through continual work on self-awareness and seeing through the "lens" of others, the clinician lays the foundation for the collaborative relationship that best supports the patient's health. Communication based on trust, respect, and a willingness to re-examine assumptions allows patients to express concerns that run counter to the dominant culture. These concerns may be associated with strong feelings such as anger or shame. You, the clinician, must be willing to listen to and validate these emotions, and not let your own feelings prevent you from exploring painful areas. You must also be willing to re-examine your beliefs about the "right approach" to clinical care in a given situation. Make every effort to be flexible and creative in your plans and respectful of patients' knowledge about their own best interests. By consciously distinguishing what is truly important to the patient's health from what is just the standard advice, you and your patients can construct an approach to their health care that is congruent with both their beliefs and effective clinical care. Remember that if the patient stops listening, fails to follow your advice, or does not return, your care has not been successful.

ADVANCED INTERVIEWING

The Challenging Patient. Interviewing patients may precipitate a number of reactions and behaviors that are challenging, difficult, and sometimes even threatening. Your ability to handle these situations will evolve throughout your career. *Always remember the importance of listening to the patient and clarifying the patient's concerns.*

The Silent Patient. Novice interviewers are often uncomfortable with periods of silence and feel obligated to keep the conversation going. Silence has many meanings and purposes. Patients frequently fall silent for short periods to collect thoughts, remember details, or decide whether you can be trusted with certain information. The period of silence usually feels much longer to the clinician than it does to the patient. Be attentive and respectful, convey encouragement to continue when the patient is ready. During periods of silence, watch the patient closely for nonverbal cues, such as difficulty controlling emotions.

Patients with depression or dementia may lose their usual spontaneity of expression, give short answers to questions, and then fall silent. If you have already tried guiding them through recent events or a typical day, try shifting your inquiry to the symptoms of depression or begin an exploratory mental status examination.

See Chapter 5, Behavior and Mental Status, pp. 141–169.

At times, silence may be the patient's response to the way you are asking questions. Are you asking too many short-answer questions in rapid succession? Have you offended the patient by signs of disapproval or criticism? Have you failed to recognize an overwhelming symptom such as pain, nausea, or dyspnea? If so, you may need to ask the patient directly, "You seem very quiet. Have I done something to upset you?"

The Confusing Patient.   Some patients present a confusing array of *multiple symptoms*. They seem to have every symptom that you ask about, or "a positive review of systems." With these patients, focus on the context of the symptom, emphasizing the patient's perspective (see pp. 68–69), and guide the interview into a psychosocial assessment.

See Chapter 5, Behavior and Mental Status, Medically Unexplained Symptoms, pp. 142–143, and Table 5-1, Somatoform Disorders: Types and Approach, pp. 165–166.

At other times, you may feel baffled, frustrated, and confused because you cannot make sense out of the patient's story. The history is vague and difficult to understand, ideas are poorly connected, and language is hard to follow. Even though you word your questions carefully, you cannot seem to get clear answers. The patient may seem peculiar, distant, aloof, or inappropriate. Symptoms may be described in bizarre terms: "My fingernails feel too heavy" or "My stomach knots up like a snake." Perhaps there is a mental status change like psychosis or delirium, a mental illness such as schizophrenia, or a neurologic disorder. Consider delirium in acutely ill or intoxicated patients and dementia in the elderly. Their histories are inconsistent and dates are hard to follow. Some may even confabulate to fill in the gaps in their memories.

See Table 20-4, Delirium and Dementia, p. 964.

When you suspect a psychiatric or neurologic disorder, do not dwell on gathering a detailed history. This can tire and frustrate both you and the patient. Shift to the mental status examination, focusing on level of consciousness, orientation, memory, and capacity to understand. You can work in the initial questions smoothly by asking, "When was your last appointment at the clinic? Let's see … that was about how long ago?" "Your address now is … ? … and your phone number?" You can check these responses in the chart or seek permission to speak with family members or friends to obtain their perspectives.

See Chapter 5, Behavior and Mental Status, The Mental Status Examination, pp. 151–152.

The Patient With Altered Capacity.   Some patients cannot provide their own histories because of delirium, dementia, or mental health conditions. Others are unable to remember certain parts of the history, such as events related to a febrile illness or a seizure. Under these circumstances, you need to determine whether the patient has *"decision-making capacity,"* which is the ability to understand information related to health, to make medical choices based on reason and a consistent set of values, and to declare preferences about treatments. The term *capacity* is preferable to the term *"competence,"* which is a legal term, although some use these terms interchangeably. Generally, clinicians make the determination of capacity and when to seek substituted consent. A recent review notes that currently there are no formal practice guidelines from professional societies for the assessment of capacity to consent to treatment, although the Mini-Mental State Examination and the MacArthur Competence Assessment Tool for Treatment have been used with some success.[52-54] If mental illness impairs decision making, psychiatric consultation is usually helpful. However, many patients with psychiatric conditions and even cognitive impairments retain their ability to make reasoned and insightful medical decisions.

For patients with capacity, even if they communicate only with facial expressions or gestures, you must maintain confidentiality and elicit their input. Assure patients that any shared history will be confidential, obtain their consent before talking with others, and clarify what you can discuss. Your knowledge about the patient can be quite comprehensive, yet others may offer surprising and important information. A spouse, for example, may report significant family strains, depressive symptoms, or drinking habits that the patient has failed to reveal. Consider dividing the interview into two segments—one with the patient and the other with both the patient and a second informant. Each interview has its own merits. Information from other sources often gives you helpful ideas for planning the patient's care, but remains confidential. Learn the tenets of the *Health Insurance Portability and Accountability Act (HIPAA)* passed by Congress in 1996, which sets strict standards for disclosure for both institutions and providers when sharing patient information.[55]

For patients with impaired capacity, you will often need to find a *surrogate informant or decision maker* to assist with the history and decision making. Check whether the patient has a *durable power of attorney for health care* or a *health care proxy*. If not, a spouse or family member, who can represent the patient's wishes, can fill this role in many cases.

Apply the basic principles of interviewing to your conversations with relatives or friends. Find a private place to talk. Introduce yourself, state your purpose, inquire how they are feeling under the circumstances, and recognize and acknowledge their concerns. As you listen to their versions of the history, assess their credibility in light of the quality of their relationship with the patient. Establish how they know the patient. For example, when a child is brought in for health care, the accompanying adult may not be the parent or caregiver, but just the most available ride. Always seek the best-informed source. Occasionally, a relative or friend insists on being with the patient during your evaluation. Try to find out why, and defer to the patient's wishes.

The Talkative Patient. The garrulous, rambling patient may be just as difficult as the silent or confused patient. Faced with limited time and the need to "get the whole story," you may grow impatient, even exasperated. Although this problem has no perfect solution, several techniques are helpful.

Give the patient free rein for the first 5 or 10 minutes, listening closely to the conversation. Perhaps the patient simply needs a good listener and is expressing pent-up concerns, or the patient's style is to tell stories. Does the patient seem obsessively detailed? Is the patient unduly anxious or apprehensive? Is there flight of ideas or a disorganized thought process that suggests a thought disorder?

Focus on what seems most important to the patient. Show your interest by asking questions in those areas. Interrupt only if necessary, but be courteous. Learn to set limits when needed. Remember that part of your task is structuring the interview to gain important information about the patient's health. A brief summary may help you change the subject yet validate any concerns. "Let me make sure that I understand. You have described many concerns. In particular, I heard about two different kinds of pain, one on your left side that goes into your groin and is fairly new, and one in your upper abdomen after you eat that you have had for months. Let's focus just on the side pain first. Can you tell me what it feels like?" Or you can ask the patient, "What is your #1 concern today?"

See Summarization, p. 62.

Finally, do not show your impatience. If time runs out, explain the need for a second meeting. Setting a time limit for the next appointment may be helpful. "I know we have much more to talk about. Can you come again next week? We will have a 30-minute visit then."

The Crying Patient.
Crying signals strong emotions, ranging from sadness to anger or frustration. Pausing, gentle probing, or responding with empathy gives the patient permission to cry. Usually crying is therapeutic, as is your quiet acceptance of the patient's distress or pain. Offer a tissue and wait for the patient to recover. Make a supportive remark like "I am glad you were able to express your feelings." Most patients will soon compose themselves and resume their story. Aside from an acute grief or loss, it is unusual for crying to escalate and become uncontrollable.

Crying makes many people uncomfortable. If this is true for you, learn how to accept displays of emotion so you can support patients at these moving and significant times.

The Angry or Disruptive Patient.
Many patients have reasons to be angry: they are ill, they have suffered a loss, they lack their accustomed control over their own lives, and they feel relatively powerless in the health care system.[21] They may direct this anger toward you. It is possible that this hostility toward you is justified . . . were you late for your appointment, inconsiderate, insensitive, or angry yourself? If so, acknowledge the fact and try to make amends. More often, however, patients displace their anger onto the clinician as a reflection of their frustration or pain.

Accept angry feelings from patients. Allow them to express their feelings without getting angry in return. Avoid joining patients in their hostility toward another provider, the clinic, or the hospital, even if you feel sympathetic. You can validate their feelings without agreeing with their reasons.

"I understand that you felt very frustrated by answering the same questions over and over. Our complex health care system can seem very unsupportive when you are not feeling well." After the patient has calmed down, help find steps that will avert such situations in the future. Rational solutions to emotional problems are not always possible, however, and people need time to express and work through their angry feelings.

Some angry patients become overtly disruptive, belligerent, or out of control. Before approaching such patients, alert the security staff; as a clinician, maintaining a safe environment is one of your responsibilities. Stay calm, appear accepting, and avoid being confrontational. Keep your posture relaxed and nonthreatening and your hands loosely open. At first, do not try to make disruptive patients lower their voices or stop haranguing you or the staff. Listen carefully. Try to understand what they are saying. Once you have established rapport, gently suggest moving to a different location that is more private.

The Patient With a Language Barrier. Nothing underscores the importance of the history more than being unable to talk with the patient, an increasingly common experience. More than 49 million Americans have a primary language other than English, and another 22 million have limited English proficiency.[56] This group is less likely to have regular primary or preventive care and more likely to report problems with care, including higher rates of adverse outcomes from medical errors.[57] Learning to work with qualified interpreters is essential for optimal health outcomes and cost-effective care.[58-60] Experts take this one step further, "If it isn't culturally and linguistically appropriate, it isn't health care."[61]

If your patient speaks a different language, make every effort to find a trained interpreter. A few broken words and gestures of medical Spanish, for example, may enhance rapport, but they are no substitute for the full story. Even being fluent in your patient's language may not transcend important cultural nuances in the meanings of actual words.[62] Recruiting family members is equally hazardous—confidentiality may be violated, meanings may be distorted, and translations may be incomplete and even harmful. Untrained interpreters may try to speed up the interview by telescoping lengthy replies into a few words, omitting details that may be significant. The ideal interpreter is a neutral person who is familiar with both languages and cultures and can serve as a "cultural navigator."[63,64] However, even interpreters with cultural fluency may not be familiar with the multiple subcultures in many countries.

As you begin working with the interpreter, establish rapport and review the information that would be most useful. Explain that you need the interpreter to translate everything, not to condense or summarize. *Make your questions clear, short, and simple.* Help the interpreter by outlining your goals for each segment of the history. After going over your plans, arrange the room so that you have easy eye contact and nonverbal communication with the patient. Then speak directly to the patient . . . "How long have you been sick?" rather than "How long has the patient been sick?" Having the interpreter close to the patient, or even behind you, keeps you from turning your head back and forth.

When available, bilingual written questionnaires are invaluable, especially for the review of systems. First, however, be sure that patients can read in their language; otherwise, ask for help from the interpreter. In some clinical settings, there are speakerphone translators; use them if there are no better options.

Guidelines for Working With an Interpreter: "INTERPRET"

I	Introductions: Make sure to introduce all the individuals in the room. During the introduction, include information as to the roles individuals will play.
N	Note Goals: Note the goals of the interview. What is the diagnosis? What will the treatment entail? Will there be any follow-up?
T	Transparency: Let the patient know that everything said will be interpreted throughout the session.
E	Ethics: Use qualified interpreters (not family members or children) when conducting an interview. Qualified interpreters allow the patient to maintain autonomy and make informed decisions about his or her care.
R	Respect Beliefs: Limited English Proficient (LEP) patients may have cultural beliefs that need to be taken into account as well. The interpreter may be able to serve as a cultural broker and help explain any cultural beliefs that may exist.
P	Patient Focus: The patient should remain the focus of the encounter. Providers should interact with the patient and not the interpreter. Make sure to ask and address any questions the patient may have prior to ending the encounter. If you don't have trained interpreters on staff, the patient may not be able to call in with questions.
R	Retain Control: It is important as the provider that you remain in control of the interaction and not let the patient or the interpreter take over the conversation.
E	Explain: Use simple language and short sentences when working with an interpreter. This will ensure that comparable words can be found in the second language and that all the information can be conveyed clearly.
T	Thanks: Thank the interpreter and the patient for their time. On the chart, note that the patient needs an interpreter and who served as an interpreter this time.

Source: U.S. Department of Health and Human Services. Interpret Tool: working with interpreters in cultural settings. Available at https: www.thinkculturalhealth.hhs.gov/pdfs/InterpretTool. pdf. Accessed June 6, 2012.

The Patient With Low Literacy or Low Health Literacy. Before giving written instructions, assess the patient's *ability to read*. Over 14% of Americans, or 30 million people, are unable to read basic documents.[47] Lack of reading skills may explain why the patient has not taken medications or followed recommendations for treatment.

To detect low literacy, ask about years completed in school. Or try practical approaches like asking "How comfortable are you about filling out health forms?" or checking how well the patient can read written instructions. Another rapid screen is to hand the patient a written text upside down—most patients will turn the page around immediately. Many patients are reluctant to disclose their problems with reading. Be sensitive to their quandary, and do not confuse their degree of literacy with level of intelligence. Explore the reasons that reading is difficult—language barriers, learning disorders, poor vision, or level of education.

Growing research shows that low *health literacy* leads to poor health outcomes and use of health services. Health literacy goes beyond just reading skills, and includes the skills needed to function effectively in the health care environment: print literacy, or the ability to interpret information in documents; numeracy, or the ability to use quantitative information for tasks like interpreting food labels or adhering to medication regimens; and oral literacy, or the ability to speak and listen effectively.[65] Over 80 million U.S. adults are thought to have limited health literacy, the focus of a major report and government and private sector action plans since 2004.[66]

The Patient With Hearing Loss. Approximately 9% of the U.S. population is deaf or hard of hearing. This population "is a heterogeneous group that includes persons who have varying degrees of hearing loss, use multiple languages, and belong to different cultures. Solutions to providing health care to one group from (this) population do not necessarily apply to the other groups. Factors that must be considered with this population include degree of hearing loss, age of onset of loss, preferred language, and psychological issues."[67] Communication and trust are special challenges and the risk of miscommunication is high. Even hearing-impaired patients who use English may not follow standard English usage.

Find out the patient's preferred method of communication. Several questions help you determine whether the patient belongs to the deaf culture or the hearing culture: when the hearing loss occurred relative to the development of speech and language; the kinds of schools the patient attended; and responses to written questionnaires. Patients may use American Sign Language, a unique language with its own syntax. These patients typically have with a low English reading level and prefer certified ASL interpreters during their visits.[67] Other patients may employ varying combinations of signs and speech. If working with an interpreter, use the principles identified earlier. Alternatively, time-consuming handwritten questions and answers may be the only solution, but be sure to assess literacy first.

Partial hearing deficits vary. If the patient has a hearing aid, find out if the patient is using it. Make sure it is working. For patients with unilateral hearing loss, sit on the hearing side. A person who is *hard of hearing* may not be aware of the problem, a situation you will have to tactfully address. Eliminate background noise as much as possible, such as television or hallway conversation. For patients who have partial hearing or who can read lips, face them directly, in good light. Patients should put on their glasses to better pick up visual cues that help them understand you. Speak at a normal volume and rate and do not let your voice trail off at the ends of sentences. Avoid covering your mouth or looking down at papers while speaking. Emphasize key points first. Remember that even the best lip readers comprehend only a percentage of what is said, so having patients repeat what you have said is important. When closing, write out any oral instructions.

The Patient With Impaired Vision. When meeting with a blind patient, shake hands to establish contact and explain who you are and why you are there. If the room is unfamiliar, orient the patient to the surroundings and report if anyone else is present. It still may be helpful to adjust the light. Encourage visually impaired patients to wear glasses whenever possible. Remember to give full explanations because postures and gestures are unseen.

The Patient With Limited Intelligence. Patients of moderately limited intelligence can usually give adequate histories. If you suspect a disability, pay special attention to the patient's schooling and ability to function independently. How far have such patients gone in school? If they didn't finish, why not? What kinds of courses have they taken? How did they do? Have they had any testing done? Are they living alone? Do they need assistance with activities such as transportation or shopping? The sexual history is equally important and often overlooked. Find out if the patient is sexually active and provide information that may be needed about pregnancy or sexually transmitted infections.

If you are unsure about the patient's level of intelligence, make a smooth transition to the mental status examination and assess simple calculations, vocabulary, memory, and abstract thinking.

See Chapter 5, Behavior and Mental Status, pp. 141–169.

For patients with severe mental retardation, turn to family or caregivers to elicit the history, but always show interest in the patient first. Establish rapport, make eye contact, and engage in simple conversation. As with children, avoid "talking down" or using affectations of speech or condescending behavior. The patient, family members, caregivers, or friends will appreciate your respect.

The Patient With Personal Problems. Patients may ask you for advice about personal problems that fall outside the range of your clinical expertise. Should the patient quit a stressful job, for example, or move out of state? Instead of responding, ask about the different approaches the patient has considered and related pros and cons, others who have provided advice, and what supports are available for different choices. Letting the patient talk through the problem with you is more valuable and therapeutic than providing the answer yourself.

The Seductive Patient. Clinicians of both genders occasionally find themselves physically attracted to their patients. Similarly, patients may make sexual overtures or exhibit flirtatious behavior toward clinicians. The emotional and physical intimacy of the clinician–patient relationship may lend itself to these sexual feelings.

If you become aware of such feelings in yourself, accept them as a normal human response, and bring them to conscious level so they will not affect your behavior. Denying these feelings makes it more likely for you to act inappropriately. *Any* sexual contact or romantic relationship with patients is *unethical;* keep your relationship with the patient within professional bounds, and seek help if you need it.[68–71]

When patients are seductive or make sexual advances, you may be tempted to ignore their behavior because you are not sure that it really happened, or you are just hoping it will go away. Calmly but firmly make it clear that your relationship is professional, not personal. If unwelcome overtures continue, leave the room and find a chaperone to continue the interview. You should also reflect on your image. Has your clothing or demeanor been unconsciously seductive? Have you been overly warm with the patient? It is your responsibility to evaluate these factors and avoid any that contribute to these problems.

Sensitive Topics

Clinicians talk with patients about many subjects that are emotionally charged. These discussions can be particularly awkward when you are inexperienced or assessing patients you do not know well. Even seasoned clinicians are affected by societal taboos enveloping certain subjects: abuse of alcohol or drugs, sexual practices, death and dying, financial concerns, racial and ethnic bias, family interactions, domestic violence, psychiatric illnesses, physical deformities, bowel function, and others. Many of these topics trigger strong personal responses related to family, cultural, and societal value systems. Mental illness, drug use during pregnancy, and same-sex practices are three obvious examples of issues that may evoke biases that can affect the patient interview. This section explores challenges to the clinician in several of these sensitive areas.

Several basic principles can help guide your response to sensitive topics:

Guidelines for Broaching Sensitive Topics

▶ *The single most important rule is to be nonjudgmental.* The clinician's role is to learn about the patient and help the patient achieve better health. Disapproval of behaviors or elements in the health history will only interfere with this goal.
▶ *Explain why you need to know certain information.* This makes patients less apprehensive. For example, say to patients, "Because sexual practices put people at risk for certain diseases, I ask all of my patients the following questions."
▶ Find opening questions for sensitive topics and learn the specific kinds of information needed for your assessments.
▶ Finally, consciously acknowledge whatever discomfort you are feeling. Denying your discomfort may lead you to avoid the topic altogether.

Look into other strategies for becoming more comfortable with sensitive areas. Examples include general reading about these topics in medical and lay literature; talking openly to selected colleagues and teachers about your concerns; taking special courses that help you explore your own feelings and reactions; and ultimately, reflecting on your own life experience. Take advantage of all these resources. Whenever possible, listen to experienced clinicians, then practice similar discussions with your own patients. The range of topics that you can explore with comfort will widen progressively.

The Sexual History.   Asking questions about sexual behavior can be life-saving. Sexual behaviors determine risks for pregnancy, sexually transmitted infections (STIs), and AIDS; good interviewing helps prevent or reduce these risks. Sexual practices may be directly related to the patient's symptoms and integral to both diagnosis and treatment. Many patients have questions or concerns about sexuality that they would discuss more freely if you ask about sexual health. Finally, sexual dysfunction may result from use of medication or from misinformation that, if recognized, can be readily addressed.

You can introduce questions about sexual behavior at multiple points in an interview. If the chief complaint involves genitourinary symptoms, include questions about sexual health as part of "expanding and clarifying" the patient's story. For women, you can ask these questions as part of the Obstetric/Gynecologic section of the Past Medical History. You can bring them into discussions about Health Maintenance, along with diet, exercise, and screening tests, or as part of the lifestyle issues or important relationships covered in the Personal and Social History. Or, in a comprehensive history, you can ask about sexual practices during the Review of Systems. Do not forget this area of inquiry just because the patient is elderly or has a disability or chronic illness.

An orienting sentence or two is often helpful. "To assess your risk for various diseases, I need to ask you some questions about your sexual health and practices" or "I routinely ask all patients about their sexual function." For more specific complaints you might state, "To figure out why you have this discharge and what we should do about it, I need to ask some questions about your sexual activity." Try to be matter-of-fact in your style; the patient will be likely to follow your lead. *Use specific language.* Refer to genitalia with explicit words such as penis or vagina and avoid phrases like "private parts." Choose words that the patient understands or explain what you mean. "By intercourse, I mean when a man inserts his penis into a woman's vagina."

In general, ask about specific sexual behaviors as well as satisfaction with sexual function. Review the examples of questions that follow. These questions are designed to help patients reveal their concerns.

See specific questions in Chapter 13, Male Genitalia and Hernias, pp. 522–524, and Chapter 14, Female Genitalia, pp. 546–547.

The Sexual History: Sample Questions

▶ "When was the last time you had intimate physical contact with someone?" Did that contact include sexual intercourse?" Using the term "sexually active" can be ambiguous. Patients have been known to reply, "No, I just lie there."

▶ "Do you have sex with men, women, or both?" Individuals may have sex with persons of the same gender, yet not consider themselves gay, lesbian, or bisexual. Some gay and lesbian patients have had sex with the opposite gender. Your questions should always be about the behaviors.

▶ "How many sexual partners have you had in the last 6 months? In the last 5 years? In your lifetime?" Again, these questions give the patient an easy opportunity to acknowledge multiple partners. Ask also about routine use of condoms. "Do you *always* use condoms?"

▶ It is important to ask all patients, "Do you have any concerns about HIV infection or AIDS?", since infection occurs even in the absence of risk factors.

Note that these questions make no assumptions about marital status, sexual preference, or attitudes toward pregnancy or contraception. Listen to each of the patient's responses, and ask additional questions as indicated. To elicit information about sexual behaviors, you will need to ask more specific and focused questions than in other parts of the interview.

The Mental Health History. Cultural constructs of mental and physical illness vary widely, leading to differences in social acceptance and attitudes. Think how easy it is for patients to talk about diabetes and taking insulin compared with discussing schizophrenia and using psychotropic medications. Ask open-ended questions initially. "Have you ever had any problem with emotional or mental illnesses?" Then move to more specific questions such as "Have you ever visited a counselor or psychotherapist?" "Have you ever been prescribed medication for emotional issues?" "Have you or has anyone in your family ever been hospitalized for an emotional or mental health problem?"

For patients with depression or thought disorders such as schizophrenia, a careful history of their illness is in order. Be sensitive to reports of mood changes or symptoms such as fatigue, unusual tearfulness, appetite or weight changes, insomnia, and vague somatic complaints. Two opening screening questions for depression are: "Over the past 2 weeks, have you felt down, depressed, or hopeless?" and "Over the past 2 weeks, have you felt little interest or pleasure in doing things?"[72] If the patient seems depressed, always ask about suicide: "Have you ever thought about hurting yourself or ending your life?" As with chest pain, you must evaluate severity—both depression and angina are potentially lethal.

Turn to Chapter 5, Behavior and Mental Status, for discussions of depression, suicidality, and psychotic disorders, pp. 141–170.

Many patients with schizophrenia or other psychotic disorders can function in the community and tell you about their diagnoses, symptoms, hospitalizations, and current medications. Investigate their symptoms and assess any effects on mood or daily activities.

Alcohol and Prescription and Illicit Drugs. Many clinicians hesitate to ask patients about excess use of alcohol and drugs, whether prescribed or illicit. The prevalence of substance abuse in persons aged 12 or older remains high: for alcohol dependence or abuse, 7.5% or 18.6 million people; for illicit drug dependence or abuse, 2.7% or 6.9 million people; and for pain relievers, 1.6 million people (2007 data).[73] An estimated 30% of the population has risky or problem drinking, and over 20% have used prescription drugs for non-medical reasons, especially opioids, sedatives and tranquillizers, and stimulants.[32,74–75]

The high prevalence of substance abuse makes it is essential to ask routinely about current and past use of alcohol and drugs, patterns of use, and family history. Be familiar with current definitions of addiction, dependence, and tolerance.

Addiction, Physical Dependence, and Tolerance

Tolerance: A state of adaptation in which exposure to a drug induces changes that result in a diminution of one or more of the drug's effects over time.

Physical Dependence: A state of adaptation that is manifested by a drug class-specific withdrawal syndrome that can be produced by abrupt cessation, rapid dose reduction, decreasing blood level of the drug, and/or administration of an antagonist.

Addiction: A primary, chronic, neurobiologic disease, with genetic, psychosocial, and environmental factors influencing its development and manifestations. It is characterized by behaviors that include one or more of the following: impaired control over drug use, compulsive use, continued use despite harm, and craving.

Source: American Pain Society. Definitions Related to the Use of Opioids for the Treatment of Pain. A consensus statement from the American Academy of Pain Medicine, the American Pain Society, and the American Society of Addiction Medicine, 2001. At http://www.partnersagainstpain.com/printouts/A7012R9.pdf. Accessed August 14, 2011.

Alcohol. Questions about alcohol and other drugs follow naturally after questions about caffeine and cigarettes. "Tell me about your use of alcohol" is an opening query that avoids the easy yes-no response. Remember that some patients do not consider wine or beer as "alcohol." Positive answers to two additional questions are highly suspicious for problem-drinking: "Have you ever had a drinking problem?"; and "When was your last drink?" especially if the night before.[76] The most widely used screening questions are the ***CAGE*** questions about ***C****utting down, ****A****nnoyance when criticized, ****G****uilty feelings, and ****E****ye-openers. The CAGE Questionnaire is readily available online.

National Institute of Alcohol Abuse annd Alcoholism Safe Drinking Levels for Adults Without Contraindications to Alcohol Use

- Men: ≤14 drinks/week and ≤4 drinks on 1 occasion
- Women: ≤7 drinks/week and ≤3 drinks on 1 occasion
- NIAAA recommends ≤1 drink/day for people ≥65 years old
- 1 drink is defined as 12 ounces of beer, 5 ounces of wine, or 1.5 ounces of spirits

Two or more affirmative answers to the CAGE Questionnaire suggest alcohol misuse and have a sensitivity that ranges from 43% to 94% and specificity that ranges from 70% to 96%.[77,78] Several well-validated short screening tests, such as the MAST and the ACEDIT, are also helpful.[79] If you detect misuse, you need to ask about blackouts (loss of memory about events during drinking), seizures, accidents or injuries while drinking, job problems, conflict in personal relationships.

Illicit Drugs. The National Institute on Drug Abuse recommends asking specifically about nonmedical use of illicit and prescription drugs: "In your lifetime have you ever used: marijuana; cocaine; prescription stimulants; methamphetamines; sedatives or sleeping pills; hallucinogens like LSD, ecstasy, mushrooms . . . ; street opioids like heroin or opium; prescription opioids like fentanyl, oxycodone, hydrocodone . . . ; or other substances." For those answering yes, a series of further questions is recommended.[80]

Another approach is to adapt the CAGE questions to screening for substance abuse by adding "or drugs" to each question. Once you identify substance abuse, continue further with questions like "Are you always able to control your use of drugs?" "Have you had any bad reactions?" "What happened . . . Any drug-related accidents, injuries, or arrests? Job or family problems?" . . . "Have you ever tried to quit? Tell me about it."

Intimate Partner Violence and Domestic Violence.

Intimate Partner Violence and Domestic Violence. Intimate partner violence is the leading cause of serious injury and the second leading cause of death among U.S. women of reproductive age.[81] Each year, women experience 4.8 million intimate partner-related physical assaults and rapes and men experience 2.9 million assaults; these are groups that experience high rates of mental health disorders and substance abuse.[82] Prevalence varies from 20% in general practice settings to over 30% in emergency rooms and orthopedic clinics.[83–87] The American Medical Association and the American College of Obstetricians and Gynecologist recommend routine screening of all women for intimate partner violence, although evidence of improved screening outcomes is still inconclusive, in part because effective interventions are still being tested.[88–90] Elders are also highly vulnerable to neglect and abuse.[91–93]

Sensitive interviewing is essential, since even with skilled inquiry only 25% of patients disclose their abuse experience.[94] The type of questioning is important. Experts recommend beginning with normalizing statements such as "Because abuse is common in many women's lives, I've begun to ask about it routinely."[95] Disclosure is more likely when probing questions lead and then in-depth direct questions follow. "Are you in a relationship where you have been hit or threatened?" with a pause to encourage the patient to respond. If the patient says no, continue with "Has anyone ever treated you badly or made you do things you don't want to?" or "Is there anyone you are afraid of?" or "Have you ever been hit, kicked, punched, or hurt by someone you know?" Following disclosure, empathic validating and nonjudgmental responses are critical but currently occur less than half the time.

Clues to Physical and Sexual Abuse.   Be alert to the unspoken clues to abuse, often present in the growing numbers of victims of human sex trafficking in the U.S and internationally, estimated at 50,000 women and children in the annually in the U.S alone.[96,97]

See also Chapter 18, Assessing Children, Infancy Through Adolescence, Table 18-11, Physical Signs of Sexual Abuse, p. 889.

Clues to Physical and Sexual Abuse

▶ Injuries that are unexplained, seem inconsistent with the patient's story, are concealed by the patient, or cause embarrassment
▶ Delay in getting treatment for trauma
▶ History of repeated injuries or "accidents"
▶ Presence of alcohol or drug abuse in patient or partner
▶ Partner tries to dominate the visit, will not leave the room, or seems unusually anxious or solicitous
▶ Pregnancy at a young age; multiple partners
▶ Repeated vaginal infections and STIs
▶ Difficulty walking or sitting due to genital/anal pain
▶ Vaginal lacerations or bruises
▶ Fear of the pelvic examination or physical contact
▶ Fear of leaving the examination room

When you suspect abuse, it is important to spend part of the encounter alone with the patient. You can use the transition to the physical examination as a reason to ask others to leave the room. If the patient is also resistant, you should not force the situation, potentially placing the victim in jeopardy. Be attuned to diagnoses that have a higher association with abuse, such as pregnancy and somatization disorder.

To begin screening for child abuse, ask parents about their approach to discipline. Ask how they cope with a baby who will not stop crying or a child who misbehaves: "Most parents get very upset when their baby cries (or their child has been naughty). How do you feel when your baby cries?" "What do you do when your baby won't stop crying?" "Do you have any fears that you might hurt your child?"

See Chapter 18, Assessing Children: Infancy Through Adolescence, pp. 765–891.

Death and the Dying Patient.   There is a growing and important emphasis in health care education on improving training related to death and dying. Many clinicians avoid talking about death because of their own discomfort and anxiety. Work through your own feelings with the help of reading and discussion. Even as beginning students, you will need to know basic concepts of care because you will come into contact with patients of all ages near the end of their lives.

For discussion of end-of-life decision making, grief and bereavement, and advance directives, turn to Chapter 20, The Older Adult, p. 935.

Kübler-Ross has described five stages in our response to loss or the anticipatory grief of impending death: denial and isolation, anger, bargaining, depression or sadness, and acceptance.[98] These stages may occur sequentially or overlap in any order or combination.[99] Be sensitive to the patient's feelings about dying; watch for cues that the patient is open to talking about them. Make openings for patients to ask questions: "I wonder if you have any concerns about the procedure? . . . your illness? . . . what it will be like when you go home?" Explore these concerns and provide whatever information the patient requests. Avoid unwarranted reassurance. If you explore and accept patients' feelings, answer their questions and demonstrate your commitment to caring for them throughout their illness, coping will grow where it really matters—within the patients themselves.

Dying patients rarely want to talk about their illnesses at each encounter, nor do they wish to confide in everyone they meet. Give them opportunities to talk, and listen receptively, but if they stay at a social level, respect their preferences. Remember that illness—even a terminal one—is only a part of the total person. A smile, a touch, an inquiry about a family member, a comment on the day's events, or even gentle humor affirms and sustains the unique individual you are caring for. Communicating effectively means getting to know the whole patient; that is part of the helping process.

Understanding the patient's wishes about treatment at the end of life is an important responsibility. Failing to establish communication about end-of-life decisions is widely viewed as a flaw in clinical care. Even if discussions of death and dying are difficult, you must learn to ask specific questions. The condition of the patient and the health care setting often determine what needs to be discussed. For patients who are acutely ill and in the hospital, discussions about what the patient wants to have done in the event of a cardiac or respiratory arrest are usually mandatory. Asking about *Do Not Resuscitate (DNR) status* is often difficult when you have no previous relationship with the patient or lack knowledge of the patient's values and life experience. Find out about the patient's frame of reference because the media give many patients an unrealistic view of the effectiveness of resuscitation. "What experiences have you had with the death of a close friend or relative?" "What do you know about cardiopulmonary resuscitation (CPR)?" Educate patients about the likely success of CPR, especially if they are chronically ill or advanced in age. Assure them that relieving pain and taking care of their spiritual and physical needs will be a priority.

In general, it is important to encourage any adult, but especially the elderly or chronically ill, to establish a *health proxy* who can act as the patient's health decision maker. This part of the interview can be a "values history" that identifies what is important to the patient and makes life worth living, and the point when living would no longer be worthwhile. Ask how patients spend their time every day, what brings them joy, and what they look forward to. Make sure to clarify the meaning of statements like, "You said that you don't want to be a burden to your family. What exactly do you mean by that?" Explore the patient's religious or spiritual frame of

See discussion of the Patient With Altered Capacity, pp. 78–79.

reference so that you and the patient can make the most appropriate decisions about health care.

 ## ETHICS AND PROFESSIONALISM

Medical ethics come into play scores of times each day in almost every patient interaction.[100-102] The potential power of clinician–patient communication calls for guidance beyond our innate sense of morality.[103] *Ethics* are a set of principles crafted through reflection and discussion to define right and wrong. *Medical ethics,* which guide our professional behavior, are neither static nor simple, but several principles have guided clinicians throughout the ages. Although in most situations your sense of right and wrong will be all that you need, even as students, you will face decisions that call for the application of ethical principles.

Some of the traditional and still fundamental maxims embedded in the healing professions are listed below. This body of ethics has been termed *"principalism."* As the field of clinical ethics expands, other ethical systems come in use: *utilitarianism,* or providing the greatest good for the greatest number, building on the work of John Stuart Mill; *feminist ethics,* which invoke problems of marginalization of social groups; *casuistry,* or the analysis of paradigmatic prior cases as relevant; and *communitarianism,* which emphasizes the interests of communities and societies over individuals and social responsibilities bearing on the need to maintain the institutions of civil society.[104]

Building Blocks of Professional Ethics in Patient Care

▸ *Nonmaleficence or primum non nocere* is commonly stated as, "First, do no harm." In the context of an interview, giving information that is incorrect or not really related to the patient's problem can do harm. Avoiding relevant topics or creating barriers to open communication can also do harm.

▸ *Beneficence* is the dictum that the clinician needs to "do good" for the patient. As clinicians, your actions need to be motivated by what is in the patient's best interest.

▸ *Autonomy* reminds us that patients have the right to determine what is in their own best interest. This principle has become increasingly important over time and is consistent with collaborative rather than paternalistic clinician–patient relationships.

▸ *Confidentiality* can be one of the most challenging principles. As a clinician, you are obligated not to repeat what you learn from or know about a patient. This privacy is fundamental to our professional relationships with patients. In the daily flurry of activity in a hospital, it is all too easy to let something slip. You must be on your guard.

As students, you are exposed to some of the ethical challenges that you will confront later as practicing clinicians. However, there are dilemmas unique to students that you will face from the time that you begin taking care of patients. The following vignettes capture some of the most common experiences. They raise a variety of interconnected ethical and practical issues.

Ethics and Professionalism: Scenario 1

You are a third-year medical student on your first clinical rotation in the hospital. It is late in the evening when you are finally assigned to the patient you are to "work up" and present the next day at preceptor rounds. You go to the patient's room and find the patient exhausted from the day's events and clearly ready to settle down for the night. You know that your intern and attending physician have already done their evaluations. Do you proceed with a history and physical that is likely to take 1 to 2 hours? Is this process only for your education? Do you ask permission before you start? What do you include?

Here you are confronted with the tension between *the need to learn by doing* and *doing no harm to patients*. There is a utilitarian ethical principle that reminds us that if clinicians-in-training do not learn, there will be no future caregivers. Yet the dictums to do no harm and prioritize what is in the patient's best interests are clearly in conflict with that future need. This dilemma will arise often while you are a student.

The means to address this ethical dilemma is to obtain *informed conscent*. Always make sure the patient realizes that you are in training and new at patient evaluation. It is impressive how often patients willingly let students be involved in their care; it is an opportunity for patients to give back to their caregivers. Even when clinical activities appear to be purely for educational purposes, there may be a benefit to the patient. Multiple caregivers provide multiple perspectives, and the experience of being heard and having a special advocate can be therapeutic.

Ethics and Professionalism: Scenario 2

It is after 10 PM, and you and your resident are on the way to complete the required advance directives form with a frail, elderly patient who was admitted earlier that day with bilateral pneumonia. The form, which includes a discussion of Do Not Resuscitate orders, must be completed before the team can sign out and leave for the day. Just then, your resident is paged to an emergency and asks you to go ahead and meet with the patient to complete the form; the resident will cosign it later. You had a lecture on advance directives and end-of-life discussions in your first year of medical school but have never seen a clinician discuss these issues with a patient. You have not yet met the patient, nor have you had a chance to really look at the form. What should you do? Do you inform the resident that you have never done this before nor even seen it done? Do you need to inform the patient that this is totally new for you? Who should decide whether you are competent to do this independently?

In this situation, you are being asked to take responsibility for clinical care that exceeds your level of comfort and perhaps your competence. This can happen in a number of situations, such as being asked to evaluate a clinical situation without proper back-up or to draw blood or start an IV before practicing under supervision. For the patient in the second scenario, you may have many of the following thoughts: "the patient needs to have this completed before going to sleep and so will benefit"; "the risk to the patient from discussing advance directives is minimal"; "you are pretty good with elderly patients and think that you might be able to do this"; "what if the patient actually arrests that night and you are responsible for what happens?"; and finally, "if you bother the resident now, he or she will be angry and that may affect your evaluation." There is educational value in being pushed to the limits of your knowledge to solve problems and to gain confidence in functioning independently. But what is the right thing to do in this situation?

The principles listed above only partially help you sort this out, because only part of your quandary relates to your relationship with the patient. Much of the tension in this scenario has to do with the dynamics of a health care team and your role on that team. You are there to help with the work of the team, but you are primarily there to learn. Current formulations of medical ethics address those issues and others. One such formulation is the Tavistock Principles.[105] These principles construct a framework for analyzing health care situations that extend beyond our direct care of individual patients to complicated choices about the interactions of health care teams and the distribution of resources for the well-being of society. A broadly representative group, which initially met in Tavistock Square in London in 1998, has continued to develop an evolving document of ethical principles for guiding health care behavior for both individuals and institutions across the health care spectrum. A current iteration of the Tavistock Principles follows.

The Tavistock Principles

Rights: People have a right to health and health care.

Balance: Care of the individual patient is central, but the health of populations is also our concern.

Comprehensiveness: In addition to treating illness, we have an obligation to ease suffering, minimize disability, prevent disease, and promote health.

Cooperation: Health care succeeds only if we cooperate with those we serve, each other, and those in other sectors.

Improvement: Improving health care is a serious and continuing responsibility.

Safety: Do no harm.

Openness: Being open, honest, and trustworthy is vital in health care.

In the second scenario, think about the Tavistock Principles of *openness and cooperation*, in addition to the balance between *do no harm* and *beneficence*. You need to work with your team in a way that is honest and reliable to do the best for the patient. You can also see that there are no clear or easy answers in such situations. What responses are available to you to address these and other quandaries?

You need to reflect on your beliefs and assess your level of comfort with a given situation. Sometimes there may be alternative solutions. For example, in Scenario 1, the patient may really be willing to have the history and physical examination done at that late hour, or perhaps you can negotiate a time for the next morning. In Scenario 2, you might find another person who is more qualified to complete the form or to supervise when you do it. Alternatively, you may choose to go ahead and complete the form, focusing on an open communication, and alerting the patient to your inexperience while obtaining the patient's consent. You will need to choose which situations warrant voicing your concerns, even at the risk of a bad evaluation.

Seek coaching on how to express your reservations in a way that ensures that they will be heard. As a clinical student, you will need settings for discussing these immediately relevant ethical dilemmas with other students and with more senior trainees and faculty. Small groups that are structured to address these kinds of issues are particularly useful in providing validation and support. Take advantage of such opportunities whenever possible.

Ethics and Professionalism: Scenario 3

You are the student on the clinical team that has been taking care of Ms. Robbins, a 64-year-old woman admitted for an evaluation of weight loss and weakness. During the hospitalization, she had a biopsy of a mass in her chest in addition to many other tests. You have gotten to know her well, spending a lot of time with her to answer questions, explain procedures, and learn about her and her family. You have discussed her fears about what "they" will find and know that she likes to know everything possible about her health and medical care. You have even heard her express frustrations with her attending physician at not always being given the "straight story." It is late Friday afternoon, but you promised Ms. Robbins that you would come by one more time before the weekend and let her know if the results of the biopsy were back yet. Just before you go to her room, the resident tells you that the pathology is back from her biopsy and shows metastatic cancer, but the attending physician does not want the team to say anything until he comes in on Monday.

What are you going to do? You feel that it is wrong to avoid the situation by not going to her room. You also believe that the patient's preference and anxiety are best served by finding out then and not waiting for 3 days. You do not want to go against the attending physician's clear instructions, however, both because you respect the fact that it is his patient and because that feels dishonest.

In this situation, telling the patient about her biopsy results is dictated by several ethical principles: the patient's best interests, autonomy, and your integrity. The other part of the ethical dilemma concerns communicating your plan to the attending. Sometimes the most challenging part of such dilemmas tests your will to follow through with the right course of action. Although it may appear to be a lose–lose situation, a respectful and honest discussion with the attending, articulating what is in the patient's best interest, will usually be heard. Enlist the support of your resident or other helpful attendings if that is possible. Learning how to navigate difficult discussions will be a useful professional skill.

Bibliography

Citations

1. Suchman AL, Matthews DA. What makes the patient doctor relationship therapeutic? Exploring the connectional dimension of medical care. Ann Intern Med 1988;108;25–130.
2. Matthews DA, Suchman AL, Branch WT. Making "connexions": enhancing the therapeutic potential of patient-clinician relationships. Ann Intern Med 1993;118:973–977.
3. Larson EB, Yao X. Clinical empathy as emotional labor in the patient-physician relationship. JAMA 2005;293:1100–1106.
4. Krasner MS, Epstein RM, Beckman H et al. Association of an educational program in mindful communication with burnout, empathy, and attitudes among primary care physicians. JAMA 2009;302:1284–1293.
5. Smith RC. Patient-Centered Interviewing: An Evidence-Based Method. Philadelphia: Lippincott Williams & Wilkins, 2002.
6. Smith RC. An evidence-based infrastructure for patient-centered interviewing. In Frankel FM, Quill TE, McDaniel SH (eds): The Biopsychosocial Approach: Past, Present, and Future. Rochester: University of Rochester Press, 2003, 149.
7. Hastings C. The lived experiences of the illness: making contact with the patient. In Benne P, Wrubel J (eds): The Primacy of Caring: Stress and Coping in Health and Illness. Menlo Park, CA: Addison-Wesley, 1989.
8. Stewart M. Questions about patient-centered care: answers from quantitative research. In Stewart M, et al (eds): Patient-centered Medicine: Transforming the Clinical Method. Abington, UK: Radcliffe Medical Press, 2003, pp. 263–268.
9. Atlas SJ, Grant RW, Ferris TG et al. Patient-physician connectedness and the quality of primary care. Ann Intern Med 2009;150:325–335.
10. Wagner EH, Austin BT, Korff MV. Organizing care for patients with chronic illness. Milbank Q 1996;74:511–544.
11. Coulehan JL, Block MR. The Medical Interview: Mastering Skills for Clinical Practice. 4th ed. Philadelphia: F.A. Davis Company, 2001
12. Halpern J. What is clinical empathy? J Gen Intern Med 2003;18:670–675.
13. Halpern J. Empathy and patient-physician conflicts. J Gen Intern Med 2007;22:696–700.
14. Spiro H. What is empathy and can it be taught? Ann Intern Med 1992;116:843–846.
15. Egnew TR. Suffering, meaning, and healing: challenges of contemporary medicine. Ann Fam Med 2009;2:170–175.
16. Lipkin M Jr, Putnam SM, Lazare A et al (eds). The Medical Interview: Clinical Care, Education, and Research. New York: Springer-Verlag, 1995.
17. Balint M. The Doctor, His Patient and the Illness, 2nd ed. New York: International Universities Press, 1964.
18. Makoul G, Zick A, Green M. An evidence-based perspective on greetings in medical encounters. Arch Int Med 2007;167:1172–1176.
19. McKinstry B. Should general practitioners call patients by their first names? BMJ 1990;301:795–796.
20. Lavin M. What doctors should call their patients. Med Ethics 1988;14;129–131.
21. Platt FW, Gaspar DL, Coulehan JL et al. "Tell me about yourself": the patient-centered interview. Ann Intern Med 2001;134:1079–1085.
22. Ventres W, Kooienga S, Vuvkovic N et al. Physicians, patients and the electronic health record: an ethnographic analysis. Ann Fam Med 2006; 4:124–131.
23. Beckman HB, Frankel RM. The effect of physician behavior on the collection of data. Ann Intern Med 1984;101:692–696.
24. White J, Levinson W, Roter D. "Oh, by the way"...: the closing moments of the medical visit. J Gen Intern Med 1994;9:24–28.
25. Kleinman A, Eisenberg L, Good B. Culture, illness, and care: clinical lessons from anthropological and cross-cultural research. Ann Intern Med 1978;88:251–258.
26. Smith RC, Lyles JS, Mettler J et al. The effectiveness of an intensive teaching experience for residents in interviewing: a randomized controlled study. Ann Intern Med 1998; 128;118–126.
27. Von Korff M, Shapiro S, Burke JD et al. Anxiety and depression in a primary care clinic. Arch Gen Psychiatry. 1987;44:152–156.
28. Bass LW, Cohen RL. Ostensible versus actual reasons for seeking pediatric attention: another look at the parental ticket of admission. Pediatrics 1982;70:870–874.
29. Lang F, Floyd MR, Beine KL. Clues to patients' explanations and concerns about their illnesses: a call for active listening. Arch Fam Med 2000;9:222–227.
30. Rollnick S, Butler CC, Kinnersly P et al. Motivational interviewing. BMJ 2010;340:1242–1245.
31. Hettema J, Steele J, Miller WR. Motivational interviewing. Ann Rev Clin Psychol 2005;1:91–111.

32. Cole S, Bogenschutz M, Hungerford M. Motivational interviewing and psychiatry: use in addiction treatment, risky drinking and routine practice. Focus 2011;IX:42–52.

33. Gaster B, Edwards K, Trinidad SB et al. Patient-centered discussions about prostate cancer screening: A real-world approach. Ann Intern Med 2010;153:661–665.

34. Kemp EC, Floyd MR, McCord-Duncan E et al. Patients prefer the method of "Tell back-collaborative inquiry" to assess understanding of medical information. J Am Board Fam Med 2008;21:24–30.

35. Epstein RM. Mindful practice. JAMA 1999;282:833–839.

36. Smedley BA, Stith AY, Nelson AR (eds): Committee on Understanding and Eliminating Racial and Ethnic Disparities in Health Care. Unequal Treatment: Confronting Racial and Ethnic Disparities in Health Care. Washington DC: Institute of Medicine, 2003.

37. Agency for Healthcare Research and Quality, U.S. Department of Health and Human Services. 2010 National Healthcare Disparities Report. Available at http://www.ahrq.gov/qual/nhdr10/nhdr10.pdf. Accessed August 19, 2011.

38. Boutin-Foster C, Foster JC, Konopasek L. Viewpoint: physician, know thyself: the professional culture of medicine as a framework for teaching cultural competence. Acad Med 2008;83:106–111.

39. Teal CR, Street RL. Critical elements of culturally competent communication in the medical encounter: a review and model. Soc Sci Med 2009;68:533–543.

40. Management Sciences for Health. The Providers' Guide to Quality and Culture. What is cultural competence. Available at http://erc.msh.org/mainpage.cfm?file=2.1.htm&module=provider&language=English. Accessed August 20, 2011.

41. Silliman J, Fried MG, Ross L, Gutierrez ER. Ch. 1, Women of Color and Their Struggles for Reproductive Justice, in Undivided Rights –Women of Color Organize for reproductive Justice. Cambridge Massachusetts: South End Press, 2004, p. 6.

42. Hunt LM. Beyond cultural competence. Park Ridge Bulletin 24: 3–4, 2001. Available at http://www.parkridgecenter.org/Page1882.html. Accessed August 20, 2011.

43. Kumas-Tan Z, Beagan B, Loppie C et al. Measures of cultural competence: examining hidden assumptions. Acad Med 2007;82:548–557.

44. Tervalon M, Murray-Garcia J. Cultural humility versus cultural competence: a critical distinction in defining physician training outcomes in multicultural education. J Health Care Poor Underserved 1998;9:117–125.

45. Tervalon M. Components of culture in health for medical students' education. Acad Med 2003;78:570–576.

46. Smith WR, Betancourt JR, Wynia MK et al. Recommendations for teaching about racial and ethnic disparities in health and health care. Ann Intern Med 2007;147:654–665.

47. National Center for Cultural Competence. Georgetown University Center for Child and Human Development. Available at http://www11.georgetown.edu/research/gucchd/nccc/index.html. See also Self Assessments at http://www11.georgetown.edu/research/gucchd/nccc/resources/assessments.html. Accessed August 20, 2011.

48. Jacobs EA, Kohrman C, Lemon M et al. Teaching physicians-in-training to address racial disparities in health: a community-hospital partnership. Public Health Rep 2003;18(4):349–356.

49. Juarez JA, Marvel K, Brezinski KL et al. Bridging the gap: a curriculum to teach residents cultural humility. Fam Med 2006;38:97–102.

50. National Consortium for Multicultural Education for Health Professionals. Available at http://culturalmeded.stanford.edu./1102. Accessed August 20, 2011.

51. Jacobs EA, Rolle I, Ferrans CE et al. Understanding African Americans' views of the trustworthiness of physicians. J Gen Intern Med 2006;21:642–647.

52. Appelbaum PS. Assessment of patients' competence to consent to treatment. N Engl J Med 2007;357:1834–1840.

53. Raymont V, Bingley W, Buchanan A et al. Prevalence of mental incapacity in medical inpatients and associated risk factors: cross-sectional study. Lancet 2004;364:1421–1427.

54. Grisso T, Appelbaum PS. MacArthur Competence Assessment Tool for Treatment (MacCAT-T). Sarasota, FL: Professional resource Press, 1998.

55. Office for Civil Rights – Health Insurance Portability and Accountability Act of 1996 (HIPAA), U.S. Department of Health and Human Services. Available at http://www.hhs.gov/ocr/privacy. Accessed August 14, 2011.

56. Flores G. Language barriers to health care in the United States. N Engl J Med 2006;355:229–230.

57. Schyve PM. Language differences as a barrier to quantity and safety in health care: the Joint Commission perspective. J Gen Int Med 2007;22(Suppl 2):360–361.

58. Jacobs EA, Shephard DS, Suya JA et al. Overcoming language barriers in health care: costs and benefits in interpreter services. Am J Public Health 2004;94:866–869.

59. Jacobs EA, Sadowski LS, Rathous PJ. The impact of enhanced interpreter service intervention on hospital costs and patient satisfaction. J Gen Intern Med 2007;22 (Suppl 2):306–311.

60. Hardt E, Jacobs EA, Chen A. Insights into the problems that language barriers may pose for the medical interview. J Gen Intern Med 2006;21:1357–1358.

61. Office of Minority Health, Department of Health and Human Services. Think Cultural Health. CLAS Standards; Communication Tools. Available at https://www.thinkculturalhealth.hhs.gov/index.asp. Accessed August 20, 2011.

62. Brady AK. Medical Spanish. Ann Intern Med 2010;152:127–128.

63. Gregg J, Saha S. Communicative competence: a framework for understanding language barriers in health care. J Gen Int Med 2007;22(Suppl 2):368–370.

64. Saha S, Fernandez A. Language barriers in health care. J Gen Int Med 2007;22(Suppl 2):381–382.

65. Berkman ND, Sheridan SL, Donahue KE et al. Low health literacy and health outcomes: an updated systematic review. Ann Intern Med 2011;155:97–107.

66. Institute of Medicine. Health literacy: a prescription to end confusion. April 2004. Available at http://www.iom.edu/Reports/2004/Health-Literacy-A-Prescription-to-End-Confusion.aspx. Accessed August 14, 2011.

67. Meador HE, Zazove P. Health care interactions with deaf culture. J Am Board Fam Pract 2005;18:218–222.

68. Committee on Ethics, American College of Obstetricians and Gynecologists. ACOG Committee Opinion No. 373: Sexual misconduct. Obstet Gynecol 2007;110(2 Pt 1):441–444.

69. Nadelson C, Notman MT. Boundaries in the doctor-patient relationship. Theor Med Bioeth 2002;23:191–201.

70. Gabbard GO, Nadelson C. Professional boundaries in the physician-patient relationship. JAMA 1995;273(18):1445–1449.

71. Council on Ethical and Judicial Affairs. American Medical Association: sexual misconduct in the practice of medicine. JAMA 1991;266:2741–2745.

72. U.S. Preventive Services Task Force. Screening for depression: recommendations and rationale. Ann Intern Med 2002;136:760–764.

73. Substance Abuse and Mental Health Services Administration, Department of Health and Human Services. Results from the 2007 National Survey on Drug Use and Health: National Findings. Updated September 2008. Available at http://oas.samhsa.gov/nsduh/2k7nsduh/2k7results.cfm#Ch7. Accessed August 14, 2011.

74. Medline Plus, National Institutes of Health. Prescription drug abuse. Available at http://www.nlm.nih.gov/medlineplus/prescriptiondrugabuse.html. Accessed August 14, 2011.

75. American Pain Society. Definitions Related to the Use of Opioids for the Treatment of Pain. A consensus statement from the American Academy of Pain Medicine, the American Pain Society, and the American Society of Addiction Medicine, 2001. Available at http://www.partnersagainstpain.com/printouts/A7012R9.pdf. Accessed August 14, 2011.

76. Cyr MG, Wartman SA. The effectiveness of routine screening questions in the detection of alcoholism. JAMA 1988;259:51–54.

77. U.S. Preventive Services Task Force. Screening and behavioral counseling interventions in primary care to reduce alcohol misuse: recommendation statement. Rockville, MD: Agency for Healthcare Research and Quality, April 2004. Available at http://www.ahrq.gov/clinic/3rduspstf/alcohol/alcomisrs.htm. Accessed August 14, 2011.

78. Ewing JA. Detecting alcoholism: the CAGE questionnaire. JAMA 1984;252:1905–1907.

79. Wilson JF. In the clinic: alcohol use. Ann Intern Med 2009;150:ITC3-1 – ITC3-16.

80. National Institute on Drug Abuse. Screening for drug use in medical settings. April 2009. Available at http://www.nida.nih.gov/nidamed/quickref/screening_qr.pdf. Accessed August 14, 2011.

81. Hewitt LN, Bhavsar P, Phelan HA. The secrets women keep: intimate partner violence screening in the female trauma patient. J Trauma 2011;70:320–323.

82. Centers for Disease Control and Prevention. Understanding intimate partner violence. Fact sheet 2011. Available at http://www.cdc.gov/ViolencePrevention/pdf/IPV_factsheet-a.pdf. Accessed August 19, 2011.

83. Ahmad F, Hogg-Johnson S, Stewart DR at al. Computer-assisted screening for intimate partner violence and control: a randomized trial. Ann Intern Med 2009;151:93–102.

84. Rees S, Silove D, Chey T et al. Lifetime prevalence of gender-based violence in women and the relationship with mental disorders and psychosocial function. JAMA 2011;306:513–521.

85. Daugherty JD, Houry DE. Intimate partner violence screening in the emergency department. J Postgrad Med. 2008 Oct-Dec;54(4):301–305.

86. Bhandari M, Sprague S, Dosanjh S et al. The prevalence of intimate partner violence across orthopaedic fracture clinics in Ontario. J Bone Joint Surg Am 2011;93:132–141.

87. Breiding MJ, Black MC, Ryan GW. Prevalence and risk factors of intimate partner violence in eighteen U.S. States/Territories, 2005. Am J Prevent Med 2008;34:112–118.

88. U.S. Preventive Services Task Force. Screening for family and intimate partner violence: recommendation statement. Rockville MD, Agency for Healthcare Research and Quality, March 2004. Available at http://www.uspreventiveservicestaskforce.org/uspstf/uspsfamv.htm. Accessed August 19, 2011.

89. MacMillan HL, wathen CN, Jamieson E et al. Screening for intimate partner violence in health care settings: a randomized trial. JAMA 2009;302:493–501.

90. Moracco KE, Cole TB. Preventing intimate partner violence. Screening is not enough. JAMA 2009;302:568–570.

91. Acierno R, Hernandez MA, Amstadter AB et al. Prevalence and correlates of emotional, physical, sexual, and financial abuse and potential neglect in the United States: the National Elder Mistreatment Study. Am J Public Health. 2010;100(2):292–7. Epub 2009 Dec 17.

92. Samaras N, Chevalley T, Samaras D, Gold G. Older patients in the emergency department: a review. Ann Emerg Med 2010; 56 261–269.

93. Mosqueda L, Dong X. Elder abuse and self-neglect: "I don't care anything about going to the doctor, to be honest…". JAMA 2011;306:532–540.

94. Alpert EJ. Addressing domestic violence: the (long) road ahead. Ann Intern Med 2007;147:666–667.

95. Rhodes KV, Frankel RM, Levinthal N et al. "You're not the victim of domestic violence, are you?" Provider-patient communication about domestic violence. Ann Intern Med 2007;147:620–627.

96. Bhandari M, Sprague S, Dosanjh S et al. The relationship of trauma to mental disorders among trafficked and sexually exploited girls and women. S Am J Public Health 2010;100:2442–2449.

97. Logan TK, Walker R, Hunt G. Understanding human trafficking in the United States. Trauma Violence Abuse 2009;10:3–30.

98. Kübler-Ross E. On Death and Dying. New York: Macmillan, 1997.

99. Maciejewski PK, Zhang B, Block SD et al. An empirical examination of the stage theory of grief. JAMA 2007;297:16–23.

100. Manthous CA. Introducing the primer of medical ethics. Chest 2006;130:1640–1641.

101. Carrese JA, Sugarman J. The inescapable relevance of bioethics for the practicing clinician. Chest 2006;1230:1864–1872.

102. Swetz KM, Crowley ME, Hook C et al. Report of 255 clinical ethics consultations and review of the literature. Mayo Clin Proc 2007;82:686–91.

103. ABIM Foundation, American Board of Internal Medicine, ACP-ASIM Foundation, American College of Physicians-American Society of Internal Medicine, European Federation of Internal Medicine. Medical professionalism in the new millenium: a physician charter. Ann Intern Med 2002;136:243–246.

104. Giordano J. The ethics of interventional pain management: basic concepts and theories: problems and practice. Presentation, Texas Tech University Health Sciences Center, Lubbock, TX, February 15, 2008.

105. Berwick D, Davidoff F, Hiatt H, et al. Refining and implementing the Tavistock principles for everybody in health care. BMJ 2001;323(7313):616–619.

Additional References

The Fundamentals of Skilled Interviewing

Côté L, Leclère H. How clinical teachers perceive the doctor-patient relationship and themselves as role models. Acad Med 2000;75:1117–1124.

Coulehan JL. The Medical Interview: Mastering Skills for Clinical Practice, 5th ed. Philadelphia: FA Davis Co, 2006.

Delbanco TL. Enriching the doctor-patient relationship by inviting the patient's perspective. Ann Intern Med 1993;116:414–418.

Egnew TR. The meaning of healing: transcending suffering. Ann Fam Med 2005;3:255–262.

Frankel RM, Quill TE, McDanial SH. The biopsychosocial approach: past, present, and future. Rochester, NY: University of Rochester Press, 2003.

Hutchinson TA, Dobkin PL. Mindful medical practice: just another fad? Can Fam Physician 2009;55:778–779.

Kurtz SM, Silverman J, Draper J et al. Teaching and learning communication skills in medicine, 2nd ed. San Francisco: Oxford/Radcliffe Pub, 2005.

Lazare A, Putnam SM, Lipkin M Jr. Three functions of the medical interview. Also Novack DH. Therapeutic aspects of the clinical encounter. In Lipkin M Jr, Putnam SM, Lazare A et al (eds): The Medical Interview: Clinical Care, Education, and Research. New York: Springer-Verlag, 1995.

Mast MS. The importance of nonverbal communication in the physician-patient interaction. Patient Educ Couns 2007; 67:315–318.

McAulay V. The changing doctor-patient relationship. Diagnoses are made from careful history and examination. BMJ 2000; 320:873–874.

Smith RC, Lyles JS, Mettler J et al. The effectiveness of an intensive teaching experience for residents in interviewing: a randomized controlled study. Ann Intern Med 1998;128:118–126.

The Sequence and Context of the Interview

Carrillo JE, Green AR, Betancourt JR. Cross-cultural primary care: a patient-based approach. Ann Intern Med 1999;130:829–834.

Csordas TJ, Storck, Strauss M. Diagnosis and distress in Navajo healing. J Nerv Ment Dis 2008;197:585–596.

Fadiman A. The Spirit Catches You and You All Fall Down. New York: Farrar, Straus and Giroux, 1997.

Makoul G. Essential elements of communication in medical encounters: the Kalamazoo consensus statement. Acad Med 2001;76:390–393.

Makoul G, Clayman MI. An integrative model of shared decision making in medical encounters. Patient Educ Couns 2006;60:301–312.

McLaughlin KA, Hatzenbuehler ML, Keyes KM. Responses to discrimination and psychiatric disorders among Black, Hispanic, female, and lesbian, gay, and bisexual individuals. Am J Public Health 2010;100:1477–1484.

Advanced Interviewing

Americans with Disabilities Act Home Page, U.S. Department of Justice. Available at http://www.ada.gov/#Anchor-47857. Accessed September 23, 2011.

Barnett S. Cross-cultural communication with patients who use American Sign Language. Fam Med 2002;34(5):376–382.

Cochran SD, Mays VM. Physical health complaints among lesbians, gay men, and bisexual and homosexually experienced heterosexual individuals: results from the California Quality of Life Survey. Am J Public Health 2007;97:2048–2055.

Doyal L. Closing the gap between professional teaching and practice. BMJ 2001;322(7288):685–686.

Easton P, Entwistle VA, Williams B. Health in the 'hidden population' of people with low literacy. A systematic review of the literature. BMC Public Health 2010;10:459–469.

Enbom JA, Parshley P, Kollath J. A follow-up evaluation of sexual misconduct complaints: the Oregon Board of Medical Examiners, 1998 through 2002. Am J Obstet Gynecol 2004;190:1642–50; discussion 1650–1653, 6A.

End of Life/Palliative Education Resource Center. Available at http://www.eperc.mcw.edu/EPERC. Accessed September 18, 2011.

Gordon AJ, Kunins HV, Rastegar DA et al. Update in addiction medicine for the generalist. J Gen Intern Med 2011;26:77–82.

Grantmakers in Health: In the right words: addressing language and culture in providing health care. Issues in Brief 2003;18:1–54.

Iezzoni LI, O'Day BL, Killeen M, et al. Communicating about health care: observations from persons who are deaf or hard of hearing. Ann Intern Med 2004;140:356–362.

Johnson CV, Mimiaga MJ, Bradford J. Health care issues among lesbian, gay, bisexual, transgender and intersex (LGBTI) populations in the United States: introduction. J Homosex 2008;54:213–224.

Kleinman A, Eisenberg L, Good B. Culture, illness, and care: clinical lessons from anthropological and cross-cultural research. Ann Intern Med 1978;88:251–258.

Lang, Clues to patients' explanations and concerns about their illnesses: a call for active listening. Arch Fam Med 2000;9:222–227.

Marcus EN. The silent epidemic–the health effects of illiteracy. N Engl J Med 2006;355:339–341.

Marlatt GA, Donovan DM. Relapse Prevention: Maintenance Strategies in the Treatment of Addictive Behaviors, 2nd ed. New York: Guilford Press, 2005.

Meador HE, Zazove P. Health care interactions with deaf culture. J Am Board Fam Pract 2005;18:218–222.

Miller WR, Rollnick S, Butler C. Motivational Interviewing in Health Care-Helping Patients Change Behavior. New York: Guilford Press, 2008.

National Center for Education Statistics, U.S. Department of Education. National Assessment of Health Literacy 2003, released January 2009. Available at http://nces.ed.gov/naal/kf_demographics.asp#2. Accessed August 14, 2011.

O'Brien CP. A 50-year old woman addicted to heroin. Review of treatment of heroin addiction. JAMA 2008;300:314–321.

O'Connor PG, Nyquist JG, McLellan AT. Integrating addiction medicine into graduate medical education in primary care: the time has come. Ann Intern Med 2011;154:56–59.

Rastegar DA, Fingerhood MI. Addiction medicine: an evidence-based handbook. Philadelphia: Lippincott Williams & Wilkins, 2005.

Rivadeneyra R, Elderkin-Thompson V, Silver RC, et al. Patient centeredness in medical encounters requiring an interpreter. Am J Med 2000;108:470–474.

Robinson GE, Stewart DE. A curriculum on physician-patient sexual misconduct and teacher-learner mistreatment. Part 1: Content. Can Med Assoc J 1996;154:643–649.

Schwartzberg JG, Cowett A, VanGeest J, Wolf MS. Communication techniques for patients with low health literacy: a survey of physicians, nurses, and pharmacists. Am J Health Behav 2007;31 (Suppl 1):S96–104.

Sudore RL, Fried TR. Redefining the "planning" in advance care planning: preparing for end-of-life decision making. Ann Intern Med 2010;153:256–261.

Vandemark LM, Mueller M. Mental health after sexual violence: the role of behavioral and demographic risk factors. Nurs Res 2008;57(3):175–81.

Ethics and Professionalism

ABIM Foundation, American Board of Internal Medicine, ACP-ASIM Foundation, American College of Physicians-American Society of Internal Medicine, European Federation of Internal Medicine. Medical professionalism in the new millenium: a physician charter. Ann Intern Med 2002;136:243–246.

Beauchamp TL, Childress JF. Principles of Biomedical Ethics, 6th ed. New York: Oxford University Press, 2008.

Benner P, Tanner CA, Chesla CA. Expertise in Nursing Practice: Caring, Clinical Judgment, and Ethics, 2nd ed. New York: Springer, 2009.

Lo B. Resolving Ethical Dilemmas: A Guide for Clinicians, 4th ed. Philadelphia: Lippincott Williams & Wilkins, 2009.

Medical professionalism in the new millennium: a physician charter. Ann Intern Med 2002;136:243–246.

Miller E, Decker MR, Silverman JG et al. Migration, sexual exploitation, and women's health: a case report from a community health center. Violence Against Women 2007;13:486–497.

Mostaghimi A, Crotty BH. Professionalism in the digital age. Ann Intern Med 2011;154:560–562.

Office for Civil Rights – Health Insurance Portability and Accountability Act of 1996 (HIPAA), U.S. Department of Health and Human Services. Available at http://www.hhs.gov/ocr/privacy. Accessed August 14, 2011.

Snyder L, for the American College of Physicians Ethics, Professionalism, and Human Rights Committee. American College of Physicians Ethics Manual, 6th ed. Ann Intern Med Suppl 2012;156(1):73–104.

The Bates' suite offers these additional resources to enhance learning and facilitate understanding of this chapter:

- *Bates' Pocket Guide to Physical Examination and History Taking,* 7th edition
- *Bates' Visual Guide to Physical Examination*
- thePoint online resources, for students and instructors: http://thepoint.lww.com

Table 3-1 **Motivational Interviewing: A Clinical Example**

The police brought a 40-year-old woman to the psychiatric emergency room because while intoxicated she threatened to kill her partner and herself. She had no history of violence or of legal or psychiatric problems. When she became sober the next day, she reported calmly that she was an alcoholic and was not violent and had no intention of hurting herself. She wanted to be discharged. The typical psychiatric approach to this problem would be a combination of education and confrontation; the psychiatrist would explain the dangers of alcoholism to the patient and encourage her to seek treatment, handing her a list of alcohol treatment centers.

In contrast, the actual MI conversation proceeded like this:

Patient: I am an alcoholic and don't want to change. I am not dangerous; just let me go home now.

Psychiatrist: OK, that's what we'll do. We can't force you to change. Can I just ask you a few questions and then we'll let you out of here?

(MI: Respect for autonomy–the psychiatrist respects the individual's right to change or not make a change; collaboration– the psychiatrist is equal to the patient in power and asks permission for further inquiry.)

Patient: OK.

Psychiatrist: I am interested in learning a little about your drinking. I understand you don't want to change. So I am assuming that the alcohol is mostly a good thing in your life. I am wondering if there is anything not so good about the alcohol in your life?

(MI: Elicit ambivalence)

Patient: Well, they said my liver is not so good anymore. It's going to fail if I don't stop drinking.

Psychiatrist: OK, so that sounds like one part of the drinking that is not so good.

(MI: Explore ambivalence)

Patient: Right.

Psychiatrist: But it doesn't sound important enough to make you want to change. I'm guessing that you don't care so much whether your liver fails or not.

(MI: Not at all sarcastic here; really respecting her autonomy)

Patient: Well, I can't live without a liver.

Psychiatrist: OK. Then it sounds like you don't care much whether you live or die.

(MI: Again, not at all sarcastic; simply reflecting content and respecting autonomy)

Patient: No way! I love life!

Psychiatrist: Well, I'm not sure I understand then. On the one hand, you are very sure that you are not going to stop drinking, yet you also say you love life and don't want your liver to fail.

(MI: Develop discrepancy. Elicit change talk.)

Patient: Well, I know I'm going to have to cut down or stop sometime. This is just not the time.

Psychiatrist: OK. I hear what you are saying. You want to stop drinking at some point, to save your liver and save your life—it's just not the right time now.

(MI: Listen, understand, express empathy, and reflect feelings; respect autonomy.)

Patient: Right.

Psychiatrist: OK. Can I ask another question or two?…If you do think you're going to stop at some point, I wonder what thoughts you've had about when and how you would like to stop drinking? Would you want or need any help if and when you decided to cut down or stop drinking?

(MI: Open questions for understanding; encourage change talk.)

Source: Cole S, Bogenschutz M, Hungerford M. Motivational interviewing and psychiatry: use in addiction treatment, risky drinking and routine practice. Focus IX:42–52, 2011.

| Table |
| 3-2 |

Brief Action Planning—A Self-Management Support Tool©

Brief Action Planning™ is structured around three core questions:

1. _____ Elicit person's preferences/desires for behavior change.

   "Is there anything you would like to do for your health in the next week or two?"

   _____ What?

   _____ Where?

   _____ When?

   _____ How often?

   _____ Elicit commitment statement

   "Just to make sure we understand each other, would you please tell me back what you've decided to do?"

2. _____ Evaluate confidence.

   "I wonder how confident you feel about carrying out your plan. Considering a scale of 0 to 10, where '0' means you are not at all confident and '10' means you are very confident, about how confident do you feel?"

   (If the confidence level is less than 7, problem solve overcoming barriers or adjusting plan. *"5 is great. A lot higher than zero. I wonder if there is any way we might modify the plan to get you to a level of '7' or more? Maybe we could make the goal a little easier, or you could ask for help from a friend or family member, or even think of something else that might help you feel more confident?"*

3. _____ Arrange a follow-up (or accountability).

   "Sounds like a plan that's going to work for you. When would you like to check in with me to review how you're doing with your plan?"

Regional Examinations

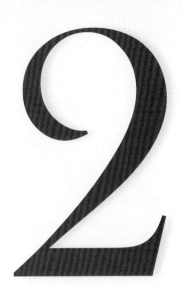

Beginning the Physical Examination: General Survey, Vital Signs, and Pain

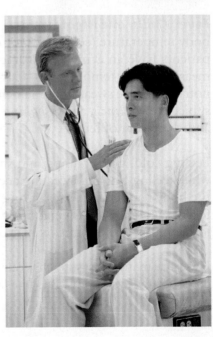

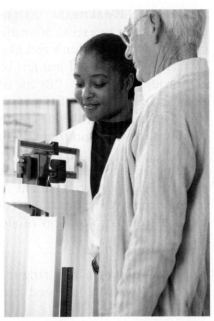

Once you understand the patient's concerns and have elicited a careful history, you are ready to begin the physical examination. At first you may feel unsure of how the patient will relate to you. With practice, your skills in physical examination will grow, and you will gain confidence. Through study and repetition, the examination will flow more smoothly, and you will soon shift your attention from technique and how to handle instruments to what you hear, see, and feel. Touching the patient's body will seem more natural, and you will learn to minimize any discomfort to the patient. As you gain proficiency, what once took between 1 and 2 hours will take considerably less time.

This chapter discusses the initial elements of your physical examination of the patient:

- *Common and Concerning Symptoms* explores constitutional symptoms like fatigue, fever and chills, and weight change.

- *Health Promotion and Counseling* focuses on key ingredients for a healthy lifestyle, namely optimal weight, nutrition, and exercise, and provides counseling tips for patients who are overweight or obese, a pandemic for all age groups in our population.

- *The General Survey* describes crystallizing your initial impressions into more systematic observations of the patient's state of health: demeanor and facial affect, posture, and gait, and review the height and weight.

- *Vital Signs* covers techniques for accurate measurements of blood pressure, heart rate, respiratory rate, and temperature.

- *Pain, the Fifth Vital Sign* provides an approach to assessing pain, a priority for compassionate care for all of the health professions.

The Health History

Common or Concerning Symptoms

▶ Fatigue and weakness
▶ Fever, chills, night sweats
▶ Weight changes
▶ Pain

Fatigue and Weakness. *Fatigue* is a nonspecific symptom with many causes. It refers to a sense of weariness or loss of energy that patients describe in various ways. "I don't feel like getting up in the morning"... "I don't have any energy"... "I just feel blah"... "I'm all done in"... "I can hardly get through the day"... "By the time I get to the office, I feel as if I've done a day's work." Because fatigue is a normal response to hard work, sustained stress, or grief, elicit the life circumstances in which it occurs. Fatigue unrelated to such situations requires further investigation.

Use open-ended questions as you listen to the attributes of the patient's fatigue. Encourage the patient to fully describe what he or she is experiencing. Important clues about etiology often emerge from a good psychosocial history, exploration of sleep patterns, and a thorough review of systems.

Weakness is different from fatigue. It denotes a demonstrable loss of muscle power and will be discussed later with other neurologic symptoms (see p. 692).

Fever, Chills, and Night Sweats. *Fever* refers to an abnormal elevation in body temperature (see p. 126 for definitions of normal). Ask about fever if patients have an acute or chronic illness. Find out whether patients have measured their temperatures. Has the patient felt feverish or unusually hot, noted excessive sweating, or felt chilly and cold? Try to distinguish between subjective *chilliness,* and a *shaking chill* with shivering throughout the body and chattering of teeth.

Feeling cold, goosebumps, and shivering accompany a rising temperature, while feeling hot and sweating accompany a falling temperature. Normally the body temperature rises during the day and falls during the night. When fever exaggerates this swing, *night sweats* occur. Malaise, headache, and pain in the muscles and joints often accompany fever.

Fever has many causes. Focus your questions on the timing of the illness and its associated symptoms. Become familiar with patterns of infectious diseases

Fatigue is a common symptom of depression and anxiety, but also consider *infections* (such as hepatitis, infectious mononucleosis, and tuberculosis); *endocrine disorders* (hypothyroidism, adrenal insufficiency, diabetes mellitus, panhypopituitarism); heart failure; chronic disease of the lungs, kidneys, or liver; electrolyte imbalance; moderate to severe anemia; malignancies; nutritional deficits; and medications.

Weakness, especially if localized in a neuroanatomical pattern, suggests possible *neuropathy* or *myopathy.*

Recurrent shaking chills suggest more extreme swings in temperature and systemic *bacteremia.*

Feeling hot and sweating also accompany menopause. Night sweats occur in *tuberculosis* and *malignancy.*

that may affect your patient. Inquire about travel, contact with sick people, or other unusual exposures. Even medications may cause fever. By contrast, recent ingestion of aspirin, acetaminophen, corticosteroids, and nonsteroidal anti-inflammatory drugs may mask fever and affect the temperature recorded at the office visit.

Weight Changes.   Weight changes result from changes in body tissues or body fluid. Good opening questions include "How often do you check your weight?" "How is it compared to a year ago?" If there are changes, ask, "Why do you think it has changed?" "What would you like to weigh?" If weight gain or loss appears to be a problem, ask about the amount of change, its timing, the setting in which it occurred, and any associated symptoms.

Weight gain occurs when caloric intake exceeds caloric expenditure over time, and typically results in increased body fat. Weight gain can also reflect abnormal accumulation of body fluids.

Patients with a body mass index (BMI) of 25 to 29 are defined as *overweight;* those with a BMI over 30 are *obese.* In patients who are overweight or obese, plan a thorough assessment to avert the high risks of associated morbidity and mortality. Ask when the weight gain began. Was the patient overweight as a child? Are the parents overweight? Ask about weight at life milestones like birth, kindergarten, high school or college graduation, military discharge, pregnancy, menopause, and retirement. Has a recent disability or surgery affected weight? Establish the patient's level of physical activity and the outcomes of any prior attempts at weight loss. Assess eating patterns and dietary preferences.

Review the patient's medications.

Explore any clinically significant *weight loss,* defined as loss of 5% or more of usual body weight over a 6-month period. Mechanisms include decreased food intake due to anorexia, depression, dysphagia, vomiting, abdominal pain, or financial difficulties; defective gastrointestinal absorption or inflammation; and increased metabolic requirements. Ask about abuse of alcohol, cocaine, amphetamines, or opiates, or withdrawal from marijuana, all associated with weight loss. Heavy smoking also suppresses appetite.

Rapid changes in weight, over a few days, suggest changes in body fluids, not tissues.

Edema from extravascular fluid retention is visible in conditions like *heart failure, nephrotic syndrome,* and *liver failure.*

See Classification of Overweight and Obesity by BMI on p. 110.

See Table 4-1, Obesity-Related Health Factors, p. 135, and discussion on pp. 108–112.

Many drugs are associated with weight gain, such as: tricyclic antidepressants; insulin and sulfonylurea; contraceptives, glucocorticoids, and progestational steroids; mirtazapine and paroxetine; gabapentin and valproate; and propranolol.

Causes of weight loss include gastrointestinal diseases; *endocrine disorders (diabetes mellitus, hyperthyroidism, adrenal insufficiency);* chronic infections, HIV/AIDS; malignancy; chronic cardiac, pulmonary, or renal failure; depression; and *anorexia nervosa or bulimia.* See Table 4-2, Eating Disorders and Excessively Low BMI, p. 136.

Try to determine whether the drop in weight is proportional to any change in food intake or whether intake has remained normal or even increased.

Pursue a thorough psychosocial history. Who cooks and shops for the patient? Where does the patient eat? With whom? Are there any problems with obtaining, storing, preparing, or chewing food? Does the patient avoid or restrict certain foods for medical, religious, or other reasons?

Check the medication history.

Throughout the history, be alert for signs of *malnutrition*. Symptoms may be subtle and nonspecific, such as weakness, easy fatigability, cold intolerance, flaky dermatitis, and ankle swelling. Securing a good diet history of eating patterns and quantities is essential. Ask general questions about intake at different times throughout the day, such as "Tell me what you typically eat for lunch." "What do you eat for a snack?" "When?"

Pain. Pain is one of the most common presenting symptoms in office practice. Each year an estimated 76 million Americans report intermittent or persistent pain.[2-4] Health care costs, lost income, and over 50 million lost workdays a year are estimated at $100 billion annually.[5] Nearly three-fifths of adults 65 years of age and older report pain lasting more than a year. Localizing symptoms, "the seven attributes of a symptom," and the psychosocial history are essential to your physical examination, assessment, and a comprehensive management plan.

Weight loss with relatively high food intake suggests *diabetes mellitus, hyperthyroidism,* or *malabsorption.* Consider also binge eating (bulimia) with clandestine vomiting.

Poverty, old age, social isolation, physical disability, emotional or mental impairment, lack of teeth, ill-fitting dentures, alcoholism, and drug abuse increase the likelihood of malnutrition.

Drugs associated with weight loss include anticonvulsants, antidepressants, levodopa, digoxin, metformin, and thyroid medication.[1]

See Table 4-3, Nutrition Screening, p. 137.

Turn to the section on Acute and Chronic Pain, pp. 127–130, at the end of this chapter for an approach to assessment and management.

Health Promotion and Counseling: Evidence and Recommendations

Important Topics for Health Promotion and Counseling

▶ Optimal weight, nutrition, and diet
▶ Exercise

Optimal Weight, Nutrition, and Diet. Fewer than half of U.S. adults maintain a healthy weight, with a BMI between 18.5 and 24.9. Obesity has increased in every segment of the U.S. population, regardless of age, gender, ethnicity, or socioeconomic status. Review the alarming statistics about the rising prevalence of obesity nationally and worldwide in the table on the next page.[6,7]

See Calculating the BMI and Measuring the Waist Circumference, p. 117.

Obesity at a Glance

- More than 68% of U.S. adults are overweight or obese (BMI >25).
- More than 17% of U.S. children and adolescents are overweight and 15% are obese.
- Health Disparities: the prevalence of overweight or obese populations is higher in certain ethnic and income groups:
  - Women: black women—77%; white women—59%
  - Women: women with an income <130% of the poverty threshold are 50% more likely to be obese than those at higher income levels
  - Men: black men—71%; white men—72%
  - Adolescents: highest prevalence in Mexican-American boys and girls (46%; 42%), black girls (46%), white boys from lower-income families
- Overweight and obesity increase risk of heart disease, numerous types of cancers, type 2 diabetes, stroke, arthritis, sleep apnea, infertility, and depression. Obesity may increase risk of death.[8,9]
- More than 85% of people with type 2 diabetes and 20% of people with hypertension or elevated cholesterol are overweight or obese.
- Obesity is increasing worldwide. In the world's poorest countries, being poor is associated with underweight and malnutrition; but being poor in a middle-income country adopting a Western lifestyle increases the risk of obesity.
- Only 64% of obese U.S. adults report that health care professionals have advised them to lose weight.

See Table 4-1, Obesity-Related Health Factors, p. 135.

Sources: Roger VL, Go AS, Lloyd-Jones DM, et al. Heart disease and stroke statistics–2011 update: a report from the American Heart Association. (Data source: National Health and Nutrition Survey (NHANES) 2005–2008; National Heart, Lung, blood Institute, and unpublished data) Circulation 123:e18–e209, 2011 At http://circ.ahajournals.org/cgi/reprint/CIR.0b013e3182009701; also Centers for Disease Control and Prevention. Obesity and overweight. Data and statistics. At http://www.cdc.gov/obesity/data/index.html. Accessed June 18 2011. Hossain P, Kawar B, El Hahas M. Obesity and diabetes in the developing world—a growing challenge. New Engl J Med 356: 213–215, 2007.

To promote optimal patient weight and nutrition, adopt the four-pronged approach outlined here. Reducing weight by even 5% to 10% can improve blood pressure, lipid levels, and glucose tolerance, and reduce the risk of diabetes or hypertension.

Four Steps to Promote Optimal Weight and Nutrition

1. Measure BMI and waist circumference; identify risk of overweight and obesity and establish additional risk factors for heart disease and obesity-related diseases.
2. Assess dietary intake.
3. Assess the patient's motivation to change.
4. Provide counseling about nutrition and exercise.

Take advantage of the excellent resources available for patient assessment and counseling summarized in the following sections. Review the role of weight in the growing prevalence of *metabolic syndrome*, present in 34% of the U.S. population.[6]

See definition and discussion of *metabolic syndrome* in Chapter 9, Cardiovasular System, pp. 357–358.

Step 1: Measure the BMI and Assess Risk Factors. Classify the BMI according to the national guidelines in the following table. If the BMI is *above 25*, assess the patient for *additional risk factors* for heart disease and other obesity-related diseases: hypertension, high LDL cholesterol, low HDL cholesterol, high triglycerides, high blood glucose, family history of premature heart disease, physical inactivity, and cigarette smoking. Patients with a BMI over 25 and two or more risk factors should pursue weight loss, especially if the waist circumference is elevated.

Classification of Overweight and Obesity by BMI

	Obesity Class	BMI (kg/m²)
Underweight		<18.5
Normal		18.5–24.9
Overweight		25.0–29.9
Obesity	I	30.0–34.9
	II	35.0–39.9
Extreme obesity	III	≥40

Source: National Institutes of Health and National Heart, Lung, and Blood Institute: Clinical Guidelines on the Identification, Evaluation, and Treatment of Overweight and Obesity in Adults: The Evidence Report. NIH Publication 98-4083. June 1998.

Step 2: Assess Dietary Intake. Take a diet history and assess the patient's eating patterns. Select a brief screening tool and be sensitive to the impact of income and cultural preferences on what the patient chooses to eat.

See Table 4-3, Nutrition Screening, p. 137.

Step 3: Assess Motivation to Change. Once you have assessed BMI, risk factors, and dietary intake, address the patient's motivation to make lifestyle changes that promote weight loss. The Prochaska model helps tailor interventions to the patient's level of motivation to adopt new eating behaviors.

See Table 4-4, Obesity: Stages of Change Model and Assessing Readiness, p. 138.

Step 4: Provide Counseling About Nutrition and Exercise. It is important to be well-informed about diet and nutrition as you counsel overweight patients, especially in light of the many and often contradictory diet options in the popular press. The U.S. Department of Agriculture released new dietary guidelines in 2010 to help clinicians and patients address the obesity epidemic more effectively. The Department's new nutrition icon, MyPlate, is appealing and easy to understand. Take the time to review the MyPlate webpage and the dietary guidelines report, as well as the resources listed in the following text. Updated clinical guidelines are available from the National Institutes of Health.

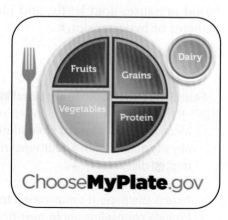

www.choosemyplate.gov/index.html

Clinician Resources on Diet and Nutrition

▶ U.S. Department of Agriculture. Dietary Guidelines for Americans 2010. At http://www.cnpp.usda.gov/Publications/DietaryGuidelines/2010/PolicyDoc/PolicyDoc.pdf

▶ National Institutes of Health and National Heart, Lung, and Blood Institute. Clinical Guidelines on the Identification, Evaluation, and Treatment of Overweight and Obesity in Adults, 1998. Update available Fall 2011. At http://www.nhlbi.nih.gov/guidelines/obesity/ob_gdlns.pdf

▶ U.S. Preventive Services Task Force. Screening for Obesity in Adults: recommendations and rationale. Rockville, MD. Agency for Healthcare Research and Quality, November 2003. At http://www.ahrq.gov/clinic/3rduspstf/obesity/obesrr.htm

A key element of effective counseling is helping the patient to set reasonable goals. Experts note that patients often have a "dream weight" as much as 30% below initial body weight.[1] However, a 5% to 10% weight loss is more realistic and still proven to reduce risk of diabetes and other obesity-associated health problems. Educate your patients about common roadblocks to sustained weight loss: hitting a plateau due to feedback physiologic systems that maintain body homeostasis; poor adherence to diet due to increasing hunger over time as weight declines; and inhibition of leptin, a protein cytokine secreted and stored in fat cells that modulates hunger.[10] Use a full array of strategies to promote weight loss. A safe goal for weight loss is ½ to 2 pounds per week.

Strategies That Promote Weight Loss

▶ The most effective diets combine realistic weight loss goals with exercise and behavioral reinforcements.

▶ Encourage patients to walk 30 to 60 minutes 5 or more days a week, or a total of at least 150 minutes a week. Pedometers help patients match distance in steps with calories burned.

▶ The total calorie goal, usually 800 to 1,200 calories a day, is more important than type of diet. Since many types of diets have been studied and appear to confer similar results, support the patient's preferences as long as they are reasonable.[11,12] Consider low-fat diets for those with dyslipidemias.

▶ Encourage behavioral habits that have been shown to assist weight loss such as portion-controlled meals, meal planning, food diaries, and activity records.

▶ Follow professional guidelines for pharmacologic therapies in patients at high weights and morbidities who do not respond to conventional treatment.[13]

If the BMI falls *below 18.5,* investigate possible anorexia, bulimia, or other serious medical conditions.

See Table 4-2, Eating Disorders and Excessively Low BMI, p. 136.

The *USDA Dietary Guidelines 2010* point out that to maintain caloric balance and achieve and sustain a healthy weight, most Americans need to lower their caloric intake and increase physical activity. The Guidelines emphasize consuming *nutrient-dense foods and beverages*[14]:

- "Americans currently consume too much sodium and too many calories from solid fats, added sugars, and refined grains. These replace nutrient-dense foods and beverages and make it difficult . . . to achieve recommended nutrient intake while controlling calorie and sodium intake."

- Added sugars consist primarily of sweeteners; solid fats refer to saturated and/or trans fats, which are usually solid at room temperature; refined grains lack whole grain contents like bran, germ, or endosperm.

- "A healthy eating pattern . . . emphasizes nutrient-dense foods and beverages–vegetables, fruits, whole grains, fat-free or low-fat milk and milk products, seafood, lean meats and poultry, eggs, beans and peas, and nuts and seeds."

Introduce your patients to the colorful "chooseMyPlate.gov" Web site and its easy-to-follow guides for selecting fruits, vegetables, grains, protein, and dairy products. Sodium intake should be less than 2,300 mg/day; saturated fatty acids should be ≤10% of total calories; and dietary cholesterol should be ≤300 mg/day.

The American Heart Association and the Institute of Medicine currently recommend restricting sodium intake to *1,500 mg/day*. See discussion below.

Americans are urged to follow simple practical tips for daily meals, the *"10 tips to a great plate"*: balance calories; eat less; avoid oversized portions; eat nutrient-dense foods more often; make half the plate fruits and vegetables; switch to fat-free or low-fat milk; make half of grain intake whole grains; eat foods high in solid fats, salt, and added sugars less often; use the Nutrition Facts label to choose lower sodium versions of foods like soup, bread, and frozen meals; and drink water or unsweetened beverages instead of sweetened soda, energy drinks, or sports drinks.

Be prepared to help adolescent females and women of childbearing age increase intake of iron, vitamin C, and folic acid. Assist adults older than 50 years to identify foods rich in vitamin B_{12}. Advise older adults and those with dark skin or low exposure to sunlight to increase intake of vitamin D.

See Table 4-5, Nutrition Counseling: Sources of Nutrients, p. 139.

Blood Pressure and Dietary Sodium. In a major report in 2010, the American Heart Association calls for limiting dietary sodium intake to *1,500 mg/day* for all Americans, an even lower target than the USDA Dietary Guidelines 2010.[15] This is roughly a *half teaspoon of salt a day*. The report cites rigorous evidence that excess dietary sodium causes hypertension and provokes cardiovascular disease. Sodium loading suppresses the renin-angiotensin-aldosterone system by inhibiting renin release and "increases oxidative stress and endothelial dysfunction and promotes . . . fibrosis in the heart, kidneys, and arteries . . . resulting in cardiac and vascular remodeling." Sodium reduction has a direct and progressive influence on blood pressure, especially below intakes of 2,300 mg/day, and dampens the age-related rise in blood pressure that leads to hypertension in 90% of U.S. adults. A recent meta-analysis concludes that a difference of 5 g of salt intake a day is linked

See Table 4-6, Patients With Hypertension: Recommended Changes in Diet, p. 139.

to a 23% difference in the rate of stroke and a 17% difference in the rate of total cardiovascular disease.[16]

Because over 75% of consumed sodium comes from processed foods and *only 10% of Americans consume 2,300 mg/day or less of recommended dietary sodium,* the American Heart Association and the Institute of Medicine have jointly recommended population-wide salt reduction measures including new government standards for manufacturers, restaurants, and foodservice operators.[15,17,18] Advise patients to read the Nutrition Facts panel on food labels closely to help them adhere to the 1,500-mg/day guideline. Urge them to consider the well-investigated Dietary Approaches to Stop Hypertension, or DASH Eating Plan, for a model diet.[19]

Exercise. Fitness is a key component of both weight control and weight loss. Americans should do 30 minutes of moderate activity, defined as walking 2 miles in 30 minutes on most days of the week or its equivalent. Patients can increase exercise by such simple measures as parking farther away from their place of work or using stairs instead of elevators.

Moderate and Vigorous Exercise

A 154-pound man (5′10″) uses up approximately the number of calories listed doing each activity below. **Those who weigh more will use more calories, and those who weigh less will use fewer.** The calorie values listed include both calories used by the activity and calories used for normal body functioning.

	Approximate Calories Used by a 154-pound Man	
	In 1 hour	In 30 minutes
Moderate Physical Activities:		
Hiking	370	185
Light gardening/yard work	330	165
Dancing	330	165
Golf (walking and carrying clubs)	330	165
Bicycling (less than 10 miles per hour)	290	145
Walking (3½ miles per hour)	280	140
Weight training (general light workout)	220	110
Stretching	180	90
Vigorous Physical Activities:		
Running/jogging (5 miles per hour)	590	295
Bicycling (more than 10 miles per hour)	590	295
Swimming (slow freestyle laps)	510	255
Aerobics	480	240
Walking (4½ miles per hour)	460	230
Heavy yard work (chopping wood)	440	220
Weight lifting (vigorous effort)	440	220
Basketball (vigorous)	440	220

Source: U.S. Department of Agriculture: Choose MyPlate.gov. Physical Activity. How many calories does physical activity use? Modified June 2011. At http://www.choosemyplate.gov/foodgroups/physicalactivity_calories_used_table.html. Accessed June 24, 2011.

The General Survey

The *General Survey* of the patient's appearance, height, and weight begins with the opening moments of the patient encounter, but you will find that your observations of the patient's appearance crystallize as you start the physical examination. The best clinicians continually sharpen their powers of observation and description. As you talk with and examine the patient, heighten your focus on the patient's mood, build, and behavior. These details enrich and deepen your emerging clinical impression. A skilled observer describes the distinguishing features of the patient's appearance so well that colleagues can spot the patient in a crowd of strangers.

Many factors contribute to the patient's body habitus: socioeconomic status, nutrition, genetic makeup, degree of fitness, mood state, early illnesses, gender, geographic location, and age cohort. Recall that the patient's nutritional status affects many of the characteristics you scrutinize during the *General Survey:* height and weight, blood pressure, posture, mood and alertness, facial coloration, dentition and condition of the tongue and gingiva, color of the nail beds, and muscle bulk, to name a few. Be sure to make the assessment of height, weight, BMI, and risk for obesity a routine part of your clinical practice.

Now is the time to recall the observations you have been making since the first moments of your interaction, refining them throughout your assessment. Does the patient hear you when greeted in the waiting room or examination room? Rise with ease? Walk easily or stiffly? If hospitalized when you first meet, what is the patient doing—sitting up and enjoying television?... or lying in bed?... What do you see on the bedside table—a magazine?... a flock of "get well" cards?... a Bible or a rosary?... an emesis basin?... or nothing at all? Each observation should raise questions or hypotheses for you to consider as your assessment unfolds.

GENERAL APPEARANCE

Apparent State of Health.   Try to make a general judgment based on observations throughout the encounter. Support it with the significant details.

Is the patient acutely or chronically ill, frail, or fit and robust?

Level of Consciousness.   Is the patient awake, alert, and responsive to you and others in the environment? If not, promptly assess the level of consciousness.

See Chapter 17, The Nervous System, Level of Consciousness, p. 735

Signs of Distress.   Does the patient show evidence of the problems listed below?

- Cardiac or respiratory distress

Is there clutching of the chest, pallor, diaphoresis, or labored breathing, wheezing, and coughing?

- Pain

  Is there wincing, sweating, protectiveness of a painful area, facial grimacing, or an unusual posture favoring one limb or body area?

- Anxiety or depression

  Are there anxious facial expressions, fidgety movements, cold and moist palms, inexpressive or flat affect, poor eye contact, or psychomotor slowing. See Chapter 5, Behavior and Mental Status, pp. 141–169.

Skin Color and Obvious Lesions.   Assess any changes in skin color, scars, plaques, or nevi.

Pallor, cyanosis, jaundice, rashes, bruises should be pursued. See Chapter 6, The Skin, Hair, and Nails, pp. 171–203.

Dress, Grooming, and Personal Hygiene.   How is the patient dressed? Is the clothing appropriate for the temperature and weather? Is it clean and appropriate to the setting?

Excess clothing may reflect the cold intolerance of *hypothyroidism*, hide skin rash or needle marks, mask anorexia, or signal personal lifestyle preferences.

Glance at the patient's shoes. Are there cut-outs or holes? Are the shoes run-down?

Cut-out holes or slippers may indicate gout, bunions, edema, or other painful foot conditions. Run-down shoes can contribute to foot and back pain, calluses, falls, and infection.

Is the patient wearing unusual jewelry? Are there body piercings?

Copper bracelets are sometimes worn for *arthritis*. Piercing may appear on any part of the body.

Note the patient's hair, fingernails, and use of cosmetics. They may be clues to the patient's personality, mood, lifestyle, and self-regard.

"Grown-out" hair and nail polish can help you estimate the length of an illness. Fingernails chewed to the quick may reflect stress.

Do personal hygiene and grooming seem appropriate to the patient's age, lifestyle, occupation, and stage of life?

Unkempt appearance may be seen in *depression* and *dementia,* but this appearance must be compared with the patient's probable norm.

Facial Expression.   Observe the facial expression at rest, during conversation about specific topics, during the physical examination, and in interaction with others. Watch for eye contact. Is it natural? Sustained and unblinking? Averted quickly? Absent?

Watch for the stare of *hyperthyroidism;* the immobile face of *parkinsonism;* the flat or sad affect of *depression*. Decreased eye contact may be cultural or may suggest anxiety, fear, or sadness.

Odors of the Body and Breath. Odors can be important diagnostic clues, like the fruity odor of diabetes or the scent of alcohol.

Breath odors can indicate the presence of alcohol, acetone (diabetes), pulmonary infections, uremia, or liver failure.

Never assume that alcohol on a patient's breath explains changes in mental status or neurologic findings.

People with alcoholism may have other serious and potentially correctable problems such as hypoglycemia, subdural hematoma, or postictal state.

Posture, Gait, and Motor Activity. What is the patient's preferred posture?

There is a preference for sitting upright in *left-sided heart failure* and for leaning forward with arms braced in *chronic obstructive pulmonary disease.*

Is the patient restless or quiet? How often does the patient change position?

Anxious patients appear agitated and restless. Patients in pain often avoid movement.

Is there any involuntary motor activity? Are some body parts immobile? Which ones?

Look for tremors, other involuntary movements, or paralysis. See Table 17-5, Tremors and Involuntary Movements, pp. 752–753.

Does the patient walk smoothly, with comfort, self-confidence, and balance, or is there a limp or discomfort, fear of falling, loss of balance, or any movement disorder?

See Table 17-10, Abnormalities of Gait and Posture, p. 759. An impaired gait increases risk of falls.

Height and Weight. Measure the patient's height in stocking feet and weigh the patient to determine the BMI.

Is the patient unusually short or tall? Is the build slender, muscular, or stocky? Is the body symmetric? Note the general body proportions.

Be aware of very short stature in *Turner's syndrome,* childhood renal failure, and *achondroplastic* and *hypopituitary dwarfism;* long limbs in proportion to the trunk in hypogonadism and *Marfan's syndrome;* height loss in *osteoporosis* and vertebral compression fractures.

Is the patient emaciated, slender, overweight, or obese? If the patient is obese, is the fat distributed evenly or concentrated over the upper torso, or around the hips?

There is generalized fat in simple obesity; truncal fat with relatively thin limbs in *Cushing's syndrome* and *metabolic syndrome.*

Weigh the patient with shoes off. Make note of any weight changes over time.

Calculating the BMI. Use your measurements of height and weight to calculate the *body mass index,* or *BMI.* Body fat consists primarily of adipose in the form of triglycerides and is stored in subcutaneous, inter-abdominal, and intramuscular fat deposits that are difficult to measure directly. The BMI incorporates estimated but more accurate measures of body fat than weight alone. The National Institutes of Health caution that people who are very muscular can have a high BMI but still be healthy. Likewise, the BMI for older adults and those with low muscle mass may appear inappropriately "normal."

There are several ways to calculate the BMI, as shown in the accompanying table. Choose the method best suited to your practice. The electronic medical record software may do this automatically.

Waist Circumference. If the BMI is 35 or greater, measure the patient's waist circumference just above the hips. Risk for diabetes, hypertension, and cardiovascular disease increases significantly if the waist circumference is *35 inches or more in women and 40 inches or more in men.*

Causes of weight loss include *malignancy, diabetes mellitus, hyperthyroidism, chronic infection, depression, diuresis,* and successful dieting.

See discussion of Optimal Weight, Nutrition and Diet, pp. 108–113.

Methods to Calculate Body Mass Index (BMI)

Unit of Measure	Method of Calculation
Weight in pounds, height in inches	(1) Body Mass Index Chart (see table on the next page)
	(2) $\left(\dfrac{\text{Weight (lbs)} \times 700^*}{\text{Height (inches)}}\right) \div \text{Height (inches)}$
Weight in kilograms, height in meters squared	(3) $\dfrac{\text{Weight (kg)}}{\text{Height (m}^2)}$
Either	(4) "BMI Calculator" at Web site www.nhlbisupport.com/bmi

*Several organizations use 704.5, but the variation in BMI is negligible. Conversion formulas:

2.2 lbs = 1 kg; 1 inch = 2.54 cm; 100 cm = 1 meter.

Source: National Institutes of Health–National Heart, Lung, and Blood Institute: Calculate Your Body Mass Index. Available at: http://www.nhlbisupport.com/bmi. Accessed June 25, 2011.

Body Mass Index Table

BMI	Normal						Overweight						Obese								
	19	20	21	22	23	24	25	26	27	28	29	30	31	32	33	34	35	36	37	38	39
Height (inches)											Body Weight (pounds)										
58	91	96	100	105	110	115	119	124	129	134	138	143	148	153	158	162	167	172	177	181	186
59	94	99	104	109	114	119	124	128	133	138	143	148	153	158	163	168	173	178	183	188	193
60	97	102	107	112	118	123	128	133	138	143	148	153	158	163	168	174	179	184	189	194	199
61	100	106	111	116	122	127	132	137	143	148	153	158	164	169	174	180	185	190	195	201	206
62	104	109	115	120	126	131	136	142	147	153	158	164	169	175	180	186	191	196	202	207	213
63	107	113	118	124	130	135	141	146	152	158	163	169	175	180	186	191	197	203	208	214	220
64	110	116	122	128	134	140	145	151	157	163	169	174	180	186	192	197	204	209	215	221	227
65	114	120	126	132	138	144	150	156	162	168	174	180	186	192	198	204	210	216	222	228	234
66	118	124	130	136	142	148	155	161	167	173	179	186	192	198	204	210	216	223	229	235	241
67	121	127	134	140	146	153	159	166	172	178	185	191	198	204	211	217	223	230	236	242	249
68	125	131	138	144	151	158	164	171	177	184	190	197	203	210	216	223	230	236	243	249	256
69	128	135	142	149	155	162	169	176	182	189	196	203	209	216	223	230	236	243	250	257	263
70	132	139	146	153	160	167	174	181	188	195	202	209	216	222	229	236	243	250	257	264	271
71	136	143	150	157	165	172	179	186	193	200	208	215	222	229	236	243	250	257	265	272	279
72	140	147	154	162	169	177	184	191	199	206	213	221	228	235	242	250	258	265	272	279	287
73	144	151	159	166	174	182	189	197	204	212	219	227	235	242	250	257	265	272	280	288	295
74	148	155	163	171	179	186	194	202	210	218	225	233	241	249	256	264	272	280	287	295	303
75	152	160	168	176	184	192	200	208	216	224	232	240	248	256	264	272	279	287	295	303	311
76	156	164	172	180	189	197	205	213	221	230	238	246	254	263	271	279	287	295	304	312	320

Source: National Institutes of Health–National Heart, Lung, and Blood Institute: Body Mass Index Table. Available at http://www.nhlbi.nih.gov/guidelines/obesity/bmi_tbl.pdf. Accessed June 25, 2011.

The Vital Signs

Now you are ready to review or measure the *Vital Signs*: blood pressure, heart rate, respiratory rate, and temperature. The vital signs provide critical initial information that often influences the direction of your evaluation. Typically they are already recorded in the record by office staff. If they are abnormal, you will often retake them during the visit.

Begin by measuring the blood pressure and the heart rate. The heart rate can be assessed by counting the radial pulse with your fingers, or the apical pulse with your stethoscope at the cardiac apex. Continue either of these techniques as you count the respiratory rate without alerting the patient—breathing patterns can change if the patient knows breaths are being

See Table 9-3, Abnormalities of the Arterial Pulse and Pressure Waves, p. 393. See Table 4-7, Abnormalities in Rate and Rhythm of Breathing, p. 140.

counted. The temperature may be taken in various sites, depending on the patient and the equipment available. Learn the techniques for ensuring the accuracy of the vital signs described in the pages to follow.

BLOOD PRESSURE

The Complexities of Measuring Blood Pressure.   Before turning to the recommended techniques for manual blood pressure measurements, it is important to review recent evidence about the correlation of office, home, and ambulatory blood pressure measurements with the "true blood pressure," the average blood pressure measured over days and weeks. Experts continue to raise concerns about the validity of routine office readings by physicians and other health professionals.[20–22] Given the prevalence of hypertension, defined as blood pressure 140/90 or higher, errors in office diagnosis pose substantial threats to clinical decision making. Observer and measurement error, natural physiologic fluctuations in blood pressure, and anxiety and situational determinants can all alter the relationship of office measurements to "true" blood pressure.

Home and ambulatory blood pressure measurements are more accurate and predictive of cardiovascular disease and end-organ damage than conventional office measurements.[23] *Ambulatory blood pressure monitoring* is fully automated and allows recording over an extended period of time. There are *automated office blood pressure devices* that sense the natural oscillations in the arterial pressure waves and estimate the systolic and diastolic pressure according to empirically derived algorithms. They can take five or more readings and display both individual and averaged measurements. These oscillometric devices hold promise for replacing manual auscultatory measurements in the office. They eliminate observer error, minimize the "white coat effect," increase the number of readings, and produce measurements that are comparable to mean ambulatory blood pressure, the current standard.[20,24,25] The cut-off for normal home, ambulatory, and automated office measurements, 135/85, is lower than for office measurements.[26–28] Currently there is no consensus on the setting, timing, or total number of blood pressure measurements needed for classifying patients or guiding treatment.

New insights based on office, home, and ambulatory blood pressure monitoring are briefly summarized here.

- Two types of hypertension based on manual office blood pressure measurements are especially important to understand: white coat hypertension and masked hypertension. In *white coat hypertension,* constituting roughly 15% to 20% of Stage 1 hypertensives, the office blood pressure is high but ambulatory pressures are normal, so cardiovascular risk is low. *Masked hypertension* is more problematic. In these patients, approximately 10% of the general population, the office blood pressure is normal but the ambulatory blood pressure is high, indicating high risk of cardiovascular disease.[23,27]

- Poor measurement technique, including rounding of measurements to zero, anxiety at the time of measurement, the presence of a physician or nurse, and even the prior diagnosis of hypertension can substantially alter manual office blood pressure readings. Studies suggest that white coat hypertension may be a conditioned anxiety response because affected individuals do not appear to have generalized anxiety.[23,29]

- Averaging several blood pressure measurements is best, regardless of the setting. There are numerous short-term biological variations in blood pressure. The accuracy of clinic and home blood pressure measurements improves significantly when at least two measurements are taken, with additional gains in accuracy up to at least four readings.[30] The variance between office and research systolic blood pressure reaches up to 15 mm Hg.

- Replacing manual office measurements with an automated office device has been shown to reduce blood pressure measurements by 5.4/2.1 mm Hg compared to ambulatory monitoring. It virtually eliminates the difference between manual and ambulatory measurements, substantially reducing the "white coat effect."[31] The patient must be seated in a quiet room for several minutes while readings are being taken for this effect to occur.

Choosing the Correct Blood Pressure Cuff (Sphygmomanometer). More than 74.5 million Americans have elevated blood pressure.[6] To detect blood pressure elevations, an accurate instrument is essential. Three types of blood pressure devices are currently used: aneroid, electronic, and "hybrid," which combines features of both electronic and ambulatory devices. In hybrid devices, the mercury column is replaced by an electronic pressure gauge; blood pressure can be displayed as a simulated mercury column, an aneroid reading, or a digital readout. All measuring instruments should be routinely tested for accuracy using international protocols.[32,33]

Mercury Blood Pressure Cuffs. Some offices continue to use mercury cuffs, although these are no longer available for sale. Experts recommend that mercury cuffs, properly maintained to avoid environmental spill, can still be used for routine office measurements and are important for evaluating the accuracy of any nonmercury device.[27]

Home Blood Pressure Monitoring. Many patients monitor their blood pressure at home. Be prepared to advise them about how to choose the best upper arm cuff for home use and have it recalibrated. Wrist and fingers monitors have become popular but introduce inaccuracies based on physiology and technique.[27] Systolic pressure increases in more distal arteries, whereas diastolic pressure falls. When not used at heart level, wrist and finger monitors also introduce errors based on the hydrostatic effect of differences in position relative to the heart.

Self-monitoring of blood pressure by well-instructed patients using approved devices improves blood pressure control, especially when it is done two times daily at the upper arm with automatic readouts.[34-36]

It is important to for clinicians and patients to choose a cuff that fits the patient's arm. Follow the guidelines outlined here for selecting the correct size.

Selecting the Correct Blood Pressure Cuff

▶ Width of the inflatable bladder of the cuff should be about 40% of upper arm circumference (about 12–14 cm in the average adult).

▶ Length of the inflatable bladder should be about 80% of upper arm circumference (almost long enough to encircle the arm).

▶ The standard cuff is 12 × 23 cm, appropriate for arm circumferences up to 28 cm.

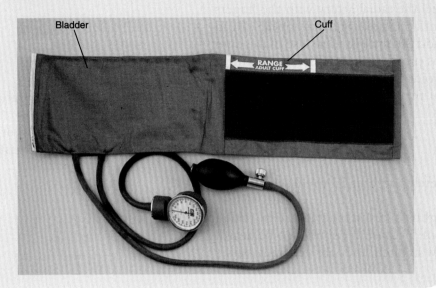

If the cuff is too *small* (narrow), the blood pressure will read *high;* if the cuff is too *large* (wide), the blood pressure will read *low* on a small arm and *high* on a large arm.

Making Accurate Blood Pressure Measurements. Before assessing the blood pressure, take several steps to make sure your measurement will be accurate. Proper technique is important and reduces the inherent variability arising from the patient or examiner, the equipment, and the procedure itself.[37]

Steps to Ensure Accurate Blood Pressure Measurement

▶ In ideal situations, instruct the patient to avoid smoking or drinking caffeinated beverages for 30 minutes before the blood pressure is measured.

▶ Check to make sure the examining room is quiet and comfortably warm.

▶ Ask the patient to sit quietly for at least 5 minutes in a chair with feet on the floor, rather than on the examining table.

▶ Make sure the arm selected is *free of clothing*. There should be no arteriovenous fistulas for dialysis, scarring from prior brachial artery cutdowns, or signs of lymphedema (seen after axillary node dissection or radiation therapy).

▶ Palpate the brachial artery to confirm that it has a viable pulse.

▶ Position the arm so that the brachial artery, at the antecubital crease, is *at heart level*—roughly level with the 4th interspace at its junction with the sternum.

▶ If the patient is seated, rest the arm on a table a little above the patient's waist; if standing, try to support the patient's arm at the midchest level.

If the brachial artery is 7 to 8 cm *below* heart level, the blood pressure will read approximately 6 cm higher; if the brachial artery is 6 to 7 cm *higher,* the blood pressure will read 5 cm lower.[38,39]

Now you are ready to measure the blood pressure.

- With the arm at heart level, center the inflatable bladder over the brachial artery. The lower border of the cuff should be about 2.5 cm above the antecubital crease. Secure the cuff snugly. Position the patient's arm so that it is slightly flexed at the elbow.

A loose cuff or a bladder that balloons outside the cuff leads to falsely high readings.

- To determine how high to raise the cuff pressure, first estimate the systolic pressure by palpation. As you feel the radial artery with the fingers of one hand, rapidly inflate the cuff until the radial pulse disappears. Read this pressure on the manometer and add 30 mm Hg to it. Use of this sum as the target for subsequent inflations prevents discomfort from unnecessarily high cuff pressures. It also avoids the occasional error caused by an *auscultatory gap*—a silent interval that may be present between the systolic and the diastolic pressures.

An unrecognized auscultatory gap may lead to serious underestimation of systolic pressure (150/98 in the example below) or overestimation of diastolic pressure.

- Deflate the cuff promptly and completely and wait 15 to 30 seconds.

- Now place the bell of a stethoscope lightly over the brachial artery, taking care to make an air seal with its full rim. Because the sounds to be heard, the *Korotkoff sounds*, are relatively low in pitch, they are generally better heard with the bell.

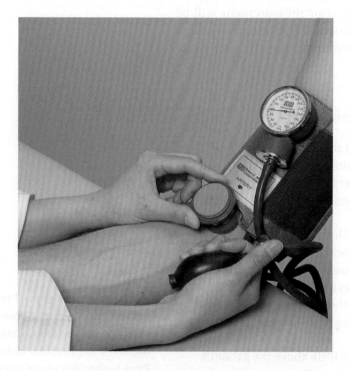

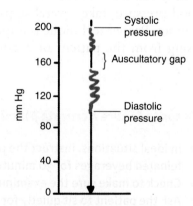

If you find an auscultatory gap, record your findings completely (e.g., 200/98 with an auscultatory gap from 170–150).

An auscultatory gap is associated with arterial stiffness and atherosclerotic disease.[40]

- Inflate the cuff rapidly again to the level just determined, and then deflate it slowly at a rate of about 2 to 3 mm Hg per second. Note the level at which you hear the sounds of at least two consecutive beats. This is the *systolic pressure*.

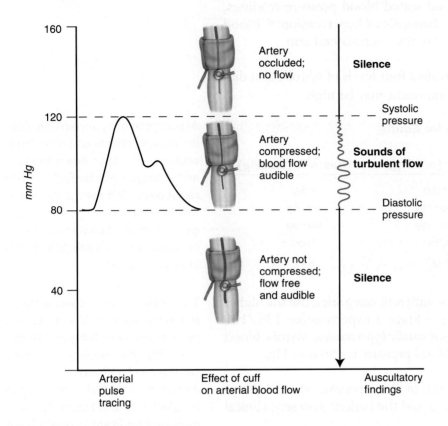

160 —

120 —

mm Hg

80 —

40 —

Artery occluded; no flow — **Silence**

Systolic pressure

Artery compressed; blood flow audible — **Sounds of turbulent flow**

Diastolic pressure

Artery not compressed; flow free and audible — **Silence**

Arterial pulse tracing

Effect of cuff on arterial blood flow

Auscultatory findings

- Continue to lower the pressure slowly until the sounds become muffled and then disappear. To confirm the disappearance of sounds, listen as the pressure falls another 10 to 20 mm Hg. Then deflate the cuff rapidly to zero. The disappearance point, which is usually only a few mm Hg below the muffling point, provides the best estimate of true *diastolic pressure* in adults.

In some people, the muffling point and the disappearance point are farther apart. Occasionally, as in aortic regurgitation, the sounds never disappear. If the difference is 10 mm Hg or greater, record both figures (e.g., 154/80/68).

- Read both the systolic and the diastolic levels to the nearest 2 mm Hg. Wait 2 or more minutes and repeat. Average your readings. If the first two readings differ by more than 5 mm Hg, take additional readings.

- When using an aneroid instrument, hold the dial so that it faces you directly. Avoid slow or repetitive inflations of the cuff, because the resulting venous congestion can cause false readings.

By making the sounds less audible, venous congestion may produce artificially low systolic and high diastolic pressures.

- Blood pressure should be taken in both arms at least once. Normally, there may be a difference in pressure of 5 mm Hg and sometimes up to 10 mm Hg. Subsequent readings should be made on the arm with the higher pressure.

Pressure difference of more than 10–15 mm Hg occurs in *subclavian steal syndrome, aortic dissection.*

Classification of Normal and Abnormal Blood Pressure. In its seventh report in 2003, the Joint National Committee on Prevention, Detection, Evaluation, and Treatment of High Blood Pressure recommended using the mean of two or more properly measured seated blood pressure readings, taken on two or more office visits, for diagnosis of hypertension.[41] Blood pressure measurement should be verified in the contralateral arm.

The Joint National Committee has identified four levels of systolic and diastolic hypertension. Note that either component may be high.

JNCVII Blood Pressure Classification for Adults		
Category	Systolic (mm Hg)	Diastolic (mm Hg)
Normal	<120	<80
Prehypertension	120–139	80–89
Stage 1 Hypertension	140–159	90–99
Stage 2 Hypertension	≥160	≥100
If Diabetes or Renal Disease	<130	<80

When the systolic and diastolic levels fall in different categories, use the higher category. For example, 170/92 mm Hg is Stage 2 hypertension; 135/100 mm Hg is Stage 1 hypertension. In *isolated systolic hypertension,* systolic blood pressure is ≥140 mm Hg, and diastolic blood pressure is <90 mm Hg.

Low Blood Pressure. Relatively low levels of blood pressure should always be interpreted in the light of past readings and the patient's present clinical state.

Orthostatic Hypotension. If indicated, assess *orthostatic hypotension,* common in older adults. Measure blood pressure and heart rate in two positions—*supine* after the patient is resting from 3 to 10 minutes, then within 3 minutes after the patient *stands up.* Normally, as the patient rises from the horizontal to the standing position, systolic pressure drops slightly or remains unchanged, while diastolic pressure rises slightly. Orthostatic hypotension is a drop in systolic blood pressure of 20 mm Hg or greater or in diastolic blood pressure of 10 mm Hg or greater within 3 minutes of standing.[43–45]

Special Situations

Weak or Inaudible Korotkoff Sounds. Consider technical problems such as erroneous placement of your stethoscope, failure to make full skin contact with the bell, and venous engorgement of the patient's arm from repeated inflations of the cuff. Also consider the possibility of shock.

When you cannot hear Korotkoff sounds at all, you may be able to estimate the systolic pressure by palpation. Alternative methods such as Doppler techniques or direct arterial pressure tracings may be necessary.

Assessment of hypertension also includes its effects on target "end organs"—the eyes, heart, brain, and kidneys. Look for hypertensive retinopathy, left ventricular hypertrophy, and neurologic deficits suggesting stroke. Renal assessment requires urinalysis and blood tests of renal function.

Treatment of *isolated systolic hypertension* in patients 60 years or older reduces total mortality and both mortality and complications from cardiovascular disease.[41,42] A pressure of 110/70 mm Hg would usually be normal but could also indicate significant hypotension if past pressures have been high.

A fall in systolic pressure of 20 mm Hg or more, especially when accompanied by symptoms and tachycardia, indicates *orthostatic (postural) hypotension.* Causes include drugs, moderate or severe blood loss, prolonged bed rest, and diseases of the autonomic nervous system.

See Chapter 20, Assessing the Older Adult, p. 945.

In rare cases, patients are pulseless due to occlusive disease in the arteries of all the limbs from *Takayasu arteritis, giant cell arteritis,* or *atherosclerosis.*

To intensify Korotkoff sounds, one of the following methods may be helpful:

- Raise the patient's arm before and while you inflate the cuff. Then lower the arm and determine the blood pressure.

- Inflate the cuff. Ask the patient to make a fist several times, and then determine the blood pressure.

White Coat Hypertension.   Try to relax the patient and remeasure the blood pressure later in the encounter. Consider automated office readings or ambulatory recordings.

See definition of white coat hypertension on p. 119.

The Obese or Very Thin Patient.   For the *obese arm,* use a cuff 15 cm in width. If the upper arm is short despite a large circumference, use a thigh cuff or a very long cuff. If the arm circumference is >50 cm and not amenable to use of a thigh cuff, wrap an appropriately sized cuff around the forearm, hold the forearm at heart level and feel for the radial pulse.[27] Other options include using a Doppler probe at the radial artery or an oscillometric device. For the *very thin arm,* consider using a pediatric cuff.

Using a small cuff overestimates systolic blood pressure in obese patients.[46]

Arrhythmias.   Irregular rhythms produce variations in pressure and therefore unreliable measurements. Ignore the effects of an occasional premature contraction. With frequent premature contractions or atrial fibrillation, determine the average of several observations and note that your measurements are approximate. Ambulatory monitoring for 2 to 24 hours is recommended.[27]

Palpation of an irregularly irregular rhythm indicates *atrial fibrillation.* For all irregular patterns, an ECG is needed to identify the type of rhythm.

The Hypertensive Patient With Unequal Blood Pressures in the Arms and Legs.   To detect coarctation of the aorta, make two further blood pressure measurements at least once in every hypertensive patient:

Coarctation of the aorta results from narrowing of the thoracic aorta, usually proximal but sometimes distal to the left subclavian artery.

- Compare blood pressures in the arms and legs. In normal patients, the systolic blood pressure should be 5 to 10 mm higher in the arms.

Coarctation of the aorta and *occlusive aortic disease* are distinguished by hypertension in the upper extremities and low blood pressure in the legs, and by diminished or delayed femoral pulses.[47]

- Compare the volume and timing of the radial or brachial and femoral pulses. Normally, volume is equal and the pulses occur simultaneously.

To determine blood pressure in the leg, use a wide, long thigh cuff that has a bladder size of 18×42 cm, and apply it to the midthigh. Center the bladder over the posterior surface, wrap it securely, and listen over the popliteal artery. If possible, the patient should be prone. Alternatively, ask the supine patient to flex one leg slightly, with the heel resting on the bed.

HEART RATE AND RHYTHM

Examine the arterial pulses, the heart rate and rhythm, and the amplitude and contour of the pulse wave.

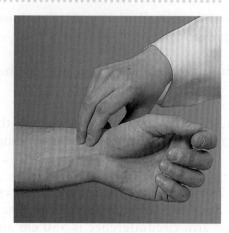

Heart Rate. The radial pulse is commonly used to assess the heart rate. With the pads of your index and middle fingers, compress the radial artery until a maximal pulsation is detected. If the rhythm is regular and the rate seems normal, count the rate for 30 seconds and multiply by 2. If the rate is unusually fast or slow count for 60 seconds. The range of normal is 50–90 beats per minute.[48]

Rhythm. To begin your assessment of rhythm, feel the radial pulse. If there are any irregularities, check the rhythm again by listening with your stethoscope at the cardiac apex. Premature beats may not be detected peripherally, and the heart rate can be seriously underestimated. Is the rhythm regular or irregular? If irregular, try to identify a pattern: (1) Do early beats appear in a basically regular rhythm? (2) Does the irregularity vary consistently with respiration? (3) Is the rhythm totally irregular?

See Table 9-1, Selected Heart Rates and Rhythms, p. 391, and Table 9-2, Selected Irregular Rhythms, p. 392.

Always check an ECG to determine the type of rhythm.

RESPIRATORY RATE AND RHYTHM

Observe the *rate, rhythm, depth,* and *effort of breathing.* Count the number of respirations in 1 minute either by visual inspection or by subtly listening over the patient's trachea with your stethoscope during your examination of the head and neck or chest. Normally, adults take approximately 20 breaths per minute in a quiet, regular pattern. An occasional sigh is normal. Check to see if expiration is prolonged.

See Table 4-7, Abnormalities in Rate and Rhythm of Breathing, p. 140.

Prolonged expiration is common in COPD.

TEMPERATURE

The average *oral temperature,* usually quoted at 37°C (98.6°F), fluctuates considerably. In the early morning hours, it may fall as low as 35.8°C (96.4°F), and in the late afternoon or evening, it may rise as high as 37.3°C (99.1°F). *Rectal temperatures* are *higher* than oral temperatures by an average of 0.4 to 0.5°C (0.7 to 0.9°F), but this difference is also quite variable. In contrast, *axillary temperatures* are *lower* than oral temperatures by approximately 1°, but take 5 to 10 minutes to register and are generally considered less accurate than other measurements.

Most patients prefer oral to rectal temperature measurements. However, taking oral temperatures is not recommended when patients are unconscious,

Fever or pyrexia refers to an elevated body temperature. *Hyperpyrexia* refers to extreme elevation in temperature, above 41.1°C (106°F), while *hypothermia* refers to an abnormally low temperature, below 35°C (95°F) rectally.

restless, or unable to close their mouths. Temperature readings may be inaccurate and thermometers broken by unexpected movements of the patient's jaws.

Oral Temperatures. For *oral temperatures,* choose a glass or an electronic thermometer. When using a *glass thermometer,* shake the thermometer down to 35°C (96°F) or below, insert it under the tongue, instruct the patient to close both lips, and wait 3 to 5 minutes. Then read the thermometer, reinsert it for a minute, and read it again. If the temperature is still rising, repeat this procedure until the reading remains stable. Note that hot or cold liquids, and even smoking, can alter the temperature reading. In these situations, it is best to delay measuring the temperature for 10 to 15 minutes. Due to breakage and mercury exposure, glass thermometers are being replaced by electronic thermometers.

If using an *electronic thermometer,* carefully place the disposable cover over the probe and insert the thermometer under the tongue. Ask the patient to close both lips, and then watch closely for the digital readout. An accurate temperature recording usually takes about 10 seconds.

Rectal Temperatures. For a *rectal temperature,* ask the patient to lie on one side with the hip flexed. Select a rectal thermometer with a stubby tip, lubricate it, and insert it about 3 cm to 4 cm (1½ inches) into the anal canal, in a direction pointing to the umbilicus. Remove it after 3 minutes, then read. Alternatively, use an electronic thermometer after lubricating the probe cover. Wait about 10 seconds for the digital temperature recording to appear.

Tympanic Membrane Temperatures. Taking the *tympanic membrane temperature* is an increasingly common practice and is quick, safe, and reliable if performed properly. Make sure the external auditory canal is free of cerumen, which lowers temperature readings. Position the probe in the canal so that the infrared beam is aimed at the tympanic membrane (otherwise the measurement will be invalid). Wait 2 to 3 seconds until the digital temperature reading appears. This method measures core body temperature, which is higher than the normal oral temperature by approximately 0.8°C (1.4°F). Tympanic measurements are more variable than oral or rectal measurements, including right and left comparisons in the same person.[49]

Acute and Chronic Pain

Understanding Acute and Chronic Pain. The International Association for the Study of Pain defines *pain* as "an unpleasant sensory and emotional experience" associated with tissue damage. The experience of pain is complex and multifactorial. Pain involves sensory, emotional, and cognitive processing but may lack a specific physical etiology.[2]

Causes of *fever* include infection, trauma such as surgery or crush injuries, malignancy, blood disorders such as acute hemolytic anemia, drug reactions, and immune disorders such as collagen vascular disease.

The chief cause of *hypothermia* is exposure to cold. Other predisposing causes include reduced movement as in paralysis, interference with vasoconstriction from sepsis or excess alcohol, starvation, hypothyroidism, and hypoglycemia. Older adults are especially susceptible to hypothermia and also less likely to develop fever.

Rapid respiratory rates tend to increase the discrepancy between oral and rectal temperatures. In these situations, rectal temperatures are more reliable.

Chronic pain may be a spectrum disorder related to mental health and somatic conditions. See Chapter 5, Behavior and Mental Status, Symptoms and Behavior, pp. 142–146.

Chronic pain is defined in several ways: pain not associated with cancer or other medical conditions that persists for more than 3 to 6 months; pain lasting more than 1 month beyond the course of an acute illness or injury; or pain recurring at intervals of months or years.[2] Chronic noncancer pain affects 5% to 33% of patients in primary care settings. More than 40% of patients report that their pain is poorly controlled.[50]

Assessing the Patient's History.   Adopt a comprehensive approach to understanding the patient's pain, carefully listening to the patient's description of the many features of pain and contributing factors. Accept the patient's self-report, which experts state is the most reliable indicator of pain.[2]

Location.   Ask the patient to point to the pain, because lay terms may not be specific enough to localize the site of origin.

Severity.   Assessing the severity of the pain is especially important. Use a consistent method to determine severity. Three scales are common: the Visual Analog Scale and two scales using ratings from 1 to 10—the Numeric Rating Scale and the Wong-Baker FACES Pain Rating Scale. Multidimensional tools like the Brief Pain Inventory are also available; these take longer to administer but address the effects of pain on the patient's activity level.[51] The FACES Pain Rating Scale is reproduced below, because it can be used by children as well as patients with language barriers or cognitive impairment.[52]

Wong-Baker FACES™ Pain Rating Scale

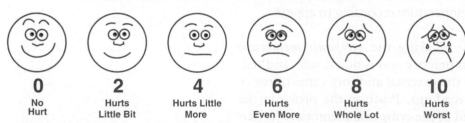

0	2	4	6	8	10
No Hurt	Hurts Little Bit	Hurts Little More	Hurts Even More	Hurts Whole Lot	Hurts Worst

Explain to the person that each face is for a person who feels happy because he has no pain (hurt) or sad because he has some or a lot of pain. Face 0 is very happy because he doesn't hurt at all. Face 2 hurts just a little bit. Face 4 hurts a little more. Face 6 hurts even more. Face 8 hurts a whole lot. Face 10 hurts as much as you can imagine, although you don't have to be crying to feel this bad. Ask the person to choose the face that best describes how he is feeling.

(From Hockenberry MJ, Wilson D: *Wong's essentials of pediatric nursing*, ed. 8, St. Louis, 2009, Mosby. Used with permission. Copyright Mosby.)

Associated Features.   Ask the patient to describe the pain and how it started. Is it related to a site of injury, movement, or time of day? What is the quality of the pain—sharp, dull, burning? Ask if the pain radiates or follows a particular pattern. What makes the pain better or worse? Pursue the seven features of pain, as you would with any symptom.

Attempted Treatments, Medications, Related Illnesses, and Impact on Daily Activities.   Ask about any treatments that the patient has tried, including medications, physical therapy, and alternative medicines. A comprehensive medication history identifies drugs that interact with analgesics and reduce their efficacy.

See Chapter 3, The Seven Attributes of a Symptom, p. 70.

Explore any comorbid conditions such as arthritis, diabetes, HIV/AIDS, substance abuse, sickle cell disease, or psychiatric disorders. These can have significant effects on the patient's experience of pain.

Chronic pain is the leading cause of disability and impaired performance at work. Inquire about the effects of pain on the patient's daily activities, mood, sleep, work, and sexual activity.

Health Disparities.　Be aware of the well-documented health disparities in pain treatment and delivery of care, which range from lower use of analgesics in emergency rooms for African-American and Hispanic patients to disparities in use of analgesics for cancer, postoperative, and low back pain.[2] Studies show that clinician stereotypes, language barriers, and unconscious clinician biases in decision making all contribute to these disparities. Critique your own communication style, seek information and best practice standards, and improve your techniques of patient education and empowerment as first steps to ensure uniform and effective pain management.

See Institute of Medicine report, *Unequal Treatment: Confronting Racial and Ethnic Disparities in Health Care*, 2002.[53]

Types of Pain.　Be familiar with recent advances in the scientific understanding of pain processes, helpfully described in several excellent modules for clinicians that are available online.[2] Review the summary of types of pain in the following box to aid in your diagnosis and management.[54,55]

Types of Pain

Nociceptive (somatic)	Nociceptive (somatic) pain is linked to tissue damage to the skin, musculoskeletal system, or viscera (visceral pain) but the sensory nervous system is intact, as in arthritis or spinal stenosis. It can be acute or chronic. It is mediated by the afferent A-delta and C-fibers of the sensory system. The involved afferent nociceptors can be sensitized by inflammatory mediators and modulated by both psychological processes and neurotransmitters like endorphins, histamines, acetylcholine, serotonin, norepinephrine, and dopamine.
Neuropathic pain	*Neuropathic pain* is a direct consequence of a lesion or disease affecting the somatosensory system. Over time, neuropathic pain may become independent of the inciting injury, becoming burning, lancinating, or shock-like in quality, It may persist even after healing from the initial injury has occured. Mechanisms postulated to evoke neuropathic pain include central nervous system brain or spinal cord injury from stroke or trauma; peripheral nervous system disorders causing entrapment or

(continued)

Types of Pain (continued)

	pressure on spinal nerves, plexuses, or peripheral nerves; and referred pain syndromes with increased or prolonged pain responses to inciting stimuli. These triggers appear to induce changes in pain signal processing through "neuronal plasticity," leading to pain that persists beyond healing from the initial injury.
Central sensitization	In *central sensitization pain*, there is alteration of central nervous system processing of sensation, leading to amplification of pain signals. There is a lower pain threshold to nonpainful stimuli, and the response to pain may be more severe than expected. Mechanisms are the subject of ongoing research. An example is fibromyalgia, which has a strong overlap with depression, anxiety, and somatization disorders and responds best to medications that modify neurotransmitters like serotonin and dopamine.[56]
Psychogenic and idiopathic pain	*Psychogenic pain* involves the many factors that influence the patient's report of pain—psychiatric conditions like anxiety or depression, personality and coping style, cultural norms, and social support systems. *Idiopathic pain* is pain without an identifiable etiology.

Pain Management. Managing pain is a complex clinical challenge. Treatment should be multidimensional, and requires sophisticated knowledge of nonopioid, opioid, and adjuvant analgesics and behavioral and physical therapy, areas that are beyond the scope of this book. Over recent decades clinicians have become increasingly attentive to chronic pain in response to numerous guidelines for treatment and care. In parallel, prescriptions for some opioids have increased more than 800% in the past 10 years.[57] Roughly a third of all patients with chronic noncancer pain, or more than 3% of U.S. adults, take opioids, primarily for arthritis and low back pain.[58,] At the same time, rates of death from opioid overdose have climbed to 148 per 100,000.[59] Recent studies show that the death rate is directly related to the maximum prescribed dose of daily opioids. Risk of overdose increases more than four- to eightfold for patients taking the highest doses, namely 100 mg/day or more.[59,60] Risk factors for fatal overdose include age 65 years or older, depression, substance abuse, and concurrent benzodiazepine treatment. To avoid such hazards, make a commitment to acquiring skills in pain assessment and therapeutics, and take advantage of the validated substance abuse screening and brief intervention protocols that have been shown to reduce substance-use–related problems.[61–64]

Focus on the *Four A's* to monitor patient outcomes:
- *Analgesia*
- *Activities of daily living*
- *Adverse effects*
- *Aberrant drug-related behaviors*

See Chapter 2, Interviewing and the Health History, for definitions of tolerance, physical dependence, and addiction.

Recording Your Findings

Your write-up of the physical examination begins with a general description of the patient's appearance, based on the General Survey. Note that initially you may use sentences to describe your findings; later you will use phrases. The style below contains phrases appropriate for most write-ups.

Recording the Physical Examination—The General Survey and Vital Signs

Choose vivid and graphic adjectives, as if you are painting a picture in words. Avoid clichés such as "well-developed" or "well-nourished" or "in no acute distress," because they could apply to any patient and do not convey the special features of the patient before you.

Record the vital signs taken at the time of your examination. They are preferable to those taken earlier in the day by other providers. (Common abbreviations for blood pressure, heart rate, and respiratory rate are self-explanatory.)

"Mrs. Scott is a young, healthy-appearing woman, well-groomed, fit, and cheerful. Height is 5′4″, weight 135 lbs, BMI 24, BP 120/80, right and left arms, HR 72 and regular, RR 16, temperature 37.5°C."

OR

"Mr. Jones is an elderly man who looks pale and chronically ill. He is alert, with good eye contact but unable to speak more than two or three words at a time due to shortness of breath. He has intercostal muscle retraction when breathing and sits upright in bed. He is thin, with diffuse muscle wasting. Height is 6′2″, weight 175 lbs, BP 160/95, right arm, HR 108 and irregular, RR 32 and labored, temperature 101.2°F."

Suggests exacerbation of chronic obstructive pulmonary disease.

Bibliography

Citations

1. Bray GA, Wilson JF. In the clinic. Obesity. Ann Intern Med 2008;154:ITC4-1–ITC4-16.
2. American Medical Association. Pain Management: The Online Series. Pathophysiology of pain and pain assessment. Module 1–Pathophysiology of pain and pain assessment. Module 3 – Pain management: Barriers to Pain Management & Pain in Special Populations. Module 7 Assessing and Treating Persistent Non-malignant Pain: An Overview. September 2007. Available at http://www.ama-cmeonline.com/pain_mgmt/. Accessed July 1, 2011.
3. Upshur CC, Luckmann RS, Savageau JA. Primary care provider concerns about management of chronic pain in community clinic populations. J Gen Int Med 2006;21:652–655.
4. Sinatra R. Opioid analgesics in primary care: challenges and new advances in the management of noncancer pain. J Am Board Fam Med 2006;19:165–167.
5. National Center for Health Statistics, Centers for Disease Prevention and Control. New report finds pain affects millions of Americans. 2006, updated 12.29.09. Available at http://www.cdc.gov/nchs/pressroom/06facts/hus06.htm. Accessed June 18, 2011.
6. Roger VL, Go AS, Lloyd-Jones DM et al. Heart disease and stroke statistics–2011 update: a report from the American Heart Association. Data source: National Health and Nutrition Survey (NHANES) 2005-2008; National Heart, Lung, blood Institute, and unpublished data. Circulation 2011;123:e18–e209. Available at http://circ.ahajournals.org/cgi/reprint/CIR.0b013e3182009701. Accessed April 13, 2011.
7. Flegal KM, Carroll MD, Ogden CL et al. Prevalence and trends in obesity among US adults, 1999–2008. JAMA 2010;303:235–241.
8. Adams KF, Schatzkin A, Harris TB et al. Overweight, obesity and morality in a large prospective cohort of persons 50 to 71 years old. N Engl J Med 2006;335:763–778.
9. Kenchaiah S, Evans JC, Levy D et al. Obesity and the risk of heart failure. N Engl J Med 2002;347:305–313.

10. Kelesidis T, Kelesidis I, Chou S et al. Narrative review: the role of leptin in human physiology: emerging clinical applications. Ann Intern Med 2010;152:93–100.

11. Foster GD, Wyatt HR, Hill JO et al. Weight and metabolic outcomes after 2 years on a low-carbohydrate versus low-fat diet: a randomized trial. Ann Intern Med 2010;153:147–157.

12. Sacks FM, Bray GA, Carey VJ et al. Comparison of weight-loss diets with different compositions of fat, protein, and carbohydrates. N Engl J Med 2009;360:859–873.

13. Snow V, Barry P, Fitterman N et al. Pharmacologic and surgical management of obesity in primary care: a clinical practice guideline from the American College of Physicians. Ann Intern Med 2005;142:525–531.

14. U.S. Department of Agriculture. Dietary Guidelines for Americans 2010. Available at http://www.cnpp.usda.gov/Publications/DietaryGuidelines/2010/PolicyDoc/PolicyDoc.pdf. Accessed June 20, 2011.

15. Appel LJ, Frohlich ED, Hall JE et al. AHA Presidential Advisory. The importance of population-wide sodium reduction as a means to prevent cardiovascular disease and stroke. A call to action from the American Heart Association. Circulation 2011;123:1138–1143. Available at http://circ.ahajournals.org/cgi/content/short/123/10/1138. Accessed June 24, 2011.

16. Strazzullo P, d'Elia L, Ngainga-Bakwin K et al. Salt intake, stroke, and cardiovascular disease: meta-analysis of prospective studies. BMJ 339:b4567.doi:10.1136/bmj.b4567. November 2009.

17. Institute of Medicine. Strategies to reduce sodium intake in the United States. Report brief. April 2010. Available at http://www.iom.edu/~/media/Files/Report%20Files/2010/Strategies-to-Reduce-Sodium-Intake-in-the-United-States/Strategies%20to%20Reduce%20Sodium%20Intake%202010%20%20Report%20Brief.ashx. Accessed June 24, 2011.

18. Gunn JP, Kuklina EV, Keenan NL et al. Sodium intake among adults—United States, 2005-2006. MMWR 2010;59:746–749.

19. National Institutes of Health and National Heart, Lung, and Blood Institute. Clinical Guidelines on the Identification, Evaluation, and Treatment of Overweight and Obesity in Adults, 1998. Update available Fall 2011. Available at http://www.nhlbi.nih.gov/guidelines/obesity/ob_gdlns.pdf. Accessed June 20, 2011.

20. Myers MG, Godwin M, Dawes M et al. Measurement of blood pressure in the office. Recognizing the problem and proposing the solution. Hypertension 2010;55:195–200.

21. Omen ES, Lipkowitz MS. The role of ambulatory BP monitoring in clinical care. Geriatrics 2007;62:11–14.

22. Brondolo E, Libby DJ, Denton EG et al. Racism and ambulatory blood pressure in a community sample. Psychosom Med 2008;70:49–56.

23. Pickering TG, Gering W, Schwartz JE et al. Franz Volhard lecture: should doctors still measure blood pressure? The missing patients with masked hypertension. J Hypertension 2008;26:2259–2267.

24. Myers MG, Valdivieso M, Chessman M at al. Can sphygmomanometers designed for self-measurement of blood pressure in the home be used in office practice? Blood Press Monit 2010;15:300–304.

25. Landgraf J, Wishner SH, Kloner RA. Comparison of automated oscillometric versus auscultatory blood pressure measurement. Am J Cardiol 2010;106:386–388.

26. Mancia G, De Backer G, Dominiczak A et al. 2007 ESH-ESC Practice Guidelines for the Management of Arterial Hypertension: ESH-ESC Task Force on the Management of Arterial Hypertension. J Hypertens 2007;25:1751–1762.

27. Pickering TG, Hall JE, Appel LJ et al. Recommendations for blood pressure measurement in humans and experimental animals. Part 1: blood pressure measurement in humans: a statement for professionals from the Subcommittee of Professional and Public Education of the American Heart Association Council on High Blood Pressure Research. Circulation 2005;111: 697–716.

28. Godwin M, Birtwhistle R, Delva D et al. Manual and automated office measurements in relation to awake ambulatory blood pressure monitoring. Family Practice 2011;28:110–117.

29. Ogedegbe G, Pickering TG, Clemow L et al. The misdiagnosis of hypertension: the role of patient anxiety. Arch Intern Med 2008;168:2459–2465.

30. Powers BJ, Olsen MK, Smith VA et al. Measuring blood pressure for decision making and quality reporting: where and how many measures? Ann Intern Med 2011;154:781–788.

31. Myers MG, Godwin M, Dawes M et al. Conventional versus automated measurement of blood pressure in primary care patients with systolic hypertension: randomised parallel design controlled trial. BMJ, 2011. Available at http://www.bmj.com/content/342/bmj.d286.full.pdf. Accessed May 6, 2011.

32. O'Brien E, Asmar R, Beilin L et al. European Society of Hypertension recommendations for conventional, ambulatory, and more blood pressure measurement. J Hypertens 2005;21:821–848.

33. O'Brien E, Pickering T, Asmar R et al. International protocol for validation of blood pressure measuring devices in adults. Blood Press Monit 2002;7:3–17.

34. Verberk WJ, Kroon AA, Kessles AGH et al. Home blood pressure measurement. A systematic review. J Am Coll Cardiol 2005;46:743–751.

35. McManus RJ, Mant J, Roalfe A et al. Targets and self-monitoring in hypertension: randomized controlled trial and cost effectiveness analysis. BMJ 331(7515):493. epub 2005.

36. Bakx JC, van der Wel MC, van Weel. Self-monitoring of high blood pressure. BMJ 2005;331(7515):466–467.

37. Chobanian AV, Bakris GL, Black HR et al. The Seventh Report of the Joint National Committee on Prevention, Detection, Evaluation, and Treatment of High Blood Pressure—The JNC 7 Report. JAMA 2003;289:2560-2572. Available at http://www.nhlbi.nih.gov/guidelines/hypertension/jnc7full.pdf. Accessed June 25, 2011.

38. McGee S. Ch. 15 Blood Pressure, in Evidence-Based Physical Diagnosis. St. Louis: Saunders, 2007. PP. 153–173.

39. Mitchell PL, Parlin RW, Blackburn H. Effect of vertical displacement of the arm on indirect blood-pressure measurements. N Engl J Med 1964;271:72–74.

40. Cavallini MC, Roman MJ, Blank SG et al. Association of the auscultatory gap with vascular disease in hypertensive patients. Ann Intern Med 1996;124:877–883.

41. Chobanian A. Isolated systolic hypertension in the elderly. N Engl J Med 2007;357:789–796.

42. Chaudhry SI, Krumholz HM, Foody JM. Systolic hypertension in older persons. JAMA 2004;292:1074–1080.

43. Freeman R. Neurogenic orthostatic hypotension. N Engl J Med 2008;358:615–624.

44. Carslon JE. Assessment of orthostatic blood pressure: measurement technique and clinical applications. South Med J 1999;92:167–173.

45. Consensus Committee of the American Autonomic Society and the American Academy of Neurology. Consensus statement on the definition of orthostatic hypotension, pure autonomic failure, and multiple system atrophy. Neurology 1996;46:1470.

46. Fonseca-Reyes S, de Alba-García JG, Parra-Carrillo JZ et al. Effect of standard cuff on blood pressure readings in patients with obese arms. How frequent are arms of a 'large circumference'? Blood Press Monit 2003;8:101–106.

47. Aboulhosn J, Child JS. Left ventricular outflow obstruction: subaortic stenosis, bicuspid aortic valve, supravalvar aortic stenosis, and coarctation of the aorta. Circulation 2006; 114(22):2412–2422.

48. Spodick DH. Normal sinus heart rate: appropriate rate thresholds for sinus tachycardia and bradycardia. South Med J 1996; 89(7): 666–667.

49. McGee S. Ch. 16 Temperature, in Evidence-Based Physical Diagnosis. St. Louis: Saunders, 2007, pp. 174–186.

50. Nicholson B, Passik SD. Management of chronic noncancer pain in the primary care setting. South Med J 2007;100:1028–1036.

51. Daut RL, Cleeland CS, Flanery RC. Development of the Wisconsin Brief Pain Questionnaire to assess pain in cancer and other diseases. Pain 1983;17:197–210.

52. Bieri D, Reeve R, Champion GD et al. The Faces Pain Scale for the self-assessment of the severity of pain experienced by children: development, initial validation and preliminary investigation for ratio scale properties. Pain 1990;41:139–150.

53. Smedley BR, Stith AY, Nelson AR, Editors, Committee on Understanding and Eliminating Racial and Ethnic Disparities in Health Care. Unequal Treatment: Confronting Racial and Ethnic Disparities in Health Care. Washington DC: National Academies Press, 2002.

54. Foley K. Opioids and chronic neuropathic pain. N Engl J Med 2003;348(13):1279–1280.

55. Haanpaa M, Attal N, Backonja M et al. NeuPSIG guidelines on neuropathic pain assessment. Pain 2011;152:14–27.

56. Abeles AM, Pilinger MH, solitary BM et al. Narrative review: the pathophysiology of fibromyalgia. Ann Intern Med 2007;146:726–734.

57. McClellan TA, Turner BJ. Chronic non-cancer pain management and opioid overdose: time to change prescribing practices. Ann Intern Med 2010;152:123–124.

58. Altman RD, Smith HS. Opioid therapy for osteoarthritis and chronic low back pain. Postgrad Med 2010;122:87–97.

59. Dunn KM, Saunders KW, Rutter CM et al. Opioid prescriptions for chronic pain and overdose. A cohort study. Ann Intern Med 2010;152:85–92.

60. Bohnert AS, Valenstein M, Bair MJ et al. Association between opioid prescribing patterns and opioid overdose-related deaths. JAMA 2011;305:1315–1321.

61. Madras BK, Compton WM, Avula D et al. Screening, brief interventions, referral to treatment (SBIRT) for illicit drug and alcohol use at multiple healthcare sites: comparison at intake and 6 months later. Drug Alcohol Depend 2009;99:280–295.

62. Gilron I, Watson PN, Cahill CM et al. Neuropathic pain: a practical guide for the clinician. CMAJ 2006;175:256–275.

63. Butler SF, Budman SH, Fernandez K et al. Validations of a screener and opioid assessment measure for patients with chronic pain. Pain 2004;112(1-2):65–75.

64. Webster LR, Webster RM. Predicting aberrant behaviors in opioid-treated patients: preliminary validation of the Opioid Risk Tool. Pain Med 2005;6:432–442.

Additional References

Weight and Nutrition

American Academy of Family Physicians. Nutrition Screening Initiative. Available at: http://www.aafp.org/afp/980301ap/edits.html. Accessed September 23, 2011.

American Medical Association. Roadmaps for Clinical Practice. Assessment and Management of Adult Obesity. A Primer for Physicians. November 2003. Available at http://www.ama-assn.org/resources/doc/public-health/booklet1.pdf. Accessed July 1, 2011.

Ashar BH, Rowland Seymour A. Advising patients who use dietary supplements. Am J Med 2008;121:91–97.

Ashen MD, Blumenthal RS. Low HDL cholesterol levels. N Engl J Med 2005;353:1252–1260.

Attia E, Walsh BT. Behavioral management for anorexia nervosa. N Engl J Med 2009;360:500–506.

Bayturan O, Tuzcu EM, Uno K et al. Comparison of rates of progression of coronary atherosclerosis in patients with diabetes mellitus versus those with the metabolic syndrome. Am J Cardiol. 2010;105:1735–1739.

Berrington de Gonzalez A, Hartge P, Cerhan JR et al. Body-mass index and mortality among 1.46 million white adults. N Engl J Med 2010;363:2211–2219.

Centers for Disease Control and Prevention. Obesity and overweight. Data and statistics, 2008. Available at http://www.cdc.gov/obesity/data/index.html. Accessed June 18, 2011.

Ford ES, Wayne G, Dietz WH et al. Prevalence of the metabolic syndrome among U.S. adults: findings from the Third National Health and Nutrition Examination Survey. JAMA 2002; 287:356–359.

Hossain P, Kawar B, El Hahas M. Obesity and diabetes in the developing world–a growing challenge. New Engl J Med 2007; 356: 213–215.

Huang HY, Caballero B, Change S et al. The efficacy and safety of multivitamins and mineral supplement use to prevent cancer and chronic disease in adults: a systematic review for a National Institutes of Health State-of-the-Science Conference. Ann Intern Med 2006;145:372–385.

Johnson WD, Kroon JJ, Greenway FL et al. Prevalence of risk factors for metabolic syndrome in adolescents: National Health and Nutrition Examination Survey (NHANES), 2001–2006. Arch Pediatr Adolesc Med 2009;163:371–377.

Lien LF, Brown AJ, Ard JD et al. Effects of PREMIER lifestyle modifications on participants with and without the metabolic syndrome. Hypertension 2007;50:609–616.

NIH Publication No. 03-4082, Facts about the DASH Eating Plan, United States Department of Health and Human Services, National Institutes of Health, National Heart, Lung, and Blood Institute, Karanja NM et al. J Am Dietetic Assoc (JADA) 1999;8:S19-27. Available at http://www.nhlbi.nih.gov/health/public/heart/hbp/dash. See also In brief: your guide to lowering your blood pressure with DASH. Available at http://www.nhlbi.nih.gov/health/public/heart/hbp/dash/dash_brief.pdf. Accessed July 1, 2011.

Office of Dietary Supplements, National Institutes of Health. Dietary Supplement Fact Sheets: Calcium; Vitamin D. Available at http://ods.od.nih.gov/factsheets/list-all/. Accessed June 24, 2011.

Post RE, Mainous AG 3rd, Gregorie SH et al. The influence of physician acknowledgement of patient's weight status on patient perceptions of overweight and obesity in the United States. Arch Intern Med 2011;171:316–321.

Sacks FM, Svetkey LP, Vollmer WM et al. Effects on blood pressure of reduced dietary sodium and the dietary approaches to stop hypertension (DASH) diet. N Engl J Med 2001;344:3–10.

Steinhausen HC, Weber S. The outcome of bulimia nervosa: findings from one-quarter century of research. Am J Psychiatry 2009;166:1331–1341.

U.S. Department of Agriculture. Choose MyPlate.gov. Modified June 2011. Available at http://www.choosemyplate.gov/index.html. Accessed June 20, 2011.

U.S. Preventive Services Task Force. Screening for Obesity in Adults: recommendations and rationale. Rockville, MD. Agency for Healthcare Research and Quality, November 2003. Available at http://www.ahrq.gov/clinic/3rduspstf/obesity/obesrr.htm. Accessed June 20, 2011.

Blood Pressure

Beevers G, Lip GY, O'Brien E. ABC of hypertension. Blood pressure measurement. Part I. Sphygmomanometry: factors common in all techniques. BMJ 2001;322:981–985.

Beevers G, Lip GY, O'Brien E. ABC of hypertension. Blood pressure measurement. Part II Conventional sphygmomanometry: technique of auscultatory blood pressure measurement. BMJ 2001;322:1043–1047.

Bobrie G, Genes N, Vaur L et al. Is isolated home hypertension as opposed to "isolated office" hypertension a sign of greater cardiovascular risk? Arch Intern Med 2001;161:2205–2011.

Hodgkinson J, Mant J, Martin U et al. Relative effectiveness of clinic and home blood pressure monitoring compared with ambulatory blood pressure monitoring in diagnosis of hypertension: systematic review. BMJ. 2011;342:d3621

Lin PH, Appel LJ, Funk K et al. The PREMIER intervention helps participants follow the Dietary Approaches to Stop Hypertension dietary pattern and the current Dietary Reference Intakes recommendations. J Am Diet Assoc 2007;107:1541–1551.

OBrien E, Waider B, Parati G et al. Blood pressure measuring devices: recommendations of the European Society of Hypertension. BMJ 2001;322(7285): 531–536.

Perry HM, Davis BR, Price TR et al, for the Systolic Hypertension in the Elderly Program Cooperative Research Group. Effect of treating isolated systolic hypertension on the risk of developing various types and subtypes of stroke: the Systolic Hypertension in the Elderly Program (SHEP). JAMA 2000;284:465–471.

Pickering TG, Hall JE, Appel L et al. Response to Recommendations for Blood Pressure Measurement in Human and Experimental Animals; Part 1: Blood pressure measurement in humans and miscuffing: A problem with new guidelines: Addendum. Hypertension 2006. Available at http://hyper.ahajournals.org/cgi/reprint/48/1/e5. Accessed May 13, 2011.

Tholl U, Forstner K, Anlauf M. Measuring blood pressure: pitfalls and recommendations. Nephrol Dial Transplant 2004;19:766.

U.S. Preventive Services Task Force. Screening for High Blood Pressure: U.S. Preventive Services Task Force Reaffirmation Recommendation Statement. AHRQ Publication No. 08-05105-EF-2, December 2007; first published in Ann Intern Med 2007;147:783–786. Agency for Healthcare Research and Quality, Rockville, MD. Available at http://www.uspreventiveservicestaskforce.org/uspstf07/hbp/hbprs.htm. Accessed September 23 2011.

Writing Group of the PREMIER Collaborative Research Group. Effects of comprehensive lifestyle modification on blood pressure control: main results of the PREMIER clinical trial. JAMA 2003;289:2083–2093.

Acute and Chronic Pain

Flor H, Turk DC. Chronic Pain–An Integrated Biobehavioral Approach. Seattle: IASP Press, 2011.

Haller DL, Acosta MC. Characteristics of pain patients with opioid-use disorder. Psychosomatics 2010;51:257–266.

International Association for the Study of Pain. Charlton JE. Core Curriculum for Professional Education in Pain, 3rd ed. Charlton JE (ed), 2005. Available at http://www.iasp-pain.org/AM/Template.cfm?Section=Publications&Template=/CM/HTMLDisplay.cfm&ContentID=2307#TOC. Accessed September 23, 2011.

National Heart Lung and Blood Institute, National Institutes of Health. Calculate your body mass index. Available at http://www.nhlbisupport.com/bmi. Accessed June 25, 2011.

The Bates' suite offers these additional resources to enhance learning and facilitate understanding of this chapter:

- Bates' Pocket Guide to Physical Examination and History Taking, 7th edition
- Bates' Visual Guide to Physical Examination
- thePoint online resources, for students and instructors: http://thepoint.lww.com

Table 4-1 Obesity-Related Health Factors

Cardiovascular
- Hypertension
- Coronary artery disease
- Atrial fibrillation
- Heart failure
- Cor pulmonale
- Varicose veins

Endocrine
- Metabolic syndrome
- Type 2 diabetes
- Dyslipidemia
- Polycystic ovarian syndrome/androgenicity
- Amenorrhea/infertility/menstrual disorders

Gastrointestinal
- Gastroesophageal reflux disease (GERD)
- Nonalcoholic fatty liver disease (NAFLD)
- Cholelithiasis
- Hernias
- Cancer: colon, pancreas, esophagus, liver

Genitourinary
- Urinary stress incontinence
- Obesity-related glomerulopathy
- Hypogonadism (male)
- Cancer: breast, cervical, ovarian, uterine
- Pregnancy complications
- Nephrolithiasis, chronic renal disease

Integument
- Striae distensae (stretch marks)
- Status pigmentation of legs
- Lymphedema
- Cellulitis
- Intertrigo, carbuncles
- Acanthosis nigricans/skin tags

Muscoloskeletal
- Hyperuricemia and gout
- Immobility
- Osteoarthritis (knees, hips)
- Low back pain

Neurologic
- Stroke
- Idiopathic intracranial hypertension
- Meralgia paresthetica

Psychological
- Depression/low self-esteem
- Body image disturbance
- Social stigmatization

Respiratory
- Dyspnea
- Obstructive sleep apnea
- Hypoventilation syndrome/Pickwickian syndrome
- Pulmonary embolism
- Asthma

Source: American Medical Association. Roadmaps for Clinical Practice—Case Studies in Disease Prevention and Health Promotion—Assessment and Management of Adult Obesity: A Primer for Physicians. Available at: http://www.ama-assn.org/ama1/pub/upload/mm/433/healthrisks.pdf. Accessed July 1, 2011.

Table 4-2 Eating Disorders and Excessively Low BMI

In the United States, an estimated 5 to 10 million women and 1 million men suffer from eating disorders. These severe disturbances of eating behavior are often difficult to detect, especially in teens wearing baggy clothes or in individuals who binge and then induce vomiting or evacuation. Be familiar with the two principal eating disorders, *anorexia nervosa* and *bulimia nervosa*. Both conditions are characterized by distorted perceptions of body image and weight. Early detection is important, because prognosis improves when treatment occurs in the early stages of these disorders.

Clinical Features

Anorexia Nervosa	Bulimia Nervosa
• Refusal to maintain minimally normal body weight (or BMI above 17.5 kg/m^2)	• Repeated binge eating followed by self-induced vomiting, misuse of laxatives, diuretics or other medications, fasting, or excessive exercise
• Afraid of appearing fat	• Often with normal weight
• Frequently starving but in denial; lacking insight	• Overeating at least twice a week during 3-month period; large amounts of food consumed in short period (~2 hrs)
• Often brought in by family members	
• May present as failure to make expected weight gains in childhood or adolescence, amenorrhea in women, loss of libido or potency in men	• Preoccupation with eating; craving and compulsion to eat; lack of control over eating; alternating with periods of starvation
• Associated with depressive symptoms such as depressed mood, irritability, social withdrawal, insomnia, decreased libido	• Dread of fatness but may be obese

• Additional features supporting diagnosis: self-induced vomiting or purging, excessive exercise, use of appetite suppressants and/or diuretics	• Subtypes of
	
	  • *Purging:* bulimic episodes accompanied by self-induced vomiting or use of laxatives, diuretics, or enemas
	
	  • *Nonpurging:* bulimic episodes accompanied by compensatory behavior such as fasting, exercise, but without purging

• Biologic complications
 	
  • *Neuroendocrine changes:* amenorrhea, increased corticotropin-releasing factor, cortisol, growth hormone, serotonin; decreased diurnal cortisol fluctuation, luteinizing hormone, follicle-stimulating hormone, thyroid-stimulating hormone
 	
  • *Cardiovascular disorders:* bradycardia, hypotension, arrhythmias, cardiomyopathy
 	
  • *Metabolic disorders:* hypokalemia, hypochloremic metabolic alkalosis, increased BUN, edema
 	
  • *Other:* dry skin, dental caries, delayed gastric emptying, constipation, anemia, osteoporosis
	• Biologic complications See changes listed for anorexia nervosa, especially weakness, fatigue, mild cognitive disorder; also erosion of dental enamel, parotitis, pancreatic inflammation with elevated amylase, mild neuropathies, seizures, hypokalemia, hypochloremic metabolic acidosis, hypomagnesemia

Sources: World Health Organization. The ICD-10 Classification of Mental and Behavioral Disorders: Diagnostic Criteria for Research. Geneva: World Health Organization, 1993. American Psychiatric Association. DSM-IV-TR: Diagnostic and Statistical Manual of Mental Disorders, 4th ed. Washington, DC: American Psychiatric Association, 1994. Halmi KA. Eating Disorders: In: Kaplan HI, Sadock BJ, eds. Comprehensive Textbook of Psychiatry, 7th ed. Philadelphia: Lippincott Williams & Wilkins, 1663–1676, 2000. Mehler PS. Bulimia nervosa. N Engl J Med 349(9):875–880, 2003.

Table 4-3 Nutrition Screening

Nutrition Screening Checklist

I have an illness or condition that made me change the kind and/or amount of food I eat.	Yes (2 pts)	_____
I eat fewer than 2 meals per day.	Yes (3 pts)	_____
I eat few fruits or vegetables, or milk products.	Yes (2 pts)	_____
I have 3 or more drinks of beer, liquor, or wine almost every day.	Yes (2 pts)	_____
I have tooth or mouth problems that make it hard for me to eat.	Yes (2 pts)	_____
I don't always have enough money to buy the food I need.	Yes (4 pts)	_____
I eat alone most of the time.	Yes (1 pt)	_____
I take 3 or more different prescribed or over-the-counter drugs each day.	Yes (1 pt)	_____
Without wanting to, I have lost or gained 10 pounds in the last 6 months.	Yes (2 pts)	_____
I am not always physically able to shop, cook, and/or feed myself.	Yes (2 pts)	_____
	TOTAL	_____

Instructions. Check "yes" for each condition that applies, then total the nutritional score. For total scores of 3–5 points (moderate risk) or ≥6 points (high risk), further evaluation is needed (especially for the elderly).

Rapid Screen for Dietary Intake

	Portions Consumed by Patient	Recommended
Grains, cereals, bread group	_____	6–11
Fruit group	_____	2–4
Vegetable group	_____	3–5
Meat/meat substitute group	_____	2–3
Dairy group	_____	2–3
Sugars, fats, snack foods	_____	—
Soft drinks	_____	—
Alcoholic beverages	_____	<2

Instructions. Ask the patient for a 24-hour dietary recall (perhaps two of these) before completing the form.

Sources: *Nutrition Screening*—American Academy of Family Physicians. The Nutrition Screening Initiative. Available at: http://www.aafp.org/afp1980301ap/edits.html. Accessed July 1, 2011; *Rapid Screen for Dietary Intake*—Nestle M. Nutrition. In Woolf SH, Jonas S, Lawrence RS, eds. Health Promotion and Disease Prevention in Clinical Practice. Baltimore: Williams & Wilkins, 1996.

Table 4-4

Obesity: Stages of Change Model and Assessing Readiness

Stage	Characteristic	Patient Verbal Cue	Appropriate Intervention	Sample Dialogue
Precontemplation	Unaware of problem, no interest in change`	"I'm not really interested in weight loss. It's not a problem."	Provide information about health risks and benefits of weight loss	"Would you like to read some information about the health aspects of obesity?"
Contemplation	Aware of problem, beginning to think of changing	"I know I need to lose weight, but with all that's going on in my life right now, I'm not sure I can."	Help resolve ambivalence; discuss barriers	"Let's look at the benefits of weight loss, as well as what you may need to change."
Preparation	Realizes benefits of making changes and thinking about how to change	"I have to lose weight, and I'm planning to do that."	Teach behavior modification; provide education	"Let's take a closer look at how you can reduce some of the calories you eat and how to increase your activity during the day."
Action	Actively taking steps toward change	"I'm doing my best. This is harder than I thought."	Provide support and guidance, with a focus on the long term	"It's terrific that you're working so hard. What problems have you had so far? How have you solved them?"
Maintenance	Initial treatment goals reached	"I've learned a lot through this process."	Relapse control	"What situations continue to tempt you to overeat? What can be helpful for the next time you face such a situation?"

Sources: American Medical Association. Roadmaps for Clinical Practice—Case Studies in Disease Prevention and Health Promotion—Assessment and Management of Adult Obesity: A Primer for Physicians. Available at: http://www.ama-assn.org/resources/doc/public-health/booklet1.pdf. Accessed July 1, 2011; Adapted from Prochaska JO, DiClemente CC. Toward a comprehensive model of change. In: Miller WR, ed. Treating Addictive Behaviors. New York: Plenum, 1986:3–27.

Table 4-5 Nutrition Counseling: Sources of Nutrients

Nutrient	Food Source
Calcium	Dairy foods such as milk, natural cheeses, and yogurt Calcium-fortified cereals, fruit juice, soy milk, and tofu Dark green leafy vegetables like collard, turnip, and mustard greens; bok choy Sardines
Iron	Lean meat, dark turkey meat, liver Clams, mussels, oysters, sardines, anchovies Iron-fortified cereals Enriched and whole grain bread Spinach, peas, lentil, turnip greens, peas, and artichokes Dried prunes and raisins
Folate	Cooked dried beans and peas Oranges, orange juice Liver Black-eyed peas, lentils, okra, chick peas, peanuts Folate-fortified cereals
Vitamin D	Vitamin D–fortified milk Cod liver oil; salmon, mackerel, tuna Egg yolks, butter, margarine Vitamin D–fortified cereals

Source: Adapted from: Dietary Guidelines Committee, 2000 Report. Nutrition and Your Health: Dietary Guidelines for Americans. Washington, DC: Agricultural Research Service, U.S. Department of Agriculture, 2000; Choose MyPlate.gov. Available at http://www.choosemyplate.gov/index.html. Accessed June 24, 2011; Office of Dietary Supplements, National Institutes of Health. Dietary Supplement Fact Sheets: Calcium; Vitamin D. At http://ods.od.nih.gov/factsheets/list-all/. Accessed June 24, 2011.

Table 4-6 Patients With Hypertension: Recommended Changes in Diet

Dietary Change	Food Source
Increase foods high in potassium	Baked white or sweet potatoes, white beans, beet greens, soybeans, spinach, lentils, kidney beans Bananas, plantains, many dried fruits, orange juice Tomato sauce, juice, and paste
Decrease foods high in sodium	Canned foods (soups, tuna fish) Pretzels, potato chips, pickles, olives Many processed foods (frozen dinners, ketchup, mustard) Batter-fried foods Table salt, including for cooking

Source: Adapted from: Dietary Guidelines Committee, 2000 Report. Nutrition and Your Health: Dietary Guidelines for Americans. Washington, DC: Agricultural Research Service, U.S. Department of Agriculture, 2000; Choose MyPlate.gov. Available at http://www.choosemyplate.gov/index.html. Accessed June 24, 2011; Office of Dietary Supplements, National Institutes of Health. Dietary Supplement Fact Sheets: Calcium; Vitamin D. At http://ods.od.nih.gov/factsheets/list-all/. Accessed June 24, 2011.

Table 4-7   Abnormalities in Rate and Rhythm of Breathing

When observing respiratory patterns, note the of rate, depth, and regularity of the patient's breathing. Traditional terms, such as tachypnea, are given below so that you will understand them, but simple descriptions are recommended.

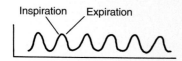

Normal

The respiratory rate is about 14–20 per min in normal adults and up to 44 per min in infants.

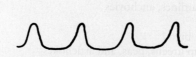

Slow Breathing (*Bradypnea*)

Slow breathing may be secondary to diabetic coma, drug-induced respiratory depression, and increased intracranial pressure.

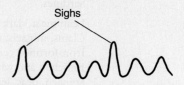

Sighing Respiration

Breathing punctuated by frequent sighs should alert you to the possibility of hyperventilation syndrome—a common cause of dyspnea and dizziness. Occasional sighs are normal.

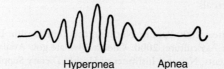

Rapid Shallow Breathing (*Tachypnea*)

Rapid shallow breathing has a number of causes, including restrictive lung disease, pleuritic chest pain, and an elevated diaphragm.

Cheyne-Stokes Breathing

Periods of deep breathing alternate with periods of apnea (no breathing). Children and aging people normally may show this pattern in sleep. Other causes include heart failure, uremia, drug-induced respiratory depression, and brain damage (typically on both sides of the cerebral hemispheres or diencephalon).

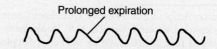

Obstructive Breathing

In obstructive lung disease, expiration is prolonged because narrowed airways increase the resistance to air flow. Causes include asthma, chronic bronchitis, and COPD.

Rapid Deep Breathing (*Hyperpnea, Hyperventilation*)

Rapid deep breathing has several causes, including exercise, anxiety, and metabolic acidosis. In the comatose patient, consider infarction, hypoxia, or hypoglycemia affecting the midbrain or pons. *Kussmaul breathing* is deep breathing due to metabolic acidosis. It may be fast, normal in rate, or slow.

Ataxic Breathing (*Biot's Breathing*)

Ataxic breathing is characterized by unpredictable irregularity. Breaths may be shallow or deep, and stop for short periods. Causes include respiratory depression and brain damage, typically at the medullary level.

Behavior and Mental Status

As clinicians, we are uniquely poised to detect and elicit patients' clues to mental illness and harmful dysfunctional behaviors through empathic listening and close observation. Nonetheless, these clues are often missed. This chapter introduces you to common symptoms and behaviors suggestive of mental health disorders; presents concepts that guide history taking and the general assessment of mental health; and highlights priorities for mental health promotion and counseling. The chapter concludes with the elements of the *mental status examination*. This examination helps you assess behavioral and mental health disorders more formally and is an integral component of the examination of the nervous system.

See Chapter 17, The Nervous System, pp. 681–762.

It is especially important for clinicians to learn the common features of mental illness given the frequency of these disorders, the shortage of psychiatrists, and the likelihood that the primary care physician will be the first to encounter the patient's distress.[1] National statistics, advisories of the Surgeon General and leading professional societies, and reports from the U.S. Preventive Services Task Force and the Centers for Disease Control and Prevention all attest to the need to promote the mental and physical health of our patients. The prevalence of mental health disorders in U.S. adults is approximately 26%, affecting 57 million people; yet only 20% to 30% receive treatment.[2–4] Even for those receiving care, adherence to treatment guidelines in primary care offices is <50% and disproportionately lower for ethnic minorities.[5–8]

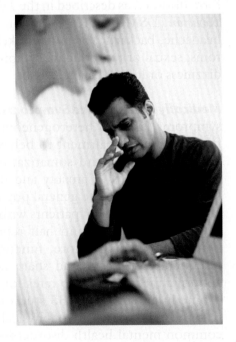

Mental health disorders are commonly masked by other conditions, calling for sensitive and careful inquiry. Experts state that "these disorders are associated with substantial psychosocial morbidity and they are all treatable."[9] Learn to look for the interaction of anxiety and depression in patients with substance abuse, termed "dual diagnosis," since both must be treated for the patient to achieve optimal function. Watch for underlying psychiatric conditions in "difficult encounters" and patients with unexplained symptoms.[10] Explore the outlook of patients with chronic medical illnesses, a group that is especially vulnerable to depression and anxiety.[11] Finally, bear in mind that nearly half of those with any mental disorder meet criteria for two or more disorders, with severity strongly related to comorbidity.[12]

Symptoms and Behavior

Patient Symptoms: What Do They Mean?

For beginning clinicians, the challenge is to sort out the array of symptoms encountered in office practice. As we have seen, symptoms may be psychological, relating to mood or anxiety, or *physical,* relating to a body sensation such as pain, fatigue, or palpitations. In mental health literature, such physical symptoms are often termed *somatic.* Studies reveal that physical symptoms prompt more than 50% of U.S. office visits.[13] Approximately 5% of these symptoms are acute, triggering immediate evaluation. Another 70% to 75% are minor or self-limited and resolve in 6 weeks. Nevertheless, approximately 25% of patients have persisting and recurrent symptoms that elude assessment through the history and physical examination and fail to improve. Overall, 30% of symptoms are *medically unexplained.* Some of them involve single complaints that appear to persist longer than others, for example, back pain, headache, or musculoskeletal complaints. Others occur in clusters presenting as *functional syndromes,* such as irritable bowel syndrome, fibromyalgia, chronic fatigue, temporomandibular joint disorder, and multiple chemical sensitivity. When patients exhibit physical symptoms that are not fully explained by a medical condition, the effects of substance abuse, or other mental health disorders, consider the diagnosis of somatoform disorder, as described in the *Diagnostic and Statistical Manual IV Text Revision* (DSM-IV-TR). Common somatic complaints include: pain from headache, backache, or musculoskeletal conditions; gastrointestinal symptoms; sexual or reproductive symptoms; and neurologic symptoms such as dizziness or loss of balance.

See Table 5-1, Somatoform Disorders, pp. 165–166, for types of somatoform disorders and guidelines for clinician management.

A *physical symptom* can be explained physically or medically or can be unexplained; a *somatoform symptom* lacks an adequate medical or physical explanation. A *somatoform disorder* meets DSM-IV-TR diagnostic criteria.[11]

Medically Unexplained Symptoms. Patients with medically unexplained symptoms fall into heterogeneous groupings on a continuum ranging from selected impairment to behaviors meeting diagnostic DSM IV-TR criteria for mood and somatization disorders.[14] Many patients do not report symptoms of anxiety and depression, the most common mental health disorders in the general population, but focus on physical concerns instead. Two-thirds of patients with depression, for example, present with physical complaints, and half report multiple unexplained or somatic symptoms.[15] Furthermore, functional syndromes have been shown to "frequently co-occur and share key symptoms and selected objective abnormalities."[16] Overlap rates for fibromyalgia and chronic fatigue syndrome in an analysis of 53 studies ranged from 34% to 70%. Failure to recognize the admixture of physical symptoms, functional syndromes, and common mental health disorders—anxiety, depression, unexplained and somatoform symptoms, and substance abuse—adds to the burden of patient undertreatment and poor quality of life. Authors of the first randomized controlled intervention trial for patients with medically unexplained symptoms advise viewing this symptom cluster as "a generalized warning sign of underlying psychological distress, of which depression is an advanced manifestation."[17]

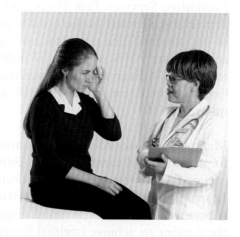

The "Difficult Encounter." Patients with unexplained and somatoform symptoms are often high users of the health care system and labeled as "difficult patients." Patient depression and anxiety "make physician ratings of difficult encounters three times more likely, and somatization increases this likelihood nine-fold."[18] A growing literature reveals that 15% to 20%, or up to three to four visits a day, of primary care visits are considered difficult.[10] In the difficult encounter dyad, clinician factors are emerging that include job stress and burnout, anxiety and depression in the clinician, and aversion to the psychosocial aspects of care.[19] In the words of an expert:

> *"Celebrate the well-navigated difficult encounter. Dealing with difficulty signifies mastery rather than weakness. Olympic dives are rated in terms of difficulty, as are mountain climbs, hiking trails, musical works, crossword puzzles, and highly technical procedures. Partnering with patients in the challenging aspects of their health, lives, or medical care is a stepping stone to surmounting together the difficult encounter."* [10]

Mental Health Disorders and Unexplained Symptoms in Primary Care Settings

Mental Health Disorders in Primary Care

- Approximately 20% of primary care outpatients have mental disorders, but 50% to 75% of these disorders are undetected and untreated.[20,21]
- Prevalence of mental disorders in primary care settings is roughly[20,22–24]:
  - Anxiety—20%
  - Mood disorders including dysthymia, depressive, and bipolar disorders—25%
  - Depression—10%
  - Somatoform disorders—10% to 15%
  - Alcohol and substance abuse—15% to 20%

Explained and Unexplained Symptoms

- Physical symptoms account for approximately 50% of office visits.
- Roughly one-third of physical symptoms are unexplained; in 20% to 25% of patients, physical symptoms become chronic or recurring.[13,15]
- In patients with *unexplained symptoms,* the prevalence of depression and anxiety exceeds 50% and increases with the total number of reported physical symptoms,[13,15] making detection and "dual diagnosis" important clinical goals.

Common Functional Syndromes

- Co-occurrence rates for *common functional syndromes* such as irritable bowel syndrome, fibromyalgia, chronic fatigue, temporomandibular joint disorder, and multiple chemical sensitivity reach 30% to 90%, depending on the disorders compared.[16]
- The prevalence of *symptom overlap* is high in the common functional syndromes: namely, complaints of fatigue, sleep disturbance, musculoskeletal pain, headache, and gastrointestinal problems.
- The common functional syndromes also overlap in rates of functional impairment, psychiatric comorbidity, and response to cognitive and antidepressant therapy.

Patient Identifiers for Selective Mental Health Screening

Unexplained conditions lasting beyond 6 weeks are increasingly recognized as common chronic disorders that should prompt screening for depression, anxiety, or both. Because screening all patients is time-consuming and expensive, experts recommend a two-tier approach: brief screening questions with high sensitivity and specificity for patients at risk, followed by more detailed investigation when indicated.

Several groups of patients warrant brief screening because of high rates of coexisting depression and anxiety. Recent studies have helped clarify these *overlap symptoms* and *functional syndromes* and provide streamlined practical screening tools, suitable for office care, for detecting mental disorders. A well-established instrument to aid in office diagnosis is the PRIME-MD (Primary Care Evaluation of Mental Disorders); however, it contains 26 questions and takes up to 10 minutes to complete. Better delineation of the current multi-item diagnostic categories in the DSM-IV-TR is highly likely over the next 5 to 8 years, and new and more effective techniques for office screening and management continue to emerge.[17,24–26]

Patient Identifiers for Mental Health Screening

▶ Medically unexplained physical symptoms—more than half indicate a depressive or anxiety disorder
▶ Multiple physical or somatic symptoms or "high symptom count"
▶ High severity of the presenting somatic symptom
▶ Chronic pain
▶ Symptoms for more than 6 weeks
▶ Physician rating as a "difficult encounter"
▶ Recent stress
▶ Low self-rating of overall health
▶ High use of health care services
▶ Substance abuse

Chronic pain may be a spectrum disorder in patients with anxiety, depression, or somatic symptoms. See Chapter 4, Beginning the Physical Examination: General Survey, Vital Signs, and Pain, pp. 105–140.

High-Yield Screening Questions and Questionnaires for Office Practice (follow-up systems for diagnosis and treatment are needed)

Depression[20,27,28]
▶ Over the past 2 weeks, have you felt down, depressed, or hopeless?
▶ Over the past 2 weeks, have you felt little interest or pleasure in doing things (anhedonia)?

Anxiety[29–32]
Anxiety disorders include generalized anxiety disorder, social phobia, panic disorder, posttraumatic stress disorder, and acute stress disorder.

▶ Over the past 2 weeks, have you been feeling nervous, anxious, or on edge?
▶ Over the past 2 weeks, have you been unable to stop or control worrying?
▶ Over the past 4 weeks, have you had an anxiety attack—suddenly feeling fear or panic?

(continued)

High-Yield Screening Questions and Questionnaires for Office Practice (follow-up systems for diagnosis and treatment are needed) (continued)

Hypochondriacal Features
- Whiteley Index: 14-item self-rating scale[25,33]

Alcohol and Substance Abuse
- CAGE questions adapted for alcohol and drug abuse—see Chapter 3, Interviewing and the Health History, pp. 88–89.

Multidimensional
- PRIME-MD (Primary Care Evaluation of Mental Disorders) for the five most common disorders in primary care: depression, anxiety, alcohol, somatoform, and eating disorders; 26-item patient questionnaire followed by clinician evaluation; takes approximately 10 minutes[33]
- PRIME-MD Patient Health Questionnaire, available as patient health questionnaire for self-rating; takes approximately 3 minutes[23]

Personality Disorders. Patients with personality disorders, formerly called *character disorders,* can also display problematic office behaviors that escape diagnosis. These disorders are characterized in the DSM IV-TR by "an enduring pattern of inner experience and behavior that deviates markedly from the expectations of the individual's culture, is pervasive and inflexible, has an onset in adolescence or early adulthood, is stable over time, and leads to distress or impairment."[14] These patients have dysfunctional interpersonal coping styles that disrupt and destabilize their relationships, including those with their health care providers. A recent study reports an overall prevalence of 9%, with prevalence of the three subcomponent clusters of: 5.7% for odd and eccentric disorders; 1.5% for dramatic, emotional, or erratic disorders; and 6% for anxious or fearful disorders.[35] Personality disorders co-occur at high frequencies with alcohol and substance abuse and with the Axis I disorders of depression, anxiety disorders, bipolar disorder, ADHD, autism spectrum disorders, anorexia nervosa, bulimia nervosa, and schizophrenia.[36] Note that classification of the personality disorders is expected to change in DSM-V, expected in 2013.[37]

Personality Disorders: DSM IV-TR

Cluster/Personality Type	Characteristic Behavior Patterns
A: Odd or Eccentric Disorders	
Paranoid	Distrust and suspiciousness
Schizoid	Detachment from social relations with a restricted emotional range
Schizotypal	Eccentricities in behavior and cognitive distortions; acute discomfort in close relationships
	(continued)

Personality Disorders: DSM IV-TR (continued)

Cluster/Personality Type	Characteristic Behavior Patterns
B: Dramatic, Emotional or Erratic Disorders	
▷ Antisocial	Disregard for the law and the rights of others; a defect in the experience of compunction or remorse for harming others
▷ Borderline	Instability in interpersonal relationships, self-image and affective regulation; impulsivity
▷ Histrionic	Emotional overreactivity, theatrical behavior, and seductiveness; attention-seeking behavior
▷ Narcissistic	Persisting grandiosity, need for admiration and lack of empathy for others
C: Anxious or Fearful Disorders	
▷ Avoidant	Social inhibition, feelings of inadequacy and hypersensitivity to negative evaluation
▷ Dependent	Submissive and clinging behavior; psychological dependence on others
▷ Obsessive-compulsive	Rigid, detail-oriented behavior, often associated with compulsions to perform tasks repetitively and unnecessarily and rigid conformity to rules

Note that these diagnostic criteria are expected to change significantly in the DSM V, expected in 2013, with reduction to six disorder types (antisocial, avoidant, borderline, narcissistic, obsessive/compulsive, and schizotypal) and emphasis on self and interpersonal functioning.[37]

Source: Schiffer RB. Ch 420, Psychiatric disorders in medical practice, in Cecil Textbook of Medicine, 22nd Ed. Philadelphia: Saunders, 2004. pp. 2628–2639. American Psychiatric Association. DSM IV-TR. Washington, DC: American Psychiatric Press, 2000.

For more detailed diagnostic criteria, beyond the scope of this book, turn to the DSM IV-TR and the DSM-V.

Borderline Personality Disorder. Interaction with patients with borderline personality disorders is especially challenging. Prevalence in primary care practices is 6%, though the diagnosis is often missed.[38,39] More than 90% of patients with this disorder meet criteria for other personality disorders. Many have co-existing mood, anxiety, and substance abuse disorders. Presenting symptoms overlap with depression, anxiety, substance abuse, and eating disorders, which complicate diagnosis. In clinical settings, over 75% of those affected are women, and the disorder shows a strong genetic and familial pattern.[40] Patients with this disorder are impulsive—more than 50% attempt suicide and cut or injure themselves. Recurrent suicidal threats or acts, combined with fear of abandonment, strongly suggest the diagnosis.[41] More than half lose their jobs because of interpersonal problems, and roughly one-third experience sexual abuse. Patients often report feeling depressed and empty, with mood swings that spiral out of control leading to feelings of rage, sadness, and anxiety. To clinicians, these patients may appear demanding, disruptive, or manipulative. Recognition of borderline features leads to better self-insight, referral for expert evaluation, and reduction in harm for the patient.

The Health History

Common or Concerning Symptoms

▶ Changes in attention, mood, or speech
▶ Changes in insight, orientation, or memory
▶ Anxiety, panic, ritualistic behavior, and phobias
▶ Delirium or dementia

Overview.   As you listen to the patient's story, you will quickly observe the patient's level of *alertness* and *orientation*, and *mood, attention,* and *memory.* While the history unfolds, you will learn about the patient's *insight* and *judgment,* as well as any *recurring or unusual thoughts or perceptions.* These and other specific components of mental function will alert you to important underlying concerns and conditions that may require more detailed follow-up, including a formal mental status examination.

Many of the terms pertinent to the mental health history and the mental status examination are familiar to you from social conversation. Take the time to learn their precise meanings in the context of the formal evaluation of mental status, as detailed in the table below.

See Techniques of Examination for the formal mental status examination on pp. 151–160.

Terminology: The Mental Status Examination

Level of Consciousness	Alertness or State of Awareness of the Environment
Attention	The ability to focus or concentrate over time on one task or activity—an inattentive or distractible person with impaired consciousness has difficulty giving a history or responding to questions.
Memory	The process of registering or recording information, tested by asking for immediate repetition of material, followed by storage or retention of information. *Recent or short-term memory* covers minutes, hours, or days; *remote or long-term memory* refers to intervals of years.
Orientation	Awareness of personal identity, place, and time; requires both memory and attention
Perceptions	Sensory awareness of objects in the environment and their interrelationships (external stimuli); also refers to internal stimuli such as dreams or hallucinations
Thought processes	The logic, coherence, and relevance of the patient's thought as it leads to selected goals; *how* people think

(continued)

Terminology: The Mental Status Examination (continued)

Level of Consciousness	Alertness or State of Awareness of the Environment
Thought content	What the patient thinks about, including level of insight and judgment
Insight	Awareness that symptoms or disturbed behaviors are normal or abnormal; for example, distinguishing between daydreams and hallucinations that seem real
Judgment	Process of comparing and evaluating alternatives when deciding on a course of action; reflects values that may or may not be based on reality and social conventions or norms
Affect	An observable, usually episodic, feeling or tone expressed through voice, facial expression, and demeanor
Mood	A more sustained emotion that may color a person's view of the world (affect is to mood as weather is to climate)
Language	A complex symbolic system for expressing, receiving, and comprehending words; as with consciousness, attention, and memory, language is essential for assessing other mental functions
Higher cognitive functions	Assessed by vocabulary, fund of information, abstract thinking, calculations, construction of objects that have two or three dimensions

Attention, Mood, Speech; Insight, Orientation, Memory. As you listen to the patient's concerns, assess *level of consciousness; general appearance; mood,* including depression or mania; and *ability to pay attention, remember, understand,* and *speak.* By placing the patient's vocabulary and general fund of information in the context of his or her cultural and educational background, you can often make a rough estimate of intelligence. Likewise, the patient's responses to illness and life circumstances often tell you about *insight and judgment.* If you suspect a problem in orientation and memory, you can ask, "Let's see, your last clinic appointment was when . . . ?" "And the date today?" The more you can integrate your exploration of mental status into taking a sensitive history, the less it will seem like an interrogation.

See Table 5-2, Disorders of Mood, p. 167, and Table 17-6, Disorders of Speech, p. 754.

Anxiety, Panic, Ritualistic Behavior, Phobias. If the patient has unusual thoughts, preoccupations, beliefs, or perceptions, explore them as they arise during the interview. For example, worries persisting over a 6-month period suggest a possible generalized *anxiety disorder,* one of the most prevalent psychiatric conditions in the United States, with a lifetime prevalence of approximately 3%.[2] Over time, you will come to recognize some of its mimics: *panic disorder,* with recurrent panic attacks followed by a period of anxiety about further attacks; *obsessive-compulsive disorder,* with intrusive thoughts

See Table 5-3, Anxiety Disorders, p. 168, and Table 5-4, Psychotic Disorders, p. 169.

and ritualistic behaviors; *posttraumatic stress disorder,* characterized by avoidance, numbing, and hyperarousal; and *social phobia,* with its marked anticipatory anxiety in social situations. For such patients, you need to supplement your interview with questions in specific areas. You may need to go further and pursue a formal mental status examination.

Delirium or Dementia.   All patients with documented or suspected brain lesions, psychiatric symptoms, or reports from family members of vague or changed behavioral symptoms need further systematic assessment. Patients may have subtle behavioral changes, difficulty taking medications properly, problems attending to household chores or paying bills, or loss of interest in their usual activities. Other patients may behave strangely after surgery or during an acute illness. Each problem should be identified as expeditiously as possible. Mental function influences the ability to hold a job and is often important in evaluating disability. These may be signs of depression or dementia.

See Table 20-4, Delirium and Dementia, p. 964.

See also discussions in Chapter 17, The Nervous System, pp. 681–762 and in Chapter 20, The Older Adult, pp. 917–966.

Health Promotion and Counseling: Evidence and Recommendations

Important Topics for Health Promotion and Counseling

- Screening for depression and suicidality
- Screening for alcohol, prescription drug, and substance abuse

Mental health disorders impose a profound burden of suffering, affecting roughly one in four U.S. adults in a given year.[2] Serious mental illness affects approximately 6% of the population. Severity of illness is strongly linked to both comorbidity and disability. For the general population, focus health promotion and counseling on depression, suicide risk, and dementia, three important conditions often overlooked. Also screen routinely for addiction to alcohol or drugs.

See Chapter 3, Interviewing and the Health History, pp. 55–102.

Mood Disorders and Depression.   Mood disorders include major depression, dysthymic disorder, and bipolar disorder and affect over 9% of the U.S. population, or 21 million people.[2] Of these, roughly 15 million Americans, or almost 7%, have major depression, often with coexisting anxiety disorders and substance abuse. Depression is twice as common in women and is a frequent companion of chronic medical illness. The prevalence of postpartum depression is 10% to 15%. Screen high-risk patients for early signs of depression that are often missed: low self-esteem, loss of pleasure in daily activities (*anhedonia*), sleep disorders, and difficulty concentrating or making decisions. Watch carefully for depression symptoms in vulnerable patients, especially those who are young, female, single, divorced or separated, seriously or chronically ill, bereaved, or have other psychiatric disorders, including substance abuse. Prior history or family history of depression also place patients at risk. However, note that risk factors alone are not sufficient to identify patients who are depressed.

The U.S. Preventive Services Task Force in 2009 reaffirmed its endorsement of screening for depression in clinical settings that can provide care supports and accurate diagnosis, treatment, and follow-up.[42] Asking two simple questions about mood and anhedonia appears to be as effective as using more detailed instruments. All positive screening tests warrant full diagnostic interviews. Failure to diagnose depression can have fatal consequences—suicide rates among patients with major depression are eight times higher than in the general population.

See screening questions on p. 144 and review screening tools readily available for office practice.[28,43-48]

Suicide. Preventing suicide is a national public health imperative. Suicide ranks as the 11th leading cause of death in the United States. It is the second leading cause of death among 25 to 34 year olds and the third leading cause of death among 15 to 24 year olds.[49] There are almost 11 completed suicides per 100,000 population annually.[50] Suicide rates are four times higher in men, who are more likely to use firearms and less likely to use poison than women. The highest suicide rates are in men 75 years of age or older: 36 per 100,000. Suicide rates reach 12 per 100,000 in young adults ages 15 to 24 years and are especially high in American Indian/Alaska natives ages 15 to 24, reaching 20 per 100,000. Suicide attempts are even higher, especially among female black and Hispanic high school students, with an estimated 8 to 25 attempts for every suicide death. In 2009, over 13% of U.S. high school students reported that they had considered attempting suicide in the prior year.

Alcohol, Prescription Drug, and Substance Abuse. As discussed, the interaction between mental disorders and alcohol and substance abuse is profound. In 2009, over 23% of the U.S. population over age 12 years, or 59 million people, reported binge drinking and over 6% reported heavy drinking.[51] Over 21 million Americans, over 8%, reported use of an illicit drug during the prior month, including 16 million marijuana users, 1.6 million cocaine users, and 7 million nonmedical prescription drug users. Twenty-two and a half (22.5) million, or 8.9%, of the population were classified with substance abuse or dependence in the past year based on DSM-IV-TR criteria. These include 15 million with dependence or abuse involving only alcohol, almost 4 million with dependence or abuse involving illicit drugs, and 3.2 million with mixed alcohol and illicit drug dependence or abuse. Rates of drug-induced deaths continue to increase and are highest among whites. The Centers for Disease Control and Prevention reports that *prescription drug abuse now kills more people than illicit drugs, reversing trends of even 10 to 15 years ago.*[52]

Screening for alcohol and substance abuse and misuse of prescription drugs should be part of *every* patient history. However, effective treatments at the primary care level have yet to emerge, although brief interventions hold promise.[53]

See discussion of screening tools in Chapter 3, Interviewing and the Health History, Alcohol and Illicit Drugs, pp. 88–89, and Chapter 11, Abdomen, Screening for Alcohol Abuse, pp. 447–448.

Techniques of Examination

The Mental Status Examination

- Appearance and behavior
- Speech and language
- Mood
- Thoughts and perceptions
- Cognition, including memory, attention, information and vocabulary, calculations, abstract thinking, and constructional ability

The interplay between mental and physical health is challenging and complex. Mental disorders often emerge as somatic complaints, and physical illnesses provoke behavioral and emotional responses. Always look carefully for pathophysiologic and pharmacologic causes as you assess changes in mental status. The patient's personality, psychodynamics, and personal experiences color assessments of mental status. By integrating your findings from the history and physical examination, selectively amplified by part or all of the formal mental status examination, you will come to understand the patient as a whole, molded by life experiences, family, and culture.

The Mental Status Examination is a central component of the clinical assessment process in psychiatric practice. Because mental status and brain structure and function are intimately intertwined, this examination is taught as an integral part of the assessment of the nervous system and is the first segment of the nervous system write-up. With dedication and practice, you will learn to describe the patient's mood, speech, behavior, and cognition, and relate these findings to your examination of the cranial nerves, motor and sensory systems, and reflexes.

See Chapter 17, Nervous System, pp. 681–762, especially pp. 699–700 and Recording Your Findings, p. 739.

At first you may hesitate to do the formal mental status examination. An insensitive examination may alarm the patient, and even a skillful review of cognition may uncover a deficit the patient is trying to ignore. As with other domains of clinical assessment, your skills and confidence will improve with experience Remember that patients appreciate an understanding listener, and some will owe their health, safety, and even their lives to your attention.

The Mental Status Examination consists of five components: appearance and behavior; speech and language; mood; thoughts and perceptions; and cognitive function, which includes orientation, attention, memory, attention, and higher cognitive functions such as information and vocabulary, calculations, abstract thinking, and constructional ability.

The format that follows should help to organize your observations, but it is not intended as a step-by-step guide. When a full examination is indicated, be flexible but thorough in your approach. In some situations, however, sequence is important. If the patient's consciousness, attention, comprehension of words, or ability to speak seem impaired, assess these deficits promptly. Such patients cannot give a reliable history, and you will not be able to test most of the other mental functions.

APPEARANCE AND BEHAVIOR

Integrate the observations you have made throughout the history and physical examination, including the following.

Level of Consciousness.   Is the patient awake and alert? Does the patient seem to understand your questions and respond appropriately and reasonably quickly, or is there a tendency to lose track of the topic and fall silent or even asleep?

See the table on Level of Consciousness (Arousal), Chapter 17, The Nervous System, p. 735.

If the patient does not respond to your questions, escalate the stimulus in steps:

- Speak to the patient by name and in a loud voice.

Lethargic patients are drowsy but open their eyes and look at you, respond to questions, and then fall asleep.

- Shake the patient gently, as if awakening a sleeper.

Obtunded patients open their eyes and look at you, but respond slowly and are somewhat confused.

If there is no response to these stimuli, promptly assess the patient for stupor or coma—severe reductions in level of consciousness.

Posture and Motor Behavior.   Does the patient lie in bed or prefer to walk around? Note body posture and the patient's ability to relax. Observe the pace, range, and character of movements. Do they seem to be under voluntary control? Are certain parts immobile? Do posture and motor activity change with topics under discussion or with activities or people around the patient?

Look for tense posture, restlessness, and anxiety fidgeting; the crying, pacing, and hand-wringing of *agitated depression;* the hopeless, slumped posture and slowed movements of *depression;* the agitated and expansive movements of a *manic episode.*

Dress, Grooming, and Personal Hygiene.   How is the patient dressed? Is clothing clean, pressed, and properly fastened? How does it compare with clothing worn by people of comparable age and social group? Note the patient's hair, nails, teeth, skin, and, if present, beard. How are they groomed? How do the person's grooming and hygiene compare with those of other people of comparable age, lifestyle, and socioeconomic group? Compare one side of the body with the other.

Grooming and personal hygiene may deteriorate in *depression, schizophrenia,* and *dementia.* Excessive fastidiousness may be seen with *obsessive–compulsive disorder.* One-sided neglect may result from a lesion in the opposite parietal cortex, usually the nondominant side.

Facial Expression.   Observe the face, both at rest and when the patient interacts with others. Watch for variations in expression related to topics under discussion. Are they appropriate? Or is the face relatively immobile throughout?

Note expressions of anxiety, depression, apathy, anger, elation, or facial immobility in parkinsonism.

Manner, Affect, and Relationship to People and Things.   Drawing on your observations of facial expressions, voice, and body movements, assess the patient's *affect*, or external expression of the inner emotional state. Does it vary appropriately with topics under discussion, or is the affect, labile, blunted, or flat? Does it seem inappropriate or extreme at certain points? If so, how? Note the patient's openness, approachability, and reactions to others and to the surroundings. Does the patient seem to hear or see things that you do not or seem to be conversing with someone who is not there?

Watch for the anger, hostility, suspiciousness, or evasiveness of patients with *paranoia;* the elation and euphoria of *mania;* the flat affect and remoteness of *schizophrenia;* the apathy (dulled affect with detachment and indifference) of *dementia;* and anxiety or depression.

▐ SPEECH AND LANGUAGE

Throughout the interview, note the characteristics of the patient's speech, including the following:

Quantity.   Is the patient talkative or relatively silent? Are comments spontaneous or only responsive to direct questions?

Rate.   Is speech fast or slow?

Volume.   Is speech loud or soft?

Note the slow speech of *depression;* the accelerated rapid, loud speech in *mania.*

Articulation of Words.   Are the words spoken clearly and distinctly? Is there a nasal quality to the speech?

Fluency.   This involves the rate, flow, and melody of speech and the content and use of words. Be alert for abnormalities of spontaneous speech such as:

Dysarthria refers to defective articulation. *Aphasia* refers to a disorder of language. See Table 17-6, Disorders of Speech, p. 754.

- Hesitancies and gaps in the flow and rhythm of words

- Disturbed inflections, such as a monotone

- Circumlocutions, in which phrases or sentences are substituted for a word the person cannot think of, such as "what you write with" for "pen"

- Paraphasias, in which words are malformed ("I write with a den"), wrong ("I write with a bar"), or invented ("I write with a dar").

These abnormalities suggest *aphasia.* The patient may have difficulty talking or understanding others.

If the patient's speech lacks meaning or fluency, proceed with further testing as outlined in the following table.

Testing for Aphasia

Word Comprehension	Ask the patient to follow a one-stage command, such as "Point to your nose." Try a two-stage command: "Point to your mouth, then your knee."
Repetition	Ask the patient to repeat a phrase of one-syllable words (the most difficult repetition task): "No ifs, ands, or buts."
Naming	Ask the patient to name the parts of a watch.
Reading Comprehension	Ask the patient to read a paragraph aloud.
Writing	Ask the patient to write a sentence.

These tests help you determine the kind of aphasia the patient may have. Remember that deficiencies in vision, hearing, intelligence, and education may also affect performance. Two common kinds of aphasia—Wernicke's and Broca's—are compared in Table 17-6, Disorders of Speech, p. 754.

A person who can write a correct sentence does not have aphasia.

MOOD

Assess mood by exploring the patient's perceptions of his or her mood. Find out about the patient's usual mood level and how it has varied with life events. "How did you feel about that?", for example, or, more generally, "How is your overall mood?" The reports of relatives and friends may be of great value.

Moods include sadness and deep melancholy; contentment, joy, euphoria, and elation; anger and rage; anxiety and worry; and detachment and indifference.

What has the patient's mood been like? How intense has it been? Has it been labile or unchanging? How long has it lasted? Is it appropriate to the patient's circumstances? In case of depression, have there also been episodes of an elevated mood, suggesting a bipolar disorder?

For depressive and bipolar disorders, see Table 5-2, Disorders of Mood, p. 167.

If you suspect depression, assess its depth and any associated risk of suicide. Pursue the following questions:

- Do you get pretty discouraged (or depressed or blue)?

- How low do you feel?

- What do you see for yourself in the future?

- Do you ever feel that life isn't worth living? Or that you would just as soon be dead?

- Have you ever thought of doing away with yourself?

- How did (do) you think you would do it?

- What do you think would happen after you were dead?

Asking about suicidal thoughts is essential and may be the only way to uncover suicidal ideation and plans. You may feel uneasy about direct questions, but most patients are relieved to discuss their thoughts and feelings.

By open discussion, you demonstrate your interest and concern for a possibly life-threatening problem.

THOUGHT AND PERCEPTIONS

Thought Processes.   Assess the logic, relevance, organization, and coherence of the patient's thought processes as revealed in the patient's words and speech throughout the interview. Does speech progress logically toward a goal? Listen for patterns of speech that suggest disorders of thought processes, as outlined in the table below.

Variations and Abnormalities in Thought Processes

Circumstantiality	Speech characterized by indirection and delay in reaching the point because of unnecessary detail, although components of the description have a meaningful connection. Many people without mental disorders speak circumstantially.	This occurs in people with obsessions.
Derailment (loosening of associations)	Speech in which a person shifts from one subject to others that are unrelated or related only obliquely without realizing that the subjects are not meaningfully connected.	Seen in *schizophrenia, manic episodes,* and other *psychotic disorders.*
Flight of Ideas	An almost continuous flow of accelerated speech in which a person changes abruptly from topic to topic. Changes are usually based on understandable associations, plays on words, or distracting stimuli, but the ideas do not progress to sensible conversation.	Most frequently noted in *manic episodes.*
Neologisms	Invented or distorted words, or words with new and highly idiosyncratic meanings	Observed in *schizophrenia, psychotic disorders,* and *aphasia.*
Incoherence	Speech that is largely incomprehensible because of illogic, lack of meaningful connections, abrupt changes in topic, or disordered grammar or word use. Shifts in meaning occur within clauses. Flight of ideas, when severe, may produce incoherence.	Observed in severe psychotic disturbances (usually *schizophrenia*).
Blocking	Sudden interruption of speech in midsentence or before completion of an idea. The person attributes this to losing the thought. Blocking occurs in normal people.	Blocking may be striking in *schizophrenia.*
Confabulation	Fabrication of facts or events in response to questions, to fill in the gaps in an impaired memory	Seen in Korsakoff's syndrome from alcoholism.
Perseveration	Persistent repetition of words or ideas	Occurs in *schizophrenia* and other *psychotic disorders.*
Echolalia	Repetition of the words and phrases of others	Occurs in manic episodes and *schizophrenia.*
Clanging	Speech in which a person chooses a word on the basis of sound rather than meaning, as in rhyming and punning speech. For example, "Look at my eyes and nose, wise eyes and rosy nose. Two to one, the ayes have it!"	Occurs in *schizophrenia* and *manic episodes.*

Thought Content.   You should assess information relevant to thought content during the interview. Follow leads suggested by the patient instead of asking stereotyped lists of questions. For example, "You mentioned a few minutes ago that a neighbor was responsible for your entire illness. Can you tell me more about that?" Or, in another situation, "What do you think about at times like these?"

You may need to make more specific inquiries. If so, use terms that are tactful and accepting. "When people are upset like this, sometimes they can't keep certain thoughts out of their minds," or ". . . things seem unreal. Have you experienced anything like this?" In these ways, find out about any of the patterns shown in the following table.

Abnormalities of Thought Content

Compulsions	Repetitive behaviors or mental acts that a person feels driven to perform in order to produce or prevent some future state of affairs, although such expectations are unrealistic	*Compulsions, obsessions, phobias,* and *anxieties* are often associated with neurotic disorders. See Table 5-3, Anxiety Disorders, p. 168.
Obsessions	Recurrent, uncontrollable thoughts, images, or impulses that a person considers unacceptable and alien	
Phobias	Persistent, irrational fears, accompanied by a compelling desire to avoid the stimulus	
Anxieties	Apprehensions, fears, tensions, or uneasiness that may be focused (phobia) or free-floating (a general sense of ill-defined dread or impending doom)	
Feelings of Unreality	A sense that things in the environment are strange, unreal, or remote	
Feelings of Depersonalization	A sense that one's self is different, changed, or unreal, or has lost identity or become detached from one's mind or body	Delusions and feelings of unreality or depersonalization are more often associated with *psychotic disorders.* See Table 5-4, Psychotic Disorders, p. 169. Delusions may also occur in delirium, severe mood disorders, and dementia.
Delusions	False, fixed, personal beliefs that are not shared by other members of the person's culture. Examples include:	
	▶ *Delusions of persecution*	
	▶ *Delusions of grandeur*	
	▶ *Delusional jealousy*	
	▶ *Delusions of reference*, in which a person believes that external events, objects, or people have a particular and unusual personal significance (e.g., that the radio or television might be giving instructions to the person)	
	▶ *Delusions of being controlled* by an outside force	
	▶ *Somatic delusions* of having a disease, disorder, or physical defect	
	▶ *Systematized delusions*, a single delusion with many elaborations or a cluster of related delusions around a single theme, all systematized into a complex network	

Perceptions.   Inquire about false perceptions. For example, "When you heard the voice speaking to you, what did it say? How did it make you feel?" Or, "After you've been drinking a lot, do you ever see things that aren't really there?" Or, "Sometimes after major surgery like this, people hear peculiar or frightening things. Have you experienced anything like that?" In these ways, find out about the following abnormal perceptions.

Abnormalities of Perception	
Illusions	Misinterpretations of real external stimuli
Hallucinations	Subjective sensory perceptions in the absence of relevant external stimuli. The person may or may not recognize the experiences as false. Hallucinations may be auditory, visual, olfactory, gustatory, tactile, or somatic. (False perceptions associated with dreaming, falling asleep, and awakening are not classified as hallucinations.)

Illusions may occur in grief reactions, *delirium,* acute and *posttraumatic stress disorders,* and *schizophrenia.*

Hallucinations may occur in *delirium, dementia* (less commonly), *posttraumatic stress disorder, schizophrenia,* and alcoholism.

Insight and Judgment.   These attributes are usually best assessed during the interview.

Insight.   Some of your very first questions to the patient often yield important information about insight: "What brings you to the hospital?" "What seems to be the trouble?" "What do you think is wrong?" More specifically, note whether the patient is aware that a particular mood, thought, or perception is abnormal or part of an illness.

Patients with psychotic disorders often lack insight into their illness. Denial of impairment may accompany some neurologic disorders.

Judgment.   You can usually assess judgment by noting the patient's responses to family situations, jobs, use of money, and interpersonal conflicts. "How do you plan to get help after leaving the hospital?" "How are you going to manage if you lose your job?" "If your husband starts to abuse you again, what will you do?" "Who will take care of your financial affairs while you are in the nursing home?"

Judgment may be poor in delirium, dementia, mental retardation, and psychotic states. Anxiety, mood disorders, intelligence, education, income, and cultural values also influence judgment.

Note whether decisions and actions are based on reality or, for example, on impulse, wish fulfillment, or disordered thought content. What values seem to underlie the patient's decisions and behavior? Allowing for cultural variations, how do these compare with a comparable mature adult? Because judgment reflects maturity, it may be variable and unpredictable during adolescence.

Disorientation is common when memory or attention is impaired, as in delirium.

COGNITIVE FUNCTIONS

Orientation.   You can usually assess the patient's orientation during the interview. For example, you can ask quite naturally for specific dates and times, the patient's address and telephone number, the names of family members, or the route taken to the hospital. At times, direct questions will be needed:

"Can you tell me what time it is now . . . and what day it is?"

Determine the patient's orientation to:

- *Time*—the time of day, day of the week, month, season, date and year, duration of hospitalization

- *Place*—the patient's residence, the names of the hospital, city, and state

- *Person*—the patient's own name, and the names of relatives and professional personnel

Attention.   These tests of attention are commonly used:

Digit Span.   Explain that you would like to test the patient's ability to concentrate, perhaps adding that this can be difficult when people are in pain, ill, or feverish. Recite a series of digits, starting with two at a time and speaking each number clearly at a rate of about one per second. Ask the patient to repeat the numbers back to you. If this repetition is accurate, try a series of three numbers, then four, and so on as long as the patient responds correctly. Jot down the numbers as you say them to ensure your own accuracy. If the patient makes a mistake, try once more with another series of the same length. Stop after a second failure in a single series.

When choosing digits, use street numbers, zip codes, telephone numbers, and other numerical sequences that are familiar to you, but avoid consecutive numbers, easily recognized dates, and sequences that are familiar to the patient.

Now, starting again with a series of two, ask the patient to repeat the numbers to you backward.

Normally, a person should be able to repeat correctly at least five digits forward and four backward.

> Causes of poor performance include *delirium, dementia, mental retardation,* and performance anxiety.

Serial 7s.   Instruct the patient, "Starting from a hundred, subtract 7, and keep subtracting 7. . . ." Note the effort required and the speed and accuracy of the responses. Writing down the answers helps you keep up with the arithmetic. Normally, a person can complete serial 7s in 1½ minutes, with fewer than four errors. If the patient cannot do serial 7s, try 3s or counting backward.

> Poor performance may result from delirium, the late stage of dementia, mental retardation, loss of calculating ability, anxiety, or depression. Also consider the possibility of limited education.

Spelling Backward.   This can substitute for serial 7s. Say a five-letter word, spell it, for example, W-O-R-L-D, and ask the patient to spell it backward.

Remote Memory.   Inquire about birthdays, anniversaries, social security number, names of schools attended, jobs held, or past historical events such as wars relevant to the patient's past.

> Remote memory may be impaired in the late stage of *dementia.*

Recent Memory.   This could involve the events of the day. Ask questions with answers you can check against other sources so that you can see if the patient is confabulating (making up facts to compensate for a defective memory). These might include the day's weather, today's appointment time, and medications or laboratory tests taken during the day.

Recent memory is impaired in *dementia* and *delirium. Amnestic disorders* impair memory or new learning ability and reduce a person's social or occupational functioning, but they do not have the global features of delirium or dementia. Anxiety, depression, and mental retardation may also impair recent memory.

New Learning Ability.   Give the patient three or four words such as "83 Water Street and blue," or "table, flower, green, and hamburger." Ask the patient to repeat them so that you know that the information has been heard and registered. This step, like digit span, tests registration and immediate recall. Then proceed to other parts of the examination. After 3 to 5 minutes, ask the patient to repeat the words. Note the accuracy of the response, awareness of whether it is correct, and any tendency to confabulate. Normally, a person should be able to remember the words.

Higher Cognitive Functions

Information and Vocabulary.   Information and vocabulary, when observed clinically, provide a rough estimate of a person's intelligence. Assess them during the interview. Ask a student, for example, about favorite courses, or inquire about work, hobbies, reading, favorite television programs, or current events. Explore such topics first with simple questions, then with more difficult ones. Note the person's grasp of information, the complexity of the ideas expressed, and the vocabulary used.

If considered in the context of cultural and educational background, information and vocabulary are fairly good indicators of intelligence. They are relatively unaffected by any but the most severe psychiatric disorders, and they may be helpful for distinguishing mentally retarded adults (whose information and vocabulary are limited) from those with mild or moderate *dementia* (whose information and vocabulary are fairly well preserved).

More directly, you can ask about specific facts such as:

The name of the president, vice president, or governor

The names of the last four or five presidents

The names of five large cities in the country

Calculating Ability.   Test the patient's ability to do arithmetical calculations, starting at the rote level with simple addition ("What is 4 + 3? . . . 8 + 7?") and multiplication ("What is 5 × 6? . . . 9 × 7?"). The task can be made more difficult by using two-digit numbers ("15 + 12" or "25 × 6") or longer, written examples.

Poor performance may be a useful sign of dementia or may accompany *aphasia,* but it must be assessed in terms of the patient's intelligence and education.

Alternatively, pose practical and functionally important questions, like: "If something costs 78 cents and you give the clerk one dollar, how much should you get back?"

Abstract Thinking.   Test the capacity to think abstractly in two ways.

Proverbs.   Ask the patient what people mean when they use some of the following proverbs:

A stitch in time saves nine.

Don't count your chickens before they're hatched.

Concrete responses are often given by people with mental retardation, *delirium,* or *dementia* but may also be a function of limited education. Patients with *schizophrenia* may respond concretely or with personal, bizarre interpretations.

The proof of the pudding is in the eating.

A rolling stone gathers no moss.

The squeaky wheel gets the grease.

Note the relevance of the answers and their degree of concreteness or abstractness. For example, "You should sew a rip before it gets bigger" is concrete, whereas "Prompt attention to a problem prevents trouble" is abstract. Average patients should give abstract or semiabstract responses.

Similarities.   Ask the patient to tell you how the following are alike:

An orange and an apple   A church and a theater

A cat and a mouse   A piano and a violin

A child and a dwarf   Wood and coal

Note the accuracy and relevance of the answers and their degree of concreteness or abstractness. For example, "A cat and a mouse are both animals" is abstract, "They both have tails" is concrete, and "A cat chases a mouse" is not relevant.

Constructional Ability.   The task here is to copy figures of increasing complexity onto a piece of blank unlined paper. Show each figure one at a time and ask the patient to copy it as well as possible.

The three diamonds below are rated poor, fair, and good (but not excellent).[54]

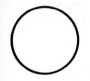 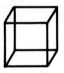 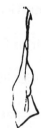 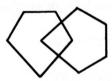 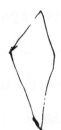 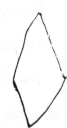

In another approach, ask the patient to draw a clock face complete with numbers and hands. The example below is rated excellent.

These three clocks are poor, fair, and good.[54]

  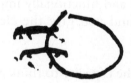 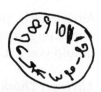

If vision and motor ability are intact, poor constructional ability suggests dementia or parietal lobe damage. Mental retardation may also impair performance.

SPECIAL TECHNIQUES

Mini-Mental State Examination (MMSE). This brief test is useful in screening for cognitive dysfunction or dementia, and following their course over time. For more detailed information regarding the MMSE, contact the Publisher, Psychological Assessment Resources, Inc., 16204 North Florida Avenue, Lutz, Florida 33549. Below are some sample questions.

MMSE Sample Items

Orientation to Time
  "What is the date?"

Registration
  "Listen carefully; I am going to say three words. You say them back after I
    stop. Ready? Here they are . . .
  HOUSE (pause), CAR (pause), LAKE (pause). Now repeat those words
    back to me." [Repeat up to five times, but score only the first trial.]

Naming
  "What is this?" [Point to a pencil or pen.]

Reading
  "Please read this and do what it says." [Show examinee the words on the
    stimulus form.]
  CLOSE YOUR EYES

Reproduced by special permission of the Publisher, Psychological Assessment Resources, Inc., 16204 North Florida Avenue, Lutz, Florida 33549, from the Mini Mental State Examination, by Marshal Folstein and Susan Folstein, Copyright 1975, 1998, 2001 by Mini Mental LLC, Inc. Published 2001 by Psychological Assessment Resources, Inc. Further reproduction is prohibited without permission of PAR, Inc.

Recording Your Findings

Recording Behavior and Mental Status

"Mental Status: The patient is alert, well-groomed, and cheerful. Speech is fluent and words are clear. Thought processes are coherent, insight is good. The patient is oriented to person, place, and time. Serial 7s accurate; recent and remote memory intact. Calculations intact."

OR

"Mental Status: The patient appears sad and fatigued; clothes are wrinkled. Speech is slow and words are mumbled. Thought processes are coherent, but insight into current life reverses is limited. The patient is oriented to person, place, and time. Digit span, serial 7s, and calculations accurate, but responses delayed. Clock drawing is good."

Suggests depression.

Bibliography

Citations

1. Rief W, Hessel A, Braehler E. Somatization symptoms and hypochondriacal features in the general population. Psychosomatic Medicine 2001;63:595–602.
2. National Institute of Mental Health. The numbers count: mental disorders in America. Updated June 26 2008. Available at http://wwwapps.nimh.nih.gov/health/publications/the-numbers-count-mental-disorders-in-america.shtml. Accessed July 22, 2011.
3. Kessler RC, Demnler O, Frank RG et al. Prevalence and treatment of mental disorders, 1990 to 2003. N Engl J Med 2005; 352:2515–2523.
4. Jackson JL, Passamonti M, Kroenke K. Outcome and impact of mental disorders in primary care at 5 years. Psychosom Med 2007;69:270–276.
5. Hepner KA, Rowe M, Rost K et al. The effect of adherence to practice guidelines on depression outcomes. Ann Int Med 2007;147:320–329.
6. Gonzalez HM, Vega WA, Williams DR et al. Depression care in the United States: too little for too few. Arch Gen Psychiatry 2010;67:37–46.
7. Williams DR, González HM, Neighbors H. Prevalence and distribution of major depressive disorder in African Americans, Caribbean blacks, and non-Hispanic whites: results from the National Survey of American Life. Arch Gen Psychiatry 2007;64:305–315.
8. U.S. Department of Health and Human Services. Mental Health: Culture, Race, and Ethnicity—A Supplement to Mental Health: A Report of the Surgeon General. Rockville, MD: U.S. Department of Health and Human Services, Substance Abuse and Mental Health Services Administration, Center for Mental Health Services, 2001.
9. Schiffer RB. Ch 420, Psychiatric disorders in medical practice. In Cecil Textbook of Medicine, 22nd Ed. Philadelphia: Saunders, 2004. pp. 2628–2639.
10. Kroenke K. Unburdening the difficult clinical encounter. Arch Intern Med 2009;169:333–334.
11. Strine TW, Mokdad AH, Balluz LS et al. Depression and anxiety in the United States: findings from the 2006 Behavioral Risk Factor Surveillance System. Psychiatr Serv 2008;59:1283–1390.
12. Kessler RC, Chiu WT, Demler O et al. Prevalence, severity, and comorbidity of twelve-month DSM-IV disorders in the National Comorbidity Survey Replication (NCS-R). Arch Gen Psych 2005;62:617–627.
13. Kroenke K. Patients presenting with somatic complaints: epidemiology, psychiatric comorbidity, and management. Int J Methods Psychiatr Res 2003;12:34–43.
14. American Psychiatric Association. Diagnostic and Statistical Manual of Mental Disorders, Fourth Edition, Text Revision. Washington, DC: American Psychiatric Press, 2000.
15. Kroenke K. The interface between physical and psychological symptoms. Primary Care Companion. J Clin Psychiatry 2003;5 (Suppl 7):11–18.
16. Aaron LA, Buchwald D. A review of the evidence for overlap among unexplained clinical conditions. Ann Intern Med 2001;134:868–881.
17. Smith RC, Lyles JS, Gardiner JC et al. Primary care clinicians treat patients with medically unexplained symptoms: a randomized controlled trial. J Gen Int Med 2006;21:671–677.
18. Jackson JL, Kroenke K. Managing somatization—medically unexplained should not mean medically ignored. J Gen Int Med 2006;21:797–799.
19. An PG, Rabatin JS, Manwell LB et al. Burden of difficult encounters in primary care: data from the Minimizing Error, Maximizing Outcomes study. Arch Intern Med 2009;169:410–414.
20. Staab JP, Datto CJ, Weinreig RM et al. Detection and diagnosis of psychiatric disorders in primary medical care settings. Med Clin N Am 2001;85:579–596.
21. Ansseau, Dierick M, Buntinkxz F et al. High prevalence of mental disorders in primary care. J Affect Disord 2004;78:49–55.
22. Kroenke K, Spitzer RL, deGruy et al. A symptom checklist for screen for somatoform disorders in primary care. Psychosomatics 1998;39:263–272.
23. Spitzer RL, Kroenke K, Williams JBW et al. Validation and utility of a self-report version of PRIME-MD—the PHQ Primary Care Study. JAMA 1999;282:1737–1744.
24. Kroenke K, Sharpe M, Sykes R. Revising the classification of somatoform disorders: key questions and preliminary recommendations. Psychosomatics 2007;48:277–285.
25. Reif W, Martin A, Rauh E et al. Evaluation of general practitioners' training: how to manage patients with unexplained physical symptoms. Psychosomatics 2006;47:304–311.
26. Houston JP, Kroenke K, Faries De et al. A provisional screening instrument for four common mental disorders in adult primary care patients. Psychosomatics 2011;52:48–55.
27. U.S. Preventive Services Task Force. Screening for depression: recommendations and rationale. Ann Int Med 2002;136:760–764.
28. Whooley MA, Avins AL, Miranda J et al. Case-finding instruments for depression. Two questions are as good as many. J Gen Intern Med 1997;12:439–445.
29. Kroenke K, Spitzer RL, Williams JB et al. An ultra-brief screening scale for anxiety and depression: the PHQ-4. Psychosomatics 2009;50:613–621.
30. Spitzer RL, Kroenke K, Williams JB et al. A brief measure for assessing generalized anxiety disorder: the GAD 7. Arch Int Med 2006;166:1092–1097.
31. Kroenke K, Spitzer RL, Williams JBW et al. Anxiety disorders in primary care: prevalence, impairment, comorbidity, and detection. Ann Int Med 2007;146:317–325.
32. Lowe B, Grafe K, Zipfel S et al. Detecting panic disorder in medical and psychosomatic outpatients—comparative validation of the Hospital Anxiety and Depression Scale, the Patient Health Questionnaire, a screening question, and physicians" diagnosis. J Psychosom Res 2003;55:515–519.
33. Pilowsky U. Dimensions of hypochondriasis. Br J Psychiatry 1967;113(494):89–93.
34. Spitzer RL, Williams JB, Kroenke K et al. Utility of a new procedure for diagnosing mental disorders in primary care. The PRIME-MD 1000 study. JAMA 1994;272;1749–1756.

35. Lenzenweger MF, Lane MC, Loranger AW et al. DSM-IV personality disorders in the National Comorbidity Survey Replication. Biol Psychiatry 2007;62:553–564.

36. Compton WM, Thomas YF, Stinson FS et al. Prevalence, correlates, disability, and comorbidity of DSM-IV drug abuse and dependence in the United States—results from the national epidemiologic survey on alcohol and related conditions. Arch Gen Psychiatry 2007;64:566–576.

37. American Psychiatric Association. DSM-5 revisions for personality disorders reflect major change. July 7 2011. Available at http://www.dsm5.org/Newsroom/Documents/DSM-5-Revisions-for-Personality-Disorders-Reflect-Major-Change-.pdf. Accessed July 22, 2011.

38. Gross R, Olfson M, Gameroff M et al. Borderline personality disorder in primary care. Arch Int Med 2002;162:53–60.

39. Grant BF, Chou SP, Goldstein RB et al. Prevalence, correlates, disability, and comorbidity of DSM-IV borderline personality disorder: results from the Wave 2 National Epidemiologic Survey on Alcohol and Related Conditions. J Clin Psychiatry 2008;69:533–545.

40. Gunderson JG. Borderline personality disorder. N Engl J Med 2011;364:2037–2042.

41. Zittel Conklin C, Westen D. Borderline personality disorder in clinical practice. Am J Psychiatry 2005;162:867–875.

42. U.S. Preventive Services Task Force. Screening for depression: recommendations and rationale. Ann Intern Med 2009; 151:784–792. See also http://www.uspreventiveservicestaskforce.org/uspstf09/adultdepression/addeprrs.htm. Accessed July 24, 2011.

43. Williams JW, Noel H, Cordes JA et al. Is this patient clinically depressed? JAMA 2002;287:1160–1170.

44. Beck AT, Steer RA. Internal consistencies of the original and revised Beck Depression Inventory. J Clin Psychol 1984;40:1365–1367.

45. Zung A A self-rating depression scale. Arch Gen Psychiatry 1965;12:63–70. Also at http://healthnet.umassmed.edu/mhealth/ZungSelfRatedDepressionScale.pdf. Accessed July 29, 2011.

46. Kroenke K, Spitzer RL, Williams JB et al. The patient health questionnaire somatic, anxiety, and depressive symptom scales: a systematic review. Gen Hosp Psychiatry 2010;32:345–359.

47. Gaynes BN, DeVeaugh-Geiss J, Weir S et al. Feasibility and diagnostic validity of the M-3 checklist: a brief, self-rated screen for depressive, bipolar, anxiety, and post-traumatic stress disorders in primary care. Ann Fam Med 2010;8:160–169.

48. Duffy FF, West JC, Fochtmann LJ et al. Performance in practice: physician practice assessment tools for the screening, assessment, and treatment of adults with substance use disorder. Focus 2011;9:31–41. (focus.psychiatryonline.org)

49. Centers for Disease Control and Prevention. Suicide Facts at a Glance. Summer 2010. Available at http://www.cdc.gov/ViolencePrevention/pdf/Suicide_DataSheet-a.pdf. Accessed July 28, 2011.

50. National Institute of Mental Health. Suicide in the U.S.: statistics and prevention. Updated June 2008. Available at http://wwwapps.nimh.nih.gov/health/publications/suicide-in-the-us-statistics-and-prevention.shtml. Accessed July 28, 2011.

51. Substance Abuse and Mental Health Services Administration. Results from the 2009 National Survey on Drug Use and Health: Volume I. Summary of National Findings (Office of Applied Studies, NSDUH Series H-38A, HHS Publication No. SMA 10-4586Findings), 2010. Rockville, MD. Also at http://www.oas.samhsa.gov/NSDUH/2k9NSDUH/2k9ResultsP.pdf. Accessed July 28, 2011.

52. Centers for Disease Control and Prevention. Morbidity and Mortality Weekly Report. CDC Health Disparities and Inequalities Report—United States, 2011. Supplement Vol 60, January 14, 2011. Available at http://www.cdc.gov/mmwr/pdf/other/su6001.pdf. Accessed July 28, 2011.

53. Polen MR, Whitlock EP, Wisdom JP et al. Screening in primary care settings for illicit drug use: staged systematic review for the U.S. Preventive Services Task Force. Evidence Synthesis No. 58, Part 1. (Prepared by the Oregon Evidence-based Practice Center under Contract No. 290-02-0024.) AHRQ Publication No. 08-05108-EF-s. Rockville, MD, Agency for Healthcare Research and Quality, January 2008.

54. Strub RL, Black FW. The Mental Status Examination in Neurology, 2nd Ed. Philadelphia: FA Davis, 1985.

Additional References

Centers for Disease Control and Prevention. National Center for Health Statistics. Fast Stats A to Z. Suicide and self-inflicted injury. Available at http://www.cdc.gov/nchs/fastats/suicide.htm. Accessed September 25, 2011.

Coffey CE, Cummings JL. American Psychiatric Publishing Textbook of Geriatric Neuropsychiatry, 3rd ed. Washington, DC: American Psychiatric Publishing, 2011.

Cottler LB, Campbell W, Krishna VAS et al. Predictors of high rates of suicidal ideation among drug users. J Nerv Ment Dis 2005;193:431–437.

Fancher T, Kravitz R. In the clinic. Depression. Ann Intern Med 2007;146:ITC5-1–ITC5-16.

Folstein M, Folstein SE, Mchugh PR. "Mini-mental state." A practical method for grading the cognitive state of patients for the clinician. J Psych Res 1975;12:189–198.

Frye MA. Bipolar disorder – a focus on depression. N Engl J Med 2011;364:51–59.

Haas LJ, Leiser JP, Magill MK. Management of the difficult patient. Am Fam Phys 2005;72:2063–2068.

Hales RE, Yudofsky SC, Gabbard GO (eds). Essentials of Psychiatry, 3rd ed. Washington, DC: American Psychiatric Publishing, 2011.

Hasin D, Katz H. Somatoform and substance use disorders. Psychosomatic Med 2007;69:870–875.

Hull SK, Broquet K. How to manage difficult patient encounters. Fam Pract Manage 14:31–34, 2007. Available at http://www.aafp.org/fpm/2007/0600/p30.html. Accessed September 25, 2011.

Manchikanti L, Giordano J, Boswell MV et al. Psychological factors as predictors of opioid abuse and illicit drug use in chronic pain patients. J Opioid Manag 2007;3:89–100.

McGrady A, Lynch DJ, Nagel RW et al. Coherence between physician diagnosis and patient self reports of anxiety and depression in primary care. Nerv Ment Dis 2010;198:420–424.

National Institute of Mental Health. Use of Mental Health Services and Treatment among Adults, 2008. Available at http://www.

nimh.nih.gov/statistics/3USE_MT_ADULT.shtml. Accessed September 25, 2011.

Sadock BJ, Sadock VA, Ruiz P et al (eds). Kaplan & Sadock's Comprehensive Textbook of Psychiatry, 9th ed. Philadelphia: Wolters Kluwer/Lippincott Williams & Wilkins, 2009.

Seaburn DB, Morse D, McDaniel S et al. Physician responses to ambiguous patient symptoms. J Gen Intern Med 2005;20:525–530.

Silber MH. Chronic insomnia. N Engl J Med 2005;353:803–810.

Turk DC, Swanson KS, Gatchel RJ. Predicting opioid misuse by chronic pain patients: a systematic review and literature synthesis. Clin J Pain 2008;24:497–508.

Unutzer J. Late-life depression. N Engl J Med 2011;357:2269–2276.

U.S. Preventive Services Task Force. Screening for suicide risk in adults. Summary of the evidence. (Gaynes BN, West SL, Ford CA et al) May 2004. Available at http://www.uspreventiveservicestaskforce.org/3rduspstf/suicide/suicidesum.htm. Accessed July 28, 2011.

The Bates' suite offers these additional resources to enhance learning and facilitate understanding of this chapter:

- *Bates' Pocket Guide to Physical Examination and History Taking*, 7th edition
- *Bates' Visual Guide to Physical Examination*
- thePoint online resources, for students and instructors: http://thepoint.lww.com

Table 5-1 Somatoform Disorders: Types and Approach to Symptoms

TYPES OF SOMATOFORM DISORDERS

Somatoform Disorders[a]

Disorder	Features
Somatization disorder	Chronic multisystem disorder characterized by complaints of pain, gastrointestinal and sexual dysfunction, and pseudoneurologic symptoms. Onset is usually early in life, and psychosocial and vocational achievements are limited.
Conversion disorder	Syndrome of symptoms of deficits mimicking neurologic or medical illness in which psychological factors are judged to be of etiologic importance
Pain disorder	Clinical syndrome characterized predominantly by pain in which psychological factors are judged to be of etiologic importance
Hypochondriasis	Chronic preoccupation with the idea of having a serious disease. The preoccupation is usually poorly amenable to reassurance
Body dysmorphic disorder	Preoccupation with an imagined or exaggerated defect in physical appearance

Other Somatoform-like Disorders

Disorder	Features
Factitious disorder	Intentional production or feigning of physical or psychological signs when external reinforcers (e.g., avoidance of responsibility, financial gain) are not clearly present
Malingering	Intentional production or feigning of physical or psychological signs when external reinforcers (e.g., avoidance of responsibility, financial gain) are present
Dissociative disorders	Disruptions of consciousness, memory, identity, or perception judged to be due to psychological factors

APPROACH TO SOMATIC AND UNEXPLAINED SYMPTOMS

Stepped Care Approach to Somatic Symptoms in Primary Care[b]

Is the somatic symptom likely to be...	Clinician action might be...
Acutely serious? (<5% of cases)	Expedited diagnostic workup
Minor/self-limited? (70%–75% of cases)	Address patient expectations
	Symptom-specific therapy
	Follow-up in 2–6 weeks
Chronic or recurrent? (20%–25% of cases)	Screen for depression and anxiety
Caused or aggravated by a depressive or anxiety disorder?	Antidepressant therapy and/or cognitive–behavioral therapy (CBT)
Due to a functional somatic syndrome?	Syndrome-specific therapy
	Antidepressant therapy and/or CBT
Persistent and medically unexplained?	Regular, time-limited clinic visits
	Consider mental health referral
	Symptom management strategies, if evidence-based (e.g., behavioral treatments, pain self-management programs, pain or other specialty clinics, complementary and alternative medicine)
	Rehabilitative rather than disability approach

(table continues on page 166)

Management Guidelines for Patients With Medically Unexplained Symptoms[c]

Is the somatic symptom likely to be...	Clinician action might be...
General Aspects	Show empathy and understanding for the complaints and frustrating experiences the patient has had so far (e.g., explain that medically unexplained symptoms are common).
	Develop a good patient–physician relationship; try to be the "coordinator" of diagnostic procedures and care.
Diagnosis	Explore not only the history of complaints and former treatments, but any impairment, anxiety, and psychosocial issues.
	Use screeners and self-report questionnaires to enhance detection; use symptom diaries to assess course and factors influencing symptoms.
	When the patient presents with a new symptom, examine the relevant organ system.
	Provide the results of investigations to give clear reassurance that there is no serious physical disease.
	Avoid unnecessary diagnostic tests or surgical procedures.
Treatment	Provide regularly scheduled visits (e.g., every 4–6 weeks), especially in the case of a history of very frequent healthcare utilization.
	Explain that treatment is coping, not curing (when pathology cannot be found or does not explain degree of complaints).
Referral	Suggest coping strategies like regular physical activity, relaxation, distraction.
	If referral is necessary to start psychotherapy or psychopharmacotherapy, prepare the patient for the treatment and provide reassurance that you will continue to be the patient's doctor.

Sources: [a]Schiffer RB. Psychiatric disorders in medical practice. In: Goldman L, Ausiello D, eds. Cecil Textbook of Medicine. 22nd ed. Philadelphia: Saunders 2004, pp. 2628–2639; [b]Kroenke K. Patients presenting with somatic complaints: epidemiology, psychiatric comorbidity, and management. Int J Methods Psychiatr Res 12(1):34–43, 2003; [c]Reif W, Martin A, Rauh E, et al. Evaluation of general practitioners' training: how to manage patients with unexplained physical symptoms. Psychosomatics 47(4):304–311, 2006.

Table
5-2   Disorders of Mood

Mood disorders may be either depressive or bipolar. A bipolar disorder can include manic, hypomanic, or depressive features. *Four types of episodes,* described below, are combined in different ways in diagnosis of mood disorders. A major depressive disorder includes only one or more major depressive episodes. A *bipolar I disorder* includes one or more manic or mixed episodes, usually accompanied by major depressive episodes. A *bipolar II disorder* includes one or more major depressive episodes accompanied by at least one hypomanic episode.

Dysthymic and *cyclothymic disorders* are chronic and less severe conditions that do not meet the criteria of the other disorders. Mood disorders due to general medical conditions or substance abuse are classified separately.

Major Depressive Episode

At least five of the symptoms listed below (including one of the first two) must be present during the same 2-week period. They must also represent a change from the person's previous state.

- Depressed mood (may be an irritable mood in children and adolescents) most of the day, nearly every day
- Markedly diminished interest or pleasure in almost all activities most of the day, nearly every day
- Significant weight gain or loss (not dieting) or increased or decreased appetite nearly every day
- Insomnia or hypersomnia nearly every day
- Psychomotor agitation or retardation nearly every day
- Fatigue or loss of energy nearly every day
- Feelings of worthlessness or inappropriate guilt nearly every day
- Inability to think or concentrate or indecisiveness nearly every day
- Recurrent thoughts of death or suicide, or a specific plan for or attempt at suicide

The symptoms cause significant distress or impair social, occupational, or other important functions. In severe cases, hallucinations and delusions may occur.

Mixed Episode

A mixed episode, which must last at least 1 week, meets the criteria for both major and manic depressive episodes.

Dysthymic Disorder

A depressed mood and symptoms for most of the day, for more days than not, over at least 2 years (1 year in children and adolescents). Freedom from symptoms lasts no more than 2 months at a time.

Manic Episode

A distinct period of abnormally and persistently elevated, expansive, or irritable mood must be present for at least a week (any duration if hospitalization is necessary). During this time, at least three of the symptoms listed below have been persistent and significant. (Four of these symptoms are required if the mood is only irritable.)

- Inflated self-esteem or grandiosity
- Decreased need for sleep (feels rested after sleeping 3 hours)
- More talkative than usual or pressure to keep talking
- Flight of ideas or racing thoughts
- Distractibility
- Increased goal-directed activity (either socially, at work or school, or sexually) or psychomotor agitation
- Excessive involvement in pleasurable high-risk activities (buying sprees, foolish business ventures, sexual indiscretions)

The disturbance is severe enough to impair social or occupational functions or relationships. It may necessitate hospitalization for the protection of self or others. In severe cases, hallucinations and delusions may occur.

Hypomanic Episode

The mood and symptoms resemble those in a manic episode but are less impairing, do not require hospitalization, do not include hallucinations or delusions, and have a shorter minimum duration—4 days.

Cyclothymic Episode

Numerous periods of hypomanic and depressive symptoms that last for at least 2 years (1 year in children and adolescents). Freedom from symptoms lasts no more than 2 months at a time.

Tables 5-2 to 5-4 are based, with permission, on the Diagnostic and Statistical Manual of Mental Disorders, 4th ed., text revision (DSM IV-TR). Washington, DC: American Psychiatric Press, 2000. For further details and criteria, the reader should consult this manual, its successor, or comprehensive textbooks of psychiatry.

Table 5-3 Anxiety Disorders

Panic Disorder	A *panic disorder* is defined by recurrent, unexpected panic attacks, at least one of which has been followed by a month or more of persistent concern about further attacks, worry over their implications or consequences, or a significant change in behavior in relation to the attacks. A *panic attack* is a discrete period of intense fear or discomfort that develops abruptly and peaks within 10 minutes. It involves at least four of the following symptoms: (1) palpitations, pounding heart, or accelerated heart rate; (2) sweating; (3) trembling or shaking; (4) shortness of breath or a sense of smothering; (5) a feeling of choking; (6) chest pain or discomfort; (7) nausea or abdominal distress; (8) feeling dizzy, unsteady, lightheaded, or faint; (9) feelings of unreality or depersonalization; (10) fear of losing control or going crazy; (11) fear of dying; (12) paresthesias (numbness or tingling); (13) chills or hot flushes. Panic disorder may occur with or without *agoraphobia*.
Agoraphobia	Agoraphobia is an anxiety about being in places or situations where escape may be difficult or embarrassing, or help unavailable. Such situations are avoided, require a companion, or cause marked anxiety.
Specific Phobia	A specific phobia is a marked, persistent, and excessive or unreasonable fear that is cued by the presence or anticipation of a specific object or situation, such as dogs, injections, or flying. The person recognizes the fear as excessive or unreasonable, but exposure to the cue provokes immediate anxiety. Avoidance or fear impairs the person's normal routine, occupational or academic functioning, or social activities or relationships.
Social Phobia	A social phobia is a marked, persistent fear of one or more social or performance situations that involve exposure to unfamiliar people or to scrutiny by others. Those afflicted fear that they will act in embarrassing or humiliating ways, as by showing their anxiety. Exposure creates anxiety and possibly a panic attack, and the person avoids precipitating situations. He or she recognizes the fear as excessive or unreasonable. Normal routines, occupational or academic functioning, or social activities or relationships are impaired.
Obsessive–Compulsive Disorder	This disorder involves obsessions or compulsions that cause marked anxiety or distress. Although they are recognized at some point as excessive or unreasonable, they are very time-consuming and interfere with the person's normal routine, occupational functioning, or social activities or relationships.
Acute Stress Disorder	The person has been exposed to a traumatic event that involved actual or threatened death or serious injury to self or others and responded with intense fear, helplessness, or horror. During or immediately after this event, the person has at least three of these dissociative symptoms: (1) a subjective sense of numbing, detachment, or absence of emotional responsiveness; (2) a reduced awareness of surroundings, as in a daze; (3) feelings of unreality; (4) feelings of depersonalization; and (5) amnesia for an important part of the event. The event is persistently re-experienced, as in thoughts, images, dreams, illusions, and flashbacks, or distress from reminders of the event. The person is very anxious or shows increased arousal and tries to avoid stimuli that evoke memories of the event. The disturbance causes marked distress or impairs social, occupational, or other important functions. The symptoms occur within 4 weeks of the event and last from 2 days to 4 weeks.
Posttraumatic Stress Disorder	The event, the fearful response, and the persistent re-experiencing of the traumatic event resemble those in acute stress disorder. Hallucinations may occur. The person has increased arousal, tries to avoid stimuli related to the trauma, and has numbing of general responsiveness. The disturbance causes marked distress, impairs social, occupational, or other important functions, and lasts for more than a month.
Generalized Anxiety Disorder	This disorder lacks a specific traumatic event or focus for concern. Excessive anxiety and worry, which the person finds hard to control, are about a number of events or activities. At least three of the following symptoms are associated: (1) feeling restless, keyed up, or on edge; (2) being easily fatigued; (3) having difficulty in concentrating or having the mind going blank; (4) irritability; (5) muscle tension; (6) difficulty in falling or staying asleep, or restless, unsatisfying sleep. The disturbance causes significant distress or impairs social, occupational, or other important functions.

Table
5-4 Psychotic Disorders

Psychotic disorders involve grossly impaired reality testing. Specific diagnoses depend on the nature and duration of the symptoms and on a cause when it can be identified. Seven disorders are outlined below.

Schizophrenia	Schizophrenia impairs major functioning, as at work or school or in interpersonal relations or self-care. For this diagnosis, performance of one or more of these functions must have decreased for a significant time to a level markedly below prior achievement. In addition, the person must manifest at least two of the following for a significant part of 1 month: (1) delusions; (2) hallucinations; (3) disorganized speech; (4) grossly disorganized or catatonic behavior;* and (5) negative symptoms such as a flat affect, alogia (lack of content in speech), or avolition (lack of interest, drive, and ability to set and pursue goals). Continuous signs of the disturbance must persist for at least 6 months.
	Subtypes of this disorder include paranoid, disorganized, and catatonic schizophrenia.
Schizophreniform Disorder	A schizophreniform disorder has symptoms similar to those of schizophrenia, but they last less than 6 months, and the functional impairment seen in schizophrenia need not be present.
Schizoaffective Disorder	A schizoaffective disorder has features of both a major mood disturbance and schizophrenia. The mood disturbance (depressive, manic, or mixed) is present during most of the illness and must, for a time, be concurrent with symptoms of schizophrenia (listed above). During the same period of time, there must also be delusions or hallucinations for at least 2 weeks without prominent mood symptoms.
Delusional Disorder	A delusional disorder is characterized by nonbizarre delusions that involve situations in real life, such as having a disease or being deceived by a lover. The delusion has persisted for at least a month, but the person's functioning is not markedly impaired, and behavior is not obviously odd or bizarre. The symptoms of schizophrenia, except for tactile and olfactory hallucinations related to the delusion, have not been present.
Brief Psychotic Disorder	In this disorder, at least one of the following psychotic symptoms must be present: delusions, hallucinations, disordered speech such as frequent derailment or incoherence, or grossly disorganized or catatonic behavior. The disturbance lasts at least 1 day but less than 1 month, and the person returns to his or her prior functional level.
Psychotic Disorder Due to a General Medical Condition	Prominent hallucinations or delusions may be experienced during a medical illness. For this diagnosis, they should not occur exclusively during the course of delirium. The medical condition should be documented and judged to be causally related to the symptoms.
Substance-Induced Psychotic Disorder	Prominent hallucinations or delusions may be induced by intoxication or withdrawal from a substance such as alcohol, cocaine, or opioids. For this diagnosis, these symptoms should not occur exclusively during the course of delirium. The substance should be judged to be causally related to the symptoms.

*Catatonic behaviors are psychomotor abnormalities that include stupor, mutism, negativistic resistance to instructions or attempts to move the person, rigid or bizarre postures, and excited, apparently purposeless activity.

The Skin, Hair, and Nails

Anatomy and Physiology

The major function of the skin is to keep the body in homeostasis despite daily assaults from the environment. The skin provides boundaries for body fluids while protecting underlying tissues from microorganisms, harmful substances, and radiation. It modulates body temperature and synthesizes vitamin D. Hair, nails, and sebaceous and sweat glands are considered appendages of the skin. The skin and its appendages undergo many changes during aging.

Turn to Chapter 20, The Older Adult, pp. 919–920, to review normal and abnormal changes of the skin with aging.

Skin.   The skin is the heaviest single organ of the body, accounting for approximately 16% of body weight and covering an area of roughly 1.2 to 2.3 meters squared. It contains three layers: the epidermis, the dermis, and the subcutaneous tissues.

The most superficial layer, the *epidermis*, is thin, devoid of blood vessels, and itself divided into two layers: an outer horny *stratum corneum* of dead keratinized cells and an inner cellular layer, the *stratum basale* and the *stratum spinosum*, also known as the malpighian layer, where both melanin and keratin are formed. Migration from the inner layer to the upper layer takes approximately 1 month.

The epidermis depends on the underlying *dermis* for its nutrition. The dermis is well supplied with blood. It contains connective tissue, sebaceous glands, sweat glands, and hair follicles. It merges below with *subcutaneous*, or *adipose, tissue*, also known as fat.

The color of normal skin depends primarily on four pigments: melanin, carotene, oxyhemoglobin, and deoxyhemoglobin. The amount of *melanin*, the brownish

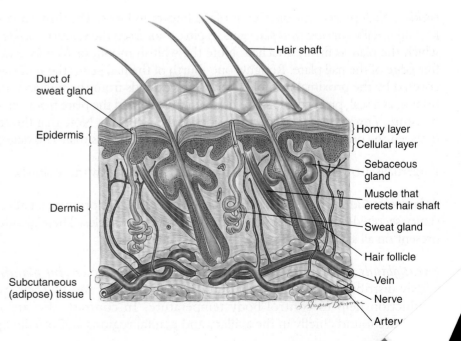

pigment of the skin, is genetically determined and is increased by exposure to sunlight. *Carotene* is a golden yellow pigment that exists in subcutaneous fat and in heavily keratinized areas such as the palms and soles.

Hemoglobin, which circulates in the red cells and carries most of the oxygen of the blood, exists in two forms. *Oxyhemoglobin,* a bright red pigment, predominates in the arteries and capillaries. An increase in blood flow through the arteries to the capillaries causes a reddening of the skin, whereas the opposite change usually produces pallor. The skin of light-colored people is normally redder on the palms, soles, face, neck, and upper chest.

As blood passes through the capillary bed, oxyhemoglobin loses its oxygen to the tissues and changes to *deoxyhemoglobin*—a darker and somewhat bluer pigment. An increased concentration of deoxyhemoglobin in cutaneous blood vessels gives the skin a bluish cast known as *cyanosis.*

Cyanosis can be either central or peripheral, depending on the oxygen level in the arterial blood. If this level is low, cyanosis is *central.* If it is normal, cyanosis is *peripheral.* Peripheral cyanosis occurs when cutaneous blood flow decreases and slows, and tissues extract more oxygen than usual from the blood. Peripheral cyanosis may be a normal response to anxiety or a cold environment.

Skin color is also affected by the scattering of light reflected back through the turbid superficial layers of the skin or vessel walls. This scattering makes the color look bluer and less red. The bluish color of a subcutaneous vein results from this effect; it is much bluer than the venous blood obtained on venipuncture.

Hair.   Adults have two types of hair: *vellus hair,* which is short, fine, inconspicuous, and relatively unpigmented; and *terminal hair,* which is coarser, thicker, more conspicuous, and usually pigmented. Scalp hair and eyebrows are examples of terminal hair.

Nails.   Nails protect the distal ends of the fingers and toes. The firm, rectangular, and usually curving *nail plate* gets its pink color from the vascular *nail bed* to which the plate is firmly attached. Note the whitish moon, or *lunula,* and the free edge of the nail plate. Roughly one-fourth of the nail plate (the *nail root*) is covered by the proximal nail fold. The *cuticle* extends from the fold and, functioning as a seal, protects the space between the fold and the plate from external moisture. *Lateral nail folds* cover the sides of the nail plate. Note that the angle between the proximal nail fold and nail plate is normally less than 180 degrees.

Fingernails grow approximately 0.1 mm daily; toenails grow more slowly.

Sebaceous Glands and Sweat Glands.   *Sebaceous glands* produce a fatty substance secreted onto the skin surface through the hair follicles. These glands are present on all skin surfaces except the palms and soles.

Sweat glands are of two types: eccrine and apocrine. The *eccrine glands* are widely distributed, open directly onto the skin surface, and by their sweat production help to control body temperature. In contrast, the *apocrine glands* are found chiefly in the axillary and genital regions and usually open

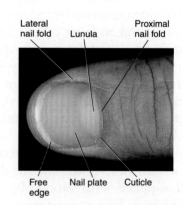

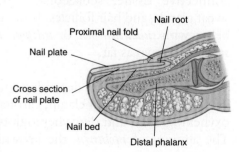

into hair follicles. Bacterial decomposition of apocrine sweat is responsible for adult body odor.

The Health History

Common or Concerning Symptoms

▶ Hair loss
▶ Rash
▶ Growths

Start your inquiry about the skin with a few open-ended questions: "Have you noticed any changes in your skin? . . . your hair? . . . your nails?" "Have you had any rashes? . . . sores? . . . lumps? . . . itching?"

Ask, "Have you noticed any growths you are concerned about? Do you have any moles or growths that have changed in size, shape, color, or sensation? What about any new moles or growths?" If patients have such growths, pursue any personal or family history of melanoma and results of any prior biopsies of the skin.

You may wish to defer further questions about the skin until the physical examination, when you inspect the skin and identify the lesions of concern.

Causes of generalized itching, without apparent rash, include dry skin, pregnancy, uremia, jaundice, lymphomas and leukemia, drug reaction, lice and, less commonly, diabetes and thyroid disease.

Approximately half of *melanomas* are initially detected by the patient.

Health Promotion and Counseling: Evidence and Recommendations

Important Topics for Health Promotion and Counseling

▶ Skin cancers: types, risk factors, and screening guidelines
▶ Avoiding excess sun exposure

Skin Cancers: Types, Risk Factors, and Screening for Melanoma. Clinicians play an essential role in educating patients about early detection of suspicious growths, protective measures for skin care, and the hazards of excessive sun exposure. Skin cancers are the most common cancers in the United States, affecting roughly one in five Americans.[1] *Basal and squamous cell skin cancers* usually arise in sun-exposed areas, particularly the head, neck, and upper limbs. *Melanomas* are associated with sun exposure but are often on nonexposed areas subject to intermittent sunburns such as the trunk and thighs.

Teach patients about these three major types of skin cancers to promote early detection, especially for melanomas, since awareness and detection continue to lag, impacting onset of treatment and the chance for cure.

- *Basal cell carcinoma.* These skin cancers consist of immature cells similar to those in the basal layer of the epidermis, and account for roughly 80% of all skin cancers. They usually arise in sun-exposed areas, especially the head and neck. Classically they appear as pearly erythematous translucent papules, but may also be subtle red macules or display even other morphologies. Basal cell carcinomas tend to grow slowly and almost never metastasize.

- *Squamous cell carcinoma.* This type consists of more mature cells usually resembling the spinous layer of the epidermis, accounting for approximately 16% of skin cancers. These cancers are often crusted hyperkeratotic lesions with a rough surface or flat reddish patches with an inflamed or ulcerated appearance. Metastasis is rare, occurring in 1% of cases.

- *Melanoma.* Melanomas arise from the pigment-producing melanocytes in the epidermis that give skin its color, and account for the remaining 4% to 5% of skin cancers. Melanomas are potentially the most lethal of the skin cancers, although almost 100% of thin, early-stage melanomas can be cured.[2] The incidence of melanomas has doubled in recent decades and is increasing more rapidly than any other cancer.[3-5] Lifetime risk is 1 in 75. Indoor tanning increases risk by 75%, and melanoma is now the most common cancer in young adults ages 25 to 29. Melanomas can spread rapidly to the lymph system and internal organs; they cause 80% of deaths from skin cancer.[6] Mortality rates are highest in white men, possibly due to lower "skin awareness" and lower rates of self-examination.

Risk Factors for Melanoma. Educate your patients about *risk factors for melanoma.* Recent data from over 364,000 people screened by the National Melanoma/Skin Cancer Screening Program of the American Academy of Dermatology validates the *HARMM model* for designating risk factors for melanoma.[7]

HARMM Melanoma Risk Model	
Risk Factor	**Increased Risk of Melanoma**
▶ **H**istory of previous melanoma	3.3
▶ **A**ge over 50	1.2
▶ **R**egular dermatologist absent	1.4
▶ **M**ole changing	2.0
▶ **M**ale gender	1.4
Number of Risk Factors	**Increased Likelihood of Melanoma**
▶ 0–1	1.0
▶ 2	1.7
▶ 3	2.5
▶ 4–5	4.5

Source: Goldberg MS, Doucette JT, Lim HW et al. Risk factors for presumptive melanoma in skin cancer screening: American Academy of Dermatology National Melanoma/Skin Cancer Screening Program experience 2001–2005. J Am Acad Dermatology 57:60–66, 2007.

Other risk factors are: ≥50 common moles; one to four atypical or unusual moles, especially if dysplastic[8,9]; red or light hair; *solar lentigines* (acquired macules on sun-exposed areas); freckles (more genetically derived brown macules); ultraviolet radiation from heavy sun exposure, sunlamps, or tanning booths; light eye or skin color, especially skin that freckles or burns easily; severe blistering sunburns in childhood; immunosuppression from HIV or from chemotherapy; and family history of melanoma. Early detection of melanoma when macular or less than 1 mm in depth greatly improves prognosis.

Screening Guidelines for Skin Cancer. Although the U.S. Preventive Services Task Force does not recommend routine screening for skin cancer in its 2009 update, citing insufficient evidence, it does advise clinicians to "remain alert for skin lesions with malignant features" during routine physical examinations and references the ABCDE nomenclature below.[10,11] The American Cancer Society and the American Academy of Dermatology recommend monthly skin self-examination as well as regular examination by a physician for people older than 50 years or those with multiple melanomas or dysplastic nevus syndrome.[12,13]

The most commonly recommended screening measure is *total body skin examination,* since melanomas can appear anywhere, especially in adults at high risk due to family history or personal history of multiple or dysplastic nevi or prior melanoma. Both new and changing nevi should be closely examined, since at least half of melanomas arise *de novo* from isolated melanocytes rather than pre-existing nevi. Evidence supporting *skin self-examination* is conflicting, but this low-cost method or patient education promotes health awareness in at-risk patients.

See Techniques for Skin Self-Examination, pp. 179–180.

Screening for Melanoma: the ABCDEs. Both clinicians and patients should apply the ABCDE method when screening moles for melanoma. The sensitivity of this mnemonic for detecting melanoma ranges from 50% to 97%, and specificity ranges from 96% to 99%.[11]

See Table 6-10, Benign and Malignant Nevi, p. 195.

The average patient has 15 to 30 moles, or *nevi.* Common types include:

- *Junctional nevi*—typically brown macules
- *Intradermal nevi*—typically skin-colored papules
- *Compound nevi*—typically brown macules

Contrast these features with the characteristics of melanomas listed below, which you can easily teach your patients with photographs readily at hand.

Watch for the "ugly duckling sign"— a mole that looks different from the typical moles seen in a given patient.[5]

Note that early melanomas may be <6 mm, and many benign nevi may be >6 mm. Nonetheless, the 6-mm cutoff has recently been revalidated.[14]

ABCDEs for Early Recognition of Possible Melanoma

- **A** for **A**symmetry of once side of mole compared to the other
- **B** for irregular **B**orders, especially ragged, notched, or blurred
- **C** for variegation in **C**olor, especially blue and black mixed with white and red (white from scarring and regression; red from inflammatory reaction to abnormal cells)
- **D** for **D**iameter ≥6 mm or different from others
- **E** for **E**volution or change in size, symptoms, or morphology

In addition to visual inspection, *dermoscopy* is an increasingly useful office practice that helps determine whether a melanocytic lesion is benign or malignant.[5] Dermoscopy is a well-established method for viewing skin lesions with a magnifier using either an oil/gel interface or cross-polarizing light filters. This method limits the amount of reflected light, making it easier to visualize deeper pigmentary or vascular structures. Regular *photomapping* and use of laser techniques also assist in diagnosis.

Avoiding Excess Sun Exposure. Urge patients to reduce sun exposure by using umbrellas and wearing protective sunglasses, hats, and clothing. Intermittent sun exposure appears to be more harmful than chronic exposure.[13] Patients should apply sunscreen with a sun protection factor (SPF) of 15 or higher to all unprotected skin. Experts recommend avoiding sunbathing, tanning beds, and sunlamps. In 2009, the International Agency for Research on Cancer upgraded their classification of indoor tanning devices to definitively "carcinogenic to humans."[12] Targeted patient messages in primary care practices have been shown to amplify these sun-protective behaviors.[15,16]

Sunscreens fall into two categories: physical blockers containing minerals like zinc oxide or titanium dioxide; and light-absorbing chemical sunscreens. Water-resistant sunscreens that remain on the skin for prolonged periods are preferable. The SPF is a rating of sunscreen effectiveness denoting the number of minutes for treated versus untreated skin to redden when exposed to ultraviolet-B. An SPF of 15 blocks over 90% of ultraviolet-B. Use of sunscreens can lull patients into a false sense of security, however, and even increase sun exposure.

Techniques of Examination

The examination of the skin, hair, and nails begins with the General Survey and continues throughout the physical examination. For a thorough skin examination, make sure the patient wears a gown that allows close inspection of the hair, anterior and posterior body surfaces, palms and soles, and web spaces between the fingers and toes. Start with natural light whenever possible, but use an intense light source whenever you need to better characterize your findings.

Artificial light can distort colors and mask jaundice.

Commit one to two minutes to *inspecting the entire surface of the skin,* and an additional one to two minutes if you plan to use dermoscopy.[17] Before starting the examination, you may wish to review the tables at the end of the chapter to better identify skin colors, and patterns and shapes of lesions that you may encounter.

Consider biopsy for any lesions that are suspicious for carcinoma or, when needed, as an aide to diagnosis.

SKIN

Inspect and palpate the skin. Note these characteristics:

Color. Patients may be the first to notice a change in their skin color. Ask them about it. Look for increased brown pigmentation, loss of pigmentation, redness, pallor, cyanosis, and yellowing of the skin.

See Table 6-1, Skin Colors, pp. 183–184. Correlate your findings with observations of the mucous membranes, since a number of disorders appear in both areas.

Assess the red color of oxyhemoglobin and the pallor in its absence where the horny layer of the epidermis is thinnest and causes the least scatter: the fingernails, the lips, and the mucous membranes, particularly those of the mouth and the palpebral conjunctiva. In dark-skinned people, inspecting the palms and soles may also be useful.

Pallor results from decreased redness in *anemia* and decreased blood flow, seen in fainting or arterial occlusion.

Central cyanosis is best identified in the lips, oral mucosa, and tongue. The lips can also turn blue in the cold, and melanin in the lips may simulate cyanosis in darker-skinned people.

Causes of *central cyanosis* include advanced lung disease, congenital heart disease, and hemoglobinopathies.

Cyanosis of the nails, hands, and feet may be central or peripheral in origin. Anxiety or a cold examining room may cause peripheral cyanosis.

The *cyanosis of heart failure* is usually peripheral, reflecting deoxygenation or impaired circulation. In *COPD* and *pulmonary edema*, hypoxia may give rise to central cyanosis.

Look for the yellow color of *jaundice* in the sclera. Jaundice may also appear in the palpebral conjunctiva, lips, hard palate, undersurface of the tongue, tympanic membrane, and skin. To see jaundice more easily in the lips, blanch out the red color by pressure with a glass slide.

Jaundice suggests liver disease or excessive hemolysis of red blood cells.

For the yellow color that accompanies high levels of carotene, look at the palms, soles, and face.

Seen in *carotenemia*

Moisture. Examples are dryness, sweating, and oiliness.

Dryness in *hypothyroidism*; oiliness in *acne*

Temperature. Use the backs of your fingers to assess skin temperature. In addition to identifying generalized warmth or coolness of the skin, note the temperature of any red areas.

Generalized warmth in fever, *hyperthyroidism*; coolness in *hypothyroidism*. Local warmth if inflammation or cellulitis

Texture. Examples are roughness and smoothness.

Roughness in *hypothyroidism*; velvety texture in *hyperthyroidism*

Mobility and Turgor. Lift a fold of skin and note how easily it lifts up (mobility) and how quickly it returns into place (turgor).

Decreased mobility in edema, *scleroderma*; decreased turgor in dehydration

Lesions. Closely inspect any lesions, noting important features such as:

- *Anatomic location and distribution* over the body. Are the lesions generalized or localized? Do they, for example, involve the exposed surfaces, the intertriginous or skin-fold areas, extensor or flexor areas, or acral areas (such as the hands and feet)? Do they involve areas exposed to specific allergens or irritants, such as wristbands or rings?

Many skin diseases have typical distributions. *Acne* affects the face, upper chest, and back; *psoriasis*, the knees and elbows (among other areas); and *Candida* infections, the intertriginous areas. See patterns in Table 6-2, Skin Lesions—Anatomic Location and Distribution, p. 185.

- *Types of skin lesions* (e.g., macules, papules, vesicles, nevi). If possible, find representative and recent lesions that have not been traumatized by scratching or otherwise altered. Inspect them carefully and feel them.

- *Color.*

See Table 6-4, Primary Skin Lesions, pp. 187–189; Table 6-5, Secondary Skin Lesions, p. 190; Table 6-6, Secondary Skin Lesions—Depressed, p. 191; Table 6-7, Acne Vulgaris—Primary and Secondary Lesions, p. 192; Table 6-8, Vascular and Purpuric Lesions of the Skin, p. 193; Table 6-9, Skin Tumors, p. 194; and Table 6-10, Benign and Malignant Nevi, p. 195.

- *Patterns and shapes.* Are the lesions linear, clustered, annular (in a ring), arciform (in an arc), geographic, or serpiginous (serpent- or worm-like)? Are they dermatomal, covering a skin band that corresponds to a sensory nerve root (see pp. 723–724)?

Vesicles in a unilateral dermatomal pattern are typical of herpes zoster.[18,19] See patterns in Table 6-3, Skin Lesions—Patterns and Shapes, p. 186.

SKIN LESIONS IN CONTEXT

Once you are familiar with the basic types of lesions, review how they look in Tables 6-11 and 6-12 and recheck their appearance in a well-illustrated dermatology textbook. Keep a good clinical dermatology book close at hand so that whenever you see a skin lesion, you can broaden your knowledge of skin disorders and related systemic diseases. Accurate description of lesions and their location and distribution, combined with the history and overall physical examination, will gradually build your clinical acumen.

See Table 6-11, Skin Lesions in Context, pp. 196–197, and Table 6-12, Diseases and Related Skin Conditions, pp. 198–199.

Evaluating the Bedbound Patient. People confined to bed, especially when they are emaciated, elderly, or neurologically impaired, are particularly susceptible to skin damage and ulceration. *Pressure sores* result from sustained compression that obliterates arteriolar and capillary blood flow

See Table 6-13, Pressure Ulcers, p. 200.

to the skin, and from shear forces created by body movements. When a person slides down in bed from a partially sitting position, for example, or is dragged rather than lifted up after being supine, rough movement can distort the soft tissues of the buttocks and close off the arteries and arterioles. Friction and moisture further increase the risk of abrasions and sores.

Assess every susceptible patient by carefully inspecting the skin that overlies the sacrum, buttocks, greater trochanters, knees, and heels. Roll the patient onto one side to see the low back and gluteal area best.

Local redness of the skin warns of impending necrosis, although some deep pressure sores develop without antecedent redness. Inspect closely for skin breaks and ulcers.

HAIR

Inspect and palpate the hair. Note its quantity, distribution, and texture.

Alopecia refers to hair loss—diffuse, patchy, or total. Sparse hair is seen in *hypothyroidism*; fine, silky hair in *hyperthyroidism*

See Table 6-14, Hair Loss, p. 201.

NAILS

Inspect and palpate the fingernails and toenails. Note their color and shape, and any lesions. Longitudinal bands of pigment may be seen in the nails of normal people who have darker skin.

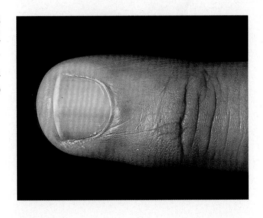

See Table 6-15, Findings in or Near the Nails, pp. 202–203.

SPECIAL TECHNIQUES

Instructions for the Skin Self-Examination. The American Academy of Dermatology recommends regular self-examination of the skin using the following techniques. The patient will need a full-length mirror, a hand-held mirror, and a well-lit room that provides privacy. Teach the patient the **ABCDE** method for assessing moles (see p. 175), and show the patient the photos of melanomas in Table 6-10 on p. 195.

Patient Instructions for the Skin Self-Examination

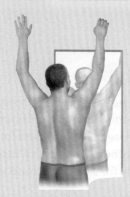

Examine your body front and back in the mirror, then look at your right and left sides with arms raised.

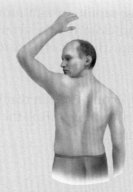

Bend elbows and look carefully at forearms, upper underarms, and palms.

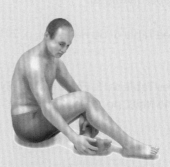

Look at the backs of your legs and feet, the spaces between your toes, and the soles.

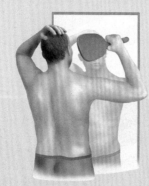

Examine the back of your neck and scalp with a hand mirror. Part hair for a closer look.

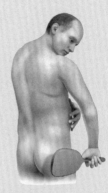

Finally, check your back and buttocks with a hand mirror.

Source: Adapted from American Academy of Dermatology. How to examine your skin. Available at http://www.aad.org/skin-conditions/skin-cancer-detection/about skin-self-exams. Assessed May 21, 2010.

Recording Your Findings

Note that initially you may use sentences to describe your findings; later you will use phrases. The style below contains phrases appropriate for most write-ups.

Recording the Physical Examination—The Skin

"Color pink. Skin warm and moist. Nails without clubbing or cyanosis. No suspicious nevi. No rash, petechiae, or ecchymoses."
OR
"Marked facial pallor, with circumoral cyanosis. Palms cold and moist. Cyanosis in nail beds of fingers and toes. One blue-black plague, 1 × 2 cm, with irregular border on right forearm. No rash."
OR
"Facial plethora. Skin icteric. Spider angioma over anterior torso. Palmar erythema. Single pearly plague with depressed center and telangiectasias, 1 × 1 cm, on posterior neck above collarline. No suspicious nevi. Nails with clubbing but no cyanosis."

Suggests central cyanosis and possible melanoma

Suggests possible liver disease and basal cell carcinoma

Bibliography

1. American Academy of Dermatology. Skin cancer. Available at http://www.aad.org/media-resources/stats-and-facts/conditions/skin-cancer/skin-cancer. Accessed May 20, 2011.
2. American Academy of Dermatology. Dermatology A to Z. Melanoma. Available at http://www.aad.org/skin-conditions/dermatology-a-to-z/melanoma. Accessed May 20, 2011.
3. National Cancer Institute. Surveillance Epidemiology and End Results (SEER). Fast Stats. Statistics stratified by end results. Melanoma of the skin. Available at http://seer.cancer.gov/faststats/selections.php?series=cancer. Accessed May 20, 2011. See also National Cancer Institute. Seer Cancer Stat Fact Sheets. Melanoma of the skin. Available at http://seer.cancer.gov/statfacts/html/skin.html. Accessed May 20, 2011.
4. Linos E, Swetter SM, Cockburn MG et al. Increasing burden of melanoma in the United States. J Invest Dermatol 2009;129:1666–1674.
5. Goodson AG, Grossman D. Strategies for early melanoma detection: approaches to the patient with nevi. J Am Acad Dermatol 2009;60:719–735. http://www.ncbi.nlm.nih.gov/pmc/articles/PMC2690513/pdf/nihms114603.pdf
6. Miller AJ, Mihm MC. Melanoma. N Engl J Med 2006;355:51–65.
7. Goldberg MS, Doucette JT, Lim HW et al. Risk factors for presumptive melanoma in skin cancer screening: American Academy of Dermatology National Melanoma/Skin Cancer Screening Program experience 2001–2005. J Am Acad Dermatology 2007;75:60–66. http://www.eblue.org/article/

PIIS0190962207004215/fulltext-article-footnote-1#article-footnote-1.
8. Naeyaert JM, Broches L. Dysplastic nevi. N Engl J Med 2003;349:2233–2240.
9. Tucker MA, Halpern A, Holly EA et al. Clinically recognized dysplastic nevi: a central risk factor for cutaneous melanoma. JAMA 1997;277:1439–1444.
10. U.S. Preventive Services Task Force. Screening for skin cancer. U.S. Preventive Services Task Force recommendation statement. Ann Intern Med 2009;150:189–193.
11. Wolff T, Tai E, Miller T. Screening for Skin Cancer: An Update of the Evidence for the U.S. Preventive Services Task Force. Evidence Synthesis No. 67. AHRQ Publication No. 09-05128-EF-1. Rockville, MD: Agency for Healthcare Research and Quality. February 2009.
12. American Cancer Society. Cancer Facts and Figures 2010, Skin, pp. 19–20. Available at http://www.cancer.org/acs/groups/content/@epidemiologysurveilance/documents/document/acspc-026238.pdf. Accessed May 21, 2011.
13. National Cancer Institute. Genetics of skin cancer. Melanoma. Updated April 20, 2011. Available at http://www.cancer.gov/cancertopics/pdq/genetics/skin/HealthProfessional/page4#Section_39. Accessed May 21, 2011.
14. Abbasi NR, Yancovitz M, Gutkowicz-Krusin D et al. Utility of lesion diameter in the clinical diagnosis of cutaneous melanoma. Arch Dermatol 2008;144:469–474. http://archderm.ama-assn.org/cgi/reprint/144/4/469.
15. Glanz K, Schoenfeld ER, Steffen A. A randomized trial of tailored skin cancer prevention messages for adults: Project SCAPE. Am J Public Health 2010;100:735–741.

16. Lin JS, Eder M, Weinmann S. Behavioral counseling to prevent skin cancer: a systematic review for the U.S. Preventive Services Task force. Ann Intern Med 2011;154:190–201.

17. Zalaudek I, Kittler H, Marghoob AA et al. Time required for a complete skin examination with and without dermoscopy: a prospective, randomized multicenter study. Arch Dermatol 2008;144:509–513.

18. Wilson JF. In the clinic. Herpes zoster. Ann Intern Med 2011;154:ITC3-1–ITC3-15.

19. Whitley RJ. A 70-year-old woman with shingles: review of herpes zoster. JAMA 2009;302:73–80.

20. Thiboutot D, Gollnick H, Bettoli V et al. New insights into the management of acne: an update from the Global Alliance to Improve Outcomes in Acne group. J Am Acad Dermatol 2009;60(5 Suppl):S1–S50.

21. Garcia AD, Thomas DR. Assessment and management of chronic pressure ulcers in the elderly. Med Clin North Am 2006;90:925–944.

22. VanGilder C, MacFarlane G, Meyer S et al. Body mass index, weight, and pressure ulcer prevalence: an analysis of the 2006–2007 International Pressure Ulcer Prevalence Surveys. J Nurs Care Qual 2009;24:127–135.

23. Spicknall KE, Zirwas MJ, English JC 3rd. Clubbing: an update on diagnosis, differential diagnosis, pathophysiology, and clinical relevance. J Am Acad Dematol 2005;52:1020–1028.

24. Fawcett RS, Hart TM, Lindford S et al. Nail abnormalities: clues to systemic diseases. Am Fam Physician 2004;69:1418–1425.

25. Hanford RR, Cobb MW, Banner NT. Unilateral Beau's lines associated with a fractured and immobilized wrist. Cutis 1995;56:263–264.

Additional References

American Academy of Dermatology. How to examine your skin. Available at http://www.aad.org/skin-conditions/skin-cancer-detection/about-skin-self-exams. Accessed May 21, 2011.

Boulton AJ, Kirsner RS, Vileikyte L. Neuropathic diabetic foot ulcers. N Engl J Med 2004;351:48–55.

Fox GN. 10 derm mistakes you don't want to make. J Fam Pract 2008;57:162–169.

Goldsmith LA, Fitzpatrick TB. Fitzpatrick's Dermatology in General Medicine, 8th ed. New York: McGraw-Hill Professional, 2012.

Habif TP, Campbell JL, Chapman S et al. Clinical Dermatology: A Color Guide to Diagnosis and Therapy, 3rd ed. New York: Saunders, 2011.

Habif TP. Clinical Dermatology, 5th ed. Philadelphia: Elsevier Mosby, 2010.

Hall JC, Hall JC, Sauer GC. Sauer's Manual of Skin Diseases, 10th ed. Philadelphia: Wolters Kluwer Health/Lippincott Williams & Wilkins, 2010.

Hordinsky M. Advances in hair diseases. Adv Dermatol 2008; 24:245–259.

Li J, Chen J, Kirsner R. Pathophysiology of acute wound healing. Clin Dermatol 2007;25:9–18.

Lyder CH. Effective management of pressure ulcers. A review of proven strategies. Adv Nurse Pract 2006;14:32–37.

Miller AJ and Mihm MC. Melanoma. N Engl J Med 2006;355:51–65.

Myers KA, Farquhar DRE. Does this patient have clubbing? JAMA 2001;286:341–347.

Olasz EB, Yancey KB. Bullous pemphigoid and related subepidermal autoimmune blistering diseases. Curr Dir Autoimmun 2008;10:141–166.

Rubin AI, Chen EH, HC, Ratner D. Basal cell carcinoma. N Engl J Med 2005;353:2262–2269.

Schon MP, Boehncke W. Psoriasis. N Engl J Med 2005;352:1899–1912.

Shapiro J. Clinical practice. Hair loss in women. N Engl J Med 2007;357:1620–1630.

Singh N, Armstrong DG, Lipsky BA. Preventing foot ulcers in patients with diabetes. JAMA 2005;293:217–228.

Spicknall KE, Zirwas MJ, English JC 3rd. Clubbing: an update on diagnosis, differential diagnosis, pathophysiology, and clinical relevance. J Am Acad Dermatol 2005;52:1020–1028.

Swartz MN. Cellulitis. N Engl J Med 2004;350:904–912.

Taïeb A, Picardo M. Clinical practice. Vitiligo. N Engl J Med 2009; 360:160–169.

Wilson J. In the clinic. Herpes zoster. Ann Intern Med 2011; 154:ITC3-1-3-15.

Wolff K, Johnson RA, Fitzpatrick TB. Fitzpatrick's Color Atlas and Synopsis of Clinical Dermatology, 6th ed. New York: McGraw-Hill Medical, 2009.

The Bates' suite offers these additional resources to enhance learning and facilitate understanding of this chapter:

- Bates' Pocket Guide to Physical Examination and History Taking, 7th edition
- Bates' Visual Guide to Physical Examination
- thePoint online resources, for students and instructors: http://thepoint.lww.com

Table 6-1 | Skin Colors

Changes in Pigmentation

A widespread increase in *melanin* may be caused by Addison's disease (hypofunction of the adrenal cortex) or some pituitary tumors. More common are local areas of increased or decreased pigment.

Café-Au-Lait Spot
A slightly but uniformly pigmented macule or patch with a somewhat irregular border, usually 0.5 to 1.5 cm in diameter; benign. Six or more such spots, each with a diameter of >1.5 cm, however, suggest neurofibromatosis (p. 197). (The small, darker macules are unrelated.)

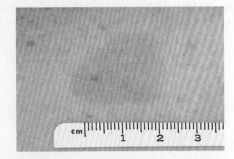

Tinea Versicolor
Common superficial fungal infection of the skin, causing hypo- or hyperpigmented ("versicolor"), slightly scaly macules on the trunk, neck, and upper arms (short-sleeved shirt distribution). They are easier to see in darker skin and may be more obvious after tanning. In lighter skin, macules may look reddish or tan instead of pale.

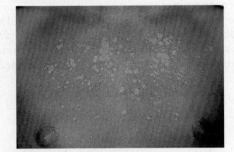 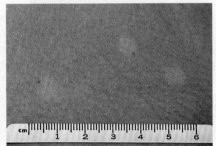

Vitiligo
In vitiligo, depigmented macules appear on the face, hands, feet, extensor surfaces, and other regions and may coalesce into extensive areas that lack melanin. The brown pigment is normal skin color; the pale areas are vitiligo. The condition may be hereditary. These changes may be distressing to the patient.

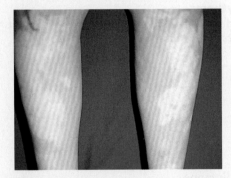 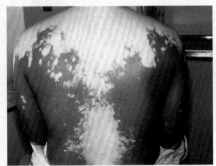

Cyanosis

Cyanosis is the somewhat bluish color that is visible in these toenails and toes. Compare this color with the normally pink fingernails and fingers of the same patient. Cyanosis, especially when slight, may be hard to distinguish from normal skin color.

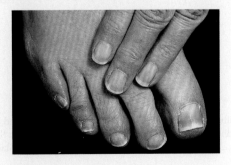

(table continues on page 184)

Table
6-1 Skin Colors *(continued)*

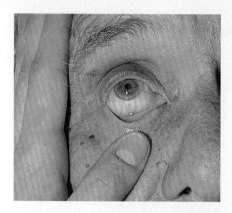

Jaundice

Jaundice makes the skin diffusely yellow. Contrast this patient's skin color with the examiner's hand. Jaundice is seen most easily and reliably in the sclera, as shown here. It may also be visible in mucous membranes. Causes include *liver disease* and *hemolysis of red blood cells.*

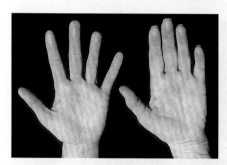

Carotenemia

The yellowish palm of carotenemia is compared with a normally pink palm, sometimes a subtle finding. Unlike jaundice, carotenemia does not affect the sclera, which remains white. The cause is a diet high in carrots and other yellow vegetables or fruits. Carotenemia is not harmful but indicates the need for assessing dietary intake.

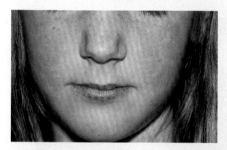

Erythema

Red hue, increased blood flow, seen here as the "slapped cheeks" of *erythema infectiosum* ("fifth disease").

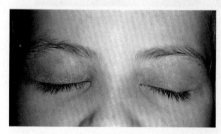

Heliotrope

Violaceous patches over the eyelids in the collagen vascular disease *dermatomyositis.*

Sources of photos: *Tinea Versicolor*—Ostler HB, Mailbach HI, Hoke AW et al. Diseases of the Eye and Skin: A Color Atlas. Philadelphia: Lippincott Williams & Wilkins, 2004; *Vitiligo, Erythema*—Goodheart HP. Goodheart's Photoguide of Common Skin Disorders: Diagnosis and Management, 2nd ed. Philadelphia: Lippincott Williams & Wilkins, 2003; *Heliotrope*—Hall JC. Sauer's Manual of Skin Diseases, 8th ed. Philadelphia: Lippincott Williams & Wilkins, 2000.

Table

6-2   **Skin Lesions—Anatomic Location and Distribution**

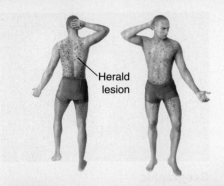

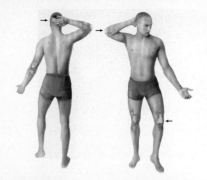

Herald lesion

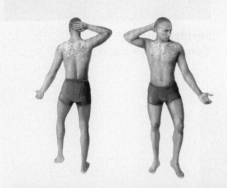

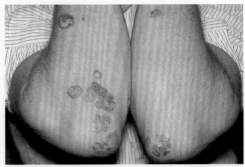

Pityriasis Rosea
Reddish oval ringworm-like papules or plagues

Psoriasis
Silvery scaly papules or plagues, mainly on the extensor surfaces

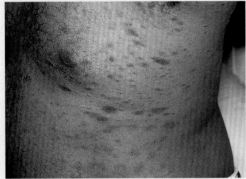

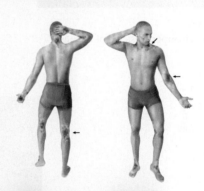

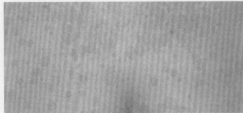

Tinea Versicolor
Tan, flat, scaly plaques

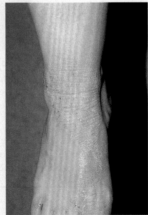

Atopic Eczema
(adult form)
Appears mainly on flexor surfaces

Source: Hall JC. *Sauer's Manual of Skin Diseases*, 8th ed. Philadelphia: Lippincott Williams & Wilkins, 2000; Photos from: Goodheart HP. Goodheart's *Photoguide of Common Skin Disorders: Diagnosis and Management*, 2nd ed. Philadelphia: Lippincott Williams & Wilkins, 2003.

Table 6-3   Skin Lesions—Patterns and Shapes

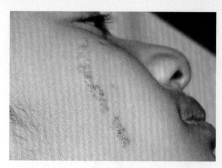

Linear
Example: Linear epidermal nevus

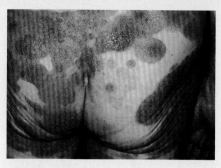

Geographic
Example: Mycosis fungoides

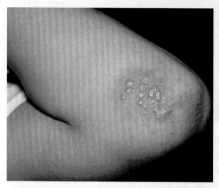

Clustered
Example: Grouped vesicles of herpes simplex

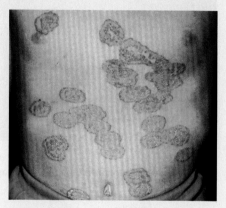

Serpiginous
Example: Tinea corporis

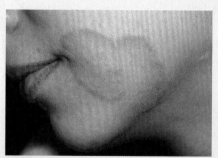

Annular, arciform
Example: Annular plaque of tinea faciale (ringworm)

Sources of photos: *Linear Epidermal Nevus, Herpes Simplex, Tinea Faciale*—Goodheart HP. Goodheart's Photoguide of Common Skin Disorders: Diagnosis and Management, 2nd ed. Philadelphia: Lippincott Williams & Wilkins, 2003; *Mycosis Fungoides, Tinea Corporis*—Hall JC. Sauer's Manual of Skin Diseases, 8th ed. Philadelphia: Lippincott Williams & Wilkins, 2000.

Table 6-4 Primary Skin Lesions *(initial presentation)*

Flat, Nonpalpable Lesions With Changes in Skin Color

Macule—Small flat spot, up to 1.0 cm

Patch—Flat spot, 1.0 cm or larger

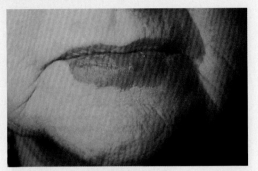

HEMANGIOMA

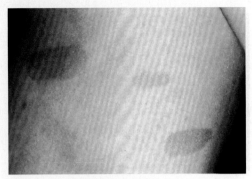

CAFÉ-AU-LAIT SPOT

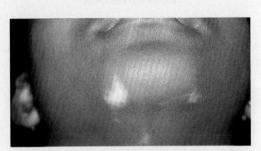

VITILIGO

Palpable Elevations: Solid Bumps

Plaque—Elevated lesion 1.0 cm or larger, often formed by coalescence of papules

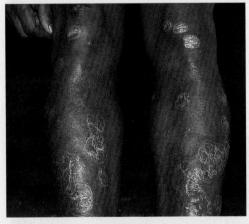

PSORIASIS

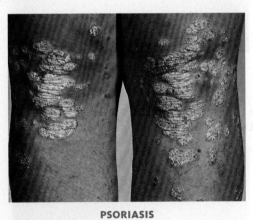

PSORIASIS

(table continues on page 188)

Table 6-4 **Primary Skin Lesions** *(initial presentation)* (*continued*)

Papule—Up to 1.0 cm

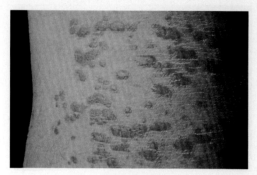

PSORIASIS

Nodule—Knot-like lesion larger than 0.5 cm, deeper and firmer than a papule

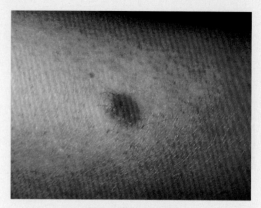

DERMATOFIBROMA

Cyst—Nodule filled with expressible material, either liquid or semisolid

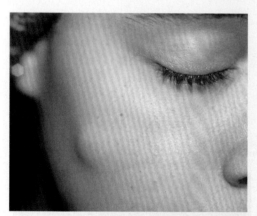

EPIDERMAL INCLUSION CYST

Wheal—A somewhat irregular, relatively transient, superficial area of localized skin edema

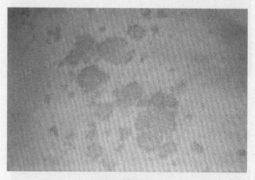

URTICARIA

Palpable Elevations With Fluid-Filled Cavities
Vesicle—Up to 1.0 cm; filled with serous fluid

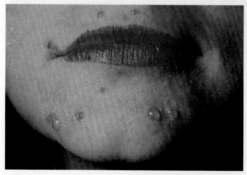

HERPES SIMPLEX

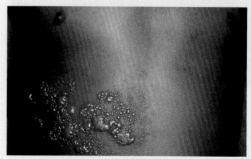

HERPES ZOSTER

Bulla—1.0 cm or larger; filled with serous fluid

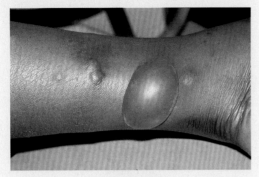

INSECT BITE

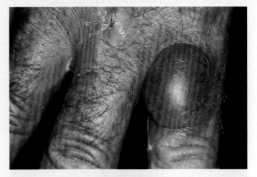

INSECT BITE

Pustule—Filled with pus (yellow proteinaceous fluid filled with neutrophils)

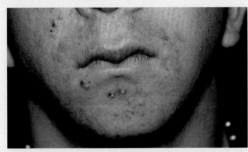

ACNE

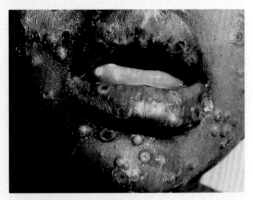

SMALL POX

Burrow (scabies)—A minute, slightly raised tunnel in the epidermis, commonly found on the finger webs and on the sides of the fingers. It looks like a short (5–15 mm), linear or curved gray line and may end in a tiny vesicle. Skin lesions include small papules, pustules, lichenified areas, and excoriations. With a magnifying lens, look for the *burrow* of the mite that causes scabies.

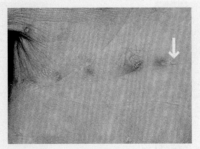

SCABIES

Sources of photos: *Hemangioma, Café-au-Lait Spot, Psoriasis* [bottom], *Dermatofibroma, Herpes Simplex, Herpes Zoster, Insect Bite* [right]—Hall JC. Sauer's Manual of Skin Diseases, 9th ed. Philadelphia: Lippincott Williams & Wilkins, 2006; *Vitiligo, Psoriasis* [top], *Epidermal Inclusion Cyst, Urticaria, Insect Bite* [left], *Acne, Scabies*—Goodheart HP, Goodheart's Photoguide of Common Skin Disorders: Diagnosis and Management, 2nd ed. Philadelphia: Lippincott Williams & Wilkins, 2003; *Small Pox*—Ostler, HB, Mailbach HI, Hoke AW et al. Diseases of the Eye and Skin: A Color Atlas. Philadelphia: Lippincott Williams & Wilkins, 2004.

Table 6-5

Secondary Skin Lesions *(seen in overtreatment, excess scratching, infection of primary lesions)*

Scale—A thin flake of dead exfoliated epidermis.

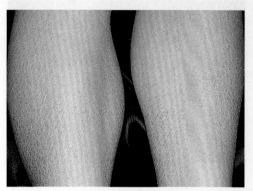

ICHTHYOSIS VULGARIS

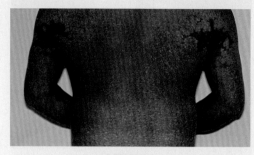

DRY SKIN

Crust—The dried residue of skin exudates such as serum, pus, or blood

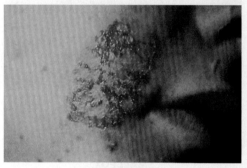

IMPETIGO

Lichenification—Visible and palpable thickening of the epidermis and roughening of the skin with increased visibility of the normal skin furrows (often from chronic rubbing)

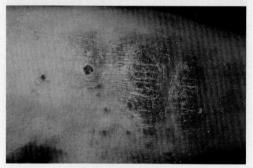

NEURODERMATITIS

Scars—Increased connective tissue that arises from injury or disease

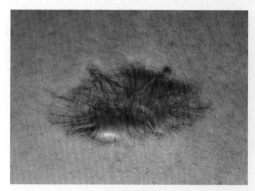

HYPERTROPHIC SCAR FROM STEROID INJECTIONS

Keloids—Hypertrophic scarring that extends beyond the borders of the initiating injury

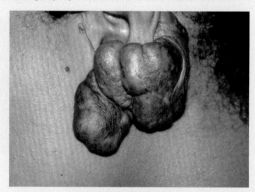

KELOID—EAR LOBE

Table 6-6 **Secondary Skin Lesions—Depressed**

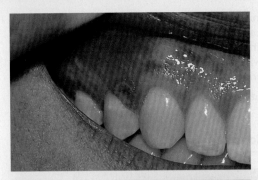

Erosion—Nonscarring loss of the superficial epidermis; surface is moist but does not bleed

    Example: Aphthous stomatitis, moist area after the rupture of a vesicle, as in chickenpox

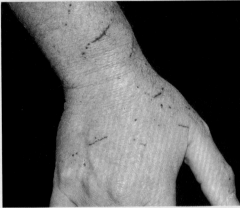

Excoriation—Linear or punctate erosions caused by scratching

    Example: Cat scratches

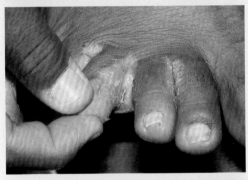

Fissure—A linear crack in the skin, often resulting from excessive dryness

    Example: Athlete's foot

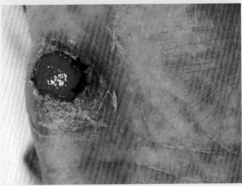

Ulcer—A deeper loss of epidermis and dermis; may bleed and scar

    Examples: Stasis ulcer of venous insufficiency, syphilitic chancre

Sources of photos: *Erosion, Excoriation, Fissure*—Goodheart HP. Goodheart's Photoguide of Common Skin Disorders: Diagnosis and Management, 2nd ed. Philadelphia: Lippincott Williams & Wilkins, 2003; *Ulcer*—Hall JC. Sauer's Manual of Skin Diseases, 8th ed. Philadelphia: Lippincott Williams & Wilkins, 2000.

Table
6-7   Acne Vulgaris—Primary and Secondary Lesions

Acne vulgaris is the most common cutaneous disorder in the United States, affecting more than 85% of adolescents.[20] Acne is a disorder of the pilosebaceous unit that involves proliferation of the keratinocytes at the opening of the follicle; increased production of sebum, stimulated by androgens, which combines with keratinocytes to plug the follicular opening; growth of *Propionibacterium acnes*, an anaerobic diphtheroid normally found on the skin; and inflammation from bacterial activity and release of free fatty acids and enzymes from activated neutrophils. Cosmetics, humidity, heavy sweating, and stress are contributing factors.

Lesions appear in areas with the greatest number of sebaceous glands, namely the face, neck, chest, upper back, and upper arms. They may be primary, secondary, or mixed.

Primary Lesions	Secondary Lesions

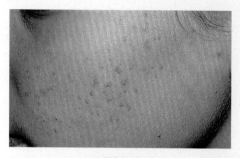

Mild Acne
Open and closed comedones, occasional papules

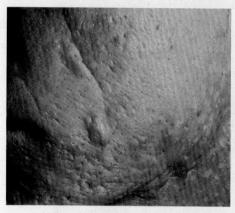

Acne With Pitting and Scars

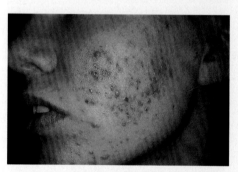

Moderate Acne
Comedones, papules, pustules

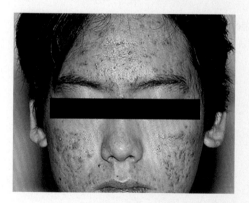

Severe Cystic Acne

Table 6-8   Vascular and Purpuric Lesions of the Skin

Vascular Lesions

	Spider Angioma*	Spider Vein*	Cherry Angioma
Color and Size	Fiery red. From very small to 2 cm	Bluish. Size variable, from very small to several inches	Bright or ruby red; may become purplish with age. 1–3 mm
Shape	Central body, sometimes raised, surrounded by erythema and radiating legs	Variable. May resemble a spider or be linear, irregular, cascading	Round, flat or sometimes raised, may be surrounded by a pale halo
Pulsatility and Effect of Pressure	Often seen in center of the spider, when pressure with a glass slide is applied. Pressure on the body causes blanching of the spider.	Absent. Pressure over the center does not cause blanching, but diffuse pressure blanches the veins.	Absent. May show partial blanching, especially if pressure applied with edge of a pinpoint
Distribution	Face, neck, arms, and upper trunk; almost never below the waist	Most often on the legs, near veins; also on the anterior chest	Trunk; also extremities
Significance	Liver disease, pregnancy, vitamin B deficiency; also occurs normally in some people	Often accompanies increased pressure in the superficial veins, as in varicose veins	None; increases in size and numbers with aging

Purpuric Lesions

	Petechia/Purpura	Ecchymosis
	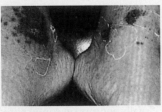	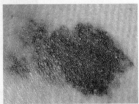
Color and Size	Deep red or reddish purple, fading away over time. Petechia, 1–3 mm; purpura are larger	Purple or purplish blue, fading to green, yellow, and brown with time. Variable size, larger than petechiae, >3 mm
Shape	Rounded, sometimes irregular; flat	Rounded, oval, or irregular; may have a central subcutaneous flat nodule (a hematoma)
Pulsatility and Effect of Pressure	Absent. No effect from pressure	Absent. No effect from pressure
Distribution	Variable	Variable
Significance	Blood outside the vessels; may suggest a bleeding disorder or, if petechiae, emboli to skin; palpable purpura in *vasculitis*	Blood outside the vessels; often secondary to bruising or trauma; also seen in bleeding disorders

*These are telangiectasias, or dilated small vessels that look red or bluish.

Sources of photos: *Spider Angioma*—Marks R. Skin Disease in Old Age. Philadelphia: JB Lippincott, 1987; *Petechia/Purpura*—Kelley WN. Textbook of Internal Medicine. Philadelphia: JB Lippincott, 1989.

Table 6-9   Skin Tumors

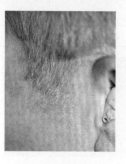
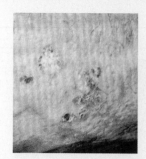

Actic Keratosis

Superficial, hyperkeratotic papules. Often multiple; can be round or irregular; pink, tan, or grayish. Appear on sun-exposed skin of older, fair-skinned people. Considered to be dysplastic or precancerous; one of every 1,000 per year develop into squamous cell carcinoma (suggested by continued growth, induration, redness at the base, and ulceration). Keratoses on face and hand, typical locations, are shown.

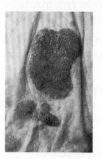
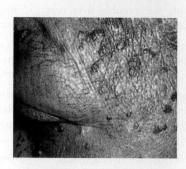

Seborrheic Keratosis

Common, benign, whitish-yellowish to brown raised papules or plaques that feel slightly greasy and velvety or warty and have a "stuck on" appearance. Typically multiple and symmetrically distributed on the trunk of older people, but may also appear on the face and elsewhere. In black people, often in younger women, may appear as small, deeply pigmented papules on the cheeks and temples (*dermatosis papulosa nigra*).

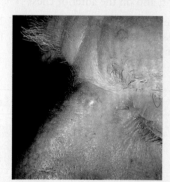

Basal Cell Carcinoma

A basal cell carcinoma, though malignant, grows slowly and almost never metastasizes. It is most common in fair-skinned adults 40 years or older, and usually appears on the face. An initial red macule or papule may develop a depressed center and a firm, elevated border. Telangiectatic vessels are often visible.

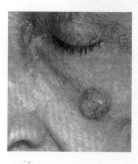
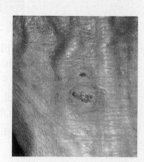

Squamous Cell Carcinoma

Usually appears on sun-exposed skin of fair-skinned adults older than 60 years. May develop in an actinic keratosis. Usually grows more quickly than a basal cell carcinoma, is firmer, and looks redder. The face and the dorsum of the hand are often affected, as shown here.

Sources of photos: *Basal Cell Carcinoma*—Rapini R. *Squamous Cell Carcinoma, Actinic Keratosis, Seborrheic Keratosis*—Hall JC. Sauer's Manual of Skin Diseases, 9th ed. Philadelphia: Lippincott, Williams & Wilkins, 2006.

Table
6-10 Benign and Malignant Nevi

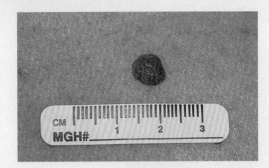

Benign Nevus

The *benign nevus*, or common mole, usually appears in the first few decades. Several nevi may arise at the same time, but their appearance usually remains unchanged. Note the following typical features and contrast them with those of atypical nevi and melanoma:

- Round or oval shape
- Sharply defined borders
- Uniform color, especially skin-colored, tan or brown
- Diameter <6 mm but >10 mm if congenital
- Flat or raised surface

Changes in these features raise the spectre of *atypical (dysplastic) nevi,* or melanoma. Atypical nevi are varied in color but often dark and larger than 6 mm, with irregular borders that fade into the surrounding skin. Look for atypical nevi primarily on the trunk. They may number more than 50 to 100.

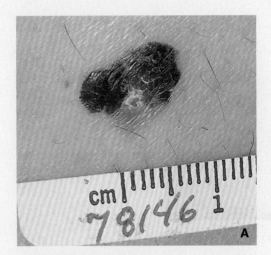

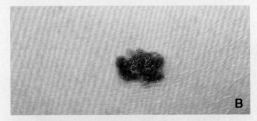

Malignant Melanoma

Learn the **ABCDEs** of melanoma from these reference standard photographs from the American Cancer Society:

- *Asymmetry* (Fig. A)
- Irregular *Borders*, especially notching (Fig. B)
- Variation in *Color*, especially mixtures of black, blue, white and red (Figs. B, C)
- *Diameter* >6 mm (Fig. C)
- *Evolution* or change in size, symptoms or morphology

Review *melanoma risk factors* such as intense year-round sun exposure, blistering sunburns in childhood, fair skin that freckles or burns easily (especially if blond or red hair), family history of melanoma, and nevi that are changing or atypical, especially if the patient is older than 50 years. Changing nevi may have new swelling or redness beyond the border, scaling, oozing, or bleeding, or sensations such as itching, burning, or pain.

On darker skin, look for melanomas under the nails, on the hands, or on the soles of the feet.

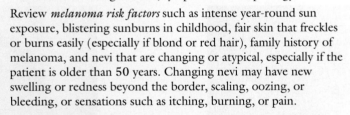

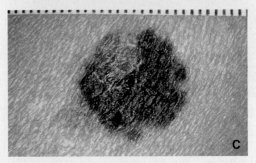

Source: Courtesy of American Cancer Society; American Academy of Dermatology

Table	
6-11	**Skin Lesions in Context**

This table shows a variety of primary and secondary skin lesions. Try to identify them, including those indicated by letters, before reading the accompanying text.

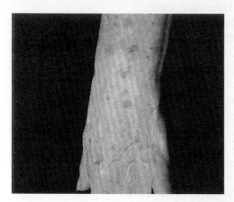

Macules on the dorsum of the hand, wrist, and forearm (*solar lentigines*)

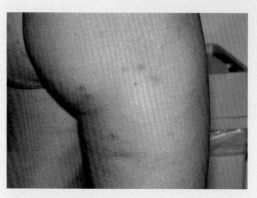

Papules and pustules (in hot tub folliculitis from *Pseudomonas*)

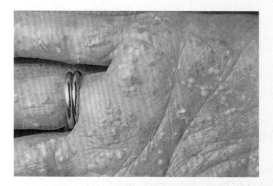

Pustules on the palm (*pustular psoriasis*)

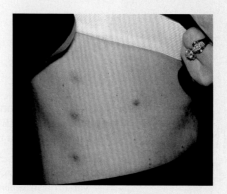

Vesicles (*chickenpox*)

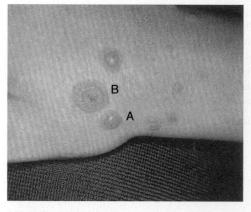

(A) Bulla, (B) target (or iris) lesion (in *erythema multiforme*)

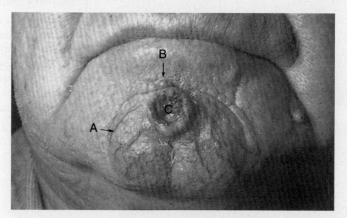

(A) Telangiectasia, (B) nodule, (C) ulcer (in *squamous cell carcinoma*)

Sources of photos: Hall JC. Sauer's Manual of Skin Diseases, 9th ed. Philadelphia: Lippincott Williams & Wilkins, 2006; *Kaposi's Sarcoma in AIDS*—DeVita VT Jr, Hellman S, Rosenberg SA, eds. AIDS: Etiology, Diagnosis, Treatment, and Prevention. Philadelphia: JB Lippincott, 1985; *Psoriasis, Papules, Vesicles [chickenpox]*—Goodheart HP. Goodheart's Photoguide of Common Skin Disorders: Diagnosis and Management, 2nd ed. Philadelphia: Lippincott Williams & Wilkins, 2003.

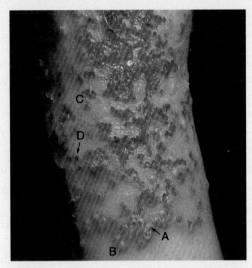

(A) Vesicle, (B) pustule, (C) erosions, (D) crust, on the back of a knee (in *infected atopic dermatitis*)

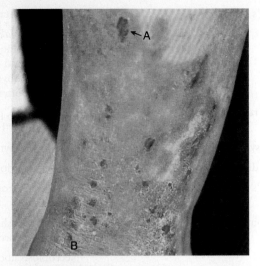

(A) Excoriation, (B) lichenification on the leg (in *atopic dermatitis*)

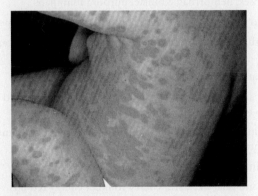

Wheals (*urticaria*) in a drug eruption in an infant

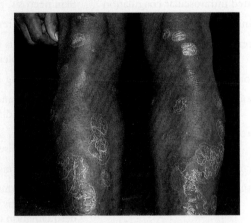

Plaques with scales on knee (*psoriasis*) and legs

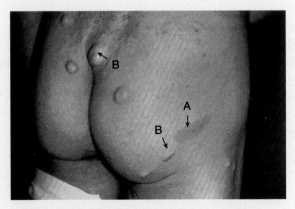

(A) Patch (café-au-lait spots), (B) nodules—a combination typical of neurofibromatosis.

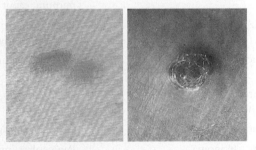

Kaposi's sarcoma in AIDS: This malignant tumor may appear in many forms: macules, papules, plaques, or nodules almost anywhere on the body. Lesions are often multiple and may involve internal structures. On left: ovoid, pinkish red plaques that typically lengthen along the skin line may become pigmented. On right: a purplish red nodule on the foot.

| Table 6-12 | Diseases and Related Skin Conditions |

Addison's disease	Hyperpigmentation of skin and mucous membranes
AIDS	*Hairy leukoplakia*, *Kaposi's sarcoma*, herpes simplex virus (HSV), human papillomavirus (HPV), cytomegalovirus (CMV), molluscum contagiosum, mycobacterial skin infections, candidiasis and other cutaneous fungal infections, oral and anal squamous cell carcinoma, acquired ichthyosis, bacterial abscesses, *psoriasis* (often severe), erythroderma, seborrheic dermatitis (often severe)
Chronic renal disease	Pallor, xerosis, pruritus, hyperpigmentation, uremic frost, metastatic calcification in the skin, calciphylaxis, "half and half" nails, hemodialysis-related skin disease
CREST syndrome	Calcinosis, Raynaud's phenomenon, sclerodactyly, *telangiectasias*
Crohn's disease	Erythema nodosum, pyoderma gangrenosum, enterocutaneous fistulas, aphthous ulcers
Cushing's disease	Striae, skin atrophy, purpura, ecchymoses, telangiectasias, acne, moon facies, buffalo hump, hypertrichosis
Dermatomyositis	Heliotrope rash, Gottron's papules, periungual telangiectasias, alopecia, poikiloderma in sun-exposed areas, Raynaud's phenomenon
Diabetes	Necrobiosis lipoidica diabeticorum, diabetic bullae, diabetic dermopathy, granuloma annulare, acanthosis nigricans, candidiasis, neuropathic ulcers, eruptive xanthomas, peripheral vascular disease
Disseminated intravascular coagulation	Skin necrosis, petechiae, ecchymoses, hemorrhagic bullae, purpura fulminans
Dyslipidemias	Xanthomas (tendon, eruptive, and tuberous), xanthelasma (may occur in healthy people)
Gonococcemia	Erythematous macules to hemorrhagic pustules; lesions in acral distribution that can involve palms and soles
Hemochromatosis	Skin bronzing and hyperpigmentation
Hypothyroidism	Dry, rough, and pale skin; coarse and brittle hair; myxedema; alopecia (lateral third of the eyebrows to diffuse); skin cool to touch; thin and brittle nails
Hyperthyroidism	Warm, moist, soft, and velvety skin; thin and fine hair; alopecia; vitiligo; pretibial myxedema (in Graves' disease); hyperpigmentation (local or generalized)
Infective endocarditis	Janeway lesions, Osler nodes, splinter hemorrhages, petechiae
Kawasaki disease	Mucosal erythema (lips, tongue, and pharynx), strawberry tongue, cherry red lips, polymorphous rash (primarily on trunk), erythema of palms and soles with later desquamation of fingertips
Liver disease	*Jaundice*, *spider angiomas* and other telangiectasias, palmar erythema, *Terry's nails*, pruritus, purpura, caput medusae
Leukemia/lymphoma	Pallor, exfoliative erythroderma, nodules, *petechiae*, ecchymoses, pruritus, vasculitis, pyoderma gangrenosum, bullous diseases
Meningococcemia	Pink macules and papules, *petechiae*, hemorrhagic petechiae, hemorrhagic bullae, purpura fulminans
Neurofibromatoses 1 (von Recklinghausen's syndrome)	*Neurofibromas*, café-au-lait spots, freckling in the axillary and inguinal areas, plexiform neurofibroma
Pancreatitis (hemorrhagic)	Grey Turner sign, Cullen's sign, panniculitis
Pancreatic carcinoma	Panniculitis, migratory thrombophlebitis

Peripheral vascular disease	Dry, scaly, shiny atrophic skin; dystrophic, brittle toenails; cool skin; hairless shins; ulcers; pallor; cyanosis; gangrene
Pregnancy (physiologic changes)	Melasma, increased pigmentation of areolae, linea nigra, palmar erythema, varicose veins, striae, *spider angiomas*, hirsutism, pyogenic granuloma
Reiter's syndrome	Psoriasis-like skin and mucous membrane lesions, keratoderma blennorrhagicum, balanitis circinata
Rheumatoid arthritis	Vasculitis, *Raynaud's phenomenon*, rheumatoid nodules, pyoderma gangrenosum, rheumatoid papules, erythematous to salmon-colored rashes
Rocky Mountain spotted fever	Erythematous rash that begins on wrists and ankles, then spreads to palms and soles; becomes more purpuric as it generalizes
Scleroderma	Thickened, taut, and shiny skin; ulcerations and pitted scars on fingertips; sclerodactyly; telangiectasias; Raynaud's phenomenon
Sickle cell	Jaundice, *leg ulcers* (malleolar regions), pallor
Syphilis	*First-degree: Chancre* (painless) (see p. 534)
	Second-degree: Rash ("the great imitator")—generalized, maculopapular rash that involves the palms and soles, pustules, condylomata lata, alopecia ("moth-eaten"), white plaques on oral and genital mucosa
	Third-degree: Gummas, granulomas
Systemic lupus erythematosus	Photosensitivity, malar (butterfly) rash, discoid rash, alopecia, vasculitis, oral ulcers, Raynaud's phenomenon
Thrombocytopenic purpura	*Petechiae, ecchymoses*
Tuberous sclerosis	Adenoma sebaceum (angiofibromas), ash-leaf spots, shagreen patch, periungal fibromas
Ulcerative colitis	*Erythema nodosum*, pyoderma gangrenosum
Viral exanthems	
Coxsackie A (hand, foot, and mouth)	Oral ulcers; macules, papules, and vesicles on hands, feet, and buttocks
Erythema infectiosum (fifth disease)	Erythema of cheeks ("slapped cheeks") followed by erythematous, pruritic, reticulated (net-like) rash that starts on trunk and proximal extremities (rash worsens with sun, fever, and temperature changes)
Roseola infantum (HSV 6)	Erythematous, maculopapular, discrete rash (often fever present) that begins on head and spreads to involve trunk and extremities, petechiae on soft palate
Rubella (German measles)	Erythematous, maculopapular, discrete less confluent rash (often fever present) that begins on head and spreads to involve trunk and extremities, petechiae on soft palate
Rubeola (measles)	Erythematous, maculopapular rash that begins on head and spreads to involve trunk and extremities (lesions become confluent on face and trunk, but are discrete on extremities), Koplik spots on buccal mucosa
Varicella (chickenpox)	Generalized, pruritic, vesicular (vesicles on an erythematous base, "dewdrop on a rose petal") rash begins on trunk and spreads peripherally, lesions appear in crops and are in different stages of healing
Herpes zoster (shingles)	Pruritic or painful vesicular rash (vesicles on an erythematous base) in a dermatomal distribution

Table
6-13   Pressure Ulcers

Pressure (*decubitus*) ulcers usually develop over bony prominences subject to unrelieved pressure, resulting in ischemic damage to underlying tissue. Prevention is important: inspect the skin thoroughly for *early warning signs of erythema that still blanches with pressure*, especially in patients with risk factors. Pressure ulcers form most commonly over the sacrum, ischial tuberosities, greater trochanters, and heels. A commonly applied staging system, based on depth of destroyed tissue, is illustrated below. Note that necrosis or eschar must be débrided before ulcers can be staged. Ulcers may not progress sequentially through the four stages.

Inspect ulcers for signs of infection (drainage, odor, cellulitis, or necrosis). Fever, chills, and pain suggest underlying **osteomyelitis**. Address the patient's overall health, including *comorbid conditions* such as vascular disease, diabetes, immune deficiencies, collagen vascular disease, malignancy, psychosis, or depression; nutritional status; pain and level of analgesia; risk for recurrence; psychosocial factors such as learning ability, social supports, and lifestyle; and evidence of polypharmacy, overmedication, or abuse of alcohol, tobacco, or illicit drugs.[21,22]

Risk Factors for Pressure Ulcers

- Decreased mobility, especially if accompanied by increased pressure or movement causing friction or shear stress
- Decreased sensation, from brain or spinal cord lesions or peripheral nerve disease

- Decreased blood flow from hypotension or microvascular disease such as diabetes or atherosclerosis
- Fecal or urinary incontinence
- Presence of fracture
- Poor nutritional status or low albumin

Stage I

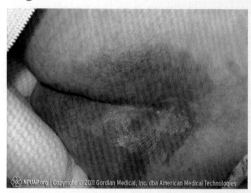

Presence of a reddened area that fails to blanche with pressure, and changes in temperature (warmth or coolness), consistency (firm or boggy), sensation (pain or itching), or color (red, blue, or purple on darker skin; red on lighter skin)

Stage II

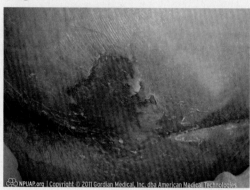

The skin forms a blister or sore. Partial-thickness skin loss or ulceration involving the epidermis, dermis, or both

Stage III

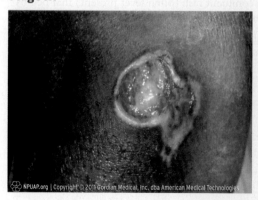

A crater appears in the skin, with full-thickness skin loss and damage to or necrosis of subcutaneous tissue that may extend to, but not through, underlying muscle

Stage IV

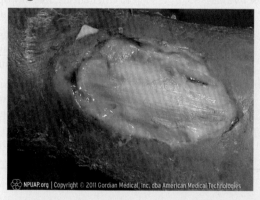

The pressure ulcer deepens. There is full-thickness skin loss, with destruction, tissue necrosis, or damage to underlying muscle, bone, and sometimes tendons and joints

Source: National Pressure Ulcer Advisory Panel, Reston, VA.

Table

6-14 | Hair Loss

Alopecia Areata

Clearly demarcated round or oval patches of hair loss, usually affecting young adults and children. There is no visible scaling or inflammation.

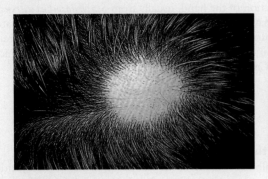
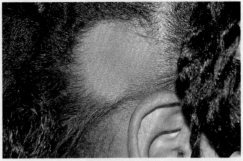

Trichotillomania (Trichotillosis)

Hair loss from pulling, plucking, or twisting hair. Hair shafts are broken and of varying lengths. More common in children, often in settings of family or psychosocial stress.

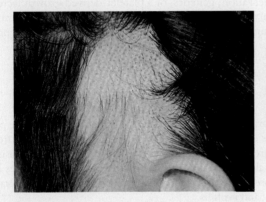
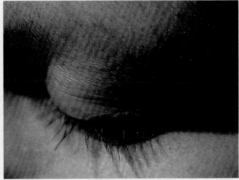

Tinea Capitis ("Ringworm")

Round scaling patches of alopecia. Hairs are broken off close to the surface of the scalp. Usually caused by fungal infection from *Trichophyton tonsurans* from humans, less commonly from *microsporum canis* from dogs or cats. Mimics seborrheic dermatitis.

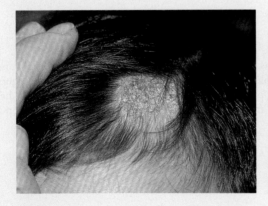
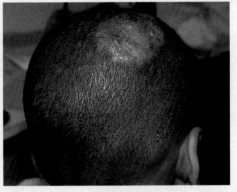

Table 6-15   **Findings in or Near the Nails**

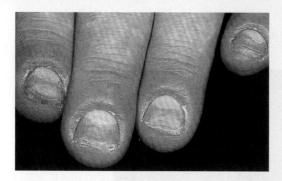

Paronychia

A superficial infection of the proximal and lateral nail folds adjacent to the nail plate. The nail folds are often red, swollen, and tender. Represents the most common infection of the hand, usually from *Staphylococcus aureus* or *Streptococcus* species, and may spread until it completely surrounds the nail plate. Creates a felon if it extends into the pulp space of the finger. Arises from local trauma due to nail biting, manicuring, or frequent hand immersion in water. Chronic infections may be related to *Candida*.

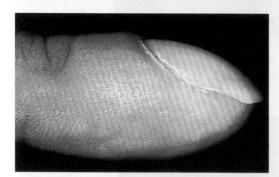

Clubbing of the Fingers

Clinically a bulbous swelling of the soft tissue at the nail base, with loss of the normal angle between the nail and the proximal nail fold. The angle increases to 180° or more, and the nail bed feels spongy or floating. The mechanism is still unknown but involves vasodilatation with increased blood flow to the distal portion of the digits and changes in connective tissue, possibly from hypoxia, changes in innervation, genetics, or a platelet-derived growth factor from fragments of platelet clumps. Seen in congenital heart disease, interstitial lung disease and lung cancer, inflammatory bowel diseases, and malignancies.[23]

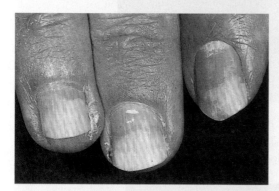

Onycholysis

A painless separation of the whitened opaque nail plate from the pinker translucent nail bed. Starts distally and progresses proximally, enlarging the free edge of the nail. Local causes include trauma from excess manicuring, psoriasis, fungal infection, and allergic reactions to nail cosmetics. Systemic causes include diabetes, anemia, photosensitive drug reactions, hyperthyroidism, peripheral ischemia, bronchiectasis, and syphilis.

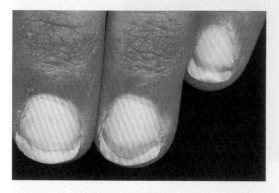

Terry's Nails

Nail plate turns white with a ground-glass appearance, a distal band of reddish brown, and obliteration of the lunula. Commonly affects all fingers, although may appear in only one finger. Seen in liver disease, usually cirrhosis, heart failure, and diabetes. May arise from decreased vascularity and increased connective tissue in nail bed.

Sources of photos: *Clubbing of the Fingers, Paronychia, Onycholysis, Terry's Nails*—Habif TP. Clinical Dermatology: A Color Guide to Diagnosis and Therapy, 2nd ed. St. Louis: CV Mosby, 1990; *White Spots, Transverse White Lines, Psoriasis, Beau's Lines*—Sams WM Jr, Lynch PJ. Principles and Practice of Dermatology. New York: Churchill Livingstone, 1990.

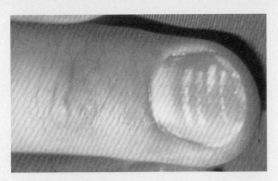

White Spots (*Leukonychia*)

Trauma to the nails is commonly followed by nonuniform white spots that grow slowly out with the nail. Spots in the pattern illustrated are typical of overly vigorous and repeated manicuring. The curves in this example resemble the curve of the cuticle and proximal nail fold.

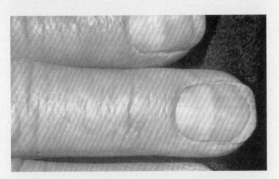

Transverse White Bands (*Mees' Lines*)

Curving transverse white bands that cross the nail parallel to the lunula. Arising from the disrupted matrix of the proximal nail, they vary in width and move distally as the nail grows out. Seen in arsenic poisoning, heart failure, Hodgkin's disease, chemotherapy, carbon monoxide poisoning, and leprosy.[24]

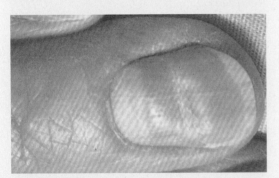

Transverse Linear Depressions (*Beau's Lines*)

Transverse depressions of the nail plates, usually bilateral, resulting from temporary disruption of proximal nail growth from systemic illness. As with Mees' lines, timing of the illness may be estimated by measuring the distance from the line to the nail bed (nails grow approximately 1 mm every 6 to 10 days). Seen in severe illness, trauma, and cold exposure if Raynaud's disease is present.[24,25]

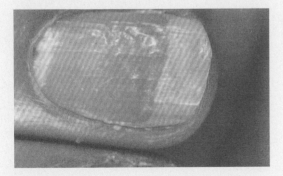

Pitting

Punctate depressions of the nail plate caused by defective layering of the superficial nail plate by the proximal nail matrix. Usually associated with psoriasis but also seen in Reiter's syndrome, sarcoidosis, alopecia areata, and localized atopic or chemical dermatitis.[24]

White Spots (Leukopathy)

Transverse White Bands (Mees' Lines)

Transverse Linear Depressions (Beau's lines)

Pitting

The Head and Neck

Guide to Chapter Organization

Many critical structures like the sensory organs, cranial nerves, and major blood vessels originate in the head and neck. To help students relate anatomy and physiology to physical examination skills, this chapter follows a unique format. Symptoms and prevention strategies for conditions of the head and neck are often interrelated, so the content for the Head and Neck in the Health History and the Health Promotion and Counseling sections remains integrated. However, for each of the individual "HEENT" (Head, Eyes, Ears, Nose, and Throat) components, Anatomy and Physiology and the relevant Techniques of Examination are grouped together, as outlined below.

Chapter Overview

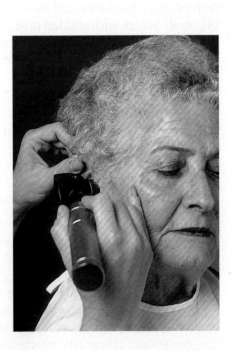

▶ Health History
▶ Health Promotion and Counseling
▶ Examination of the Head and Neck: Anatomy and Physiology and Techniques of Examination are combined for:

   Head—pp. 214–215
   Eyes—pp. 215–232
   Ears—pp. 232–238
   Nose and Paranasal Sinuses—pp. 238–241
   Mouth and Pharynx—pp. 242–246
   Neck—pp. 247–254

▶ Recording Your Findings
▶ Bibliography
▶ Tables

The Health History

Common or Concerning Symptoms

- Headache
- Change in vision: hyperopia, presbyopia, myopia, scotomas
- Double vision, or diplopia
- Hearing loss, earache, tinnitus
- Vertigo
- Nosebleed, or epistaxis
- Sore throat, hoarseness
- Swollen glands
- Goiter

THE HEAD

Headache is one of the most common symptoms in clinical practice, with a lifetime prevalence of 30% in the general population.[1-3] Among types of headaches, *migraine* predominates, approaching 80% with careful diagnosis. Headaches are generally classified as primary or secondary. However, every headache warrants careful evaluation for life-threatening causes such as meningitis, subarachnoid hemorrhage, or mass lesion. Elicit a full description of every headache and its seven attributes (see p. 70). Is it unilateral or bilateral? Severe with sudden onset, like a thunderclap? Steady or throbbing? Continuous or intermittent (comes and goes)?

See Tables 7-1 and 7-2 on Primary Headaches and Secondary Headaches; Cranial Neuralgias on pp. 259–261.

Primary headaches include migraine, tension, cluster, and chronic daily headaches; *secondary headaches* arise from underlying structural, systemic, or infectious causes such as meningitis or subarachnoid hemorrhage and may be life-threatening.[4]

Look for important signs ("red flags") that warn of headaches needing prompt investigation.

The *International Classification of Headache Disorders*, now in its second iteration, continues to evolve.[5-8]

Headache Warning Signs

- Progressively frequent or severe over a 3-month period
- Sudden onset like a "thunderclap" or "the worst headache of my life"
- New onset after age 50 years
- Aggravated or relieved by change in position
- Precipitated by Valsalva maneuver
- Associated symptoms of fever, night sweats, or weight loss
- Presence of cancer, HIV infection, or pregnancy
- Recent head trauma
- Associated papilledema, neck stiffness, or focal neurologic deficits

Thunderclap headaches reaching maximal intensity over several minutes occur in 70% of patients with *subarachnoid hemorrhage,* and are often preceded by a *sentinel leak headache* from a vascular leak into the subarachnoid space.[9]

The most important attributes of headache are its *severity* and *chronologic pattern*. Is the headache severe and of sudden onset? Does it intensify over several hours? Is it episodic? Chronic and recurring? Is there a recent change in pattern? Does the headache recur at the same time every day?

If headache is severe and of sudden onset, consider *subarachnoid hemorrhage* or *meningitis*.[9]

Migraine and *tension headaches* are episodic and tend to peak over several hours. New and persisting, progressively severe headaches raise concerns of *tumor*, *abscess*, or *mass lesion*.

After your usual open-ended assessment, ask the patient to *point to the area of pain or discomfort*.

Unilateral headache occurs in *migraine and cluster headaches*.[1,4] Tension headaches often arise in the temporal areas; cluster headaches may be retro-orbital.

Ask about associated symptoms such as nausea and vomiting.

Nausea and vomiting are common with *migraine* but also occur with *brain tumors* and *subarachnoid hemorrhage*.

Is there a prodrome of unusual feelings such as euphoria, craving for food, fatigue, or dizziness? Does the patient report an aura with neurologic symptoms, such as change in vision, numbness, or weakness?

Note that, due to increased risk of ischemic stroke and cardiovascular disease, the World Health Association advises women with migraines over age 35 and women with migraines with aura avoid use of estrogen-progestin contraceptives.[10–13]

Approximately 60% to 70% of patients with *migraine* have a symptom prodrome prior to onset. About a third experience a visual aura, such as spark photopsias (flashes of light), fortifications (zig-zag arcs of light), and scotomata (area of visual loss with surrounding normal vision).

Ask if coughing, sneezing, or changing the position of the head affects the headache.

Valsalva maneuvers may increase pain from *acute sinusitis* or from mass lesion due to changing intracranial pressure.

Is there any overuse of analgesics, ergotamines, or triptans?

Medication for overuse headache is indicated if present ≥15 days a month for three months and reverts to <15 days a month when the medication is discontinued.[14]

Ask about family history.

Genetic inheritance appears to be present in 30% to 50% of patients with migraine.[15]

THE EYES

Begin with open-ended questions such as "How is your vision?" and "Have you had any trouble with your eyes?" If the patient reports a change in vision, pursue the related details.

- Is vision worse during close work or at distances?

Difficulty with close work suggests *hyperopia* (farsightedness) or *presbyopia* (aging vision); with distances, *myopia* (nearsightedness).

- Is there blurred vision? If yes, is the onset sudden or gradual? If sudden and unilateral, is the visual loss painless or painful?

If sudden *unilateral* visual loss is *painless,* consider vitreous hemorrhage from diabetes or trauma, *macular degeneration, retinal detachment, retinal vein occlusion,* or *central retinal artery occlusion.* If *painful,* causes are usually in the cornea and anterior chamber as in *corneal ulcer, uveitis, traumatic hyphema,* and *acute glaucoma.*[16] *Optic neuritis* from multiple sclerosis may also be painful.[17] Immediate referral is warranted.[18]

- Sudden bilateral visual loss is rare.

If *bilateral and painless,* medications that change refraction such as cholinergics, anticholinergics, and steroids may contribute. If bilateral and painful, consider chemical or radiation exposures.

- Is the onset of bilateral visual loss gradual?

This usually arises from *cataracts* or *macular degeneration.*

- Location of visual loss may also be helpful. Is there blurring of the entire field of vision or only parts of it?

- If the visual field defect is partial, is it central, peripheral, or on only one side?

Slow central loss occurs in nuclear cataract (p. 268), *macular degeneration*[19] (p. 232); peripheral loss in advanced *open-angle glaucoma* (p. 262); one-sided loss in *hemianopsia* and *quadrantic defects* (p. 265).

- Are there specks in the vision or areas where the patient cannot see (*scotomas*)? If so, do they move around in the visual field with shifts in gaze or are they fixed?

Moving specks or strands suggest vitreous floaters; fixed defects, or *scotomas,* suggest lesions in the retina or visual pathways.

- Has the patient seen lights flashing across the field of vision? Vitreous floaters may accompany this symptom.

Flashing lights or new vitreous floaters suggest detachment of vitreous from retina. Prompt eye consultation is indicated.

- Does the patient wear glasses?

Ask about *pain* in or around the eyes, *redness,* and *excessive tearing or watering.*

See Table 7-3, Red Eyes, p. 262.

Check for *diplopia,* or double vision. If present, find out whether the images are side by side (horizontal diplopia) or on top of each other (vertical diplopia). Does diplopia persist with one eye closed? Which eye is affected?

One kind of horizontal diplopia is physiologic. Hold one finger upright approximately 6 inches in front of your face, a second at arm's length. When you focus on either finger, the image of the other is double. A patient who notices this phenomenon can be reassured.

Diplopia is seen in lesions in the brainstem or cerebellum, or weakness or paralysis of one or more extraocular muscles, as in horizontal diplopia from palsy of cranial nerve (CN) III or VI, or vertical diplopia from palsy of CN III or IV. Diplopia in one eye, with the other closed, suggests a problem in the cornea or lens.

THE EARS

Opening questions are "How is your hearing?" and "Have you had any trouble with your ears?" If the patient has noticed a *hearing loss,* does it involve one or both ears? Did it start suddenly or gradually? What are the associated symptoms, if any?

Hearing loss may also be congenital, from single gene mutations.[20]

Distinguish the type of hearing impairment: *conductive loss,* which results from problems in the external or middle ear, or *sensorineural loss,* from problems in the inner ear, the cochlear nerve, or its central connections in the brain.

Two questions may be helpful: Does the patient have special difficulty understanding people as they talk? What happens in a noisy environment?

People with *sensorineural loss* have particular trouble understanding speech, often complaining that others mumble; noisy environments make hearing worse. In *conductive loss,* noisy environments may help.

Pursue symptoms associated with hearing loss, such as earache or vertigo; these help sort out likely causes. Ask about medications that might affect hearing and about sustained exposure to loud noise.

Medications that affect hearing include aminoglycosides, aspirin, NSAIDs, quinine, and furosemide.

Complaints of *earache,* or *pain in the ear,* are especially common. Ask about associated fever, sore throat, cough, and concurrent upper respiratory infection.

Pain occurs in the external canal in *otitis externa* and, if respiratory infection, in the inner ear in *otitis media.*[21] It may also be referred from other structures in the mouth, throat, or neck.

Ask about *discharge from the ear,* especially if associated with earache or trauma.

Unusually soft wax, debris from inflammation or rash in the ear canal, or discharge through a perforated eardrum is present in *acute* or *chronic otitis media.*

Tinnitus is a perceived sound that has no external stimulus—commonly a musical ringing or a rushing or roaring noise in one or both ears. Tinnitus may accompany hearing loss and often remains unexplained. Occasionally, popping sounds originate in the temporomandibular joint, or vascular noises from the neck may be audible.

Tinnitus is a common symptom, increasing in frequency with age. When associated with hearing loss and vertigo, it suggests *Ménière's disease.*

Vertigo refers to the perception that the patient or the environment is rotating or spinning. These sensations point primarily to a problem in the labyrinths of the inner ear, peripheral lesions of CN VIII, or lesions in its central pathways or nuclei in the brain.

See Table 7-4, Dizziness and Vertigo, p. 263.

Complaints of *dizziness* and *light-headedness* are challenging because they are often non-specific and can signify a spectrum of conditions ranging from vertigo to presyncope, weakness, unsteadiness and disequilibrium. Clarify by asking what the patient means by dizziness. Then ask, "Do you feel as if the room is spinning or tilting (vertigo)? Do your symptoms get worse when you move your head?" *Vertigo* is the sensation of true rotational movement of the patient or the surroundings.[22] Ask, "Do you feel as if you are going to fall or pass out (*presyncope*)? . . . Or do you feel you are unsteady or losing your balance (*disequilibrium*)?"

If there is true vertigo, distinguish peripheral from central neurologic causes. Establish the time-course of symptoms. Check for nausea, vomiting, double vision, and gait disturbance. Review the patient's medications. Proceed with a careful neurologic examination focusing on presence of nystagmus and focal neurologic signs.

See Table 7-4, Dizziness and Vertigo, p. 263, for distinguishing symptoms and time-course.

Vertigo represents vestibular disease, usually from peripheral causes in the inner ear such as *benign positional vertigo, labyrinthitis,* and *Ménière's disease.* Ataxia, diplopia, and dysarthria signal central neurologic causes in the cerebellum or brainstem such as cerebral vascular disease or posterior fossa tumor; also consider *migraine.*[22] Feeling light-headed, weak in the legs, or about to faint points to *presyncope* from arrhythmia, orthostatic hypotension, or vasovagal stimulation.

THE NOSE AND SINUSES

Rhinorrhea refers to drainage from the nose and is often associated with *nasal congestion,* a sense of stuffiness or obstruction. These symptoms are frequently accompanied by sneezing, watery eyes, and throat discomfort, and itching in the eyes, nose, and throat.[23]

Causes include viral infections, *allergic rhinitis* ("hay fever"), and *vasomotor rhinitis.* Itching favors an allergic cause.

Do symptoms occur when colds are prevalent and last less than seven days? Do they occur seasonally when pollens are in the air? Are symptoms triggered by specific animal or environmental exposures?

Seasonal onset or environmental triggers suggest *allergic rhinitis.*

What remedies has the patient used? For how long? And how well do they work?

Drug-induced rhinitis occurs in excessive use of decongestants, or use of cocaine.

Is nasal or sinus congestion preceded by a viral upper respiratory tract infection (URI)? Is there purulent nasal discharge, loss of smell, tooth pain or facial pain made worse by bending forward, ear pressure, cough, or fever?

Acute bacterial sinusitis is unlikely until viral URI symptoms persist more than 7 days; both purulent drainage and facial pain should be present for diagnosis (sensitivity and specificity are above 50%).[24–28]

Ask about drugs that may induce nasal stuffiness.

Ask about oral contraceptives, reserpine, guanethidine, alcohol, cocaine.

Is the nasal congestion only on one side?

Consider a deviated nasal septum, nasal polyp, foreign body, granuloma (Wegener's), or carcinoma.

Epistaxis is bleeding from the nasal passages. Bleeding can also originate in the paranasal sinuses or nasopharynx. Note that bleeding from posterior nasal structures may pass into the throat instead of out the nostrils. Ask the patient to pinpoint the source of the bleeding. Is it from the nose, or has the patient actually coughed up or vomited blood, termed *hematemesis* and *hemoptysis*? These conditions have very different causes.

Local causes of epistaxis include trauma (especially nose-picking), inflammation, drying and crusting of the nasal mucosa, tumors, and foreign bodies.

Is epistaxis a recurrent problem? Has there been easy bruising or bleeding elsewhere in the body?

Anticoagulants, NSAIDs, and coagulopathies can contribute to epistaxis.

THE MOUTH, THROAT, AND NECK

Sore throat or *pharyngitis* is a frequent complaint, usually associated with an acute URI.

Centor's clinical prediction rule for *streptococcal* and *Fusobacterium necrophorum pharyngitis* helps guide diagnosis and treatment of bacterial infection: fever history, tonsillar exudates, swollen tender anterior cervical adenopathy, and absence of cough.[29–31]

A *sore tongue* may result from local lesions as well as from systemic illness.

Aphthous ulcers (p. 245); sore smooth tongue of nutritional deficiency (p. 289).

Bleeding from the gums, especially when brushing teeth, is a common symptom. Ask about local lesions and any tendency to bleed or bruise elsewhere.

Bleeding gums are most often caused by *gingivitis* (p. 287).

Hoarseness refers to a change in voice quality, often described as husky, rough, harsh, or lower-pitched than usual. Causes range from diseases of the larynx to extralaryngeal lesions that press on the laryngeal nerves.[32] Ask the patient about environmental allergies, acid reflux, smoking, and inhalation of fumes or other irritants.

If hoarseness is acute, voice overuse and *acute viral laryngitis* are the most likely causes.

Is the problem chronic, lasting more than 2 weeks? Is there prolonged tobacco or alcohol use, cough or hemoptysis, weight loss, or unilateral throat pain?

If hoarseness lasts more than 2 weeks, refer for laryngoscopy and consider causes such as hypothyroidism, reflux, vocal cord nodules, head and neck cancers, and neurologic disorders like *Parkinson disease, amyotrophic lateral sclerosis,* or *myasthenia gravis.*

Ask "Have you noticed any swollen glands or lumps in your neck?" because patients are more familiar with the lay terms than with "*lymph nodes.*"

Enlarged tender lymph nodes commonly accompany *pharyngitis.*

Assess thyroid function and ask about any evidence of an enlarged thyroid gland or *goiter.* To evaluate thyroid function, ask about *temperature intolerance* and *sweating.* Opening questions include, "Do you prefer hot or cold weather?" "Do you dress more warmly or less warmly than other people?"

With *goiter,* thyroid function may be increased, decreased, or normal.

"What about blankets . . . do you use more or fewer than others at home?" "Do you perspire more or less than others?" "Any new palpitations or change in weight?" Note that as people grow older, they sweat less, have less tolerance for cold, and tend to prefer warmer environments.

Intolerance to cold, preference for warm clothing and many blankets, and decreased sweating suggest *hypothyroidism*; the opposite symptoms, palpitations, and involuntary weight loss suggest *hyperthyroidism* (p. 291).

Health Promotion and Counseling: Evidence and Recommendations

Important Topics for Health Promotion and Counseling

▶ Loss of vision: cataracts, macular degeneration, glaucoma
▶ Hearing loss
▶ Oral health

Vision and hearing, critical senses for experiencing the world around us, are two areas of special importance for health promotion and counseling. Oral health, often overlooked, also merits clinical attention.

Loss of Vision. Vision disorders in healthy young adults are usually refractive errors. In older adults, eye disorders become more serious. Almost 10% of adults 60 years of age and older have impaired visual acuity; the prevalence of refractive errors, cataracts, macular degeneration, glaucoma, and blindness rises sharply over subsequent decades. These disorders reduce awareness of the social and physical environment and contribute to falls and injuries. Because onset can be gradual, those affected may not recognize their visual decline. The U.S. Preventive Services Task Force in 2009 found insufficient evidence to recommend screening despite numerous effective treatments.[33,34] Nonetheless, visual screening and early detection are standard components of older adult health care. Roughly 50% of cases of visual impairment are correctable, and about one-fourth are preventible.[35,36] Ask patients about any problems with face recognition, reading, or performing regular tasks, and test acuity with the Snellen chart or a handheld card. Refer patients with an impairment of ≥20/50 or a one-line difference between the eyes. Examine the lens and fundi to detect additional disorders.

See Chapter 20, Older Adult, pp. 917–966.

See techniques for testing acuity and using the Snellen eye chart on p. 221.

See pp. 221–232 for examination techniques. Look for clouding of the lens (*cataracts*), mottling of the macula, variations in retinal pigmentation, subretinal hemorrhage or exudates (*macular degeneration*), and change in color and size of the optic disc (*glaucoma*).

Risk factor surveillance for primary open-angle glaucoma (POAG) is especially important. However, in 2005, the U.S. Preventive Services Task Force found insufficient evidence for general screening because of the complexities of diagnosis and treatment.[37] Glaucoma is the leading cause of blindness in African Americans and the second leading cause of blindness overall. Approximately 2.5 million Americans are affected, and more than half are unaware of having the disease. In POAG, there is gradual loss of vision as a result of the loss of retinal ganglion cell axons, initial loss of peripheral visual fields, and pallor and increasing size of the optic cup, which enlarges to more than half the diameter of the optic disc. Blindness occurs in 5% of those with the disease. Risk factors include age older than 65 years, family history, African American descent, diabetes, myopia, and ocular hypertension (IOP ≥21 mm Hg). Not all people with POAG have elevated IOP, however, so tonometry is no longer recommended for screening. Diagnosis of optic disc enlargement is variable, even among experts, and the benefits of treatment, which may cause cataract formation, are unclear. Attention to risk factors and referral to eye specialists remain important tools for clinical care.

Hearing Loss. More than a third of adults older than 65 years have detectable hearing deficits, contributing to emotional isolation and social withdrawal.[38] These losses may go undetected. Unlike vision prerequisites for driving, there is no mandate for widespread hearing testing, and many seniors avoid using hearing aids. The U.S. Preventive Task Force recommends screening adults 50 years of age and older.[38] Questionnaires and handheld audioscopes work well for periodic screening. Less sensitive are the clinical "whisper test," rubbing fingers, or use of the tuning fork. Groups at risk are those with a history of congenital or familial hearing loss, syphilis, rubella, meningitis, or exposure to hazardous noise levels at work or on the battlefield.

Oral Health. Clinicians should play an active role in promoting oral health: up to half of all children 5 to 17 years have from one to eight cavities, and the average U.S. adult has 10 to 17 teeth that are decayed, missing, or filled.[39] In adults, the prevalence of gingivitis and periodontal disease is 50% and 80%, respectively. In the United States, more than half of all adults older than 65 years have no teeth at all. Effective screening begins with careful examination of the mouth. Inspect the oral cavity for decayed or loose teeth, inflammation of the gingiva, and signs of periodontal disease (bleeding, pus, recession of the gums, and bad breath). Inspect the mucous membranes, the palate, the oral floor, and the surfaces of the tongue for ulcers and leukoplakia, warning signs for oral cancer and HIV disease.

To improve oral health, counsel patients to adopt daily hygiene measures. Use of fluoride-containing toothpastes reduces tooth decay, and brushing and flossing retard periodontal disease by removing bacterial plaques. Urge patients to seek dental care at least annually to receive the benefits of more specialized preventive care such as scaling, planing of roots, and topical fluorides.

Diet, tobacco and alcohol use, changes in salivary flow from medication, and proper use of dentures should also be addressed. As with children, adults should avoid excessive intake of foods high in refined sugars such as sucrose, which enhance attachment and colonization of cariogenic bacteria. Use of all tobacco products and excessive alcohol, the principal risk factors for oral cancers, should be avoided.

Saliva cleanses and lubricates the mouth. Many medications reduce salivary flow, increasing risk for tooth decay, mucositis, and gum disease from xerostomia, especially for the elderly. For those wearing dentures, recommend removal and cleaning each night to reduce bacterial plaque and risk of malodor. Regular massage of the gums relieves soreness and pressure from dentures on the underlying soft tissue.

Anatomy and Physiology and Techniques of Examination

THE HEAD

Anatomy and Physiology

Regions of the head take their names from the underlying bones of the skull, for example, the frontal area. Knowing this anatomy helps to locate and describe physical findings.

Two paired salivary glands lie near the mandible: the *parotid gland,* superficial to and behind the mandible (both visible and palpable when enlarged), and the *submandibular gland,* located deep to the mandible. Feel for the latter as you bow and press your tongue against your lower incisors. Its lobular surface can often be felt against the tightened muscle. The openings of the parotid and submandibular ducts are visible within the oral cavity (see p. 244).

The *superficial temporal artery* passes upward just in front of the ear, where it is readily palpable. In many normal people, especially thin and elderly ones, the tortuous course of one of its branches can be traced across the forehead.

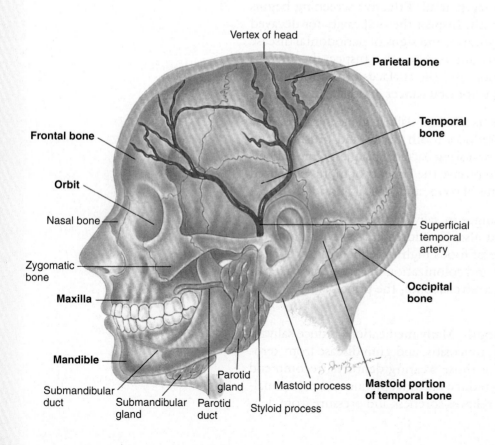

Vertex of head
Parietal bone
Temporal bone
Frontal bone
Orbit
Nasal bone
Zygomatic bone
Maxilla
Mandible
Submandibular duct
Submandibular gland
Parotid duct
Parotid gland
Styloid process
Mastoid process
Superficial temporal artery
Occipital bone
Mastoid portion of temporal bone

Techniques of Examination

Because abnormalities covered by the hair are easily missed, ask if the patient has noticed anything wrong with the scalp or hair. If you detect a hairpiece or wig, ask the patient to remove it.

Examine:

The Hair.   Note its quantity, distribution, texture, and any pattern of loss. You may see loose flakes of dandruff.

Fine hair is seen in *hyperthyroidism*; coarse hair in *hypothyroidism*. Tiny white ovoid granules that adhere to hairs may be nits (lice eggs).

The Scalp.   Part the hair in several places and look for scaliness, lumps, nevi, or other lesions.

Look for redness and scaling that may indicate *seborrheic dermatitis or psoriasis;* soft lumps that may be *pilar cysts* (wens); pigmented nevi.

The Skull.   Observe the general size and contour of the skull. Note any deformities, depressions, lumps, or tenderness. Learn to recognize the irregularities in a normal skull, such as those near the suture lines between the parietal and occipital bones.

An enlarged skull may signify *hydrocephalus* or *Paget's disease* of bone. Palpable tenderness or step-offs may be present after head trauma.

The Face.   Note the patient's facial expression and contours. Observe for asymmetry, involuntary movements, edema, and masses.

See Table 7-5, Selected Facies, p. 264.

The Skin.   Observe the skin, noting its color, pigmentation, texture, thickness, hair distribution, and any lesions.

Acne is found in many adolescents. *Hirsutism* (excessive facial hair) occurs in some women with *polycystic ovary syndrome.*

THE EYES

Anatomy and Physiology

Identify the structures illustrated at the right. Note that the upper eyelid covers a portion of the iris but does not normally overlay the pupil. The opening between the eyelids is called the *palpebral fissure.* The white sclera may look somewhat buff-colored at its periphery. Do not mistake this color for jaundice, which is a deeper yellow.

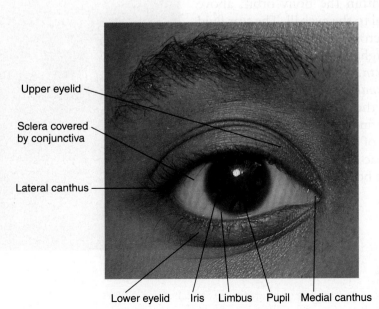

Upper eyelid

Sclera covered by conjunctiva

Lateral canthus

Lower eyelid   Iris   Limbus   Pupil   Medial canthus

The *conjunctiva* is a clear mucous membrane with two easily visible components. The *bulbar conjunctiva* covers most of the anterior eyeball, adhering loosely to the underlying tissue. It meets the cornea at the *limbus*. The *palpebral conjunctiva* lines the eyelids. The two parts of the conjunctiva merge in a folded recess that permits movement of the eyeball.

Within the eyelids lie firm strips of connective tissue called *tarsal plates*. Each plate contains a parallel row of *meibomian glands,* which open on the lid margin. The *levator palpebrae,* the muscle that raises the upper eyelid, is innervated by the oculomotor nerve, CN III. Smooth muscle, innervated by the sympathetic nervous system, also contributes to lid elevation.

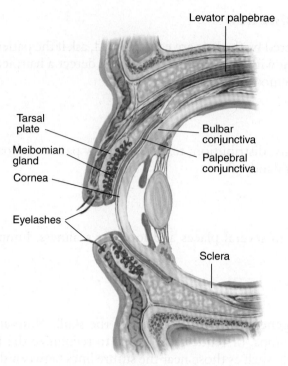

SAGITTAL SECTION OF ANTERIOR EYE WITH LIDS CLOSED

A film of tear fluid protects the conjunctiva and cornea from drying, inhibits microbial growth, and gives a smooth optical surface to the cornea. This fluid comes from the meibomian glands, conjunctival glands, and lacrimal gland. The *lacrimal gland* lies mostly within the bony orbit, above and lateral to the eyeball. The tear fluid spreads across the eye and drains medially through two tiny holes called *lacrimal puncta*. The tears then pass into the *lacrimal sac* and on into the nose through the *nasolacrimal duct*. You can easily find a *punctum* atop the small elevation of the lower lid medially. The lacrimal sac rests in a small depression inside the bony orbit and is not visible.

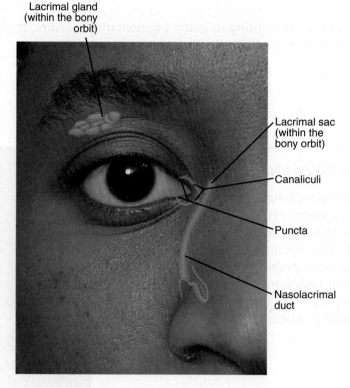

The eyeball is a spherical structure that focuses light on the neurosensory elements within the retina. The muscles of the iris control pupillary size. Muscles of the *ciliary body* control the thickness of the lens, allowing the eye to focus on near or distant objects.

A clear liquid called *aqueous humor* fills the anterior and posterior chambers of the eye. Aqueous humor is produced by the *ciliary body*, circulates from the posterior chamber through the pupil into the anterior chamber, and drains out through the *canal of Schlemm*. This circulatory system helps to control the pressure inside the eye.

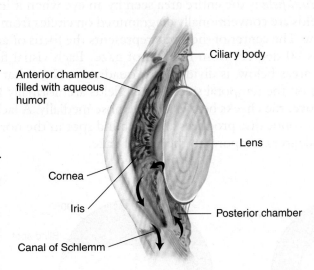

CIRCULATION OF AQUEOUS HUMOR

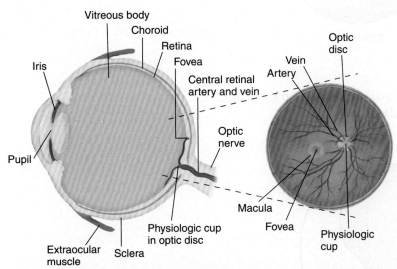

CROSS-SECTION OF THE RIGHT EYE SHOWING A PORTION OF THE FUNDUS COMMONLY SEEN WITH THE OPHTHALMOSCOPE

The posterior part of the eye that is seen through an ophthalmoscope is often called the *fundus* of the eye. Structures here include the retina, choroid, fovea, macula, optic disc, and retinal vessels. The optic nerve with its retinal vessels enters the eyeball posteriorly. You can find it with an ophthalmoscope at the *optic disc*. Lateral and slightly inferior to the disc, there is a small depression in the retinal surface that marks the point of central vision. Around it is a darkened circular area called the *fovea*. The roughly circular *macula* (named for a microscopic yellow spot) surrounds the fovea but has no discernible margins. You do not usually see the normal *vitreous body,* a transparent mass of gelatinous material that fills the eyeball behind the lens. It helps to maintain the shape of the eye.

Visual Fields. A *visual field* is the entire area seen by an eye when it looks at a central point. Fields are conventionally diagrammed on circles from the patient's point of view. The center of the circle represents the focus of gaze. The circumference is 90 degrees from the line of gaze. Each visual field, shown by the white areas below, is divided into quadrants. Note that the fields extend farthest on the temporal sides. Visual fields are normally limited by the brows above, the cheeks below, and the nose medially. A lack of retinal receptors at the optic disc produces an oval blind spot in the normal field of each eye, 15 degrees temporal to the line of gaze.

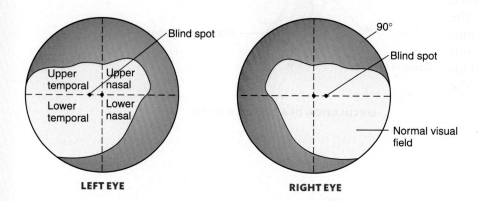

When a person is using both eyes, the two visual fields overlap in an area of binocular vision. Laterally, vision is monocular.

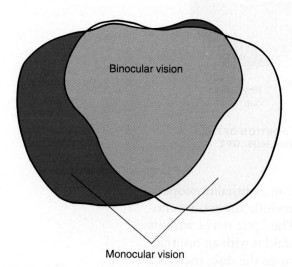

Visual Pathways. To see an image, light reflected from the image must pass through the pupil and be focused on sensory neurons in the retina. The image projected there is upside down and reversed right to left. An image from the upper nasal visual field thus strikes the lower temporal quadrant of the retina.

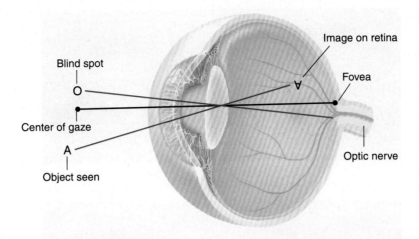

Nerve impulses, stimulated by light, are conducted through the retina, optic nerve, and optic tract on each side, then on through a curving tract called the *optic radiation*. This ends in the visual cortex, a part of the occipital lobe.

Pupillary Reactions. Pupillary size changes in response to light and to the effort of focusing on a near object.

The Light Reaction. A light beam shining onto one retina causes pupillary constriction in both that eye, termed the *direct reaction* to light, and in the opposite eye, the *consensual reaction*. The initial sensory pathways are similar to those described for vision: retina, optic nerve, and optic tract. The pathways diverge in the midbrain, however, and impulses are transmitted through the oculomotor nerve, CN III, to the constrictor muscles of the iris of each eye.

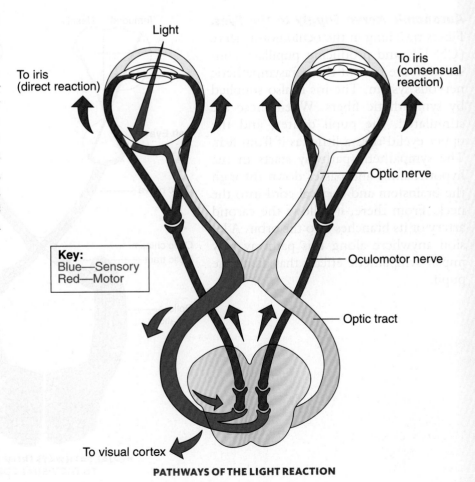

Key:
Blue—Sensory
Red—Motor

PATHWAYS OF THE LIGHT REACTION

The Near Reaction. When a person shifts gaze from a far object to a near one, the pupils constrict. This response, like the light reaction, is mediated by the oculomotor nerve (CN III). Coincident with this *pupillary constriction*, but not part of it, are (1) *convergence* of the eyes, an extraocular movement; and (2) *accommodation*, an increased convexity of the lenses caused by contraction of the ciliary muscles. This change in shape of the lenses brings near objects into focus but is not visible to the examiner.

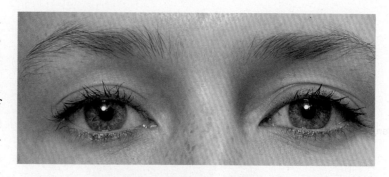

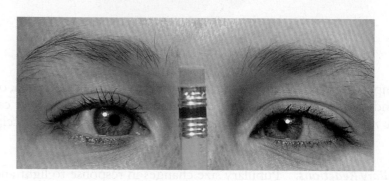

Autonomic Nerve Supply to the Eyes. Fibers travelling in the oculomotor nerve (CN III) and producing pupillary constriction are part of the parasympathetic nervous system. The iris is also supplied by sympathetic fibers. When these are stimulated, the pupil dilates, and the upper eyelid rises a little, as if from fear. The sympathetic pathway starts in the hypothalamus and passes down through the brainstem and cervical cord into the neck. From there, it follows the carotid artery or its branches into the orbit. A lesion anywhere along this pathway may impair sympathetic effects that dilate the pupil.

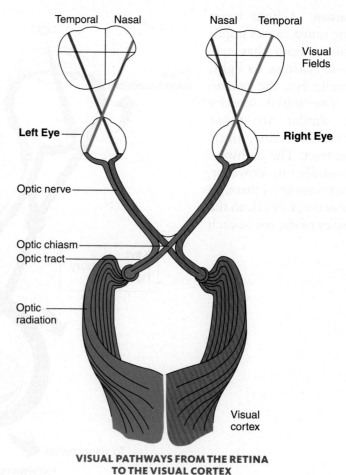

VISUAL PATHWAYS FROM THE RETINA TO THE VISUAL CORTEX

Extraocular Movements.   The coordinated action of six muscles, the four rectus and two oblique, control the eye. You can test the function of each muscle and the cranial nerve that supplies it by asking the patient to move the eye in the direction controlled by that muscle. There are six such *cardinal directions,* indicated by the lines on the figure below. When a person looks down and to the right, for example, the right inferior rectus (CN III) is principally responsible for moving the right eye, whereas the left superior oblique (CN IV) is principally responsible for moving the left eye. If one of these muscles is paralyzed, the eye will deviate from its normal position in that direction of gaze and the eyes will no longer appear conjugate, or parallel.

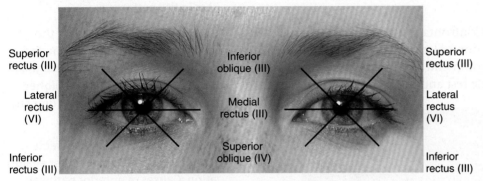

CARDINAL DIRECTIONS OF GAZE

Techniques of Examination

Important Areas of Examination

▶ Visual acuity
▶ Visual fields
▶ Conjunctiva and sclera
▶ Cornea, lens, and pupils
▶ Extraocular movements

▶ Fundi, including:
Optic disc and cup
Retina
Retinal vessels

Visual Acuity.   To test the acuity of central vision, use a well-lit Snellen eye chart, if possible. Position the patient 20 feet from the chart. Patients who use glasses other than for reading should wear them. Ask the patient to cover one eye with a card (to prevent peeking through the fingers) and to read the smallest line of print possible. Coaxing to attempt the next line may improve performance. A patient who cannot read the largest letter should be positioned closer to the chart; note the intervening distance. Determine the smallest line of print from which the patient can identify more than half the letters. Record the visual acuity designated at the side of this line, along with use of glasses, if any. Visual acuity is expressed as two numbers (e.g., 20/30): the first indicates the distance of the patient from the chart, and the second, the distance at which a normal eye can read the line of letters.

Vision of 20/200 means that at 20 feet the patient can read print that a person with normal vision could read at 200 feet. The larger the second number, the worse the vision. "20/40 corrected" means the patient could read the 40 line with glasses (a correction).

Myopia is impaired far vision.

Testing near vision with a special hand-held card helps identify the need for reading glasses or bifocals in patients older than 45 years. You can also use this card to test visual acuity at the bedside. Held 14 inches from the patient's eyes, the card simulates a Snellen chart. You may, however, let patients choose their own distance.

If you have no charts, screen visual acuity with any available print. If patients cannot read even the largest letters, test their ability to count your upraised fingers and distinguish light (such as your flashlight) from dark.

Presbyopia is impaired near vision, found in middle-aged and older people. A presbyopic person often sees better when the card is farther away.

In the United States, a person is usually considered legally blind when vision in the better eye, corrected by glasses, is 20/200 or less. Legal blindness also results from a constricted field of vision: 20 degrees or less in the better eye.

Visual Fields by Confrontation. Confrontation testing of the visual fields is a valuable technique for early detection of lesions in the anterior and posterior visual pathway. Recent studies recommend combining two tests to achieve the best results: the static finger wiggle test and the kinetic red target test.[40,41]

Sensitivity and specificity of the two tests compared to automated perimetry is 78% and 90%; diagnostic accuracy improves with higher density and severity of field defects, irrespective of diagnosis.[40]

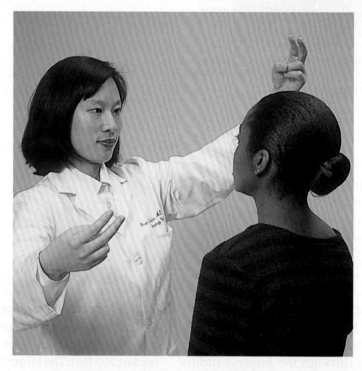

Patients with visual field defects should be referred for further evaluation. Causes of anterior pathway defects include glaucoma, optic neuropathy, optic neuritis, and glioma. Posterior pathway defects include stroke and chiasmal tumors.

Field defects that are all or partly temporal include:

Homonymous Hemianopsia

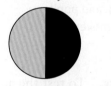
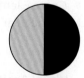

Bitemporal Hemianopsia

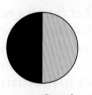
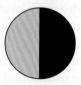

Quadrantic Defects

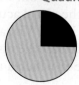
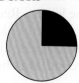

Review these patterns in Table 7-6, Visual Field Defects, p. 265.

Static Finger Wiggle Test. Imagine that the patient's visual fields are projected onto a glass bowl that encircles the patient's head, with the base of the bowl facing you. Ask the patient to look with both eyes into your eyes. As you return the patient's gaze, place you hands about 2 feet apart, lateral to the patient's ears. Wiggle both your fingers simultaneously, and bring them slowly forward, curving inward along the imaginary surface of the bowl toward the central vision line. At each position, ask the patient to tell you as soon as he or she sees the finger movement. Based these reports, map out the maximum lateral extent of the left and right monocular visual fields. Because your fingers are still in the horizontal plane at the level of the patient's ears, you will pick up some of both the superior and inferior quadrants.

Further Testing. If you find a defect, try to establish its boundaries. Test one eye at a time. If you suspect a temporal defect in the left visual field, for example, ask the patient to cover the right eye and, with the left one, to look into your eye directly opposite. Then slowly move your wiggling fingers from the defective area toward the better vision, noting where the patient first responds. Repeat this at several levels to define the border.

When the patient's left eye repeatedly does not see your fingers until they have crossed the line of gaze, a left *temporal hemianopsia* is present. It is diagrammed from the patient's viewpoint.

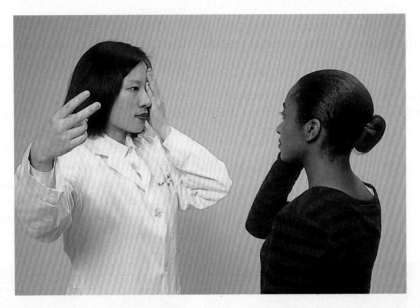

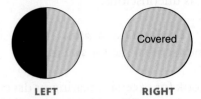

LEFT **RIGHT**

A left *homonymous hemianopsia* may thus be established.

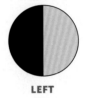

LEFT **RIGHT**

A temporal defect in the visual field of one eye suggests a nasal defect in the other eye. To test this hypothesis, examine the other eye in a similar way, again moving from the anticipated defect toward the better vision.

Kinetic Red Target Test. Facing the patient, move a 5 mm red-topped pin inward from beyond the boundary of each quadrant along a line bisecting the horizontal and vertical meridians. Ask the patient when the pin first appears to be red.

An enlarged blind spot occurs in conditions affecting the optic nerve such as *glaucoma, optic neuritis,* and *papilledema.*[18]

Position and Alignment of the Eyes. Stand in front of the patient and survey the eyes for position and alignment. If one or both eyes seem to protrude, assess them from above (see p. 254).

Inward or outward deviation of the eyes; abnormal protrusion in *Graves' disease* or ocular tumors.

Eyebrows. Inspect the eyebrows, noting their quantity and distribution and any scaliness of the underlying skin.

Scaliness in *seborrheic dermatitis;* lateral sparseness in *hypothyroidism.*

Eyelids. Note the position of the lids in relation to the eyeballs. Inspect for the following:

See Table 7-7, Variations and Abnormalities of the Eyelids, p. 266.

● Width of the palpebral fissures

Upstarting palpebral fissures in *Down syndrome.*

● Edema of the lids

● Color of the lids

Red inflamed lid margins in *blepharitis,* often with crusting.

- Lesions

- Condition and direction of the eyelashes

- Adequacy of eyelid closure. Look for this especially when the eyes are unusually prominent, when there is facial paralysis, or when the patient is unconscious.

Failure of the eyelids to close exposes the corneas to serious damage.

Lacrimal Apparatus. Briefly inspect the regions of the lacrimal gland and lacrimal sac for swelling.

Look for excessive tearing or dryness of the eyes. Assessment of dryness may require special testing by an ophthalmologist. To test for nasolacrimal duct obstruction, see p. 254.

See Table 7-8, Lumps and Swellings in and Around the Eyes, p. 267.

Excessive tearing may be from increased production or impaired drainage. In the first condition, causes include *conjunctival inflammation* and *corneal irritation*; in the second, *ectropion* (p. 266) and *nasolacrimal duct obstruction*. Dryness may occur from impaired secretion in *Sjögren's syndrome*.

Conjunctiva and Sclera. Ask the patient to look up as you depress both lower lids with your thumbs, exposing the sclera and conjunctiva. Inspect the sclera and palpebral conjunctiva for color, and note the vascular pattern against the white scleral background. Look for any nodules or swelling.

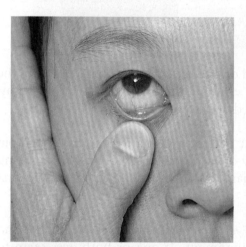

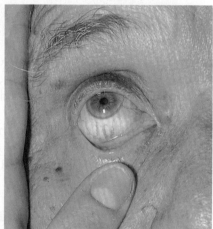

If you need a fuller view of the eye, rest your thumb and finger on the bones of the cheek and brow, respectively, and spread the lids.

Ask the patient to look to each side and down. This technique gives you a good view of the sclera and bulbar conjunctiva, but not of the palpebral conjunctiva of the upper lid. For this you need to evert the lid (see pp. 254–255).

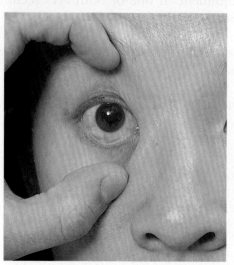

A yellow sclera indicates jaundice.

The local redness below is from *nodular episcleritis*, also seen in *rheumatoid arthritis* and *lupus erythematosus*.

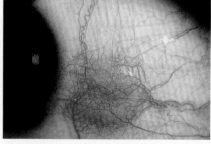

For comparisons, see Table 7-3, Red Eyes, p. 262.

Cornea and Lens.   With oblique lighting, inspect the cornea of each eye for opacities and note any opacities in the lens that may be visible through the pupil.

Iris.   At the same time, inspect each iris. The markings should be clearly defined. With your light shining directly from the temporal side, look for a crescentic shadow on the medial side of the iris. Because the iris is normally fairly flat and forms a relatively open angle with the cornea, this lighting casts no shadow.

See Table 7-9, Opacities of the Cornea and Lens, p. 268.

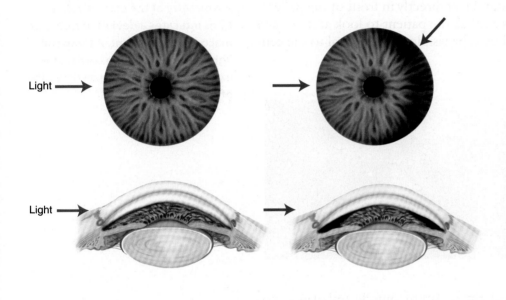

Occasionally the iris bows abnormally far forward, forming a very narrow angle with the cornea. The light then casts a crescentic shadow.

This narrow angle increases the risk for acute *narrow-angle glaucoma*—a sudden increase in intraocular pressure when drainage of the aqueous humor is blocked.

In *open-angle glaucoma*, the common form of glaucoma, the normal spatial relation between iris and cornea is preserved and the iris is fully lit.

Pupils.   Inspect the *size, shape,* and *symmetry* of the pupils. If the pupils are large (>5 mm), small (<3 mm), or unequal, measure them. Use a card with black circles of varying sizes to measure pupillary size.

Miosis refers to constriction of the pupils, *mydriasis* to dilation.

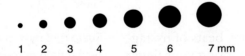

Simple *anisocoria,* or a difference in pupillary size of 0.04 mm or greater, is visible in approximately 35% of healthy people. If pupillary reactions are normal, anisocoria is considered benign.[41]

Compare benign anisocoria with *Horner's syndrome, oculomotor nerve paralysis,* and *tonic pupil.* See Table 7-10, Pupillary Abnormalities, p. 269.

Test the *pupillary reaction to light.* Ask the patient to look into the distance, and shine a bright light obliquely into each pupil in turn. Both the distant gaze and the oblique lighting help to prevent a near reaction. Look for:

● The *direct reaction* (pupillary constriction in the same eye)

● The *consensual reaction* (pupillary constriction in the opposite eye)

Always darken the room and use a bright light before deciding that a light reaction is absent.

If the reaction to light is impaired or questionable, test the *near reaction* in normal room light. Testing one eye at a time makes it easier to concentrate on pupillary responses, without the distraction of extraocular movement. Hold your finger or pencil about 10 cm from the patient's eye. Ask the patient to look alternately at it and into the distance directly behind it. Watch for pupillary constriction with near effort.

Testing the near reaction is helpful in diagnosing *Argyll Robertson* and *tonic (Adie's) pupils* (see p. 269).

Extraocular Muscles.   From about 2 feet directly in front of the patient, shine a light onto the patient's eyes and ask the patient to look at it. *Inspect the reflections in the corneas.* They should be visible slightly nasal to the center of the pupils.

Asymmetry of the corneal reflections indicates a deviation from normal ocular alignment. A temporal light reflection on one cornea, for example, indicates a nasal deviation of that eye.

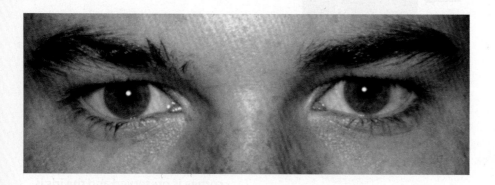

A *cover–uncover test* may reveal a slight or latent muscle imbalance not otherwise seen (see p. 270).

Now *assess the extraocular movements,* looking for:

- The normal *conjugate movements* of the eyes in each direction, or any *deviation* from normal.

See Table 7-11, Dysconjugate Gaze, p. 270.

- *Nystagmus,* a fine rhythmic oscillation of the eyes. A few beats of nystagmus on extreme lateral gaze are normal. If you see this, bring your finger in to within the field of binocular vision and look again.

Sustained nystagmus within the binocular field of gaze is seen with various neurologic conditions. See Table 17-7, Nystagmus, pp. 755–756.

- *Lid lag* as the eyes move from up to down.

In lid lag of *hyperthyroidism*, a rim of sclera is visible above the iris with downward gaze.

To *test the six extraocular movements (EOMs), ask the patient to follow your finger or pencil* as you sweep through the six cardinal directions of gaze. Making a wide H in the air, lead the patient's gaze (1) to the patient's extreme right, (2) to the right and upward, and (3) down on the right; then (4) without pausing in the middle, to the extreme left, (5) to the left and upward, and (6) down on the left. Pause during upward and lateral gaze to detect nystagmus. Move your finger or pencil at a comfortable distance from the patient. Because middle-aged or older people may have difficulty focusing on near objects, make this distance greater for them than for young people. Some patients move their heads to follow your finger. If necessary, hold the head in the proper midline position.

In paralysis of the CN VI, illustrated below, the eyes are conjugate in right lateral gaze but not in left lateral gaze.

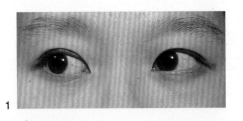
1

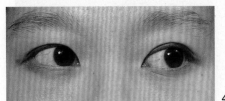
4

LOOKING RIGHT

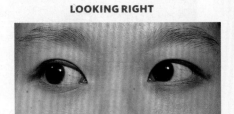

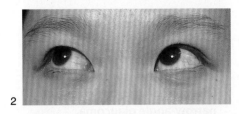
2

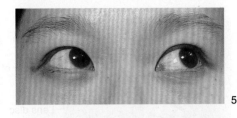
5

LOOKING LEFT

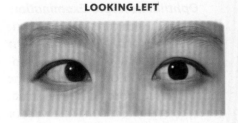

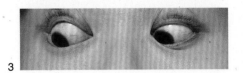
3

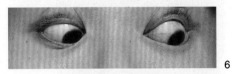
6

If you suspect lid lag or hyperthyroidism, ask the patient to follow your finger again as you move it slowly from up to down in the midline. The lid should overlap the iris slightly throughout this movement.

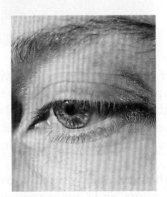

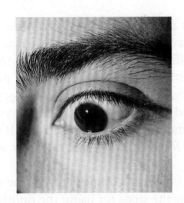

Note the rim of sclera from *proptosis*, an abnormal protrusion of the eyeballs in *hyperthyroidism*, leading to a characteristic "stare" on frontal gaze. If unilateral, consider an orbital tumor or retrobulbar hemorrhage from trauma.

Finally, test for *convergence*. Ask the patient to follow your finger or pencil as you move it in toward the bridge of the nose. The converging eyes normally follow the object to within 5 cm to 8 cm of the nose.

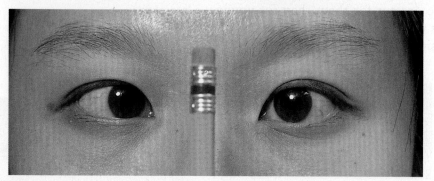

CONVERGENCE

Ophthalmoscopic Examination. In general health care, examine your patients' eyes *without dilating their pupils*. Your view is, therefore, limited to the posterior structures of the retina. To see more peripheral structures, to evaluate the macula well, or to investigate unexplained visual loss, ophthalmologists dilate the pupils with mydriatic drops unless this is contraindicated.

Aperture

Indicator of diopters

Lens disc

Contraindications for mydriatic drops include (1) head injury and coma, in which continuing observations of pupillary reactions are essential, and (2) any suspicion of narrow-angle glaucoma.

At first, using the ophthalmoscope may seem awkard, and it may be difficult to visualize the fundus. With patience and practice of proper technique, the fundus will come into view, and you will be able to assess important structures such as the optic disc and the retinal vessels. Remove your glasses unless you have marked nearsightedness or severe astigmatism. (If the patient's refractive errors make it difficult to focus on the fundi, however, it may be easier to keep your glasses on.)

Review the components of the ophthalmoscope pictured above. Then follow the steps for using the ophthalmoscope, and your examination skills will improve over time.

Steps for Using the Ophthalmoscope

▶ Darken the room. Switch on the ophthalmoscope light and turn the lens disc until you see the large round beam of white light.* Shine the light on the back of your hand to check the type of light, its desired brightness, and the electrical charge of the ophthalmoscope.

▶ Turn the lens disc to the 0 diopter. (A diopter is a unit that measures the power of a lens to converge or diverge light.) At this diopter, the lens neither

(continued)

Steps for Using the Ophthalmoscope (*continued*)

converges nor diverges light. Keep your finger on the edge of the lens disc so you can turn the disc to focus the lens when you examine the fundus.

▶ Hold the ophthalmoscope *in your right hand and use your right eye to examine the patient's right eye;* hold it *in your left hand and use your left eye to examine the patient's left eye*. This keeps you from bumping the patient's nose and gives you more mobility and closer range for visualizing the fundus. At first, you may have difficulty using your nondominant eye, but this will abate with practice.

▶ Hold the ophthalmoscope firmly braced against the medial aspect of your bony orbit, with the handle tilted laterally at about a 20-degree slant from the vertical. Check to make sure you can see clearly through the aperture. Instruct the patient to look slightly up and over your shoulder at a point directly ahead on the wall.

▶ Place yourself about 15 inches away from the patient and at an angle *15 degrees lateral to the patient's line of vision*. Shine the light beam on the pupil and look for the orange glow in the pupil—the *red reflex*. Note any opacities interrupting the red reflex.

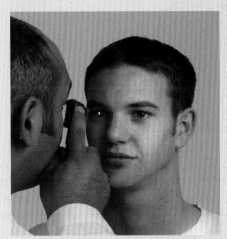

EXAMINER AT 15-DEGREE ANGLE FROM PATIENT'S LINE OF VISION, ELICITING RED REFLEX

▶ Now, place the thumb of your other hand across the patient's eyebrow. (This technique helps keep you steady but is not essential.) Keeping the light beam focused on the red reflex, move in with the ophthalmoscope on the 15-degree angle toward the pupil until you are very close to it, almost touching the patient's eyelashes.

Try to keep both eyes open and relaxed, as if gazing into the distance, to help minimize any fluctuating blurriness as your eyes attempt to accommodate.

You may need to lower the brightness of the light beam to make the examination more comfortable for the patient, avoid *hippus* (spasm of the pupil), and improve your observations.

Absence of a *red reflex* suggests an opacity of the lens (cataract) or possibly of the vitreous. Less commonly, a *detached retina* or, in children, a *retinoblastoma* may obscure this reflex. Do not be fooled by an artificial eye, which has no red reflex.

---

*Some clinicians like to use the large round beam for large pupils, and the small round beam for small pupils. The other beams are rarely helpful. The slitlike beam is sometimes used to assess elevations or concavities in the retina, the green (or red-free) beam to detect small red lesions, and the grid to make measurements. Ignore the last three lights and practice with the large or small round white beam.

Now you are ready to inspect the *optic disc* and the *retina*. You should be seeing the optic disc—a yellowish orange to creamy pink oval or round structure that may fill your field of gaze. The ophthalmoscope magnifies the normal retina about 15 times and the normal iris about 4 times. The optic disc actually measures about 1.5 mm. Follow the next steps for this important segment of the physical examination.

When the lens has been removed surgically, its magnifying effect is lost. Retinal structures then look much smaller than usual, and you can see a much larger expanse of the fundus.

Steps for Examining the Optic Disc and the Retina

The Optic Disc

▶ First, *locate the optic disc*. Look for the round yellowish-orange structure described above. If you do not see it at first, follow a blood vessel centrally until you do. You can tell which direction is central by noting the angles at which vessels branch—the vessel size becomes progressively larger at each junction as you approach the disc.

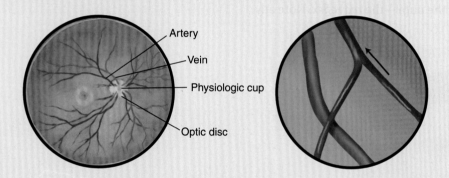

Artery
Vein
Physiologic cup
Optic disc

▶ Now, *bring the optic disc into sharp focus* by adjusting the lens of your ophthalmoscope. If both you and the patient have no refractive errors, the retina should be in focus at o diopters. If structures are blurred, rotate the lens disc until you find the sharpest focus.

   For example, if the patient is myopic (nearsighted), rotate the lens disc counterclockwise to the minus diopters; in a hyperopic (farsighted) patient, move the disc clockwise to the plus diopters. You can correct your own refractive error in the same way.

▶ *Inspect the optic disc*. Note the following features:

   ▶ *The sharpness or clarity of the disc outline*. The nasal portion of the disc margin may be somewhat blurred, a normal finding.

   ▶ *The color of the disc*, normally yellowish orange to creamy pink. White or pigmented crescents may ring the disc, a normal finding.

   ▶ *The size of the central physiologic cup*, if present. It is usually yellowish white. The horizontal diameter is usually less than half the horizontal diameter of the disc.

   ▶ *The comparative symmetry* of the eyes and findings in the fundi.

In a *refractive error*, light rays from a distance do not focus on the retina. In *myopia*, they focus anterior to the retina; in *hyperopia*, posterior to it. Retinal structures in a myopic eye look larger than normal.

See Table 7-12, Normal Variations of the Optic Disc, p. 271, and Table 7-13, Abnormalities of the Optic Disc, p. 272.

An enlarged cup suggests *chronic open-angle glaucoma*.

Detecting Papilledema. *Papilledema* describes swelling of the optic disc and anterior bulging of the physiologic cup. Increased intracranial pressure is transmitted to the optic nerve, causing stasis of axoplasmic flow, intra-axonal

(continued)

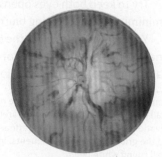

PAPILLEDEMA

Steps for Examining the Optic Disc and the Retina (*continued*)

edema, and swelling of the optic nerve head. Papilledema often signals serious disorders of the brain, such as meningitis, subarachnoid hemorrhage, trauma, and mass lesions, so searching for this important disorder is a priority during all your funduscopic examinations.

Inspect the fundus for spontaneous venous pulsations (SVPs), rhythmic variations in the caliber of the retinal veins as they cross the fundus (narrower in systole; wider in diastole), present in 90% of normal patients.

Loss of SVPs occurs with high intracranial pressures (above 190 mm H_2O) that change the pressure gradient between cerebral spinal fluid pressure and intraocular pulse pressure in the optic disc.[42,43]

The Retina—Arteries, Veins, Fovea, and Macula

▶ *Inspect the retina*, including arteries and veins as they extend to the periphery, arteriovenous crossings, the fovea, and the macula. Distinguish arteries from veins based on the features listed below.

	Arteries	Veins
Color	Light red	Dark red
Size	Smaller (⅔ to ¾ the diameter of veins)	Larger
Light Reflex (*reflection*)	Bright	Inconspicuous or absent

▶ *Follow the vessels peripherally in each of four directions*, noting their relative sizes and the character of the arteriovenous crossings.

Identify any lesions of the surrounding *retina* and note their size, shape, color, and distribution. As you search the retina, *move your head and instrument as a unit*, using the patient's pupil as an imaginary fulcrum. At first, you may lose your view of the retina because your light falls out of the pupil. You will improve with practice.

Lesions of the retina can be measured in terms of "disc diameters" from the optic disc.

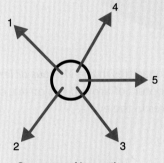

Sequence of inspection from disc to macula
LEFT EYE

See Table 7-14, Retinal Arteries and Arteriovenous Crossings: Normal and Hypertensive, p. 273; Table 7-15, Red Spots and Streaks in the Fundi, p. 274; Table 7-16, Ocular Fundi: Normal and Hypertensive Retinopathy, p. 275; Table 7-17, Ocular Fundi: Diabetic Retinopathy, p. 276; Table 7-18, Light-Colored Spots in the Fundi, p. 277.

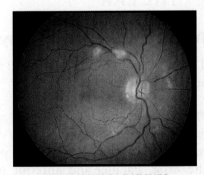

COTTON-WOOL PATCHES

Note the irregular patches between 11 and 12 o'clock, 1 to 2 disc diameters from the disc. Each measures about one-half by one-half disc diameters.

(*continued*)

Steps for Examining the Optic Disc and the Retina (*continued*)

▶ Inspect the *fovea* and surrounding *macula*. Direct your light beam laterally or by asking the patient to look directly into the light. In younger people, the tiny bright reflection at the center of the fovea helps to orient you; shimmering light reflections in the macular area are common.

Macular degeneration is an important cause of poor central vision in older adults. Types include *dry atrophic* (more common but less severe) and *wet exudative,* or neovascular. Undigested cellular debris, called *drusen,* may be hard and sharply defined, as seen below, or soft and confluent with altered pigmentation (see p. 277).

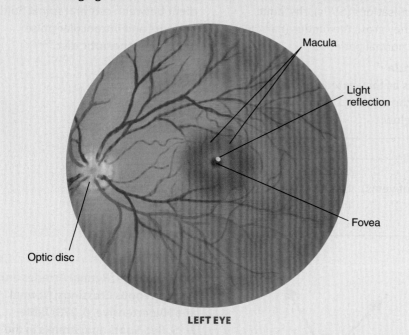

LEFT EYE

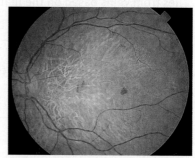

Photo from Tasman W, Jaeger E (eds). The Wills Eye Hospital Atlas of Clinical Ophthalmology, 2nd ed. Philadelphia, Lippincott Williams & Wilkins, 2001.

▶ *Inspect the anterior structures.* Look for opacities in the *vitreous or lens.* Rotate the lens disc progressively to diopters of around +10 or +12, so you can focus on the more anterior structures in the eye.

Vitreous floaters may be seen as dark specks or strands between the fundus and the lens. Cataracts are densities in the lens (see p. 268).

THE EAR

Anatomy and Physiology

The ear has three compartments: the external ear, the middle ear, and the inner ear.

The External Ear. The *external ear* comprises the auricle and ear canal. The *auricle* consists chiefly of cartilage covered by skin and has a firm elastic consistency. Its prominent curved outer ridge is the *helix*. Parallel and anterior to the helix is another curved prominence, the *antihelix*. Inferiorly is the fleshy projection of the earlobe, or *lobule*. The ear canal opens behind the *tragus,* a nodular protuberance that points backward over the entrance to the canal.

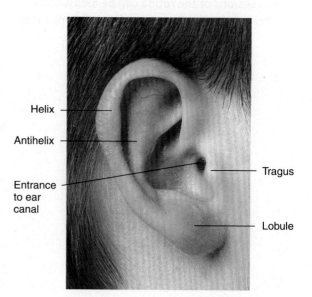

The *ear canal* curves inward and is approximately 24 mm long. Cartilage surrounds its outer portion. The skin in this portion is hairy and contains glands that produce cerumen (wax). The inner portion of the canal is surrounded by bone and lined by thin, hairless skin. Pressure on this latter area causes pain—a point to remember when you when you examine the ear. At the end of the ear canal lies the lateral *tympanic membrane*, or eardrum, marking the lateral limit of the external ear. The external ear captures sound waves for transmission into the middle and inner ear.

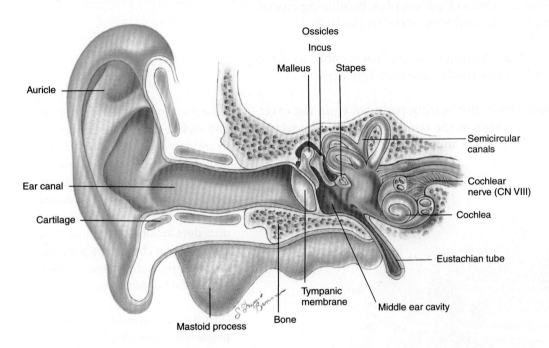

Behind and below the ear canal is the mastoid portion of the temporal bone. The lowest portion of this bone, the *mastoid process*, is palpable behind the lobule.

The Middle Ear. In the air-filled middle ear, the *ossicles*—the malleus, the incus, and the stapes—transform sound vibrations into mechanical waves for the inner ear. The proximal end of the *eustachian tube* connects the middle ear to the nasopharynx.

Two of the ossicles are visible through the tympanic membrane, and are angled obliquely and held inward at its center by the *malleus*. Find the *handle* and the *short process* of the malleus, the two chief landmarks. From the *umbo*, where the eardrum meets the tip of the malleus, a light reflection called the *cone of light* fans downward and anteriorly. Above the short process lies a small portion of the eardrum called the *pars flaccida*. The remainder of the drum is the *pars tensa*.

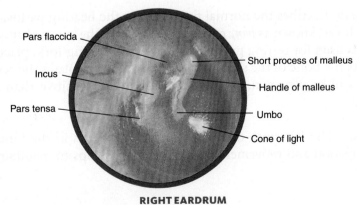

RIGHT EARDRUM

Anterior and posterior malleolar folds, which extend obliquely upward from the short process, separate the pars flaccida from the pars tensa but are usually invisible unless the eardrum is retracted. A second ossicle, the *incus,* can sometimes be seen through the drum.

The Inner Ear. The inner ear includes the *cochlea,* the *semicircular canals,* and the distal end of the *auditory nerve (CN VIII).* Movements of the stapes vibrate the perilymph in the labyrinth of the semicircular canals and the hair cells and endolymph in the ducts of the cochlea, producing electrical nerve impulses transmitted by the auditory nerve to the brain.

Much of the middle ear and all of the inner ear are inaccessible to direct examination. Assess their condition by testing auditory function.

Hearing Pathways. The first part of the hearing pathway, from the external ear through the middle ear, is known as the *conductive phase.* The second part of the pathway, involving the cochlea and cochlear nerve, is the *sensorineural phase.*

Hearing disorders of the external and middle ear cause *conductive hearing loss.* External ear causes include infection *(otitis externa),* trauma, squamous cell carcinoma, and benign bony growths such as *exostoses or osteomas.* Middle ear disorders include congenital conditions, benign cholesteatomas and otosclerosis, tumors, and perforation of the tympanic membrane.

Disorders of the inner ear cause *sensorineural hearing loss* from congenital and hereditary conditions, *presbycusis,* viral infections such as *rubella* and *cytomegalovirus,* *Ménière's disease,* noise exposure, and *acoustic neuroma.*[44]

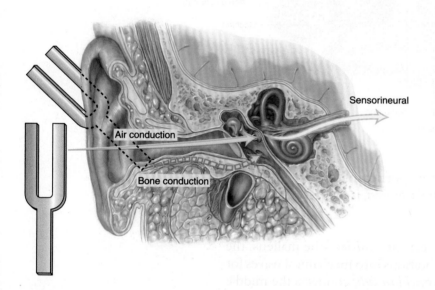

Air conduction describes the normal first phase in the hearing pathway. An alternate pathway, known as *bone conduction,* bypasses the external and middle ear and is used for testing purposes. A vibrating tuning fork, placed on the head, sets the bone of the skull into vibration and stimulates the cochlea directly. In a normal person, air conduction is more sensitive than bone conduction.

Equilibrium. The labyrinth of three semicircular canals in the inner ear senses the position and movements of the head and helps to maintain balance.

Techniques of Examination

The Auricle. Inspect the auricle and surrounding tissue for deformities, lumps, or skin lesions.

If ear pain, discharge, or inflammation is present, move the auricle up and down, press the tragus, and press firmly just behind the ear.

Ear Canal and Drum. To see the ear canal and drum, use an otoscope with the largest ear speculum that the canal will accommodate. Position the patient's head so that you can see comfortably through the instrument. To straighten the ear canal, grasp the auricle firmly but gently and pull it upward, backward, and slightly away from the head.

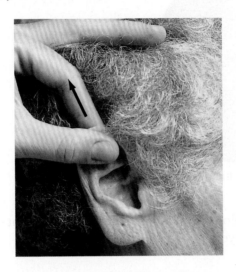

Holding the otoscope handle between your thumb and fingers, brace your hand against the patient's face. Your hand and instrument can then follow unexpected movements by the patient. (If you are uncomfortable switching hands for the left ear, as shown below, you may reach over that ear to pull it up and back with your left hand and rest your otoscope-holding right hand on the head behind the ear.)

Insert the speculum gently into the ear canal, directing it somewhat down and forward and through the hairs, if any.

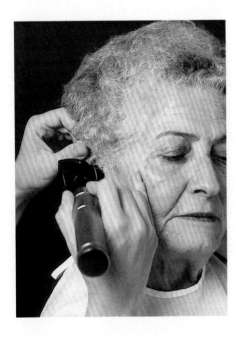

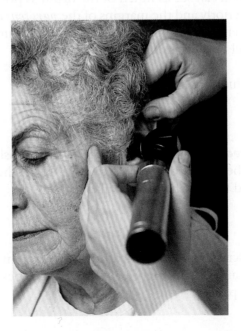

See Table 7-19, Lumps on or Near the Ear, p. 278.

Movement of the auricle and tragus (the "tug test") is painful in acute *otitis externa* (inflammation of the ear canal), but not in *otitis media* (inflammation of the middle ear). Tenderness behind the ear may be present in *otitis media*.

Nontender nodular swellings covered by normal skin deep in the ear canals suggest *exostoses*. These are nonmalignant overgrowths which may obscure the drum.

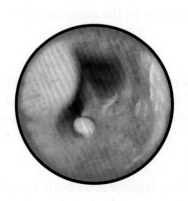

Inspect the ear canal, noting any discharge, foreign bodies, redness of the skin, or swelling. Cerumen, which varies in color and consistency from yellow and flaky to brown and sticky or even to dark and hard, may wholly or partly obscure your view.

In acute *otitis externa,* shown below, the canal is often swollen, narrowed, moist, pale, and tender. It may be reddened.

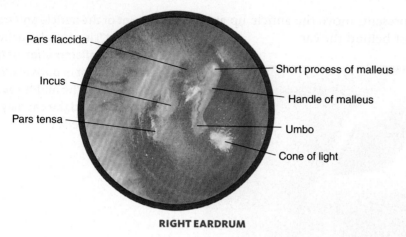

Pars flaccida

Incus

Pars tensa

Short process of malleus

Handle of malleus

Umbo

Cone of light

RIGHT EARDRUM

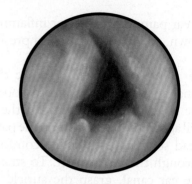

In *chronic otitis externa,* the skin of the canal is often thickened, red, and itchy.

Inspect the eardrum, noting its color and contour. The cone of light—usually easy to see—helps to orient you.

Look for the red bulging drum of acute purulent *otitis media*[21]; the amber drum of a serous effusion. See Table 7-20, Abnormalities of the Eardrum, p. 279.

Identify the *handle of the malleus,* noting its position, and inspect the *short process of the malleus.*

An unusually prominent short process and a prominent handle that looks more horizontal suggest a retracted drum.

Gently move the speculum so that you can see as much of the drum as possible, including the *pars flaccida* superiorly and the margins of the *pars tensa.* Look for any perforations. The anterior and inferior margins of the drum may be obscured by the curving wall of the ear canal.

Mobility of the eardrum can be evaluated with a pneumatic otoscope.

A serous effusion, a thickened drum, or purulent *otitis media* may decrease mobility.

Testing Auditory Acuity—Whispered Voice Test. To begin screening, ask the patient "Do you feel you have a hearing loss or difficulty hearing?" If the patient reports hearing loss, proceed to the whispered voice test.

Patients who answer "yes" are twice as likely to have a hearing deficit; for patients who report normal hearing the likelihood of moderate to severe hearing impairment is only 0.13.[45]

The *whispered voice test* is a reliable screening test for hearing loss if examiners use a standard method of testing and exhales before whispering. For best results, follow the steps on the next page.

Sensitivity is 90% to 100% and specificity 70% to 87%.[46–48] This test detects significant hearing loss of greater than 30 decibels.

Whispered Voice Test for Auditory Acuity[46]

▶ Stand 2 feet behind the seated patient so the patient cannot read your lips.

▶ Occlude the nontest ear with a finger and gently rub the tragus in a circular motion to prevent transfer of sound to the nontest ear.

▶ Exhale a full breath before whispering to ensure a quiet voice.

▶ Whisper a combination of three numbers and letters, such as 3-U-1. Use a different number/letter combination for the other ear.

▶ Interpretation:
  ▶ *Normal:* Patient repeats initial sequence correctly.
  ▶ *Normal:* Patient responds incorrectly, so test a second time with a different number/letter combination; patient repeats at least three out of the possible six numbers and letters correctly.
  ▶ *Abnormal:* Four of the six possible numbers and letters are incorrect. Conduct further testing by audiometry. (Weber and Rinne tests are less accurate and precise.)[45]

Note that older adults with *presbycusis* have higher frequency hearing loss, making them more likely to miss consonants, which have higher frequency sounds than vowels.

Testing for Conductive vs. Neurosensory Hearing Loss: Tuning Fork Tests.

For patients failing the whispered voice test, tuning fork tests may help determine if the hearing loss is conductive or neurosensory in origin. However, their precision, or test–retest reproducibility, and their accuracy compared to air-bone gap reference standards have been questioned.[45]

Note also that tuning fork tests do not distinguish normal hearing from bilateral neurosensory loss or from mixed conductive and neurosensory loss. Sensitivity and specificity of the Rinne test are 60% to 90% and 95% to 98%. Sensitivity of the Weber test is about 55%; specificity for neurosensory loss is about 79% and for conductive loss, 92%.[41]

To conduct these tests, make sure the room is quiet, and select a tuning fork of 256 Hz, or possibly 512 Hz. These frequencies fall within the range of conversational speech, namely 500 to 3,000 Hz and between 45 and 60 decibels.

Set the fork into light vibration by briskly stroking it between the thumb and index finger ($\longrightarrow$) or by tapping it on your knuckles.

● *Test for lateralization* (Weber test). Place the base of the lightly vibrating tuning fork firmly on top of the patient's head or on the midforehead.

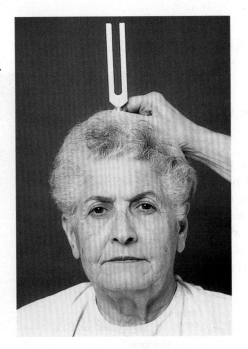

In unilateral *conductive hearing loss*, sound is heard in (lateralized to) the impaired ear. Explanations include *otosclerosis otitis media*, perforation of the eardrum, and cerumen. See Table 7-21, Patterns of Hearing Loss, p. 281.

Ask where the patient hears the sound: on one side or both sides? Normally the vibration is heard in the midline or equally in both ears. If nothing is heard, try again, pressing the fork more firmly on the head. Restrict this test to patients with unilateral hearing loss since patients with normal hearing may lateralize, and patients with bilateral conductive or sensorineural deficits will not lateralize.

In unilateral *sensorineural hearing loss*, sound is heard in the good ear.

- *Compare air conduction (AC) and bone conduction (BC) (Rinne test)*. Place the base of a lightly vibrating tuning fork on the mastoid bone, behind the ear and level with the canal. When the patient can no longer hear the sound, quickly place the fork close to the ear canal and ascertain whether the sound can be heard again. Here the "U" of the fork should face forward, thus maximizing its sound for the patient. Normally the sound is heard longer through air than through bone (AC > BC).

In *conductive hearing loss*, sound is heard through bone as long as or longer than it is through air (BC = AC or BC > AC). In *sensorineural hearing loss*, sound is heard longer through air (AC > BC).

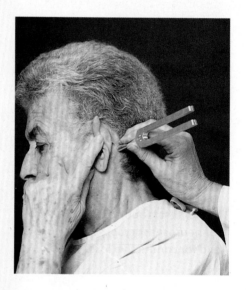
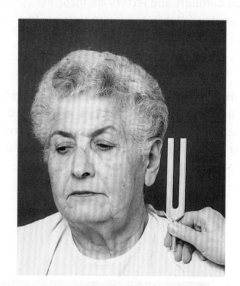

THE NOSE AND PARANASAL SINUSES

Anatomy and Physiology

Review the terms used to describe the external anatomy of the nose.

Approximately the upper third of the nose is supported by bone, the lower two thirds by cartilage. Air enters the nasal cavity by way of the *anterior naris* on either side, then passes into a widened area known as the *vestibule* and on through the narrow nasal passage to the nasopharynx.

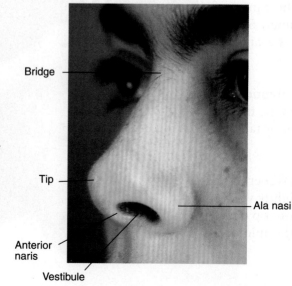

Bridge

Tip

Ala nasi

Anterior naris

Vestibule

The medial wall of each nasal cavity is formed by the *nasal septum*, which, like the external nose, is supported by both bone and cartilage. It is covered by a mucous membrane well supplied with blood. The vestibule, unlike the rest of the nasal cavity, is lined with hair-bearing skin, not mucosa.

Laterally, the anatomy is more complex. Curving bony structures, the *turbinates*, covered by a highly vascular mucous membrane, protrude into the nasal cavity. Below each turbinate is a groove, or meatus, each named according to the turbinate above it. The nasolacrimal duct drains into the inferior meatus; most of the paranasal sinuses drain into the middle meatus. Their openings are not usually visible.

The additional surface area provided by the turbinates and the mucosa covering them aids the nasal cavities in their principal functions: cleansing, humidification, and temperature control of inspired air.

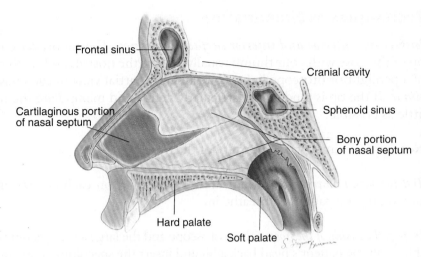

MEDIAL WALL—LEFT NASAL CAVITY (MUCOSA REMOVED)

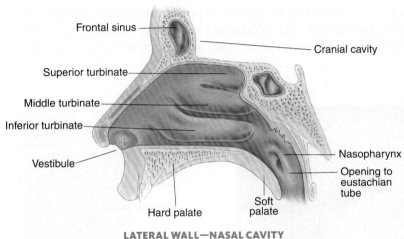

LATERAL WALL—NASAL CAVITY

The *paranasal sinuses* are air-filled cavities within the bones of the skull. Like the nasal cavities into which they drain, they are lined with mucous membrane. Their locations are diagrammed below. Only the frontal and maxillary sinuses are readily accessible to clinical examination.

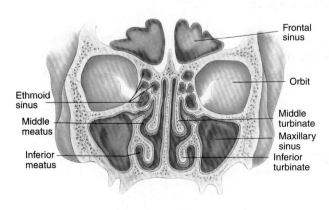

CROSS-SECTION OF NASAL CAVITY—ANTERIOR VIEW

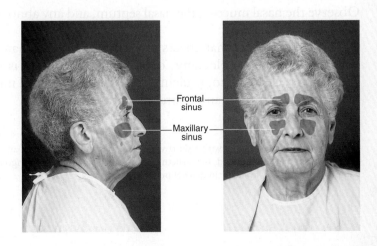

Techniques of Examination

Inspect the anterior and inferior surfaces of the nose. Gentle pressure on the tip of the nose with your thumb usually widens the nostrils and, with the aid of a penlight or otoscope light, you can get a partial view of each nasal *vestibule*. If the tip is tender, be particularly gentle and manipulate the nose as little as possible.

Note any asymmetry or deformity of the nose.

Test for nasal obstruction, if indicated, by pressing on each ala nasi in turn and asking the patient to breathe in.

Inspect the inside of the nose with an otoscope and the largest ear speculum available.[‡] Tilt the patient's head back a bit and insert the speculum gently into the vestibule of each nostril, avoiding contact with the sensitive nasal septum. Hold the otoscope handle to one side to avoid the patient's chin and improve your mobility. By directing the speculum posteriorly, then upward in small steps, try to see the inferior and middle turbinates, the nasal septum, and the narrow nasal passage between them. Some asymmetry of the two sides is normal.

Tenderness of the nasal tip or alae suggests local infection such as a furuncle.

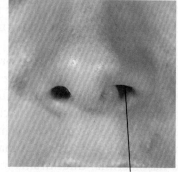

Vestibule

Deviation of the lower septum is common and may be easily visible, as illustrated. Deviation seldom obstructs air flow.

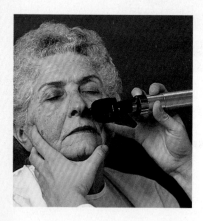

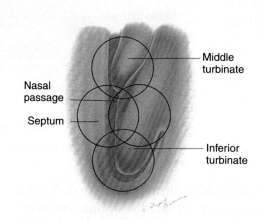

Middle turbinate

Nasal passage

Septum

Inferior turbinate

Observe the nasal mucosa, the nasal septum, and any abnormalities. Inspect:

- The *nasal mucosa* that covers the septum and turbinates. Note its color and any swelling, bleeding, or exudate. If exudate is present, note its character: clear, mucopurulent, or purulent. The nasal mucosa is normally somewhat redder than the oral mucosa.

In *viral rhinitis,* the mucosa is reddened and swollen; in *allergic rhinitis,* it may be pale, bluish, or red.

[‡]A nasal illuminator, equipped with a short wide nasal speculum but lacking an otoscope's magnification, may also be used, but structures look much smaller. Otolaryngologists use special equipment not widely available in general practice.

- The *nasal septum*. Note any deviation, inflammation, or perforation of the septum. The lower anterior portion of the septum (where the patient's finger can reach) is a common source of *epistaxis* (nosebleed).

Fresh blood or crusting may be seen. Causes of septal perforation include trauma, surgery, and intranasal use of cocaine or amphetamines, which also cause septal ulceration.

- Any *abnormalities* such as ulcers or polyps.

Nasal polyps are pale saclike growths of inflamed tissue that can obstruct the air passage or sinuses. Conditions conducive to polyps include allergic rhinitis, aspirin sensitivity, asthma, chronic sinus infections, and cystic fibrosis.[28]

Inspection of the nasal cavity through the anterior naris is usually limited to the vestibule, the anterior portion of the septum, and the lower and middle turbinates. Examination of posterior abnormalities requires a nasopharyngeal mirror and technique is beyond the scope of this book.

Place all nasal and ear specula outside your instrument case after use; then discard or clean and disinfect them appropriately. Check the policies of your institution.

Palpate for sinus tenderness. Press up on the *frontal sinuses* from under the bony brows, avoiding pressure on the eyes. Then press up on the *maxillary sinuses*.

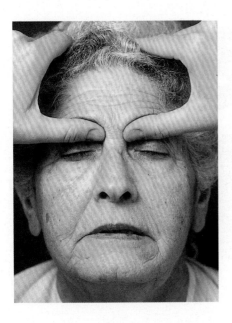
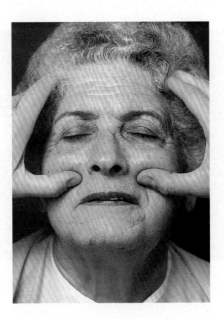

Local tenderness, together with symptoms such as pain, fever, and nasal discharge, suggest *acute sinusitis* involving the frontal or maxillary sinuses.[25,49] Transillumination may be diagnostically useful. For this technique, see p. 255.

MOUTH AND PHARYNX

Anatomy and Physiology

The *lips* are muscular folds that surround the entrance to the mouth. When opened, the gums (gingiva) and teeth are visible. Note the scalloped shape of the *gingival margins* and the pointed *interdental papillae*.

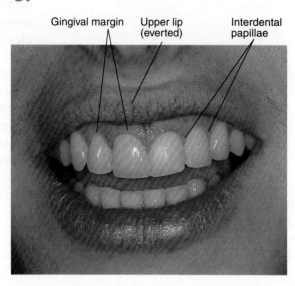

Gingival margin   Upper lip (everted)   Interdental papillae

The *gingiva* is firmly attached to the teeth and to the maxilla or mandible in which they are seated. In lighter-skinned people, the gingiva is pale or coral pink and lightly stippled. In darker-skinned people, it may be diffusely or partly brown, as shown below. A midline mucosal fold, called a *labial frenulum*, connects each lip with the gingiva. A shallow *gingival sulcus* between the gum's thin margin and each tooth is not readily visible (but is probed and measured by dentists). Adjacent to the gingiva is the *alveolar mucosa*, which merges with the *labial mucosa* of the lip.

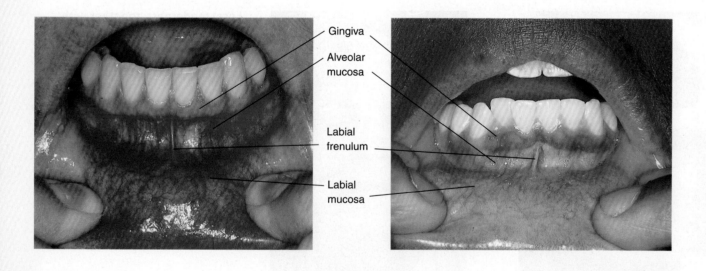

Gingiva

Alveolar mucosa

Labial frenulum

Labial mucosa

Each tooth, composed chiefly of dentin, lies rooted in a bony socket with only its enamel-covered crown exposed. Small blood vessels and nerves enter the tooth through its apex and pass into the pulp canal and pulp chamber.

Note the terms designating the 32 adult teeth, 16 in each jaw.

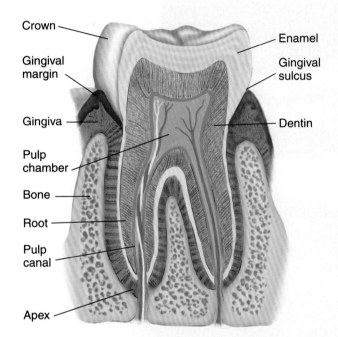

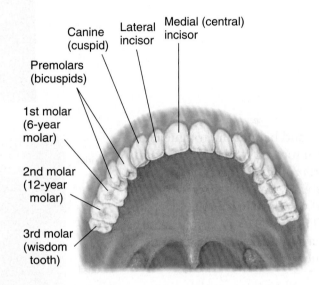

The dorsum of the *tongue* is covered with papillae, giving it a rough surface. Some of these papillae look like red dots, which contrast with the thin white coat that often covers the tongue.

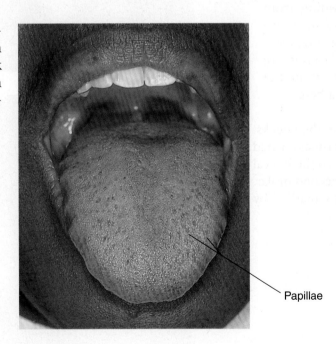

The undersurface of the tongue has no papillae. Note the midline *lingual frenulum* that connects the tongue to the floor of the mouth. At the base of the tongue, the *ducts of the submandibular gland* (Wharton's ducts) pass forward and medially. They open on papillae that lie on each side of the lingual frenulum.

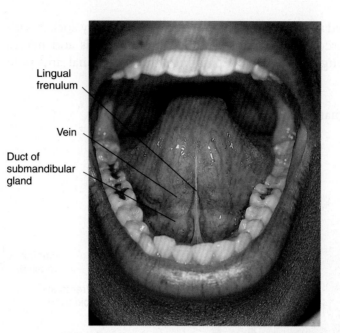

Above and behind the tongue rises an arch formed by the *anterior* and *posterior pillars*, the *soft palate*, and the *uvula*. A meshwork of small blood vessels may web the soft palate. The *pharynx* is visible in the recess behind the soft palate and tongue.

In the adjacent photograph, note the right tonsil protruding from the hollowed *tonsillar fossa*, or cavity, between the anterior and posterior pillars. In adults, tonsils are often small or absent, as in the empty left tonsillar fossa here.

The *buccal mucosa* lines the cheeks. Each *parotid duct,* sometimes termed *Stensen's duct,* opens onto the buccal mucosa near the upper second molar. Its location is frequently marked by its own small papilla.

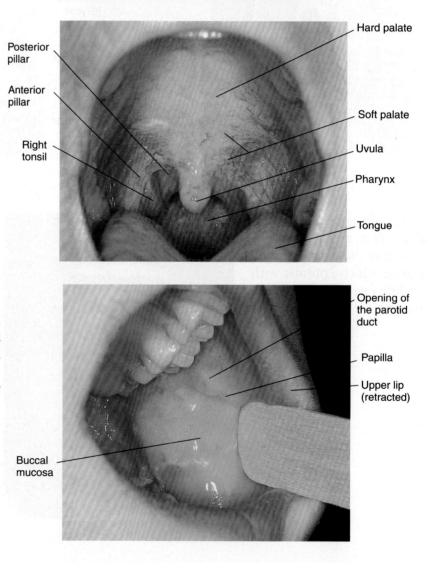

Techniques of Examination

If the patient wears dentures, offer a paper towel and ask the patient to remove them so that you can see the mucosa underneath. If you detect any suspicious ulcers or nodules, put on a glove and palpate any lesions, noting any thickening or infiltration of the tissues that might suggest malignancy.

Inspect the following:

The Lips. Observe their color and moisture, and note any lumps, ulcers, cracking, or scaliness.

The Oral Mucosa. Look into the patient's mouth and, with a good light and the help of a tongue blade, inspect the oral mucosa for color, ulcers, white patches, and nodules. The wavy white line on the adjacent buccal mucosa developed where the upper and lower teeth meet, related to irritation from sucking or chewing.

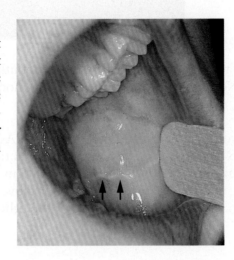

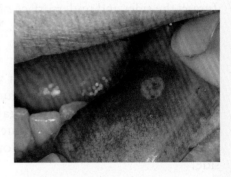

The Gums and Teeth. Note the color of the gums, normally pink. Brown patches may be present, especially but not exclusively in black people.

Inspect the gum margins and the interdental papillae for swelling or ulceration.

Inspect the teeth. Are any of them missing, discolored, misshapen, or abnormally positioned? Check for looseness with your gloved thumb and index finger.

The Roof of the Mouth. Inspect the color and architecture of the hard palate.

Bright red edematous mucosa underneath a denture suggests denture sore mouth. There may be ulcers or papillary granulation tissue.

Cyanosis, pallor. See Table 7-22, Abnormalities of the Lips, pp. 282–283.

This patient has an *aphthous ulcer* on the labial mucosa.

See Table 7-23, Findings in the Pharynx, Palate, and Oral Mucosa, pp. 284–286.

Redness of *gingivitis*, black line of *lead poisoning*

Swollen interdental papillae in *gingivitis*. See Table 7-24, Findings in the Gums and Teeth, pp. 287–288.

Torus palatinus, a benign midline lump (see p. 285)

The Tongue and the Floor of the Mouth. Ask the patient to put out his or her tongue. Inspect it for symmetry—a test of the hypoglossal nerve (CN XII).

Note the color and texture of the dorsum of the tongue.

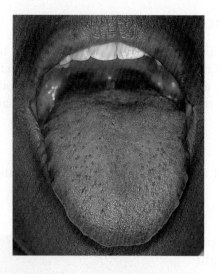

Asymmetric protrusion suggests a lesion of CN XII, as shown below.

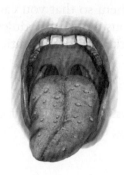

Inspect the sides and undersurface of the tongue and the floor of the mouth, areas where cancer often develops. Note any white or reddened areas, nodules, or ulcerations.

Palpate any lesions. Explain what you plan to do and put on gloves. Ask the patient to protrude the tongue. With your right hand, grasp the tip of the tongue with a square of gauze and gently pull it to the patient's left. Inspect the side of the tongue, and then palpate it with your gloved left hand, feeling for any induration. Reverse the procedure for the other side.

Tongue cancer is a common oral cancer, especially in men older than 50 years, smokers, tobacco chewers, and alcohol drinkers, and usually appears on the side or base of the tongue.[50] Any persistent nodule or ulcer, red or white, is suspect, especially if indurated. These discolored lesions represent *erythroplakia* and *leukoplakia* and should be biopsied.

A carcinoma on the left side of a tongue:

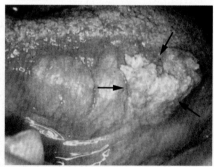

(Photo reprinted by permission of the *New England Journal of Medicine*, 328:186, 1993—arrows added)

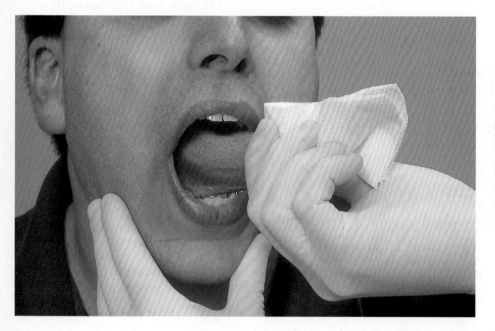

See Table 7-25, Findings in or Under the Tongue, pp. 289–290.

The Pharynx. With the patient's mouth open but the tongue not protruded, ask the patient to say "ah" or yawn. This action may let you see the pharynx well. If not, press a tongue blade firmly down upon the midpoint of the arched tongue—far enough back to visualize the pharynx but not so far that you cause gagging. Simultaneously, ask for an "ah" or a yawn. Note the rise of the soft palate—a test of CN X (the vagal nerve).

In CN X paralysis, the soft palate fails to rise and the uvula deviates to the opposite side.

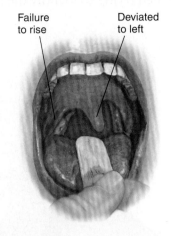

Inspect the soft palate, anterior and posterior pillars, uvula, tonsils, and pharynx. Note their color and symmetry and look for exudate, swelling, ulceration, or tonsillar enlargement. If possible, palpate any suspicious area for induration or tenderness. Tonsils have crypts, or deep infoldings of squamous epithelium. Whitish spots of normal exfoliating epithelium may sometimes be seen in these crypts.

Tonsillar exudates are common in *streptococcal pharyngitis.*[29]

Discard your tongue blade after use.

See Table 7-23, Findings in the Pharynx, Palate, and Oral Mucosa, pp. 284–286.

THE NECK

Anatomy and Physiology

For descriptive purposes, divide each side of the neck into two triangles bounded by the sternomastoid muscle. Visualize the borders of the two triangles as follows:

- For the *anterior triangle:* the mandible above, the sternomastoid laterally, and the midline of the neck medially

- For the *posterior triangle:* the sternomastoid muscle, the trapezius, and the clavicle. Note that a portion of the omohyoid muscle crosses the lower portion of this triangle and can be mistaken for a lymph node or mass.

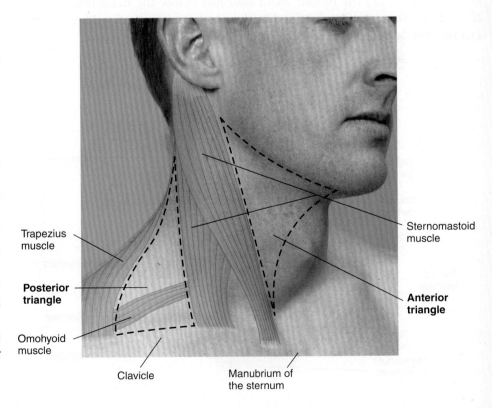

Great Vessels.   Deep to the sternomastoids run the great vessels of the neck: the *carotid artery* and the *internal jugular vein*. The *external jugular vein* passes diagonally over the surface of the sternomastoid and may be helpful when trying to identify the jugular venous pressure (see pp. 361–365).

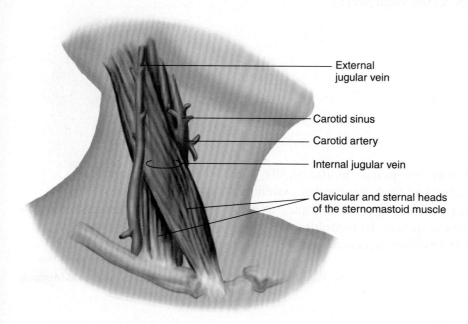

External jugular vein

Carotid sinus

Carotid artery

Internal jugular vein

Clavicular and sternal heads of the sternomastoid muscle

Midline Structures and Thyroid Gland.   Now identify the following midline structures: (1) the mobile *hyoid bone* just below the mandible, (2) the *thyroid cartilage,* readily identified by the notch on its superior edge, (3) the *cricoid cartilage,* (4) the *tracheal rings,* and (5) the *thyroid gland.*

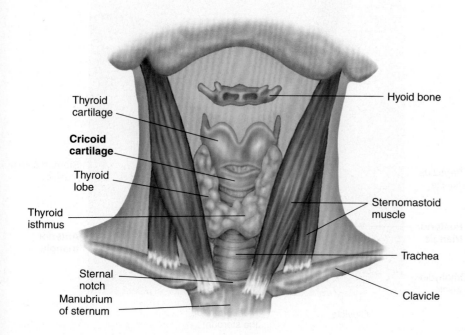

Thyroid cartilage

Cricoid cartilage

Thyroid lobe

Thyroid isthmus

Sternal notch

Manubrium of sternum

Hyoid bone

Sternomastoid muscle

Trachea

Clavicle

The thyroid gland is usually located above the suprasternal notch. The thyroid isthmus spans the second, third, and fourth tracheal rings just below the cricoid cartilage. The lateral lobes of the thyroid curve posteriorly around the sides of the trachea and the esophagus; each is about 4 cm to 5 cm in length. Except in the midline, the thyroid gland is covered by thin straplike muscles anchored to the hyoid bone and more laterally, by the sternomastoids; only the sternomastoids are visible.

Lymph Nodes. The *lymph nodes* of the head and neck are classified in a variety of ways. One classification is shown here, together with the directions of lymphatic drainage. The deep cervical chain is largely obscured by the overlying sternomastoid muscle, but at its two extremes, the tonsillar node and supraclavicular nodes may be palpable. The submandibular nodes lie superficial to the submandibular gland, and should be differentiated. Nodes are normally round or ovoid, smooth, and smaller than this gland. The gland is larger and has a lobulated, slightly irregular surface (see p. 244).

Note that the tonsillar, submandibular, and submental nodes drain portions of the mouth and throat as well as the face.

Knowledge of the lymphatic system is important. When you detect a malignant or inflammatory lesion, look for enlargement of the regional lymph nodes that drain it; when a node is enlarged or tender, look for a source such as infection in its nearby drainage area.

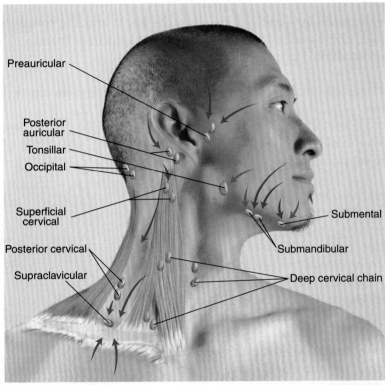

External lymphatic drainage
Internal lymphatic drainage (from mouth and throat)

Techniques of Examination

Inspect the neck, noting its symmetry and any masses or scars. Look for enlargement of the parotid or submandibular glands, and note any visible lymph nodes.

A scar of past thyroid surgery is often a clue to unsuspected thyroid disease.

The Lymph Nodes. *Palpate the lymph nodes.* Using the pads of your index and middle fingers, move the skin over the underlying tissues in each area. The patient should be relaxed, with neck flexed slightly forward and, if needed, turned slightly toward the side being examined. You can usually examine both sides at once. For the submental node, however, it is helpful to feel with one hand while bracing the top of the head with the other.

Feel in sequence for the following nodes:

1. *Preauricular*—in front of the ear

2. *Posterior auricular*—superficial to the mastoid process

3. *Occipital*—at the base of the skull posteriorly

4. *Tonsillar*—at the angle of the mandible

5. *Submandibular*—midway between the angle and the tip of the man-dible. These nodes are usually smaller and smoother than the lobulated submandibular gland against which they lie.

6. *Submental*—in the midline a few centimeters behind the tip of the man-dible

7. *Superficial cervical*—superficial to the sternomastoid

8. *Posterior cervical*—along the anterior edge of the trapezius

9. *Deep cervical chain*—deep to the sternomastoid and often inaccessible to examination. Hook your thumb and fingers around either side of the sternomastoid muscle to find them.

10. *Supraclavicular*—deep in the angle formed by the clavicle and the ster-nomastoid

A "tonsillar node" that pulsates is really the carotid artery. A small, hard, tender "tonsillar node" high and deep between the mandible and the sternomastoid is probably a styloid process.

Enlargement of a supraclavicular node, especially on the left, sug-gests possible metastasis from a thoracic or an abdominal malig-nancy.

→ External lymphatic drainage
→ Internal lymphatic drainage (e.g., from mouth and throat)

Note their size, shape, delimitation (discrete or matted together), mobil-ity, consistency, and any tenderness. Small, mobile, discrete, nontender nodes, sometimes termed "shotty," are frequently found in normal people.

- Using the pads of the second and third fingers, palpate the *preau-ricular nodes* with a gentle rotary motion. Then examine the posterior auricular and occipital lymph nodes.

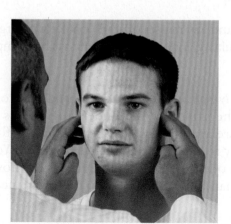

Tender nodes suggest inflamma-tion; hard or fixed nodes suggest malignancy.

Describe enlarged nodes in two dimensions, maximal length and width, for example, 1 cm × 2 cm.

- Palpate the *anterior superficial and deep cervical chains*, located anterior and superficial to the sternomastoid. Then palpate the *posterior cervical chain* along the trapezius (anterior edge) and along the sternomastoid (posterior edge). Flex the patient's neck slightly forward toward the side being examined. Examine the supraclavicular nodes in the angle between the clavicle and the sternomastoid.

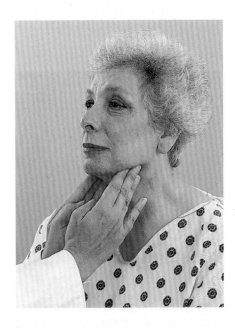 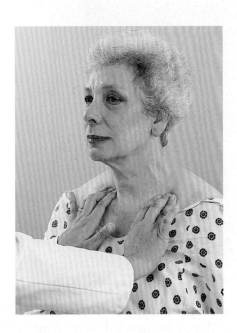

Enlarged or tender nodes, if unexplained, call for (1) re-examination of the regions they drain and (2) careful assessment of lymph nodes elsewhere so that you can distinguish between regional and generalized lymphadenopathy.

Generalized lymphadenopathy is seen in HIV or AIDS, *infectious mononucleosis, lymphoma, leukemia,* and *sarcoidosis.*

Occasionally you may mistake a band of muscle or an artery for a lymph node. You should be able to roll a node in two directions: up and down, and side to side. Neither a muscle nor an artery will pass this test.

The Trachea and the Thyroid Gland. To orient yourself to the neck, identify the thyroid and cricoid cartilages and the trachea below them.

- *Inspect the trachea* for any deviation from its usual midline position. Then *feel for any deviation.* Place your finger along one side of the trachea and note the space between it and the sternomastoid. Compare it with the other side. The spaces should be symmetric.

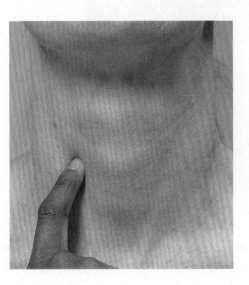

Masses in the neck may push the trachea to one side. Tracheal deviation may also signify important problems in the thorax, such as a mediastinal mass, atelectasis, or a large pneumothorax (see pp. 330–331).

- *Inspect the neck for the thyroid gland.* Tip the patient's head back a bit. Using tangential lighting directed downward from the tip of the patient's chin, *inspect the region below the cricoid cartilage* for the gland. The lower shadowed border of the thyroid glands shown here is outlined by arrows.

The patient below has a *goiter*, defined as enlargement of the thyroid gland to twice its normal size. Goiters may be simple, without nodules, or multinodular, and are usually euthyroid.[51–53]

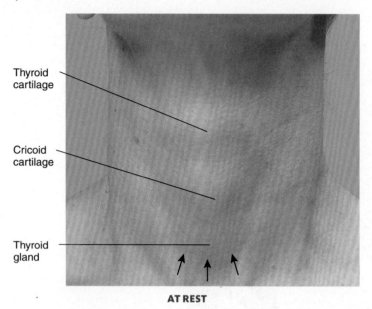

Thyroid cartilage

Cricoid cartilage

Thyroid gland

AT REST

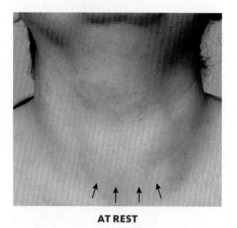

AT REST

- *Observe the patient swallowing.* Ask the patient to sip some water and to extend the neck again and swallow. Watch for upward movement of the thyroid gland, noting its contour and symmetry. The thyroid cartilage, the cricoid cartilage, and the thyroid gland all rise with swallowing and then fall to their resting positions.

With swallowing, the lower border of this large gland rises and looks less symmetric.

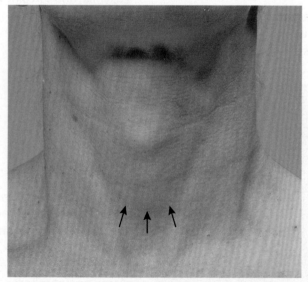

SWALLOWING

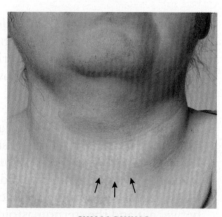

SWALLOWING

Confirm your visual observations by palpating the gland outlines as you stand facing the patient. This helps prepare you for the more systematic palpation to follow.

See Table 7-26, Thyroid Enlargement and Function, p. 291.

● *Palpate the thyroid gland.* This may seem difficult at first. Use the cues from visual inspection. Find your landmarks—the notched thyroid cartilage and the cricoid cartilage below it. Locate the *thyroid isthmus,* usually overlying the second, third, and fourth tracheal rings.

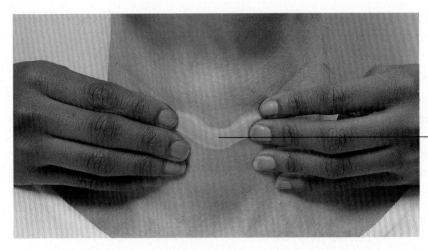

Cricoid cartilage

Develop good technique by adopting the steps below, which outline the posterior approach to palpation. The anterior approach is similar and yields comparable findings.[52] The thyroid gland is usually easier to palpate in a long slender neck. In shorter necks, hyperextension of the neck may be helpful. If the lower pole of the thyroid gland is not palpable, suspect a retrosternal location.

When the thyroid gland is retrosternal, below the suprasternal notch, it is often not palpable. *Retrosternal goiters* can cause hoarseness, shortness of breath, stridor, or dysphagia from tracheal compression; neck hyperextension and arm elevation may cause flushing from dilatation of the external jugular veins and obstruction of the thoracic inlet. Usually they present in the fifth decade; over 85% are benign.[51,41]

Steps for Palpating the Thyroid Gland (Posterior Approach)

▶ Ask the patient to flex the neck slightly forward to relax the sternomastoid muscles.

▶ Place the fingers of both hands on the patient's neck so that your index fingers are just below the cricoid cartilage.

▶ Ask the patient to sip and swallow water as before. Feel for the thyroid isthmus rising up under your finger pads. It is often, but not always, palpable.

▶ Displace the trachea to the right with the fingers of the left hand; with the right-hand fingers, palpate laterally for the right lobe of the thyroid in the space between the displaced trachea and the relaxed sternomastoid. Find the lateral margin. In a similar fashion, examine the left lobe.

   The lobes are somewhat harder to feel than the isthmus, so practice is needed. The anterior surface of a lateral lobe is approximately the size of the distal phalanx of the thumb and feels somewhat rubbery.

▶ Note the *size, shape,* and *consistency* of the gland and identify any *nodules* or *tenderness.*

▶ If the thyroid gland is enlarged, listen over the lateral lobes with a stethoscope to detect a *bruit,* a sound similar to a cardiac murmur but of noncardiac origin.

Although physical characteristics of the thyroid gland, such as size, shape, and consistency, are important, assessment of thyroid function depends upon symptoms, signs elsewhere in the body, and on laboratory tests.[54–57]

Soft in *Graves' disease*; firm in *Hashimoto's thyroiditis,* malignancy. Benign and malignant nodules,[53,58,59] tenderness in thyroiditis.

A localized systolic or continuous bruit may be heard in *hyperthyroidism.*

The Carotid Arteries and Jugular Veins. Defer a detailed examination of the neck vessels until you begin examining the cardiovascular system when the patient is supine with the head elevated to 30 degrees. Jugular venous distention may be visible when the patient is in the sitting position and should be promptly assessed. Also be alert to unusually prominent arterial pulsations.

See Chapter 9, Cardiovascular System, pp. 333–403.

Jugular venous distention is common in *heart failure.*

Note that many clinicians would examine the *cranial nerves* at this point while facing the seated patient.

See Chapter 17, Nervous System, pp. 681–762.

SPECIAL TECHNIQUES

Eye Protrusion (Proptosis or Exophthalmos). For eyes that seem unusually prominent, stand behind the seated patient and inspect from above. Draw the upper lids gently upward, then compare the protrusion of the eyes and the relationship of the corneas to the lower lids. For objective measurement, use an exophthalmometer. This instrument measures the distance between the lateral angle of the orbit and an imaginary line across the most anterior point of the cornea. The upper limits of normal are 20 mm to 22 mm.[60–61]

When protrusion exceeds normal, further evaluation by ultrasound or computerized tomography scan often follows.[63]

Exophthalmos is present in approximately 60% of patients with Graves' ophthalmopathy, and seen in half of patients with Graves' disease from autoimmune hyperthyroidism. Common symptoms of Graves' ophthalmopathy are diplopia and tearing, grittiness, and pain from corneal exposure. Eyelid retraction (91%), extraocular muscle dysfunction (43%), ocular pain (30%), and lacrimation (23%) are also common physical findings.[63,64] See also Table 7-27, Symptoms and Signs of Thyroid Disorders, p. 291.

Nasolacrimal Duct Obstruction. This test helps identify the cause of excessive tearing. Ask the patient to look up. Press on the lower lid close to the medial canthus, just inside the rim of the bony orbit; this compresses the lacrimal sac. Look for fluid regurgitated out of the puncta into the eye. Avoid this test if the area is inflamed and tender.

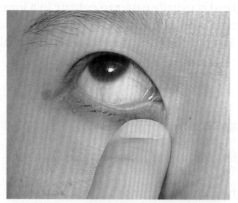

Discharge of mucopurulent fluid from the puncta suggests an obstructed nasolacrimal duct.

Upper Palpebral Conjunctiva. To search thoroughly for a foreign body in the eye, evert the upper lid following the steps below.

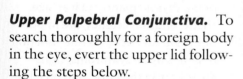

- Ask the patient to look down and relax the eyes. Be reassuring and use gentle deliberate movements. Raise the upper eyelid slightly so the lashes protrude, then grasp the upper eyelashes and pull them gently down and forward.

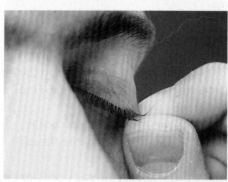

- Place a small stick such as an applicator or a tongue blade at least 1 cm above the lid margin at the upper border of the tarsal plate. Push down on the stick as you raise the edge of the lid, thus everting the eyelid or turning it "inside out." Do not press on the eyeball itself.

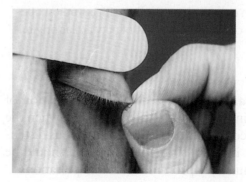

- Secure the upper lashes against the eyebrow with your thumb and inspect the palpebral conjunctiva. After your inspection, grasp the upper eyelashes and pull them gently forward. Ask the patient to look up. The eyelid will return to its normal position.

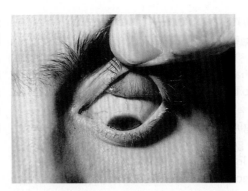

This view allows you to see the upper palpebral conjunctiva and look for a foreign body that might be lodged there.

Swinging Flashlight Test. The swinging flashlight test is a clinical test for functional impairment in the optic nerves. In dim light, note the size of the pupils. After asking the patient to gaze into the distance, swing the beam of a penlight first into one pupil, then into the other. Normally, each illuminated eye constricts promptly. The opposite eye also constricts consensually.

If left-sided optic nerve damage is present, the pupils usually react as follows: When the light beam shines into the normal right eye, there is brisk constriction of both pupils (direct response on the right and consensual response on the left). When the light swings over to the abnormal left eye, partial dilation of both pupils will occur. The afferent stimulus on the left is reduced so the efferent signals to both pupils are also reduced and a net dilation occurs. This demonstrates an afferent pupillary defect, sometimes termed as a *Marcus Gunn pupil*, the most common pupillary abnormality.

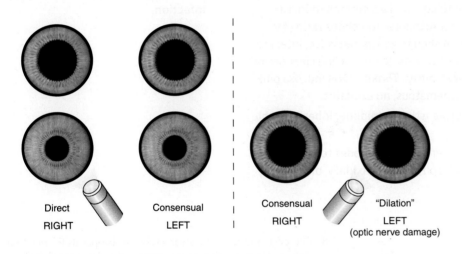

Direct RIGHT   Consensual LEFT   Consensual RIGHT   "Dilation" LEFT (optic nerve damage)

Transillumination of the Sinuses. To assess sinusitis, this test may be helpful but is not highly sensitive or specific. The room should be dark. Using a strong, narrow light source, place the light snugly deep under each brow, close to the nose. Shield the light with your hand. Look for a dim red glow as light is transmitted through the air-filled frontal sinus to the forehead.

Ask the patient to tilt his or her head back with mouth opened wide. (An upper denture should first be removed.) Shine the light downward from just below the inner aspect of each eye. Look through the open mouth at the hard palate. A reddish glow indicates a normal air-filled maxillary sinus.

Absence of glow suggests a thickened mucosa or secretions in the frontal sinus, but it may also result from developmental absence of one or both sinuses.

Absence of glow suggests thickened mucosa or secretions in the maxillary sinus.

Recording Your Findings

Initially you may use sentences to describe your findings; later you will use phrases. The style on the next page contains phrases appropriate for most write-ups.

Recording the Physical Examination—The Head, Eyes, Ears, Nose, and Throat (HEENT)

HEENT: Head—The skull is normocephalic/atraumatic (NC/AT). Hair with average texture. *Eyes*—Visual acuity 20/20 bilaterally. Sclera white, conjunctiva pink. Pupils are 4 mm constricting to 2 mm, equally round and reactive to light and accommodations. Disc margins sharp; no hemorrhages or exudates, no arteriolar narrowing. *Ears*—Acuity good to whispered voice. Tympanic membranes (TMs) with good cone of light. Weber midline. AC > BC. *Nose*—Nasal mucosa pink, septum midline; no sinus tenderness. *Throat (or Mouth)*—Oral mucosa pink, dentition good, pharynx without exudates.
Neck—Trachea midline. Neck supple; thyroid isthmus palpable, lobes not felt.
Lymph Nodes—No cervical, axillary, epitrochlear, inguinal adenopathy.

OR

Head—The skull is normocephalic/atraumatic. Frontal balding. *Eyes*— Visual acuity 20/100 bilaterally. Sclera white; conjunctiva injected. Pupils constrict 3 mm to 2 mm, equally round and reactive to light and accommodation. Disc margins sharp; no hemorrhages or exudates. Arteriolar-to-venous ratio (AV ratio) 2:4; no AV nicking. *Ears*—Acuity diminished to whispered voice; intact to spoken voice. TMs clear. *Nose*—Mucosa swollen with erythema and clear drainage. Septum midline. Tender over maxillary sinuses. *Throat*—Oral mucosa pink, dental caries in lower molars, pharynx erythematous, no exudates.

Neck—Trachea midline. Neck supple; thyroid isthmus midline, lobes palpable but not enlarged.

Lymph Nodes—Submandibular and anterior cervical lymph nodes tender, 1×1 cm, rubbery and mobile; no posterior cervical, epitrochlear, axillary, or inguinal lymphadenopathy.

Suggests myopia and mild arteriolar narrowing. Also upper respiratory infection.

Bibliography

Citations

1. Taylor FR. Diagnosis and classification of headache. Primary Care: Clinics in Office Practice 2004;31:243–259.
2. Lipton RB, Stewart WF, Seymour D et al. Prevalence and burden of migraine in the United States: data from the American Migraine Study II. Headache 2001;41:646–657.
3. Lipton RB, Bigal ME, Diamond M et al. Migraine prevalence, disease burden, and the need for preventative therapy. Neurology 2007;68:343–349.
4. Lipton RB, Bigal ME, Steiner TJ et al. Classification of primary headaches. Neurology 2004;63:427–435.
5. Headache Classification Subcommittee of the International Headache Society. The International Classification of Headache Disorders, 2nd edition. Cephalalgia 2004;24 (Suppl 1): 9–160.
6. Sun-Edelstein C, Bigal ME, Rappoport AM. Chronic migraine and medication overuse headache: clarifying the current International Headache Society classification criteria. Cephalalgia 2009;29:445–452.
7. Fumal A, Schoenen J. Tension-type headache: current research and clinical management. Lancet Neurol 2008;7:70–83.
8. Olesen J, Steiner T, Bousser MG et al. Proposals for new standardized general diagnostic criteria for the secondary headaches. Cephalalgia 2009;29:1331–1336.
9. SchwedtTJ, Matharu MS, Dodick DW. Thunderclap headache. Lancet Neurol 2006;5:621–631.
10. Spector JT, Kahn SR, Jones MR et al. Migraine headache and ischemic stroke risk: an updated meta-analysis. Am J Med 2010; 123:612–624.
11. Chang CL, Donaghy M, Poulter N. Migraine and stroke in young women: case-control study. The World Health Organisation Collaborative Study of Cardiovascular Disease and Steroid Hormone Contraception. BMJ 1999;318(7175):13–18.
12. Kurth T, Slomke MA, Kase CS et al. Migraine, headache, and the risk of stroke in women: a prospective study. Neurology 2005;64:1020–1026.
13. World Health Organization. Medical eligibility criteria for contraceptive use. 3rd ed. Geneva, World Health Organization, 2004. Available at: www.who.int/reproductivehealth/publications/family_planning/9241562668index/en/index.html. Accessed March 5, 2011.
14. Dodick DW. Chronic daily headache. N Engl J Med 2006;354: 158–165.
15. Honkasalo ML, Kaprio J, Winter T et al. Migraine and concomitant symptoms among 8167 adult twin pairs. Headache 1995;35:70–78.

16. Shingleton BJ, O'Donoghue MW. Blurred vision. N Engl J Med 2000;343(8):556–562.

17. Coleman AC. Glaucoma. Lancet 1999;20:1803–1810.

18. Balcer LJ. Optic neuritis. N Engl J Med 2006;354:1273–1280.

19. De Jong PT. Age-related macular degeneration. N Engl J Med 2006;355:1474–1485.

20. Willems PJ. Genetic causes of hearing loss. N Engl J Med 2000;342:1101–1109.

21. Hendley JO. Otitis media. N Engl J Med 2002;347:1169–1174.

22. Chan Y. Differential diagnosis of dizziness. Curr Opin Otolaryngol Head Neck Surg 2009;17:200–203.

23. Plaut M, Valentine MD. Allergic rhinitis. N Engl J Med 2005; 353:1934–1944.

24. Wilson JF. In the clinic. Acute sinusitis. Ann Intern Med 2010; 163:ITC3–1–ITC3–16.

25. Piccirillo JF. Acute bacterial sinusitis. N Engl J Med 2004; 351:902–910.

26. Rosenfeld RM, Andes d, Bhattacharya N et al. Clinical practice guideline: adult sinusitis. Otolaryngol Head Neck Surg 2007;137(3 Suppl):S1–S31.

27. Small CB, Bachert C, Lund VJ et al. Judicious antibiotic use and intranasal corticosteroids in acute rhinosinusitis. Am J Med 2007;120:289–294.

28. Dykewicz MS, Hamilos DL. Rhinitis and sinusitis. J Allergy Clin Immunol 2010;125(2 Suppl 2):S103–S115.

29. Centor RM. Perspective: Expand the pharyngitis paradigm for adolescents and young adults. Ann Intern Med 2009;151:812–815.

30. Centor RM, Allison JJ, Cohen SJ. Pharyngitis management: defining the controversy. J Gen Intern Med 2007;22:127–130.

31. Snow V, Mottur-Pilson C, Cooper RJ et al. American Academy of Family Physicians; American College of Physicians-American Society of Internal Medicine; Centers for Disease Control. Principles of appropriate antibiotic use for acute pharyngitis in adults. Ann Intern Med 2001;134:506–508.

32. Schwartz SR, Cohen SM, Dailey SH et al. Clinical practice guideline: hoarseness (dysphonia). Otolaryngol Head Neck Surg 2009;141(3 Suppl 2):S1–S31.

33. U.S. Preventive Services Task Force. Screening for impaired visual acuity in older adults: U.S. Preventive Services Task Force recommendation statement. Ann Intern Med 2009;151:37–43.

34. Chou R, Dana T, Bougatsos C. Screening older adults for impaired visual acuity: a review of the evidence for the U.S. Preventive Services Task Force. Ann Intern Med 2009;151:44–58.

35. Rosenberg EA, Sperazza LC. The visually impaired patient. Am Fam Physician 2008;15:77:1431–1436.

36. Kaufman SR. Developments in age-related macular degeneration: diagnosis and treatment. Geriatrics 2009;64:16–19.

37. U.S. Preventive Services Task Force. Screening for glaucoma: recommendation statement. AHRQ Publication No. 04–0548–A. Agency for Health Care Quality and Research. Available at http://www.uspreventiveservicestaskforce.org/uspstf05/glaucoma/glaucrs.htm. Accessed April 15, 2011.

38. U.S. Preventive Services Task Force. Screening for hearing loss in older adults. March 2011. Available at http://www.uspreventiveservicestaskforce.org/upstf/usphear.htm. Accessed May 27, 2012.

39. U.S. Preventive Services Task Force. Counseling to prevent dental and periodontal disease. In Guide to Clinical Preventive Services, 2nd ed. Baltimore: Williams & Wilkins, 1996: 711.

40. Kerr NM, Chew SSL, Eady EK et al. Diagnostic accuracy of confrontation visual field tests. Neurology 2010;74:1184–1190

41. McGee S. Evidence Based Physical Diagnosis. St. Louis: Elsevier, 2007.

42. Levin BE. The clinical significance of spontaneous pulsations of the retinal vein. Arch Neurol 1978;35:37–40.

43. Jacks AS, Miller NR. Spontaneous retinal venous pulsation: aetiology and significance. J Neurol Neurosurg Psychiatry 2004;74:7–9.

44. Weber PC, Klein AJ. Otolaryngology for the internist. Med Clin N Am 1999;83:125–137.

45. Bagai A, Thavendiranathan P, Detsky AS. Does this patient have hearing impairment? JAMA 2006;295:416–428.

46. Pirozzo S, Papinczak T, Glasziou P. Whispered voice test for screening for hearing impairment in adults and children: systematic review. BMJ 2003;327:967–971.

47. Eekhof JA, de Bock GH, de Laat JA et al. The whispered voice: the best test for screening for hearing impairment in general practice? Br J Gen Pract 1996;46:473–474.

48. Swan IR, Browning GG. The whispered voice as a screening test for hearing impairment. J R Coll Gen Pract 1985;35:197.

49. Williams JW, Simel DL, Roberts L et al. Clinical evaluation for sinusitis: making the diagnosis by history and physical examination. Ann Intern Med 1992;117:705–710.

50. Gupta R, Pery M. Digital examination for oral cancer. BMJ 1999;319:1113–1114.

51. Hashmi SM, Premachandra DJ, Bennett AMD et al. Management of retrosternal goiters: results of early surgical intervention to prevent airway morbidity, and a review of the english literature. J Laryng Otol 2006;120:644–649.

52. Siminoski K. Does this patient have a goiter? JAMA 1995;273: 813–817.

53. Hegedus L. The thyroid nodule. N Engl J Med 2004;351: 1764–1771.

54. Devdhar M, Ousman YH, Burman KD. Hypothyroidism. Endocinrinol Metab Clin North Am 2007;36:595–615.

55. McDermott MT. In the clinic: hypothyroidism. Ann Intern Med 2009;151: ITC6–1–ITC6–16.

56. Nyack B, Hodak SP. Hyperthyroidism. Endocrinol Metab Clin North Am 2007;36:617–656.

57. Franklyn JA. Subclinical thyroid disorders—consequences and implications for treatment. Ann Endocrinol 2007;68: 229–230.

58. Hegedus L, Bonnema SJ, Bennedeck FN. Management of simple nodular goiter: current status and future perspectives. Endocr Rev 2003;24:102–132.

59. Castro MR, Gharib H. Controversies in the management of thyroid nodules. Ann Intern Med 2005;142:926–931.

60. Gladstone GJ. Ophthalmologic aspects of thyroid-related orbitopathy. Endocrinol Metab Clin North Am 1998;27:91–100.

61. Bartley GB, Fatourechi V, Kadrmas EF et al. Clinical features of Graves' ophthalmopathy in an incidence cohort. Am J Ophthalmol 1996;121:284–290.

62. Alsuhaibani AH, Nerad JA. Thyroid-associated orbitopathy. Semin Plast Surg 2007;21:65–73.

63. Bartalama L, Tanda ML. Graves' ophthalmopathy. N Engl J Med 2009;360:994–1001.

64. Brent GA. Graves' disease. N Engl J Med 2008;358:2594–2605.

65. Birkholz ES, Oetting TA. Kayser Fleischer Ring: A systems based review of the ophthalmologist's role in the diagnosis of Wilson's Disease. EyeRounds.org. July 28 2009. Available at

http://www.EyeRounds.org/cases/97–kayser-fleischer-ring-Wilsons-Disease.htm. Accessed March 19, 2011.

66. Sullivan CA, Chopdar A, Shun-Shin GA. Dense Kayser-Fleischer ring in asymptomatic Wilson's disease (hepatolenticular degeneration). Br J Ophthalmol 2002;86:114.

Additional References

The Head

Bendtsen L, Jensen R. Tension-type headache. Neurol Clinic 2009;27:525–535.

Cady RK, Dodick DW, Levine HL et al. Sinus headache: a neurology, otolaryngology, allergy, and primary care consensus on diagnosis and treatment. Mayo Clin Proc 2005;80:908–916.

Katsarava Z, Holle D, Diener HC. Medication overuse headache. Curr Neurol Neurosci Rep 2009;9:115–119.

Martin VT, Behbehani M. Ovarian hormones and migraine headache: understanding mechanisms and pathogenesis—part I. Headache 2006;46:3–23.

Schürks M, Rist PM, Bigal ME et al. Migraine and cardiovascular disease: systematic review and meta-analysis. BMJ 2009; 339:b3914.

Straus SE, Thorpe KE, Holroyd-Leduc J. How do I perform a lumbar puncture and analyze the results to diagnose bacterial meningitis? JAMA 2006;296:2012–2022.

U.S. Headache Consortium Guidelines. Available at http://www.americanheadachesociety.org/professionalresources/USHeadacheConsortiumGuidelines.asp. Accessed October 8, 2011.

Van Gijn J, Kerr RS, Rinkel GJ. Subarachnoid haemorrhage. Lancet 2007;369:306–318.

The Eye

Albert DM, Miller JW, Azar DT. Albert & Jakobiec's Principles and Practice of Ophthalmology, 3rd ed. Philadelphia: Saunders/Elsevier, 2008.

Gold DH, Lewis RA. Clinical eye atlas, 2nd ed. New York: Oxford University Press, 2011.

Ehlers JP, Shah CP, Chirag P et al (eds). The Wills Eye Manual: Office and Emergency Room Diagnosis and Treatment of Eye Disease. Philadelphia: Wolters Kluwer/Lippincott Williams & Wilkins, 2008.

Gordon-Bennett P, Ung T, Stephenson C et al. Misdiagnosis of angle closure glaucoma. BMJ 2006;333:1157–1158.

Lin AP, Orengo-Nania S, Braun UK. The PCP's role in chronic open-angle glaucoma. 2009;64:20–28.

Moore FC, Chalk C. The essential neurologic examination: what should medical students be taught? Neurology 2009;72:2020:2023.

Paulus YM, Gariano RF. Diabetic retinopathy: a growing concern in an aging population. Geriatrics 2009;64:16–20.

Mohamed Q, Gillies MC, Wong TY. Management of diabetic retinopathy. JAMA 2007;298:902–916.

Spoor TC (ed). Atlas of Neuro-ophthalmology. New York: Taylor & Francis, 2004.

Rosenberg EA, Sperazza LC. The visually impaired patient. Am Fam Physician 2008;77:1431–1436.

Wong TY, Klein R, Sharrett AR et al. Retinal arteriolar diameter and risk for hypertension. Ann Intern Med 2004;140:248–255.

Yanoff M, Duker JS. Ophthalmology, 3rd ed. St. Louis: Mosby, 2009.

The Ears, Nose, and Throat

Bagai A, Thavendiranathan P, Detsky AS. Does this patient have hearing impairment? JAMA 2006;295:416–428.

Bull TR, Almeyda JS. Color Atlas of ENT Diagnosis, 5th ed. New York: Thieme, 2010.

Greenberg MS, Glick M, Ship JA et al. Burket's Oral Medicine, 11th ed. Hamilton, Ont: BC Decker, 2008.

Houck WA, Soares-Welch CV, Montori VM, Li JT. Learning the thyroid examination--a multimodality intervention for internal medicine residents. Teach Learn Med 2002;14:24–28.

Ip S, Fu L, Balk E et al. Update on acute bacterial rhinosinusitis. Evidence Report/Technology Assessment No. 124. (Prepared by Tufts-New England Medical Center Evidence-based Practice Center under Contract No. 290–02–0022). AHRQ Publication No. 05–E020–2. Rockville, MD: Agency for Healthcare Research and Quality. June 2005.

Olivencia-Simmons I. Wegener's granulomatosis: symptoms, diagnosis, and treatment. J Am Acad Nurse Pract 2007; 19:315–320.

Patil SP, Schneider H, Schwartz AR, Smith PL. Adult obstructive sleep apnea: pathophysiology and diagnosis. Chest 2007; 132:325–337.

Langlais RP, Miller CS, Nield-Gerhig JS. Color Atlas of Common Oral Diseases, 4th ed. Philadelphia: Wolters/Kluwer Lippincott Williams & Wilkins, 2009.

Newman MF, Takei H, Klokkevold PR et al. Carranza's Clinical Periodontology, 11th ed. St. Louis: Saunders Elsevier, 2012.

Radtke A, von Brevern M, Tiel-Wilck K et al. Self-treatment with a modified epley procedure resolved positional vertigo self-treatment of benign paroxysmal positional vertigo: Semont maneuver vs. Epley procedure. Neurology 2004;63:150–152.

Regezi JA, Sciubba JJ, Jordan RCK. Oral Pathology: Clinical Pathologic Correlations, 6th ed. St. Louis: Elsevier/Saunders, 2008.

Tan T, Little P, Stokes T. Guideline Development Group. Antibiotic prescribing for self limiting respiratory tract infections in primary care: summary of NICE guidance. BMJ 2008;23;337:a437.

The Neck

Bliss SJ, Flanders SA, Saint S. A pain in the neck. N Engl J Med 2004;350:1037–1042.

Dorshimer GW, Kelly M. Cervical pain in the athlete: common conditions and treatment. Prim Care 2005;32:231–243.

Henry PH, Long DL. Enlargement of the lymph nodes and spleen. In Longo DL, Fauci AS, Kasper DL et al (eds). Harrison's Principles of Internal Medicine, 18th ed. New York: McGraw-Hill, 2011.

Rosenberg TL, Brown JJ, Jefferson GD. Evaluating the adult patient with a neck mass. Med Clin North Am 2010;94: 1017–1029.

> **The Bates' suite offers these additional resources to enhance learning and facilitate understanding of this chapter:**
>
> - Bates' Pocket Guide to Physical Examination and History Taking, 7th edition
> - Bates' Visual Guide to Physical Examination
> - thePoint online resources, for students and instructors: http://thepoint.lww.com

Table
7-1 Primary Headaches

	Migraines	Tension	Cluster
Process	Neuronal dysfunction, possibly of brainstem origin, involving low serotonin, spreading cortical depression and trigemino-vascular activation. Types: with aura; without aura; variants.	Unclear—possibly heightened CNS pain sensitivity. Involves pericranial muscle tenderness. Etiology also unclear.	Unclear—possibly hypothalamic then trigemino-autonomic activation.
Location	Unilateral in ~70%; bifrontal or global in ~30%	Usually bilateral; may be generalized or localized to the back of the head and upper neck or to the frontotemporal area	Unilateral, usually behind or around the eye or temple
Quality and Severity	Throbbing or aching, variable in severity.	Steady; pressing or tightening; nonthrobbing. Mild to moderate intensity	Deep, continuous, severe
Timing			
Onset	Fairly rapid, reaching a peak in 1–2 hours	Gradual	Abrupt; peaks within minutes
Duration	4–72 hours	30 minutes to 7 days	Up to 3 hours
Course	Peak incidence early to mid-adolescence; prevalence is ~6% in men and ~15% in women. Recurrent—usually monthly, but weekly in ~10%	Episodic; may be chronic; Annual prevalence ~40%	Episodic, clustered in time, with several each day for 4–8 weeks and then relief for 6–12 months; prevalence <1%, more common in men.
Associated Factors	Nausea, vomiting, photophobia, phonophobia, aura in 30%, either visual (flickering, zig-zagging lines), motor (paresthesias of hand, arm, or face, or language dysfunction).	Sometimes photophobia, phonophobia; nausea absent	Autonomic symptoms: lacrimation, rhinorrhea, miosis, ptosis, eyelid edema, conjunctival infection
Factors That Aggravate or Provoke	Alcohol, certain foods, or stress may provoke; also menses, high altitude; aggravated by noise and bright light	Sustained muscle tension, as in driving or typing	During attack, sensitivity to alcohol may increase
Factors That Relieve	Quiet, dark room; sleep; sometimes transient relief from pressure on the involved artery	Possibly massage, relaxation	

Sources: Taylor FR. Diagnosis and classification of headache. Primary Care: Clinics in Office Practice 2004;31:243–259; Lipton RB, Stewart WF, Seymour D et al. Prevalence and burden of migraine in the United States: data from the American Migraine Study II. Headache 2001;41:646–657; Lipton RB, Bigal ME, Steiner TJ et al. Classification of primary headaches. Neurology 2004;63:427–435; Headache Classification Subcommittee of the International Headache Society. The International Classification of Headache Disorders, 2nd ed. Cephalalgia 2004;24 (Suppl 1):9–160; Sun-Edelstein C, Bigal ME, Rappoport AM. Chronic migraine and medication overuse headache: clarifying the current International Headache Society classification criteria. Cephalalgia 2009;29:445–452; Fumal A, Schoenen J. Tension-type headache: current research and clinical management. Lancet Neurol 2008;7:70–83; Schwedt TJ, Matharu MS, Dodick DW. Thunderclap headache. Lancet Neurol 2006;5:621–631.

| Table 7-2 | **Secondary Headaches and Cranial Neuralgias** |

Type	Process	Location	Quality and Severity
Secondary Headaches			
Analgesic Rebound	Withdrawal of medication	Previous headache pattern	Variable
Headaches From Eye Disorders			
Errors of Refraction (farsightedness and astigmatism, but not nearsightedness)	Probably the sustained contraction of the extraocular muscles, and possibly of the frontal, temporal, and occipital muscles	Around and over the eyes; may radiate to the occipital area	Steady, aching, dull
Acute Glaucoma	Sudden increase in intraocular pressure (see p. 262)	In and around one eye	Steady, aching, often severe
Headache From Sinusitis	Mucosal inflammation of the paranasal sinuses	Usually above the eye (frontal sinus) or over the maxillary sinus	Aching or throbbing, variable in severity; consider possible migraine
Meningitis	Infection of the meninges surrounding the brain and spinal cord	Generalized	Steady or throbbing, very severe
Subarachnoid Hemorrhage	Bleeding, most often from a ruptured intracranial aneurysm	Generalized	Very severe, "the worst of my life"
Brain Tumor	Displacement of or traction on pain-sensitive arteries and veins or pressure on nerves	Varies with the location of the tumor	Aching, steady, variable in intensity
Giant Cell (Temporal) Arteritis	Vasculitis from cell-mediated immune response to elastic lamina of artery	Localized near the involved artery, most often the temporal, but also the occipital; age related	Throbbing, generalized, persistent; often severe
Postconcussion Headache	Follows acceleration-deceleration traumatic brain injury	May be localized to the injured area, but not necessarily	Generalized, dull, aching, constant; may have features of tension and migraine headaches
Cranial Neuralgias			
Trigeminal Neuralgia (CNV)	Compression of CN V, often by aberrant loop of artery or vein, usually near entry to pons	Cheek, jaws, lips, or gums; trigeminal nerve divisions 2 and 3 > 1	Shocklike, stabbing, burning; severe

Note: Blanks appear in this table when the categories are not applicable or not usually helpful in assessing the problem.

Sources: Lipton RB, Bigal ME, Steiner TJ et al. Classification of primary headaches. Neurology 2004;63:427–435; Headache Classification Subcommittee of the International Headache Society. The International Classification of Headache Disorders, 2nd ed. Cephalalgia 2004;24 Suppl 1:9–160; Van de Beek D, de Gans J, Spanjaard L et al. Clinical features and prognostic factors in adults with bacterial meningitis. N Engl J Med 2004;351:1849–1859; Salvarini C, Cantini F, Hunder GG. Polymyalgia rheumatica and giant cell arteritis. Lancet 2008;372:234–245; Smetana GW, Shmerling RH. Does this patient have temporal arteritis? JAMA 2002;287:92–101; Ropper AH, Gorson KC. Clinical practice. Concussion. N Engl J Med 2007;356:166–172.

| Timing | | | | Factors That | |
Onset	Duration	Course	Associated Factors	Aggravate or Provoke	Factors That Relieve
Variable	Depends on prior headache pattern	Depends on frequency of "mini-withdrawals"	Depends on prior headache pattern	Fever, carbon monoxide, hypoxia, withdrawal of caffeine, other headache triggers	Depends on cause
Gradual	Variable	Variable	Eye fatigue, "sandy" sensations in the eyes, redness of the conjunctiva	Prolonged use of the eyes, particularly for close work	Rest of the eyes
Often rapid	Variable, may depend on treatment	Variable, may depend on treatment	Diminished vision, sometimes nausea and vomiting	Sometimes provoked by drops that dilate the pupils	
Variable	Often several hours at a time, recurring over days or longer	Often recurrent in a repetitive daily pattern	Local tenderness, nasal congestion, discharge, and fever	May be aggravated by coughing, sneezing, or jarring the head	Nasal decongestants, antibiotics
Fairly rapid, usually <24 hours	Variable, usually days	A persistent headache in an acute illness	Fever, stiff neck, change in mental status		Immediate antibiotics until determined if bacterial or viral
Usually abrupt, severe with prodromal symptoms	Variable, usually days	A persistent headache in an acute illness	Nausea, vomiting, possibly loss of consciousness, neck pain		Subspecialty treatments
Variable	Often brief	Often intermittent but progressive		May be aggravated by coughing, sneezing, or sudden movements of the head	Subspecialty treatments
Gradual or rapid	Variable	Recurrent or persistent over weeks to months	Tenderness of the adjacent scalp; fever (in ~50%), fatigue, weight loss; new headache (~60%), jaw claudication (~50%), visual loss or blindness (~15%–20%), polymyalgia rheumatica (~50%)	Movement of neck and shoulders	
Within 7 days of the injury up to 3 months	Weeks, months, or even years	Tends to diminish over time	Poor concentration, problems with memory, vertigo, irritability, restlessness, fatigue	Mental and physical exertion, straining, stooping, emotional excitement, alcohol	Rest; medication
Abrupt, paroxysmal	Each jab lasts seconds but recurs at intervals of seconds or minutes	May last for months, then disappear for months, but often recurs. It is uncommon at night.	Exhaustion from recurrent pain	Touching certain areas of the lower face or mouth; chewing, talking, brushing teeth	Medication; neurovascular decompression

Table 7-3 Red Eyes

	Conjunctivitis	**Subconjunctival Hemorrhage**
	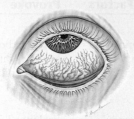	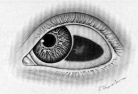
Pattern of Redness	Conjunctival injection: diffuse dilatation of conjunctival vessels with redness that tends to be maximal peripherally	Leakage of blood outside of the vessels, producing a homogeneous, sharply demarcated, red area that resolves over 2 weeks
Pain	Mild discomfort rather than pain	Absent
Vision	Not affected except for temporary mild blurring due to discharge	Not affected
Ocular Discharge	Watery, mucoid, or mucopurulent	Absent
Pupil	Not affected	Not affected
Cornea	Clear	Clear
Significance	Bacterial, viral, and other infections; highly contagious; allergy; irritation	Often none. May result from trauma, bleeding disorders, or sudden increase in venous pressure, as from cough

	Corneal Injury or Infection	**Acute Iritis**	**Acute Angle Closure Glaucoma**
	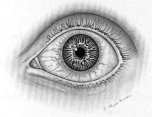	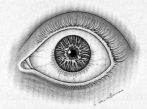	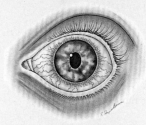
Pattern of Redness	Ciliary injection: dilation of deeper vessels that are visible as radiating vessels or a reddish violet flush around the limbus. Ciliary injection is an important sign of these three conditions but may not be apparent. The eye may be diffusely red instead. Other clues of these more serious disorders are pain, decreased vision, unequal pupils, and a clouded cornea.		
Pain	Moderate to severe, superficial	Moderate, aching, deep	Severe, aching, deep
Vision	Usually decreased	Decreased; photophobia	Decreased
Ocular Discharge	Watery or purulent	Absent	Absent
Pupil	Not affected unless iritis develops	Small and irregular	Dilated, fixed
Cornea	Changes depending on cause	Clear or slightly clouded; injection confined to corneal limbus	Steamy, cloudy
Significance	Abrasions, and other injuries; viral and bacterial infections	Associated with systemic infection, Herpes zoster, tuberculosis; refer promptly	Acute increase in intraocular pressure constitutes an emergency

Source: Leibowitz HM. The red eye. N Engl J Med 2000;342:345–351.

Table

7-4   **Dizziness and Vertigo**

"Dizziness" is a nonspecific term used by patients encompassing several disorders that clinicians must carefully sort out. A detailed history usually identifies the primary etiology. It is important to learn the specific meanings of the following terms or conditions:

- *Vertigo*—a spinning sensation accompanied by nystagmus and ataxia; usually from *peripheral vestibular dysfunction* (~40% of "dizzy" patients) but may be from a *central brainstem lesion* (~10%; causes include atherosclerosis, multiple sclerosis, vertebrobasilar migraine, or TIA)
- *Presyncope*—a near faint from "feeling faint or lightheaded"; causes include orthostatic hypotension, especially from medication, arrhythmias, and vasovagal attacks (~5%)
- *Disequilibrium*—unsteadiness or imbalance when walking, especially in older patients, causes include fear of walking, visual loss, weakness from musculoskeletal problems, and peripheral neuropathy (up to 15%)
- *Psychiatric*—causes include anxiety, panic disorder, hyperventilation, depression, somatization disorder, alcohol, and substance abuse (~10%)
- *Multifactorial or unknown*—(up to 20%)

Peripheral and Central Vertigo

	Onset	Duration and Course	Hearing	Tinnitus	Additional Features
Peripheral Vertigo					
Benign Positional Vertigo	Sudden, on rolling onto affected side or tilting head up	Onset a few seconds to <1 minute Lasts a few weeks, may recur	Not affected	Absent	Sometimes nausea, vomiting, nystagmus
Vestibular Neuronitis (acute labyrinthitis)	Sudden	Onset hours to up to 2 weeks May recur over 12–18 months	Not affected	Absent	Nausea, vomiting, nystagmus
Ménière's Disease	Sudden	Onset several hours to ≥1 day Recurrent	Sensorineural hearing loss—recurs, eventually progresses	Present, fluctuating	Pressure or fullness in affected ear; nausea, vomiting, nystagmus
Drug Toxicity	Insidious or acute—linked to loop diuretics, aminoglycosides, salicylates, alcohol	May or may not be reversible Partial adaptation occurs	May be impaired	May be present	Nausea, vomiting
Acoustic Neuroma	Insidious from CN VIII compression, vestibular branch	Variable	Impaired, one side	Present	May involve CN V and VII
Central Vertigo	Often sudden (see causes above)	Variable but rarely continuous	Not affected	Absent	Usually with other brainstem deficits—dysarthria, ataxia, crossed motor and sensory deficits

Sources: Chan Y. Differential diagnosis of dizziness. Curr Opin Otolaryngol Head Neck Surg 2009;17:200–203; Kroenke K, Lucas CA, Rosengerg ML et al. Causes of persistent dizziness: a prospective study of 100 patients in ambulatory care. Ann Intern Med 1992;117:898–904; Tusa RJ. Vertigo. Neurol Clin 2001;19:23–55; Lockwood AH, Salvi RJ, Burkard RF. Tinnitus. N Engl J Med 2002;347:904–910.

Table	
7-5	**Selected Facies**

FACIAL SWELLING

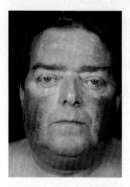

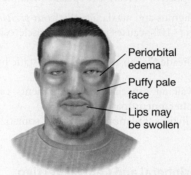

Periorbital edema
Puffy pale face
Lips may be swollen

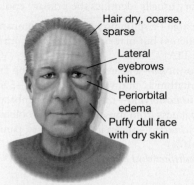

Hair dry, coarse, sparse
Lateral eyebrows thin
Periorbital edema
Puffy dull face with dry skin

Cushing's Syndrome

The increased adrenal cortisol production of Cushing's syndrome produces a round or "moon" face with red cheeks. Excessive hair growth may be present in the mustache and sideburn areas and on the chin.

Nephrotic Syndrome

The face is edematous and often pale. Swelling usually appears first around the eyes and in the morning. The eyes may become slitlike when edema is severe.

Myxedema

The patient with severe hypothyroidism (*myxedema*) has a dull, puffy facies. The edema, often pronounced around the eyes, does not pit with pressure. The hair and eyebrows are dry, coarse, and thinned. The skin is dry.

OTHER FACIES

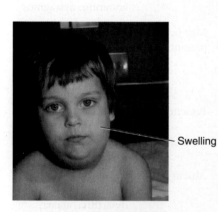

Swelling

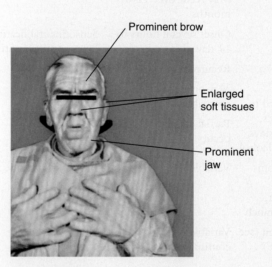

Prominent brow
Enlarged soft tissues
Prominent jaw

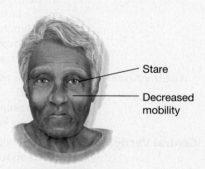

Stare
Decreased mobility

Parotid Gland Enlargement

Chronic bilateral asymptomatic parotid gland enlargement may be associated with obesity, diabetes, cirrhosis, and other conditions. Note the swellings anterior to the ear lobes and above the angles of the jaw. Gradual unilateral enlargement suggests neoplasm. Acute enlargement is seen in mumps.

Acromegaly

The increased growth hormone of acromegaly produces enlargement of both bone and soft tissues. The head is elongated, with bony prominence of the forehead, nose, and lower jaw. Soft tissues of the nose, lips, and ears also enlarge. The facial features appear generally coarsened.

Parkinson's Disease

Decreased facial mobility blunts expression. A masklike face may result, with decreased blinking and a characteristic stare. Since the neck and upper trunk tend to flex forward, the patient seems to peer upward toward the observer. Facial skin becomes oily, and drooling may occur.

Table
7-6 Visual Field Defects

Visual Field Defects

1 Horizontal Defect Occlusion of a branch of the central retinal artery may cause a horizontal (altitudinal) defect. Ischemia of the optic nerve can produce a similar defect.

2 Blind Right Eye (right optic nerve) A lesion of the optic nerve and, of course, of the eye itself, produces unilateral blindness.

3 Bitemporal Hemianopsia (optic chiasm) A lesion at the optic chiasm, may involve only fibers crossing over to the opposite side. Since these fibers originate in the nasal half of each retina, visual loss involves the temporal half of each field.

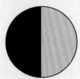

4 Left Homonymous Hemianopsia (right optic tract) A lesion of the optic tract, interrupts fibers originating on the same side of both eyes. Visual loss in the eyes is, therefore, similar (homonymous) and involves half of each field (hemianopsia).

5 Homonymous Left Superior Quadrantic Defect (right optic radiation, partial) A partial lesion of the optic radiation in the temporal lobe, may involve only a portion of the nerve fibers, producing, for example, a homonymous quadrantic defect.

 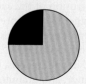

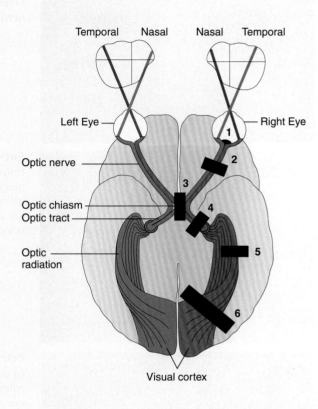

6 Left Homonymous Hemianopsia (right optic radiation) A complete interruption of fibers in the optic radiation, produces a visual defect similar to that produced by a lesion of the optic tract.

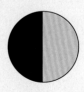

Table 7-7 | Variations and Abnormalities of the Eyelids

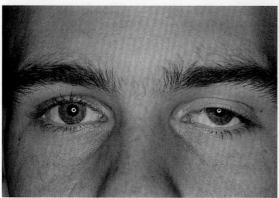

Ptosis

Ptosis is a drooping of the upper lid. Causes include myasthenia gravis, damage to the oculomotor nerve, and damage to the sympathetic nerve supply (*Horner's syndrome*). A weakened muscle, relaxed tissues, and the weight of herniated fat may cause senile ptosis. Ptosis may also be congenital.

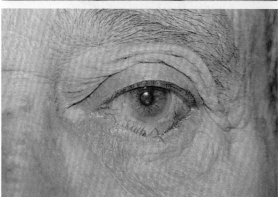

Entropion

Entropion, more common in the elderly, is an inward turning of the lid margin. The lower lashes, which are often invisible when turned inward, irritate the conjunctiva and lower cornea. Ask the patient to squeeze the lids together and then open them; then check for an entropion that is not obvious.

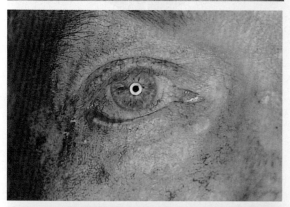

Ectropion

In ectropion, the margin of the lower lid is turned outward, exposing the palpebral conjunctiva. When the punctum of the lower lid turns outward, the eye no longer drains well, and tearing occurs. Ectropion is also more common in the elderly.

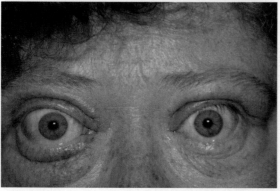

Lid Retraction and Exophthalmos

A wide-eyed stare suggests retracted eyelids. Note the rim of sclera between the upper lid and the iris. Retracted lids and "lid lag" when eyes move from up to down markedly increase the likelihood of hyperthyroidism, especially when accompanied by a fine tremor, moist skin, and heart rate >90 beats per minute.[41]

Exophthalmos describes protrusion of the eyeball, a common feature of Graves' ophthalmopathy, triggered by autoreactive T lymphocytes. In this disorder, there are a spectrum of eye changes, ranging from lid retraction to extraocular muscle dysfunction, ocular pain, and lacrimation. Changes do not always progress. In unilateral exophthalmos, consider Graves' disease (usually bilateral), trauma, orbital tumor, and granulomatous disorders.[63]

Source of photos: Ptosis, Ectropion, Entropion—Tasman W, Jaeger E, eds. The Wills Eye Hospital Atlas of Clinical Ophthalmology, 2nd ed. Philadelphia: Lippincott Williams & Wilkins, 2001.

Table 7-8
Lumps and Swellings in and Around the Eyes

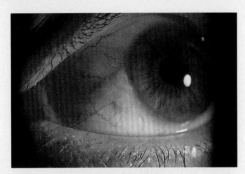

Pinguecula

A harmless yellowish triangular nodule in the bulbar conjunctiva on either side of the iris. Appears frequently with aging, first on the nasal and then on the temporal side.

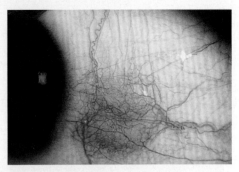

Episcleritis

A localized ocular inflammation of the episcleral vessels. Vessels appear movable over the scleral surface. May be nodular or show only redness and dilated vessels. Seen in rheumatoid arthritis, Sjögren's syndrome, and herpes zoster.

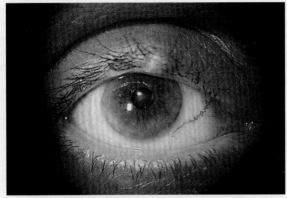

Sty

A painful, tender, red infection in a gland at the margin of the eyelid.

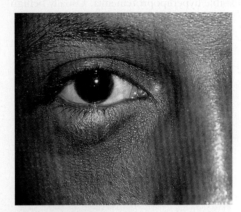

Chalazion

A subacute nontender, usually painless nodule involving a blocked meibomian gland. May become acutely inflamed but, unlike a sty, usually points inside the lid rather than on the lid margin.

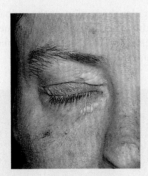

Xanthelasma

Slightly raised, yellowish, well-circumscribed plaques that appear along the nasal portions of one or both eyelids. May accompany lipid disorders.

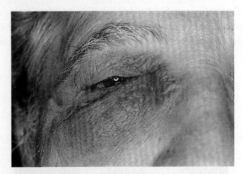

Inflammation of the Lacrimal Sac (Dacryocystitis)

A swelling between the lower eyelid and nose. An *acute* inflammation (illustrated) is painful, red, and tender. *Chronic* inflammation is associated with obstruction of the nasolacrimal duct. Tearing is prominent, and pressure on the sac produces regurgitation of material through the puncta of the eyelids.

Source of photos: Tasman W, Jaeger E, eds. The Wills Eye Hospital Atlas of Clinical Ophthalmology, 2nd ed. Philadelphia: Lippincott Williams & Wilkins, 2001.

Table	
7-9	**Opacities of the Cornea and Lens**

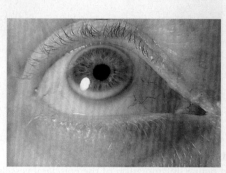

Corneal Arcus. A thin grayish white arc or circle not quite at the edge of the cornea. Accompanies normal aging but also seen in younger people, especially African Americans. In young people, suggests possible hyperlipoproteinemia. Usually benign.

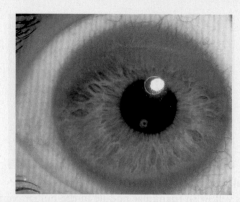

Kayser-Fleischer Ring. A golden to red brown ring, sometimes shading to green or blue, from copper deposition in the periphery of the cornea found in Wilson's disease. Due to a rare autosomal recessive mutation of the ATO7B gene on chromosome 13 causing abnormal copper transport, reduced biliary copper excretion, and abnormal accumulation of copper in the liver and tissues throughout the body. Patients present with liver disease, renal failure, and neurologic symptoms of tremor, dystonia, and psychiatric disorders ranging from behavior changes to depression and schizophrenia.[65,66]

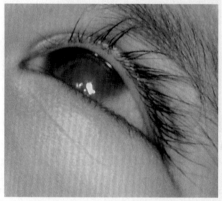

Corneal Scar. A superficial grayish white opacity in the cornea, secondary to an old injury or to inflammation. Size and shape are variable. Do not confuse with the opaque lens of a cataract, visible on a deeper plane and only through the pupil.

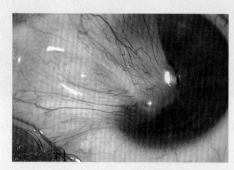

Pterygium. A triangular thickening of the bulbar conjunctiva that grows slowly across the outer surface of the cornea, usually from the nasal side. Reddening may occur. May interfere with vision as it encroaches on the pupil.

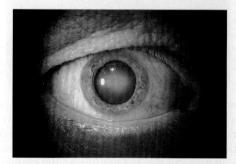

Cataracts. Opacities of the lenses visible through the pupil. Risk factors are older age, smoking, diabetes, corticosteroid use.

Nuclear cataract. A nuclear cataract looks gray when seen by a flashlight. If the pupil is widely dilated, the gray opacity is surrounded by a black rim.

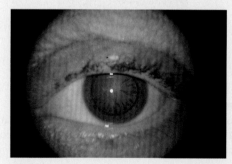

Peripheral contact. Produces spokelike shadows that point—gray against black, as seen with a flashlight, or black against red with an ophthalmoscope. A dilated pupil, as shown here, facilitates this observation.

Table 7-10   Pupillary Abnormalities

Unequal Pupils (*Anisocoria*)—When anisocoria is greater in bright light than in dim light, the larger pupil cannot constrict properly. Causes include blunt trauma to the eye, open-angle glaucoma (p. 262), and impaired parasympathetic nerve supply to the iris, as in tonic pupil and oculomotor nerve paralysis. When anisocoria is greater in dim light, the smaller pupil cannot dilate properly, as in Horner's syndrome, caused by an interruption of the sympathetic nerve supply. See also Table 17-13, Pupils in Comatose Patients, p. 761.

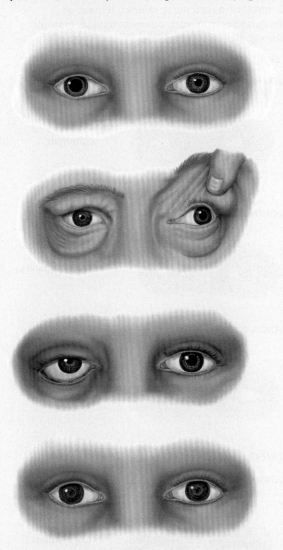

Tonic Pupil (*Adie's Pupil*). Pupil is large, regular, and usually unilateral. Reaction to light is severely reduced and slowed, or even absent. Near reaction, although very slow, is present. Slow accommodation causes blurred vision. Deep tendon reflexes are often decreased.

Oculomotor Nerve (CN III) Paralysis. The dilated pupil is fixed to light and near effort. Ptosis of the upper eyelid and lateral deviation of the eye are almost always present.

Horner's Syndrome. The affected pupil, though small, reacts briskly to light and near effort. Ptosis of the eyelid is present, perhaps with loss of sweating on the forehead. In congenital Horner's syndrome, the involved iris is lighter in color than its fellow (*heterochromia*).

Small, Irregular Pupils. Small, irregular pupils that accommodate but do not react to light indicate *Argyll Robertson pupils*. Seen in central nervous system syphilis.

Equal Pupils and One Blind Eye. Unilateral blindness does not cause anisocoria as long as the sympathetic and parasympathetic innervation to both irises is normal. A light directed into the seeing eye produces a direct reaction in that eye and a consensual reaction in the blind eye. A light directed into the blind eye, however, causes no response in either eye.

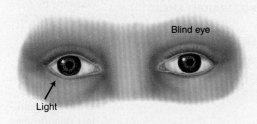

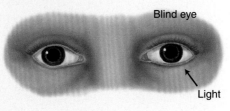

Table
7-11

Dysconjugate Gaze

There are a variety of gaze abnormality patterns that give clinicians clues about developmental disorders and cranial nerve abnormalities.

Developmental Disorders

Developmental dysconjugate gaze is caused by an imbalance in ocular muscle tone. This imbalance has many causes, may be hereditary, and usually appears in early childhood. These gaze deviations are classified according to direction:

Esotropia   *Exotropia*

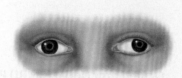

Disorders of Cranial Nerves

New onset of dysconjugate gaze in adult life is usually the result of cranial nerve injuries, lesions, or abnormalities from such causes as trauma, multiple sclerosis, syphilis, and others.

A Left Cranial Nerve VI Paralysis

LOOKING TO THE RIGHT

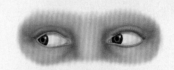

Eyes are conjugate.

Cover–Uncover Test

A cover–uncover test may be helpful. Here is what you would see in the right monocular esotropia illustrated above.

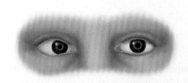

Corneal reflections are asymmetric.

LOOKING STRAIGHT AHEAD

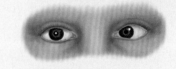

Esotropia appears.

COVER

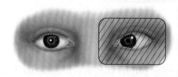

The right eye moves outward to fix on the light. (The left eye is not seen but moves inward to the same degree.)

LOOKING TO THE RIGHT

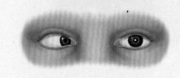

Esotropia is maximum.

A Left Cranial Nerve IV Paralysis

LOOKING DOWN AND TO THE RIGHT

UNCOVER

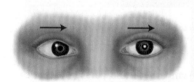

The left eye moves outward to fix on the light. The right eye deviates inward again.

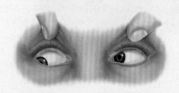

The left eye cannot look down when turned inward. Deviation is maximum in this direction.

A Left Cranial Nerve III Paralysis

LOOKING STRAIGHT AHEAD

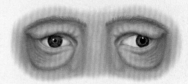

The eye is pulled outward by action of the CN VI. Upward, downward, and inward movements are impaired or lost. Ptosis and pupillary dilation may be associated.

Table	
7-12	**Normal Variations of the Optic Disc**

Physiologic Cupping

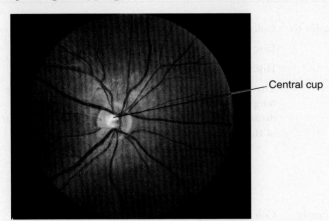

Central cup

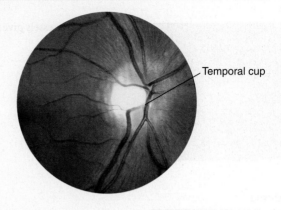

Temporal cup

The physiologic cup is a small whitish depression in the optic disc, the entry point for the retinal vessels. Although sometimes absent, the cup is usually visible either centrally or toward the temporal side of the disc. Grayish spots are often seen at its base.

Rings and Crescents

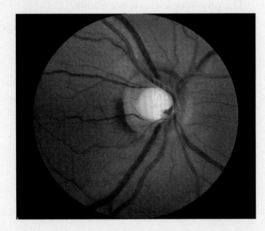

Medullated Nerve Fibers

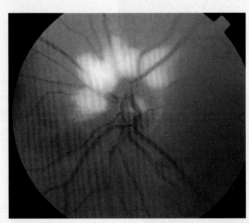

Rings and crescents are often seen around the optic disc. These are developmental variations that appear as either white sclera, black retinal pigment, or both, especially along the temporal border of the disc. Rings and crescents are not part of the disc itself and should not be included in your estimate of disc diameter.

Medullated nerve fibers are a much less common but dramatic finding. Appearing as irregular white patches with feathered margins, they obscure the disc edge and retinal vessels. They have no pathologic significance.

Table 7-13 Abnormalities of the Optic Disc

	Process	Appearance
Normal 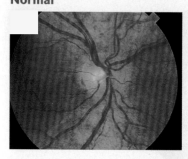	Tiny disc vessels give normal color to the disc.	Color yellowish orange to creamy pink Disc vessels tiny Disc margins sharp (except perhaps nasally) The physiologic cup is located centrally or somewhat temporally. It may be conspicuous or absent. Its diameter from side to side is usually less than half that of the disc.
Papilledema 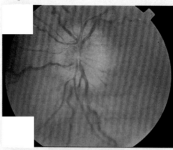	Elevated intracranial pressure causes intraaxonal edema along the optic nerve, leading to engorgement and swelling of the optic disc.	Color pink, hyperemic Often with loss of venous pulsations Disc vessels more visible, more numerous, curve over the borders of the disc Disc swollen with margins blurred The physiologic cup is not visible. Seen in intracranial mass, lesion, or hemorrhage, meningitis
Glaucomatous Cupping 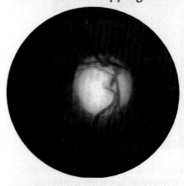	Increased pressure within the eye leads to increased cupping (backward depression of the disc) and atrophy. The base of the enlarged cup is pale.	The physiologic cup is enlarged, occupying more than half of the disc's diameter, at times extending to the edge of the disc. Retinal vessels sink in and under it, and may be displaced nasally.
Optic Atrophy 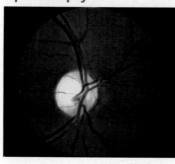	Death of optic nerve fibers leads to loss of the tiny disc vessels.	Color white Tiny disc vessels absent Seen in optic neuritis, multiple sclerosis, temporal arteritis

Sources of photos for Normal—Tasman W, Jaeger E, eds. The Wills Eye Hospital Atlas of Clinical Ophthalmology, 2nd ed. Philadelphia: Lippincott Williams & Wilkins, 2001; Papilledema, Glaucomatous Cupping, Optic Atrophy—Courtesy of Ken Freedman, MD.

Normal Retinal Artery and Arteriovenous (AV) Crossing

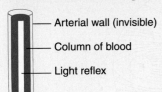

- Arterial wall (invisible)
- Column of blood
- Light reflex

The normal arterial wall is transparent; only the column of blood can usually be seen. The normal light reflex is *narrow—about one-fourth the diameter of the blood column.* Because the arterial wall is transparent, a vein crossing beneath the artery can be seen right up to the column of blood on either side.

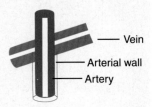

- Vein
- Arterial wall
- Artery

Retinal Arteries in Hypertension

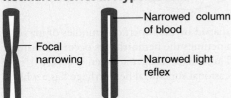

- Focal narrowing
- Narrowed column of blood
- Narrowed light reflex

In hypertension, the arteries may show areas of focal or generalized narrowing. The light reflex is also narrowed. The arterial wall thickens and becomes less transparent.

Copper Wiring

Sometimes the arteries, especially those close to the disc, become full and somewhat tortuous and develop an increased light reflex with a bright coppery luster.

Silver Wiring

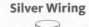

Occasionally a portion of a narrowed artery develops such an opaque wall that no blood is visible within it. It is then called a silver wire artery.

Arteriovenous Crossing

When the arterial walls lose their transparency, changes appear in the arteriovenous crossings. Decreased transparency of the retina probably also contributes to the first two changes shown below.

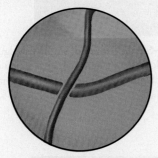

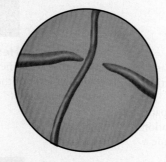

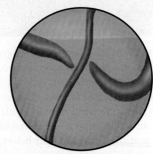

Concealment or AV nicking. The vein appears to stop abruptly on either side of the artery.

Tapering. The vein appears to taper down on either side of the artery.

Banking. The vein is twisted on the distal side of the artery and forms a dark, wide knuckle.

Table 7-15   Red Spots and Streaks in the Fundi

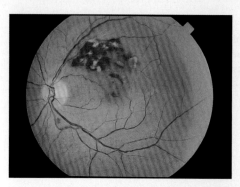

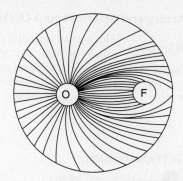

Superficial Retinal Hemorrhages—Small, linear, flame-shaped, red streaks in the fundi, shaped by the superficial bundles of nerve fibers that radiate from the optic disc in the pattern illustrated (O = optic disc; F = fovea). Sometimes the hemorrhages occur in clusters and look like a larger hemorrhage but can be identified by the linear streaking at the edges. These hemorrhages are seen in severe hypertension, papilledema, and occlusion of the retinal vein, among other conditions. An occasional superficial hemorrhage has a white center consisting of fibrin. White-centered retinal hemorrhages have many causes.

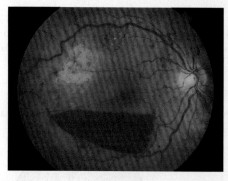

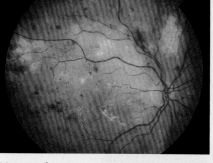

Preretinal Hemorrhage—Develops when blood escapes into the potential space between the retina and vitreous. This hemorrhage is typically larger than retinal hemorrhages. Because it is anterior to the retina, it obscures any underlying retinal vessels. In an erect patient, red cells settle, creating a horizontal line of demarcation between plasma above and cells below. Causes include a sudden increase in intracranial pressure.

Deep Retinal Hemorrhages—Small, rounded, slightly irregular red spots that are sometimes called dot or blot hemorrhages. They occur in a deeper layer of the retina than flame-shaped hemorrhages. Diabetes is a common cause.

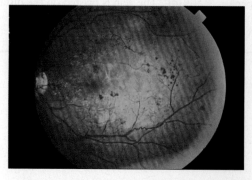

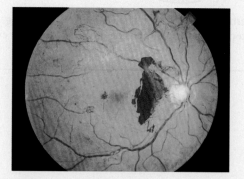

Microaneurysms—Tiny, round, red spots commonly seen in and around the macular area. They are minute dilatations of very small retinal vessels; the vascular connections are too small to be seen with an ophthalmoscope. A hallmark of diabetic retinopathy.

Neovascularization—Refers to the formation of new blood vessels. They are more numerous, more tortuous, and narrower than other blood vessels in the area and form disorderly looking red arcades. A common feature of the proliferative stage of diabetic retinopathy. The vessels may grow into the vitreous, where retinal detachment or hemorrhage may cause loss of vision.

Source of photos: Tasman W, Jaeger E, eds. The Wills Eye Hospital Atlas of Clinical Ophthalmology, 2nd ed. Philadelphia: Lippincott Williams & Wilkins, 2001.

Table 7-16 | Ocular Fundi: Normal and Hypertensive Retinopathy

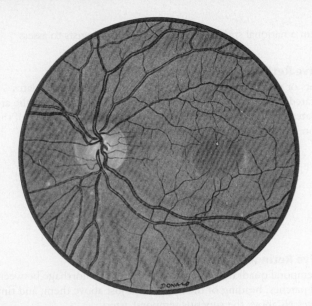

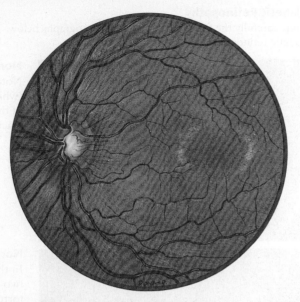

Normal Fundus of a Light-Skinned Person

Inspect the optic disc. Follow the major vessels in four directions, noting their relative sizes and any arteriovenous crossings—both normal here. Inspect the macular area. The slightly darker fovea is just discernible; no light reflex is visible in this subject. Look for any lesions in the retina. Note the striped, or tessellated, character of the fundus, especially in the lower field, that comes from normal underlying choroidal vessels. The fundus of a light-skinned person with brunette coloring is redder.

Normal Fundus of a Dark-Skinned Person

Again, inspect the disc, vessels, macula, and retina. The ring around the fovea is a normal light reflection. The color of the fundus has a grayish brown, almost purplish cast, which comes from pigment in the retina and the choroid that characteristically obscures the choroidal vessels; no tessellation is visible.

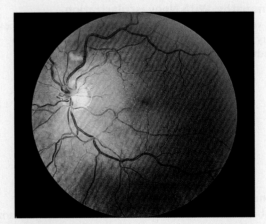

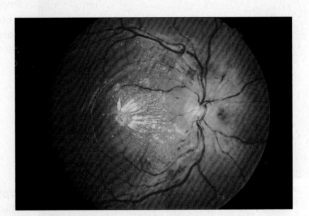

Hypertensive Retinopathy

Marked arteriolar-venous crossing changes are seen, especially along the inferior vessels. Copper wiring of the arterioles is present. A cotton-wool spot is seen just superior to the disc. Incidental disc drusen are also present but are unrelated to hypertension.

Hypertensive Retinopathy With Macular Star

Punctate exudates are readily visible: some are scattered; others radiate from the fovea to form a macular star. Note the two small, soft exudates about 1 disc diameter from the disc. Find the flame-shaped hemorrhages sweeping toward 7 o'clock and 8 o'clock; a few more may be seen toward 10 o'clock. These two fundi show changes typical of accelerated (malignant) hypertension and are often accompanied by papilledema (pp. 230–231).

Source of photos: Hypertensive Retinopathy, Hypertensive Retinopathy With Macular Star—Tasman W, Jaeger E, eds. The Wills Eye Hospital Atlas of Clinical Ophthalmology, 2nd ed. Philadelphia: Lippincott Williams & Wilkins, 2001.

Source: Wong TY, Mitchell P. Hypertensive retinopathy. N Engl J Med 2004;351:2310–2317.

Table 7-17 Ocular Fundi: Diabetic Retinopathy

Diabetic Retinopathy

Study carefully the fundi in the series of photographs below. They represent a national standard used by ophthalmologists to assess diabetic retinopathy.

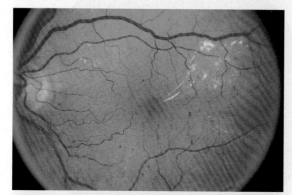

Nonproliferative Retinopathy, Moderately Severe

Note tiny red dots or microaneurysms. Note also the ring of hard exudates (white spots) located superotemporally. Retinal thickening or edema in the area of the hard exudates can impair visual acuity if it extends into the center of the macula. Detection requires specialized stereoscopic examination.

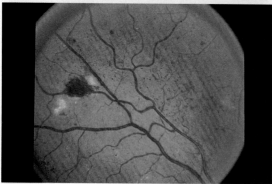

Nonproliferative Retinopathy, Severe

In the superior temporal quadrant, note the large retinal hemorrhage between two cotton-wool patches, beading of the retinal vein just above them, and tiny tortuous retinal vessels above the superior temporal artery.

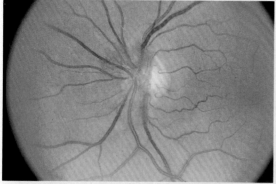

Proliferative Retinopathy, With Neovascularization

Note new preretinal vessels arising on the disc and extending across the disc margins. Visual acuity is still normal, but the risk for visual loss is high. Photocoagulation reduces this risk by >50%.

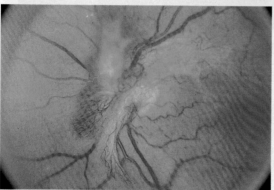

Proliferative Retinopathy, Advanced

This is the same eye, but 2 years later and without treatment. Neovascularization has increased, now with fibrous proliferations, distortion of the macula, and reduced visual acuity.

Source of photos: Nonproliferative Retinopathy, Moderately Severe; Proliferative Retinopathy, With Neovascularization; Nonproliferative Retinopathy, Severe; Proliferative Retinopathy, Advanced—Early Treatment Diabetic Retinopathy Study Research Group. Courtesy of MF Davis, MD, University of Wisconsin, Madison. Source: Frank RB. Diabetic retinopathy. N Engl J Med 2004;350:48–58.

Table
7-18   **Light-Colored Spots in the Fundi**

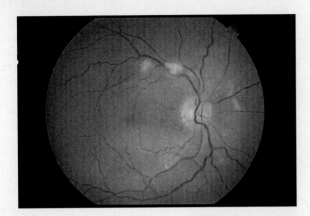

Soft Exudates: Cotton-Wool Patches

Cotton-wool patches are white or grayish, ovoid lesions with irregular "soft" borders. They are moderate in size but usually smaller than the disc. They result from infarcted nerve fibers. Seen in hypertension and many other conditions.

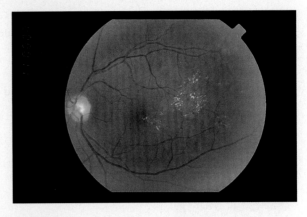

Hard Exudates

Hard exudates are creamy or yellowish, often bright, lesions with well-defined "hard" borders. They are small and round but may coalesce into larger irregular spots. They often occur in clusters or in circular, linear, or star-shaped patterns. Causes include diabetes and hypertension.

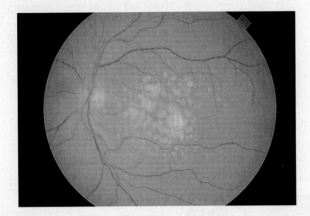

Drusen

Drusen are yellowish round spots that vary from tiny to small. The edges may be soft, as here, or hard (p. 232). They are haphazardly distributed but may concentrate at the posterior pole between the optic disc and the macula. Drusen appear in normal aging but may also accompany various conditions, including age-related macular degeneration.

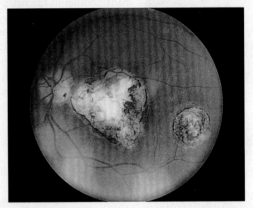

Healed Chorioretinitis

Here inflammation has destroyed the superficial tissues to reveal a well-defined, irregular patch of white sclera marked with dark pigment. Size varies from small to very large. *Toxoplasmosis* is illustrated. Multiple, small, somewhat similar-looking areas may be due to laser treatments. Here there is also a temporal scar near the macula.

Source of photos: Cotton-Wool Patches, Drusen, Healed Chorioretinitis—Tasman W, Jaeger E, eds. The Wills Eye Hospital Atlas of Clinical Ophthalmology, 2nd ed. Philadelphia: Lippincott Williams & Wilkins, 2001; Hard Exudates—Courtesy of Ken Freedman, MD.

Table 7-19	Lumps on or Near the Ear

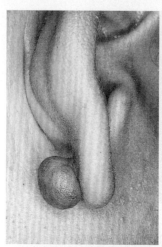

Keloid. A firm, nodular, hypertrophic mass of scar tissue extending beyond the area of injury. It may develop in any scarred area but is most common on the shoulders and upper chest. A keloid on a pierced earlobe may have troublesome cosmetic effects. Keloids are more common in darker-skinned people. Recurrence may follow treatment.

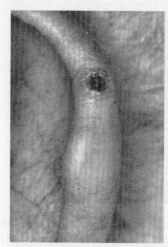

Chondrodermatitis Helicis. This chronic inflammatory lesion starts as a painful, tender papule on the helix or antihelix. Here the upper lesion is at a later stage of ulceration and crusting. Reddening may occur. Biopsy is needed to rule out carcinoma.

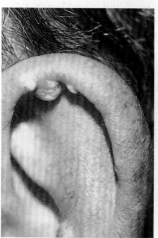

Tophi. A deposit of uric acid crystals characteristic of chronic tophaceous gout. It appears as hard nodules in the helix or antihelix and may discharge chalky white crystals through the skin. It also may appear near the joints, hands (p. 675), feet, and other areas. It usually develops after chronic sustained high blood levels of uric acid.

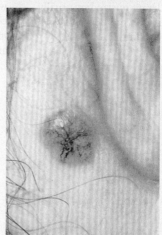

Basal Cell Carcinoma. This raised nodule shows the lustrous surface and telangiectatic vessels of basal cell carcinoma, a common slow-growing malignancy that rarely metastasizes. Growth and ulceration may occur. These are more frequent in fair-skinned people overexposed to sunlight.

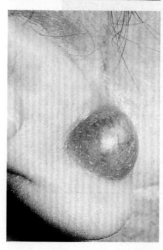

Cutaneous Cyst. Formerly called a *sebaceous cyst,* a dome-shaped lump in the dermis forms a benign closed firm sac attached to the epidermis. A dark dot (blackhead) may be visible on its surface. Histologically, it is usually either (1) an *epidermoid* cyst, common on the face and neck, or (2) a *pilar (trichilemmal)* cyst, common in the scalp. Both may become inflamed.

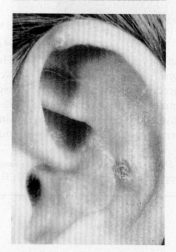

Rheumatoid Nodules. In chronic rheumatoid arthritis, look for small lumps on the helix or antihelix and additional nodules elsewhere on the hands, along the surface of the ulna distal to the elbow (p. 674), and on the knees and heels. Ulceration may result from repeated injuries. Such nodules may antedate the arthritis.

Sources of photos: Keloid—Sams WM Jr, Lynch PJ, eds. Principles and Practice of Dermatology. Edinburgh: Churchill Livingstone, 1990; Tophi—du Vivier A. Atlas of Clinical Dermatology, 2nd ed. London, UK: Gower Medical Publishing, 1993; Cutaneous Cyst, Chondrodermatitis Helicis—Young EM, Newcomer VD, Kligman AM. Geriatric Dermatology: Color Atlas and Practitioner's Guide. Philadelphia: Lea & Febiger, 1993; Basal Cell Carcinoma—N Engl J Med, 326:169–170, 1992; Rheumatoid Nodules—Champion RH, Burton JL, Ebling FJG, eds. Rook/Wilkinson/Ebling Textbook of Dermatology, 5th ed. Oxford, UK: Blackwell Scientific, 1992.

Table 7-20   Abnormalities of the Eardrum

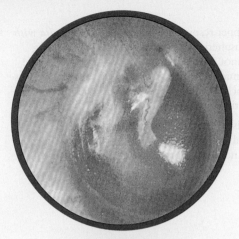

Normal Eardrum (Right)

This normal right eardrum (tympanic membrane) is pinkish gray. Note the malleus lying behind the upper part of the drum. Above the short process lies the *pars flaccida*. The remainder of the drum is the *pars tensa*. From the umbo, the bright cone of light fans anteriorly and downward. Posterior to the malleus, part of the incus is visible behind the drum. The small blood vessels along the handle of the malleus are normal.

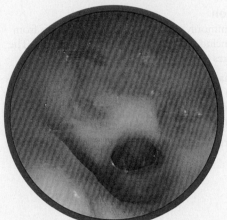

Perforation of the Drum

Perforations are holes in the eardrum, usually from purulent infections of the middle ear. They are classified as *central* perforations, which do not extend to the margin of the drum, and *marginal* perforations, which do involve the margin.

The more common central perforation is illustrated here. A reddened ring of granulation tissue surrounds the perforation, indicating chronic infection. The eardrum itself is scarred, and no landmarks are visible. Discharge from the infected middle ear may drain out through the perforated opening. A perforation often closes in the healing process, as in the next photo. The membrane covering the hole may be exceedingly thin and transparent.

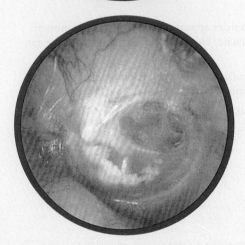

Tympanosclerosis

In the inferior portion of this left eardrum, there is a large, chalky white patch with irregular margins. It is typical of tympanosclerosis: a deposition of hyaline material within the layers of the tympanic membrane that sometimes follows a severe episode of otitis media. It does not usually impair hearing and is seldom clinically significant.

Other abnormalities in this eardrum include a *healed perforation* (the large oval area in the upper posterior drum) and signs of a *retracted drum*. A retracted drum is pulled medially, away from the examiner's eye, and the malleolar folds are tightened into sharp outlines. The short process often protrudes sharply, and the handle of the malleus, pulled inward at the umbo, looks foreshortened and more horizontal.

Sources of photos: Normal Eardrum—Hawke M, Keene M, Alberti PW. Clinical Otoscopy: A Text and Colour Atlas. Edinburgh: Churchill Livingstone, 1984; Perforation of the Drum, Tympanosclerosis—Courtesy of Michael Hawke, MD, Toronto, Canada.

(table continues on page 280)

Table 7-20

Abnormalities of the Eardrum (*continued*)

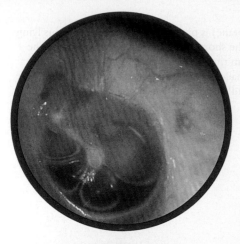

Serous Effusion

Serous effusions are usually caused by viral upper respiratory infections (*otitis media with serous effusion*) or by sudden changes in atmospheric pressure as from flying or diving (*otitic barotrauma*). The eustachian tube cannot equalize the air pressure in the middle ear and outside air. Air is absorbed from the middle ear into the bloodstream, and serous fluid accumulates there instead. Symptoms include fullness and popping sensations in the ear, mild conduction hearing loss, and, sometimes, pain.

Amber fluid behind the eardrum is characteristic, as in this patient with otitic barotrauma. A fluid level, a line between air above and amber fluid below, can be seen on either side of the short process. Air bubbles (not always present) can be seen here within the amber fluid.

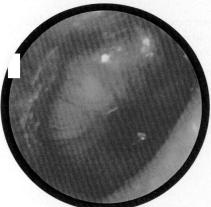

Acute Otitis Media With Purulent Effusion

Acute otitis media with purulent effusion is commonly caused by bacterial infection from *S. pneumoniae* and *H. influenzae*. Symptoms include earache, fever, and hearing loss. The eardrum reddens, loses its landmarks, and bulges laterally, toward the examiner's eye.

Here the eardrum is bulging, and most landmarks are obscured. Redness is most obvious near the umbo, but dilated vessels can be seen in all segments of the drum. A diffuse redness of the entire drum often develops. Spontaneous rupture (perforation) of the drum may follow, with discharge of purulent material into the ear canal.

Hearing loss is the conductive type. Acute purulent otitis media is much more common in children than in adults.

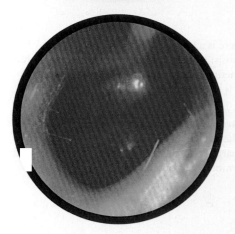

Bullous Myringitis

In bullous myringitis, painful hemorrhagic vesicles appear on the tympanic membrane, the ear canal, or both. Symptoms include earache, blood-tinged discharge from the ear, and conductive hearing loss.

In this right ear, at least two large vesicles (bullae) are discernible on the drum. The drum is reddened, and its landmarks are obscured.

This condition is caused by mycoplasma, viral, and bacterial otitis media.

Sources of photos: Serous Effusion—Hawke M, Keene M, Alberti PW. Clinical Otoscopy: A Text and Colour Atlas. Edinburgh: Churchill Livingstone, 1984; Acute Otitis Media, Bullous Myringitis—The Wellcome Trust, National Medical Slide Bank, London, UK.

Table 7-21   Patterns of Hearing Loss

	Conductive Loss	Sensorineural Loss
	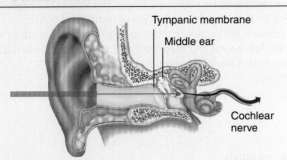	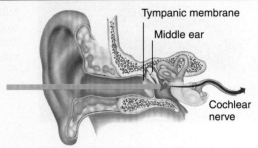
Pathophysiology	External or middle ear disorder impairs sound conduction to inner ear. Causes include foreign body, *otitis media*, perforated eardrum, and otosclerosis of ossicles.	Inner ear disorder involves cochlear nerve and neuronal impulse transmission to the brain. Causes include loud noise exposure, inner ear infections, trauma, acoustic neuroma, congenital and familial disorders, and aging.
Usual Age of Onset	Childhood and young adulthood, up to age 40	Middle or later years
Ear Canal and Drum	Abnormality usually visible, except in otosclerosis	Problem not visible
Effects	• Little effect on sound • Hearing seems to improve in noisy environment • Voice remains soft because inner ear and cochlear nerve are intact	• Higher registers are lost, so sound may be distorted • Hearing worsens in noisy environment • Voice may be loud because hearing is difficult
Weber Test (in unilateral hearing loss)	• Tuning fork at vertex • Sound lateralizes to *impaired ear*—room noise not well heard, so detection of vibrations *improves*.	• Tuning fork at vertex • Sound lateralizes to *good ear*—inner ear or cochlear nerve damage impairs transmission to affected ear.
Rinne Test	• Tuning fork at external auditory meatus; then on mastoid bone • Bone conduction longer than or equal to air conduction (BC ≥ AC). While air conduction through the external or middle ear is impaired, vibrations through bone bypass the problem to reach the cochlea.	• Tuning fork at external auditory meatus; then on mastoid bone • Air conduction longer than bone conduction (AC > BC). The inner ear or cochlear nerve is less able to transmit impulses regardless of how the vibrations reach the cochlea. The normal pattern prevails.

Table 7-22 Abnormalities of the Lips

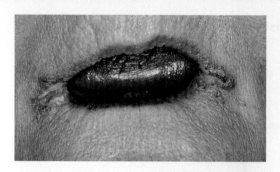

Angular Cheilitis

Angular cheilitis starts with softening of the skin at the angles of the mouth, followed by fissuring. It may be due to nutritional deficiency or, more commonly, to overclosure of the mouth, seen in people with no teeth or with ill-fitting dentures. Saliva wets and macerates the infolded skin, often leading to secondary infection with *Candida*, as seen here.

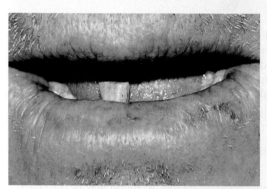

Actinic Cheilitis

Actinic cheilitis results from excessive exposure to sunlight and affects primarily the lower lip. Fair-skinned men who work outdoors are most often affected. The lip loses its normal redness and may become scaly, somewhat thickened, and slightly everted. Because solar damage predisposes to carcinoma of the lip, examine such skin lesions carefully.

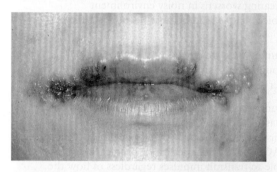

Herpes Simplex (*Cold Sore, Fever Blister*)

The herpes simplex virus (HSV) produces recurrent and painful vesicular eruptions of the lips and surrounding skin. A small cluster of vesicles first develops. As these break, yellow-brown crusts form. Healing takes 10 to 14 days. Both new and erupted vesicles are visible here.

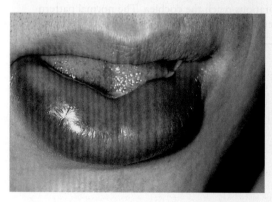

Angioedema

Angioedema is a localized subcutaneous or submucosal swelling caused by leakage of intravascular fluid into interstitial tissue. Two types are common. When vascular permeability is triggered by mast cells in allergic and NSAID reactions, look for associated urticaria and pruritus. These are uncommon in angioedema from bradykinin and complement-derived mediators, the mechanism in ACE-inhibitor reactions. Angioedema is usually benign and resolves within 24 to 48 hours. It can be life threatening when it involves the larynx, tongue, or upper airway or develops into anaphylaxis.

Sources of photos: Angular Cheilitis, Herpes Simplex, Angioedema—Neville B et al. Color Atlas of Clinical Oral Pathology. Philadelphia: Lea & Febiger, 1991; Used with permission; Actinic Cheilitis—Langlais RP, Miller CS. Color Atlas of Common Oral Diseases. Philadelphia: Lea & Febiger, 1992. Used with permission.

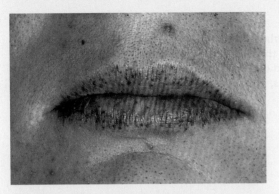

Hereditary Hemorrhagic Telangiectasia (Osler-Weber-Rendu syndrome)

Multiple small red spots on the lips strongly suggest hereditary hemorrhagic telangiectasia, an autosomal dominant endothelial disorder causing vascular fragility and arteriovascular malformations (AVMs). Telangiectasias are also visible on the oral mucosa and fingertips. Nosebleeds, gastrointestinal bleeding, and iron deficiency anemia are common. AVMs in the lungs and brain can cause life-threatening hemorrhage and embolic disease.

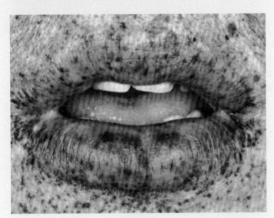

Peutz-Jeghers Syndrome

Look for prominent small brown pigmented spots in the dermal layer of the lips, buccal mucosa, and perioral area. These spots may also appear on the hands and feet. In this autosomal dominant syndrome, these characteristic skin changes accompany numerous intestinal polyps. The risk of gastrointestinal and other cancers ranges from 40% to 90%. Note that these spots rarely appear around the nose and mouth.

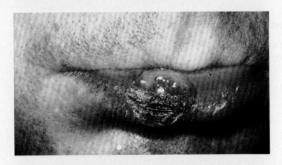

Chancre of Primary Syphilis

This ulcerated papule with an indurated edge usually appears after 3 to 6 weeks of incubating infection from the spirochete *Treponema pallidum*. These lesions may resemble a carcinoma or crusted cold sore. Similar primary lesions are common in the pharynx, anus, and vagina but may escape detection since they are painless, nonsuppurative, and usually heal spontaneously in 3 to 6 weeks. Wear gloves during palpation since these chancres are infectious.

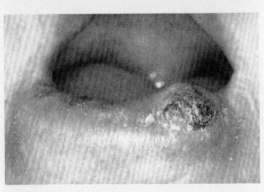

Carcinoma of the Lip

Like actinic cheilitis, squamous cell carcinoma usually affects the lower lip. It may appear as a scaly plaque, as an ulcer with or without a crust, or as a nodular lesion, illustrated here. Fair skin and prolonged exposure to the sun are common risk factors.

Sources of photos: Hereditary Hemorrhagic Telangiectasia—Langlais RP, Miller CS. Color Atlas of Common Oral Diseases. Philadelphia: Lea & Febiger, 1992; Used with permission; Peutz-Jeghers Syndrome—Robinson HBG, Miller AS. Colby, Kerr, and Robinson's Color Atlas of Oral Pathology. Philadelphia: JB Lippincott, 1990; Chancre of Syphilis—Wisdom A. A Colour Atlas of Sexually Transmitted Diseases, 2nd ed. London: Wolfe Medical Publications, 1989; Carcinoma of the Lip—Tyldesley WR. A Colour Atlas of Orofacial Diseases, 2nd ed. London: Wolfe Medical Publications, 1991.

Table 7-23

Findings in the Pharynx, Palate, and Oral Mucosa

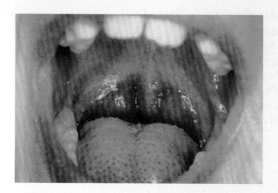

Large Normal Tonsils

Normal tonsils may be large without being infected, especially in children. They may protrude medially beyond the pillars and even to the midline. Here they touch the sides of the uvula and obscure the pharynx. Their color is pink. The white marks are light reflections, not exudate.

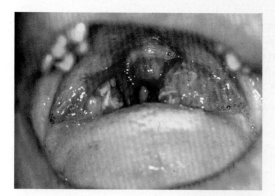

Exudative Tonsillitis

This red throat has a white exudate on the tonsils. This, together with fever and enlarged cervical nodes, increases the probability of *group A streptococcal infection* or *infectious mononucleosis*. Anterior cervical lymph nodes are usually enlarged in the former, posterior nodes in the latter.

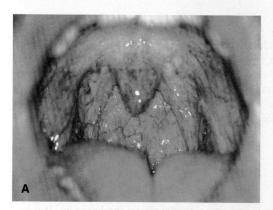

Pharyngitis

These two photos show reddened throats without exudate.

In **A**, redness and vascularity of the pillars and uvula are mild to moderate.

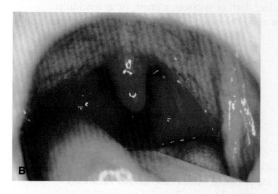

In **B**, redness is diffuse and intense. Each patient would probably complain of a sore throat, or at least a scratchy one. Causes are both viral and bacterial. If the patient has no fever, exudate, or enlargement of cervical lymph nodes, the chances of infection by either of two common causes—*group A streptococci* and *Epstein-Barr virus* (infectious mononucleosis)—are small.

Sources of photos: Large Normal Tonsils, Exudative Tonsillitis, Pharyngitis [A and B]—The Wellcome Trust, National Medical Slide Bank, London, UK.

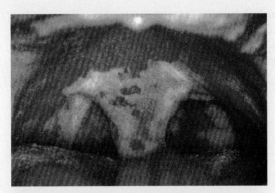

Diphtheria

Diphtheria, an acute infection caused by *Corynebacterium diphtheriae*, is now rare but still important. Prompt diagnosis may lead to life-saving treatment. The throat is dull red, and a gray exudate (pseudomembrane) is present on the uvula, pharynx, and tongue. The airway may become obstructed.

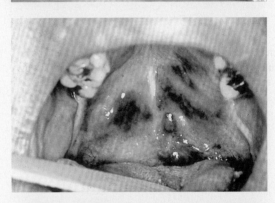

Thrush on the Palate (Candidiasis)

Thrush is a yeast infection from *Candida* species. Shown here on the palate, it may appear elsewhere in the mouth (see p. 289). Thick, white plaques are somewhat adherent to the underlying mucosa. Predisposing factors include (1) prolonged treatment with antibiotics or corticosteroids and (2) AIDS.

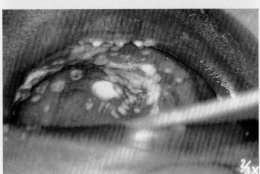

Kaposi's Sarcoma in AIDS

The deep purple color of these lesions suggests Kaposi's sarcoma, a low-grade vascular tumor associated with human herpesvirus 8. The lesions may be raised or flat. About a third of patients with Kaposi's sarcoma have lesions in the oral cavity; other affected sites are the gastrointestinal tract and the lungs. Antiretroviral therapy has markedly reduced the prevalence of this disease.

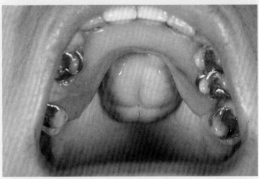

Torus Palatinus

A torus palatinus is a midline bony growth in the hard palate that is fairly common in adults. Its size and lobulation vary. Although alarming at first glance, it is harmless. In this example, an upper denture has been fitted around the torus.

Sources of photos: Diphtheria—Harnisch JP et al. Diphtheria among alcoholic urban adults. Ann Intern Med 1989;111:77; Thrush on the Palate—The Wellcome Trust, National Medical Slide Bank, London, UK; Kaposi's Sarcoma in AIDS—Ioachim HL. Textbook and Atlas of Disease Associated With Acquired Immune Deficiency Syndrome. London: Gower Medical Publishing, 1989.

(table continues on page 286)

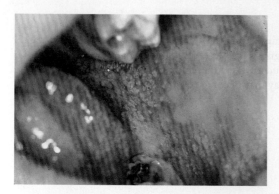

Fordyce Spots (*Fordyce Granules*)

Fordyce spots are normal sebaceous glands that appear as small yellowish spots in the buccal mucosa or on the lips. Here they are seen best anterior to the tongue and lower jaw. These spots are usually not numerous.

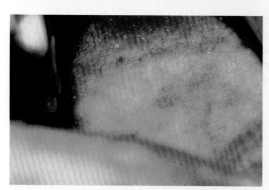

Koplik's Spots

Koplik's spots are an early sign of measles (rubeola). Search for small white specks that resemble grains of salt on a red background. They usually appear on the buccal mucosa near the first and second molars. In this photo, look also in the upper third of the mucosa. The rash of measles appears within a day.

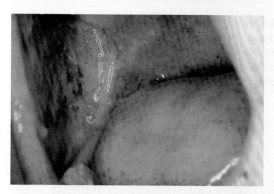

Petechiae

Petechiae are small red spots caused by blood that escapes from capillaries into the tissues. Petechiae in the buccal mucosa, as shown, are often caused by accidentally biting the cheek. Oral petechiae may be due to infection or decreased platelets, as well as trauma.

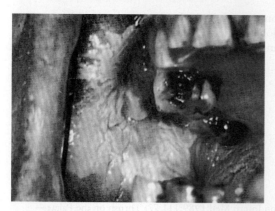

Leukoplakia

A thickened white patch (*leukoplakia*) may occur anywhere in the oral mucosa. The extensive example shown on this buccal mucosa resulted from frequent chewing of tobacco, a local irritant. This benign reactive process of the squamous epithelium may lead to cancer and should be biopsied. Another risk factor is human papillomavirus infection.

Sources of photos: Fordyce Spots—Neville B et al. Color Atlas of Clinical Oral Pathology. Philadelphia: Lea & Febiger, 1991; Used with permission; Koplik's Spots, Petechiae—The Wellcome Trust, National Medical Slide Bank, London, UK; Leukoplakia—Robinson HBG, Miller AS. Colby, Kerr, and Robinson's Color Atlas of Oral Pathology. Philadelphia: JB Lippincott, 1990.

Table
7-24   Findings in the Gums and Teeth

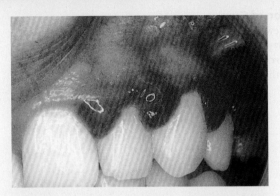

Marginal Gingivitis

Marginal gingivitis is common among teenagers and young adults. The gingival margins are reddened and swollen, and the interdental papillae are blunted, swollen, and red. Brushing the teeth often makes the gums bleed. *Plaque*—the soft white film of salivary salts, protein, and bacteria that covers the teeth and leads to gingivitis—is not readily visible.

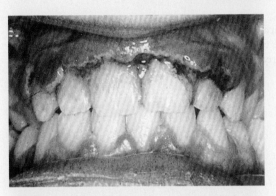

Acute Necrotizing Ulcerative Gingivitis

This uncommon form of gingivitis occurs suddenly in adolescents and young adults and is accompanied by fever, malaise, and enlarged lymph nodes. Ulcers develop in the interdental papillae. Then the destructive (necrotizing) process spreads along the gum margins, where a grayish pseudomembrane develops. The red, painful gums bleed easily; the breath is foul.

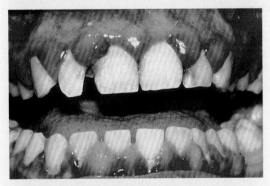

Gingival Hyperplasia

Gums enlarged by hyperplasia are swollen into heaped-up masses that may even cover the teeth. The redness of inflammation may coexist, as in this example. Causes include phenytoin therapy (as in this case), puberty, pregnancy, and leukemia.

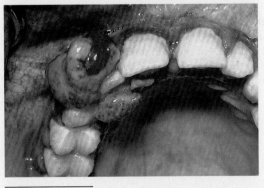

Pregnancy Tumor (also termed Pregnancy Epulis or Pyogenic Granuloma)

Red purple papules of granulation tissue form in the gingival interdental papillae, and sometimes on the fingers. They are red, soft, painless, and usually bleed easily. They occur in 1% to 5% of pregnancies and usually regress after delivery. Note the accompanying gingivitis.

Sources of photos: Marginal Gingivitis, Acute Necrotizing Ulcerative Gingivitis—Tyldesley WR. A Colour Atlas of Orofacial Diseases, 2nd ed. London: Wolfe Medical Publications, 1991; Gingival Hyperplasia—Courtesy of Dr. James Cottone; Pregnancy Tumor—Langlais RP, Miller CS. Color Atlas of Common Oral Diseases. Philadelphia: Lea & Febiger, 1992. Used with permission.

(table continues on page 288)

Table 7-24 **Findings in the Gums and Teeth** (*continued*)

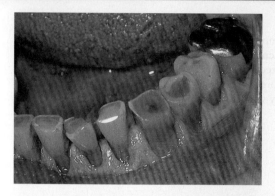

Attrition of Teeth; Recession of Gums

In many elderly people, the chewing surfaces of the teeth are worn down by repetitive use so that the yellow-brown dentin becomes exposed—a process called *attrition*. Note also the *recession of the gums*, which has exposed the roots of the teeth, giving a "long in the tooth" appearance.

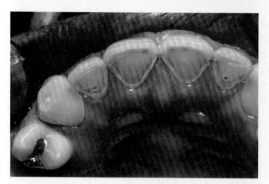

Erosion of Teeth

Teeth may be eroded by chemical action. Note here the erosion of the enamel from the lingual surfaces of the upper incisors, exposing the yellow-brown dentin. This results from recurrent regurgitation of stomach contents, as in bulimia.

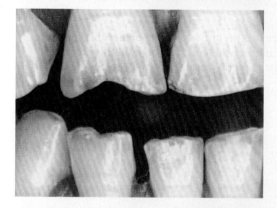

Abrasion of Teeth With Notching

The biting surface of the teeth may become abraded or notched by recurrent trauma, such as holding nails or opening bobby pins between the teeth. Unlike Hutchinson's teeth, the sides of these teeth show normal contours; size and spacing of the teeth are unaffected.

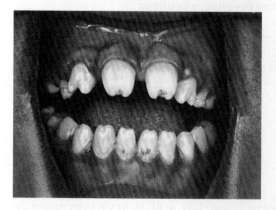

Hutchinson's Teeth in Congenital Syphilis

Hutchinson's teeth are smaller and more widely spaced than normal and are notched on their biting surfaces. The sides of the teeth taper toward the biting edges. The upper central incisors of the permanent (not the deciduous) teeth are most often affected. These teeth are a sign of congenital syphilis.

Sources of photos: Attrition of Teeth, Erosion of Teeth—Langlais RP, Miller CS. Color Atlas of Common Oral Diseases. Philadelphia: Lea & Febiger, 1992. Used with permission; Abrasion of Teeth, Hutchinson's Teeth—Robinson HBG, Miller AS. Colby, Kerr, and Robinson's Color Atlas of Oral Pathology. Philadelphia: JB Lippincott, 1990.

Table 7-25 Findings in or Under the Tongue

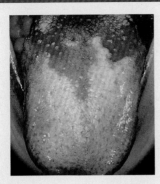

Geographic Tongue. In this benign condition, the dorsum shows scattered smooth red areas denuded of papillae. Together with the normal rough and coated areas, they give a maplike pattern that changes over time.

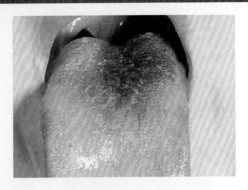

Hairy Tongue. Note the "hairy" yellowish to brown and black elongated papillae on the tongue's dorsum. This benign condition is associated with antibiotic therapy, *Candida* infection, and poor dental hygiene. It also may occur spontaneously.

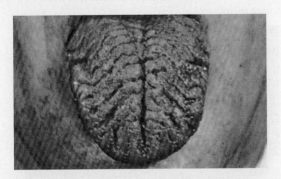

Fissured Tongue. Fissures appear with increasing age, sometimes termed *scrotal tongue*. Food debris may accumulate in the crevices and become irritating, but a fissured tongue is benign.

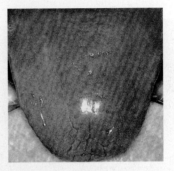

Smooth Tongue (Atrophic Glossitis). A smooth and often sore tongue that has lost its papillae suggests a deficiency in riboflavin, niacin, folic acid, vitamin B_{12}, pyridoxine, or iron, or treatment with chemotherapy.

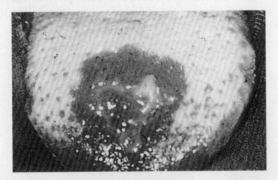

Candidiasis. Note the thick white coating from *Candida* infection. The raw red surface is where the coat was scraped off. Infection may also occur without the white coating. It is seen in immunosuppression from chemotherapy or prednisone therapy.

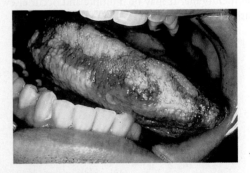

Hairy Leukoplakia. These whitish raised areas with a feathery or corrugated pattern most often affect the sides of the tongue. Unlike candidiasis, these areas cannot be scraped off. They are seen in HIV and AIDS infection.

(table continues on page 290)

Table 7-25 Findings in or Under the Tongue (continued)

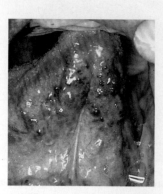

Varicose Veins. Small purplish or blue-black round swellings appear under the tongue with age. These dilatations of the lingual veins have no clinical significance.

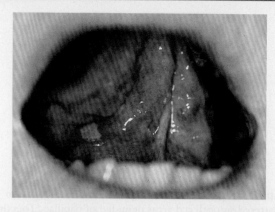

Aphthous Ulcer (Canker Sore). A painful, round or oval ulcer that is white or yellowish gray and surrounded by a halo of reddened mucosa. It may be single or multiple. It heals in 7–10 days, but may recur.

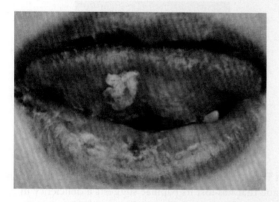

Mucous Patch of Syphilis. This painless lesion of secondary syphilis is highly infectious. It is slightly raised, oval, and covered by a grayish membrane. It may be multiple and occur elsewhere in the mouth.

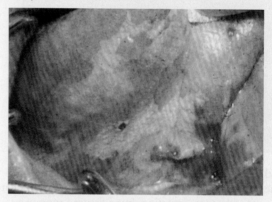

Leukoplakia. With this persisting painless white patch in the oral mucosa, the undersurface of the tongue appears painted white. Patches of any size raise the possibility of squamous cell carcinoma and require biopsy.

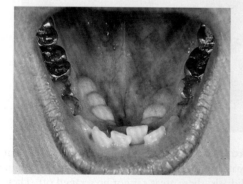

Tori Mandibulares. Rounded bony growths on the inner surfaces of the mandible are typically bilateral, asymptomatic, and harmless.

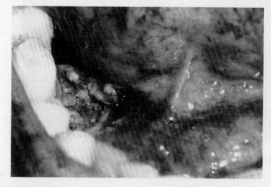

Carcinoma, Floor of the Mouth. This ulcerated lesion is in a common location for carcinoma. Medially, note the reddened area of mucosa, called *erythroplakia,* also suspicious for malignancy.

Table 7-26 | Thyroid Enlargement and Function

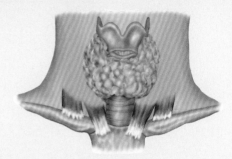

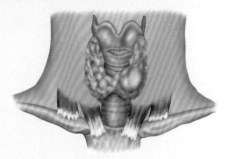

Diffuse Enlargement. Includes the isthmus and lateral lobes; there are no discretely palpable nodules. Causes include Graves' disease, Hashimoto's thyroiditis, and endemic goiter.

Single Nodule. May be a cyst, a benign tumor, or one nodule within a multinodular gland. It raises the question of malignancy. Risk factors are prior irradiation, hardness, rapid growth, fixation to surrounding tissues, enlarged cervical nodes, and occurrence in men.

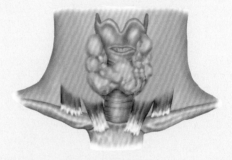

Multinodular Goiter. An enlarged thyroid gland with two or more nodules suggests a metabolic rather than a neoplastic process. Positive family history and continuing nodular enlargement are additional risk factors for malignancy.

Table 7-27 | Symptoms and Signs of Thyroid Dysfunction

	Hyperthyroidism	Hypothyroidism
Symptoms	Nervousness Weight loss despite increased appetite Excessive sweating and heat intolerance Palpitations Frequent bowel movements Tremor and proximal muscle weakness	Fatigue, lethargy Modest weight gain with anorexia Dry, coarse skin and cold intolerance Swelling of face, hands, and legs Constipation Weakness, muscle cramps, arthralgias, paresthesias, impaired memory and hearing
Signs	Warm, smooth, moist skin With Graves' disease, eye signs such as stare, lid lag, and exophthalmos Increased systolic and decreased diastolic blood pressures Tachycardia or atrial fibrillation Hyperdynamic cardiac pulsations with an accentuated S_1 Tremor and proximal muscle weakness	Dry, coarse, cool skin, sometimes yellowish from carotene, with nonpitting edema and loss of hair Periorbital puffiness Decreased systolic and increased diastolic blood pressures Bradycardia and, in late stages, hypothermia Sometimes decreased intensity of heart sounds Impaired memory, mixed hearing loss, somnolence, peripheral neuropathy, carpal tunnel syndrome

Sources: Siminoski K. Does this patient have a goiter? JAMA 1995;273:813–817; Hegedus L. The thyroid nodule. N Engl J Med 2004;351:1764–1771; Devdhar M, Ousman YH, Burman KD. Hypothyroidism. Endocinrinol Metab Clin North Am 2007;36:595–615; McDermott MT. In the clinic: hypothyroidism. Ann Intern Med 151: ITC6-1–ITC6-16, 2009; Nyack B, Hodak SP. Hyperthyroidism. Endocrinol Metab Clin North Am 2007; 36:617–656; Franklyn JA. Subclinical thyroid disorders—consequences and implications for treatment. Ann Endocrinol 2007;68:229–230.

The Thorax and Lungs

Anatomy and Physiology

Study the *anatomy of the chest wall,* identifying the structures illustrated. Note that the interspace between two ribs is numbered by the rib above it.

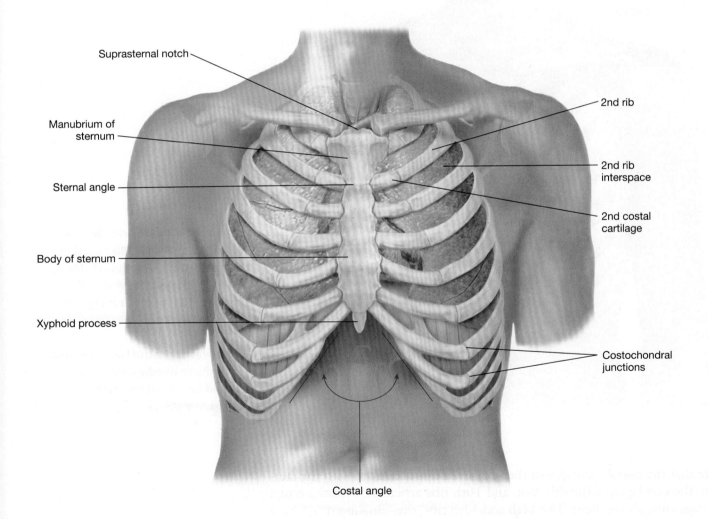

Suprasternal notch

Manubrium of sternum

Sternal angle

Body of sternum

Xyphoid process

2nd rib

2nd rib interspace

2nd costal cartilage

Costochondral junctions

Costal angle

Locating Findings on the Chest. Describe chest findings in two dimensions: *along the vertical axis* and *around the circumference of the chest.*

Vertical Axis. Practice counting the ribs and interspaces. The *sternal angle,* also termed the angle of Louis, is the best guide. Place your finger in the hollow curve of the suprasternal notch, then move your finger down approximately 5 cm to the horizontal bony ridge joining the manubrium to the body of the sternum. Move your finger laterally and find the adjacent 2nd rib and costal cartilage. From here, using two fingers, "walk down" the interspaces, one space at a time, on an oblique line, illustrated by the red numbers below. Do not try to count interspaces along the lower edge of the sternum; the ribs there are too close together. To find the interspaces in a woman, displace the breast laterally or palpate a little more medially. Avoid pressing too hard on tender breast tissue.

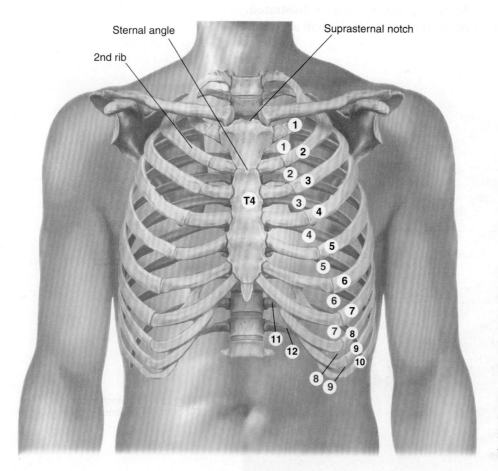

Sternal angle

Suprasternal notch

2nd rib

T4

Note special landmarks: 2nd intercostal space for needle insertion for tension pneumothorax; 4th intercostal space for chest tube insertion; T4 for lower margin of endotracheal tube on a chest x-ray.

Neurovascular structures run under each rib, so needles and tubes should be placed just superior to the rib margins.

Note that the costal cartilages of the first seven ribs articulate with the sternum; the cartilages of the 8th, 9th, and 10th ribs articulate with the costal cartilages just above them. The 11th and 12th ribs, the "floating ribs," have no anterior attachments. The cartilaginous tip of the 11th rib usually can be felt laterally, and the 12th rib may be felt posteriorly. When palpated, costal cartilages and ribs feel identical.

Posteriorly, the 12th rib is another possible starting point for counting ribs and interspaces. It helps locate findings on the lower posterior chest and, when needed, provides an alternative to the anterior approach. With the fingers of one hand, press in and up against the lower border of the 12th rib; then "walk up" the interspaces numbered in red below, or follow a more oblique line up and around to the front of the chest.

The inferior tip of the scapula is another useful bony landmark; it usually lies at the level of the 7th rib or interspace.

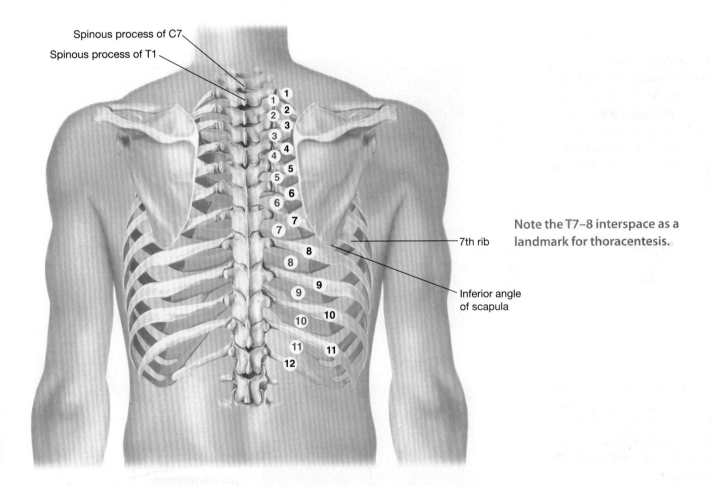

Note the T7–8 interspace as a landmark for thoracentesis.

The spinous processes of the vertebrae are also useful anatomical landmarks. When the neck is flexed forward, the most protruding process is usually the vertebra of C7. If two processes are equally prominent, they are C7 and T1. You can often palpate and count the processes below them, especially when the spine is flexed.

Circumference of the Chest. Visualize a series of vertical lines as shown in the adjacent illustrations. The *midsternal* and *vertebral lines* are precise; the others are estimated. The *midclavicular line* drops vertically from the midpoint of the clavicle. To find it, accurately identify both ends of the clavicle (see p. 615).

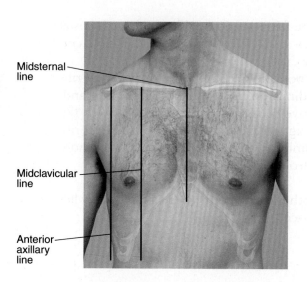

Midsternal line

Midclavicular line

Anterior axillary line

The *anterior* and *posterior axillary lines* drop vertically from the anterior and posterior axillary folds, the muscle masses that border the axilla. The *midaxillary line* drops from the apex of the axilla.

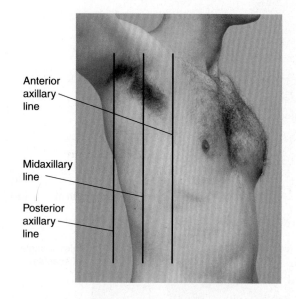

Anterior axillary line

Midaxillary line

Posterior axillary line

Posteriorly, the *vertebral line* overlies the spinous processes of the vertebrae. The scapular line drops from the inferior angle of the scapula.

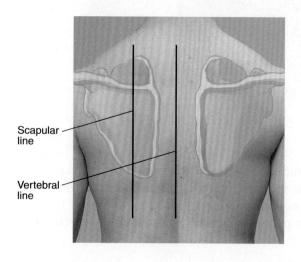

Scapular line

Vertebral line

Lungs, Fissures, and Lobes. Picture the lungs and their fissures and lobes on the chest wall. Anteriorly, the apex of each lung rises approximately 2 cm to 4 cm above the inner third of the clavicle. The lower border of the lung crosses the 6th rib at the midclavicular line and the 8th rib at the midaxillary line. Posteriorly, the lower border of the lung lies at about the level of the T10 spinous process. On inspiration, it descends farther.

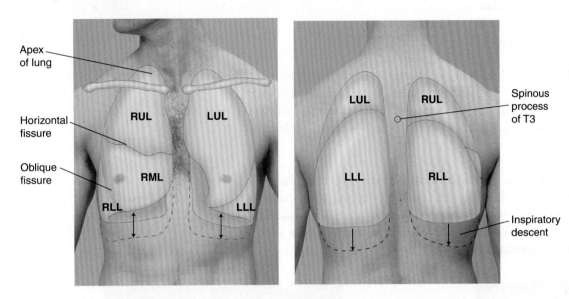

Each lung is divided roughly in half by an *oblique (major) fissure.* This fissure may be approximated by a string that runs from the T3 spinous process obliquely down and around the chest to the 6th rib at the midclavicular line. The right lung is further divided by the *horizontal (minor) fissure.* Anteriorly, this fissure runs close to the 4th rib and meets the oblique fissure in the midaxillary line near the 5th rib. The *right lung* is thus divided into *upper, middle,* and *lower lobes.* The *left lung* has only *two lobes,* upper and lower.

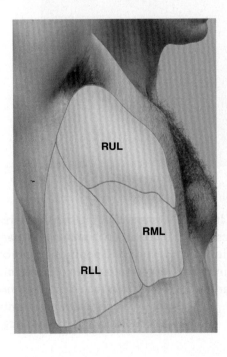

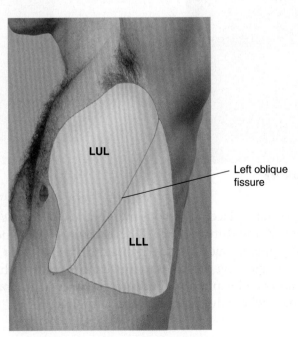

Locations on the Chest. Learn the general anatomical terms used to locate chest findings:

Supraclavicular—above the clavicles
Infraclavicular—below the clavicles
Interscapular—between the scapulae
Infrascapular—below the scapulae
Bases of the lungs—the lowermost portions
Upper, middle, and lower lung fields

You can infer which lobes of the lungs are involved in underlying abnormal findings. Signs in the right upper lung field, for example, almost certainly originate in the right upper lobe. Signs found laterally in the right middle lung field, however, could come from any of three different lobes.

The Trachea and Major Bronchi. Breath sounds over the trachea and bronchi have a different quality than breath sounds over the lung parenchyma. Be sure you know the location of these structures. The trachea bifurcates into its mainstem bronchi at the levels of the sternal angle anteriorly and the T4 spinous process posteriorly.

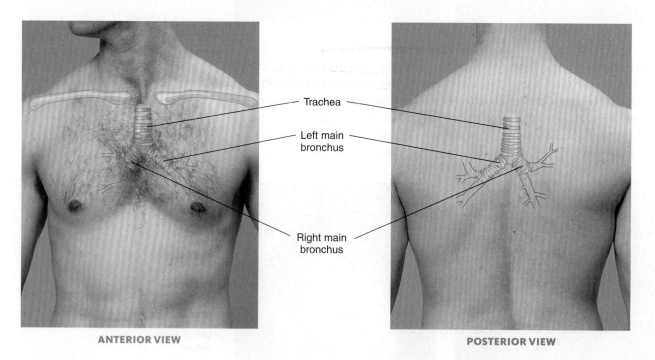

Trachea

Left main bronchus

Right main bronchus

ANTERIOR VIEW   POSTERIOR VIEW

The Pleurae. Two pleural surfaces, or serous membranes, cover the lung. The *visceral pleura* covers the outer surface. The *parietal pleura* lines the inner rib cage and the upper surface of the diaphragm. *Pleural fluid* lubricates the pleural surfaces, allowing the lungs to move more easily within the rib cage during inspiration and expiration. Between the visceral and parietal pleura is a potential space where fluid sometimes accumulates.

Pleural effusions may be transudates, seen in atelectasis, heart failure, and nephrotic syndrome, or exudates, seen in numerous conditions including pneumonia, tuberculosis, pulmonary embolus, pancreatitis, and malignancy.

Breathing. Breathing is primarily automatic, controlled by respiratory centers in the brainstem that produce the neuronal drive for the muscles of respiration. The principal muscle of inspiration is the *diaphragm*. During inspiration, the diaphragm contracts, descends in the chest, and expands the thoracic cavity, compressing the abdominal contents and pushing out the abdominal wall. The muscles in the rib cage also expand the thorax, especially the *scalenes*, which run from the cervical vertebrae to the first two ribs, and the parasternal intercostal muscles, or *parasternals*, which cross obliquely from the sternum to the ribs. As the thorax expands, intrathoracic pressure decreases, drawing air through the tracheobronchial tree into the *alveoli*, or distal air sacs, filling the expanding lungs. Oxygen diffuses into the adjacent pulmonary capillaries as carbon dioxide exchanges from the blood into the alveoli.

During expiration, the chest wall and lungs recoil and the diaphragm relaxes and rises passively. As air flows outward, the chest and abdomen return to their resting positions.

Normal breathing is quiet and easy—barely audible near the open mouth as a faint whish. When a healthy person lies supine, the breathing movements of the thorax are relatively slight. By contrast, the abdominal movements are usually easy to see. In the sitting position, movements of the thorax become more prominent.

During exercise and in certain diseases, extra work is required to breathe, and accessory muscles are recruited; the sternomastoids and the scalenes may become visible. Abdominal muscles assist in expiration.

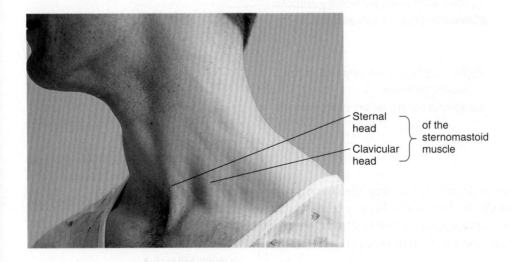

Sternal head ⎤
              ⎥ of the
Clavicular   ⎬ sternomastoid
head   ⎦ muscle

The Health History

Common or Concerning Symptoms

- Chest pain
- Shortness of breath (dyspnea)
- Wheezing
- Cough
- Blood-streaked sputum (hemoptysis)

Chest Pain. Complaints of *chest pain* or *chest discomfort* raise concern about heart disease but often arise from structures in the thorax and lungs as well. To assess this symptom, you must pursue a dual investigation of both thoracic and cardiac causes. Sources of chest pain are listed below. For this important symptom, you must keep all of these in mind:

See Table 8-1, Chest Pain, pp. 322–323.

Sources of Chest Pain and Related Causes

The myocardium	*Angina pectoris, myocardial infarction, myocarditis*
The pericardium	*Pericarditis*
The aorta	*Dissecting aortic aneurysm*
The trachea and large bronchi	*Bronchitis*
The parietal pleura	*Pericarditis, pneumonia, pneumothorax, pleural effusion, pulmonary embolus*
The chest wall, including the musculoskeletal system and skin	*Costochondritis, herpes zoster*
The esophagus	*Reflux esophagitis, esophageal spasm, esophageal tear*
Extrathoracic structures such as the neck, gallbladder, and stomach	*Cervical arthritis, biliary colic, gastritis*

This section focuses on *pulmonary complaints*, including chest symptoms, dyspnea, wheezing, cough, and hemoptysis. For health history topics such as exertional chest pain, palpitations, orthopnea, paroxysmal nocturnal dyspnea, and edema, see Chapter 9, The Cardiovascular System (see pp. 345–347).

Your initial questions should be as open-ended as possible. "Do you have any discomfort or unpleasant feelings in your chest?" Ask the patient to point to location of the pain in the chest. Watch for any gestures as the patient describes the pain. Elicit all seven attributes of this symptom to distinguish among the various causes of chest pain (see p. 70).

A clenched fist over the sternum suggests *angina pectoris;* a finger pointing to a tender area on the chest wall suggests *musculoskeletal pain;* a hand moving from neck to epigastrium suggests *heartburn.*

Lung tissue has no pain fibers. Pain in conditions such as pneumonia or pulmonary infarction usually arises from inflammation of the adjacent parietal pleura. Muscle strain from prolonged recurrent coughing may also be responsible. The pericardium also has few pain fibers. The pain of pericarditis stems from inflammation of the adjacent parietal pleura. Chest pain is commonly also associated with anxiety, but the mechanism remains obscure.

Anxiety is the most frequent cause of chest pain in children; *costochondritis* is also common.

Shortness of Breath (Dyspnea) and Wheezing. *Dyspnea*, commonly termed *shortness of breath*, is a painless but uncomfortable awareness of breathing that is inappropriate to the level of exertion.[1] Thoroughly assess this prominent symptom of cardiac and pulmonary disease.

The degree of dyspnea in patients with *chronic obstructive pulmonary disease (COPD)* predicts 5-year survival better than forced expiratory volume in one second (FEV1).[2,3]

Ask, "Have you had any difficulty breathing?" Find out when the symptom occurs, at rest or with exercise, and how much exertion produces onset. Because of variations in age, body weight, and physical fitness, there is no absolute scale for quantifying dyspnea. Instead, make every effort *to determine its severity based on the patient's daily activities*. How many steps or flights of stairs can the patient climb before pausing for breath? What about carrying bags of groceries, mopping the floor, or making the bed? Has dyspnea altered the patient's lifestyle and daily activities? How? Carefully elicit the timing and setting, any associated symptoms, and relieving or aggravating factors.

See Table 8-2, Dyspnea, pp. 324–325.

Most patients relate shortness of breath to their level of activity. Anxious patients present a different picture. They may describe difficulty taking a deep enough breath, a smothering sensation with inability to get enough air, *paresthesias,* or sensations of tingling or "pins and needles" around the lips or in the extremities.

Anxious patients may have episodic dyspnea during both rest and exercise, and also *hyperventilation,* or rapid, shallow breathing.

Wheezes are musical respiratory sounds that may be audible to the patient and to others.

Wheezing occurs in partial airway obstruction from secretions and tissue inflammation in asthma, or from a foreign body.

Cough. *Cough* is a common symptom that ranges in significance from trivial to ominous. Typically, cough is a reflex response to stimuli that irritate receptors in the larynx, trachea, or large bronchi. These stimuli include mucus, pus, and blood, as well as external agents such as dust, foreign bodies, or even extremely hot or cold air. Other causes include inflammation of the respiratory mucosa and pressure or tension in the air passages from a tumor or enlarged peribronchial lymph nodes. Although cough typically signals a problem in the respiratory tract, it may also be cardiovascular in origin.

See Table 8-3, Cough and Hemoptysis, p. 326.

Cough can be a symptom of *left-sided heart failure.*

For complaints of cough, a thorough assessment is in order. Duration of the cough is important: is the cough *acute,* lasting less than 3 weeks; *subacute,* lasting 3 to 8 weeks; or *chronic,* more than 8 weeks?

Viral upper respiratory infections are the most common cause of *acute cough.* Also consider acute bronchitis, pneumonia, left ventricular heart failure, asthma, or a foreign body. Postinfectious cough, bacterial sinusitis, asthma occur in *subacute cough;* postnasal drip, asthma, gastroesophageal reflux, chronic bronchitis, bronchiectasis in *chronic cough.*[4-6]

Ask whether the cough is dry or produces sputum, or phlegm.

Ask the patient to describe the volume of any sputum and its color, odor, and consistency.

To help patients quantify volume, try a multiple-choice question. "How much do you think you cough up in 24 hours: a teaspoon, tablespoon, quarter cup, half cup, cupful?" If possible, ask the patient to cough into a tissue; inspect the phlegm and note its characteristics. The symptoms associated with a cough often lead you to its cause.

Hemoptysis.   *Hemoptysis* is the coughing up of blood from the lungs; it may vary from blood-streaked phlegm to frank blood. For patients reporting hemoptysis, assess the volume of blood produced as well as the other sputum attributes; ask about the related setting and activity and any associated symptoms.

Before using the term "hemoptysis," try to confirm the source of the bleeding. Blood or blood-streaked material may originate in the mouth, pharynx, or gastrointestinal tract and is easily mislabeled. When vomited, it probably originates in the gastrointestinal tract. Occasionally, however, blood from the nasopharynx or the gastrointestinal tract is aspirated and then coughed out.

Mucoid sputum is translucent, white, or gray; *purulent* sputum is yellow or green

Foul-smelling sputum is present in anaerobic *lung abscess;* tenacious sputum in cystic fibrosis

Large volumes of purulent sputum are present in *bronchiectasis* or *lung abscess*

Diagnostically helpful symptoms include fever, chest pain, dyspnea, orthopnea, and wheezing.

See Table 8-3, Cough and Hemoptysis, p. 326. Hemoptysis is rare in infants, children, and adolescents, although common in *cystic fibrosis.*

Blood originating in the stomach is usually darker than blood from the respiratory tract and may be mixed with food particles.

Health Promotion and Counseling: Evidence and Recommendations

Important Topics for Health Promotion and Counseling

▶ Tobacco cessation
▶ Immunizations

Tobacco Cessation.   Despite declines in smoking over the past several decades, 21% of U.S. adults continue to smoke.[7,8] Approximately 80% of smokers start by age 18 years.[9] Although rates of smoking in youths declined from 1997 to 2003, rates have remained relatively stable in recent years. Smoking accounts for one in five U.S. deaths each year, and half of all long-term smokers die of smoking-related diseases.[10] Counsel smokers about the high risk of related diseases and death.

Adverse Effects of Smoking on Health and Disease

Condition	Increased Risk Compared With Nonsmokers
▶ Coronary artery disease	2–4 times higher
▶ Stroke	2–4 times higher
▶ Peripheral vascular disease	10 times higher
▶ COPD mortality	12–13 times higher
▶ Lung cancer mortality	23 times higher in men
	13 times higher in women

Source: Centers for Disease Control and Prevention, DHHS. Smoking and tobacco use. Fact sheet. Health effects of cigarette smoking. Available at: http://www.cdc.gov/tobacco/data_statistics/Factsheets/health_cig_smoking/index.htm. Accessed March 20, 2011.

In addition, smoking contributes to at least 15 types of cancer and increases risk of infertility, preterm birth, low birth weight, and sudden infant death syndrome. Nonsmokers exposed to smoke also have increased risk of lung cancer, ear and respiratory infections, asthma, and residential fires.

Smoking is the leading preventable cause of death. Although a number of tests, such as helical computerized tomography, have been studied, screening for lung cancer is currently not recommended.[11] Instead, clinicians should focus on prevention and cessation, especially in teenagers and pregnant women.[12] Because 70% of smokers see a physician each year and 70% of those express interest in quitting, the benefits of brief counseling interventions are considerable.[8,13] Advising smokers to quit during every visit raises quit rates by 30%.[14] Use the "5 As" framework or the Stages of Change model to assess readiness to quit.[12,15]

Assessing Readiness to Quit Smoking: Brief Interventions Models

5 As Model	Stages of Change Model
▶ **Ask** about tobacco use	▶ **Precontemplation**—"I don't want to quit."
▶ **Advise** to quit	
▶ **Assess** willingness to make a quit attempt	▶ **Contemplation**—"I am concerned but not ready to quit now."
▶ **Assist** in quit attempt	▶ **Preparation**—"I am ready to quit."
▶ **Arrange** follow-up	▶ **Action**—"I just quit."
	▶ **Maintenance**—"I quit 6 months ago."

Nicotine is highly addicting, comparable to heroin and cocaine, and quitting is difficult. More than 80% of smokers who try to quit on their own resume smoking within 30 days and only 3% of smokers quit successfully each year.[16] Stimulation of the nicotinic cholinergic receptors in the brain increases release of dopamine, which enhances pleasure and modulates mood. Daily smokers inhale enough nicotine to achieve almost complete receptor saturation. The inhaled nicotine reaches the brain in seconds, causing a powerful and reinforcing rush effect. Use cognitive therapy techniques to help smokers recognize and design strategies to combat the features of addiction: craving, triggers such as stress or environmental cues, and signs of withdrawal like irritability, poor concentration, anxiety, and depressed mood. Quit rates roughly double when counseling is combined with pharmacotherapies such as nicotine replacement, bupropion, and, more recently, varencycline.[17,18]

Immunizations (Adults).   *Influenza* claims more than 36,000 deaths and 200,000 hospitalizations annually, especially during the late fall and winter, peaking in February. The CDC Advisory Committee on Immunization Practices updates its recommendations for vaccination annually. Two types of vaccine are available: the "flu shot," an inactivated vaccine containing killed virus, and a nasal-spray vaccine containing attenuated live viruses, approved only for healthy people between 5 and 49 years. Because influenza viruses change from year to year, each vaccine contains three vaccine strains and is modified yearly. Annual vaccination is recommended for all people aged 6 months and older, especially the groups listed below.[19]

Summary of CDC Influenza Vaccine Recommendations 2010—Adults

- Adults with chronic pulmonary conditions and chronic medical conditions; adults who are immunosuppressed or morbidly obese
- Women who are or who will be pregnant during influenza season
- Residents of nursing homes and chronic care facilities
- American Indians and Alaska natives
- Health care personnel
- Household contacts and caregivers of children 5 years of age and younger (especially infants age 6 months and younger) and of adults 50 years of age and older with medical conditions placing them at higher risk for complications of influenza

Streptococcus pneumonia causes pneumonia and meningitis and can lead to sepsis and death. Since the introduction in 1998 of routine vaccination for infants and children, the overall incidence of pneumococcal infections in all age groups has decreased 45%. In 2009, invasive pneumococcal disease still accounted for 43,500 cases and 5,000 deaths. For adults, use the 23-valent inactivated pneumococcal polysaccharide vaccine for the groups listed on the next page; for children, use the 7-valent conjugate vaccine, also inactivated.[20,21]

Techniques of Examination

It is helpful to examine the posterior thorax and lungs while the patient is sitting, and the anterior thorax and lungs with the patient supine. Proceed in an orderly fashion: inspect, palpate, percuss, and auscultate. Try to visualize the underlying lobes, and compare one side to the other, so asymmetries are more easily identified. For men, arrange the patient's gown so that you can see the chest fully. For women, cover the anterior chest when you examine the back; for the anterior examination, drape the gown over each half of the chest as you examine the other half.

● *With the patient sitting,* examine the posterior thorax and lungs. The patient's arms should be folded across the chest with hands resting, if possible, on the opposite shoulders. This position swings the scapulae laterally and increases access to the lung fields. Then ask the patient to lie down.

● *With the patient supine,* examine the anterior thorax and lungs. It is easier to examine women in this position because the breasts can be gently displaced. Some authorities prefer to examine both the back and the front of the chest with the patient sitting. This technique is also satisfactory.

● *For patients who cannot sit up,* get help so that you can examine the posterior chest in the sitting position. If this is not possible, roll the patient to one side and then to the other. Percuss the upper lung, and auscultate both lungs in each position. Because ventilation is relatively greater in the dependent lung, your chances of hearing abnormal wheezes or crackles are greater on the dependent side (see p. 314).

INITIAL SURVEY OF RESPIRATION AND THE THORAX

Even though you may have already recorded the respiratory rate when you took the vital signs, it is wise to again *observe the rate, rhythm, depth, and effort of breathing*. A healthy resting adult breathes quietly and regularly about 14 to 20 times a minute. Note whether expiration lasts longer than usual.

See Table 4-7, Abnormalities in Rate and Rhythm of Breathing, p. 140.

Always inspect the patient for any signs of respiratory difficulty.

- *Assess the patient's color* for cyanosis. Recall any relevant findings from earlier parts of your examination, such as the shape of the fingernails.

Cyanosis signals hypoxia. Clubbing of the nails (see p. 202) occurs in *bronchiectasis, congenital heart disease, pulmonary fibrosis, cystic fibrosis, lung abscess, and malignancy*

- *Listen to the patient's breathing.* Is there *audible wheezing*? If so, where does it fall in the respiratory cycle?

Audible *stridor*, a high-pitched wheeze, is an ominous sign of upper airway obstruction in the larynx or trachea.

- *Inspect the neck.* During inspiration, is there contraction of the accessory muscles, namely the sternomastoid and scalene muscles, or supraclavicular retraction? Is the trachea midline?

Accessory muscle use in COPD signals difficulty breathing. Lateral displacement of the trachea occurs in *pneumothorax, pleural effusion*, or *atelectasis*

Also *observe the shape of the chest*. The anteroposterior (AP) diameter may increase with aging, compared with the lateral chest diameter.

The AP diameter also may increase in *chronic obstructive pulmonary disease* (COPD), although evidence is conflicting.[22]

EXAMINATION OF THE POSTERIOR CHEST

Inspection

From a midline position behind the patient, note the *shape of the chest* and *how the chest moves*, including:

See Table 8-4, Deformities of the Thorax, p. 327.

- Deformities or asymmetry in chest expansion

Asymmetric expansion in pleural effusion

- Abnormal retraction of the interspaces during inspiration. Retraction is most apparent in the lower interspaces.

Retraction occurs in severe *asthma*, *COPD*, or upper airway obstruction

- Impaired respiratory movement on one or both sides or a unilateral lag (or delay) in movement.

Unilateral impairment or lagging indicates pleural disease from asbestosis or silicosis; it is also seen in phrenic nerve damage or trauma

Palpation

As you palpate the chest, focus on areas of tenderness and abnormalities in the overlying skin, respiratory expansion, and fremitus.

- *Identify tender areas.* Carefully palpate any area where pain has been reported or where lesions or bruises are evident.

- *Assess any visible abnormalities* such as masses or sinus tracts (blind, inflammatory, tubelike structures opening onto the skin).

- *Test chest expansion.* Place your thumbs at about the level of the 10th ribs, with your fingers loosely grasping and parallel to the lateral rib cage. As you position your hands, slide them medially just enough to raise a loose fold of skin on each side between your thumb and the spine.

  Ask the patient to inhale deeply. Watch the distance between your thumbs as they move apart during inspiration, and feel for the range and symmetry of the rib cage as it expands and contracts. This is sometimes termed lung excursion.

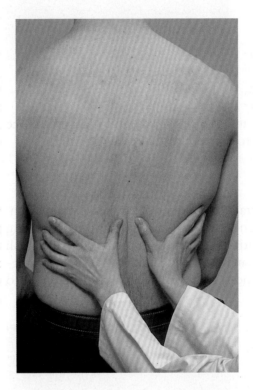

- *Feel for tactile fremitus.* Fremitus refers to the palpable vibrations transmitted through the bronchopulmonary tree to the chest wall as the patient is speaking. To detect fremitus, use either the ball (the bony part of the palm at the base of the fingers) or the ulnar surface of your hand to optimize the vibratory sensitivity of the bones in your hand. Ask the patient to repeat the words "ninety-nine" or "one-one-one." If fremitus is faint, ask the patient to speak more loudly or in a deeper voice.

  Use one hand until you have learned the feel of fremitus. Some clinicians find using one hand more accurate. Using both hands to compare sides increases your speed and may facilitate detection of differences.

Note intercostal tenderness over inflamed pleura.

Look for bruises over a fractured rib.

Although rare, sinus tracts indicate infection of the underlying pleura and lung (as in *tuberculosis, actinomycosis*).

Unilateral decrease or delay in chest expansion occurs in *chronic fibrosis* of the underlying lung or pleura, *pleural effusion, lobar pneumonia,* pleural pain with associated splinting, and unilateral bronchial obstruction.

Fremitus is decreased or absent when the voice is higher pitched or soft or when the transmission of vibrations from the larynx to the surface of the chest is impeded by a thick chest wall, an obstructed bronchus, *COPD*, or pleural changes from *effusion,* fibrosis, air (*pneumothorax*), or an infiltrating tumor.

- *Palpate and compare symmetric areas of the lungs* in the pattern shown in the photograph. Identify and locate any areas of increased, decreased, or absent fremitus. Fremitus is typically more prominent in the interscapular area than in the lower lung fields and is often more prominent on the right side than on the left. It disappears below the diaphragm.

Tactile fremitus is a somewhat imprecise assessment tool, but as a scouting technique, it directs your attention to possible abnormalities. Later in the examination, confirm any suggested findings by listening for underlying breath sounds, voice sounds, and whispered voice sounds. All these attributes tend to increase or decrease together.

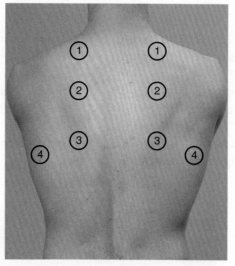

LOCATIONS FOR FEELING FREMITUS

Asymmetric *decreased* fremitus occurs in unilateral pleural effusion, pneumothorax, neoplasm due to decreased transmission of low frequency sounds; asymmetric *increased* fremitus occurs in unilateral pneumonia from increased transmission through consolidated tissue.[22]

Percussion

Percussion is one of the most important techniques of physical examination. Percussion sets the chest wall and underlying tissues in motion, producing audible sound and palpable vibrations. Percussion helps you establish whether the underlying tissues are air-filled, fluid-filled, or solid. It penetrates only 5 cm to 7 cm into the chest, however, and will not help you to detect deep-seated lesions.

The technique of percussion can be practiced on any surface. As you practice, listen for changes in percussion notes over different types of materials or different parts of the body. The key points for good technique, described for a right-handed person, are as follows:

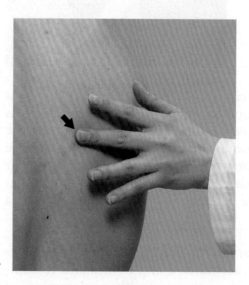

- Hyperextend the middle finger of your left hand, known as the *pleximeter finger*. Press its distal interphalangeal joint firmly on the surface to be percussed. *Avoid surface contact by any other part of the hand, because this dampens out vibrations.* Note that the thumb and 2nd, 4th, and 5th fingers are not touching the chest.

- Position your right forearm quite close to the surface, with the hand cocked upward. The middle finger should be partially flexed, relaxed, and poised to strike.

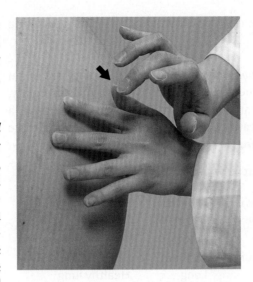

- With a *quick, sharp but relaxed wrist motion,* strike the pleximeter finger with the right middle finger, or plexor finger. Aim at your distal interphalangeal joint. You are trying to transmit vibrations through the bones of this joint to the underlying chest wall. Use the same force for each percussion strike and the same pleximeter pressure to avoid changes in the percussion note related to your technique rather than patient findings.

- Strike using the *tip of the plexor finger,* not the finger pad. Your finger should be almost at right angles to the pleximeter. A short fingernail is recommended to avoid injuring your knuckle.

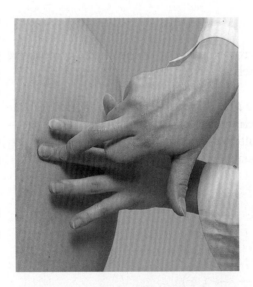

- Withdraw your striking finger quickly to avoid damping the vibrations you have created.

In summary, the movement is at the wrist. It is directed, brisk yet relaxed, and a bit bouncy.

Percussion Notes. With your plexor or tapping finger, use the lightest percussion that produces a clear note. A thick chest wall requires stronger percussion than a thin one. However, if a *louder* note is needed, apply more pressure with the *pleximeter* finger (this is more effective for increasing percussion note volume than tapping harder with the plexor finger).

- *When percussing the lower posterior chest,* stand somewhat to the side rather than directly behind the patient. This allows you to place your pleximeter finger more firmly on the chest and your plexor is more effective, making a better percussion note.

- *When comparing two areas,* use the same percussion technique in both areas. Percuss or strike twice in each location. It is easier to detect differences in percussion notes by comparing one area with another than by striking repetitively in one place.

- *Learn to identify five percussion notes.* You can practice four of them on yourself. These notes differ in their basic qualities of sound: intensity, pitch, and duration. Train your ear by concentrating on one quality at a time as you percuss first in one location, then in another. Review the table below. Healthy lungs are *resonant.*

Percussion Notes and Their Characteristics

	Relative Intensity	Relative Pitch	Relative Duration	Example of Location	Pathologic Examples
Flat	Soft	High	Short	Thigh	Large pleural effusion
Dull	Medium	Medium	Medium	Liver	Lobar pneumonia
Resonant	Loud	Low	Long	Healthy lung	Simple chronic bronchitis
Hyperresonant	Very loud	Lower	Longer	Usually none	COPD, pneumothorax
Tympanitic	Loud	High*	Longer	Gastric air bubble or puffed-out cheek	Large pneumothorax

*Distinguished mainly by its musical timbre.

While the patient keeps both arms crossed in front of the chest, percuss the thorax in symmetric locations on each side from the apex to the base.

- *Percuss one side of the chest and then the other at each level* in a ladderlike pattern, as shown by the numbers below. Omit the areas over the scapulae—the thickness of muscle and bone alters the percussion notes over the lungs. Identify and locate the area and quality of any abnormal percussion note.

Dullness replaces resonance when fluid or solid tissue replaces air-containing lung or occupies the pleural space beneath your percussing fingers. Examples include: *lobar pneumonia,* in which the alveoli are filled with fluid and blood cells; and pleural accumulations of serous fluid (*pleural effusion*), blood (*hemothorax*), pus (*empyema*), fibrous tissue, or tumor. Dullness makes pneumonic and pleural effusion 5 and 18 times more likely, respectively.[22]

Generalized hyperresonance may be heard over the hyperinflated lungs of COPD or *asthma. Unilateral hyperresonance* suggests a large pneumothorax or possibly a large air-filled bulla in the lung.

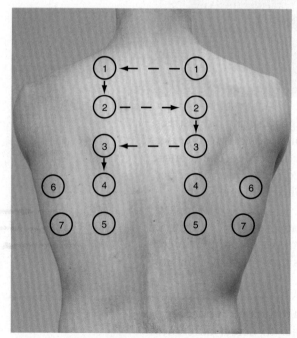

"LADDER" PATTERN FOR PERCUSSION AND AUSCULTATION

- *Identify the descent of the diaphragm, or diaphragmatic excursion.* First, *determine the level of diaphragmatic dullness* during quiet respiration. Holding the pleximeter finger *above and parallel* to the expected level of dullness, percuss downward in progressive steps until dullness clearly replaces resonance. Confirm this level of change by percussion near the middle of the hemothorax and also more laterally.

This maneuver tends to overestimate actual movements of the diaphragm.[22]

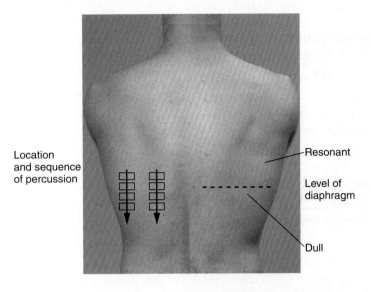

Location and sequence of percussion

Resonant

Level of diaphragm

Dull

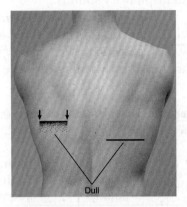

Dull

An abnormally high level suggests *pleural effusion*, or a high diaphragm as in *atelectasis* or *phrenic nerve paralysis*.

Note that with this technique, you are identifying the boundary between the resonant lung tissue and the duller structures below the diaphragm. You are not percussing the diaphragm itself. You can infer the probable location of the diaphragm from the level of dullness.

Now, *estimate the extent of diaphragmatic excursion* by determining the distance between the level of dullness on full expiration and the level of dullness on full inspiration, normally about 3 to 5.5 cm.[23]

Auscultation

Auscultation is the most important examination technique for assessing air flow through the tracheobronchial tree. Together with percussion, it also helps the clinician assess the condition of the surrounding lungs and pleural space. Auscultation involves (1) listening to the sounds generated by breathing, (2) listening for any adventitious (added) sounds, and (3) if abnormalities are suspected, listening to the sounds of the patient's spoken or whispered voice as they are transmitted through the chest wall.

Sounds from bedclothes, paper gowns, and the chest itself can generate confusion in auscultation. Hair on the chest may cause crackling sounds. Either press harder or wet the hair.

Breath Sounds (Lung Sounds). Learn to identify patterns of breath sounds by their intensity, their pitch, and the relative duration of their inspiratory and expiratory phases. Normal breath sounds are:

- *Vesicular,* or soft and low pitched. They are heard through inspiration, continue without pause through expiration, and then fade away about one third of the way through expiration.

If the patient is cold or tense, you may hear muscle contraction sounds—muffled, low-pitched rumbling or roaring noises. A change in the patient's position may eliminate this noise. You can reproduce this sound on yourself by doing a Valsalva maneuver (straining down) as you listen to your own chest.

- *Bronchovesicular,* with inspiratory and expiratory sounds about equal in length, at times separated by a silent interval. Detecting differences in pitch and intensity is often easier during expiration.

- *Bronchial,* or louder, harsher and higher in pitch, with a short silence between inspiratory and expiratory sounds. Expiratory sounds last longer than inspiratory sounds.

The characteristics of these three kinds of breath sounds are summarized below. Also shown are the *tracheal* breath sounds—very loud, harsh sounds that are heard by listening over the trachea in the neck.

Characteristics of Breath Sounds

	Duration of Sounds	Intensity of Expiratory Sound	Pitch of Expiratory Sound	Locations Where Heard Normally
Vesicular*	Inspiratory sounds last longer than expiratory sounds.	Soft	Relatively low	Over most of both lungs
Broncho-vesicular	Inspiratory and expiratory sounds are about equal.	Intermediate	Intermediate	Often in the 1st and 2nd interspaces anteriorly and between the scapulae
Bronchial	Expiratory sounds last longer than inspiratory ones.	Loud	Relatively high	Over the manubrium, (larger proximal airways)
Tracheal	Inspiratory and expiratory sounds are about equal.	Very loud	Relatively high	Over the trachea in the neck

Silent gap (handwritten note in Bronchial row)

*The thickness of the bars indicates intensity; the steeper their incline, the higher the pitch.

Sources: Loudon R and Murphy LH. Lungs sounds. Am Rev Respir Dis 1994;130:663–673; Wilkins RL, Dexter JR, Murphy RLH et al. Lung sound nomenclature survey, Chest 1990;98:886–889; Schreur HJW, Sterk PJ, Vanderschoot JW et al. Lung sound intensity in patients with emphysema and in normal subjects at standardised airflows. Thorax 1992;47:674–679; Bettancourt PE, DelBono EA, Speigelman D, et al. Clinical utility of chest auscultation in common pulmonary disease. Am J Resp Crit Care Med 1994;150:1921.

If bronchovesicular or bronchial breath sounds are heard in locations distant from those listed, suspect that air-filled lung has been replaced by fluid-filled or solid lung tissue.

See Table 8-5, Normal and Altered Breath and Voice Sounds, p. 328.

Listen to the breath sounds with the diaphragm of a stethoscope after instructing the patient to breathe deeply through an open mouth. Use the ladder pattern suggested for percussion, moving from one side to the other and comparing symmetric areas of the lungs. If you hear or suspect abnormal sounds, auscultate adjacent areas to assess the extent of any abnormality. Listen to at least one full breath in each location. If the patient becomes light-headed from hyperventilation, allow the patient to take a few normal breathes.

Note the *intensity* of the breath sounds, which reflects the air flow rate at the mouth. Breath sounds are usually louder in the lower posterior lung fields. Their intensity may vary from one area to another. If the breath sounds seem faint, ask the patient to breathe more deeply. Shallow breathing or a thick chest wall can both alter breath sound intensity.

Breath sounds may be decreased when air flow is decreased (as in obstructive lung disease or muscular weakness) or when the transmission of sound is poor (as in *pleural effusion, pneumothorax,* or *COPD*).

Is there a *silent gap* between the inspiratory and expiratory sounds?

A gap suggests bronchial breath sounds.

Listen for the *pitch, intensity, and duration of the expiratory and inspiratory sounds.* Are vesicular breath sounds distributed normally over the chest wall? Or are there bronchovesicular or bronchial breath sounds in unexpected places? If so, where are they?

Adventitious (Added) Sounds.   Listen for any added, or adventitious, sounds that are superimposed on the usual breath sounds. Detection of adventitious sounds—*crackles* (sometimes called *rales*), *wheezes,* and *rhonchi*—is an important part of your examination, often leading to diagnosis of cardiac and pulmonary conditions. The most common kinds of these sounds are described on the next page.

For further discussion and other added sounds, see Table 8-6, Adventitious (Added) Lung Sounds: Causes and Qualities, p. 329.

If you hear *crackles,* especially those that do not clear after coughing, listen carefully for the following characteristics.[24–27] These are clues to the underlying condition:

- Loudness, pitch, and duration, summarized as fine or coarse crackles

Fine late inspiratory crackles that persist from breath to breath suggest abnormal lung tissue.

- Number, few to many.

- Timing in the respiratory cycle

- Location on the chest wall

- Persistence of their pattern from breath to breath

- Any change after a cough or change in the patient's position

Clearing of crackles, wheezes, or rhonchi after coughing or position change suggests inspissated secretions, seen in *bronchitis* or *atelectasis.*

Adventitious or Added Breath Sounds

Crackles (or Rales)	Wheezes and Rhonchi
▶ **Discontinuous**	▶ **Continuous**
▶ Intermittent, nonmusical, and brief	▶ ≥250 msec, musical, prolonged (but not necessarily persisting throughout the respiratory cycle)
▶ Like dots in time	▶ Like dashes in time
▶ *Fine crackles:* soft, high-pitched, very brief (5–10 msec)	▶ *Wheezes:* relatively high-pitched (≥400 Hz) with hissing or shrill quality
· · · · ·	‿‿‿‿‿‿
▶ *Coarse crackles:* somewhat louder, lower in pitch, brief (20–30 msec)	▶ *Rhonchi:* relatively low-pitched (≤200 Hz) with snoring quality
• • • • •	‿‿‿

Source: Loudon R and Murphy LH. Lungs sounds. Am Rev Respir Dis 130:663–673, 1994.

Crackles may be from abnormalities of the lungs (*pneumonia, fibrosis, early heart failure*) or of the airways (bronchitis, bronchiectasis).

Wheezes suggest narrowed airways, as in *asthma, COPD,* or *bronchitis.*

Rhonchi suggest secretions in large airways.

In some normal people, crackles may be heard at the anterior lung bases after maximal expiration. Crackles in dependent portions of the lungs may also occur after prolonged recumbency.

If you hear *wheezes* or *rhonchi,* note their timing and location. Do they change with deep breathing or coughing?

Findings predictive of *COPD* include combinations of symptoms and signs, especially wheezing by self-report or examination, plus a history of smoking, age, and decreased breath sounds. Diagnosis requires spirometry and often further pulmonary testing.[28–34]

Transmitted Voice Sounds. If you hear abnormally located bronchovesicular or bronchial breath sounds, assess transmitted voice sounds. With a stethoscope, listen in symmetric areas over the chest wall as you assess any abnormal vocal resonances suspicious for pneumonia or pleural effusion.

Increased transmission of voice sounds suggests that air-filled lung has become airless. See Table 8-5, Normal and Altered Breath and Voice Sounds, p. 328.

- Ask the patient to say "ninety-nine." Normally the sounds transmitted through the chest wall are muffled and indistinct.

Louder voice sounds are called *bronchophony.*

- Ask the patient to say "ee." You will normally hear a muffled long E sound.

If "ee" sounds like "A," an E-to-A change, or *egophony,* is present, seen in lobar consolidation from *pneumonia.* The "A" has a nasal bleating quality, and should be localized. In patients with fever and cough, the presence of bronchial breath sounds and egophony more than triples the likelihood of pneumonia.[22]

- Ask the patient to whisper "ninety-nine" or "one-two-three." The whispered voice is normally heard faintly and indistinctly, if at all.

Louder, clearer whispered sounds are called *whispered pectoriloquy*.

EXAMINATION OF THE ANTERIOR CHEST

When examined in the supine position, the patient should lie comfortably with arms somewhat abducted. Examine a patient having difficulty breathing in the sitting position or with the head of the bed elevated to a comfortable level.

Persons with severe *COPD* may prefer to sit leaning forward, with lips pursed during exhalation and arms supported on their knees or a table.

Inspection

Observe *the shape of the patient's chest* and *the movement of the chest wall*. Note:

- Deformities or asymmetry

See Table 8-4, Deformities of the Thorax, p. 327.

- Abnormal retraction of the lower interspaces during inspiration. Supraclavicular retraction is often present.

Abnormal retraction occurs in severe *asthma, COPD,* or upper airway obstruction

- Local lag or impairment in respiratory movement

Underlying disease of lung or pleura

Palpation

Palpation has four potential uses:

- *Identification of tender areas*

Tender pectoral muscles or costal cartilages suggest, but do not prove, that chest pain has a musculoskeletal origin.

- *Assessment of observed abnormalities*

- *Further assessment of chest expansion.* Place your thumbs along each costal margin, your hands along the lateral rib cage. As you position your hands, slide them medially a bit to raise loose skin folds between your thumbs. Ask the patient to inhale deeply. Observe how far your thumbs diverge as the thorax expands, and feel for the extent and symmetry of respiratory movement.

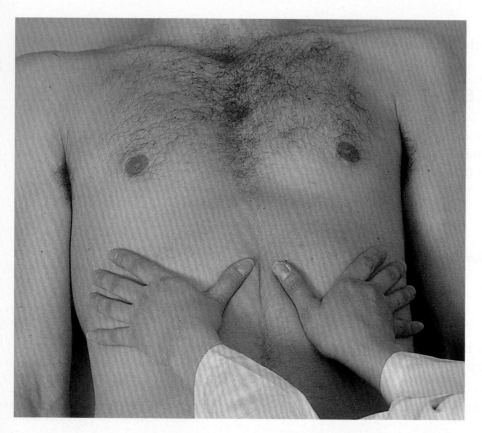

- *Assessment of tactile fremitus.* Compare both sides of the chest, using the ball or ulnar surface of your hand. Fremitus is usually decreased or absent over the precordium. When examining a woman, gently displace the breasts as necessary.

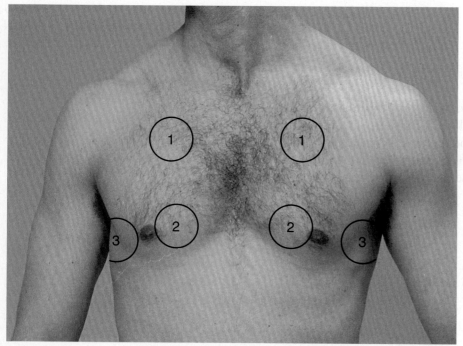

LOCATIONS FOR FEELING FREMITUS

Percussion

Percuss the anterior and lateral chest, again comparing both sides. The heart normally produces an area of dullness to the left of the sternum from the 3rd to the 5th interspaces. Percuss the left lung lateral to the area of dullness.

Dullness replaces resonance when fluid or solid tissue replaces air-containing lung or occupies the pleural space. Because pleural fluid usually sinks to the lowest part of the pleural space (posteriorly in a supine patient), only a very large effusion can be detected anteriorly.

The hyperresonance of *COPD* may totally replace cardiac dullness.

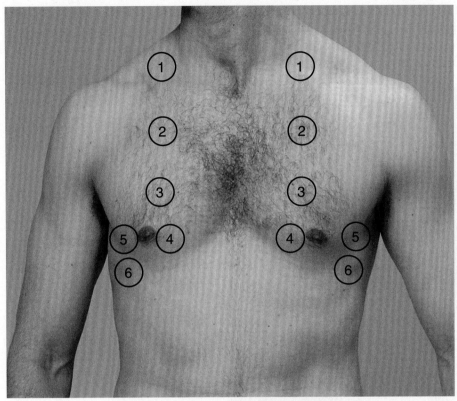

LOCATIONS FOR PERCUSSION AND AUSCULTATION

In a woman, to enhance percussion, gently displace the breast with your left hand while percussing with the right.

The dullness of right middle lobe pneumonia typically occurs behind the right breast. Unless you displace the breast, you may miss the abnormal percussion note.

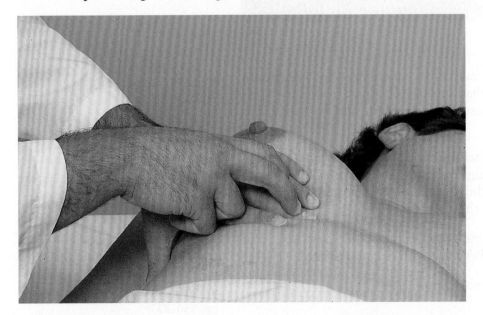

Alternatively, you may ask the patient to move her breast for you.

Identify and locate any area with an abnormal percussion note.

With your pleximeter finger above and parallel to the expected upper border of liver dullness, percuss in progressive steps downward in the right midclavicular line. Identify the upper border of liver dullness. Later, during the abdominal examination, you will use this method to estimate the size of the liver. As you percuss down the chest on the left, the resonance of normal lung usually changes to the tympany of the gastric air bubble.

A lung affected by *COPD* often displaces the upper border of the liver downward and lowers the level of diaphragmatic dullness posteriorly.

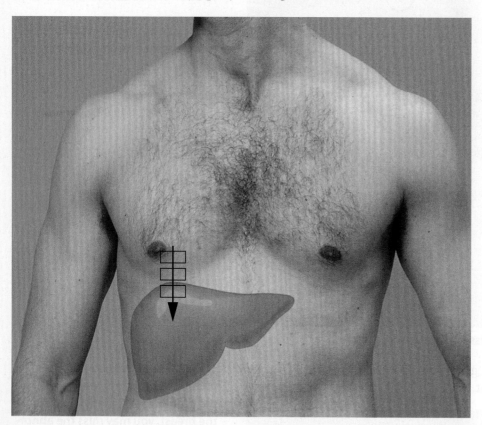

Auscultation

Listen to the chest anteriorly and laterally as the patient breathes with mouth open, and somewhat more deeply than normal. Compare symmetric areas of the lungs, using the pattern suggested for percussion and extending it to adjacent areas if indicated.

Listen to the breath sounds, noting their intensity and identifying any variations from normal vesicular breathing. Breath sounds are usually louder in the upper anterior lung fields. Bronchovesicular breath sounds may be heard over the large airways, especially on the right.

Identify any adventitious sounds, time them in the respiratory cycle, and locate them on the chest wall. Do they clear with deep breathing?

If indicated, *listen for transmitted voice sounds.*

See Table 8-6, Adventitious (Added) Lung Sounds: Causes and Qualities, p. 329, and Table 8-7, Physical Findings in Selected Chest Disorders, pp. 330–331.

SPECIAL TECHNIQUES

Clinical Assessment of Pulmonary Function. Walk tests are practical, simple ways to assess cardiopulmonary function commonly used in rehabilitation and pre- and postoperative settings. In 2002, the American Thoracic Society issued guidelines to standardize the 6-minute walk test based on a review of the relevant literature.[35] The test is easy to administer and requires only a 100-foot hallway. It measures "the distance that a patient can quickly walk on a flat, hard surface in a period of 6 minutes" and provides a global evaluation of the pulmonary and cardiovascular systems, neuromuscular units, and muscle metabolism. Review the specifics of testing, which should be done on two occasions and include taking the medical history and vital signs. Shorter tests continue to be evaluated.[36]

Forced Expiratory Time. This test assesses the expiratory phase of breathing, which is typically slowed in obstructive pulmonary disease. Ask the patient to take a deep breath in and then breathe out as quickly and completely as possible with mouth open. Listen over the trachea with the diaphragm of a stethoscope and time the audible expiration. Try to get three consistent readings, allowing a short rest between efforts if necessary.

Patients older than 60 years with a forced expiratory time of 6 to 8 seconds are twice as likely to have COPD; if more than 8 seconds, the likelihood increases to 4.[37]

Identification of a Fractured Rib. Local pain and tenderness of one or more ribs raise the question of fracture. By anteroposterior compression of the chest, you can help to distinguish a fracture from soft-tissue injury. With one hand on the sternum and the other on the thoracic spine, squeeze the chest. Is this painful, and where?

An increase in the local pain (distant from your hands) suggests rib fracture rather than just soft-tissue injury.

Recording Your Findings

Note that initially you may use sentences to describe your findings; later you will use phrases. The style below contains phrases appropriate for most write-ups.

Recording the Physical Examination—The Thorax and Lungs

"Thorax is symmetric with good expansion. Lungs resonant. Breath sounds vesicular; no rales, wheezes, or rhonchi. Diaphragms descend 4 cm bilaterally."
OR
"Thorax symmetric with moderate kyphosis and increased anteroposterior (AP) diameter, decreased expansion. Lungs are hyperresonant. Breath sounds distant with delayed expiratory phase and scattered expiratory wheezes. Fremitus decreased; no bronchophony, egophony, or whispered pectoriloquy. Diaphragms descend 2 cm bilaterally."

These findings suggest *COPD*.

Bibliography

Citations

1. American Thoracic Society. Dyspnea—mechanisms, assessment, and management: a consensus statement. Am J Respir Crit Care Med 1999;159(1):321–340.

2. Nishimura K, Izumi T, Tsukino M et al. Dyspnea is a better predictor of 5-year survival than airway obstruction in patients with COPD. Chest 2002;121:1434–1440.

3. Celli BR, Cote CG, Marin JM et al. The body-mass index, airflow obstruction, dyspnea, and exercise capacity index in chronic obstructive pulmonary disease. N Engl J Med 2004; 350:1005–1012.

4. Irwin RS and Madison JM. The diagnosis and treatment of cough. N Engl J Med 2000;343(23):1715–1721.

5. Barker A. Bronchiectasis. N Engl J Med 2002;346(18):1383–1393.

6. Wenzel RP, Fowler AA. Acute bronchitis. N Engl J Med 2006;355(20):2125–2130.

7. Centers for Disease Control and Prevention. Smoking and Tobacco Use. Tables, Charts and Graphs. Prevalence of Current Smoking among Adults Aged 18 Years and Over: United States, 1997-2009. Available at http://www.cdc.gov/nchs/data/nhis/earlyrelease/earlyrelease201006.pdf#page=52. Accessed February 26, 2011.

8. Centers for Disease Control and Prevention. Smoking and tobacco use. Fact sheet. Health effects of cigarette smoking. Updated March 2011. Available at http://www.cdc.gov/tobacco/data_statistics/fact_sheets/health_effects/effects_cig_smoking/index.htm. Accessed March 20, 2011.

9. Centers for Disease Control and Prevention. Smoking and tobacco use. Children and adolescents. youth tobacco prevention. Youth and tobacco use: current estimates. Available at http://www.cdc.gov/tobacco/data_statistics/fact_sheets/youth_data/tobacco_use/index.htm. Accessed February 26, 2011.

10. Office of the Surgeon General. How tobacco smoke causes disease: the biology and behavioral basis for smoking-attributable disease: a report of the Surgeon General. – Rockville, MD. Dept. of Health and Human Services, Public Health Service, Office of Surgeon General, 2010. Available at http://www.surgeongeneral.gov/library/tobaccosmoke/report/index.html. Accessed February 26, 2011.

11. U.S. Preventative Services Task Force. Lung cancer screening: recommendation statement. Rockville, MD, Agency for Healthcare Research and Quality, May 2004. Available at http://www.uspreventiveservicestaskforce.org/3rduspstf/lungcancer/lungcanrs.htm. Accessed February 26, 2011.

12. U.S. Preventative Services Task Force. Counseling to prevent tobacco use and tobacco-caused disease: recommendation statement. Rockville, MD, Agency for Healthcare Research and Quality, May 2004. Available at http://www.uspreventiveservicestaskforce.org/3rduspstf/tobacccoun/tobcounrs.pdf. Accessed February 26, 2011.

13. Rigotti N. Treatment of tobacco use and dependence. N Engl J Med 2002;346:506–512.

14. Ranney L, Melvin C, Lux L et al. Systematic review: smoking cessation intervention strategies for adults and adults in special populations. Ann Int Med 2006;145:845–856.

15. Norcross JC, Prochaska JO. Using the stages of change. Harvard Mental Health Letter May 2002, pp. 5–7.

16. Benowitz NL. Nicotine addiction. N Engl J Med 2010; 362:2295–2303.

17. Wilson JF. In the clinic: tobacco cessation. Ann Intern Med 2007;146:!TC2-1 – ITC 2–16.

18. Hays JT, Ebbert JO. Varenicline for tobacco dependence. N Engl J Med 2008;359:2018–2024.

19. Centers for Disease Control and Prevention, DHHS. Seasonal Influenza. Health Professionals. Vaccine Recommendations (ACIP). 2010-2011 ACIP Recommendations. Summary of Influenza Recommendations 2010. Available at http://www.cdc.gov/flu/professionals/acip/flu_vax1011.htm#box1. Accessed February 26, 2011.

20. Centers for Disease Control and Prevention. Updated Recommendations for Prevention of Invasive Pneumococcal Disease Among Adults Using 23-Valent Pneumococcal Polysaccharide Vaccine. MMWR 2010;59(34):1102–1105.

21. Centers for Disease Control and Prevention. Prevention of Pneumococcal Disease among Infants and Children: Use of 13-Valent Pneumococcal Conjugate Vaccine and 23-Valent Pneumococcal Polysaccharide Vaccine. MMWR 2010;59(RR-11):1–29.

22. McGee S. Evidence-based Physical Diagnosis, 2nd ed. Philadelphia: Saunders, 2007.

23. Wong CL, Holroyd-Leduc J, Straus SE. Does this patient have a pleural effusion? JAMA 2009;301:309–317.

24. Loudon R and Murphy LH. Lungs sounds. Am Rev Respir Dis 1994;130:663–673.

25. Epler GR, Carrrington CB, Gaensler EA. Crackles (rales) in the interstitial pulmonary diseases. Chest 1978;73:333–339.

26. Nath AR, Capel LH. Inspiratory crackles and mechanical events of breathing. Thorax 1974;29:695–698.

27. Nath AR and Capel LH. Lung crackles in bronchiectasis. Thorax 1980;35:694–699.

28. Badgett RG, Tanaka DJ, Hunt DK et al. Can moderate chronic obstructive pulmonary disease be diagnosed by historical and physical findings alone? Am J Med 1993;94:188–196.

29. Holleman DR, Simel DL. Does the clinical examination predict airflow limitation. JAMA 1995;273:63–68.

30. Straus SE, McAlister FA, Sackett DL et al. The accuracy of patient history, wheezing, and laryngeal measurements in diagnosing obstructive airway disease. JAMA 2000;283:1853–1857.

31. Panettieri RA. In the clinic: asthma. Ann Intern Med 2007; 146:ITC6-1–ITC6-16.

32. Littner M. In the clinic: chronic obstructive pulmonary disease. Ann Intern Med 2008;148:ITC3-1–ITC3-16.

33. Neiwoehner DR. Outpatient management of severe COPD. N Engl J Med 2010;362:1407–1436.

34. Pauwels RA, Buist AS, Calverley PM et al. GOLD Scientific Committee. Global strategy for the diagnosis, management, and prevention of chronic obstructive pulmonary disease: NHLBI/WHO Global Initiative for Chronic Obstructive Lung Disease (GOLD) workshop summary. Am J Resp Crit Care Med 2001;163:125–1276.

35. American Thoracic Society Committee on Proficiency Standards for Clinical Pulmonary Function Laboratories. ATS statement: guidelines for the six-minute walk test. Am J Respir Crit Care Med 2002;166:111–117.

36. Solway S, Brooks D, Lacasse Y et al. A qualitative systematic overview of the measurement properties of functional walk tests used in the cardiorespiratory domain. Chest 2001; 119:256–270.

37. Schapira RM, Schapira MM, Funahashi A et al. The value of the forced expiratory time in the physical diagnosis of obstructive airways disease. JAMA 1993;270:731–736.

Additional References

Examination of the Lungs

Graffelman AW, le Cessie S, Knuistingh Neven A et al. Can history and exam alone reliably predict pneumonia? J Fam Pract 2007;56:465–470.

Holleman DR, Simel DL, Goldberg JS. Diagnosis of obstructive airways disease from the clinical examination. J Gen Intern Med 1993;8:63–68.

Hurst JR, Vestbo J, Anzueto A et al. Susceptibility to exacerbation of chronic obstructive pulmonary disease. N Engl J Med 2010;363:1128–1138.

Lichtenstein D, Goldstein I, Mourgeon E et al. Comparative diagnostic performance of auscultation, chest radiography, and lung ultrasonography in acute respiratory distress syndrome. Anesthesiology 2004;10:9–15.

Loudon RG. The lung exam. Clin Chest Med 1987;8:265–272.

McFadden ER, Kiser R, deGroot WJ. Acute bronchial asthma. Relations between clinical and physiologic manifestations. N Engl J Med 1973;288:221–225,.

Meslier N, Charbonneau G, Racineux JL. Wheezes. Eur Respir J 1995;8: 1942–1948. doi:10.1183/09031936.95.08111942. PMID 8620967. Available at http://erj.ersjournals.com/cgi/pmidlookup?view=long&pmid=8620967. Accessed October 10, 2011.

Nici L, Donner C, Wouters WE et al on behalf of the ATS/ERS Pulmonary Rehabilitation Writing Committee. American Thoracic Society/European Respiratory Society Statement on Pulmonary Rehabilitation. Am J Respir Crit Care Med 2006;173: 1390–1413.

Pulmonary Conditions

Benowitz NL. Nicotine addiction. N Engl J Med 2010;362:2295–2303.

Carey MA, Card JW, Voltz JW et al. It's all about sex: male-female differences in lung development and disease. Trends Endocrinol Metab 2007;18:308–313.

Centers for Disease Control and Prevention. Tuberculosis. Updated October 2011. Available at http://www.cdc.gov/tb. Accessed October 10, 2011.

Chung KF, Pavord ID. Prevalence, pathogenesis, and causes of chronic cough. Lancet. 2008;371(9621):1364–74.

Eder W, Ege MJ, Mutius E. The asthma epidemic. New Engl J Med 2006;355:2226–2235.

Fiore MC, Jaén CR, Baker TB et al. Treating tobacco use and dependence: 2008 update. Rockville, MD: US Dept of Health and Human Services; May 2008. http://www.ahrq.gov/path/tobacco.htm#Clinic. Accessed October 10, 2011.

Global Strategy for the Diagnosis, Management and Prevention of COPD, Global Initiative for Chronic Obstructive Lung Disease (GOLD) 2010. Available at http://www.goldcopd.org. Accessed October 10, 2011.

Iannuzzi MC, Rybicki BA, Tierstein AS. Sarcoidosis. N Engl J Med 2007;357:2153–2165.

Konstantinides S. Acute pulmonary embolism. N Engl J Med 2008;359:2804–2813.

Nathanson E, Nunn P, Uplekar M et al. MDR tuberculosis—critical steps for prevention and control. N Engl J Med 2010; 363:1050–1058.

Qaseem A, Snow V, Shekelle P et al. Diagnosis and management of stable chronic obstructive pulmonary disease: a clinical practice guideline from the American College of Physicians. Ann Intern Med 2007;147:633–638.

Silverman EK, Sandhaus RA. Alpha1-antitripsin deficiency. N Engl J Med 2009;360:2749–2757.

Somers VK, White DP, Amin R et al. Sleep apnea and cardiovascular disease. An American Heart Association/American College of Cardiology Foundation Scientific Statement from the American Heart Association Council for High Blood Pressure Research Professional Education Committee, Council on Clinical Cardiology, Stroke Counsel, and Council on Cardiovascular Nursing. J Am Coll Cardiology 2008;52:686–717.

Ware LB, Matthay MA. Acute pulmonary edema. N Engl J Med 2005;353:2788–2796.

Weinberger SE, Cockrill BA, Mandel J. Principles of Pulmonary Medicine, 5th ed. Philadelphia: Saunders/Elsevier, 2008.

Wilson J. In the clinic. Smoking cessation. Ann Intern Med 2007;146: ITC2-1–ITC2-16.

Witt TJ, Niewoehner D, Macdonald R et al. Management of stable chronic obstructive pulmonary disease: a systematic review for a clinical practice guideline. Ann Intern Med 2007;147:639–653.

The Bates' suite offers these additional resources to enhance learning and facilitate understanding of this chapter:

- Bates' Pocket Guide to Physical Examination and History Taking, 7th edition
- Bates' Visual Guide to Physical Examination
- thePoint online resources, for students and instructors: http://thepoint.lww.com

Table

8-1   Chest Pain

Problem	Process	Location	Quality	Severity
Cardiovascular				
Angina Pectoris	Temporary myocardial ischemia, usually secondary to coronary atherosclerosis	Retrosternal or across the anterior chest, sometimes radiating to the shoulders, arms, neck, lower jaw, or upper abdomen	Pressing, squeezing, tight, heavy, occasionally burning	Mild to moderate, sometimes perceived as discomfort rather than pain
Myocardial Infarction	Prolonged myocardial ischemia, resulting in irreversible muscle damage or necrosis	Same as in angina	Same as in angina	Often but not always a severe pain
Pericarditis	• Irritation of parietal pleura adjacent to the pericardium	Retrosternal or left precordial, may radiate to the tip of left shoulder	Sharp, knifelike	Often severe
	• Mechanism unclear	Retrosternal	Crushing	Severe
Dissecting Aortic Aneurysm	A splitting within the layers of the aortic wall, allowing passage of blood to dissect a channel	Anterior chest, radiating to the neck, back, or abdomen	Ripping, tearing	Very severe
Pulmonary				
Tracheobronchitis	Inflammation of trachea and large bronchi	Upper sternal or on either side of the sternum	Burning	Mild to moderate
Pleuritic Pain	Inflammation of the parietal pleura, as in pleurisy, pneumonia, pulmonary infarction, or neoplasm	Chest wall overlying the process	Sharp, knifelike	Often severe
Gastrointestinal and Other				
Reflex Esophagitis	Inflammation of the esophageal mucosa by reflux of gastric acid	Retrosternal, may radiate to the back	Burning, may be squeezing	Mild to severe
Diffuse Esophageal Spasm	Motor dysfunction of the esophageal muscle	Retrosternal, may radiate to the back, arms, and jaw	Usually squeezing	Mild to severe
Chest Wall Pain, Costochondritis	Variable, often unclear	Often below the left breast or along the costal cartilages.	Stabbing, sticking, or dull, aching	Variable
Anxiety	Unclear	Precordial, below the left breast, or across the anterior chest	Stabbing, sticking, or dull, aching	Variable

Note: Remember that chest pain may be referred from extrathoracic structures such as the neck (*arthritis*) and abdomen (*biliary colic, acute cholecystitis*). Pleural pain may be from abdominal conditions such as *subdiaphragmatic abscess.*

Timing	Factors That Aggravate	Factors That Relieve	Associated Symptoms
Usually 1–3 min but up to 10 min. Prolonged episodes up to 20 min	Exertion, especially in the cold; meals; emotional stress. May occur at rest	Rest, nitroglycerin	Sometimes dyspnea, nausea, sweating
20 min to several hours			Dyspnea, nausea, vomiting, sweating, weakness
Persistent	Breathing, changing position, coughing, lying down, sometimes swallowing	Sitting forward may relieve it.	Seen in autoimmune disorders, post–myocardial infarction, viral infection, chest irradiation
Persistent			Of the underlying illness
Abrupt onset, early peak, persistent for hours or more	Hypertension		If thoracic, hoarseness, dysphagia, also syncope, hemiplegia, paraplegia
Variable	Coughing	Lying on the involved side may relieve it.	Cough
Persistent	Deep inspiration, coughing, movements of the trunk		Of the underlying illness
Variable	Large meal; bending over, lying down	Antacids, sometimes belching	Sometimes regurgitation, dysphagia
Variable	Swallowing of food or cold liquid; emotional stress	Sometimes nitroglycerin	Dysphagia
Fleeting to hours or days	Movement of chest, trunk, arms		Often local tenderness
Fleeting to hours or days	May follow effort, emotional stress		Breathlessness, palpitations, weakness, anxiety

Table 8-2 | Dyspnea

Problem	Process	Timing
Left-Sided Heart Failure (*left ventricular failure or mitral stenosis*)	Elevated pressure in pulmonary capillary bed with transudation of fluid into interstitial spaces and alveoli, decreased compliance (increased stiffness) of the lungs, increased work of breathing	Dyspnea may progress slowly, or suddenly as in acute pulmonary edema.
Chronic Bronchitis	Excessive mucus production in bronchi, followed by chronic obstruction of airways	Chronic productive cough followed by slowly progressive dyspnea
Chronic Obstructive Pulmonary Disease (COPD)	Overdistention of air spaces distal to terminal bronchioles, with destruction of alveolar septa, alveolar enlargement and limitation of expiratory air flow	Slowly progressive dyspnea; relatively mild cough later
Asthma	Reversible bronchial hyperresponsiveness involving release of inflammatory mediators, increased airway secretions, and bronchoconstriction	Acute episodes, separated by symptom-free periods. Nocturnal episodes common
Diffuse Interstitial Lung Diseases (*such as sarcoidosis, widespread neoplasms, asbestosis, and idiopathic pulmonary fibrosis*)	Abnormal and widespread infiltration of cells, fluid, and collagen into interstitial spaces between alveoli. Many causes	Progressive dyspnea, which varies in its rate of development with the cause
Pneumonia	Inflammation of lung parenchyma from the respiratory bronchioles to the alveoli	An acute illness, timing varies with the causative agent
Spontaneous Pneumothorax	Leakage of air into pleural space through blebs on visceral pleura, with resulting partial or complete collapse of the lung	Sudden onset of dyspnea
Acute Pulmonary Embolism	Sudden occlusion of all or part of pulmonary arterial tree by a blood clot that usually originates in deep veins of legs or pelvis	Sudden onset of dyspnea
Anxiety With Hyperventilation	Overbreathing, with resultant respiratory alkalosis and fall in arterial partial pressure of carbon dioxide (pCO_2)	Episodic, often recurrent

Sources: American Thoracic Society. Dyspnea—mechanisms, assessment, and management: a consensus statement. Am J Respir Crit Care Med 1999;159(1):321–340; Wenzel RP and Fowler AA. Acute bronchitis. N Engl J Med 2006;355(20):2125–2130; Badgett RG, Tanaka DJ, Hunt DK et al. Can moderate chronic obstructive pulmonary disease be diagnosed by historical and physical findings alone? Am J Med 1993;94:188–196; Holleman DR and Simel DL. Does the clinical examination predict airflow limitation. JAMA 1995;273:63-68; Straus SE, McAlister FA, Sackett DL et al. The accuracy of patient history, wheezing, and laryngeal measurements in diagnosing obstructive airway disease. JAMA 2000;283:1853–1857; Panettieri RA. In the clinic: asthma. Ann Intern Med 2007;146:ITC6-1–ITC6-16; Littner M. In the clinic: chronic obstructive pulmonary disease. Ann Intern Med 2008;148:ITC3-1–ITC3-16; Neiwoehner DR. Outpatient management of severe COPD. N Engl J Med 2010;362:1407–1436; Pauwels RA, Buist AS, Calverley PM et al. GOLD Scientific Committee. Global strategy for the diagnosis, management, and prevention of chronic obstructive pulmonary disease: NHLBI/WHO Global Initiative for Chronic Obstructive Lung Disease (GOLD) workshop summary. Am J Resp Crit Care Med 2001;163:125–1276; Metlay JP, Kapoor WN, Fine MJ. Does this patient have community-acquired pneumonia? Diagnosing pneumonia by history and physical examination. JAMA 1997;378(17):1440–1445; Neiderman M. In the clinic: community-acquired pneumonia. Ann Intern Med 2009;151:ITC4-1–ITC4-16; Agnelli G, Becattini C. Acute pulmonary embolism. N Engl J Med 2010;363:266–274.

Factors That Aggravate	Factors That Relieve	Associated Symptoms	Setting
Exertion, lying down	Rest, sitting up, though dyspnea may become persistent	Often cough, orthopnea, paroxysmal nocturnal dyspnea; sometimes wheezing	History of heart disease or its predisposing factors
Exertion, inhaled irritants, respiratory infections	Expectoration; rest, though dyspnea may become persistent	Chronic productive cough, recurrent respiratory infections; wheezing may develop	History of smoking, air pollutants, recurrent respiratory infections
Exertion	Rest, though dyspnea may become persistent	Cough, with scant mucoid sputum	History of smoking, air pollutants, sometimes a familial deficiency in alpha$_1$-antitrypsin
Variable, including allergens, irritants, respiratory infections, exercise, and emotion	Separation from aggravating factors	Wheezing, cough, tightness in chest	Environmental and emotional conditions
Exertion	Rest, though dyspnea may become persistent	Often weakness, fatigue. Cough less common than in other lung diseases	Varied. Exposure to trigger substances.
		Pleuritic pain, cough, sputum, fever, though not necessarily present	Varied
		Pleuritic pain, cough	Often a previously healthy young adult
		Often none. Retrosternal oppressive pain if the occlusion is massive. Pleuritic pain, cough, and hemoptysis may follow an embolism if pulmonary infarction ensues. Symptoms of anxiety (see below).	Postpartum or postoperative periods; prolonged bed rest; heart failure, chronic lung disease, and fractures of hip or leg; deep venous thrombosis (often not clinically apparent)
Often occurs at rest. An upsetting event may not be evident.	Breathing in and out of a paper or plastic bag may help	Sighing, lightheadedness, numbness or tingling of the hands and feet, palpitations, chest pain	Other manifestations of anxiety may be present, such as chest pain diaphoresis, palpitations

Table 8-3

Cough and Hemoptysis

Problem	Cough and Sputum	Associated Symptoms and Setting
Acute Inflammation		
Laryngitis	Dry cough (without sputum), may become productive of variable amounts of sputum	An acute, fairly minor illness with hoarseness. Often associated with viral nasopharyngitis
Tracheobronchitis	Dry cough, may become productive	An acute, often viral illness, with burning retrosternal discomfort
Mycoplasma and Viral Pneumonias	Dry hacking cough, often becoming productive of mucoid sputum	An acute febrile illness, often with malaise, headache, and possibly dyspnea
Bacterial Pneumonias	Pneumococcal: sputum mucoid or purulent; may be blood-streaked, diffusely pinkish, or rusty	An acute illness with chills, high fever, dyspnea, and chest pain. Often preceded by acute upper respiratory infection
	Klebsiella: similar; or sticky, red, and jellylike	Typically occurs in older alcoholic men
Chronic Inflammation		
Postnasal Drip	Chronic cough; sputum mucoid or mucopurulent	Repeated attempts to clear the throat. Postnasal discharge may be seen in posterior pharynx. Associated with allergic rhinitis, with or without sinusitis
Chronic Bronchitis	Chronic cough; sputum mucoid to purulent, may be blood-streaked or even bloody	Often long history of cigarette smoking. Recurrent superimposed infections. Wheezing and dyspnea may develop.
Bronchiectasis	Chronic cough; sputum purulent, often copious and foul-smelling; may be blood-streaked or bloody	Recurrent bronchopulmonary infections common; sinusitis may coexist.
Pulmonary Tuberculosis	Cough dry or sputum that is mucoid or purulent; may be blood-streaked or bloody	Early, no symptoms. Later, anorexia, weight loss, fatigue, fever, and night sweats
Lung Abscess	Sputum purulent and foul-smelling; may be bloody	A febrile illness. Often poor dental hygiene and a prior episode of impaired consciousness
Asthma	Cough, with thick mucoid sputum, especially near end of an attack	Episodic wheezing and dyspnea, but cough may occur alone. Often a history of allergy
Gastroesophageal Reflux	Chronic cough, especially at night or early in the morning	Wheezing, especially at night (often mistaken for asthma), early morning hoarseness, and repeated attempts to clear the throat. Often a history of heartburn and regurgitation
Neoplasm		
Cancer of the Lung	Cough dry to productive; sputum may be blood-streaked or bloody	Usually a long history of cigarette smoking. Dyspnea, weight loss.
Cardiovascular Disorders		
Left Ventricular Failure or Mitral Stenosis	Often dry, especially on exertion or at night; may progress to the pink frothy sputum of pulmonary edema or to frank hemoptysis	Dyspnea, orthopnea, paroxysmal nocturnal dyspnea
Pulmonary Emboli	Dry to productive; may be dark, bright red, or mixed with blood	Dyspnea, anxiety, chest pain, fever; factors that predispose to deep venous thrombosis
Irritating Particles, Chemicals, or Gases	Variable. There may be a latent period between exposure and symptoms.	Exposure to irritants. Eyes, nose, and throat may be affected.

Sources: Irwin RS, Madison JM. The diagnosis and treatment of cough. N Engl J Med 2000;343(23):1715–1721; Metlay JP, Kapoor WN, Fine MJ. Does this patient have community-acquired pneumonia? Diagnosing pneumonia by history and physical examination. JAMA 1997;378(17):1440–1445; Neiderman M. In the clinic: community-acquired pneumonia. Ann Intern Med 2009;151:ITC4-1–ITC4-16; Barker A. Bronchiectasis. N Engl J Med. 346(18):1383–1393, 2002; Wenzel RP, Fowler AA. Acute bronchitis. N Engl J Med 2006;355(20):2125–2130; Panettieri RA. In the clinic: asthma. Ann Intern Med 2007;146:ITC6-1–ITC6-16; Escalante P. In the clinic: tuberculosis. Ann Intern Med 2009;150:ITC6-1–ITC6-16; Agnelli G, Becattini C. Acute pulmonary embolism. N Engl J Med 2010;363:266–274.

Table 8-4   Deformities of the Thorax

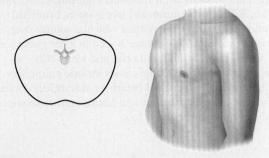

Normal Adult

The thorax in the normal adult is wider than it is deep. Its lateral diameter is larger than its anteroposterior diameter.

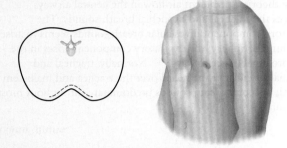

Funnel Chest *(Pectus Excavatum)*

Note depression in the lower portion of the sternum. Compression of the heart and great vessels may cause murmurs.

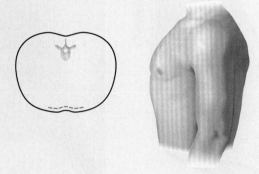

Barrel Chest

There is an increased anteroposterior diameter. This shape is normal during infancy, and often accompanies aging and chronic obstructive pulmonary disease.

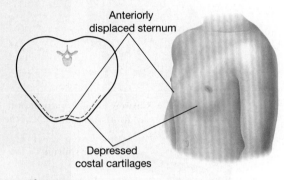

Anteriorly displaced sternum

Depressed costal cartilages

Pigeon Chest *(Pectus Carinatum)*

The sternum is displaced anteriorly, increasing the anteroposterior diameter. The costal cartilages adjacent to the protruding sternum are depressed.

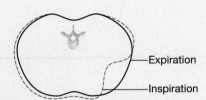

Expiration

Inspiration

Traumatic Flail Chest

Multiple rib fractures may result in paradoxical movements of the thorax. As descent of the diaphragm decreases intrathoracic pressure, on inspiration the injured area caves inward; on expiration, it moves outward.

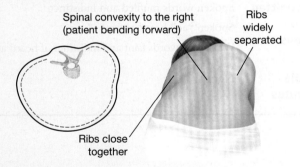

Spinal convexity to the right (patient bending forward)

Ribs widely separated

Ribs close together

Thoracic Kyphoscoliosis

Abnormal spinal curvatures and vertebral rotation deform the chest. Distortion of the underlying lungs may make interpretation of lung findings very difficult.

Table 8-5 Normal and Altered Breath and Voice Sounds

The origins of breath sounds are still unclear. According to leading theories, turbulent air flow in the central airways produces the tracheal and bronchial breath sounds. The inspiratory component if vesicular breath sounds seems to arise in the lung periphery; the expiratory component arises in the more proximal larger airways.[22,24] Normally, tracheal and bronchial sounds may be heard over the trachea and mainstem bronchi; vesicular breath sounds predominate throughout most of the lungs.

When lung tissue loses its air, it transmits high-pitched sounds much better. If the tracheobronchial tree is open, bronchial breath sounds may replace the normal vesicular sounds over airless areas of the lung. This change is seen in lobar pneumonia when the alveoli fill with fluid, red cells, and white cells—a process called *consolidation*. Other causes include pulmonary edema or hemorrhage. Bronchial breath sounds usually correlate with an increase in tactile fremitus and transmitted voice sounds. These findings are summarized below.

	Normal Air-Filled Lung	**Airless Lung, as in Lobar Pneumonia**
	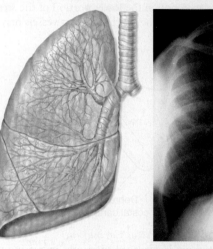	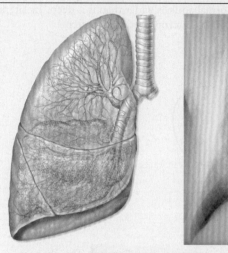
Breath Sounds	Predominantly vesicular	Bronchial or bronchovesicular over the involved area
Transmitted Voice Sounds	Spoken words muffled and indistinct Spoken "ee" heard as "ee" Whispered words faint and indistinct, if heard at all	Spoken words louder (*bronchophony*) Spoken "ee" heard as "ay" (*egophony*) Whispered words louder, clearer (*whispered pectoriloquy*)
Tactile Fremitus	Normal	Increased

Table 8-6   Adventitious (Added) Lung Sounds: Causes and Qualities

Crackles

Crackles have two leading explanations. (1) They result from a series of tiny explosions when small airways, deflated during expiration, pop open during inspiration. This mechanism probably explains the late inspiratory crackles of interstitial lung disease and early heart failure. (2) Crackles result from air bubbles flowing through secretions or lightly closed airways during respiration. This mechanism probably explains at least some coarse crackles.

Inspiration   Expiration

Late inspiratory crackles may begin in the first half of inspiration but must continue into late inspiration. They are usually fine, fairly profuse, and persist from breath to breath. They appear first at the bases of the lungs, spread upward as the condition worsens, and shift to dependent regions with changes in posture. Causes include *interstitial lung disease* (such as pulmonary fibrosis) and early *heart failure*.

Early inspiratory crackles appear and end soon after the start of inspiration. They are often coarse and relatively few in number. Expiratory crackles are sometimes associated. Causes include *chronic bronchitis* and *asthma*.

Midinspiratory and expiratory crackles are heard in *bronchiectasis* but are not specific for this diagnosis. Wheezes and rhonchi may be associated.

Wheezes and Rhonchi

Wheezes occur when air flows rapidly through bronchi that are narrowed nearly to the point of closure. They are often audible at the mouth as well as through the chest wall. Causes of wheezes throughout the chest include *asthma, chronic bronchitis, COPD,* and *heart failure* (cardiac asthma). In *asthma,* wheezes may be heard only in expiration or in both phases of the respiratory cycle. Rhonchi suggest secretions in the larger airways. In chronic bronchitis, wheezes and rhonchi often clear with coughing.

Occasionally in severe obstructive pulmonary disease, the patient is unable to force enough air through the narrowed bronchi to produce wheezing. The resulting *silent chest* is ominous and warrants immediate attention.

Persistent localized wheezing suggests partial obstruction of a bronchus, seen with a tumor or foreign body. It may be inspiratory, expiratory, or both.

Stridor

A wheeze that is entirely or predominantly inspiratory is called *stridor*. It is often louder in the neck than over the chest wall. It indicates a partial obstruction of the larynx or trachea, and demands immediate attention.

Pleural Rub

Inflamed and roughened pleural surfaces grate against each other as they are momentarily and repeatedly delayed by increased friction. These movements produce creaking sounds known as a *pleural rub* (or pleural friction rub), usually during expiration.

Pleural rubs resemble crackles acoustically, although they are produced by different pathologic processes. The sounds may be discrete, but sometimes are so numerous that they merge into a seemingly continuous sound. A rub is usually confined to a relatively small area of the chest wall, and typically is heard in both phases of respiration. When inflamed pleural surfaces are separated by fluid, the rub often disappears.

Mediastinal Crunch
(Hamman's Sign)

A *mediastinal crunch* is a series of precordial crackles synchronous with the heart beat, not with respiration. Best heard in the left lateral position, it is due to mediastinal emphysema (*pneumomediastinum*).

Sources: McGee S. Evidence-based Physical Diagnosis, 2nd ed. Philadelphia: Saunders, 2007; Loudon R, Murphy LH. Lungs sounds. Am Rev Respir Dis 1994;130:663–673; Epler GR, Carrrington CB, Gaensler EA. Crackles (rales) in the interstitial pulmonary diseases. Chest 1978;73:333–339; Nath AR, Capel LH. Inspiratory crackles and mechanical events of breathing. Thorax 1974;29:695–698; Nath AR, Capel LH. Lung crackles in bronchiectasis. Thorax 1980;35:694–699.

Table 8-7

Physical Findings in Selected Chest Disorders

The red boxes in this table suggest a framework for clinical assessment. Start with the three boxes under Percussion Note: resonant, dull, and hyperresonant. Then move from each of these to other boxes that emphasize some of the key differences among various conditions. The changes described vary with the extent and severity of the disorder. Abnormalities deep in the chest usually produce fewer signs than superficial ones, and may cause no signs at all. Use the table for the direction of typical changes, not for absolute distinctions.

Condition	Percussion Note	Trachea	Breath Sounds	Adventitious Sounds	Tactile Fremitus and Transmitted Voice Sounds
Normal The tracheobronchial tree and alveoli are clear; pleurae are thin and close together; mobility of the chest wall is unimpaired.	**Resonant**	Midline	Vesicular, except perhaps bronchovesicular and bronchial sounds over the large bronchi and trachea, respectively	None, except perhaps a few transient inspiratory crackles at the bases of the lungs	Normal
Chronic Bronchitis The bronchi are chronically inflamed and a productive cough is present. Airway obstruction may develop.	**Resonant**	Midline	Vesicular (normal)	None; or scattered coarse *crackles* in early inspiration and perhaps expiration; or *wheezes* or *rhonchi*	Normal
Left-Sided Heart Failure (Early) Increased pressure in the pulmonary veins causes congestion and interstitial edema (around the alveoli); bronchial mucosa may become edematous.	**Resonant**	Midline	Vesicular	*Late inspiratory crackles* in the dependent portions of the lungs; possibly *wheezes*	Normal
Consolidation Alveoli fill with fluid or blood cells, as in pneumonia, pulmonary edema, or pulmonary hemorrhage.	**Dull** over the airless area	Midline	*Bronchial* over the involved area	*Late inspiratory crackles* over the involved area	*Increased* over the involved area, with *bronchophony, egophony,* and *whispered pectoriloquy*
Atelectasis (Lobar Obstruction) When a plug in a mainstem bronchus (as from mucus or a foreign object) obstructs air flow, affected lung tissue collapses into an airless state.	**Dull** over the airless area	May be *shifted toward involved side*	*Usually absent* when bronchial plug persists. Exceptions include right upper lobe atelectasis, where adjacent tracheal sounds may be transmitted.	None	*Usually absent* when the bronchial plug persists. In exceptions (e.g., right upper lobe atelectasis) may be increased

Condition	Percussion Note	Trachea	Breath Sounds	Adventitious Sounds	Tactile Fremitus and Transmitted Voice Sounds
Pleural Effusion Fluid accumulates in the pleural space, separates air-filled lung from the chest wall, blocking the transmission of sound.	**Dull** to flat over the fluid	*Shifted toward opposite side* in a large effusion	*Decreased to absent,* but bronchial breath sounds may be heard near top of large effusion.	None, except a *possible pleural* rub	*Decreased to absent, but may be increased* toward the top of a large effusion
Pneumothorax When air leaks into the pleural space, usually unilaterally, the lung recoils from the chest wall. Pleural air blocks transmission of sound.	**Hyperresonant** or tympanitic over the pleural air	*Shifted toward opposite side* if much air	*Decreased to absent* over the pleural air	None, except a *possible pleural* rub	*Decreased to absent* over the pleural air
Chronic Obstructive Pulmonary Disease (COPD) Slowly progressive disorder in which the distal air spaces enlarge and lungs become hyperinflated. Chronic bronchitis is often associated.	Diffusely **hyperresonant**	Midline	*Decreased to absent*	None, or the crackles, wheezes, and rhonchi of associated chronic bronchitis	*Decreased*
Asthma Widespread narrowing of the tracheobronchial tree diminishes air flow to a fluctuating degree. During attacks, air flow decreases further, and lungs hyperinflate.	**Resonant** to diffusely **hyperresonant**	Midline	*Often obscured by wheezes*	*Wheezes, possibly crackles*	*Decreased*

The Cardiovascular System

Listening to the heart has come to epitomize the art of bedside diagnosis. Mastering the skills of cardiac examination requires patience, practice, and repetition—a process especially vulnerable to evolving technology and the time constraints of clinical practice.[1,2] Many reports attest to the current decline in physical examination skills, well-documented for the cardiovascular system at all levels of training.[3-9] As you study this chapter, combining your knowledge of anatomy and physiology with hands-on practice of inspection, palpation, and auscultation brings rewards of proven diagnostic value. Take advantage of the numerous new visual and auditory learning modalities that can reinforce your growing clinical acumen.[10-14]

SURFACE PROJECTIONS OF THE HEART AND GREAT VESSELS

To begin, visualize the underlying structures of the heart as you inspect the anterior chest. Note that the *right ventricle* occupies most of the anterior cardiac surface. This chamber and the pulmonary artery form a wedgelike structure behind and to the left of the sternum, outlined in black.

The inferior border of the right ventricle lies below the junction of the sternum and the xiphoid process. The right ventricle narrows superiorly and joins the pulmonary artery at the level of the sternum or "*base of the heart,*" a clinical term that

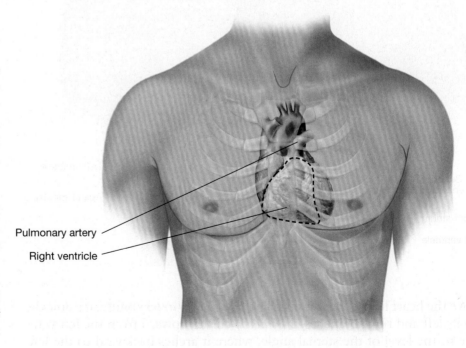

Pulmonary artery

Right ventricle

refers to the superior aspect of the heart at the right and left 2nd inter-spaces next to the sternum.

The *left ventricle*, behind the right ventricle and to the left, forms the left lateral margin of the heart, as outlined below. Its tapered inferior tip is often termed the *cardiac "apex."* It is clinically important because it produces the apical impulse, identified during palpation of the precordium as the *point of maximal impulse,* or *PMI.* This impulse locates the left border of the heart and is normally found in the 5th interspace 7 cm to 9 cm lateral to the midsternal line, typically at or just medial to the left midclavicular line. The PMI is not always palpable, even in a healthy patient with a normal heart.

- In supine patients the *diameter of the PMI* may be as large as a quarter, approximately 1 to 2.5 cm.

- Note that, in some patients, the most prominent precordial impulse may not be at the apex of the left ventricle. For example, in patients with chronic obstructive pulmonary disease, the most prominent palpable impulse or PMI may be in the xiphoid or epigastric area as a result of *right ventricular hypertrophy.*

A PMI greater than 2.5 cm is evidence of *left ventricular hypertrophy (LVH),* or enlargement, seen in *hypertension* and *aortic stenosis.*

Similarly, *displacement of the PMI* lateral to the midclavicular line or greater than 10 cm lateral to the midsternal line also suggests *LVH.*

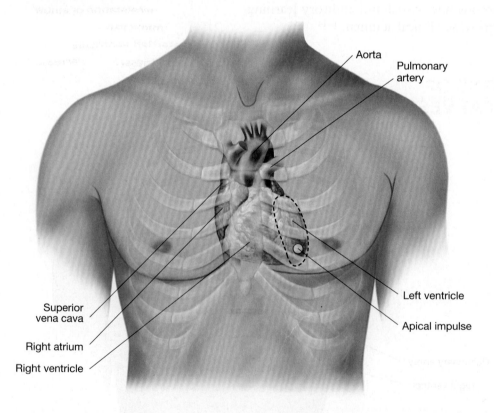

Aorta

Pulmonary artery

Left ventricle

Apical impulse

Superior vena cava

Right atrium

Right ventricle

Above the heart lie the *great vessels.* The *pulmonary artery* bifurcates quickly into its left and right branches. The *aorta* curves upward from the left ventricle to the level of the sternal angle, where it arches backward to the left and then downward. On the medial border, the *superior* and *inferior venae cavae* channel venous blood from the upper and lower portions of the body into the right atrium.

CARDIAC CHAMBERS, VALVES, AND CIRCULATION

Circulation through the heart is diagrammed below. Identify the cardiac chambers, valves, and direction of blood flow. Because of their location, the *tricuspid* and *mitral valves* are often called *atrioventricular valves*. The *aortic* and *pulmonic valves* are called *semilunar valves* because each of their leaflets is shaped like a half moon. Although in this diagram all the valves are in an open position, they do not open simultaneously in the living heart.

As the heart valves close, the heart sounds of S_1 and S_2 arise from vibrations emanating from the leaflets, the adjacent cardiac structures, and the flow of blood. Study carefully the positions and movements of the atrioventricular and semilunar valves in relation to events in the cardiac cycle. This knowledge will improve your diagnostic accuracy when you auscultate the heart.

In most adults over age 40 years, the diastolic sounds of S_3 and S_4 are pathologic, and are highly correlated with heart failure and acute myocardial ischemia.[13,15,16] In recent studies an S_3 corresponds to a abrupt deceleration of inflow across the mitral valve, and an S_4 to increased left ventricular and diastolic stiffness which decreases compliance.[17–19]

Course of oxygenated blood → Course of deoxygenated blood →
RA = Right atrium; LA = Left atrium; RV = Right ventricle; LV = Left ventricle

EVENTS IN THE CARDIAC CYCLE

The heart serves as a pump that generates varying pressures as its chambers contract and relax. *Systole is the period of ventricular contraction.* In the diagram below, pressure in the left ventricle rises from less than 5 mm Hg in its resting state to a normal peak of 120 mm Hg. After the ventricle ejects much of its blood into the aorta, the pressure levels off and starts to fall. *Diastole is the period of ventricular relaxation.* Ventricular pressure falls further to below 5 mm Hg, and blood flows from atrium to ventricle. Late in diastole, ventricular pressure rises slightly during inflow of blood from atrial contraction.

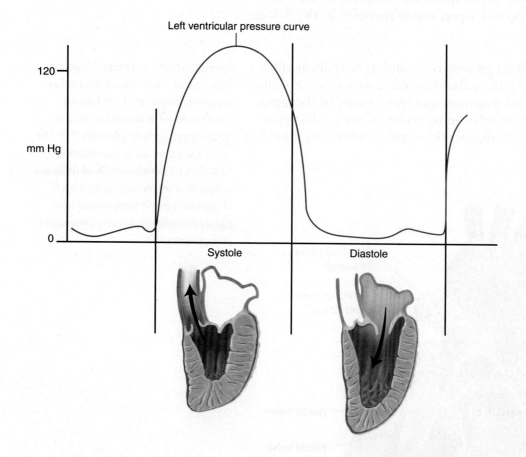

Left ventricular pressure curve

120

mm Hg

0

Systole

Diastole

Note that during *systole* the aortic valve is open, allowing ejection of blood from the left ventricle into the aorta. The mitral valve is closed, preventing blood from regurgitating back into the left atrium. In contrast, during *diastole* the aortic valve is closed, preventing regurgitation of blood from the aorta back into the left ventricle. The mitral valve is open, allowing blood to flow from the left atrium into the relaxed left ventricle. At the same time, during systole the pulmonic valve opens and the tricuspid valve closes as blood is ejected from the right ventricle into the pulmonary artery. During diastole, the pulmonic valve closes and the tricuspid valve opens as blood flows into the right atrium.

Understanding the interrelationships of the pressure gradients in the left heart (the left atrium, left ventricle, and aorta), together with the position and movement of the four heart valves, is fundamental to understanding heart sounds. An extensive literature explores how heart sounds are generated. Possible explanations include closure of the valve leaflets; tensing of related structures, leaflet positions, and pressure gradients at the time of atrial and ventricular systole; and the acoustic effects of moving columns of blood.

Trace the changing left ventricular pressures and sounds through one cardiac cycle. Note that the first and second heart sounds define the duration of systole and diastole. The corresponding events on the right side of the heart occur at pressures that are usually lower than those on the left. The explanations given here are oversimplified, but retain clinical usefulness.

During *diastole,* pressure in the blood-filled left atrium slightly exceeds that in the relaxed left ventricle, and blood flows from left atrium to left ventricle across the open mitral valve. Just before the onset of ventricular systole, atrial contraction produces a slight pressure rise in both chambers.

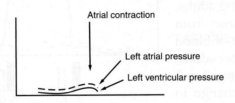

During *systole,* the left ventricle starts to contract and ventricular pressure rapidly exceeds left atrial pressure, shutting the mitral valve. *Closure of the mitral valve produces the first heart sound, S_1.*

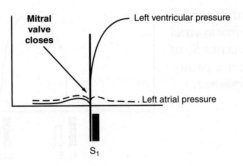

As left ventricular pressure continues to rise, it quickly exceeds the pressure in the aorta and forces the aortic valve open. In some pathologic conditions, an early systolic ejection sound (Ej) accompanies the opening of the aortic valve. *Normally, maximal left ventricular pressure corresponds to systolic blood pressure.*

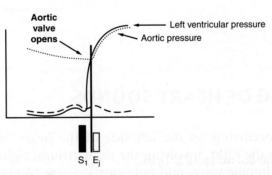

As the left ventricle ejects most of its blood, ventricular pressure begins to fall. When left ventricular pressure drops below aortic pressure, the aortic valve shuts. *Aortic valve closure produces the second heart sound, S_2, and another diastole begins.*

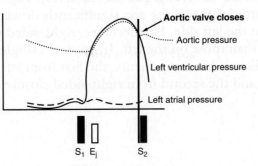

In *diastole*, left ventricular pressure continues to drop and falls below left atrial pressure. The mitral valve opens. This event is usually silent, but may be audible as a pathologic opening snap (OS) if valve leaflet motion is restricted, as in mitral stenosis.

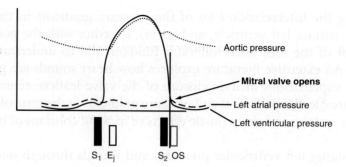

Aortic pressure
Mitral valve opens
Left atrial pressure
Left ventricular pressure

S_1 E_j S_2 OS

After the mitral valve opens, there is a period of rapid ventricular filling as blood flows early in diastole from left atrium to left ventricle. In children and young adults, a third heart sound, S_3, may arise from rapid deceleration of the column of blood against the ventricular wall. In older adults, an S_3, sometimes termed "an S_3 gallop," usually indicates a pathologic change in ventricular compliance.

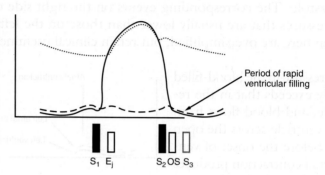

Period of rapid ventricular filling

S_1 E_j S_2 OS S_3

Finally, although not often heard in normal adults, a fourth heart sound, S_4, marks atrial contraction. It immediately precedes S_1 of the next beat and can also reflect a pathologic change in ventricular compliance.

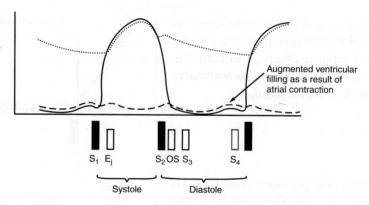

Augmented ventricular filling as a result of atrial contraction

S_1 E_j S_2 OS S_3 S_4

Systole   Diastole

THE SPLITTING OF HEART SOUNDS

While these events are occurring on the left side of the heart, similar changes are occurring on the right, involving the right atrium, right ventricle, tricuspid valve, pulmonic valve, and pulmonary artery. Right ventricular and pulmonary arterial pressures are significantly lower than corresponding pressures on the left side. Furthermore, right-sided events usually occur slightly later than those on the left. Instead of a single heart sound, you may hear two discernible components, the first from left-sided aortic valve closure, or A_2, and the second from right-sided closure of the pulmonic valve, or P_2.

Consider the second heart sound, S_2, and its two components, A_2 and P_2, caused primarily by closure of the aortic and pulmonic valves, respectively. During inspiration, the right heart filling time is increased, which increases right ventricular stroke volume and the duration of right ventricular ejection compared with the neighboring left ventricle. This delays the closure of the pulmonic valve, P_2, splitting S_2 into its two audible components. During expiration, these two components fuse into a single sound, S_2. Note that because walls of veins contain less smooth muscle, the venous system has more capacitance than the arterial system and lower systemic pressure. Distensibility and impedance in the pulmonary vascular bed contribute to the "hangout time" that delays P_2.[20]

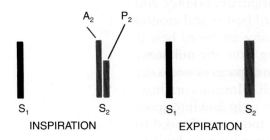

Of the two components of the S_2, A_2 is normally louder, reflecting the high pressure in the aorta. It is heard throughout the precordium. P_2, in contrast, is relatively soft, reflecting the lower pressure in the pulmonary artery. It is heard best in its own area, the 2nd and 3rd left interspaces close to the sternum. It is here that you should search for the splitting of S_2.

S_1 also has two components, an earlier mitral and a later tricuspid sound. The mitral sound, its principal component, is much louder, again reflecting the high pressures on the left side of the heart. It can be heard throughout the precordium and is loudest at the cardiac apex. The softer tricuspid component is heard best at the lower left sternal border; it is here that you may hear a split S_1. The earlier, louder mitral component may mask the tricuspid sound, however, and splitting is not always detectable. Splitting of S_1 does not vary with respiration.

HEART MURMURS

Heart murmurs are distinguishable from heart sounds by their longer duration. They are attributed to turbulent blood flow and may be diagnostic of valvular heart disease, or "innocent" flow murmurs, especially in young adults. A *stenotic valve* has an abnormally narrowed valvular orifice that obstructs blood flow, as in *aortic stenosis*, and causes a characteristic murmur. So does a valve that fails to fully close, as in *aortic regurgitation* or *insufficiency*. Such a valve allows blood to leak backward in a retrograde direction and produces a *regurgitant* murmur.

To identify murmurs accurately, you must learn the chest wall location where they are best heard, their timing in systole or diastole, and their descriptive qualities. In the Techniques of Examination section, you will learn to integrate several characteristics, including murmur intensity, pitch, duration, and direction of radiation (see pp. 379–382).

RELATION OF AUSCULTATORY FINDINGS TO THE CHEST WALL

The locations on the chest wall where you hear heart sounds and murmurs help to identify the valve or chamber where they originate. Sounds and murmurs arising from the mitral valve are usually heard best at and around the cardiac apex. Those originating in the tricuspid valve are heard best at or near the lower left sternal border. Murmurs arising from the pulmonic valve are usually heard best in the 2nd and 3rd left interspaces close to the sternum, but may also be heard at higher or lower levels. Murmurs originating in the aortic valve may be heard anywhere from the right 2nd interspace to the apex. *These areas overlap*, as illustrated below, and you will need to correlate auscultatory findings with other cardiac examination findings to identify sounds and murmurs accurately.

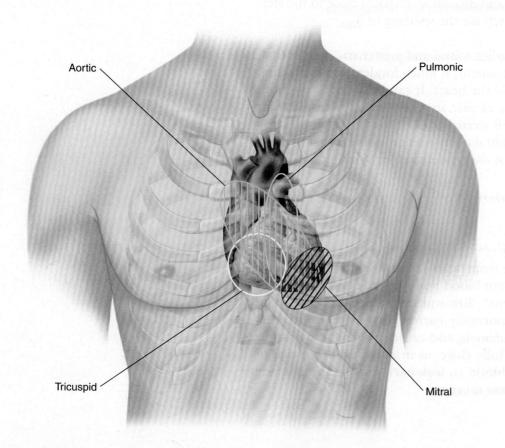

Aortic

Pulmonic

Tricuspid

Mitral

THE CONDUCTION SYSTEM

An electrical conduction system stimulates and coordinates the contraction of cardiac muscle.

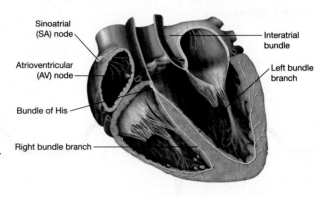

Each normal electrical impulse is initiated in the *sinus node*, a group of specialized cardiac cells located in the right atrium near the junction of the vena cava. The sinus node acts as the cardiac pacemaker and automatically discharges an impulse about 60 to 100 times a minute. This impulse travels through both atria to the *atrioventricular node*, a specialized group of cells located low in the atrial septum. Here the impulse is delayed before passing down the bundle of His and its branches to the ventricular myocardium. Muscular contraction follows: first the atria, then the ventricles. The normal conduction pathway is diagrammed here in simplified form.

The electrocardiogram, or ECG, records these events. Contraction of cardiac smooth muscle produces electrical activity, resulting in a series of waves on the ECG. The ECG consists of *six limb leads* in the *frontal plane* and *six chest or precordial leads* in the *transverse plane*.

- Electrical vectors approaching a lead cause a *positive, or upward, deflection*.

- Electrical vectors moving away from the lead cause a *negative, or downward, deflection*.

- When positive and negative vectors balance, they are *isoelectric*, appearing as a straight line.

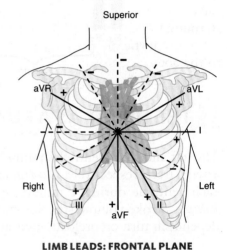

LIMB LEADS: FRONTAL PLANE

The components of the *normal ECG* and their duration are briefly summarized here, but you will need further instruction and considerable practice to interpret recordings from patients. Note:

- The small *P wave* of atrial depolarization (duration up to 80 milliseconds; *PR interval* 120 to 200 milliseconds)

- The larger *QRS complex* of ventricular depolarization (up to 100 milliseconds), consisting of one or more of the following:

  - the Q *wave*, a downward deflection from septal depolarization
  - the R *wave*, an upward deflection from ventricular depolarization
  - the S *wave*, a downward deflection following an R wave

- A *T wave* of ventricular repolarization, or recovery (duration relates to QRS)

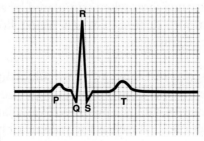

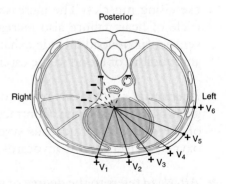

CHEST LEADS: TRANSVERSE PLANE

The electrical impulse slightly precedes the myocardial contraction that it stimulates. The relation of electrocardiographic waves to the cardiac cycle is shown below.

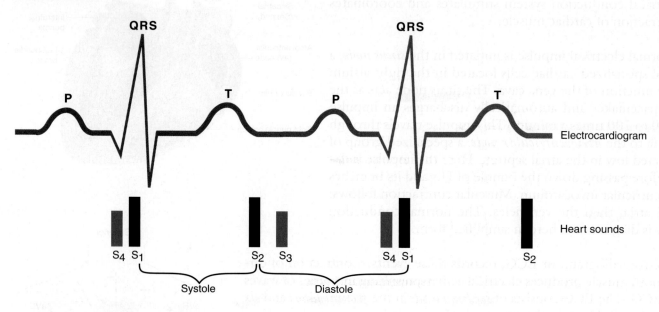

THE HEART AS A PUMP

The left and right ventricles pump blood into the systemic and pulmonary arterial trees, respectively. *Cardiac output,* the volume of blood ejected from each ventricle during 1 minute, is the product of *heart rate* and *stroke volume.* Stroke volume (the volume of blood ejected with each heartbeat) depends in turn on preload, myocardial contractility, and afterload.

- *Preload* refers to the load that stretches the cardiac muscle before contraction. The volume of blood in the right ventricle at the end of diastole constitutes its preload for the next beat. Right ventricular preload is increased by increasing venous return to the right heart. Physiologic causes include inspiration and the increased volume of blood flow from exercising muscles. The increased blood volume in a dilated right ventricle of heart failure also increases preload. Causes of decreased right ventricular preload include exhalation, decreased left ventricular output, and pooling of blood in the capillary bed or the venous system.

- *Myocardial contractility* refers to the ability of the cardiac muscle, when given a load, to shorten. Contractility increases when stimulated by action of the sympathetic nervous system and decreases when blood flow or oxygen delivery to the myocardium is impaired.

- *Afterload* refers to the degree of vascular resistance to ventricular contraction. Sources of resistance to left ventricular contraction include the tone in the walls of the aorta, the large arteries, and the peripheral vascular tree (primarily the small arteries and arterioles), as well as the volume of blood already in the aorta.

Pathologic increases in preload and afterload, called *volume overload* and *pressure overload,* respectively, produce changes in ventricular function that may be clinically detectable. These changes include alterations in ventricular impulses, detectable by palpation, and in normal heart sounds. Pathologic heart sounds and murmurs may also develop.

The term *heart failure* is now preferred over "congestive heart failure" because not all patients have volume overload on initial presentation.[21]

ARTERIAL PULSES AND BLOOD PRESSURE

With each contraction, the left ventricle ejects a volume of blood into the aorta and on into the arterial tree. The ensuing pressure wave moves rapidly through the arterial system, where it is felt as the *arterial pulse.* Although the pressure wave travels quickly, many times faster than the blood itself, a palpable delay between ventricular contraction and peripheral pulses makes the pulses in the arms and legs unsuitable for timing events in the cardiac cycle.

Blood pressure in the arterial system varies during the cardiac cycle, peaking in systole and falling to its lowest trough in diastole. These are the levels that are measured with the blood pressure cuff, or sphygmomanometer. The difference between systolic and diastolic pressures is known as the *pulse pressure.*

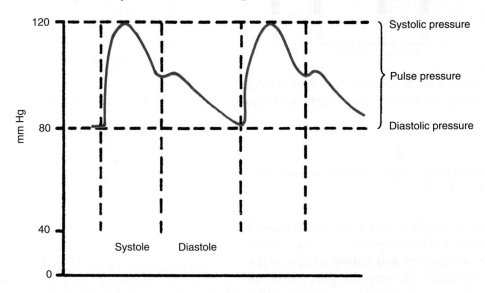

Factors Influencing Arterial Pressure

▶ Left ventricular stroke volume
▶ Distensibility of the aorta and the large arteries
▶ Peripheral vascular resistance, particularly at the arteriolar level
▶ Volume of blood in the arterial system

Changes in any of these four factors alter systolic pressure, diastolic pressure, or both. Blood pressure levels fluctuate strikingly throughout any 24-hour period, varying with physical activity, emotional state, pain, noise, environmental temperature, use of coffee, tobacco, and other drugs, and even time of day.

JUGULAR VENOUS PRESSURE (JVP) AND PULSATIONS

The jugular veins provide an important index of right heart pressures and cardiac function. *Jugular venous pressure (JVP)* reflects right atrial pressure, which in turn equals central venous pressure and right ventricular end-diastolic pressure. The JVP is best estimated from the *right internal jugular vein*, which has the most direct channel into the right atrium. Some affirm that the right external jugular vein can also be used.[22] Since the jugular veins lie deep to the sternomastoid muscles, you must learn to identify the pulsations they transmit to the surface of the neck, briefly described below, and measure their highest point of oscillation.

See pp. 361–368 for detailed descriptions and images of the techniques of examination needed to assess the JVP.

Changing pressures in the right atrium during diastole and systole produce oscillations of filling and emptying in the jugular veins, or *jugular venous pulsations*. Atrial contraction produces an *a wave* in the jugular veins just before S1 and systole, followed by the *x descent* of atrial relaxation. As right atrial pressure begins to rise with inflow from the vena cava during right ventricular systole, there is a second elevation, the *v wave*, followed by the *y descent* as blood passively empties into the right ventricle during early and mid diastole.

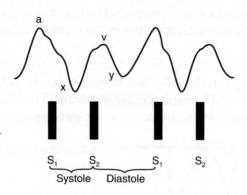

CHANGES OVER THE LIFE SPAN

Aging may affect the location of the apical impulse, the pitch of heart sounds and murmurs, the stiffness of the arteries, and blood pressure. For example, the *apical impulse* is usually felt easily in children and young adults; as the chest deepens in its anteroposterior diameter, the impulse gets harder to find. For the same reason, *splitting of S2* may be harder to hear in older people as its pulmonic component becomes less audible. Furthermore, at some time during the life span, almost everyone has a *heart murmur*. Most murmurs occur without other evidence of cardiovascular abnormality and may, therefore, be considered normal variants. These common murmurs vary with age, and knowing their patterns helps you to distinguish normal from abnormal.

Turn to pp. 765–891, Chapter 18, Assessing Children: Infancy Through Adolescence, and to p. 907, Chapter 19, The Pregnant Woman, for information on how to distinguish these innocent murmurs.

Murmurs may originate in large blood vessels as well as in the heart. The *jugular venous hum*, which is common in children, may still be heard through young adulthood (see pp. 844–845). A second, more important example is the *cervical systolic murmur* or *bruit*, which may be innocent in children but suspicious for atherosclerotic disease in adults.

The Health History

Common or Concerning Symptoms

▶ Chest pain
▶ Palpitations
▶ Shortness of breath: dyspnea, orthopnea, or paroxysmal nocturnal dyspnea
▶ Swelling or edema

Assessing Cardiac Symptoms—Overview and Comparison With Baseline Activity Levels. This section approaches chest symptoms from a *cardiac standpoint*, and includes the important symptoms of chest pain, palpitations, shortness of breath from orthopnea or paroxysmal dyspnea (PND), and peripheral swelling from edema. For chest symptoms, make a habit of thinking through the range of possible cardiac, pulmonary, and extrathoracic etiologies. Study the various sources of *chest pain, dyspnea, wheezing, cough*, and even *hemoptysis*, because these symptoms can be cardiac as well as pulmonary in origin.

When assessing cardiac symptoms, it is important to *quantify the patient's baseline level of activity*. For example, in patients with chest pain, does the pain occur with climbing stairs? How many flights? How about with walking—50 feet, one block, more? What about carrying groceries or doing housework (e.g., making beds, vacuuming)? How does this compare with these activities in the past? When did the symptoms appear or change? If the patient is short of breath, does this occur at rest, during exercise, or after climbing stairs? Sudden shortness of breath is more serious in an athlete than in a person who only walks from one room to another. Quantifying the baseline level of activity helps establish both the severity of the patient's symptoms and their significance as you consider the next steps for management.

Chest Pain. *Chest pain* is one of the most serious of all patient complaints. It is the most common symptom of coronary heart disease (CHD), which affects over 16 million Americans. In 2008, 9 million Americans reported angina pectoris and 7.9 million had a myocardial infarction.[23] Coronary heart disease is the leading killer of both men and women. In 2007, CHD accounted for one in every six U.S. deaths. Death rates remain highest for black men and black women compared to other ethnic groups.

As you elicit your patient's story of chest pain, always consider life-threatening diagnoses such as angina pectoris, myocardial infarction, dissecting aortic aneurysm, and pulmonary embolus.[25–27] Learn to distinguish cardiovascular causes from disorders of the pericardium, trachea and bronchi, parietal pleura, esophagus, and chest wall, and from extrathoracic causes in the neck, shoulder, gall bladder, and stomach.

Review the Health History section of Chapter 8, The Thorax and Lungs, pp. 300–302; Table 8-1, Chest Pain, pp. 322–323; and Table 8-2, Dyspnea, pp. 324–325.

Classic exertional pain, pressure, or discomfort in the chest, shoulder, back, neck, or arm in *angina pectoris*, is seen in 50% of patients with acute myocardial infarction; atypical descriptors also are common, such as cramping, grinding, pricking or, rarely, tooth or jaw pain.[24] Annual incidence of *exertional angina* is 1 per 1,000 in the population 30 years or older.

Acute coronary syndrome is increasingly used to refer to any of the clinical syndromes caused by acute myocardial ischemia, including *unstable angina, non-ST elevation myocardial infarction,* and *ST elevation infarction.*[28]

Note that recent studies show that although both men and women with *acute coronary syndrome* usually present with the classic symptoms of exertional angina, women, particularly those over age 65, are more likely to report atypical symptoms that may go unrecognized, such as upper back, neck, or jaw pain, shortness of breath, paroxysmal nocturnal dyspnea, nausea or vomiting, and fatigue, making careful history taking ever more important.[29–31] Failure to identify cardiac causes of chest pain can have dire consequences. Inappropriate discharge from the emergency room results in a 25% mortality rate.[26]

Your initial queries should be open-ended . . . "Please tell me about any symptoms you might be having in your chest." Following this, explore the patient's concerns more specifically. Ask the patient to point to the pain and describe all seven of the dimensions of the symptom. Move on to more specific questions such as "Is the pain related to exertion?" and "What kinds of activities bring on the pain?" Also "How intense is the pain, on a scale of 1 to 10?" . . . "Does it radiate into the neck, shoulder, back, or down your arm?" . . . "Are there any associated symptoms like shortness of breath, sweating, palpitations, or nausea?" . . . "Does it ever wake you up at night?" . . . "What do you do to make it better?"

Palpitations. *Palpitations* involve an unpleasant awareness of the heartbeat. When describing palpitations, patients use terms such as skipping, racing, fluttering, pounding, or stopping of the heart. Palpitations may result from an irregular heartbeat, from rapid acceleration or slowing of the heart, or from increased forcefulness of cardiac contraction. Anxious and hyperthyroid patients may report palpitations. Palpitations do not necessarily mean heart disease. In contrast, the most serious dysrhythmias, such as ventricular tachycardia, often do not produce palpitations.

You may ask directly about palpitations, but if the patient does not understand your question, reword it. "Are you ever aware of your heartbeat? What is it like?" Ask the patient to tap out the rhythm with a hand or finger. Was it fast or slow? Regular or irregular? How long did it last? If there was an episode of rapid heartbeats, did they start and stop suddenly or gradually? For this group of symptoms, an ECG is indicated.

It is helpful to teach selected patients how to make serial measurements of their pulse rates in case they have further episodes.

Shortness of Breath. *Shortness of breath* is a common patient concern and may represent *dyspnea, orthopnea,* or *paroxysmal nocturnal dyspnea. Dyspnea* is an uncomfortable awareness of breathing that is inappropriate to a given level of exertion. This complaint is common in patients with cardiac or pulmonary problems.

Orthopnea is dyspnea that occurs when the patient is lying down and improves when the patient sits up. Classically, it is quantified according to the number of pillows the patient uses for sleeping, or by the fact that the patient needs to sleep sitting up. Make sure that the reason the patient uses extra pillows or sleeps upright is shortness of breath and not other causes.

Causes of chest pain in the absence of coronary artery disease on angiogram include *microvascular coronary dysfunction* and *abnormal cardiac nocioception,* which require specialized testing.[32,33] Roughly half of women with chest pain and normal angiograms have microvascular coronary dysfunction.

Anterior chest pain, often tearing or ripping, and often radiating into the back or neck, occurs in *acute aortic dissection.*[27,34]

See Table 9-1, Selected Heart Rates and Rhythms, and Table 9-2, Selected Irregular Rhythms, for selected heart rates and rhythms (pp. 391–392).

Symptoms or signs of irregular heart action warrant an ECG. *Atrial fibrillation,* which is "irregularly irregular," can often be identified at the bedside.

Clues in the history include transient skips and flip-flops (possible *premature contractions*), rapid regular beating of sudden onset and offset (possible *paroxysmal supraventricular tachycardia*), a rapid regular rate of <120 beats per minute, especially if starting and stopping more gradually (possible *sinus tachycardia*).

Sudden dyspnea occurs in *pulmonary embolus, spontaneous pneumothorax,* anxiety.
See Chapter 8, The Thorax and Lungs, pp. 293–331.

Orthopnea occurs in *left ventricular heart failure* or *mitral stenosis;* also in *obstructive lung disease.*

Paroxysmal nocturnal dyspnea, or *PND,* describes episodes of sudden dyspnea and orthopnea that awaken the patient from sleep, usually 1 or 2 hours after going to bed, prompting the patient to sit up, stand up, or go to a window for air. There may be associated wheezing and coughing. The episode usually subsides but may recur at about the same time on subsequent nights.

PND occurs in *left ventricular heart failure* or *mitral stenosis;* may be mimicked by *nocturnal asthma attacks.*

Edema.   *Edema* refers to the accumulation of excessive fluid in the extravascular interstitial space. Interstitial tissue can absorb several liters of fluid, accommodating up to a 10% weight gain before pitting edema appears.[35] Causes vary from local to systemic. Focus your questions on the location, timing, and setting of the swelling, and on associated symptoms. "Have you had any swelling anywhere? Where? . . . Anywhere else? When does it occur? Is it worse in the morning or at night? Do your shoes get tight?"

Dependent edema appears in the lowest body parts: the feet and lower legs when sitting, or the sacrum when bedridden. Causes may be cardiac (*heart failure*), nutritional (*hypoalbuminemia*), or positional.

Continue with "Are the rings tight on your fingers? Are your eyelids puffy or swollen in the morning? Have you had to let out your belt?" Also, "Have your clothes gotten too tight around the middle?" It is useful to ask patients who retain fluid to record daily morning weights, because edema may not be obvious until several liters of extra fluid have accumulated.

Edema occurs in renal and liver disease, notably periorbital puffiness, tight rings in *nephrotic syndrome;* enlarged waistline from *ascites* and *liver failure.*

Health Promotion and Counseling: Evidence and Recommendations

Important Topics for Health Promotion and Counseling

▶ The challenges of cardiovascular disease (CVD) screening
▶ Special populations at risk: women and African Americans
▶ Screening for cardiovascular risk factors
  ▶ *Step 1:* Screen for global risk factors
  ▶ *Step 2:* Calculate 10-Year and long-term CVD risk using online calculators
  ▶ *Step 3:* Track individual risk factors—hypertension, diabetes, dyslipidemias, metabolic syndrome, smoking, family history, and obesity
▶ Promoting lifestyle and risk factor modification

Cardiovascular disease, which consists primarily of hypertension, coronary heart disease, heart failure, stroke, and congenital heart disease, affects over 82 million U.S. adults.[23] It is the leading cause of death in the United States and strikes a disproportionate number of African Americans and women. There has been notable success in reaching the Healthy People 2010 goals of reducing death from heart disease, both through major declines in cardiovascular risk factors, or *primary prevention,* and through improvement in treatment of existing heart disease such as heart attack and heart failure, or *secondary prevention.* But many challenges lie ahead.[36] Obesity, diabetes, and tobacco abuse threaten to undo the important gains of recent decades and are key targets for Healthy People 2020.

Health promotion to prevent cardiovascular disease includes screening for important risk factors, but also entails developing critical interviewing and counseling skills to nurture healthier lifestyles and behaviors. As emerging clinicians, your task will be threefold:

1. To understand important demographic data about cardiovascular disease and prevention

2. To identify cardiovascular risk factors

3. To form partnerships to help patients reduce cardiovascular risk by changing adverse behaviors and adopting pharmacologic treatments

The information presented in the Health Promotion and Counseling section is designed to improve your ability to identify and assess important cardiovascular risk factors and to promote "heart-healthy" lifestyles for your patients.

The Challenges of Cardiovascular Disease (CVD) Screening. As new studies refine our knowledge of the epidemiology of cardiovascular disease, screening guidelines become more complex in order to accommodate more customized approaches to specific risk groups. For example, guidelines for prescribing aspirin for primary prevention now differ by sex, age, and risk of coronary heart disease versus stroke.[38,39] Increasingly, clinicians are advised to pursue "shared decision making" with individual patients when risks and benefits of screening interventions are similar or equivocal. Fortunately, risk factors are increasingly interrelated, major professional societies of related disciplines are now issuing joint guidelines, and online calculators for rapid assessment of risk for cardiovascular disease and stroke are readily available. The Health Promotion and Counseling section provides an *approach* to screening and prevention, but you should review the excellent reports listed below for a deeper understanding of the evidence behind recent recommendations

- Heart disease and stroke statistics—2011 update: a report from the American Heart Association.[23]

- 2010 ACCF/AHA guideline for assessment of cardiovascular risk in asymptomatic adults: A report of the American College of Cardiology Foundation/American Heart Association Task Force on Practice Guidelines.[40]

- Effectiveness-based guidelines for the prevention of cardiovascular disease in women—2011 update: A guideline from the American Heart Association.[41]

- Management of high blood pressure in blacks. An update of the International Society on Hypertension in Blacks consensus Statement 2010.[42]

- Guidelines for the Primary Prevention of Stroke. A Guideline for Healthcare Professionals from the American Heart Association/American Stroke Association 2011.[43]

See Promoting Lifestyle and Risk Factor Modification on pp. 358–360 for discussion of assessing patient readiness to make health-promoting behavior changes; see also Chapter 3, Interviewing and the Health History (p. 72) for a discussion of motivational interviewing.[37]

Screening Early.   Heart disease has "a long asymptomatic latent period," so clinicians are now urged to assess *lifetime risk* in asymptomatic patients as early as age 20.[40] Furthermore, over half of all coronary deaths lack prior warning signs or cardiac diagnoses. Earlier risk assessment can lower this burden of asymptomatic disease by starting needed interventions earlier.

The Magnitude of Risk Factor Reduction.   In its goals for 2020, the American Heart Association[23] has advanced a new concept to promote cardiovascular health, "*ideal cardiovascular health*," defined as:

> The absence of clinically manifest cardiovascular disease and the simultaneous presence of optimal levels of all 7 health behaviors (lean body mass, avoidance of smoking, participation in physical activity, and healthy dietary intake) ... and health factors (untreated total cholesterol <200 mg/dL, untreated blood pressure <120/<80 mm Hg, and fasting blood glucose <100 mg/dL).

The graph below, based on data available in 2011, shows that significant portions of the U.S. population fail to reach ideal cardiovascular health. Among U.S. adults age 20 years and older, the age-standardized prevalence of ideal levels of cardiovascular health behaviors and factors ranges widely: for the healthy diet score—only 0.2%; weight—only 33%; blood pressure—only 42%; physical activity—only 45%; cholesterol—47%; fasting glucose—61%; and never smoked or stopped smoking for more than 12 month—72%. *Only 3% of U.S. adults have all 7 criteria at ideal levels.*

American Heart Association Prevalence Estimates for Poor, Intermediate, and Ideal Cardiovascular Health U.S. Adults 2010

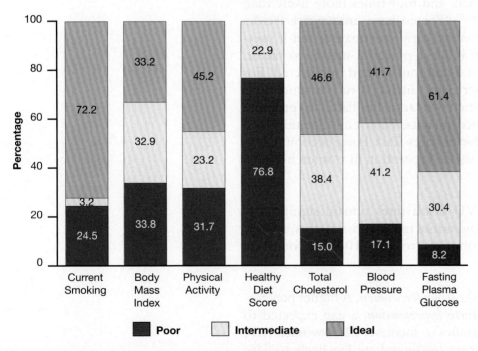

Source: National Health and Nutrition Examination Survey (NHANES) 2005—2006), in Roger VL, Go AS, Lloyd-Jones DM, et al. Heart disease and stroke statistics--2011 update: a report from the American Heart Association. Circulation 123:e18–e209, 2011. At http://circ.ahajournals.org/cgi/reprint/CIR.0b013e3182009701 . Accessed April 13, 2011.

The goals of the American Heart Association for 2020 are ambitious: to improve cardiovascular health for all Americans by 20% and to reduce deaths from cardiovascular disease and stroke by 20%.

Special Populations at Risk: Women and African Americans

Women. Although mortality rates for coronary heart disease for women have declined 50% since 1980, and awareness, treatment, and prevention of cardiovascular disease have substantially improved, cardiovascular disease (CVD) is still the leading cause of death for women (as well as for men). In its 2011 Guideline for the Prevention of Cardiovascular Disease in Women, the American Heart Association (AHA) reports that "reversing a trend of the past 4 decades, coronary heart disease death rates in US women 35 to 54 years of age now actually appear to be increasing," attributed to the effects of obesity.[41] There is evidence that while men's cardiovascular risk scores have improved in recent years, they have remained stable or worsened for women, especially younger women.[44,45] The statistics below illuminate concerning trends for cardiovascular health in women.

- For women, stroke accounts for a higher proportion of cardiovascular deaths, namely 60%, than heart disease. (For men, the ratio is reversed.) Higher lifetime risk of stroke in women is linked to the increased risk of stroke with age, the larger number of women over age 65, and their greater life expectancy, lower awareness of heart disease and stroke symptoms, and changing CVD risk factors, detailed below.

- Recent data show that self-reported stroke prevalence in women ages 45 to 54 years is double that of men, and four times more likely than in women ages 35 to 44 years.[23,46,47] Women have unique risk factors for stroke: pregnancy, hormone therapy, early menopause, and if present, preeclampsia. Atrial fibrillation is also a powerful stroke risk factor, increasing risk fivefold, and is often asymptomatic and undetected. For these reasons, the 2011 AHA expert panel included recommendations for prevention of stroke among women with atrial fibrillation to promote recognition and treatment with anticoagulants. These considerations also are part of the 2009 U.S. Preventive Services Task Force recommendations on use of aspirin for primary stroke prevention in women between the ages of 55 and 79.[38]

- Data from 2007 indicate that CVD death rates remain significantly higher for black women related to disparities in CVD risk factors, namely 286/100,000 for black women compared to 205/100,000 for white women.

- There are *adverse trends in CVD risk factors for women.* A higher percentage of women over age 65 years have *hypertension*, a gap expected to widen as longevity for women continues to increase. Black women have the highest prevalence of hypertension (44%) and are less likely to have their hypertension controlled. More than two-thirds of all U.S. women are now *overweight or obese*, contributing to the epidemic of type 2 diabetes, which greatly increases risk of myocardial infarction and stroke.

In 2011, the American Heart Association, recognizing the special cardiovascular risk faced by women, adopted a more aggressive CVD classification for women with more specific definitions of risks. Addressing the fact that 50% of women have a lifetime risk of developing heart disease, the AHA recommends placing women into one of three categories: *high risk, at risk,* and *"ideal cardiovascular health."*[41]

American Heart Association Cardiovascular Risk Categories for Women 2011

▶ **High risk**
  ▶ ≥1 high-risk states, including: existing CHD, CVD, peripheral arterial disease, abdominal aortic aneurysm, diabetes mellitus, or end-stage or chronic renal disease
  ▶ **10-year predicted risk of >10%** (a significant change from the 2007 cutoff of 20%)
▶ **At risk**
  ▶ ≥1 major risk factors including: smoking, BP ≥120/≥80 or treated hypertension, total cholesterol ≥200 mg/dL, HDL-c <50 mg/dL, or treated dyslipidemia, obesity, poor diet, physical inactivity, family history of premature CVD
  ▶ Evidence of advanced subclinical atherosclerosis (e.g., coronary calcification, carotid plaque, intima-media thickness), metabolic syndrome, or poor exercise capacity
  ▶ Systemic autoimmune collagen-vascular disease (e.g., lupus or rheumatoid arthritis)
  ▶ History or preeclampsia, gestational diabetes, or pregnancy-induced hypertension
▶ **Ideal cardiovascular health (all of these)**
  ▶ Total cholesterol <200 mg/dL (untreated)
  ▶ BP <120/<80 (untreated)
  ▶ Fasting glucose <100 mg/dL (untreated)
  ▶ Body mass index <25 kg/m²
  ▶ Abstinence from smoking
  ▶ Physical activity at goal: ≥150 min/wk moderate intensity, ≥75 min/wk vigorous intensity, or combination
  ▶ Healthy diet

Source: Mosca L, Benjamin EJ, Berra K et al. Effectiveness-based guidelines for the prevention of cardiovascular disease in women—2011 update: A guideline from the American Heart Association. Circulation 2011;123:1243–1262.

African Americans. As noted above, CVD death rates for blacks remain inordinately high compared to whites for both men and women. CVD death rates for men in 2007 were 406/100,000 for black men compared to

294/100,000 for white men; and 286/100,000 for black women compared to 206/100,000 for white women.[23] Of the seven "ideal cardiovascular health" indicators, 61% of white adults have three or fewer indicators at ideal levels compared to 71% of blacks and Mexican Americans. CVD disparities are most striking for coronary heart disease, hypertension, stroke, diabetes, and overweight and obesity, as shown in the table below.

Cardiovascular Diseases and Risk Factors: Prevalence in U.S. White and Black Adults (2007–2009)

	Men		Women	
	White	Black	White	Black
Coronary Heart Disease	8.5%	7.9%	5.8%	7.6%
Hypertension	33.9%	43.0%	31.3%	45.7%
Stroke	2.4%	4.5%	3.3%	4.4%
Diabetes	6.8%	14.3%	6.5%	4.7%
Overweight/ Obesity	72.3%	70.8%	59.3%	77.7%
Cholesterol ≥200 mg/dL	41.2%	37.0%	47.0%	41.2%
Smoking	25.0%	22.9%	20.7%	18.8%
Physical Activity	37.4%		29.3%	

Source: Roger VL, Go AS, Lloyd-Jones DM, et al. Heart disease and stroke statistics—2011 update: a report from the American Heart Association. Circulation 2011;123:e18–e209. Tables 23-1, 23-2. Available at http://circ.ahajournals.org/cgi/reprint/CIR.0b013e3182009701. Accessed April 13, 2011.

The prevalence of high cholesterol, obesity, and diabetes in Mexican Americans places them at similar risk to blacks.

Screening for Cardiovascular Risk Factors.

Step 1: Screen for Global Risk Factors. Begin routine screening at age 20 for individual risk factors or "global" risk of CVD and for any family history of premature heart disease. Recommended screening intervals are listed below.

Major Cardiovascular Risk Factors and Screening Frequency

Risk Factor	Screening Frequency	Goal
Family history of pre-mature CVD (at age <55 years in first-degree male relatives and age <65 years in first-degree female relatives)	Update regularly	

(continued)

Major Cardiovascular Risk Factors and Screening Frequency (*continued*)

Risk Factor	Screening Frequency	Goal
Cigarette smoking	At each visit	Cessation
Poor diet	At each visit	Improved overall eating pattern
Physical inactivity	At each visit	30 min moderate intensity daily
Obesity, especially central adiposity	At each visit	BMI 20–25 kg/m²; Waist circumference: 40 inches in men, ≤35 inches in women
Hypertension	At each visit	<140/90 <135/85 if black with HTN and without end-organ disease or CVD <130/80 if diabetes or black with HTN and end-organ disease or CVD <125/75 if renal disease
Dyslipidemias	Every 5 years if low risk Every 2 years if risk factors	See ATP III guidelines
Diabetes	Every 3 years beginning at age 45 More frequently at any age if risk factors	HgA1C ≥6.5%, at risk if 5.7%–6.4%
Pulse	At each visit	Identify and treat atrial fibrillation

Source: Adapted from: Pearson TA, Blair SN, Daniels SR et al. AHA Guidelines for Primary Prevention of Cardiovascular Disease and Stroke: 2002 Update. Consensus Panel Guide to Comprehensive Risk Reduction for Adult Patients without Coronary or Other Atherosclerotic Vascular Diseases. Circulation 2002;106:388–391; Flack JM, Sica DA, Bakris G et al. Management of high blood pressure in blacks. An update of the International Society on Hypertension in Blacks Consensus Statement. Hypertension 2010;56:780–800; American Diabetes Association. Standards of medical care in diabetes—2011. Diabetes Care 2011;34:S1–S61.

Step 2: Calculate 10-Year and Long-Term CVD Risk Using Online Calculators. Assemble individual risk factor data and calculate multivariable global risk assessment. This is easily accomplished by accessing well-validated online calculators. These are usually based on Framingham data that is most appropriate for individuals age 40 years and older. Many of these calculators provide 10-year CVD risk assessments that can also be used to guide treatment of dyslipidemias. Some, listed on the next page, provide 30-year assessments. A 10-year risk of 20% is generally considered poor or high risk, but this cutoff is in flux and has already been dropped to 10% for women, as shown in the table on p. 351.[40,41] Try out the calculators on the next page and check your own risk profile.

- Framingham 10-year and 30-year risk calculator: http://www.framinghamheartstudy.org/risk/gencardio.html

- Stroke risk calculator (Cleveland Clinic): http://my.clevelandclinic.org/p2/stroke-risk-calculator.aspx

You have now completed Step 2 of cardiovascular risk assessment.

Be aware, however, that due to the intense burden of CVD on the population that begins early in life, experts champion *lifetime risk assessment*, currently under development, as a powerful tool for public and individual patient education.[40,48] The presence of even one risk factor at age 50 dramatically increases lifetime risk and life expectancy. For example, at age 50 years, men with optimal risk factors have a 5.2% lifetime risk for developing CVD by age 75; for women at age 50 years with optimal risk factors, lifetime risk is 8.2%. Even one elevated risk factor raises these CVD risk figures to a 26% lifetime risk for men and a 15% lifetime risk for women, with associated declines in life expectancy.[48] By far the most potent risk factor at age 50 years is diabetes, which increases CVD risk at age 75 years to 67% for men and 57% for women.

Step 3: Track Individual Risk Factors—Hypertension, Diabetes, Dyslipidemias, Metabolic Syndrome, Obesity, Smoking, Family History.

Hypertension. According to the U.S. Preventive Services Task Force, hypertension accounts for "35% of all myocardial infarctions and strokes, 49% of all episodes of heart failure, and 24% of all premature deaths."[49] The Task Force strongly recommends *screening all people 18 years or older for high blood pressure*. Recent long-term population-based studies have fueled a dramatic shift in national strategies to prevent and reduce blood pressure (BP). The Seventh Report of the Joint National Committee on Prevention, Detection, Evaluation, and Treatment of High Blood Pressure, known as JNC 7, the National High Blood Pressure Education Program, and clinical investigators have issued several key messages for prevention.[50,51] These findings underlie the tougher and simpler blood pressure classification of JNC 7, reaffirmed by the U.S. Preventive Service Task Force in 2007.[52,53] (For new guidelines pending at the time of publication, see Joint National Commission 8 information available at http://www.nhlbi.nih.gov/guidelines/hypertension/jnc8/index.htm Accessed April 24, 2010.)

JNC 7: Classification and Management of Blood Pressure for Adults

▶ Normal	<120/80 mm Hg
▶ Prehypertension	120–139/80–89 mm Hg
▶ Stage 1 Hypertension	140–159/90–99 mm Hg
▶ Stage 2 Hypertension	>160/>100 mm Hg
▶ If diabetes or kidney disease	<130/80 mm Hg

Source: Chobanion AV, Bakris GL, Black HR, et al. The Seventh Report of the Joint National Committee on Prevention, Detection, Evaluation, and Treatment of High Blood Pressure—The JNC 7 Report. JAMA 2003;289:2560–2572. Also at http://www.nhlbi.nih.gov/guidelines/hypertension/jncintro.htm. Accessed May 6, 2011.

The average 55-year-old has a 90% lifetime risk of developing hypertension. Important risk factors for developing hypertension include: physical inactivity, excessive alcohol use, excessive dietary sodium intake, insufficient dietary potassium intake, family history of premature CVD, and renal disease. Hypertension may be caused by many medications and disease states. Unfortunately, 50% of adults older than 60 years suffer from hypertension and, of these, as many as two-thirds have hypertension that is poorly controlled. The consequences of hypertension for cardiovascular disease are profound; each increment of 20 mm Hg systolic or 10 mm Hg diastolic above 115/75 doubles the risk of CVD. Treatment remains critically important and represents a key contributor to achieving and exceeding Health People 2010 goals for reducing cardiovascular disease.[50,54]

Diabetes. Diabetes wreaks ever more devastating consequences to health in the United States and worldwide. The dramatic increase in obesity coupled with physical inactivity has created a public health epidemic of enormous significance. In 2011, diabetes affected over 11.5% of U.S. adults, or 25.4 million people.[23] This figure includes over 7 million adults yet to be diagnosed. *Prediabetes* affects an additional 81 million adults, or 37% of the population. The total prevalence of diabetes in the United States is expected to double by 2050.

The health disparities in diabetes prevalence remain striking: 6% to 7% of whites and Asian Americans compared to 10% to 11% of Hispanics and blacks, rising to 17% of American Indian/Alaska Natives under age 35. Unfortunately, as shown in the adjacent diagram, only 22% of those affected are treated and controlled, and diabetes continues to double the risk of developing and dying from CVD.

See Chapter 4, Beginning the Physical Examination: General Survey, Vital Signs, and Pain, pp. 112–113, for discussion of the benefits of restricting dietary sodium to <1,500 mg/day in reducing risk of CVD and controlling hypertension.[55]

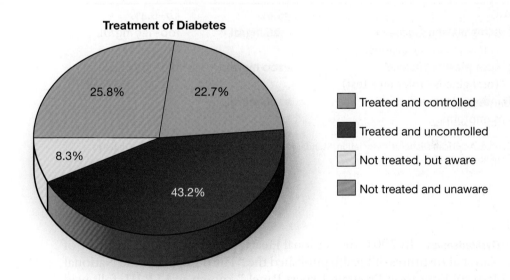

Source: National Health and Nutrition Examination Survey (NHANES) 2005–2008 in Roger VL, Go AS, Lloyd-Jones DM, et al. Heart disease and stroke statistics–2011 update: a report from the American Heart Association. Circulation 2011;123:e18–e209. Available at http://circ.ahajournals.org/cgi/reprint/CIR.0b013e3182009701. Accessed April 13, 2011.

Despite the fact that diabetes unequivocally increases the risk of CVD, early detection and treatment has not been firmly established to improve cardiovascular outcomes. This notwithstanding, 2011 guidelines support diagnosis if fasting glucose is ≥126 mg/dL and HgA1C values fall above 6.5%.[56] Diagnostic criteria for diabetes and prediabetes, as well as screening guidelines, are shown on the next page. Screening should be initiated at age 45 years and repeated at 3-year intervals. Screening should be initiated at any age for adults having a BMI of 25 or greater and additional risk factors.

American Diabetes Association 2011: Criteria for Diabetes Screening and Diagnosis

Screening Criteria

Healthy adults with no risk factors: begin at age 45 years, repeat at 3-year intervals

Adults with BMI ≥25 and additional risk factors:

▶ Physical inactivity
▶ First-degree relative with diabetes
▶ Members of a high-risk ethnic population—African American, Latino American, Asian American, Pacific Islander
▶ Mothers of infants ≥9 lb or diagnosed with GDM
▶ Hypertension ≥140/90 mm Hg or on therapy for hypertension
▶ HDL cholesterol <35 mg/dL and/or triglycerides >250 mg/dL
▶ Women with polycystic ovary syndrome
▶ A1C ≥5.7%, impaired glucose tolerance, or impaired fasting glucose on previous testing
▶ Other conditions associated with insulin resistance such as severe obesity, acanthosis nigricans
▶ History of cardiovascular disease

Diagnostic Criteria	Diabetes	Prediabetes
A1C	≤6.5%	5.7–6.4%
Fasting plasma glucose (on at least 2 occasions)	≥126 mg/dL	100–125 mg/dL
2-hour plasma glucose (oral glucose tolerance test)	≥200 mg/dL	140–199 mg/dL
Random glucose if classic symptoms	≥200 mg/dL	

Source: American Diabetes Association. Standards of medical care in diabetes—2011. Diabetes Care 2011;34:S1–S61.

Dyslipidemias.   In 2001, the National Heart, Lung, and Blood Institute of the National Institutes of Health published the "Third Report of the National Cholesterol Education Program Expert Panel," known as ATP III, followed by the full NCEP report in 2002.[57] These reports provide evidence-based recommendations on the management of high cholesterol and related lipid disorders, and document that "epidemiological surveys have shown that serum cholesterol levels are continuously correlated with CHD risk over a broad range of cholesterol values" in many of the world's populations.[58]

The ATP III guidelines, shown on the next page, incorporate the patient's lipid profile, the presence of coronary heart disease equivalents like diabetes, and major CAD risk factors into treatment goals based on 10-year risk categories. Note that for those at high risk, the NCEP recommends an

LDL goal of ≤70 mg/dL and intensive therapy as a therapeutic option, citing data that high-risk patients benefit from a further 30% to 40% drop in LDL even when the LDL is <100 mg/dL. The U.S. Preventive Services Task Force recommends routine lipid screening for men over age 35 and women over age 45.[59] Screening should occur at age 20 in both sexes if CHD risk factors are present.

ATP III Guidelines: 10-Year Risk and LDL Goals

10-Year Risk Category	LDL Goal (mg/dL)	Consider Drug Therapy if LDL (mg/dL)
High risk (>20%)	<100 *Optional goal: <70*	>100 <100: consider drug options, including further 30%–40% reduction in LDL
Moderately high risk (10%–20%)	<130 *Optional goal: <100*	>130 100–129: consider drug options to achieve goal of <100
Moderate risk (<10%)	<130	>160
Lower risk (0–1 risk factor)	<160	>190; (160–189: drug therapy *optional*)

Source: Adapted from Grundy SM, Cleeman JI, Merz NB, et al, for the Coordinating Committee of the National Cholesterol Education Program. Implications of recent clinical trials for the National Cholesterol Education Adult Treatment Panel III guidelines. Circulation 2004;110:227–239.

Use the CVD risk calculators to establish 10-year risk. Experts now recommend initiating interventions based on risk rather than absolute LDL level.[60,61] A low LDL is not a reason to withhold statin therapy for patients at significant risk. Studies continue to show that CVD risk drops 20% each time the LDL declines by 40 mg/dL regardless of the presenting level of LDL.[62] Given the efficacy, safety, and lower cost of statins,[63,64] some even advocate using age-based guidelines.[65] More aggressive screening efforts are needed; roughly a third of patients with high LDL levels are not screened, and two-thirds of high-risk patients do not receive medication.[61] Lifestyle changes alone, combining a low-fat diet, increased physical activity, and weight control, can decrease cholesterol levels by 20% to 30%.

The Metabolic Syndrome. The *metabolic syndrome* consists of a cluster of risk factors that create an increased risk of both CVD and diabetes. In 2009, the International Diabetes Association, the National Heart Lung blood Institute, the American Heart Association, and other societies established diagnostic criteria as the presence of three or more of the five risk factors listed on the next page.[66] The prevalence of this syndrome in U.S. adults 20 years of age and older is approximately 34%.[23]

Metabolic Syndrome: 2009 Diagnostic Criteria— Must Meet 3 or More of 5

Waist circumference	Men ≥102 cm, women ≥88 cm
Fasting plasma glucose	≥100 mg/dL, or being treated for elevated glucose
HDL cholesterol	Men <40 mg/dL, women <50 mg/dL, or being treated
Triglycerides	≥150 mg/dL, or being treated
Blood pressure	≥130/≥85, or being treated

Source: Alberti K, Eckel RH, Grundy SM et al. Harmonizing the metabolic syndrome: a joint interim statement of the Internal Diabetes Federation Task Force on Epidemiology and Prevention; National Heart, Lung, and Blood Institute; American Heart Association; World Heart Federation; Internal Atherosclerosis Society; and Internal Association for the Study of Obesity. Circulation 2009;120:1640–1645.

Other Risk Factors: Smoking, Family History, and Obesity. In adult smokers, 33% of deaths are related to CVD. *Smoking* increases the risk of coronary heart disease by two- to fourfold. Among adults, 13% report a *family history* of heart attack or angina before age 50, which roughly doubles the risk of heart attack. *Obesity*, or BMI over 30, contributed to 112,000 excess adult deaths compared to those of normal weight in recent data and was associated with 13% of CVD deaths in 2004.[23]

Promoting Lifestyle Change and Risk Factor Modification

Motivating behavior change is a challenge for all clinicians, and is the essence of risk factor reduction. Promoting cardiovascular health is a high priority for *Healthy People 2020*; 4 of the 24 objectives relate specifically to cardiovascular health—reducing hypertension, tobacco use, obesity, and coronary heart disease deaths, and improving physical activity.[67] The well-known Prochaska model is a useful tool for assessing patient "readiness to change" and tailoring advice to the patient's level of motivation.[68] Recommendations for pertinent lifestyle modifications are briefly summarized below.

See Table 4-4, Obesity: Stages of Change Model and Assessing Readiness, p. 138, and Chapter 8, Thorax and Lungs, pp. 293–331, for examples of how this model can be applied to clinical counseling.

Hypertension. Lifestyle modifications can lower systolic blood pressure from 2 to 20 mm Hg.[50] Encourage your patients to adopt the habits listed in the following table.

Lifestyle Modifications to Prevent or Manage Hypertension

- Optimal weight, or BMI of 18.5–24.9
- Intake of <6 g of sodium chloride or 2.4 g of sodium per day
- Regular aerobic exercise such as brisk walking for at least 30 minutes per day, most days of the week
- Moderate alcohol consumption per day of 2 drinks or fewer for men and 1 drink or fewer for women (2 drinks = 1 oz ethanol, 24 oz beer, 10 oz wine, or 2–3 oz whiskey)
- Dietary intake of more than 3,500 mg of potassium
- Diet rich in fruits, vegetables, and low-fat dairy products with reduced content of saturated and total fat

Source: Whelton PK, He J, Appel LJ, et al. Primary prevention of hypertension. Clinical and Public Health Advisory from the National High Blood Pressure Education Program. JAMA 2002;288:1882–1888.

Tobacco Use. Ask every patient two questions: "Do you smoke?" and "Do you want to quit smoking?" Use the "5As" framework and the Stages of Change model described in Chapter 8 to develop strategies for quitting. Encourage patients to use services that increase quit rates like the National Smoking Cessation Hotline: 1-800-QUIT NOW.[69]

See discussion on Tobacco Cessation, Chapter 8, Thorax and Lungs, pp. 302–304.

Obesity: Healthy Eating and Weight Loss. Begin with a dietary history to explore the patient's eating habits, then target the importance of foods low in cholesterol and total fat, especially foods with fewer saturated and *trans* fats. Foods with mono- and polyunsaturated fats and the omega-3 fatty acids found in fish oils help lower serum cholesterol. Review the food sources of these healthy and unhealthy fats in the table below.

See discussion of Optimal Weight, Nutrition, and Diet, Chapter 4, Beginning the Physical Examination: General Survey, Vital Signs, and Pain, pp. 108–112.

Food Sources of Healthy and Unhealthy Fats

Healthy Fats
- *Foods high in monounsaturated fat:* nuts, such as almonds, pecans, and peanuts; sesame seeds; avocados; canola oil; olive and peanut oil; peanut butter
- *Foods high in polyunsaturated fat:* corn, safflower, cottonseed, and soybean oil; walnuts; pumpkin or sunflower seeds; soft (tub) margarine; mayonnaise; salad dressings
- *Foods high in omega-3 fatty acids:* albacore tuna, herring, mackerel, rainbow trout, salmon, sardines

Unhealthy Fats
- *Foods high in cholesterol:* dairy products, egg yolks, liver and organ meats, high-fat meat and poultry
- *Foods high in saturated fat:* high-fat dairy products—cream, cheese, ice cream, whole and 2% milk, butter, and sour cream; bacon; chocolate; coconut oil; lard and gravy from meat drippings; high-fat meats like ground beef, bologna, hot dogs, and sausage
- *Foods high in* trans *fat:* snacks and baked goods with hydrogenated or partially hydrogenated oil, stick margarines, shortening, french fries

Reports from Healthy People 2010 state that "dietary factors are associated with 4 of the 10 leading causes of death—coronary heart disease, some types of cancer, stroke, and type 2 diabetes—as well as with high blood pressure and osteoporosis. Overall, the data on the three Healthy People 2010 objectives for the weight status of adults and children reflect a trend for the worse."[70]

Counseling about weight has become a clinician imperative. Assess BMI as described in Chapter 4. Discuss the principles of healthy eating; patients with a high fat intake are more likely to accumulate body fat than those with diets high in protein and carbohydrate. Help the patient to set realistic goals for diet and exercise that promote healthy eating habits *for life.*

Physical Activity. Regular exercise was the #1 health indicator for Healthy People 2010 and is #4 of the 24 objectives for Healthy People 2020. Poor diet coupled with lack of exercise has been the second leading actual cause of death. The gap between this risk factor and the leading cause, tobacco use, has continued to narrow.[71] Healthy People 2010 recommends at least 30 minutes of moderate activity 5 or more days per week, or 20 minutes of vigorous activity 3 or more times per week. Spur motivation by emphasizing the immediate benefits to health and well-being. Markers that help patients recognize the onset of aerobic metabolism include deep breathing, sweating in cool temperatures, and pulse rates exceeding 60% of the maximum normal age-adjusted heart rate, or 220 minus the person's age. Be sure to assess any pulmonary, cardiac, or musculoskeletal conditions that may limit the patient's exercise capacity.

Techniques of Examination

You are now ready to learn the classic techniques for examining the heart and great vessels. A sound knowledge of cardiac anatomy and physiology is key to understanding the hemodynamics of this closed-pump forward-flow system. It is only through diligent repetition, however, that you will gain confidence in the accuracy of your clinical findings.[12] Examine each patient carefully and methodically. Repeated examination of normal patients will help you recognize important cardiac pathology. Knowing how well these findings, by themselves or in concert with others, predict the presence or absence of cardiac conditions and diseases is vitally important. As in other chapters, the "test characteristics" of cardiac findings such as sensitivity, specificity, and likelihood ratios, are provided when pertinent and available. Students can also turn to several excellent resources for more detailed information.[16,72]

To obtain the most value from your examination, remember to examine the patient in a quiet, comfortable room where noise that interferes with auscultation is at a minimum. The general appearance of the patient provides many clues to cardiac illness, so pay special attention to the patient's color, respiratory rate, and level of anxiety, in addition to blood pressure and heart rate.

Blood Pressure and Heart Rate. As you begin the cardiovascular examination, review the blood pressure and heart rate recorded at the start of the physical examination. If you need to repeat these measurements, or if they have not already been done, take the time to measure the blood pressure and heart rate using optimal technique.[73-76]

See Chapter 4, Beginning the Physical Examination: General Survey, Vital Signs, and Pain, especially pp. 119–124.

After letting the patient rest for at least 5 minutes in a quiet setting, choose a correctly sized cuff and position the patient's arm at heart level, either resting on a table, if seated, or supported at midchest level, if standing. Make sure the bladder of the cuff is centered over the brachial artery. Inflate the cuff approximately 30 mm Hg above the pressure at which the brachial or radial pulse disappears. As you deflate the cuff, listen first for the sounds of at least two consecutive heartbeats; these mark the *systolic* pressure. Then listen for the disappearance point of the heartbeats, which marks the *diastolic* pressure. For *heart rate*, measure the radial pulse using the pads of your

A growing literature suggests that in office practice automated blood pressure measurement, taken when the patient rests alone in a quiet room, is the most accurate way to eliminate the "white coat" effect and correlates best with the current standard, 24-hour blood pressure monitoring.[77-81]

index and middle fingers, or auscultate the apical pulse with your stethoscope if heart rate is irregular.

Basic Cardiac Examination Skills: Objectives for Mastery. As you study this chapter and practice the cardiac examination, be sure you are proficient in the basic objectives listed below.

- Describe the chest wall anatomy and identify the key listening areas.

- Evaluate the jugular venous pulse, the carotid upstroke, and presence or absence of carotid bruits.

- Correctly identify and describe the point of maximal impulse (PMI).

- Correctly identify the first and second sounds (S_1 and S_2) at the base and apex.

- Recognize the effect of the P-R interval on the intensity of S_1.

- Identify physiologic and paradoxical splitting of S_2.

- Recognize key abnormal sounds in *early diastole*, including the third heart sound (S_3), pericardial knock, and opening snap of mitral stenosis.

- Recognize a fourth heart sound (S_4) *later in diastole*.

- Evaluate the timing of murmurs and correctly identify systolic and diastolic murmurs, as well as friction rubs.

- Evaluate and interpret pulsus paradoxus.

- Correctly identify the physical findings of a normal heart examination, including rate, rhythm, and characteristics of the heart sounds.

- Correctly identify heart murmurs, using maneuvers when needed.

JUGULAR VENOUS PRESSURE AND PULSATIONS

Jugular Venous Pressure (JVP). Estimating the JVP is one of the most important and frequently used skills of physical examination. As you have learned, the JVP reflects pressure in the right atrium, or central venous pressure, and is best assessed from pulsations in the *right internal jugular vein.* Contrary to widely held views, a recent study has reaffirmed inspection of the *right external jugular vein* as an accurate method for estimating central venous pressure.[22,82,83] Note that the jugular veins and pulsations are difficult to see in children under 12 years of age, so inspection is not useful in this age group.

Pressure changes from right atrial filling, contraction, and emptying cause fluctuations in the JVP and its waveforms that are visible to the examiner. Careful observation of these fluctuations yields clues about volume status, right and left ventricular function, patency of the tricuspid and pulmonary valves, pressures in the pericardium, and arrhythmias such as junctional rhythms and atrioventricular blocks. For example, JVP falls with loss of blood and increases with right or left heart failure, pulmonary hypertension, tricuspid stenosis, and pericardial compression or tamponade.

The internal jugular veins lie deep to the sternomastoid muscles in the neck and are not directly visible, so the clinician must learn to identify the *pulsations* of the *internal jugular vein* or *external jugular vein* that are transmitted to the surface of the neck, being careful to distinguish these venous pulsations from pulsations of the carotid artery.

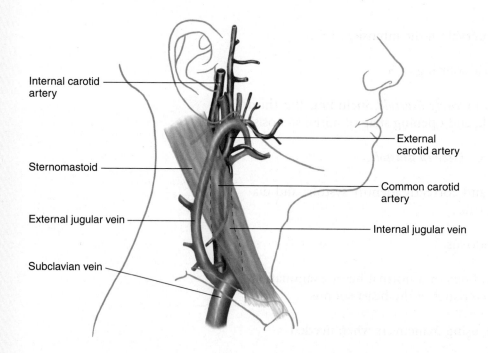

To estimate the level of the JVP, you will learn to find the *highest point of oscillation in the internal jugular vein* or, if necessary, the point above which the external jugular vein appears collapsed. The JVP is usually measured in vertical distance above the *sternal angle*, the bony ridge adjacent to the second rib where the manubrium joins the body of the sternum.

Study carefully the illustrations on the next page. Note that regardless of the patient's position, the sternal angle remains roughly 5 cm above the right atrium. In this patient, however, the pressure in the internal jugular vein is somewhat elevated.

- In *Position A*, the head of the bed is raised to the usual level, approximately 30 degrees, but the JVP cannot be measured because the meniscus, or level of oscillation, is above the jaw and, therefore, not visible.

- In *Position B*, the head of the bed is raised to 60 degrees. The "top" of the internal jugular vein is now easily visible, so the vertical distance from the sternal angle or right atrium can now be measured.

- In *Position C*, the patient is upright and the veins are barely discernible above the clavicle, making measurement untenable.

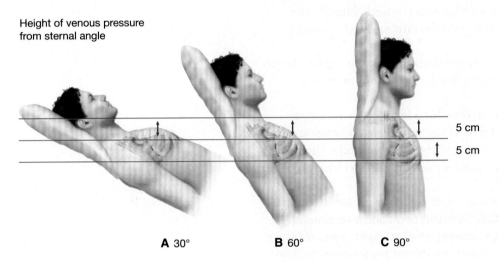

Height of venous pressure
from sternal angle

5 cm

5 cm

A 30°   **B** 60°   **C** 90°

Note that the height of the venous pressure as measured from the sternal angle is the *same* in all three positions, but your ability to *measure* the height of the column of venous blood, or JVP, differs according to how you position the patient. Jugular venous pressure measured at more than 4 cm above the sternal angle, or more than 9 cm above the right atrium, is considered elevated or abnormal.

To help you learn this portion of the cardiac examination, steps for assessing the JVP are outlined below. As you begin your assessment, consider the patient's volume status and how you may need to alter the elevation of the head of the bed or examining table.

- The usual starting point for assessing the JVP is to elevate the head of the bed to 30 degrees. Identify the external jugular vein on each side, then find the internal jugular venous pulsations transmitted from deep in the neck to the overlying soft tissues. The JVP is the highest oscillation point, or meniscus, of the jugular venous pulsations that is usually evident in euvolemic patients.

- In patients who are *hypovolemic*, you may anticipate that *the JVP will be low*, causing you to *lower the head of the bed*, sometimes even to 0 degrees, to see the point of oscillation best.

A hypovolemic patient may have to lie flat before you see the neck veins. In contrast, when jugular venous pressure is increased, elevating the patient's head to 60 degrees or even 90 degrees may be required. In all these positions, the sternal angle usually remains about 5 cm above the right atrium, as diagrammed above.

- Likewise, in volume-overloaded or *hypervolemic* patients, you may anticipate that *the JVP will be high*, causing you to *raise the head of the bed.*

Steps for Measuring the Jugular Venous Pressure

▶ Make the patient comfortable. *Raise the head slightly on a pillow* to relax the sternomastoid muscles.

▶ *Raise the head of the bed or examining table to about 30 degrees. Turn the patient's head slightly away from the side you are inspecting.*

▶ Use *tangential lighting* and examine both sides of the neck. Identify the external jugular vein on each side, then find the internal jugular venous pulsations.

▶ *If necessary, raise or lower the head of the bed* until you can see the oscillation point or meniscus of the internal jugular venous pulsations in the lower half of the neck.

▶ Focus on the *right internal jugular vein.* Look for pulsations in the suprasternal notch, between the attachments of the sternomastoid muscle on the sternum and clavicle, or just posterior to the sternomastoid. The table below helps you distinguish internal jugular pulsations from those of the carotid artery.

▶ *Identify the highest point of pulsation in the right jugular vein.* Extend a long rectangular object or card horizontally from this point and a centimeter ruler vertically from the sternal angle, making an exact right angle. Measure the vertical distance in centimeters above the sternal angle where the horizontal object crosses the ruler and add to this distance 4 cm, the distance from the sternal angle to the center of the right atrium. *The sum is the JVP.*

The following features help to distinguish jugular from carotid artery pulsations.[82]

Distinguishing Internal Jugular and Carotid Pulsations

Internal Jugular Pulsations	Carotid Pulsations
Rarely palpable	Palpable
Soft, biphasic, undulating quality, usually with two elevations and two troughs per heart beat	A more vigorous thrust with a *single outward component*
Pulsations eliminated by light pressure on the vein(s) just above the sternal end of the clavicle	Pulsations not eliminated by this pressure
Height of pulsations changes with position, dropping as the patient becomes more upright	Height of pulsations unchanged by position
Height of pulsations usually falls with inspiration	Height of pulsations not affected by inspiration

Establishing the true vertical and horizontal lines to measure the JVP is difficult. Place your ruler on the sternal angle and line it up with something in the room that you know to be vertical. Then place a card or rectangular object at an exact right angle to the ruler. This constitutes your horizontal line. Move it up or down—still horizontal—so that the lower edge rests at the top of the jugular pulsations, and read the vertical distance on the ruler. Round your measurement off to the nearest centimeter.

Increased jugular venous pressure is highly correlated with both acute and chronic right and left-sided heart failure.[16,84-87] It is also seen in tricuspid stenosis, chronic pulmonary hypertension, superior vena obstruction, and pericardial disease such as tamponade and constrictive pericarditis.[88-91]

In patients with obstructive lung disease, venous pressure may appear elevated on expiration only; the veins collapse on inspiration. This finding does not indicate heart failure.

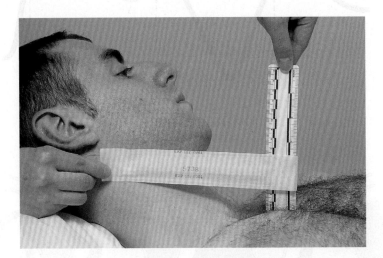

Venous pressure measured at >3 cm, or possibly 4 cm, above the sternal angle, or more than 8 cm or 9 cm in total distance above the right atrium, is considered elevated *above normal*.

An elevated JVP is 98% specific for an increased left ventricular end diastolic pressure and low left ventricular ejection fraction, and increases risk of death from heart failure.[16,86]

If you cannot see pulsations in the internal jugular vein, look for them in the external jugular vein. If you see no pulsation, use *the point above which the external jugular veins appear to collapse*. Make this observation on each side of the neck. Measure the vertical distance of this point from the sternal angle.

Local kinking or obstruction is the usual cause of unilateral distention of the external jugular vein.

The highest point of venous pulsations may lie below the level of the sternal angle. Under these circumstances, venous pressure is not elevated and seldom needs to be measured.

Jugular Venous Pulsations. Oscillations in the internal jugular vein, and often in the external jugular vein, reflect changing pressures in the right atrium. Careful inspection reveals that these undulations are composed of two quick peaks and two troughs, diagrammed on the next page.

Considerable practice and experience are required to master jugular venous pulsations. A beginner is advised to concentrate first on jugular venous pressure.

- The first elevation, the presystolic *a wave*, reflects the slight rise in atrial pressure that accompanies atrial contraction. It occurs just before S_1 and before the carotid pulse.

- The following trough, the *x descent*, starts with atrial relaxation. It continues as the right ventricle, contracting during systole, pulls the floor of the atrium downward. During ventricular systole, blood continues to flow into the right atrium from the venae cavae.

- The tricuspid valve is closed, the chamber begins to fill, and right atrial pressure begins to rise again, creating the second elevation, the *v wave*. When the tricuspid valve opens early in diastole, blood in the right atrium flows passively into the right ventricle, and right atrial pressure falls again, creating the second trough, or *y descent*.

- To remember these four oscillations in an oversimplified way, think of the following sequence: atrial contraction, atrial relaxation, atrial filling, and atrial emptying. You can think of the *a* wave as *a*trial contraction and the *v* wave as *v*enous filling. To the naked eye, the two descents are the most obvious events in the normal jugular pulse. Of the two, the sudden collapse of the *x* descent late in systole is more prominent, occurring just before S_2. The *y* descent follows S_2 early in diastole.

Jugular Venous Pulsations

a wave	x descent	v wave	y descent
Atrial contraction, tricuspid valve open	Atrial relaxation then filling, tricuspid valve closed	Venous filling, atrium tense, tricuspid closed	Atrial emptying, tricuspid open

Source: National Health and Nutrition Examination Survey (NHANES) 2005–2006), in Roger VL, Go AS, Lloyd-Jones DM, et al. Heart disease and stroke statistics—2011 update: a report from the American Heart Association. Circulation 2011;123:e18–e209. Available at http://circ.ahajournals.org/cgi/reprint/CIR.0b013e3182009701. Accessed April 13, 2011.

Observe the amplitude and timing of the jugular venous pulsations. To time them, feel the left carotid artery with your right thumb or listen to the heart simultaneously. The *a* wave just precedes S_1 and the carotid pulse, the *x* descent can be seen as a systolic collapse, the *v* wave almost coincides with S_2, and the *y* descent follows early in diastole. Look for absent or unusually prominent waves.

Prominent *a waves* occur in increased resistance to right atrial contraction, as in *tricuspid stenosis;* also in first-degree atrioventricular block, supraventricular tachycardia, junctional rhythms, *pulmonary hypertension,* and *pulmonic stenosis.*

Absent *a waves occur* in atrial fibrillation. Large *v waves occur* in *tricuspid regurgitation, and constrictive pericarditis*

THE CAROTID PULSE

After you measure the JVP, move on to assessment of the *carotid pulse*. The carotid pulse provides valuable information about cardiac function and is especially useful for detecting stenosis or insufficiency of the aortic valve. Take the time to assess the quality of the carotid upstroke, its amplitude and contour, and presence or absence of any overlying *thrills* or *bruits*.

For irregular rhythms, see Table 9-1, Selected Heart Rates and Rhythms, p. 391, and Table 9-2, Selected Irregular Rhythms, p. 392.

To assess *amplitude and contour,* the patient should be lying down with the head of the bed elevated to about 30 degrees. When feeling for the carotid artery, first inspect the neck for carotid pulsations. These may be visible just medial to the sternomastoid muscles. Then place your index and middle fingers (or left thumb) on the right carotid artery in the lower third of the neck, press posteriorly, and feel for pulsations.

A tortuous and kinked carotid artery may produce a unilateral pulsatile bulge.

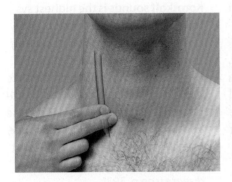 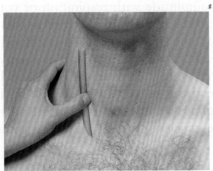

Causes of decreased pulsations include decreased stroke volume and local factors in the artery such as atherosclerotic narrowing or occlusion.

Press just inside the medial border of a relaxed sternomastoid muscle, roughly at the level of the cricoid cartilage. Avoid pressing on the *carotid sinus,* which lies level to the top of the thyroid cartilage. For the left carotid artery, use your right fingers or thumb. Never press both carotids at the same time. This may decrease blood flow to the brain and induce syncope.

Pressure on the carotid sinus may cause a reflex drop in pulse rate or blood pressure.

Slowly increase pressure until you feel a maximal pulsation; then slowly decrease pressure until you best sense the arterial pressure and contour. Aim to assess:

See Table 9-3, Abnormalities of the Arterial Pulse and Pressure Waves, p. 393.

- The *amplitude of the pulse.* This correlates reasonably well with the pulse pressure.

Small, thready, or weak pulse occurs in *cardiogenic shock; bounding* pulse in *aortic insufficiency* (see p. 393)

- The *contour of the pulse wave,* namely the speed of the upstroke, the duration of its summit, and the speed of the downstroke. The normal upstroke is *brisk.* It is smooth, rapid, and follows S_1 almost immediately. The summit is smooth, rounded, and roughly midsystolic. The downstroke is less abrupt than the upstroke.

The carotid upstroke is delayed in *aortic stenosis.*

- Any *variations in amplitude,* either from beat to beat or with respiration.

Pulsus alternans and bigeminal pulse vary beat to beat; *paradoxical pulse* varies with respiration, described on the next page.

- *The timing of the carotid upstroke in relation to S_1 and S_2.* Note that the normal carotid upstroke follows S_1 and precedes S_2. This relationship is very helpful in correctly identifying S_1 and S_2, especially when the heart rate is increased and the duration of diastole, normally shorter than systole, is shortened and approaches the duration of systole.

Pulsus Alternans. In *pulsus alternans,* the rhythm of the pulse remains regular, but the *force* of the arterial pulse alternates because of alternating strong and weak ventricular contractions. *Pulsus alternans* almost always indicates severe left-sided heart failure and is usually best felt by applying light pressure on the radial or femoral arteries. Use a blood pressure cuff to confirm your finding. After raising the cuff pressure, lower it slowly to the systolic level. The initial Korotkoff sounds are the strong beats. As you lower the cuff, you will hear the softer sounds of the alternating weak beats.

Alternately loud and soft Korotkoff sounds or a sudden doubling of the apparent heart rate as the cuff pressure declines indicates a *pulsus alternans* (see p. 393).

Placing the patient in the upright position may accentuate this finding.

Paradoxical Pulse. This is a greater than normal drop in systolic pressure during inspiration. If the pulse varies in amplitude with respiration or you suspect pericardial tamponade (because of increased jugular venous pressure, a rapid and diminished pulse, and dyspnea, for example), use a blood-pressure cuff to check for a *paradoxical pulse.* As the patient breathes quietly, lower the cuff pressure to the systolic level. Note the pressure level at which the first sounds can be heard. Then drop the pressure very slowly until sounds can be heard throughout the respiratory cycle. Again note the pressure level. The difference between these two levels is normally no greater than 3 or 4 mm Hg.

The level identified at first hearing Korotkoff sounds is the highest systolic pressure during the respiratory cycle. The level identified at hearing sounds throughout the cycle is the lowest systolic pressure. A difference between these levels of more than 10 mm Hg indicates a paradoxical pulse and suggests *pericardial tamponade,* possible *constrictive pericarditis,* but most commonly *obstructive airway disease* (see p. 393).

Thrills and Bruits. As you palpate the carotid artery, you may detect humming vibrations, or *thrills,* like the throat vibrations in a cat when it purrs.

As you assess the neck vessels, especially if you feel a thrill, listen over both the carotid arteries for a *bruit,* a murmurlike sound arising from turbulent arterial blood flow. Ask the patient to stop breathing for a few seconds, then listen with the diaphragm of the stethoscope, which generally detects the higher frequency sounds of arterial bruits better than the bell.[92] Note that higher-grade stenoses may have lower frequency or even absent sounds, more amenable to detection with the bell. Place the diaphragm near the upper end of the thyroid cartilage below the angle of the jaw, the area where the common carotid artery bifurcates into the internal carotid artery. A bruit in this location is less likely to be confused with a transmitted murmur from the heart or subclavian or vertebral artery bruits.

Although usually caused by atherosclerotic narrowing of the internal carotid artery, bruits can also arise from a tortuous carotid artery with intraluminal turbulence, external carotid arterial disease, aortic stenosis, the hypervascularity of hyperthyroidism, and external compression from thoracic outlet syndrome.

Listen for bruits in older patients and patients with suspected cerebrovascular disease.

The prevalence of asymptomatic carotid bruits increases with age, reaching 8% in adults 75 years of age and older. The sensitivity and specifity of carotid bruits for carotid stenosis vary widely, roughly 30% and 90%, but the associated risk of TIA, stroke, and CAD doubles in most studies.[93–95] Since the presence of a bruit does not correlate with the degree of underlying stenosis, pursue further investigation.[96]

The Brachial Artery. In patients with carotid obstruction, kinking, or thrills, assess the pulse in the *brachial artery*, applying the techniques described previously for determining amplitude and contour.

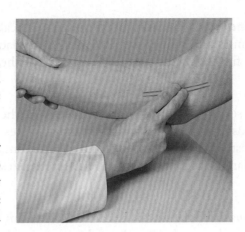

Use the index and middle fingers or thumb of your opposite hand. Cup your hand under the patient's elbow and feel for the pulse just medial to the biceps tendon. The patient's arm should rest with the elbow extended, palm up. With your free hand, you may need to flex the elbow to a varying degree to get optimal muscular relaxation.

 ## THE HEART

Positioning the Patient. For most of the cardiac examination, the patient should be *supine*, with the upper body and head of the bed or examining table raised to about 30 degrees. To bring the ventricular apex closer to the chest wall so you can assess the PMI, you should also ask the patient to *turn to the left side*, termed the *left lateral decubitus position*. To bring the left ventricular outflow tract closer to the chest wall to better listen for aortic insufficiency, have the patient *sit up, lean forward, and exhale. The examiner should stand at the patient's left side.*

The table below summarizes patient positions and a suggested sequence for the examination.

Sequence of the Cardiac Examination

Patient Position	Examination	Accentuated Findings
Supine, with the head elevated 30 degrees	Inspect and palpate the precordium: the 2nd right and left interspaces; the right ventricle; and the left ventricle, including the apical impulse (diameter, location, amplitude, duration).	
Left lateral decubitus	Palpate the apical impulse, if not previously detected. Listen at the apex with the *bell* of the stethoscope.	Low-pitched extra sounds such as an S_3, opening snap, diastolic rumble of *mitral stenosis*
Supine, with the head elevated 30 degrees	Listen at the 2nd right and left interspaces, along the left sternal border, across to the apex with the *diaphragm*.	
Sitting, leaning forward, after full exhalation	Listen at the right sternal border for tricuspid murmurs and sounds with the *bell*.	Soft decrescendo higher-pitched diastolic murmur of *aortic insufficiency*

Location and Timing of Cardiac Findings. Identify both the anatomical location of heart sounds and murmurs and where they fall in the cardiac cycle. Remember to correlate your findings with the characteristics of the patient's JVP and carotid upstroke.

- Note the *anatomical location* of sounds in terms of interspaces and the distance of the PMI from the midsternal, midclavicular, or axillary lines. The midsternal line offers the most reliable zero point for measurement, but some feel that the midclavicular line accommodates the different sizes and shapes of patients.

- Identify the *timing of impulses or sounds* in relation to the cardiac cycle. Timing of sounds is often possible through auscultation alone. In most people with normal or slow heart rates, it is easy to identify the paired heart sounds marking systole or diastole. S_1 is the first of these sounds; S_2 is the second. The relatively long diastolic interval separates one pair from the next.

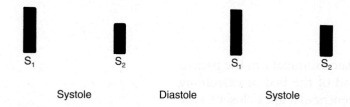

The relative intensity of these sounds is also helpful. *S_1 is usually louder than S_2 at the apex; S_2 is usually louder than S_1 at the base.*

Even experienced clinicians are sometimes uncertain about the timing of heart sounds, especially extra sounds and murmurs. "Inching" can then be helpful. Return to a place on the chest, most often the base, where it is easy to identify S_1 and S_2. Get their rhythm clearly in mind. Then inch your stethoscope down the chest in steps until you hear the new sound.

In some circumstances, auscultation alone does not suffice. The intensities of S_1 and S_2 may be abnormal, or, at rapid heart rates, the duration of diastole may shorten, making the durations of systole and diastole indistinguishable. *Palpation of the carotid artery during auscultation is an invaluable aide to timing the sound or murmur.* Since the carotid upstroke always occurs in systole immediately after S_1, sounds or murmurs coinciding with the upstroke are systolic; sounds or murmurs occurring after completion of the upstroke are diastolic.

For example, S_1 is diminished in *first-degree heart block*; S_2 is diminished in *aortic stenosis*.

Inspection and Palpation

Overview. Careful inspection of the anterior chest may reveal the location of the *apical impulse or point of maximal impulse (PMI)*, or less commonly, the ventricular movements of a left-sided S_3 or S_4. Shining a tangential light across the chest wall over the cardiac apex makes these movements more visible. If identified on inspection, palpate the PMI to

See p. 394 for how to characterize the PMI as tapping, sustained, or diffuse.

confirm its characteristics. Keep in mind the surface anatomy of the heart diagrammed below.

Palpation can also reveal thrills, the timing of S_1 and S_2, and the ventricular movements of S_3 or S_4. Begin with general palpation of the chest wall. In women, keeping the right chest draped, gently lift the breast with your left hand or ask the woman to do this to assist you.

- Palpate for *heaves, lifts,* or *thrills* using your palm and/or your fingerpads held flat or obliquely against the chest. *Lifts* and *heaves* are sustained impulses usually produced by an enlarged right or left ventricle or atrium and occasionally by ventricular aneurysms. If present you will feel the impulse rhythmically lift your fingers.

- For *thrills*, press the ball of your hand (the padded area of your palm near the wrist) firmly on the chest to check for a buzzing or vibratory sensation from underlying vascular turbulence from heart murmurs. If present, auscultate this area for murmurs. Thrills are more easily palpated in the patient position that accentuates the murmur, such as the leaning forward to enhance detection of aortic insufficiency.

- To palpate for S_1 *and* S_2, using firm pressure, place your right hand on the chest wall. With your left index and middle fingers, palpate the carotid artery in the lower third of the neck. Identify S_1 just before the carotid upstroke and S_2 just after the upstroke. This may take practice due to the upstroke's rapid rise and fall, but over time you will succeed in detecting S_1 and S_2 by palpation as well as auscultation. To palpate for S_3 *and* S_4, apply lighter pressure at the cardiac apex to determine the presence of any extra movements.

On rare occasions a patient may have *dextrocardia*, a heart situated in the right chest cavity with a right-sided apical impulse, seen in genetically transmitted transpositions present at birth. Use percussion to help locate the heart border, the liver, and stomach. In full *situs inversus*, the heart, tri-lobed lung, stomach, and spleen are on the right and the liver and gall bladder are on the left.

The presence of a thrill changes the grading of the murmur, as described on pp. 382.

Successful palpation is less likely in patients with a thickened chest wall or increased anteroposterior diameter.

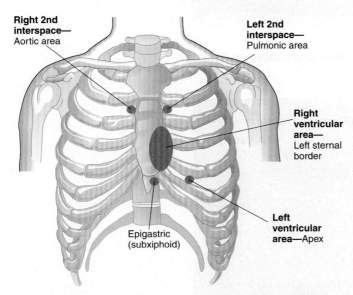

Right 2nd interspace—Aortic area

Left 2nd interspace—Pulmonic area

Right ventricular area—Left sternal border

Left ventricular area—Apex

Epigastric (subxiphoid)

- Be sure to assess the *right ventricle* by palpating the right ventricular area at the lower left sternal border and in the subxiphoid area, the pulmonary artery in the left 2nd interspace, and the aortic area in the right 2nd interspace (see p. 374).

Left Ventricular Area—The Apical Impulse or Point of Maximal Impulse (PMI). The apical impulse represents the brief early pulsation of the left ventricle as it moves anteriorly during contraction and touches the chest wall. Note that, in most examinations, the apical impulse is the point of maximal impulse, or PMI; however, some pathologic conditions, such as an enlarged right ventricle, a dilated pulmonary artery, or an aneurysm of the aorta, may produce a pulsation that is more prominent than the apex beat.

If you cannot identify the apical impulse with the patient supine, ask the patient to roll partly onto the left side; this is the *left lateral decubitus* position. Palpate again, using the palmar surfaces of several fingers. If you cannot find the apical impulse, ask the patient to exhale fully and stop breathing for a few seconds. When examining a woman, it may be helpful to displace the left breast upward or laterally as necessary, or ask her to do this for you.

The apex beat is palpable in only 25% to 40% of healthy adults in the supine position and in 50% of healthy adults in the left lateral decubitus position, especially those who are thin.[16]

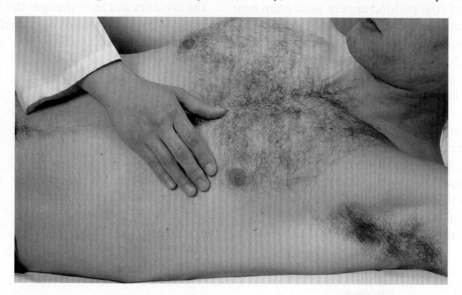

Once you have found the apical impulse, make finer assessments with your fingertips, and then with one finger.

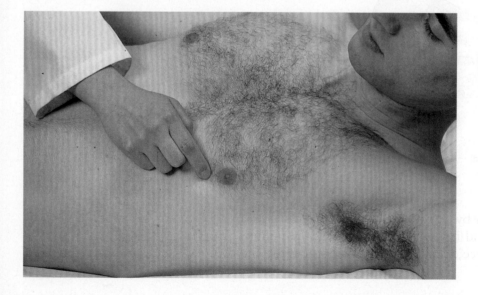

With experience, you will learn to feel the apical impulse in a high percentage of patients. Obesity, a very muscular chest wall, or an increased anteroposterior diameter of the chest, however, may obscure detection. Some apical impulses hide behind the rib cage, despite positioning.

Now assess the location, diameter, amplitude, and duration of the apical impulse. You may wish to have the patient breathe out and briefly stop breathing to check your findings.

See Table 9-4, Variations and Abnormalities of the Ventricular Impulses, p. 394.

- *Location.* Try to assess location with the patient *supine*, because the left lateral decubitus position displaces the apical impulse to the left. Locate two points: the interspaces, usually the 5th or possibly the 4th, which give the vertical location; and the distance in centimeters from the *midclavicular line*, which gives the horizontal location. Use a ruler to mark the midpoint between the sternoclavicular and acromioclavicular joints; otherwise, use of this line is less reproducible because clinicians vary in their estimates of the midpoint of the clavicle. Some clinicians use the midsternal line because it is fixed and measurement to the apical impulse has less variation.

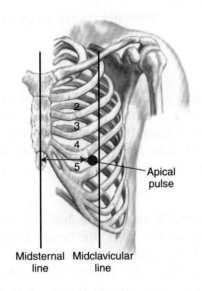

Midsternal line   Midclavicular line

Pregnancy or a high left diaphragm may displace the apical impulse upward and to the left.

Lateral displacement from cardiac enlargement is seen in *heart failure, cardiomyopathy,* and *ischemic heart disease.* Displacement also occurs from deformities of the thorax and mediastinal shift.

Lateral displacement outside the midclavicular line makes cardiac enlargement and a low left ventricular ejection fraction 3–4 and 10 times more likely, respectively.[16]

- *Diameter.* Palpate the diameter of the apical impulse. In the supine patient, it usually measures less than 2.5 cm, about the size of a quarter, and occupies only one interspace. It may feel larger in the left lateral decubitus position.

In the left lateral decubitus position, a *diffuse* PMI with a diameter greater than 3 cm indicates left ventricular enlargement.[97] If PMI is greater than 4 or 5 cm when the patient is supine, left ventricular overload is almost five times more likely.[16]

- *Amplitude.* Estimate the amplitude of the impulse. It is usually small and feels *brisk* and *tapping.* Some young adults have an increased amplitude, or hyperkinetic impulse, especially when excited or after exercise; its duration, however, is normal.

Increased amplitude may also reflect *hyperthyroidism, severe anemia,* pressure overload of the left ventricle (as in *aortic stenosis*), or volume overload of the left ventricle (as in *mitral regurgitation*).

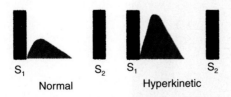

S_1 S_2 S_1 S_2

Normal   Hyperkinetic

- *Duration.* Duration is the most useful characteristic of the apical impulse for identifying hypertrophy of the left ventricle. To assess duration, listen to the heart sounds as you feel the apical impulse, or watch the movement

A *sustained,* high-amplitude impulse that is normally located suggests left ventricular hypertrophy from

of your stethoscope as you listen at the apex. Estimate the proportion of systole occupied by the apical impulse. Normally it lasts through the first two-thirds of systole, or often less, but does not continue to the second heart sound.

pressure overload (as in *hypertension*). If such an impulse is displaced laterally, consider volume overload.

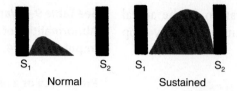

S₁ — Normal — S₂   S₁ — Sustained — S₂

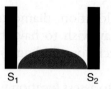

S₁ — S₂

A sustained low-amplitude (hypokinetic) impulse is seen in *dilated cardiomyopathy*.

S₃ and S₄.   By inspection and palpation, you may detect ventricular movements that are synchronous with pathologic third and fourth heart sounds. For the left ventricular impulses, feel the apical beat gently with one finger. The patient should lie partly on the left side, breathe out, and briefly stop breathing. By inking an X on the apex, you may be able to see these movements.

A brief middiastolic impulse indicates an S₃; an impulse just before the systolic apical beat itself indicates an S₄.

Right Ventricular Area—The Left Sternal Border in the 3rd, 4th, and 5th Interspaces.   The patient should be supine with the head elevated to 30 degrees. Place the tips of your curved fingers in the 3rd, 4th, and 5th interspaces and try to feel the systolic impulse of the right ventricle. Again, asking the patient to breathe out and then briefly stop breathing can improve detection.

If an impulse is palpable, assess its location, amplitude, and duration. A brief systolic tap of low or slightly increased amplitude is sometimes felt in thin or shallow-chested people, especially when stroke volume is increased by conditions such as anxiety.

A marked increase in amplitude with little or no change in duration occurs in chronic volume overload of the right ventricle, which can occur in *atrial septal defect*.

An impulse with increased amplitude and duration occurs with pressure overload of the right ventricle, as in *pulmonic stenosis* or *pulmonary hypertension*.

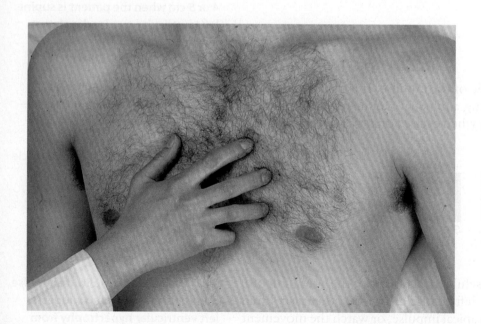

The diastolic movements of *right-sided S₃ and S₄* may be felt occasionally. Feel for them in the 4th and 5th left interspaces. Time them by auscultation or carotid palpation.

In patients with an increased anteroposterior diameter, palpation of the *right ventricle* in the *epigastric* or *subxiphoid area* is also useful. With your hand flattened, press your index finger just under the rib cage and up toward the left shoulder and try to feel right ventricular pulsations.

In obstructive pulmonary disease, hyperinflated lung may prevent palpation of an enlarged right ventricle in the left parasternal area. The impulse is felt easily, however, high in the epigastrium where heart sounds are also more audible.

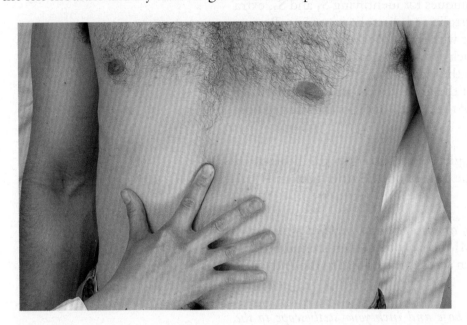

Asking the patient to inhale and briefly stop breathing is helpful. The inspiratory position moves your hand well away from the pulsations of the abdominal aorta, which might otherwise confuse your findings. The diastolic movements of S₃ and S₄, if present, may also be felt here.

Pulmonic Area—The Left 2nd Interspace. This interspace overlies the *pulmonary artery*. As the patient holds expiration, look and feel for an impulse and feel for transmitted heart sounds. In thin or shallow-chested patients, the pulsation of a pulmonary artery may sometimes be felt here, especially if patients are excited or examined after exercise.

A prominent pulsation here often accompanies dilatation or increased flow in the pulmonary artery. A palpable S₂ suggests increased pressure in the pulmonary artery (*pulmonary hypertension*).

Aortic Area—The Right 2nd Interspace. This interspace overlies the aortic outflow tract. Search for pulsations and palpable heart sounds.

A palpable S₂ suggests systemic *hypertension*. A pulsation here suggests a dilated or aneurysmal aorta.

Percussion

Palpation has replaced percussion in the estimation of cardiac size. When you cannot feel the apical impulse, however, percussion may be your only option, although it is not always reliable. Under these circumstances, cardiac dullness can occupy a large area. Starting well to the left on the chest, percuss from resonance toward cardiac dullness in the 3rd, 4th, 5th, and possibly 6th interspaces.

A markedly dilated failing heart may have a hypokinetic apical impulse that is displaced far to the left. A large pericardial effusion may make the impulse undetectable.

Auscultation

Overview. Auscultation of heart sounds and murmurs is an important skill in the physical examination that leads directly to important clinical diagnoses. The American College of Cardiology and the American Heart Association advocate cardiac auscultation as "the most widely used method of screening for valvular heart disease."[98]

In this section, you will learn the techniques for identifying S_1 and S_2, extra sounds in systole and diastole, and systolic and diastolic murmurs. Review the auscultatory areas on the next page with the following caveats: (1) many authorities discourage use of names such as "aortic area," because murmurs may be loudest in other areas; and (2) these areas may not apply to patients with cardiac enlargment, anomalies of the great vessels, or dextrocardia. It is best to use locations such as "base of the heart," apex, or parasternal border to describe your findings.

"Inching" Your Stethoscope. In a quiet room, listen to the heart with your stethoscope, starting at either the base or apex. Either pattern is satisfactory.

● Some experts recommend *starting at the apex and inching to the base*: Move the stethoscope from the PMI medially to the left sternal border, superiorly to the 2nd interspace, then across the sternum to the 2nd interspace at the right sternal border.

● Alternatively, you can *start at the base and inch your stethoscope to the apex*: with your stethoscope in the right 2nd interspace close to the sternum, move along the left sternal border in each interspace from the 2nd through the 5th, and then to the apex.

The Importance of Timing S_1 and S_2. Regardless of the direction you move your stethoscope, keep your left index and middle fingers on the right carotid artery in the lower third of the neck to facilitate correct identification of S_1, just before the carotid upstroke, and S_2, which follows the carotid upstroke. Be sure to compare the intensities of S_1 and S_2 as you move your stethoscope through the listening areas above.

● At the base, you will note that S_2 is louder than S_1 and may split with respiration. At the apex, S_1 is usually louder than S_2 unless the PR interval is prolonged.

● By carefully noting the intensities of S_1 and S_2, you will confirm each of these sounds and thereby correctly identify *systole*, the interval between S_1 and S_2, and *diastole*, the interval between S_2 and S_1.

As you will observe when listening to the extra sounds of S_3 and S_4 and to murmurs, timing systole and diastole is an absolute prerequisite to the correct identification of these events in the cardiac cycle.

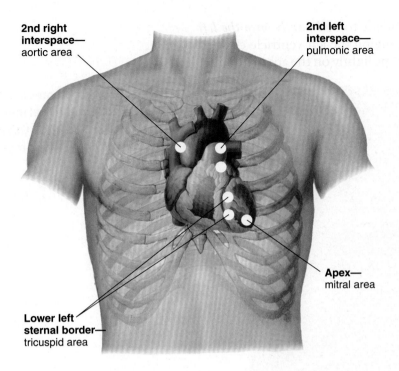

2nd right interspace—aortic area

2nd left interspace—pulmonic area

Apex—mitral area

Lower left sternal border—tricuspid area

Heart sounds and murmurs that originate in the four valves radiate widely, as illustrated below. Use anatomical location rather than valve area to describe where murmurs and sounds are best heard.

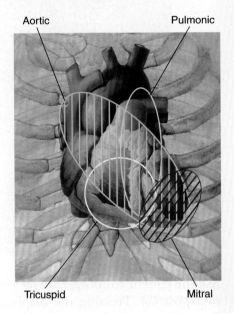

Aortic   Pulmonic

Tricuspid   Mitral

Know Your Stethoscope! It is important to understand the uses of both the diaphragm and the bell.

- *The diaphragm.* The diaphragm is better for picking up the relatively high-pitched sounds of S_1 and S_2, the murmurs of aortic and mitral regurgitation, and pericardial friction rubs. *Listen throughout the precordium* with the diaphragm, pressing it firmly against the chest.

- *The bell.* The bell is more sensitive to the low-pitched sounds of S_3 and S_4 and the murmur of mitral stenosis. Apply the bell lightly, with just enough pressure to produce an air seal with its full rim. *Use the bell at the apex, then move medially along the lower sternal border.* Resting the heel of your hand on the chest like a fulcrum may help you to maintain light pressure.

Pressing the bell firmly on the chest makes it function more like the diaphragm by stretching the underlying skin. Low-pitched sounds such as S_3 and S_4 may disappear with this technique—an observation that may help to identify them. In contrast, high-pitched sounds such as a midsystolic click, an ejection sound, or an opening snap will persist or get louder.

Listen to the entire precordium with the patient supine. For new patients and patients needing a complete cardiac examination, use two other maneuvers to listen for mitral stenosis and aortic regurgitation.

A wide array of stethoscopes are available. Learn about the various types before you purchase this expensive instrument. Some are "tunable," allowing you to vary the pressure on the diaphragm to alter its acoustic characteristics; others are electronic and can amplify and even digitally record auscultatory events.

Two Important Maneuvers.   Ask the patient to *roll partly onto the left side into the left lateral decubitus position*, bringing the left ventricle close to the chest wall. Place the bell of your stethoscope lightly on the apical impulse.

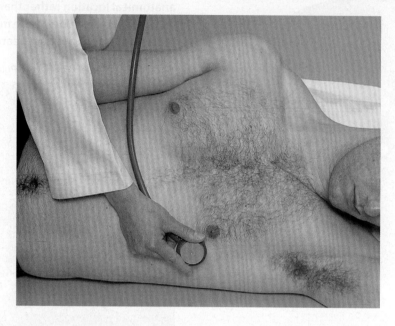

This position accentuates a left-sided S_3 and S_4 and mitral murmurs, especially *mitral stenosis*. Otherwise, you may miss these important findings.

Ask the patient to *sit up, lean forward, exhale completely, and stop breathing in expiration*. Pressing the diaphragm of your stethoscope on the chest, listen along the left sternal border and at the apex, pausing periodically so the patient may breathe.

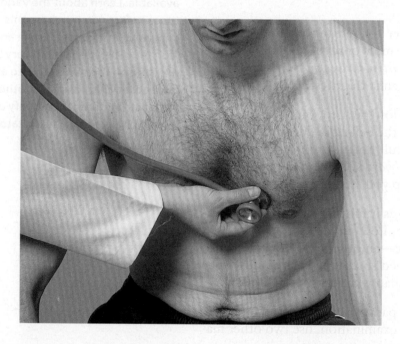

This position accentuates aortic murmurs. You may easily miss the soft diastolic murmur of *aortic regurgitation* unless you listen at this position.

Listening for Heart Sounds.   Throughout your examination, take your time at each auscultatory area. Concentrate on each of the events in the cardiac cycle, listening carefully to S_1, then S_2, then events occurring in systole and diastole. These events are described in the pages that follow.

Correctly Identifying Heart Murmurs.   Correctly identifying heart murmurs is a diagnostic challenge. A logical and systematic approach, a thorough understanding of cardiac anatomy and physiology, and, *above all, your dedication to the study, practice, and mastery of techniques of examination and the tables in this chapter will lead to your success.* Whenever possible, compare your findings with those of an experienced clinician to improve your clinical acumen. Review the tips for identifying heart murmurs summarized in the following table, and then study the following sections carefully for more detail. Reinforce your learning by listening to heart sound recordings, a proven method for increasing accurate identification of heart murmurs.[12]

Auscultatory Sounds

Heart Sounds	Guides to Auscultation
S_1	Note its intensity and any apparent splitting. Normal splitting is detectable along the lower left sternal border.
S_2	Note its intensity.
Split S_2	Listen for splitting of this sound in the 2nd and 3rd left interspaces. Ask the patient to breathe quietly, and then slightly more deeply than normal. Does S_2 split into its two components, as it normally does? If not, ask the patient to (1) breathe a little more deeply, or (2) sit up. Listen again. A thick chest wall may make the pulmonic component of S_2 inaudible.
	Width of split. How wide is the split? It is normally quite narrow.
	Timing of split. When in the respiratory cycle do you hear the split? It is normally heard late in inspiration.
	Does the split disappear as it should, during exhalation? If not, listen again with the patient sitting up.
	Intensity of A_2 and P_2. Compare the intensity of the two components, A_2 and P_2; A_2 is usually louder.
Extra Sounds in Systole	Such as ejection sounds or systolic clicks
	Note their location, timing, intensity, and pitch, and the effects of respiration on the sounds.
Extra Sounds in Diastole	Such as S_3, S_4, or an opening snap
	Note the location, timing, intensity, and pitch, and the effects of respiration on the sounds. An S_3 or S_4 in athletes is a normal finding.
Systolic and Diastolic Murmurs	Murmurs are differentiated from S_1, S_2 and extra sounds by their longer duration.

See Table 9-5, Variations in the First Heart Sound—S_1, p. 395. Note that S_1 is louder at more rapid heart rates, and PR intervals are shorter.

See Table 9-6, Variations in the Second Heart Sound—S_2, p. 396.

When either A_2 or P_2 is absent, as in disease of the respective valves, S_2 is persistently single.

Expiratory splitting suggests an abnormality (p. 396).

Persistent splitting results from delayed closure of the pulmonic valve or early closure of the aortic valve.

A loud P_2 suggests pulmonary hypertension.

The systolic click of mitral valve prolapse is the most common of these sounds. See Table 9-7, Extra Heart Sounds in Systole, p. 397.

See Table 9-8, Extra Heart Sounds in Diastole, p. 398.

See Table 9-9, Pansystolic (Holosystolic) Murmurs, p. 399; Table 9-10, Midsystolic Murmurs, pp. 400–401; and Table 9-11, Diastolic Murmurs, p. 402.

- *Timing.* First decide if you are hearing a *systolic murmur*, falling between S_1 and S_2, or a *diastolic murmur*, falling between S_2 and S_1. Palpating the carotid pulse as you listen can help you with timing. *Murmurs that coincide with the carotid upstroke are systolic.*

Systolic murmurs are usually *midsystolic* or *pansystolic*. Late systolic murmurs may also be heard. Early systolic murmurs are uncommon and are not depicted below.

Diastolic murmurs usually indicate valvular heart disease. Systolic murmurs may indicate valvular disease but often occur when the heart valves are normal.

Murmurs detected during pregnancy should be promptly evaluated for possible risk to the pregnancy and the need for termination, especially from *aortic stenosis* and *pulmonary hypertension*.

Tips for Identifying Heart Murmurs

▶ Time the murmur—is it in systole or diastole?
▶ Locate where the murmur is loudest on the precordium—at the base, along the sternal border, at the apex?
▶ Conduct any necessary maneuvers, such as having the patient lean forward and exhale or turn to the left lateral decubitus position.
▶ Determine the shape of the murmur—for example, is it crescendo or decrescendo, is it holosystolic?
▶ Grade the intensity of the murmur from 1 to 6.
▶ Identify associated features such as the quality of S_1 and S_2, the presence of extra sounds such as S_3, S_4, or an opening snap, or the presence of additional murmurs.
▶ Be sure you are listening in a quiet room!

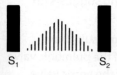

A *midsystolic murmur* begins after S_1 and stops before S_2. Brief gaps are audible between the murmur and the heart sounds. Listen carefully for the gap just before S_2. It is heard more easily and, if present, usually confirms the murmur as midsystolic, not pansystolic.

Midsystolic murmurs typically arise from blood flow across the semilunar (aortic and pulmonic) valves. See Table 9-10, Midsystolic Murmurs, pp. 400–401.

A *pansystolic (holosystolic) murmur* starts with S_1 and stops at S_2, without a gap between murmur and heart sounds.

Pansystolic murmurs often occur with regurgitant (backward) flow across the atrioventricular valves. See Table 9-9, Pansystolic (Holosystolic) Murmurs, p. 399.

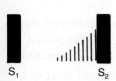

A *late systolic murmur* usually starts in mid- or late systole and persists up to S_2.

This is the murmur of mitral valve prolapse and is often, but not always, preceded by a systolic click (see p. 397).

Diastolic murmurs may be *early diastolic, middiastolic,* or *late diastolic.*

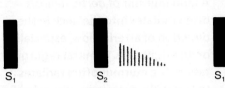

An *early diastolic murmur* starts immediately after S₂, without a discernible gap, and then usually fades into silence before the next S₁.

Early diastolic murmurs typically accompany regurgitant flow across incompetent semilunar valves.

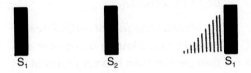

A *middiastolic murmur* starts a short time after S₂. It may fade away, as illustrated, or merge into a late diastolic murmur.

Middiastolic and presystolic murmurs reflect turbulent flow across the atrioventricular valves. See Table 9-11, Diastolic Murmurs, p. 402.

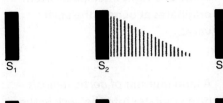

A *late diastolic (presystolic) murmur* starts late in diastole and typically continues up to S₁.

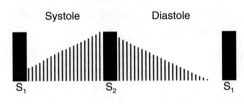

A *continuous murmur* begins in systole and extends into all or part of diastole.

Congenital *patent ductus arteriosus* and *AV fistulas,* common in dialysis patients, produce continuous murmurs. Neither is valvular in origin. Venous hums and pericardial friction rubs also have both systolic and diastolic components. See Table 9-12, Cardiovascular Sounds with Both Systolic and Diastolic Components, p. 403.

- *Shape.* The shape or configuration of a murmur is determined by its intensity over time.

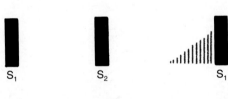

A *crescendo murmur* grows louder.

Note the presystolic murmur of *mitral stenosis* in normal sinus rhythm.

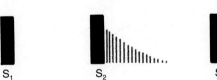

A *decrescendo murmur* grows softer.

Note the early diastolic murmur of *aortic regurgitation.*

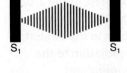

A *crescendo–decrescendo murmur* first rises in intensity, then falls.

Listen for the midsystolic murmur of *aortic stenosis* and *innocent flow murmurs.*

A *plateau murmur* has the same intensity throughout.

Note the pansystolic murmur of *mitral regurgitation.*

● *Location of Maximal Intensity.* This is determined by the site where the murmur originates. Find the location by exploring the area where you hear the murmur. Describe where you hear it best in terms of the interspace and its relation to the sternum, the apex, or the midsternal, the midclavicular, or one of the axillary lines.

For example, a murmur best heard in the 2nd right interspace often originates at or near the aortic valve.

● *Radiation or Transmission From the Point of Maximal Intensity.* This reflects not only the site of origin but also the intensity of the murmur, the direction of blood flow, and bone conduction in the thorax. Explore the area around a murmur and determine where else you can hear it.

A loud murmur of *aortic stenosis* often radiates into the neck in the direction of arterial flow, especially on the right side. In mitral regurgitation, the murmur often radiates to the axilla, suggesting the role of bone conduction.[99]

● *Intensity.* This is usually graded on a 6-point scale and expressed as a fraction. The numerator describes the intensity of the murmur wherever it is loudest; the denominator indicates the scale you are using. Intensity is influenced by the thickness of the chest wall and the presence of intervening tissue.

An identical degree of turbulence would cause a louder murmur in a thin person than in a very muscular or obese person. Emphysematous lungs may diminish the intensity of murmurs.

Learn to grade murmurs using the 6-point scale below. Note that grades 4 through 6 require the added presence of a palpable thrill.

Gradations of Murmurs

Grade	Description
Grade 1	Very faint, heard only after listener has "tuned in"; may not be heard in all positions
Grade 2	Quiet, but heard immediately after placing the stethoscope on the chest
Grade 3	Moderately loud
Grade 4	Loud, with *palpable thrill*
Grade 5	Very loud, with *thrill*. May be heard when the stethoscope is partly off the chest
Grade 6	Very loud, with *thrill*. May be heard with stethoscope entirely off the chest

● *Pitch.* This is categorized as high, medium, or low.

● *Quality.* This is described in terms such as blowing, harsh, rumbling, and musical.

A fully described murmur might be: a "medium-pitched, grade 2/6, blowing decrescendo diastolic murmur, heard best in the 4th left interspace, with radiation to the apex" (*aortic regurgitation*).

Other useful characteristics of murmurs, and also heart sounds, include variation with respiration, with the position of the patient, or with other special maneuvers.

Murmurs originating in the right side of the heart tend to vary with respiration more than left-sided murmurs.

INTEGRATING CARDIOVASCULAR ASSESSMENT

A good cardiovascular examination requires more than observation. You need to think about the possible meanings of your individual observations, fit them together in a logical pattern, and correlate your cardiac findings with the patient's blood pressure, arterial pulses, venous pulsations, jugular venous pressure, the remainder of your physical examination findings, and the patient's history.

Evaluating the common systolic murmur illustrates this point. In examining an asymptomatic teenager, for example, you might hear a grade 2/6 mid-systolic murmur in the 2nd and 3rd left interspaces. Because this suggests a murmur of pulmonic origin, you should assess the size of the right ventricle by carefully palpating the left parasternal area. Because pulmonic stenosis and atrial septal defects can occasionally cause such murmurs, listen carefully to the splitting of the second heart sound and for any ejection sounds. Listen to the murmur after the patient sits up. Look for evidence of anemia, hyperthyroidism, or pregnancy that could produce such a murmur by increasing the flow across the aortic or the pulmonic valve. If all your findings are normal, your patient probably has an *innocent* or *functional murmur*— one with no pathologic significance.

Functional murmurs are short, early, midsystolic murmurs that decrease in intensity with maneuvers that reduce left ventricular volume, such as standing, sitting up, and straining during the Valsalva maneuver. These murmurs are often heard in healthy patients and are not pathologic.

In a 60-year-old person with angina, you might hear a harsh 3/6 mid-systolic crescendo–decrescendo murmur in the right 2nd interspace radiating to the neck. These findings suggest *aortic stenosis* but could arise from *aortic sclerosis* (leaflets sclerotic but not stenotic), a dilated aorta, or increased flow across a normal valve. Assess any delay in the carotid upstroke and the intensity of A_2 for evidence of *aortic stenosis*. Check the apical impulse for left ventricular hypertrophy. Listen for *aortic regurgitation* as the patient leans forward and exhales.

Put all this information together to make a hypothesis about the origin of the murmur.

SPECIAL TECHNIQUES

Maneuvers to Identify Systolic Murmurs and Heart Failure. Earlier in this chapter, you learned how to improve your auscultation of heart sounds and murmurs by placing the patient in different positions. Two additional maneuvers help you distinguish the murmurs of mitral valve prolapse and hypertrophic cardiomyopathy from aortic stenosis.

(1) Standing and Squatting. When a person stands, venous return to the heart decreases, as does peripheral vascular resistance. Arterial blood pressure, stroke volume, and the volume of blood in the left ventricle all decline. When squatting, changes occur in the opposite direction. These changes help (1) to identify a prolapsed mitral valve and (2) to distinguish hypertrophic cardiomyopathy from aortic stenosis.

Secure the patient's gown so that it will not interfere with your examination, and prepare yourself for prompt auscultation. Instruct the patient to squat next to the examining table and hold on to it for balance. Listen to the heart with the patient in the squatting position and again in the standing position.

Maneuvers to Identify Systolic Murmurs

Maneuver	Cardiovascular Effect	Effect on Systolic Sounds and Murmurs		
		Mitral Valve Prolapse	Hypertrophic Cardiomyopathy	Aortic Stenosis
Squatting; Valsalva: Release Phase	Increased left ventricular volume from ↑ venous return to heart	↓ prolapse of mitral valve	↓ outflow obstruction	↑ blood volume ejected into aorta
	Increased vascular tone: ↑ arterial blood pressure; ↑ peripheral vascular resistance	Delay of click and murmur shortens	↓ intensity of murmur	↑ intensity of murmur
Standing; Valsalva: Strain Phase	Decreased left ventricular volume from ↓ venous return to heart	↑ prolapse of mitral valve	↑ outflow obstruction	↓ blood volume ejected into aorta
	Decreased vascular tone: ↓ arterial blood pressure	Click moves earlier in systole and murmur lengthens	↑ intensity of murmur	↓ intensity of murmur

(2) Valsalva Maneuver. The Valsalva maneuver involves forcible exhalation against a closed glottis causing increased intrathoracic pressure. The normal blood pressure response follows four phases: (1) transient increase during onset of the "strain" phase when the patient bears down; (2) normalization during the "strain" phase; (3) drop of both blood pressure and left ventricular volume during the "release" phase; and (4) "overshoot" several seconds later. This maneuver has several uses at the bedside.

To distinguish the murmur of *hypertrophic cardiomyopathy*, ask the supine patient to "bear down," or place one hand on the midabdomen and ask the patient to strain against it. Use you other hand to place your stethoscope on the patient's chest and listen in the area of the lower left sterna border.

The murmur of *hypertrophic cardiomyopathy* is the only systolic murmur that increases during the "strain phase" of the Valsalva maneuver due to increased outflow tract obstruction.[100]

The Valsalva maneuver can also identify *heart failure* and *pulmonary hypertension*. Inflate the blood pressure cuff to 15 mm Hg greater than the systolic blood pressure and ask the patient to perform the Valsalva maneuver for 10 seconds, then resume normal respiration. Keep the cuff pressure locked at 15 mm Hg above the baseline systolic pressure during the entire maneuver and for 30 seconds afterward. Listen for Korotkoff sounds over the brachial artery throughout. Typically only phases 2 and 4 are significant, since phases 1 and 3 are too short for clinical detection. *In healthy patients, phase 2, the "strain" phase, is silent and Korotkoff sounds are heard after straining is released, or during phase 4.*

In patients with *severe heart failure*, Korotkoff sounds are heard during the phase 2 strain phase, but not during phase 4 release, termed *"the square wave" response.* This response is highly correlated with volume overload and elevated left ventricular end-diastolic pressure and pulmonary capillary wedge pressure, in some studies outperforming brain natriuretic peptide.[101,102]

(3) Isometric Handgrip. Isometric handgrip increases the systolic murmurs of mitral regurgitation, aortic regurgitation, and ventricular septal defect, and also the diastolic murmurs of pulmonic stenosis and mitral stenosis.[98]

(4) Transient Arterial Occlusion. Transient compression of both arms by bilateral blood pressure cuff inflation to 20 mm Hg greater that peak systolic blood pressure augments the murmurs of mitral regurgitation, aortic regurgitation, and ventricular septal defect.[98]

Recording Your Findings

Note that initially you may use sentences to describe your findings; later you will use phrases. The style below contains phrases appropriate for most write-ups.

Recording the Physical Examination—The Cardiovascular Examination

"The jugular venous pulse (JVP) is 3 cm above the sternal angle with the head of bed elevated to 30 degrees. Carotid upstrokes are brisk, without bruits. The point of maximal impulse (PMI) is tapping, 7 cm lateral to the midsternal line in the 5th intercostal space. Crisp S_1 and S_2. At the base, S_2 is greater than S_1 and physiologically split, with $A_2 > P_2$. At the apex, S_1 is greater than S_2 and constant. No murmurs or extra sounds."

OR

"The JVP is 5 cm above the sternal angle with the head of bed elevated to 50 degrees. Carotid upstrokes are brisk; a bruit is heard over the left carotid artery. The PMI is diffuse, 3 cm in diameter, palpated at the anterior axillary line in the 5th and 6th intercostal spaces. S_1 and S_2 are soft. S_3 present at the apex. High-pitched harsh 2/6 holosystolic murmur best heard at the apex, radiating to the axilla."

This suggests *heart failure with volume overload* with possible *left carotid occlusion* and *mitral regurgitation*.[84,103,104]

Bibliography

Citations

1. Markel H. The stethoscope and the art of listening. N Engl J Med 2006;354:551–552.
2. Simel DS. Time, now, to recover the fun in the physical examination rather than abandon it. Arch Intern Med 2006;166(6):603–604.
3. Mangione S. Cardiac auscultatory skills of physicians-in-training: a comparison of three English-speaking countries. Am J Med 2001;110(3):210–216.
4. Mangione S. Cardiac auscultatory skills of internal medicine and family practice trainees. A comparison of diagnostic proficiency. JAMA 1997;278(9):717–722.
5. Mangione S. The teaching and practice of cardiac auscultation during internal medicine and cardiology training. Ann Intern Med 1993;119(1):47–54.
6. RuDusky BM. Auscultation and Don Quixote. Chest 2005;127:1869–1870.
7. Marcus G, Vessey J, Jordan MV et al. Relationship between accurate auscultation of a clinically useful third heart sound and level of experience. Arch Intern Med 2006;166:617–622.
8. Vukanovic-Criley JM, Criley S, Warde CM et al. Competency in cardiac examination skills in medical students, trainees,

physicians, and faculty. A multicenter study. Arch Intern Med 2006;166:610–616.

9. Wayne DB, Butter J, Cohen ER et al. Setting defensible standards for cardiac auscultation skills in medical students. Acad Med 2009;84(10 Suppl):S94–S96.

10. Saxena A, Barrett MJ, Patel AR et al. Merging old school methods with new technology to improve skills in cardiac auscultation. Semin Med Pract 2008;11:21–26.

11. Vukanovic-Criley JM, Boker JR, Criley SR et al. Using virtual patients to improve cardiac examination competency in medical students. Clin Cardiol 2008;31:334–339.

12. Barrett MJ, Lacey CS, Sekara AE et al. Mastering cardiac murmurs. The power of repetition. Chest 2004;126:470–475.

13. Michaels AD, Khan FU, Moyers B. Experienced clinicians improve detection of third and fourth heart sounds by viewing acoustic cardiography. Clin Cardiol 2010;33:E36–E42.

14. University of Washington Department of Medicine. Advanced physical diagnosis. Examination for heart sounds and lung sounds. Available at http://depts.washington.edu/physdx/heart/index.html. Accessed May 24, 2011.

15. Lee E, Michaels AD, Selvester RH et al. Frequency of diastolic third and fourth heart sounds with myocardial ischemia induced during percutaneous coronary intervention. J Electrocardiol 2009;42:39–45.

16. McGee S. Evidence-Based Physical Diagnosis. St. Louis: Saunders, 2007.

17. Shah SJ, Michaels AD. Hemodynamic correlates of the third heart sound and systolic time intervals. CHF 2006;12 (4 suppl 1):8–13.

18. Shah SJ, Marcus GM, Gerber IL et al. Physiology of the third heart sound: novel insights from tissue Doppler imaging. J Am Soc Echocardiogr 2008;21394–400.

19. Shah SJ, Nakamura K, Marcus GM et al. Association of the fourth heart sound with increased left ventricular end-diastolic stiffness. J Card Fail 2008;14:431–436.

20. O'Rourke RA, Braunwald E. Ch 209, Physical examination of the cardiovascular system in Harrison's Principles of Internal Medicine, 16th ed. New York: McGraw-Hill, 2005, p.1307.

21. Hunt SA, Abraham WT, Chin MH et al. ACC/AHA 2005 guideline update for the diagnosis and management of chronic heart failure in the adult—summary article. Circulation 2005;112:154–235.

22. Vinayak AG, Levitt J, Gehlbach B et al. Usefulness of the external jugular vein examination in detecting abnormal central venous pressure in critically ill patients. Arch Int Med 2006;166:2132–2137.

23. Roger VL, Go AS, Lloyd-Jones DM et al. Heart disease and stroke statistics–2011 update: a report from the American Heart Association. Circulation 2011;123:e18–e209. Available at http://circ.ahajournals.org/cgi/reprint/CIR.0b013e3182009701. Accessed April 13, 2011.

24. Abrams J. Chronic stable angina. N Engl J Med 2005;352:2524–2533.

25. Woo KM, Schneider JI. High-risk chief complaints I: chest pain–the big three. Emerg Med Clin North Am 2009;27:685–712.

26. Goldman L, Kirtane AJ. Triage of patient with acute chest syndrome and possible cardiac ischemia: the elusive search for diagnostic perfection. Ann Intern Med 2003;139:987–995.

27. Khan IA, Nair CK. Clinical, diagnostic, and management perspectives of aortic dissection. Chest 2002;122:311–328.

28. Eagle KA, Lim MJ, Dabbous OH et al. GRACE Investigators. A validated prediction model for all forms of acute coronary syndrome: estimating the risk of 6-month postdischarge death in an international registry. JAMA 2004;291:2727–2733.

29. Dey S, Flather MD, Devlin GP et al. Sex-related differences in the presentation, treatment and outcomes among patients with acute coronary syndromes. Heart 2009;95:20–26.

30. McSweeney JC, Cleves MA, Zhao W et al. cluster analysis of women's prodromal and acute myocardial infarction symptoms by race and other characteristics. J Cardiovasc Nurs 2010;25:311–322.

31. Canto JG, Goldberg RJ, Hand MM et al. Symptom presentation of women with acute coronary syndromes: myth vs. reality. Arch Intern Med 2007;167:2405–2413.

32. Phan A, Shyfelt C, Merz CN. Persistent chest pain and no obstructive coronary artery disease. JAMA 2009;301:1468–1474.

33. Carnici PG, Crea F. Coronary microvascular dysfunction. N Engl J Med 2007;356:830–840.

34. Klompas M. Does this patient have an acute thoracic aortic dissection? JAMA 2002;287(17):2262–2272.

35. Cho S, Atwood JE. Peripheral edema. Am J Med 2002;113:580–586.

36. Koh H. A 2020 vision for healthy people. N Engl J Med 2010;362;1653–1656.

37. Hettema J, Steele J, Miller WR. Motivational Interviewing. Ann Rev Clin Psych 2005;1:91–111.

38. U.S. Preventive Services Task Force. Aspirin for the primary prevention of cardiovascular disease: A U.S. Preventive Services Task Force recommendation statement. Ann Intern Med 2009;150:396–404.

39. Wolff T, Miller T, Ko S. Aspirin for the primary prevention of cardiovascular events: An update of the evidence for the U.S. Preventive Services Task Force. Ann Intern Med 2009;150:405–410.

40. Greenland PAlpert JS, Beller GA et al. 2010 ACCF/AHA guideline for assessment of cardiovascular risk in asymptomatic adults: A report of the American College of Cardiology Foundation/American Heart Association Task Force on Practice Guidelines. J Am Coll Cardiol 2010; 56:e50.

41. Mosca L, Benjamin EJ, Berra K et al. Effectiveness-based guidelines for the prevention of cardiovascular disease in women—2011 update: A guideline from the American Heart Association. Circulation 2011;123:1243–1262.

42. Flack JM, Sica DA, Bakris G et al. Management of high blood pressure in blacks. An update of the International Society on Hypertension in Blacks Consensus Statement. Hypertension 2010;56:780–800.

43. Goldstein LB, Bushnell CD, Adams RJ et al on behalf of the American Heart Association Stroke Council, Council on Cardiovascular Nursing Council on Epidemiology and Prevention Council for High Blood Pressure Research, Council on Peripheral Vascular Disease, and Interdisciplinary Council on Quality of Care and Outcomes Research. AHA/ASA

Guideline. Guidelines for the Primary Prevention of Stroke. A Guideline for Healthcare Professionals from the American Heart Association/American Stroke Association. Stroke 2011;42:517–584.

44. Towfighi A, Zheng L, Ovbiagele B. Sex-specific trends in midlife coronary heart disease risk and prevalence. Arch Intern Med 2009;169:1762–1766.

45. Vaccarino V, Parsons L, Peterson ED et al. Sex differences in mortality after acute myocardial infarction. Changes from 1994 to 2006. Arch Intern Med 2009;169:1767–1774.

46. Towfighi A, Markovic D, Ovbiagele B. Persistent sex disparity in midlife stroke prevalence in the United States. Cerebrovasc Dis 2011;31:322–328.

47. Towfighi A, Saver JL, Engelhardt R, Ovbiagele B. A midlife stroke surge among women in the United States. Neurology 2007;69:1898–1904.

48. Lloyd-Jones DM, Leip EP, Larson MG, et al. Prediction of lifetime risk for cardiovascular disease by risk factor burden at 50 years of age. Circulation 2006;(6):791–798.

49. U.S. Preventive Services Task Force. Screening for high blood pressure: recommendations and rationale. Am J Prev Med 2003;25:159–164.

50. Chobanion AV, Bakris GL, Black HR et al. The Seventh Report of the Joint National Committee on Prevention, Detection, Evaluation, and Treatment of High Blood Pressure—The JNC 7 Report. JAMA 2003;289:2560–2572. Available at http://www.nhlbi.nih.gov/guidelines/hypertension. Accessed April 24, 2011.

51. Whelton PK, He J, Appel LJ et al. Primary prevention of hypertension. Clinical and public health advisory from the National High Blood Pressure Education Program. JAMA 2002;288:1882–1888.

52. U.S. Preventive Services Task Force. Screening for high blood pressure: U.S. Preventive Services Task Force reaffirmation recommendation statement. Ann Intern Med 2007;147:783–786.

53. Wolff T, Miller T. Evidence for the reaffirmation of the U.S. Preventive Services Task Force recommendation on screening for high blood pressure. Ann Intern Med 2007;147:787–791.

54. Vasan RS, Larson MG, Leip EP et al. Impact of high-normal blood pressure on the risk of cardiovascular disease. N Engl J Med 2001;345:1291–1297.

55. Appel LJ, Frohlich ED, Hall JE, Pearson TA, Sacco RL, Seals DR, Sacks FM, Smith SC Jr, Vafiadis DK, Van Horn LV. The importance of population-wide sodium reduction as a means to prevent cardiovascular disease and stroke: a call to action from the American Heart Association. Circulation 2011;123:1138–1143.

56. American Diabetes Association. Standards of medical care in diabetes—2011. Diabetes Care 2011;34:S1–S61.

57. National Cholesterol Education Panel. Third Report of the National Cholesterol Education Program (NCEP) Expert Panel on detection, evaluation, and treatment of high blood cholesterol in adults (Adult Treatment Panel III) final report. Circulation 2002;106:3143–3421. Also available at http://www.nhlbi.nih.gov/guidelines/cholesterol/atp3_rpt.htm. Accessed May 6 2011.

58. Grundy SM, Cleeman JI, Merz NB et al, for the Coordinating Committee of the National Cholesterol Education Program. Implications of recent clinical trials for the National Cholesterol Education Program Adult Treatment Panel III guidelines. Circulation 2004;110:227–239.

59. U.S. Preventive Services Task Force. Screening for lipid disorders in adults. June 2008. Avalable at http://www.uspreventiveservicestaskforce.org/uspstf/uspschol.htm. Accessed May 6 2011.

60. Gaziano JM, Gaziano TA. Simplifying the approach to the management of dyslipidemia. JAMA 2009;302:2148–2149.

61. Kuklina EV, Yoon PW, Keenan NL. Trends in high levels of low-density lipoprotein cholesterol in the United States, 1999–2006. JAMA 2009;302:2104–2110.

62. Cheung BMY and Lam KSL. Is intensive LDL-cholesterol lowering beneficial and safe? Lancet 2010;376:1622–1624.

63. Cholesterol Treatment Trialists' (CTT) Collaboration. Efficacy and safety of more intensive lowering of LDL cholesterol: A meta-analysis of data from 170,000 participants in 26 randomised trials. Lancet2010;376:1670–1681.

64. Study of the Effectiveness of Additional Reductions in Cholesterol and Homocysteine (SEARCH) Collaborative Group. Intensive lowering of LDL cholesterol with 80 mg versus 20 mg simvastatin daily in 12,064 survivors of myocardial infarction: A double-blind randomised trial. Lancet 2010;376:1658–1669.

65. Hingorani AD, Psaty BM. Primary prevention of cardiovascular disease. Time to get more or less personal? JAMA 2009;302:2144–2145.

66. Alberti K, Eckel RH, Grundy SM et al. Harmonizing the metabolic syndrome: a joint interim statement of the Internal Diabetes Federation Task Force on Epidemiology and Prevention; National Heart, Lung, and Blood Institute; American Heart Association; World Heart Federation; Internal Atherosclerosis Society; and Internal Association for the Study of Obesity. Circulation 2009;120:1640–1645.

67. Institute of Medicine. Leading health indicators for Healthy People 2020. March 2011. Available at http://www.iom.edu/~/media/Files/Report%20Files/2011/Leading-Health-Indicators-for-Healthy-People-2020/Leading%20Health%20Indicators%202011%20Report%20Brief.pdf. Accessed May 6, 2011.

68. Norcross JC and Prochaska JO. Using the stages of change. Harvard Mental Health Letter, May 2002, pp. 5–7.

69. Fiore MC, Jaen CS, Baker TM et al. Treating tobacco use and dependence: 2008 update. Clinical Practice Guidelines. Rockville, MD. US Dept of Health and Human Services. Public Health Service. May 2008.

70. Healthy People 2010. Progress review—nutrition and overweight. U.S. Department of Health and Human Services—Public Health Service. January 21, 2004. Available at: http://www.healthypeople.gov/data/2010prog/focus19/default.htm. Accessed November 27, 2007.

71. Healthy People 2010. Progress review—physical activity and fitness. U.S. Department of Health and Human Services—Public Health Service. April 14, 2004. Available at: http://www.healthypeople.gov/data/2010prog/focus22/. Accessed November 27, 2007.

72. The Rational Clinical Examination Series, JAMA. Available at http://jama.ama-assn.org/cgi/collection/rational_clinical_exam. Accessed May 6, 2011.

73. Beevers G, Lip GY, O'Brien E. ABC of hypertension. Blood pressure measurement. Part I. Sphygmomanometry: factors common in all techniques. BMJ 2001;322:981–985.

74. Beevers G, Lip GY, O'Brien E. ABC of hypertension. Blood pressure measurement. Part II Conventional sphygmomanometry: technique of auscultatory blood pressure measurement. BMJ 2001;322:1043–1047.

75. McAlister FA, Straus SE. Evidence-based treatment of hypertension. Measurement of blood pressure: an evidence based review. BMJ 2001;322:908–911.

76. Tholl U, Forstner K, Anlauf M. Measuring blood pressure: pitfalls and recommendations. Nephrol Dial Transplant 2004; 19:766–770.

77. Myers MG, Godwin M, Dawes M et al. Measurement of blood pressure in the office—recognizing the problem and proposing the solution. Hypertension 2010;55:195–200.

78. Myers MG. Recent advances in automated blood pressure measurement. Curr Hypertens Rep 2008;10:355–358.

79. Landgraf J, Wishner SH, Kloner RA. Comparison of automated oscillometric versus auscultatory blood pressure measurement. Am J Cardiol 2010;106:386–388.

80. Ogedegbe G, Pickering TG, Clemow L et al. the misdiagnosis of hypertension: the role of patient anxiety. Arch Intern Med 2008;168:2459–2465.

81. Pickering TG, Hall JE, Appel LJ et al. Recommendations for blood pressure measurement in humans and experimental animals: part 1: blood pressure measurement in humans: a statement for professionals from the Subcommittee of Professional and Public Education of the American Heart Association Council on High Blood Pressure Research. Circulation 2005;111:697–716.

82. Cook DJ, Simel DL. Does this patient have abnormal central venous pressure? JAMA 1996;275:630–654.

83. Davison R, Cannon R. Estimation of central venous pressure by examination of jugular veins. Am Heart J 1974;87:279–282.

84. Hunt SA, Abraham WT, Chin MH et al. 2009 focused update incorporated into the ACC/AHA 2005 Guidelines for the Diagnosis and Management of Heart Failure in Adults: a report of the American College of Cardiology Foundation/American Heart Association Task Force on Practice Guidelines: developed in collaboration with the International Society for Heart and Lung Transplantation. Circulation 2009;119:e391–e479.

85. Drazner MH, Hellkamp AS, Leier CV et al. Value of clinician assessment of hemodynamics in advanced heart failure: the ESCAPE trial. Circ Heart Fail 2008;1:170–177.

86. Drazner MH, Rame E, Stevenson LW et al. Prognostic importance of elevated jugular venous pressure and a third heart sound in patients with heart failure. N Engl J Med 2001;345(8):574–581.

87. Badgett RG, Lucey CR, Muirow CD. Can the clinical examination diagnose left-sided heart failure in adults? JAMA 1997;277(21):1712–1719.

88. Khandaker MH, Espinosa RE, Nishimura RA et al. Pericardial disease: diagnosis and management. Mayo Clin Proc 2010;85:572–593.

89. Lange RA, Hillis LD. Acute pericarditis. N Engl J Med 2004; 351(21):2195–2202.

90. Wilson LD, Detterbeck FC, Yahalom J. Clinical practice. Superior vena cava syndrome with malignant causes. N Engl J Med 2007;356:1862–1869.

91. Leung CC, Moondra V, Catherwood E et al. Prevalence and risk factors of pulmonary hypertension in patients with elevated pulmonary venous pressure and preserved ejection fraction. Am J Cardiol 2010;106:284–286.

92. Sandercock PAG, Kavvadia E. The carotid bruit. Pract Neurol 2002;2:221–224.

93. Paraskevas KI, Hamilton G, Mikhailidis DP. Clinical significance of carotid bruits: an innocent finding or a useful warning sign? Neurol Res 2008;30:523–530.

94. Pickett CA, Jackson JL, Hemann BA et al. Carotid bruits and cerebrovascular disease risk: A meta-analysis. Stroke 2010;41: 2295–2302.

95. Pickett CA, Jackson JL, Hemann BA et al. Carotid bruits as a prognostic indicator of cardiovascular death and myocardial infarction: a meta-analysis. Lancet 2008;371(9624):1587–1594.

96. Sauve JS, Laupacis A, Feagan B et al. Does this patient have a clinically important carotid bruit? JAMA 1993;270:2843–2845.

97. Dans AL, Bossone EF, Guyatt GH et al. Evaluation of the reproducibility and accuracy of apex beat measurement in the detection of echocardiographic left ventricular dilation. Can J Cardiol 1995;11:493–407.

98. American College of Cardiology/American Heart Association Task Force on Practice Guidelines; Society of Cardiovascular Anesthesiologists; Society for Cardiovascular Angiography and Interventions; Society of Thoracic Surgeons et al. ACC/AHA 2006 guidelines for the management of patients with valvular heart disease: a report of the American College of Cardiology/ American Heart Association Task Force on Practice Guidelines (writing committee to revise the 1998 Guidelines for the Management of Patients With Valvular Heart Disease): developed in collaboration with the Society of Cardiovascular Anesthesiologists: endorsed by the Society for Cardiovascular Angiography and Interventions and the Society of Thoracic Surgeons. Circulation 2006;114:e84–e231.

99. McGee S. Etiology and diagnosis of systolic murmurs in adults. Am J Med 2010;123:913–921.

100. Lembo NJ, Dell'Italia LJ, Crawford MH et al. Bedside diagnosis of systolic murmurs. N Engl J Med 1988;318:1572–1578.

101. Felker GM, Cuculich PS, Gheorghiade M. The Valsalva maneuver: a bedside "biomarker" for heart failure. Am J Med 2006;119:117–122.

102. Opotowsky AR, Ojeda J, Rogers F et al. Blood pressure response to the Valsalva maneuver. A simple bedside test to determine the hemodynamic basis of pulmonary hypertension. Am Coll Cardiol 2010;56:1352–1353.

103. Fonarow GC. Epidemiology and risk stratification in acute heart failure. Am Heart J 2008;155:200–207.

104. McMurray JJ. Systolic heart failure. N Engl J Med 2010;362:228–238.

105. Siu SC, Silversides CK. Bicuspid aortic valve disease. J Am Coll Cardiol 2010;55:2789–2800.

106. Hayek E, Gring CN, Griffin BP. Mitral valve prolapse. Lancet 365:507–518, 2005.

107. Foster E. Mitral regurgitation due to degenerative mitral-valve disease. N Engl J Med 2010;363:156–165.

108. Enriquez-Sarano M, Akins CW, Vahanian A. Mitral regurgitation. Lancet 2009;373(9672):1382–1394.

109. Pierard LA, Lancellotti P. The role of ischemic mitral regurgitation in the pathogenesis of acute pulmonary edema. N Engl J Med 2004;351:1627–1634.

110. Otto CM. Evaluation and management of chronic mitral regurgitation. N Engl J Med 2001;345:740–746.

111. Etchells E, Bell C, and Robb K. Does this patient have an abnormal systolic murmur? JAMA 1997;277(7):564–571.

112. Etchells E, Glenns, Shadowitz S et al. A bedside clinical prediction rule for detecting moderate or severe aortic stenosis. J Gen Int Med 1998;13(10):699–704.

113. Ramaraj R, Sorrell VL. Degenerative aortic stenosis. BMJ 2008;336:550–556.

114. Iung B. Management of asymptomatic aortic stenosis. Heart 2011;97:253–259.

115. Ho CY, Seidman CE. A contemporary approach to hypertrophic cardiomyopathy. Circulation 2006;113:e858–e862.

116. Enriquez-Serano M, Tajik AJ. Aortic regurgitation. N Engl J Med 2004;351:1539–1546.

Additional References

Awtry EH, Philippides GJ. Alcoholic and cocaine-associated cardiomyopathies. Prog Cardiovasc Dis 2010;52:289–299.

Braunwald E, Bonow RO. Braunwald's Heart Disease: A Textbook of Cardiovascular Medicine, 9th ed. Philadelphia: Elsevier/Saunders, 2012.

Butman SM, Gordon AE, Standen JR et al. Bedside cardiovascular examination in patients with severe chronic heart failure: Importance of rest or inducible jugular venous distention. J Am Coll Cardiol 1993;22:968–974.

Cha K, Falk RH. Images in clinical medicine. Pulsus alternans. N Engl J Med 1996;334(13):834.

Chiuve SE, Fung TE, Rexrode KM et al. Adherence to a low-risk, healthy lifestyle and risk of sudden cardiac death among women. JAMA 2011;306:62–60.

Denardo SJ, Gong Y, Bucgiks FH et al. Blood pressure and outcomes in very old hypertensive coronary artery disease patients: An INVEST substudy. Am J Med 2010;123:719–726.

Devereux RB, Wachtell K, Gerdts E et al. Prognostic significance of left ventricular mass change during treatment of hypertension. JAMA 2004;292:2350–2356.

Emerging Risk Factors Collaboration, Kaptoge S, Di Angelantonio E et al. C-reactive protein concentration and risk of coronary heart disease, stroke, and mortality: an individual participant meta-analysis. Lancet 2010;375(9709):132–140.

Etchells E, Bell C, Robb K. Does this patient have an abnormal systolic murmur? JAMA 1997;277:564–571.

Goldberg LR. In the clinic: Heart failure. Ann Intern Med 2010;152:ITC6-1–ITC6-16.

Gupta S, Michaels AD. Relationship between accurate auscultation of the fourth heart sound and the level of physician experience. Clin Cardiol 2009;32:69–75.

Hansson GK. Inflammation, atherosclerosis, and coronary artery disease. N Engl J Med 2005;352(16):1685–1695.

Ho CY, Seidman CE. A contemporary approach to hypertrophic cardiomyopathy. Circulation 2006;113:e858–e862.

Hurst JW, Fuster V, Walsh RA et al. Hurst's The Heart, 13th ed. New York: McGraw-Hill, 2011.

Klein LW. Atherosclerosis regression, vascular remodeling, and plaque stabilization. J Am Coll Cardiol 2007;49: 271–273.

Kuperstein R, Feinberg MS, Eldar M et al. Physical determinants of systolic murmur intensity in aortic stenosis. Am J Cardiol 2005;95:774–776.

Leung CC, Moondra V, Catherwood E et al. Prevalence and risk factors of pulmonary hypertension in patients with elevated pulmonary venous pressureand preserved ejection fraction. Am J Cardiol 2010;106:284–286.

Lin JS, O'Connor E, Whitlock EP et al. Behavioral counseling to promote physical activity and a healthful diet to prevent cardiovascular disease in adults: a systematic review for the U.S. Preventive Services task Force. Ann Intern Med 2010;153:736–750.

Maron BJ, Thompson PD, Ackerman MJ et al. American Heart Association Council on Nutrition, Physical Activity, and Metabolism. Recommendations and considerations related to preparticipation screening for cardiovascular abnormalities in competitive athletes: 2007 update: a scientific statement from the American Heart Association Council on Nutrition, Physical Activity, and Metabolism: endorsed by the American College of Cardiology Foundation. Circulation 2007;115:1643–1655. Am J Cardiol 2010;106:284–286.

Medical College of Wisconsin. Coronary Heart Disease Risk Calculator. Available at http://www.mcw.edu/calculators/CoronaryHeartDiseaseRisk.htm. Accessed October 21, 2011.

Myers MG, Godwin M, Dawes M et al. Conventional versus automated measurement of blood pressure in primary care patients with systolic hypertension: randomised parallel design controlled trial. BMJ 342, 2011. Available at http://www.bmj.com/content/342/bmj.d286.full.pdf. Accessed May 6, 2011.

National Cholesterol Education Panel. Third Report of the National Cholesterol Education Program (NCEP) Expert Panel on detection, evaluation, and treatment of high blood cholesterol in adults (Adult Treatment Panel III) final report. Circulation 2002;106:3143–3421.

National Cholesterol Education Program. Framingham Risk Score: 10-Year Coronary Heart Disease Risk Score. Available at http://hp2010.nhlbihin.net/atpiii/calculator.asp?usertype=prof. Accessed October 21, 2011.

Neubauer S. The failing heart — an engine out of fuel. New Engl J Med 2007;356:1140–1151.

Pearson TA, Blair SN, Daniels SR et al. AHA Guidelines for Primary Prevention of CardiovascularDisease and Stroke: 2002 Update. Consensus Panel Guide to Comprehensive Risk Reduction for AdultPatients without Coronary or Other Atherosclerotic Vascular Diseases. Circulation 2002;106:388–391.

Sebastian T, Palmeri JB, Kostis L et al. Heart rate and blood pressure response in adult men and women during exercise and sexual activity. Am J Cardiol 2007;100:1795–1801.

Selvanayagam J, De Pasquale C, Arnolda L. Usefulness of clinical assessment of the carotid pulse in the diagnosis of aortic stenosis. Am J Cardiol 2004;93:493–495.

Sinisalo J, Rapola J, Rossinen J et al. Simplifying the estimation of jugular venous pressure. Am J Cardiol 2007;100:1779–1781.

Third Report of the National Cholesterol Education Program (NCEP) Expert Panel. Detection, evaluation, and treatment of high blood cholesterol in adults—executive summary. National Cholesterol Education Program, National Heart, Lung, and

Blood Institute, National Institutes of Health. NIH Publication No. 01-3670. May 2001. Also at http://www.nhlbi.nih.gov/guidelines/cholesterol/atp3_rpt.htm. Accessed May 6 2011.

Thomas JT, Kelly RF, Thomas SJ et al. Utility of history, physical examination, electrocardiogram, and chest radiograph for differentiating normal from decreased systolic function in patients with heart failure. Am J Med 2002;112:437–445.

U.S. Preventive Services Task Force. Screening for high blood pressure: U.S. Preventive Services Task Force reaffirmation recommendation statement. Ann Intern Med 2007;147:783–786. See also Wolff T, Miller T. Evidence for the reaffirmation of the U.S. Preventive Services Task Force recommendation on screening for high blood pressure. Ann Intern Med 2007;147:787–791. For new guidelines pending at the time of publication, see Joint National Commission 8 information available at http://www.nhlbi.nih.gov/guidelines/hypertension/jnc8/index.htm Accessed April 24, 2010.

The Bates' suite offers these additional resources to enhance learning and facilitate understanding of this chapter:

- *Bates' Pocket Guide to Physical Examination and History Taking,* 7th edition
- *Bates' Visual Guide to Physical Examination*
- thePoint online resources, for students and instructors: http://thepoint.lww.com

Table
9-1
Selected Heart Rates and Rhythms

Cardiac rhythms may be classified as *regular or irregular*. When rhythms are irregular or rates are fast or slow, obtain an ECG to identify the origin of the beats (sinus node, AV node, atrium, or ventricle) and the pattern of conduction. Note that with AV (atrioventricular) block, arrhythmias may have a fast, normal, or slow ventricular rate. Some authors consider 90 beats/minute the upper limit of normal.

	ECG Pattern	Usual Resting Rate
WHAT IS THE RATE?		
FAST (>100)	Sinus tachycardia	100–180
	Supraventricular (atrial or nodal) tachycardia	150–250
	Atrial flutter with a regular ventricular response	100–175
	Ventricular tachycardia	110–250
OR		
NORMAL (60–100)	Normal sinus rhythm	60–90
	Second-degree AV block	60–100
	Atrial flutter with a regular ventricular response	75–100
OR		
SLOW (<60)	Sinus bradycardia	<60
	Second-degree AV block	30–60
	Complete heart block	<40

REGULAR

IS THE RHYTHM REGULAR OR IRREGULAR?

IRREGULAR

WHAT IS THE PATTERN OF IRREGULARITY?

	ECG Pattern	Usual Resting Rate
SPORADIC	Premature or extra beats at random intervals, but normal underlying rhythm: i.e., atrial or ventricular premature contractions, sinus arrhythmia	See Table 9-2
OR **REGULARLY IRREGULAR**	Regular pattern of cadences: i.e., ventricular trigeminy	
OR **IRREGULARLY IRREGULAR**	No discernible regularity: i.e., atrial fibrillation, atrial flutter	

Table
9-2   Selected Irregular Rhythms

Type of Rhythm	ECG Waves and Heart Sounds	

SPORADIC

Sinus Arrhythmia

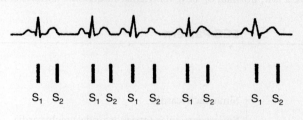

INSPIRATION   EXPIRATION

Rhythm. The heart varies cyclically, usually speeding up with inspiration and slowing down with expiration.

Heart Sounds. Normal, although S_1 may vary with the heart rate.

Atrial or Nodal Premature Contractions
(Supraventricular)

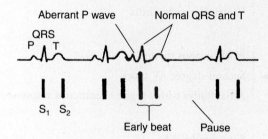

Rhythm. A beat of atrial or nodal origin comes earlier than the next expected normal beat. A pause follows, and then the rhythm resumes.

Heart Sounds. S_1 may differ in intensity from the S_1 of normal beats, and S_2 may be decreased.

SPORADIC OR REGULARLY IRREGULAR

Ventricular Premature Contractions
(Ventricular bigeminy or trigeminy)

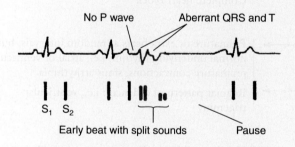

Rhythm. A beat of ventricular origin comes earlier than the next expected normal beat. A pause follows, and the rhythm resumes.

Heart Sounds. S_1 may differ in intensity from the S_1 of the normal beats, and S_2 may be decreased. Both sounds are likely to be split.

IRREGULARLY IRREGULAR

Atrial Fibrillation and Atrial Flutter With Varying AV Block

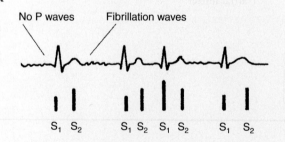

Rhythm. The ventricular rhythm is totally irregular, although short runs of the irregular ventricular rhythm may seem regular.

Heart Sounds. S_1 varies in intensity.

Table 9-3
Abnormalities of the Arterial Pulse and Pressure Waves

Normal

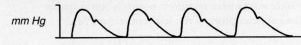

mm Hg

The pulse pressure is approximately 30–40 mm Hg. The pulse contour is smooth and rounded. (The notch on the descending slope of the pulse wave is not palpable.)

Small, Weak Pulses

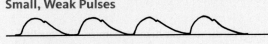

The pulse pressure is diminished, and the pulse feels weak and small. The upstroke may feel slowed, the peak prolonged. Causes include (1) decreased stroke volume, as in heart failure, hypovolemia, and severe aortic stenosis; and (2) increased peripheral resistance, as in exposure to cold and severe heart failure.

Large, Bounding Pulses

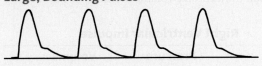

The pulse pressure is increased, and the pulse feels strong and bounding. The rise and fall may feel rapid, the peak brief. Causes include (1) increased stroke volume, decreased peripheral resistance, or both, as in fever, anemia, hyperthyroidism, aortic regurgitation, arteriovenous fistulas, and patent ductus arteriosus; (2) increased stroke volume because of slow heart rates, as in bradycardia and complete heart block; and (3) decreased compliance (increased stiffness) of the aortic walls, as in aging or atherosclerosis.

Bisferiens Pulse

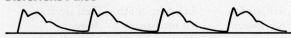

A bisferiens pulse is an increased arterial pulse with a double systolic peak. Causes include pure aortic regurgitation, combined aortic stenosis and regurgitation, and, though less commonly palpable, hypertrophic cardiomyopathy.

Pulsus Alternans

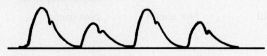

The pulse alternates in amplitude from beat to beat even though the rhythm is basically regular (and must be for you to make this judgment). When the difference between stronger and weaker beats is slight, it can be detected only by sphygmomanometry. Pulsus alternans indicates left ventricular failure and is usually accompanied by a left-sided S_3.

Bigeminal Pulse

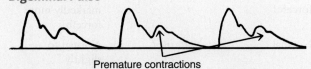

Premature contractions

This disorder of rhythm may mimic pulsus alternans. A bigeminal pulse is caused by a normal beat alternating with a premature contraction. The stroke volume of the premature beat is diminished in relation to that of the normal beats, and the pulse varies in amplitude accordingly.

Paradoxical Pulse

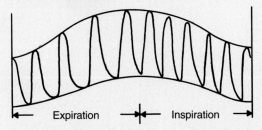

Expiration | Inspiration

A paradoxical pulse may be detected by a palpable decrease in the pulse's amplitude on quiet inspiration. If the sign is less pronounced, a blood pressure cuff is needed. Systolic pressure decreases by more than 10 mm Hg during inspiration. A paradoxical pulse is found in pericardial tamponade and frequently in exacerbations of asthma and COPD. It is sometimes noted in constrictive pericarditis.

Table 9-4

Variations and Abnormalities of the Ventricular Impulses

In the healthy heart, the *left ventricular impulse* is usually the *point of maximal impulse,* or *PMI*. This brief impulse is generated by the movement of the ventricular apex against the chest wall during contraction. The *right ventricular impulse* is normally not palpable beyond infancy, and its characteristics are indeterminate. In contrast, learn the classical descriptors of the left ventricular PMI:

- *Location:* in the 4th or 5th interspace, at the midclavicular line.
- *Diameter: discrete,* or ≤2 cm
- *Amplitude: brisk* and *tapping*
- *Duration:* ≤2/3 of systole

Careful examination of the ventricular impulse gives you important clues about underlying cardiovascular hemodynamics. The quality of the ventricular impulse changes as the left and right ventricles adapt to high-output states (anxiety, hyperthyroidism, and severe anemia) and to the more pathologic conditions of chronic pressure or volume overload. Note below the distinguishing features of three types of ventricular impulses: the *hyperkinetic ventricular impulse* from transiently increased stroke volume—this change does not necessarily indicate heart disease; the *sustained* ventricular impulse of ventricular hypertrophy from chronic pressure load, known as *increased afterload* (see p. 373); and the *diffuse* ventricular impulse of ventricular dilation from chronic volume overload, or *increased preload.*

| | **Left Ventricular Impulse** | | | **Right Ventricular Impulse** | | |
	Hyperkinetic	**Pressure Overload**	**Volume Overload**	**Hyperkinetic**	**Pressure Overload**	**Volume Overload**
Examples of Causes	Anxiety, hyperthyroidism, severe anemia	Aortic stenosis, hypertension	Aortic or mitral regurgitation; cardiomyopathy	Anxiety, hyperthyroidism, severe anemia	Pulmonic stenosis, pulmonary hypertension	Atrial septal defect
Location	Normal	Normal	Displaced to the left and possibly downward	3rd, 4th, or 5th left interspaces	3rd, 4th, or 5th left interspaces, also subxiphoid	Left sternal border, extending toward the left cardiac border, also subxiphoid
Diameter	~2 cm, though increased amplitude may make it seem larger	>2 cm	>2 cm	Not useful	Not useful	Not useful
Amplitude	More forceful tapping	More forceful tapping	*Diffuse*	Slightly more forceful	More forceful	Slightly to markedly more forceful
Duration	<2/3 systole	*Sustained* (up to S_2)	Often slightly sustained	Normal	*Sustained*	Normal to slightly sustained

Table
9-5
Variations in the First Heart Sound—S₁

Normal Variations

S₁ is softer than S₂ at the *base* (right and left 2nd interspaces).

S₁ is often but not always louder than S₂ at the *apex*.

Accentuated S₁

S₁ is accentuated in (1) tachycardia, rhythms with a short PR interval, and high cardiac output states (e.g., exercise, anemia, hyperthyroidism) and (2) mitral stenosis. In these conditions, the mitral valve is still open wide at the onset of ventricular systole and then closes quickly.

Diminished S₁

S₁ is diminished in first-degree heart block (delayed conduction from atria to ventricles). Here the mitral valve has had time after atrial contraction to float back into an almost closed position before ventricular contraction shuts it. It closes more quietly. S₁ is also diminished (1) when the mitral valve is calcified and relatively immobile, as in mitral regurgitation and (2) when left ventricular contractility is markedly reduced, as in heart failure or coronary heart disease.

Varying S₁

S₁ varies in intensity (1) in complete heart block, when atria and ventricles are beating independently of each other and (2) in any totally irregular rhythm (e.g., atrial fibrillation). In these situations, the mitral valve is in varying positions before being shut by ventricular contraction. Its closure sound, therefore, varies in loudness.

Split S₁

S₁ may be split normally along the lower left sternal border where the tricuspid component, often too faint to be heard, becomes audible. This split may sometimes be heard at the apex, but consider also an S₄, an aortic ejection sound, and an early systolic click. Abnormal splitting of both heart sounds may be heard in right bundle branch block and in premature ventricular contractions.

Table 9-6

Variations in the Second Heart Sound—S_2

	Inspiration	Expiration	

Physiologic Splitting

S_1 A_2 P_2 S_2 S_1 S_2

Listen for *physiologic splitting* of S_2 in the *2nd or 3rd left interspace*. The pulmonic component of S_2 is usually too faint to be heard at the apex or aortic area, where S_2 is a single sound derived from aortic valve closure alone. Normal splitting is *accentuated by inspiration* and usually *disappears on expiration*. In some patients, especially younger ones, S_2 may not become single on expiration. It may merge when the patient sits up.

Pathologic Splitting
(involves splitting during expiration and suggests heart disease)

S_1 S_2 S_1 S_2

Wide splitting of S_2 refers to an increase in the usual splitting that persists throughout the respiratory cycle. Wide splitting can be caused by delayed closure of the pulmonic valve (as in pulmonic stenosis or right bundle branch block). As illustrated here, right bundle branch block also causes splitting of S_1 into its mitral and tricuspid components. Wide splitting can also be caused by early closure of the aortic valve, as in mitral regurgitation.

S_1 S_2 S_1 S_2

Fixed splitting refers to wide splitting that does not vary with respiration. It occurs in atrial septal defect and right ventricular failure.

S_1 S_2 S_1 P_2 A_2 S_2

Paradoxical or reversed splitting refers to splitting that appears on expiration and disappears on inspiration. Closure of the aortic valve is abnormally delayed so that A_2 follows P_2 in expiration. Normal inspiratory delay of P_2 makes the split disappear. The most common cause of paradoxical splitting is left bundle branch block.

Increased Intensity of A_2 in the Right 2nd Interspace
(where only A_2 can usually be heard) occurs in systemic hypertension because of the increased pressure load. It also occurs when the aortic root is dilated, probably because the aortic valve is then closer to the chest wall.

Increased Intensity of P_2. When P_2 is equal to or louder than A_2, suspect pulmonary hypertension. Other causes include a dilated pulmonary artery and an atrial septal defect. When a split S_2 is heard widely, even at the apex and the right base, P_2 is accentuated.

Decreased or Absent A_2 in the Right 2nd Interspace is noted in calcific aortic stenosis because of valve immobility. If A_2 is inaudible, no splitting is heard.

Decreased or Absent P_2 is usually from the increased anteroposterior diameter of the chest associated with aging. It can also result from pulmonic stenosis. If P_2 is inaudible, no splitting is heard.

Table

9-7   **Extra Heart Sounds in Systole**

There are two kinds of extra heart sounds in systole: (1) early ejection sounds and (2) clicks, commonly heard in mid- and late systole.

Early Systolic Ejection Sounds

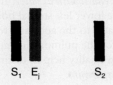

S₁ Eⱼ   S₂

Early systolic ejection sounds occur shortly after S₁, coincident with opening of the aortic and pulmonic valves. They are relatively high in pitch, have a sharp, clicking quality, and are heard better with the diaphragm of the stethoscope. An ejection sound indicates cardiovascular disease.

Listen for an *aortic ejection sound* at both the base and apex. It may be louder at the apex and usually does not vary with respiration. An aortic ejection sound may accompany a dilated aorta, or aortic valve disease from congenital stenosis or a bicuspid aortic valve.[105]

A *pulmonic ejection sound* is heard best in the 2nd and 3rd left interspaces. When S₁, usually relatively soft in this area, appears to be loud, you may be hearing a pulmonic ejection sound. Its intensity often *decreases with inspiration*. Causes include dilatation of the pulmonary artery, pulmonary hypertension, and pulmonic stenosis.

Systolic Clicks

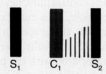

S₁   C₁ S₂

Systolic clicks are usually caused by *mitral valve prolapse*—an abnormal systolic ballooning of part of the mitral valve into the left atrium from both leaflet redundancy and elongation of the chordae tendineae. The clicks are usually mid- or late systolic. Prolapse of the mitral valve is a common cardiac condition, affecting about 2% to 3% of the general population. There is equal prevalence in men and women.[106,107]

Squatting

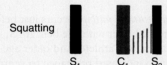

S₁   C₁ S₂

The click is usually single, but you may hear more than one, usually *at or medial to the apex,* but also *at the lower left sternal border.* It is high-pitched, so listen with the diaphragm. The click is often followed by a late systolic murmur from mitral regurgitation. The murmur usually crescendos up to S₂. Auscultatory findings are notably variable. Most patients have only a click, some have only a murmur, and some have both. Systolic clicks may also be of extracardial or mediastinal origin.

Standing

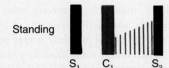

S₁   C₁   S₂

In *mitral valve prolapse,* findings vary from time to time and often change with body position. Several positions are recommended to identify the syndrome: supine, seated, squatting, and standing. *Squatting delays the click and murmur; standing moves them closer to S₁.*

Table	
9-8	**Extra Heart Sounds in Diastole**

Opening Snap

S_1 S_2 OS S_1

The *opening snap* is a very early diastolic sound usually produced by the opening of a *stenotic mitral valve*. It is heard best just medial to the apex and along the lower left sternal border. When it is loud, an opening snap radiates to the apex and to the pulmonic area, where it may be mistaken for the pulmonic component of a split S_2. Its high pitch and snapping quality help to distinguish it from an S_2. It is heard better with the *diaphragm*.

S_3

S_1 S_2 S_3 S_1

You will detect *physiologic* S_3 frequently in children and in young adults to the age of 35 or 40. It is common during the last trimester of pregnancy. Occurring early in diastole during rapid ventricular filling, it is later than an opening snap, dull and low in pitch, and heard best at the apex in the left lateral decubitus position. The *bell* of the stethoscope should be used with very light pressure.

A *pathologic* S_3 or *ventricular gallop* sounds like a physiologic S_3. An S_3 in a adults over age 40 is usually pathologic, arising from high pressures and abrupt deceleration of inflow across the mitral valve at the end of the rapid filling phase of diastole.[17,18] Causes include decreased myocardial contractility, heart failure, and volume overloading of a ventricle, as in mitral or tricuspid regurgitation. A *left-sided S3* is heard typically at the apex in the left lateral decubitus position. A *right-sided S3* is usually heard along the lower left sternal border or below the xiphoid with the patient supine, and is louder on inspiration. The term *gallop* comes from the cadence of three heart sounds, especially at rapid heart rates, and sounds like "Kentucky."

S_4

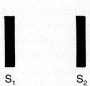

S_1 S_2 S_4 S_1

An S_4 (*atrial sound* or *atrial gallop*) occurs just before S_1. It is dull, low in pitch, and heard better with the bell. An S_4 is occasionally normal, especially in trained athletes and older age groups. More commonly, it is due to increased resistance to ventricular filling following atrial contraction. This increased resistance is related to decreased compliance (increased stiffness) of the ventricular myocardium.[19]

Causes of a left-sided S_4 include hypertensive heart disease, myocardial ischemia , aortic stenosis, and cardiomyopathy. A *left-sided S4* is heard best at the apex in the left lateral position; it may sound like "Tennessee." The less common *right-sided S4* is heard along the lower left sternal border or below the xiphoid. It often gets louder with inspiration. Causes include pulmonary hypertension and pulmonic stenosis.

An S_4 may also be associated with delayed conduction between the atria and ventricles. This delay separates the normally faint atrial sound from the louder S_1 and makes it audible. An S_4 is never heard in the absence of atrial contraction, which occurs with atrial fibrillation.

Occasionally, a patient has both an S_3 and an S_4, producing a *quadruple rhythm* of four heart sounds. At rapid heart rates, the S_3 and S_4 may merge into one loud extra heart sound, called a *summation gallop*.

Table
9-9

Pansystolic (Holosystolic) Murmurs

Pansystolic (holosystolic) murmurs are pathologic, arising from blood flow from a chamber with high pressure to one of lower pressure, through a valve or other structure that should be closed. The murmur begins immediately with S_1 and continues up to S_2.

	Mitral Regurgitation[108–110]	Tricuspid Regurgitation	Ventricular Septal Defect
Murmur	*Location.* Apex	*Location.* Lower left sternal border	*Location.* 3rd, 4th, and 5th left interspaces
	Radiation. To the left axilla, less often to the left sternal border	*Radiation.* To the right of the sternum, to the xiphoid area, and perhaps to the left midclavicular line, but not into the axilla	*Radiation.* Often wide
	Intensity. Soft to loud; if loud, associated with an apical thrill	*Intensity.* Variable	*Intensity.* Often very loud, with a thrill
	Pitch. Medium to high	*Pitch.* Medium	*Pitch.* High, holosystolic
	Quality. Harsh, holosystolic	*Quality.* Blowing, holosystolic	*Quality.* Often harsh
	Aids. Unlike tricuspid regurgitation, it does not become louder in inspiration.	*Aids.* Unlike mitral regurgitation, the intensity may increase slightly with inspiration.	
Associated Findings	S_1 normal (75%), loud (12%), soft (12%) An apical S_3 reflects volume overload of the left ventricle. The apical impulse is increased in amplitude (diffuse), laterally displaced, and may be sustained.	The right ventricular impulse is increased in amplitude and may be sustained. An S_3 may be audible along the lower left sternal border. The jugular venous pressure is often elevated, with large v waves in the jugular veins.	S_2 may be obscured by the loud murmur. Findings vary with the severity of the defect and with associated lesions.
Mechanism	When the *mitral valve fails to close fully in systole,* blood regurgitates from left ventricle to left atrium, causing a murmur. This leakage creates volume overload on the left ventricle, with subsequent dilatation. Several structural abnormalities cause this condition, and findings may vary accordingly.	When the *tricuspid valve fails to close fully in systole,* blood regurgitates from right ventricle to right atrium, producing a murmur. The most common cause is right ventricular failure and dilatation, with resulting enlargement of the tricuspid orifice, often initiated by pulmonary hypertension or left ventricular failure.	A ventricular septal defect is a congenital abnormality in which *blood flows from the relatively high-pressure left ventricle into the low-pressure right ventricle through a hole.* The defect may be accompanied by other abnormalities, but an uncomplicated lesion is described here.

Table
9-10   **Midsystolic Murmurs**

Midsystolic ejection murmurs are the most common kind of heart murmur. They may be (1) *innocent*—without any detectable physiologic or structural abnormality; (2) *physiologic*—from physiologic changes in body metabolism; or (3) *pathologic*—arising from a structural abnormality in the heart or great vessels.[99,100,101,111–113] Midsystolic murmurs tend to peak near midsystole and usually stop before S_2. The crescendo–decrescendo or "diamond" shape is not always audible, but the gap between the murmur and S_2 helps to distinguish midsystolic from pansystolic murmurs.

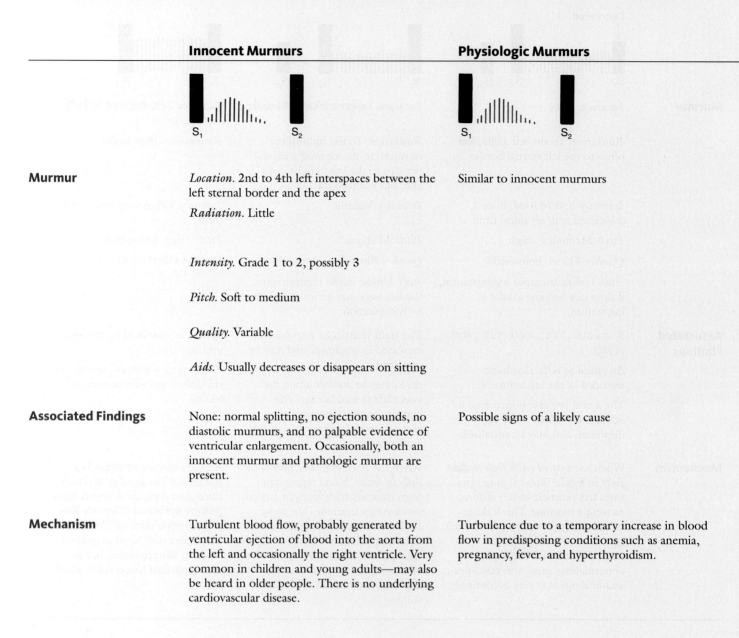

	Innocent Murmurs	**Physiologic Murmurs**
Murmur	*Location.* 2nd to 4th left interspaces between the left sternal border and the apex	Similar to innocent murmurs
	Radiation. Little	
	Intensity. Grade 1 to 2, possibly 3	
	Pitch. Soft to medium	
	Quality. Variable	
	Aids. Usually decreases or disappears on sitting	
Associated Findings	None: normal splitting, no ejection sounds, no diastolic murmurs, and no palpable evidence of ventricular enlargement. Occasionally, both an innocent murmur and pathologic murmur are present.	Possible signs of a likely cause
Mechanism	Turbulent blood flow, probably generated by ventricular ejection of blood into the aorta from the left and occasionally the right ventricle. Very common in children and young adults—may also be heard in older people. There is no underlying cardiovascular disease.	Turbulence due to a temporary increase in blood flow in predisposing conditions such as anemia, pregnancy, fever, and hyperthyroidism.

Pathologic Murmurs

Aortic Stenosis[112-114]

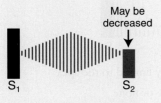

May be decreased →

S_1 S_2

Location. Right 2nd interspace

Radiation. Often to the carotids, down the left sternal border, even to the apex

Intensity. Sometimes soft but often loud, with a thrill

Pitch. Medium, harsh; crescendo–decrescendo may be higher at the apex

Quality. Often harsh; may be more musical at the apex

Aids. Heard best with the patient sitting and leaning forward

As aortic stenosis worsens A_2 decreases and the murmur peaks later in diastole. A_2 may be delayed and merge with P_2 → single S_2 on expiration or paradoxical S_2 split. Carotid upstroke may be *delayed*, with slow rise and small amplitude. Hypertrophied left ventricle may → *sustained* apical impulse and an S_4 from decreased compliance.

Significant aortic valve stenosis impairs blood flow across the valve, causing turbulence, and increases left ventricular afterload. Causes are congenital, rheumatic, and degenerative calcification of the leaflets; findings may differ with each cause. Other conditions mimic aortic stenosis without obstructing flow: *aortic sclerosis*, a stiffening of aortic valve leaflets associated with aging; a *bicuspid aortic valve*, a congenital condition that may not be recognized until adulthood; *a dilated aorta*, as in arteriosclerosis, syphilis, or Marfan's syndrome; *pathologically increased flow across the aortic valve* during systole can accompany aortic regurgitation.

Hypertrophic Cardiomyopathy[115]

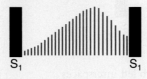

S_1 S_1

Location. 3rd and 4th left interspaces

Radiation. Down the left sternal border to the apex, possibly to the base, but not to the neck

Intensity. Variable

Pitch. Medium

Quality. Harsh

Aids. Decreases with squatting, increases with straining down from Valsalva and standing

S_3 may be present. An S_4 is often present at the apex (unlike mitral regurgitation). The apical impulse may be *sustained* and have two palpable components. The carotid pulse rises *quickly*, unlike the pulse in aortic stenosis.

Massive ventricular hypertrophy is associated with unusually rapid ejection of blood from the left ventricle during systole. Outflow tract obstruction of flow may coexist. Accompanying distortion of the mitral valve may cause mitral regurgitation.

Pulmonic Stenosis

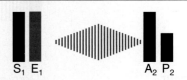

S_1 E_1 A_2 P_2

Location. 2nd and 3rd left interspaces

Radiation. If loud, toward the left shoulder and neck

Intensity. Soft to loud; if loud, associated with a thrill

Pitch. Medium; crescendo–decrescendo

Quality. Often harsh

In severe stenosis, S_2 is widely split, and P_2 is diminished or inaudible. An early pulmonic ejection sound is common. May hear a right-sided S_4. Right ventricular impulse often increased in amplitude and *sustained*.

Pulmonic valve stenosis impairs flow across the valve, increasing right ventricular afterload. Congenital and usually found in children. In an *atrial septal defect*, the systolic murmur from pathologically increased flow across the pulmonic valve may mimic pulmonic stenosis.

Table	
9-11	**Diastolic Murmurs**

Diastolic murmurs almost always indicate heart disease. There are two basic types. *Early decrescendo diastolic murmurs* signify regurgitant flow through an incompetent semilunar valve, more commonly the aortic. *Rumbling diastolic murmurs in mid- or late diastole* suggest stenosis of an atrioventricular valve, usually the mitral. Diastolic murmurs are far less common than systolic murmurs and are often more difficult to hear. A meticulous examination is therefore needed.

	Aortic Regurgitation[98,116]	**Mitral Stenosis**
	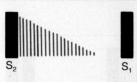 S_2 S_1	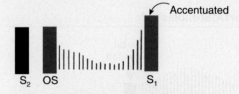 Accentuated S_2 OS S_1
Murmur	*Location.* 2nd to 4th left interspaces *Radiation.* If loud, to the apex, perhaps to the right sternal border *Intensity.* Grade 1 to 3 *Pitch.* High. *Use the diaphragm.* *Quality.* Blowing decrescendo; may be mistaken for breath sounds *Aids.* The murmur is heard best with the *patient sitting, leaning forward,* with breath held after exhalation.	*Location.* Usually limited to the apex *Radiation.* Little or none *Intensity.* Grade 1 to 4 *Pitch.* Decrescendo low-pitched rumble. *Use the bell.* *Aids.* Placing the bell exactly on the apical impulse, turning the patient into a *left lateral position,* and mild exercise all help to make the murmur audible. It is heard better in exhalation.
Associated Findings	An ejection sound may be present. An S_3 or S_4, if present, suggests severe regurgitation. Progressive changes in the apical impulse include increased amplitude, displacement laterally and downward, widened diameter, and increased duration. The pulse pressure increases, and *arterial pulses are often bounding.* A midsystolic flow murmur or a mitral diastolic (*Austin Flint*) murmur suggests large regurgitant flow.	S_1 is accentuated and may be palpable at the apex. An opening snap (OS) often follows S_2 and initiates the murmur. If pulmonary hypertension develops, P_2 is accentuated, and the right ventricular impulse becomes palpable. Mitral regurgitation and aortic valve disease may be associated with mitral stenosis.
Mechanism	The leaflets of the aortic valve fail to close completely during diastole, and blood regurgitates from the aorta back into the left ventricle. Volume overload on the left ventricle results. Two other murmurs may be associated: (1) a midsystolic murmur from the resulting increased forward flow across the aortic valve and (2) a mitral diastolic (*Austin Flint*) murmur, attributed to diastolic impingement of the regurgitant flow on the anterior leaflet of the mitral valve.	When the leaflets of the mitral valve thicken, stiffen, and become distorted from the effects of rheumatic fever, the *mitral valve fails to open sufficiently in diastole.* The resulting murmur has two components: (1) middiastolic (during rapid ventricular filling) and (2) presystolic (during atrial contraction). The latter disappears if atrial fibrillation develops, leaving only a middiastolic rumble.

Some cardiovascular sounds extend beyond one phase of the cardiac cycle. Three examples, all nonvalvular in origin, are: (1) a *venous hum*, a benign sound produced by turbulence of blood in the jugular veins—common in children; (2) a *pericardial friction rub*, produced by inflammation of the pericardial sac; and (3) *patent ductus arteriosus*, a congenital abnormality in which an open channel persists between the aorta and pulmonary artery. *Continuous murmurs* begin in systole and extend through S_2 into all or part of diastole, as in *patent ductus arteriosus*. Arteriovenous fistulas, common in dialysis patients, also produce continuous murmurs.

	Venous Hum	**Pericardial Friction Rub**	**Patent Ductus Arteriosus**
Timing	Continuous murmur without a silent interval. Loudest in diastole	May have three short components, each associated with friction from cardiac movement in the pericardial sac: (1) atrial systole, (2) ventricular systole, and (3) ventricular diastole. Usually the first two components are present; all three make diagnosis easy; only one (usually the systolic) invites confusion with a murmur.	Continuous murmur in both systole and diastole, often with a silent interval late in diastole. Loudest in late systole, obscures S_2, and fades in diastole
Location	Above the medial third of the clavicles, especially on the right	Variable, but usually heard best in the 3rd interspace to the left of the sternum	Left 2nd interspace
Radiation	1st and 2nd interspaces	Little	Toward the left clavicle
Intensity	Soft to moderate. Can be obliterated by pressure on the jugular veins	Variable. May increase when the patient leans forward, exhales, and holds breath (in contrast to pleural rub)	Usually loud, sometimes associated with a thrill
Quality	Humming, roaring	Scratchy, scraping	Harsh, machinery-like
Pitch	Low (heard better with the *bell*)	High (heard better with the *diaphragm*)	Medium

The Breasts and Axillae

Anatomy and Physiology

THE FEMALE BREAST

The female breast lies against the anterior thoracic wall, extending from the clavicle and 2nd rib down to the 6th rib, and from the sternum across to the midaxillary line. Its surface area is generally rectangular rather than round.

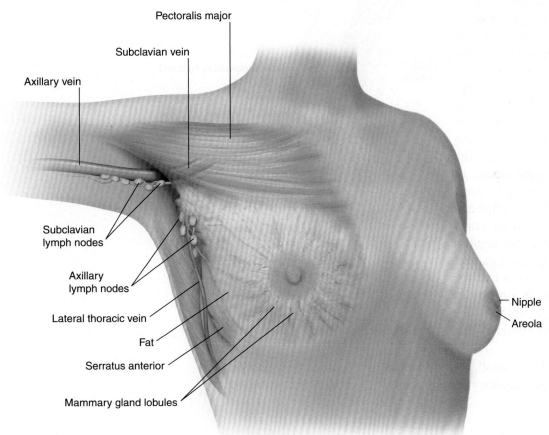

Pectoralis major

Subclavian vein

Axillary vein

Subclavian lymph nodes

Axillary lymph nodes

Lateral thoracic vein

Fat

Serratus anterior

Mammary gland lobules

Nipple

Areola

The breast overlies the pectoralis major and, at its inferior margin, the serratus anterior.

To describe clinical findings, the breast is often divided into four quadrants based on horizontal and vertical lines crossing at the nipple. A fifth area, an axillary tail of breast tissue sometimes termed the "tail of Spence," extends laterally across the anterior axillary fold. Alternatively, findings can be localized as the time on the face of a clock (e.g., 3 o'clock) and the distance in centimeters from the nipple.

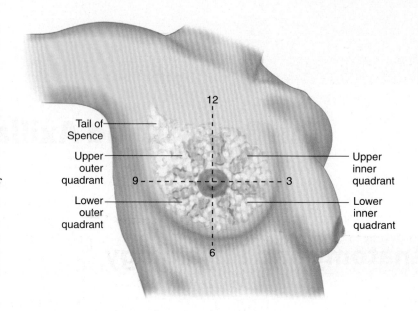

The breast is hormonally sensitive tissue, responsive to the changes of monthly cycling and aging. *Glandular tissue*, namely secretory tubuloalveolar glands and ducts, forms 15 to 20 septated *lobes* radiating around the nipple. Within each lobe are many smaller *lobules*. These drain into milk-producing ducts and sinuses that open onto the surface of the *areola*, or nipple. *Fibrous connective tissue* provides structural support in the form of fibrous bands or suspensory ligaments connected to both the skin and the underlying fascia. *Adipose tissue*, or fat, surrounds the breast, predominantly in the superficial and peripheral areas. The proportions of these components vary with age, the general state of nutrition, pregnancy, exogenous hormone use, and other factors. After menopause, there is atrophy of glandular tissue, and a notable decrease in the number of lobules.

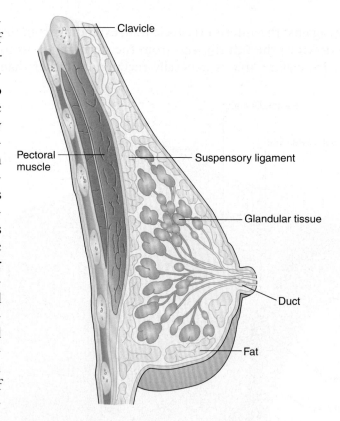

The surface of the areola has small, rounded elevations formed by sebaceous glands, sweat glands, and accessory areolar glands. A few hairs are often seen on the areola.

Both the nipple and the areola are supplied with smooth muscle that contracts to express milk from the ductal system during breast-feeding. Rich sensory innervation, especially in the nipple, triggers "milk letdown" following neurohormonal stimulation from infant sucking. Tactile stimulation of the area, including the breast examination, makes the nipple smaller, firmer, and more erect, whereas the areola puckers and wrinkles. These smooth muscle reflexes are normal and should not be mistaken for signs of breast disease.

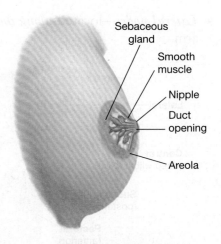

The adult breast may be soft, but it often feels granular, nodular, or lumpy. This uneven texture is normal and may be termed *physiologic nodularity*. It is often bilateral. It may be evident throughout the breast or only in parts of it. The nodularity may increase before menses, a time when breasts often enlarge and become tender or even painful. For breast changes during adolescence and pregnancy, see pp. 863–864 and p. 894.

Occasionally, one or more extra or supernumerary nipples are located along the "milk line," illustrated on the right. Only a small nipple and areola are usually present, often mistaken for a common mole. There may be underlying glandular tissue. An extra nipple has no pathologic significance.

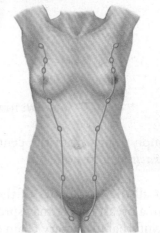

THE MALE BREAST

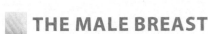

The male breast consists chiefly of a small nipple and areola. These overlie a thin disc of undeveloped breast tissue consisting primarily of ducts. Lacking estrogen and progesterone stimulation, ductal branching and development of lobules are minimal.[1] It may be difficult to distinguish male breast tissue from the surrounding muscles of the chest wall. A firm button of breast tissue 2 cm or more in diameter has been described in roughly one of three adult men.

LYMPHATICS

Lymphatics from most of the breast drain toward the axilla. Of the axillary lymph nodes, the *central nodes* are palpable most frequently. They lie along the chest wall, usually high in the axilla and midway between the anterior and posterior axillary folds. Into them drain channels from three other groups of lymph nodes, which are seldom palpable:

- *Pectoral nodes—anterior*, located along the lower border of the pectoralis major inside the anterior axillary fold. These nodes drain the anterior chest wall and much of the breast.

- *Subscapular nodes—posterior*, located along the lateral border of the scapula; palpated deep in the posterior axillary fold. They drain the posterior chest wall and a portion of the arm.

- *Lateral nodes*—located *along the upper humerus*. They drain most of the arm.

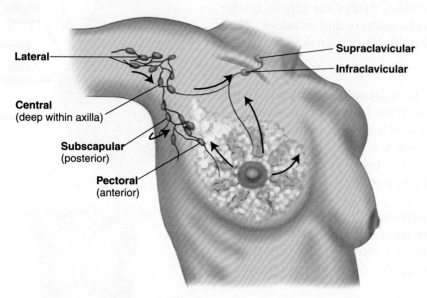

Lateral

Central
(deep within axilla)

Subscapular
(posterior)

Pectoral
(anterior)

Supraclavicular

Infraclavicular

ARROWS INDICATE DIRECTION OF LYMPH FLOW

Lymph drains from the central axillary nodes to the *infraclavicular* and *supraclavicular* nodes.

Not all the lymphatics of the breast drain into the axilla. Malignant cells from a breast cancer may spread directly to the infraclavicular nodes or into the internal mammary chain of lymph nodes within the chest.

The Health History

Common or Concerning Symptoms

> ▶ Breast lump or mass
> ▶ Breast pain or discomfort
> ▶ Nipple discharge

You can ask about the breasts during the history or later during the physical examination. Ask "Do you examine your breasts?" . . . "How often?" For a menstruating woman, ask when she examines her breast during her monthly cycle: self-examination is best done when estrogen stimulation is lowest, approximately 5 to 7 days after onset of menses. Ask whether she has any *discomfort*, *pain*, or *lumps* in her breasts. About 50% of women have palpable lumps or nodularity, and premenstrual enlargement and tenderness are common.[2] If your patient reports a lump or mass, ask about the precise location, how long it has been present, and

Lumps may be physiologic or pathologic, ranging from cysts and fibroadenomas to breast cancer. See Table 10-1, Common Breast Masses, p. 430, and Table 10-2, Visible Signs of Breast Cancer, p. 431.

any change in size or variation within the menstrual cycle. Ask about any change in breast contour, dimpling, swelling, or puckering of the skin over the breasts.

Ask about any *discharge from the nipples* and when it occurs. Does the discharge appear only after compression of the nipple, or is it spontaneous? Physiologic hypersecretion is seen in pregnancy, lactation, chest wall stimulation, sleep, and stress. If spontaneous, what is the color, consistency, and quantity? Is the color milky, brown or greenish, or bloody? Ask if the discharge is unilateral or bilateral.

Galactorrhea, or the inappropriate discharge of milk-containing fluid, is abnormal if it occurs 6 or more months after childbirth or cessation of breast-feeding.

Health Promotion and Counseling: Evidence and Recommendations

Important Topics for Health Promotion and Counseling

▶ Palpable masses of the breast
▶ Assessing risk of breast cancer
▶ Breast cancer screening

Women may experience a wide range of changes in breast tissue and sensation, from cyclic swelling and nodularity to a distinct lump or mass. The examination of the breast provides an important opportunity for exploring key concerns for women's health—what to do if a lump or mass is detected, risk factors for breast cancer, and screening measures such as breast self-examination, the clinical breast examination (CBE) by a skilled clinician, and mammography. Women will frequently seek information during the clinical encounter.

Palpable Masses of the Breast and Breast Symptoms. Breast cancer occurs in up to 4% of women with breast complaints, in approximately 5% of women reporting a nipple discharge, and in up to 11% of women specifically complaining of a breast lump or mass.[1,2] Breast masses show marked variation in etiology, from fibroadenomas and cysts seen in younger women, to abscess or mastitis, to primary breast cancer. On initial assessment, the woman's age and physical characteristics of the mass provide clues about its etiology, as shown in the next table on Palpable Masses of the Breast, but definitive diagnosis should be pursued. All breast masses require careful diagnostic assessment.

Assessing Risk of Breast Cancer. Women are increasingly interested in information about breast cancer. Be familiar with the literature detailing the epidemiology of and risk factors for breast cancer that support recommendations for screening. Key facts and figures are presented here, but further reading will enhance your counseling of women patients.

Palpable Masses of the Breast

Age	Common Lesion	Characteristics
15–25	Fibroadenoma	Usually smooth, rubbery, round, mobile, nontender
25–50	Cysts	Usually soft to firm, round, mobile; often tender
	Fibrocystic changes	Nodular, ropelike
	Cancer	Irregular, firm, may be mobile or fixed to surrounding tissue
Over 50	Cancer until proven otherwise	As above
Pregnancy/lactation	Lactating adenomas, cysts, mastitis, and cancer	As above

Adapted from Schultz MZ, Ward BA, Reiss M. Breast diseases. In Noble J, Greene HL, Levinson W, et al. (eds). Primary Care Medicine, 2nd ed. St. Louis, Mosby, 1996. See also Venet L, Strax P, Venet W, et al. Adequacies and inadequacies of breast examinations by physicians in mass screenings. Cancer 1971;28(6):1546–1551.

Breast Cancer Facts and Figures. Breast cancer is the most common cause of cancer in women worldwide, accounting for more than 10% of cancers in women. In the United States, a woman born now has a 12%, or 1 in 8, lifetime risk of developing breast cancer.[3] Ninety-five percent of new breast cancer cases occur after age 40. The probability of diagnosis over the next 10 years of a woman's life increases by decade.

Age-Specific Probabilities of Developing Invasive Breast Cancer*

If Current Age Is:	The Probability of Developing Breast Cancer in the Next 10 Years Is:	or 1 in:
20	0.06%	1,760
30	0.44%	229
40	1.44%	69
50	2.39%	42
60	3.40%	29
70	3.73%	27
Lifetime risk	12.08%	8

*Among those free of cancer at beginning of age interval. Based on cases diagnosed 2004–2006. Percentages and "1 in" numbers may not be numerically equivalent due to rounding.

Source: American Cancer Society. Breast Cancer Facts and Figures 2009–2010, p. 12. Available at: http://www.cancer.org/acs/groups/content/anho/documents/document/f861009final90809pdf.pdf. Accessed November 14, 2010.

Breast cancer is the second leading cause of cancer death in women. Five-year survival rates range from 98% for local disease to 23% for metastatic disease. In its annual report, *Breast Cancer Facts and Figures 2009–2010*, the American Cancer Society highlights important trends in breast cancer statistics.

- *Declines in new cases of invasive breast cancer since 2000.* These declines reflect a drop in use of hormone replacement therapy (HRT) in women over age 50, and a decrease in mammography screening, which means that fewer cancers are detected earlier, but are not actually a true decrease in disease occurrence.

- *More advanced breast cancer at an earlier age in African American women.* Compared to white women, African American women have a higher incidence of breast cancer before age 45, are more likely to have larger tumors at the time of diagnosis, and are more likely to die from breast cancer at every age. This discrepancy in breast cancer death rates has been growing since 1980. Although overall mortality has been decreasing by 2% per year since 1990, death rates for African American women were 38% higher than for white women by 2006. This major health disparity is attributed to the presence of coexisting illness, lack of health insurance, unequal access to care, differences in treatment, and more aggressive tumor characteristics. Clinicians should offer information and screening mammograms to African American women well before age 40, take prompt action to investigate breast masses, and advocate better insurance options and access to care.

Assessing Risk Factors for Breast Cancer.   Be familiar with the breast cancer risk factors and their relative risk, as listed on p. 412, and discuss them with your patients.[3,4] *Modifiable risk factors* include: postmenopausal obesity, use of HRT, alcohol ingestion, physical inactivity, choices about breast-feeding, and type of contraception. The most important risk factor for breast cancer is age. Other *nonmodifiable risk factors* are family history, breast tissue density, proliferative lesions with atypia on breast biopsy, duration of unopposed estrogen exposure related to early menarche, age of first full-term pregnancy, and late menopause. Note that a history of radiation to the chest also places women at high risk. Nonetheless, over 50% of women with breast cancer have no familial or reproductive risk factors.[5]

Breast Cancer in Women: Factors That Increase Relative Risk

Relative Risk	Factor
>4.0	▶ Female
	▶ Age (65+ versus <65 years, although risk increases across all ages until age 80)
	▶ Certain inherited genetic mutations for breast cancer (BRCA1 and/or BRCA2)
	▶ Two or more first-degree relatives with breast cancer diagnosed at an early age
	▶ Personal history of breast cancer
	▶ High breast tissue density
	▶ Biopsy-confirmed atypical hyperplasia
2.1–4.0	▶ One first-degree relative with breast cancer
	▶ High-dose radiation to chest
	▶ High bone density (postmenopausal)
1.1–2.0 Factors that affect circulating hormones	▶ Late age at first full-term pregnancy (>30 years)
	▶ Early menarche (<12 years)
	▶ Late menopause (>55 years)
	▶ No full-term pregnancies
	▶ Never breast-fed a child
	▶ Recent oral contraceptive use
	▶ Recent and long-term use of hormone replacement therapy
	▶ Obesity (postmenopausal)
Other factors	▶ Personal history of endometrium, ovary, or colon cancer
	▶ Alcohol consumption
	▶ Height (tall)
	▶ High socioeconomic status
	▶ Jewish heritage

Adapted with permission from Hulka et al., 2001.

Source: American Cancer Society. Breast Cancer Facts and Figures 2009–2010, p. 11. Available at: http://www.cancer.org/acs/groups/content/anho/documents/document/f861009final90809pdf.pdf. Accessed November 14, 2010.

Male breast cancer constitutes 1% of breast cancer cases, peaking in frequency around age 71.[3,6] Risk factors are BRCA2 mutations, obesity, family history of male or female breast cancer, testicular disorders, and work exposure to high temperatures and exhaust emission.

Using Breast Cancer Risk Assessment Tools. In addition to risk factor tables, several risk assessment tools can help you clarify breast cancer risk for your patients. The Gail and Claus models estimate absolute lifetime risk of breast cancer and are the most commonly used. They assess risk based on large population data sets; however, they do not predict disease in a single individual.[7-10] The BRCAPRO model is used for predicting risk of BRCA1 or BRCA2. For more detailed discussion of these and other models, turn to the National Cancer Institute's review of the Genetics of Breast and Ovarian Cancer and reports of the American Cancer Society.[11,12] Currently, no single model addresses all of the known risk factors or includes all of the genetic details of personal and family history, so devising data-based personalized management strategies is an on-going focus for research.

The *Breast Cancer Risk Assessment Tool*, often called the Gail model, at http://www.cancer.gov/bcrisktool, updated in 2007, provides 5-year and lifetime estimates of *risk for invasive breast cancer.*[7] It incorporates age, race, first-degree relatives with breast cancer, previous breast biopsies and presence of hyperplasia, age at menarche, and age at first delivery. The Gail model is best used for individuals over age 50 who have either no family history of breast cancer or one affected first-degree relative, and who have annual screening mammograms. It should not be used for women with a past history of breast cancer or radiation exposure, or those who are 35 years of age or younger. It does not determine risk for noninvasive breast cancer and does not take paternal history or disease in second-degree relatives into account, or age of onset of disease. This model has recently been updated to include breast density, but depends on use of digital mammography and special software, making it more difficult to use.[13]

The *Claus Model* assesses risk for high-risk women and incorporates family history for both female and male first- and second-degree relatives, including age of onset.[14] It is based on the woman's current age. It is best used for individuals with no more than two first- or second-degree relatives with breast cancer.[11] An expanded version includes family members with ovarian cancer. This model does not include personal, lifestyle, or reproductive risk factors. Discrepancies in risk assessment between published tables and the computerized program have been reported.[9]

The *BRCAPRO Model* at http://astor.som.jhmi.edu/BayesMendel/brcapro. html is used for high-risk women to assess risk of BRCA1 and BRCA2 mutation in a given family. It incorporates published BRCA1 and BRCA2 mutation frequencies, cancer penetration in affected carriers, and age of onset in first- and second-degree female and male relatives. It does not include non-hereditary risk factors.[15]

Selected Risk Factors That Affect Screening Decisions

BRCA1 and BRCA2 Mutations. Begin evaluating a woman's breast cancer risk as early as her 20s by asking about family history. A pattern of breast or ovarian cancer in maternal or paternal family members is suspicious for autosomal dominant genetic mutations. Look especially for a positive history of: age 50 years or younger at diagnosis, breast cancer in two or more individuals in the same lineage (paternal or maternal), multiple primary or ovarian tumors in one person, breast cancer in a male relative, Ashkenazi Jewish ancestry, or a family member with a known predisposing gene. The BRCA1 and BRCA2 gene mutations represent roughly half of familial breast cancers; they also confer increased risk for ovarian cancer. These mutations occur in <1% of the population but account for roughly 5% of breast cancers.[11] For BRCA1 mutations, the risk of developing breast cancer by age 70 is estimated at 57%, and for BRCA2, the estimated risk is 49%.[16] If family history is suspect, the next steps for clinicians include using the BRCAPRO calculator, conducting genetic testing, considering MRI for screening in addition to mammography, and making appropriate specialty referrals. (See p. 417 for recommendations on use of MRI in high-risk women.)

In Situ Breast Disorders With Proliferative Changes on Biopsy.

Since the 1980s, increased screening with mammography has resulted in rapid increases in detection of small in situ breast disorders with a subsequent biopsy. There disorders fall into two main types: *ductal carcinoma in situ (DCIS)*, found in about 80% of these disorders; and *lobular carcinoma in situ (LCIS)*, found in roughly 12%. But are these lesions precancerous? Less than half of DCIS lesions, for example, progress to invasive disease. Since the biology of which lesions will progress is still unclear, most of these cases are treated, leading to overdiagnosis. Currently, in situ lesions are classified by degree of cellular proliferation on biopsy. Presence of proliferative changes indicate small to moderate increases in risk, depending of the absence or presence of atypia, as shown in the table below.[1,17]

Risk of Breast Cancer and Histology of Benign Breast Lesions

▶ *No increased risk,* relative risk ~1.3	*Nonproliferative changes:* including cysts and ductal ectasia, mild hyperplasia, simple fibroadenoma, mastitis, granuloma, diabetic mastopathy
▶ *Small increased risk,* or relative risk 1.5–2.0	*Proliferative without atypia:* including usual ductal hyperplasia, complex fibroadenoma, papilloma
▶ *Moderate increased risk,* or relative risk >2.0 to ~4.2	*Proliferative with atypia:* including atypical ductal hyperplasia and atypical lobular hyperplasia

Source: Santen RJ, Mansel R. Benign breast disorders. N Engl J Med 2005;353:275–285; Hartmann LC, Sellers TA, Frost MH et al. Benign breast disorders and the risk of breast cancer. N Engl J Med 2005;353:229–237.

Breast Density.

Breast density on mammogram has been termed "the most undervalued and underused risk factor" in studies of breast cancer.[18] Dense breast tissue appears lighter on mammograms, and can mask detection of underlying cancers. Even after adjusting for the masking effect, however, density remains a strong independent risk factor.[10] Studies show that if there is radiologic density in 60% to 75% of breast tissue, the relative risk of breast cancer increases four- to sixfold.[10,18,19] Note that mammograms have a sensitivity and specificity of 88% and 96% in women with predominantly fatty tissue, dropping to 62% and 89% in women with high density from stromal and epithelial glandular elements.[18] Breast density appears to have an inherited component; additional links to levels of estrogen exposure are under investigation.[20,21]

Counseling women about breast density is important, as many women are not aware of this risk factor and the need for regular surveillance. You can find comments on breast density in mammography reports from centers using digital technology. These comments may affect patient decisions about using HRT.

Recommendations for Breast Cancer Screening and Chemoprevention

Individualized Screening. Discussions about risk factors for breast cancer can begin at any age. Screen all women for risk factors, including *genetic syndromes*, using the risk factor tables and assessment models described above. Be sure to include questions about ovarian cancer.

As you will see in the discussion to follow, there is disagreement among professional groups about when to start screening and the correct interval. Decisions about how and when to screen for breast cancer involve several issues, and bear thoughtful review of the balance of benefits and risks. Many studies use mortality and life-years gained as their primary endpoints, and have not addressed the benefits of earlier treatment on reduced morbidity, avoidance of chemotherapy, and increased chance of breast conservation. Changes in the recommended guidelines underscore the need for clinicians to be well informed as they counsel individual patients.

Mammography
   Women Ages 40 to 50. Use of *mammography* for screening women in this age group has been controversial due to lower sensitivity and specificity, possibly related to heterogeneous estrogen exposure in women still premenopausal; high numbers of false positives, approaching 9 out of 100 women;[5] and the high rate of resulting invasive procedures. Citing concerns about the net benefit in reduction of mortality, in 2009 the U.S. Preventive Services Task Force (USPSTF) changed its recommendation for women under age 50 in support of *individual decision making* rather than *routine* biennial screening, stating that "the decision to start regular, biennial screening mammography before the age of 50 should be an individual one and take patient context into account, including the patient's values regarding specific benefits and harms."[22] The American College of Physicians makes the same recommendation.[23] The American Cancer Society and the American Medical Association recommend annual mammography beginning at age 40.[3]

Women 50 to 74 Years. In 2009, the USPSTF made a second change in its recommendations, namely to endorse *biennial screening* for *women ages 50 to 74*. The USPSTF stated that changing from annual to biennial screening would reduce the harms of mammography screening by nearly half. Biennial screening appears to preserve 80% of the benefits of annual screening and averts about 40% of the false-positive results of annual testing, with similar late-stage disease rates at diagnosis and similar 10-year breast cancer-specific survival rates.[5] The American Cancer Society and the American Medical Association recommend annual mammography; the World Health Organization recommends mammography every 1 to 2 years. Mammography screening performs best in this age group, with a sensitivity of 77% to 95% and specificity of 94% to 97%.[22] Digital mammography appears to perform better in younger women and women with higher breast density.

Women Over Age 75. The USPSTF concluded that data are insufficient to make a firm recommendation, stating that "no women 75 years or older have been included in the multiple randomized clinical trials of breast cancer screening." The USPSTF noted three factors that alter the benefits of screening for this age group: the benefits of screening actually occur several years after the test and might be curtailed by lower survival; cancers are more likely to be estrogen-receptor positive and more easily treated; and women are more likely to die of other conditions not affected by screening for breast cancer. The USPSTF, the American Cancer Society, and the American Geriatrics Society support *individualized decisions* about continued screening, depending on coexisting conditions and anticipated 5-year survival.

Clinical Breast Examination (CBE). In 2009, the USPSTF determined that evidence supporting CBE is insufficient for establishing the balance of benefits and harms. This is also the position of the World Health Organization. In contrast, the American Cancer Society recommends the CBE every 3 years for women ages 20 to 39, and annually, preferably before mammography, beginning at age 40. The Society notes that the CBE provides an opportunity for patient education, but cautions that a thorough CBE may take up to 10 minutes. The American College of Obstetrics and Gynecology also recommends CBE. Standardization of CBE technique would be helpful for both further research and practice. Sensitivity and specificity of CBE are 40% and 88% to 99%, and heavily influenced by the technique of the examiner.[2,22]

Breast Self-Examination (BSE). In 2009, the USPSTF recommended against teaching BSE due to evidence that it does not reduce mortality and may lead to a higher rate of benign breast biopsies.[24–26] However, mortality reduction may not be the only benefit to consider. The American Cancer Society advocates BSE in conjunction with mammography and CBE to promote health awareness and advises clinicians to teach and review the patient's technique. Recent trials outside the United States show no reduction in mortality, but several reports from countries where routine screening mammography is not widely available, and one report from the United States, suggest that women performing BSE are more likely to pursue mammography.[27-30] Some subgroups may be more likely to benefit from SBE and earlier detection, such as women at high risk.[31]

Few studies have investigated how women actually practice BSE. Several studies report BSE sensitivity in the range of 12% to 41%.[32] Current evidence suggests that the duration and frequency of BSE is inadequate.[27] Clinicians should instruct interested patients in proper technique, detailed on p. 427. Monthly BSE 5 to 7 days after onset of menses can be taught to women as early as their 20s.

Magnetic Resonance Imaging (MRI). Studies of contrast-enhanced MRI for *screening* have focused only on high-risk populations; breast MRI has not yet been evaluated for screening in the general population. Sensitivity is reported at 77%, almost double that of mammograms, but there are twice the number of false positives.[5,22] The American Cancer Society convened an expert panel in 2007, which issued new screening recommendations for use of MRI for women at high risk for breast cancer.[12] The Society recommends annual screening with MRI and mammogram for women at high lifetime risk of breast cancer, above 20%, as defined by the criteria below. Women at a moderate lifetime risk, or 15% to 20%, are urged to discuss MRI screening with their provider. In 2009, the USPSTF concluded that evidence is insufficient to determine the utility of MRI for screening. Expertise in reading MRIs varies across centers and should be considered when making recommendations about this test.

American Cancer Society Criteria for Adjunct MRI in High-Risk Women

High Risk, or 20%–25%	Moderate Risk, or 15%–20%
▹ Lifetime risk 20%–25% using assessment tools	▹ Lifetime risk 15%–20% using risk assessment tools
▹ Known BRCA1 or BRCA2 mutation	▹ History of breast cancer, ductal or lobular carcinoma in situ, atypical ductal or lobular hyperplasia
▹ Known first-degree relative, including father, brother, with BRCA1 or BRCA2 mutation, but woman not tested	▹ Extremely dense breasts or unevenly dense breasts on mammograms
▹ History of chest radiation between ages 10 and 30	
▹ Has high-risk genetic syndrome or first-degree relative with high-risk syndrome	

Source: American Cancer Society. Breast Cancer Facts and Figures 2009–2010. pp 13–14. Available at: http://www.cancer.org/acs/groups/content/anho/documents/document/f861009final90809pdf.pdf. Accessed November 17, 2010.

Chemoprevention. A growing literature documents both the efficacy and the underutilization of the selective estrogen receptor modulators (SERMs) tamoxifen and raloxifene for reducing risk of invasive breast cancer in breast-cancer-free women at high risk. High risk is usually based on a 5-year Gail risk score ≥1.66%. Tomoxifen is approved for use in all women, and raloxifene for postmenopausal women. In 2002 and reaffirmed in 2009, the USPSTF recommended discussion of chemoprevention with these agents for women at high risk of breast cancer and low risk of associated adverse events.[22] Tamoxifen and raloxifene have been shown to reduce incidence for estrogen-receptor positive cancers by 30% to 50%. Studies and meta-analyses show limited impact on incidence of estrogen-receptor negative breast cancer, noninvasive cancers, or mortality.[5,33,34] The STAR trial, which compared tamoxifen directly with raloxifene and was updated in 2010, showed comparable reduction of incidence of invasive breast cancer, but a trend toward higher incidence of noninvasive breast cancer for patients receiving raloxifen.[35,36] Raloxifene has lower associated side effects such as endometrial cancer, hysterectomies, thromboembolic events, and cataracts.

It is important for clinicians to be well informed about the benefits of chemoprevention as primary prevention of breast cancer. An estimated 2 million U.S. women would benefit from chemoprevention;[3] however, the prevalence of chemoprevention use in eligible women in the United States is exceptionally low, perhaps due to concerns about side effects.[37]

Another class of drugs that holds promise for chemoprevention is currently under investigation—the aromatase inhibitors. In postmenopausal women, these drugs inhibit or inactivate the adrenal enzyme aromatase, which catalyzes the final step in tissue synthesis of estradiol from precursor androgens.

Counseling Women About Breast Cancer

The Challenges of Communicating Risks and Benefits. As breast cancer screening and prevention options become more complex, clinicians should consider how best to express statistics on risks and benefits in terms that patients can easily understand. Framing, or presenting the same information in terms of either increased benefit or decreased harm, is one of several ways of presenting data that can compromise informed consent. For example, Elmore[38] recommends that, instead of reporting a Gail model risk of diagnosis of breast cancer in 5 years as 1.1%, explaining that only 11 out of 1,000 women would get such a diagnosis is easier for patients to grasp. Likewise, using the notion of *absolute risk* may be preferable to using *relative risk* to increase patients' comprehension. For example, relative risk of developing breast cancer among women using combined estrogen and progesterone has been reported as 1.26, or a 26% increased risk in users compared to non-users.[3,39] Among 10,000 users over 5.2 years, the expected number of breast cancers is 38, compared to 30 in 10,000 nonusers. The 26% increased risk results in a total of 8 additional cases of breast cancer over 5.2 years.

Web Sites for Breast Cancer Information. Encourage your patients to pursue breast cancer–related information from recommended sources to help them make informed choices during shared decision making.

Breast Cancer Web Sites

Calculators for risk of a breast cancer diagnosis and death:
   http://www.cancer.gov/bcrisktool/ (Gail Model; updated for African
      American women)
   http://astor.som.jhmi.edu/BaysMendel/brcapro.html (model that predicts
      the probability of carrying a *BRCA1* or *BRCA2* mutation)
   http://www.diseaseriskindex.harvard.edu/update/

Breast Self-Examination Tutorials
   http://ww5.komen.org/breast-cancer/breatselfawareness.html
   http://www.breastselfexam.ca

National Guidelines for Breast Cancer Screening
   http://www.guidelines.gov

Randomized Clinical Trials of New Modalities in Breast Cancer Screening
   http://www.clinicaltrials.gov
   http://www.acrin.org/protocolsummarytable.aspx

All Web sites accessed November 21, 2010.

Techniques of Examination

THE FEMALE BREAST

The clinical breast examination provides an important opportunity to identify breast masses and to teach techniques for self-examination to the patient. Clinical investigation has shown, however, that variations in examiner experience and technique affect the value of the clinical breast examination. Clinicians are advised to adopt a more standardized approach, especially for palpation, and to use a systemic and thorough search pattern, varying palpation pressure, and a circular motion with the fingerpads.[2] These techniques are discussed in more detail in the following pages. Inspection is routinely recommended, but its value in breast cancer detection is less well studied.

As you begin the examination, be reassuring and adopt a courteous and gentle approach. Let the patient know that you are about to examine her breasts. This may be a good time to ask if she has noticed any lumps or other problems and if she performs a monthly breast self-examination. If she does not, teach her good technique and watch as she repeats the steps of examination after you, giving helpful correction as needed.

An adequate inspection initially requires full exposure of the chest, but later in the examination, cover one breast while you are palpating the other. Because breasts tend to swell and become more nodular before menses as a result of increasing estrogen stimulation, the best time for examination is 5 to 7 days *after* the onset of menstruation. Nodules appearing during the premenstrual phase should be re-evaluated at this later time.

Risk factors for breast cancer include previous breast cancer, an affected mother or sister, biopsy showing atypical hyperplasia, increasing age, early menarche, late menopause, late or no pregnancies, and previous radiation to the chest wall. See table on Breast Cancer in Women: Factors That Increase Relative Risk, p. 412.

See Patient Instructions for the Breast Self-Examination, p. 427.

Inspection

Inspect the breasts and nipples with the patient in the sitting position and disrobed to the waist. A thorough examination of the breast includes careful inspection for skin changes, symmetry, contours, and retraction in four views—arms at sides, arms over head, arms pressed against hips, and leaning forward. When examining an adolescent girl, assess her breast development according to Tanner's sex maturity ratings described on pages 863–864.

Arms at Sides. Note the clinical features listed below.

- The *appearance of the skin*, including:

  - Color

    Redness may be from local infection or inflammatory carcinoma.

  - Thickening of the skin and unusually prominent pores, which may accompany lymphatic obstruction

    Thickening and prominent pores suggest breast cancer.

- The *size and symmetry of the breasts*. Some difference in the size of the breasts, including the areolae, is common and usually normal, as shown in the photograph below.

- The *contour of the breasts*. Look for changes such as masses, dimpling, or flattening. Compare one side with the other.

  Flattening of the normally convex breast suggests cancer. See Table 10-2, Visible Signs of Breast Cancer, p. 431.

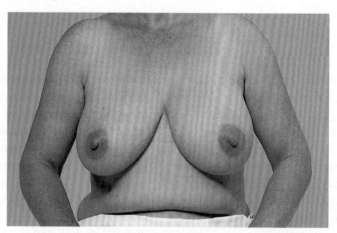

ARMS AT SIDES

- The *characteristics of the nipples*, including *size and shape*, *direction* in which they point, any *rashes* or *ulceration*, or any *discharge*.

  Asymmetry of directions in which nipples point suggests an underlying cancer. Rash or ulceration occurs in Paget's disease of the breast.[13] (See p. 431.)

Occasionally, the shape of the nipple is *inverted*, or depressed below the areolar surface. It may be enveloped by folds of areolar skin, as illustrated. Long-standing inversion is usually a normal variant of no clinical consequence, except for possible difficulty when breast-feeding.

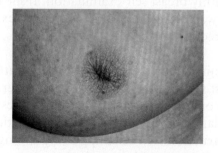

Recent or fixed flattening or depression of the nipple suggests nipple retraction. A retracted nipple may also be broadened and thickened, suggesting an underlying cancer.

Arms Over Head; Hands Pressed Against Hips; Leaning Forward. To bring out dimpling or retraction that may otherwise be invisible, ask the patient to raise her arms over her head, then press her hands against her hips to contract the pectoral muscles. Inspect the breast contours carefully in each position. If the breasts are large or pendulous, it may be useful to have the patient stand and lean forward, supported by the back of the chair or the examiner's hands.

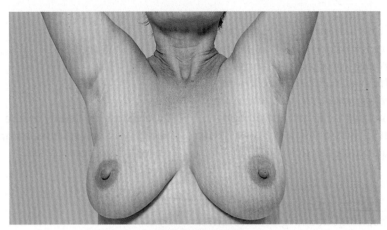

ARMS OVER HEAD

Dimpling or retraction of the breasts in these positions suggests an underlying cancer. When a cancer or its associated fibrous strands are attached to both the skin and the fascia overlying the pectoral muscles, pectoral contraction can draw the skin inward, causing dimpling.

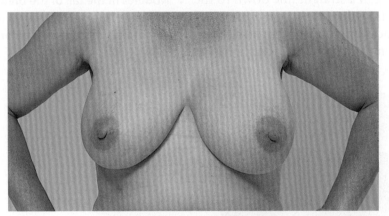

HANDS PRESSED AGAINST HIPS

Occasionally, these signs may be associated with benign lesions such as posttraumatic fat necrosis or mammary duct ectasia, but they must always be further evaluated.

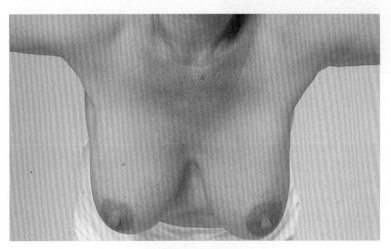

LEANING FORWARD

This position may reveal an asymmetry of the breast or nipple not otherwise visible. Retraction of the nipple and areola suggests an underlying cancer. See Table 10-2, Visible Signs of Breast Cancer, p. 431.

Palpation

The Breast. Palpation is best performed when the breast tissue is flattened. The patient should be supine. Plan to palpate a rectangular area extending from the clavicle to the inframammary fold or bra line, and from the midsternal line to the posterior axillary line and well into the axilla for the tail of the breast.

A thorough examination will take 3 minutes for each breast. Use the *fingerpads* of the 2nd, 3rd, and 4th fingers, keeping the fingers slightly flexed. It is important to be *systematic*. Although a circular or wedge pattern can be used, the *vertical strip pattern* is currently the best validated technique for detecting breast masses.[2] Palpate in *small, concentric circles* at each examining point, if possible applying light, medium, and deep pressure. You will need to press more firmly to reach the deeper tissues of a large breast. Your examination should cover the entire breast, including the periphery, tail, and axilla.

- To examine *the lateral portion of the breast*, ask the patient to roll onto the opposite hip, placing her hand on her forehead but keeping the shoulders pressed against the bed or examining table. This flattens the lateral breast tissue. Begin palpation in the axilla, moving in a straight line down to the bra line, then move the fingers medially and palpate in a vertical strip up the chest to the clavicle. Continue in vertical overlapping strips until you reach the nipple, then reposition the patient to flatten the medial portion of the breast.

- To examine *the medial portion of the breast*, ask the patient to lie with her shoulders flat against the bed or examining table, placing her hand at her neck and lifting up her elbow until it is even with her shoulder. Palpate in a straight line down from the nipple to the bra line, then back to the clavicle, continuing in vertical overlapping strips to the midsternum.

When pressing deeply on the breast, you may mistake a normal rib for a hard breast mass.

Nodules in the tail of the breast in the axilla (the tail of Spence) are sometimes mistaken for enlarged axillary lymph nodes.

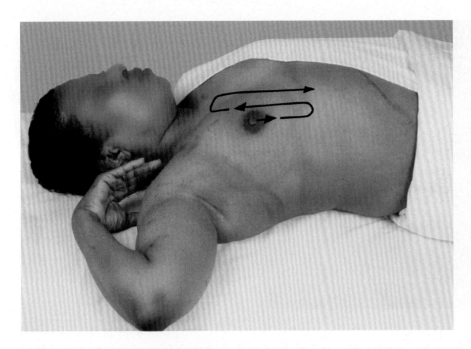

Examine the breast tissue carefully for:

- *Consistency* of the tissues. Normal consistency varies widely, depending in part on the relative proportions of firmer glandular tissue and soft fat. Physiologic nodularity may be present, increasing before menses. There may be a firm transverse ridge of compressed tissue along the lower margin of the breast, especially in large breasts. This is the normal inframammary ridge, not a tumor.

  Tender cords suggest *mammary duct ectasia,* a benign but sometimes painful condition of dilated ducts with surrounding inflammation, sometimes with associated masses.

- *Tenderness*, as in premenstrual fullness

- *Nodules.* Palpate carefully for any lump or mass that is qualitatively different from or larger than the rest of the breast tissue. This is sometimes called a dominant mass and may reflect a pathologic change that requires evaluation by mammogram, aspiration, or biopsy. Assess and describe the characteristics of any nodule:

  See Table 10-1, Common Breast Masses, p. 430.

  Location—by quadrant or clock, with centimeters from the nipple

  Hard, irregular, poorly circumscribed nodules, fixed to the skin or underlying tissues, strongly suggest cancer.

  Size—in centimeters

  Shape—round or cystic, disclike, or irregular in contour

  Consistency—soft, firm, or hard

  Delimitation—well circumscribed or not

  Tenderness

  Check for cysts and inflamed areas; some cancers may be tender.

  Mobility—in relation to the skin, pectoral fascia, and chest wall. Gently move the breast near the mass and watch for dimpling.

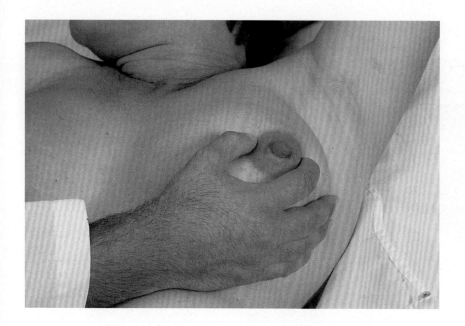

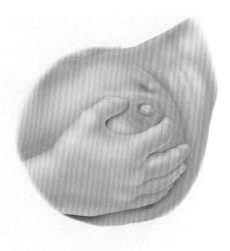

● Next, try to move the mass itself while the patient relaxes her arm and then while she presses her hand against her hip.

A mobile mass that becomes fixed when the arm relaxes is attached to the ribs and intercostal muscles; if fixed when the hand is pressed against the hip, it is attached to the pectoral fascia.

The Nipple. Palpate each nipple, noting its elasticity. Press more firmly if there is a history of nipple discharge (see p. 426).

Thickening of the nipple and loss of elasticity suggest an underlying cancer.

THE MALE BREAST

Examination of the male breast may be brief but is important. *Inspect the nipple and areola* for nodules, swelling, or ulceration. *Palpate the areola and breast tissue* for nodules. If the breast appears enlarged, distinguish between the soft fatty enlargement of obesity and the firm disc of glandular enlargement, called *gynecomastia*.

Gynecomastia arises from an imbalance of estrogens and androgens, sometimes drug related. A hard, irregular, eccentric, or ulcerating nodule suggests *breast cancer*.[40,41]

THE AXILLAE

Although the axillae may be examined with the patient lying down, a sitting position is preferable.

Inspection

Inspect the skin of each axilla, noting evidence of:

- Rash

- Infection

- Unusual pigmentation

Deodorant and other rashes may be found.

Sweat gland infection (*hidradenitis suppurativa*) may be found.

Deeply pigmented, velvety axillary skin suggests *acanthosis nigricans*—one form is associated with internal malignancy.

Palpation

To examine the left axilla, ask the patient to relax with the left arm down. Help by supporting the left wrist or hand with your left hand. Cup together the fingers of your right hand and reach as high as you can toward the apex of the axilla. Warn the patient that this may feel uncomfortable. Your fingers should lie directly behind the pectoral muscles, pointing toward the mid-clavicle. Now press your fingers in toward the chest wall and slide them downward, trying to feel the central nodes against the chest wall. Of the axillary nodes, these are the most often palpable. One or more soft, small (<1 cm), nontender nodes are frequently felt.

Use your left hand to examine the right axilla.

If the central nodes feel large, hard, or tender, or if there is a suspicious lesion in the drainage areas for the axillary nodes, feel for the other groups of axillary lymph nodes:

- *Pectoral nodes*—grasp the anterior axillary fold between your thumb and fingers, and with your fingers, palpate inside the border of the pectoral muscle.

- *Lateral nodes*—from high in the axilla, feel along the upper humerus.

- *Subscapular nodes*—step behind the patient and, with your fingers, feel inside the muscle of the posterior axillary fold.

Also, feel for infraclavicular nodes and re-examine the supraclavicular nodes.

Enlarged axillary nodes may result from infection of the hand or arm, recent immunizations or skin tests in the arm, or generalized lymph-adenopathy. Check the epitrochlear nodes and other groups of lymph nodes.

Nodes that are large (≥1 cm) and firm or hard, matted together, or fixed to the skin or to underlying tissues suggest malignancy.

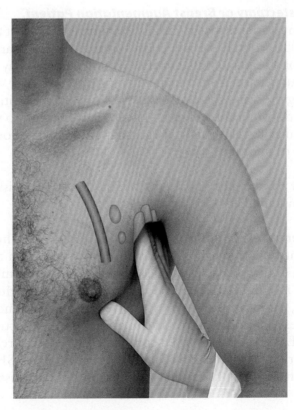

SPECIAL TECHNIQUES

Assessment of Spontaneous Nipple Discharge.   If there is a history of spontaneous nipple discharge, try to determine its origin by compressing the areola with your index finger, placed in radial positions around the nipple. Watch for discharge appearing through one of the duct openings on the nipple's surface. Note the color, consistency, and quantity of any discharge and the exact location where it appears.

Milky discharge unrelated to a prior pregnancy and lactation is *nonpuerperal galactorrhea*. Causes include *hypothyroidism*, pituitary *prolactinoma*, and drugs that are dopamine agonists, including many psychotropic agents and phenothiazines.

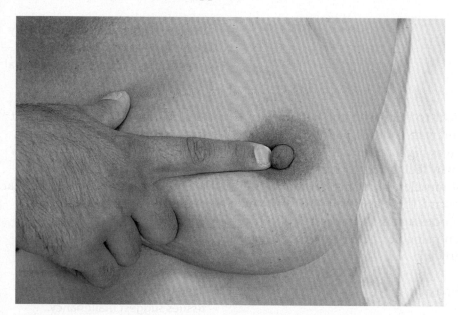

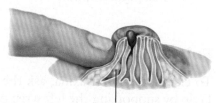
Papilloma

Spontaneous unilateral bloody discharge from one or two ducts warrants further evaluation for intraductal *papilloma*, shown above, *ductal carcinoma in situ*, or *Paget's disease of the breast*. Clear, serous, green, black, or nonbloody discharges that are multiductal are usually benign.[1]

Examination of the Mastectomy or Breast Augmentation Patient.   The woman with a mastectomy warrants special care on examination. Inspect the mastectomy scar and axilla carefully for any masses or unusual nodularity. Note any change in color or signs of inflammation. Lymphedema may be present in the axilla and upper arm from impaired lymph drainage after surgery. Palpate gently along the scar—these tissues may be unusually sensitive. Use a circular motion with two or three fingers. Pay special attention to the upper outer quadrant and axilla. Note any enlargement of the lymph nodes or signs of inflammation or infection.

Masses, nodularity, and change in color or inflammation, especially in the incision line, suggest recurrence of breast cancer.

It is especially important to carefully palpate the breast tissue and incision lines of women with breast augmentation or reconstruction.

Instructions for the Breast Self-Examination (BSE).   The office or hospital visit is an important time to teach your patient how to perform the BSE. A high proportion of breast masses are detected by women examining their own breasts. Although BSE has not been shown to reduce breast cancer mortality, monthly BSE is inexpensive and may promote stronger health awareness and more active self-care. For early detection of breast cancer, the BSE is most useful when coupled with regular breast examination by an experienced clinician and mammography. The BSE is best timed just after menses, when hormonal stimulation of breast tissue is low.

Patient Instructions for the Breast Self-Examination (BSE)

Lying Supine

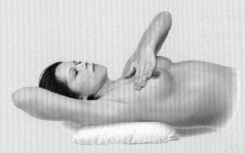
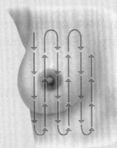

1. Lie down with a pillow under your right shoulder. Place your right arm behind your head.
2. Use the finger pads of the three middle fingers on your left hand to feel for lumps in the right breast. The finger pads are the top third of each finger.
3. Press firmly enough to know how your breast feels, using firmer pressure for tissue closest to the chest and ribs. A firm ridge in the lower curve of each breast is normal. If you're not sure how hard to press, talk with your health care provider, or try to copy the way the doctor or nurse does it.*

4. Press firmly on the breast in an up-and-down or "strip" pattern. You can also use a circular or wedge pattern, but be sure to use the same pattern every time. Check the entire breast area, from the underarm to the sternum and from the collarbone to the ribs below the breast. Remember how your breast feels from month to month.
5. Repeat the examination on your left breast, using the finger pads of the right hand.
6. If you find any masses, lumps, or skin changes, see your doctor right away.

Standing

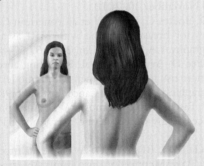
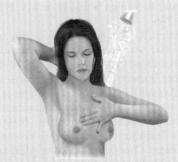

1. While standing in front of a mirror with your hands pressing firmly down on your hips, look at your breasts for any changes of size, shape, contour, or dimpling, or redness or scaliness of the nipple or breast skin. (The pressing down on the hips position contracts the chest wall muscles and enhances any breast changes.)

2. Examine each underarm while sitting up or standing and with your arm only slightly raised so you can easily feel in this area. Raising your arm straight up tightens the tissue in this area and makes it harder to examine.

Adapted from the American Cancer Society, updated September 2010. Available at http://www.cancer.org/Cancer/BreastCancer/MoreInformation/BreastCancerEarlyDetection/breast-cancer-early-detection-a-c-s-recs-b-s-e. Accessed December 3, 2010.

Recording Your Findings

Note that initially you may use sentences to describe your findings; later you will use phrases. The style below contains phrases appropriate for most write-ups.

Recording the Physical Examination—Breasts and Axillae

"Breasts symmetric and smooth without masses. Nipples without discharge."
(Axillary adenopathy usually included after Neck in section on Lymph Nodes; see p. 256.)

OR

"Breasts pendulous with diffuse fibrocystic changes. Single firm 1 × 1 cm mass, mobile and nontender, with overlying peau d'orange appearance in right breast, upper outer quadrant at 11 o'clock, 2 cm from the nipple."

Suggests possible breast cancer.

Bibliography

Citations

1. Santen RJ, Mansel R. Benign breast disorders. N Engl J Med 2005;353:275–285.
2. Barton MB, Harris R, Fletcher SW. Does this patient have breast cancer? The screening clinical breast examination: should it be done? How? JAMA 1999;282:1270–1280.
3. American Cancer Society. Breast Cancer Facts and Figures 2009–2010. Available at http://www.cancer.org/acs/groups/content/@nho/documents/document/f861009final90809pdf.pdf. Accessed November 14, 2010.
4. National Cancer Institute. Breast Cancer Prevention. Health Professional Version. Overview and Description of Evidence. Updated October 22, 2010. Available at http://www.cancer.gov/cancertopics/pdq/prevention/breast/healthprofessional/allpages/print. Accessed November 14, 2010.
5. Nattinger A. In the clinic: breast cancer screening and prevention. Ann Intern Med 2010;152:ITC4–1ITC16.
6. Gómez-Raposo C, Zambrana Tévar F, Sereno Moyano M et al. Male breast cancer. Cancer Treat Rev 2010;36:451–457.
7. National Cancer Institute. Breast Cancer Risk Assessment Tool. Updated 2007. Available at http://www.cancer.gov/bcrisktool. Accessed November 14, 2010.
8. Gail MH, Costantino JP, Pee D et al. Projecting individualized absolute invasive breast cancer risk in African American women. J Natl Cancer Inst 2007;99(23):1782–1792.
9. Evans DGR and Howell A. Review: breast cancer risk-assessment tools. Breast Cancer Res 2007;9:213–221.
10. Tice JA, Cummings SR, Smith-Bindman R et al. Using clinical factors and mammographic breast density to estimate breast cancer risk: development and validation of a new predictive model. Ann Intern Med 2008;148:337–347.
11. National Cancer Institute. Genetics of Breast and Ovarian Cancer. Health Professional Version. Updated October 25, 2010. Available at http://www.cancer.gov/cancertopics/pdq/genetics/breast-and-ovarian/HealthProfessional. Accessed November 20, 2010.
12. Saslow D, Boetes C, Burke W et al. American Cancer Society guidelines for breast screening with MRI as an adjunct to mammography. CA Cancer J Clin 2007;57:57–89.
13. Chen J, Pee D, Ayyagari R et al. Projecting absolute invasive breast cancer risk in white women with a model that includes mammographic density. J Natl Cancer Inst 2006;98:1215–1226.
14. Claus EB, Risch N, and Thompson WD. Autosomal dominant inheritance of early-onset breast cancer. Cancer 1994;73:643–651.
15. BaysMendel Lab. BRCAPRO. Available at http://astor.som.jhmi.edu/BayesMendel/brcapro.html. Accessed November 19, 2010.
16. Chen S, Parmigiani G. Meta-analysis of BRCA1 and BRCA2 penetrance. J Clin Oncol 2007;25:1329–1333.
17. Hartmann LC, Sellers TA, Frost MH et al. Benign breast disorders and the risk of breast cancer. N Engl J Med 2005;353:229–237.
18. Carney PA, Miglioretti DL, Yankaskas et al. Individual and combined effects of age, breast density, and hormone replacement therapy use on the accuracy of screening mammography. Ann Intern Med 2005;138:168–175.
19. Boyd NF, Guo H, Li M et al. Mammographic density and the risk and detection of breast cancer. N Engl J Med 2007;356:227–236.
20. Vachon CM, Sellers TA, Carlson EE et al. Strong evidence of a genetic determinant for mammographic density, a major risk factor for breast cancer. Cancer Res 2007;67:8412–8418.
21. Yager JD, Davidson NE. Mechanisms of disease: estrogen carcinogenesis in breast cancer. N Engl J Med 2006;354:270–282.

BIBLIOGRAPHY

22. U.S. Preventive Services Task Force. Screening for breast cancer: U.S. Preventive Services Task Force recommendation statement. Ann Intern Med 2009;151:716–726.

23. Qaseem A, Snow SV, Aronson M et al. Screening mammography for women 40 to 49 years of age: a clinical practice guideline from the American College of Physicians. Ann Intern Med 2007;146:511–515.

24. Nelson HD, Tyne K, Haik A et al. Screening for breast cancer: an update for the U.S. Preventive Services Task Force. Ann Intern Med 2009;151:727–737.

25. Semiglazov VF, Manikhas AG, Moseenko VM et al. Results of a prospective randomized investation (Russia/St. Petersburg/WHO) to evaluate the significance of self-examination for the early detection of breast cancer. Vopr Onko. 2003;49:434–441. As cited in Nelson HD, 2009.

26. Thomas DV, Bao DL, Ray RM et al. Randomized trial of breast self-examination in Shanghai: final results. J Natl Cancer Institute 2002;94:1445–1457.

27. Tu SP, Reisch LM, Taplin SH et al. Breast self-examination: self-reported frequency, quality, and associated outcomes. J Cancer Educ 2006;21:175–181.

28. Kagawa-Singer M, Tanjasiri SP, Valdez A et al. Outcomes of a breast health project for Hmong women and men in California. Am J Public Health 2009;99(Suppl 2):S467–473.

29. Parsa P, Kandiah M. Predictors of adherence to clinical breast examination and mammography screening among Malaysian women. Asian Pac J Cancer Prev 2010;11:681–688.

30. Dunn RA, Tan A, Samad I. Does performance of breast self-exams increase the probability of using mammography: evidence from Malaysia. Asian Pac J Cancer Prev 2010;11:417–421.

31. Wilke LG, Broadwater G, Rabiner S et al. Breast self-examination: defining a cohort still in need. Am J Surg 2009;198:575–579.

32. Humphrey LL, Helfand M, Chan BK et al. Breast cancer screening: a summary for the U.S. Preventive Services Task Force. Ann Intern Med 2002;137:347–360.

33. U.S. Preventive Services Task Force. Chemoprevention of breast cancer: recommendations and rationale. July 2002. Available at http://www.uspreventiveservicestaskforce.org/3rduspstf/breastchemo/breastchemorr.htm. Accessed November 21, 2010.

34. Nelson HD, Fu R, Griffin JC et al. Systematic review: comparative effectiveness of medication to reduce risk for primary breast cancer. Ann Intern Med 2009;151:703–715.

35. Vogel VG, Constantino JP, Wickerham Dl et al. Effects of tamoxiphen vs raloxifene on the risk of developing invasive breast cancer and other disease outcomes: the NSABP study of tamoxifen and raloxifene (STAR) P-2 trial. JAMA 2006; 295:2727–2741.

36. Vogel VG, Constantino JP, Wickerham D et al. Update of the National Surgical Adjuvant Breast and Bowel Project Study of Tamoxiphen and Raloxfene (STAR) P-2 Trail. Cancer Prev Res 2010;3:696–706.

37. Waters EA, Cronin KA, Graubard BI et al. Prevalence of tamoxifen use for breast dancer chemoprevention among U.S. women. Cancer Epidemiol Biomarkers Prev 2010;19:443–446.

38. Elmore JG, Gigerenzer G. Benign breast disease: the risks of communicating risk (editorial). N Engl J Med 2005;353:297–298.

39. Roussouw JE, Anderson GL, Prentice RL et al. Risks and benefits of estrogen plus progestin in healthy postmenopausal women: principal results from the Women's Health Initiative randomized controlled trial. JAMA 2002;288:321–333.

40. Johnson RE, Murad MH. Gynecomastia: pathophysiology, evaluation, and management. Mayo Clin Proc 2009;84:1010–1015.

41. Hines Sl, Larson JM, Thompson KM et al. A practical approach to guide clinicians in the evaluation of male patients with breast masses. Geriatrics 2008;63:19–24.

Additional References

Baer HJ, Collins LC, Connolly JL et al. Lobule type and subsequent breast cancer risk: results from the Nurses' Health Studies. Cancer 2009;115:1404–1411.

Bland KI, Beenken SW, Copeland EM. Ch. 17, The Breast. In Brunicardi FC, Andersen DK, Billiar TM et al (eds). Schwartz's Principles of Surgery, 9th ed. New York: McGraw-Hill Medical, 2010.

Fisher B, Costantino JP, Wickerham DL, et al. Tamoxifen for the prevention of breast cancer: current status of the National Surgical Adjuvant Breast and Bowel Project P-1 study. J Natl Cancer Inst 2005;97:1652–1662.

Goldhirsch A, Wood WC, Gilber RD et al. Progress and promise: highlights of the international expert consensus on the primary therapy of early breast cancer 2007. Ann Oncol 2007;18:1133–1144.

Harlan LC, Zujewski JA, Goodman MT et al. Breast cancer in men in the United States: a population-based study of diagnosis, treatment, and survival. Cancer 2010;116:3558–3568.

Harvard School of Public Health. Disease Risk Index-Breast Cancer. Available at http://www.diseaseriskindex.harvard.edu/update/hccpquiz.pl?lang=english&func=home&quiz=breast. Accessed October 22, 2011.

Hines SL, Tan W, Larson JM et al. A practical approach to guide clinicians in the evaluation of male patients with breast masses. Geriatrics 2008;63:19–24.

Maruthur NM, Bolen S, Brancati FL et al. Obesity and mammography: a systematic review and meta-analysis. J Gen Intern Med 2009;24:665–677.

McKian KP, Reynolds CA, Visscher DW et al. Novel breast tissue feature strongly associated with risk of breast cancer. J Clin Oncol 2009;27(35):5893–5898.

Robson M, Offit K. Clinical practice. Management of an inherited predisposition to breast cancer. N Engl J Med 2007;357:154–162.

Smith-Bindman R, Miglioretti DL, Lurie N, et al. Does utilization of screening mammography explain racial and ethnic differences in breast cancer? Ann Intern Med 2006;144:541–553.

Thorncroft K, Forsyth L, Desmond S et al. The diagnosis and management of diabetic mastopathy. Breast J 2007;13:607–613.

> The Bates' suite offers these additional resources to enhance learning and facilitate understanding of this chapter:
>
> - Bates' Pocket Guide to Physical Examination and History Taking, 7th edition
> - Bates' Visual Guide to Physical Examination
> - thePoint online resources, for students and instructors: http://thepoint.lww.com

Table

10-1   **Common Breast Masses**

The three most common kinds of breast masses are *fibroadenoma* (a benign tumor), *cysts*, and *breast cancer*. The clinical characteristics of these masses are listed below. However, any breast mass should be carefully evaluated and usually warrants further investigation by ultrasound, aspiration, mammography, or biopsy. The masses depicted below are large for purposes of illustration. Ideally, breast cancer should be identified early, when the mass is small. *Fibrocystic changes*, not illustrated, are also commonly palpable as nodular, ropelike densities in women ages 25–50. They may be tender or painful. They are considered benign and are not viewed as a risk factor for breast cancer.

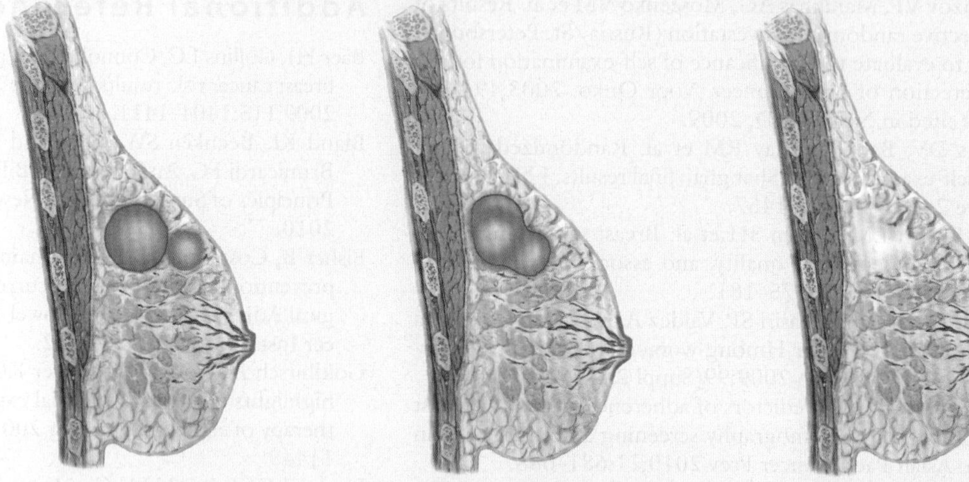

	Fibroadenoma	**Cysts**	**Cancer**
Usual Age	15–25, usually puberty and young adulthood, but up to age 55	30–50, regress after menopause except with estrogen therapy	30–90, most common over age 50
Number	Usually single, may be multiple	Single or multiple	Usually single, although may coexist with other nodules
Shape	Round, disclike, or lobular	Round	Irregular or stellate
Consistency	May be soft, usually firm	Soft to firm, usually elastic	Firm or hard
Delimitation	Well delineated	Well delineated	Not clearly delineated from surrounding tissues
Mobility	Very mobile	Mobile	May be fixed to skin or underlying tissues
Tenderness	Usually nontender	Often tender	Usually nontender
Retraction Signs	Absent	Absent	May be present

Table 10-2 | Visible Signs of Breast Cancer

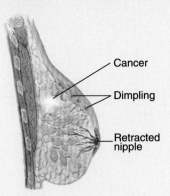

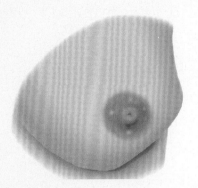

Retraction Signs

As breast cancer advances, it causes fibrosis (scar tissue). Shortening of this tissue produces *dimpling, changes in contour,* and *retraction or deviation of the nipple.* Other causes of retraction include fat necrosis and mammary duct ectasia.

Abnormal Contours

Look for any variation in the normal convexity of each breast, and compare one side with the other. Special positioning may again be useful. Shown here is marked flattening of the lower outer quadrant of the left breast.

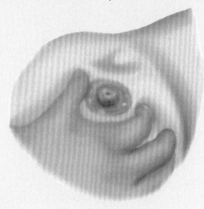

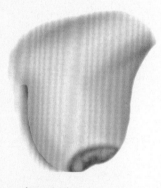

Skin Dimpling

Look for this sign with the patient's arm at rest, during special positioning, and on moving or compressing the breast, as illustrated here.

Nipple Retraction and Deviation

A retracted nipple is flattened or pulled inward, as illustrated here. It may also be broadened, and feels thickened. When involvement is radially asymmetric, the nipple may deviate or point in a different direction from its normal counterpart, typically toward the underlying cancer.

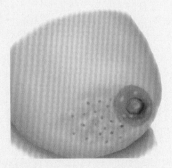

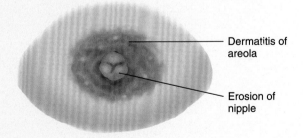

Edema of the Skin

Edema of the skin is produced by lymphatic blockade. It appears as thickened skin with enlarged pores—the so-called *peau d'orange* (orange peel) *sign.* It is often seen first in the lower portion of the breast or areola.

Paget's Disease of the Nipple

This uncommon form of breast cancer usually starts as a scaly, eczemalike lesion that may weep, crust, or erode. A breast mass may be present. Suspect Paget's disease in any persisting dermatitis of the nipple and areola. Can present with invasive breast cancer or ductal carcinoma in situ.

The Abdomen

Anatomy and Physiology

Visualize or palpate the landmarks of the abdominal wall and pelvis, as illustrated. The rectus abdominis muscles become more prominent when the patient raises the head and shoulders from the supine position.

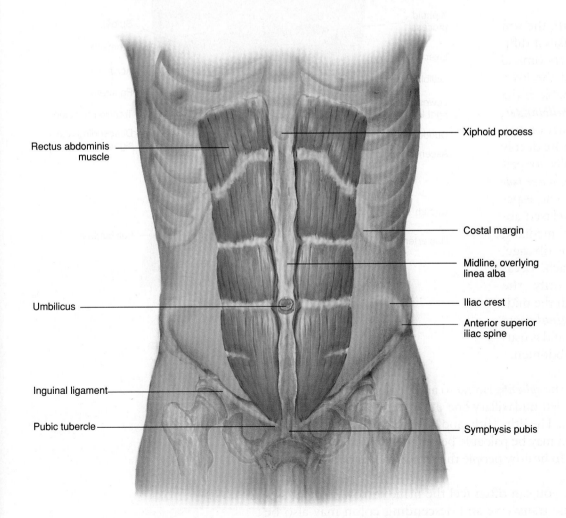

Rectus abdominis muscle

Umbilicus

Inguinal ligament

Pubic tubercle

Xiphoid process

Costal margin

Midline, overlying linea alba

Iliac crest

Anterior superior iliac spine

Symphysis pubis

For descriptive purposes, the abdomen is often divided by imaginary lines crossing at the umbilicus, forming the right upper, right lower, left upper, and left lower quadrants. Another system divides the abdomen into nine sections. Terms for three of them are commonly used: epigastric, umbilical, and hypogastric or suprapubic.

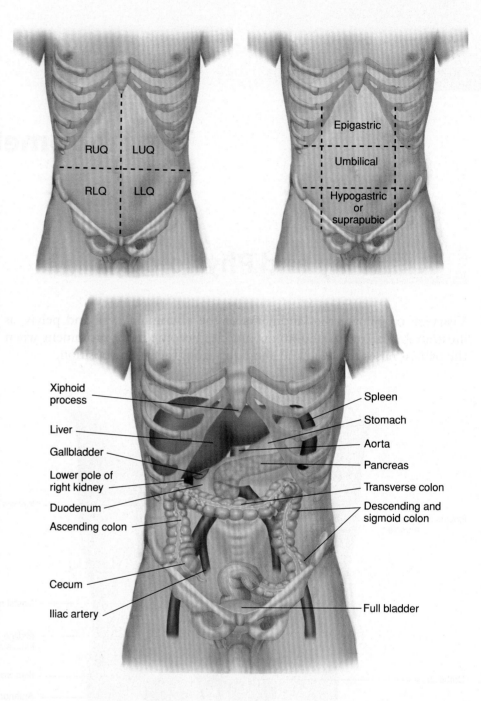

Examine the abdomen, moving in a clockwise rotation; several organs are often palpable. Exceptions are the stomach and much of the liver and spleen. The abdominal cavity extends up under the rib cage to the dome of the diaphragm, placing these organs in a protected location, beyond the reach of the palpating hand.

In the *right upper quadrant*, the soft consistency of the *liver* makes it difficult to feel through the abdominal wall. The lower margin of the liver, the liver edge, is often palpable at the right costal margin. The *gallbladder*, which rests against the inferior surface of the liver, and the more deeply lying *duodenum* are generally not palpable. At a deeper level, the *lower pole of the right kidney* may be felt, especially in thin people with relaxed abdominal muscles. Moving medially, the examiner encounters the rib cage, which protects the stomach; occasionally patients misidentify the stony hard *xiphoid process* in the midline as a tumor. The *abdominal aorta* often has visible pulsations and is usually palpable in the upper abdomen.

In the *left upper quadrant*, the *spleen* is lateral to and behind the stomach, just above the left kidney in the left midaxillary line. Its upper margin rests against the dome of the diaphragm. The 9th, 10th, and 11th ribs protect most of the spleen. The tip of the spleen may be palpable below the left costal margin in a small percentage of adults. In healthy people the *pancreas* cannot be detected.

In the *left lower quadrant*, you can often feel the firm, narrow, tubular sigmoid *colon*. Portions of the transverse and descending colon may also be palpable. In the lower midline are the *bladder*, the *sacral promontory*, the bony anterior edge of the S1 vertebra, sometimes mistaken for a tumor, and, in women, the *uterus* and *ovaries*.

In the *right lower quadrant* are bowel loops and the *appendix* at the tail of the cecum near the junction of the small and large intestines. In healthy people, these are not palpable.

A distended *bladder* may be palpable above the symphysis pubis. The bladder accommodates roughly 300 mL of urine filtered by the kidneys into the renal pelvis and the ureters. Bladder expansion stimulates contraction of bladder smooth muscle, the *detrusor muscle*, at relatively low pressures. Rising pressure in the bladder triggers the conscious urge to void.

Increased intraurethral pressure can overcome rising pressures in the bladder and prevent incontinence. Intraurethral pressure is related to smooth muscle tone in the internal urethral sphincter, the thickness of the urethral mucosa, and, in women, sufficient support to the bladder and proximal urethra from pelvic muscles and ligaments to maintain proper anatomical relationships. Striated muscle around the urethra can also contract voluntarily to interrupt voiding.

Neuroregulatory control of the bladder functions at several levels. In infants, the bladder empties by reflex mechanisms in the sacral spinal cord. Voluntary control of the bladder depends on higher centers in the brain and on motor and sensory pathways between the brain and the reflex arcs of the sacral spinal cord. When voiding is inconvenient, higher centers in the brain can inhibit detrusor contractions until the capacity of the bladder, approximately 400 to 500 mL, is exceeded. The integrity of the sacral nerves that innervate the bladder can be tested by assessing perirectal and perineal sensation in the S2, S3, and S4 dermatomes (see p. 731).

The *kidneys* are posterior organs. The ribs protect their upper poles. The *costovertebral angle*, formed by the lower border of the 12th rib and the transverse processes of the upper lumbar vertebrae, defines where to examine for kidney tenderness, termed costovertebral angle tenderness, or CVAT.

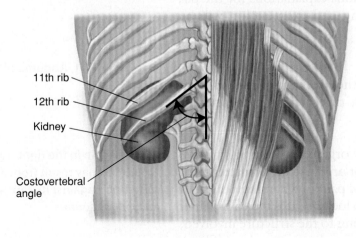

11th rib
12th rib
Kidney
Costovertebral angle

POSTERIOR VIEW

The Health History

Common or Concerning Symptoms

Gastrointestinal Disorders	Urinary and Renal Disorders
▶ Abdominal pain, acute and chronic	▶ Suprapubic pain
▶ Indigestion, nausea, vomiting including blood, loss of appetite, early satiety	▶ Dysuria, urgency, or frequency
	▶ Hesitancy, decreased stream in males
▶ Dysphagia and/or odynophagia	▶ Polyuria or nocturia
▶ Change in bowel function	▶ Urinary incontinence
▶ Diarrhea, constipation	▶ Hematuria
▶ Jaundice	▶ Kidney or flank pain
	▶ Ureteral colic

Gastrointestinal complaints rank high among reasons for office and emergency room visits. You will encounter a wide variety of upper gastrointestinal symptoms, including abdominal pain, heartburn, nausea and vomiting, difficulty or pain with swallowing, vomiting of stomach contents or blood, loss of appetite, and jaundice. Abdominal pain alone accounted for more than 13 million office visits and 4 million emergency room visits in 2007.[1,2] Lower gastrointestinal complaints are also common: diarrhea, constipation, change in bowel habits, and blood in the stool, often described as either bright red or dark and tarry.

Numerous symptoms also originate in the *genitourinary tract*: difficulty urinating, urgency and frequency, hesitancy and decreased stream in men, high urine volume, urinating at night, incontinence, blood in the urine, and flank pain and colic from renal stones or infection.

Often you will need to cluster several findings from both the patient's story and your examination as you sort through various explanations for the patient's symptoms. Your skills in history taking and examination will be needed for sound clinical reasoning.

Patterns and Mechanisms of Abdominal Pain. Before exploring gastrointestinal and genitourinary symptoms, review the mechanisms and clinical patterns of abdominal pain. Be familiar with three broad categories of abdominal pain:

See Table 11-1, Abdominal Pain, pp. 472–473.

- *Visceral pain* occurs when hollow abdominal organs such as the intestine or biliary tree contract unusually forcefully or are distended or stretched. Solid organs such as the liver can also become painful when their capsules are stretched. Visceral pain may be difficult to localize. It is typically palpable near the midline at levels that vary according to the structure involved, as illustrated on the next page. Ischemia also stimulates visceral pain fibers.

Visceral pain in the right upper quadrant may result from liver distention against its capsule in *alcoholic hepatitis*.

Visceral pain varies in quality and may be gnawing, burning, cramping, or aching. When it becomes severe, it may be associated with sweating, pallor, nausea, vomiting, and restlessness.

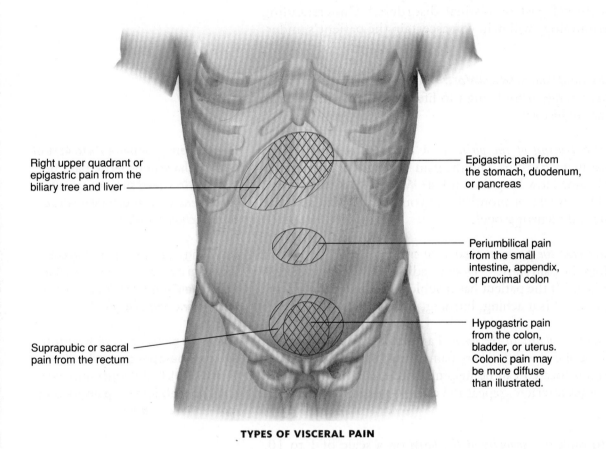

Right upper quadrant or epigastric pain from the biliary tree and liver

Epigastric pain from the stomach, duodenum, or pancreas

Periumbilical pain from the small intestine, appendix, or proximal colon

Suprapubic or sacral pain from the rectum

Hypogastric pain from the colon, bladder, or uterus. Colonic pain may be more diffuse than illustrated.

TYPES OF VISCERAL PAIN

- *Parietal pain* originates from inflammation in the parietal peritoneum. It is a steady, aching pain that is usually more severe than visceral pain and more precisely localized over the involved structure. It is typically aggravated by movement or coughing. Patients with this type of pain usually prefer to lie still.

- *Referred pain* is felt in more distant sites, which are innervated at approximately the same spinal levels as the disordered structures. Referred pain often develops as the initial pain becomes more intense and thus seems to radiate or travel from the initial site. It may be felt superficially or deeply but is usually localized.

Pain may also be referred to the abdomen from the chest, spine, or pelvis, thus complicating the assessment of abdominal pain.

Pain of duodenal or pancreatic origin may be referred to the back; pain from the biliary tree, to the right shoulder or the right posterior chest.

Pain from *pleurisy* or *inferior wall myocardial infarction* may be referred to the epigastric area.

THE GASTROINTESTINAL TRACT

Upper Abdominal Pain, Discomfort, and Heartburn. The prevalence of recurrent upper abdominal discomfort or pain is approximately 25% in the United States and other Western countries.[3] In recent years, consensus statements from expert societies have clarified the definitions and classification of numerous abdominal symptoms, particularly the Rome III criteria for functional gastrointestinal disorders.[4] Understanding carefully defined terminology will help you ascertain the patient's underlying condition.

Studies suggest that neuropeptides, such as 5-hydroxytryptophan and substance P, mediate interconnected symptoms of pain, bowel dysfunction, and stress.[4]

Acute Upper Abdominal Pain or Discomfort. For patients complaining of abdominal pain, causes range from benign to life threatening, so take the time to conduct a careful history.

- First determine the *timing of the pain*. Is it *acute or chronic?* Acute abdominal pain has many patterns. Did the pain start suddenly or gradually? When did it begin? How long does it last? What is its pattern over a 24-hour period? Over weeks or months? Are you dealing with an acute illness or a chronic and recurring one?

In emergency rooms, 40% to 45% of patients have nonspecific pain, but 15% to 30% need surgery, usually for *appendicitis*, intestinal obstruction, or *cholecystitis*.[5]

- Ask patients to *describe the pain in their own words*. Pursue important details: "Where does the pain start?" "Does it radiate or travel anywhere?" "What is the pain like?" If the patient has trouble describing the pain, try offering several choices: "Is it aching, burning, gnawing . . . ?"

Doubling over with cramping colicky pain indicates *renal stone*. Sudden knifelike epigastric pain occurs in *gallstone pancreatitis*.[6,7]

- Then ask the patient to *point to the pain*. Patients are not always clear when they try to describe in words where pain is most intense. The quadrant where the pain is located can be helpful. Often, underlying organs are involved. If clothes interfere, repeat the question during the physical examination.

Epigastric pain occurs with *gastritis* and gastroesophageal reflex disease (*GERD*). Right upper quadrant and upper abdominal pain are common in *cholecystitis*.[8]

- Ask the patient to rank the *severity of the pain* on a scale of 1 to 10. Note that severity does not always help you to identify the cause. Sensitivity to abdominal pain varies widely and tends to diminish in older patients, masking acute abdominal conditions. Pain thresholds and how patients accommodate to pain during daily activities also affect ratings of severity.

- As you explore *factors that aggravate or relieve the pain*, pay special attention to any association with meals, alcohol, medications (including aspirin and aspirinlike drugs and any over-the-counter medications), stress, body position, and use of antacids. Ask if indigestion or discomfort is related to exertion and relieved by rest.

Note that angina from inferior wall coronary artery disease may present as "indigestion," but is precipitated by exertion and relieved by rest. See Table 8-1, Chest Pain, pp. 322–323.

Chronic Upper Abdominal Discomfort or Pain. *Dyspepsia* is defined as chronic or recurrent discomfort or pain centered in the upper abdomen.[3] *Discomfort* is defined as a subjective negative feeling that is nonpainful. It can include various symptoms such as bloating, nausea, upper abdominal fullness, and heartburn.

- Note that bloating, nausea, or belching can occur alone and can be seen in other disorders. When these conditions occur alone, they do not meet the criteria for dyspepsia.

- Many patients with upper abdominal discomfort or pain will have *functional, or nonulcer, dyspepsia*, defined as a 3-month history of nonspecific upper abdominal discomfort or nausea not attributable to structural abnormalities or peptic ulcer disease. Symptoms are usually recurring and typically present for more than 6 months.[3]

Many patients with chronic upper abdominal discomfort or pain complain primarily of *heartburn, acid reflux*, or *regurgitation*. If patients report these symptoms more than once a week, they are likely to have *gastroesophageal reflux disease (GERD)* unless proven otherwise.[3,9]

- *Heartburn* is a rising retrosternal burning pain or discomfort occurring weekly or more often. It is typically aggravated by food such as alcohol, chocolate, citrus fruits, coffee, onions, and peppermint; or positions like bending over, exercising, lifting, or lying supine.

- Some patients with GERD have *atypical respiratory symptoms* such as cough, wheezing, and aspiration pneumonia. Others complain of *pharyngeal symptoms*, such as hoarseness chronic sore throat, and laryngitis.[10]

- Some patients may have *"alarm symptoms,"* such as difficulty swallowing (*dysphagia*), pain with swallowing (*odynophagia*), recurrent vomiting, evidence of gastrointestinal bleeding, weight loss, anemia, or risk factors for gastric cancer, a palpable mass, or jaundice.

Bloating may occur with *inflammatory bowel disease*; belching from *aerophagia*, or swallowing air.

Multifactorial causes include delayed gastric emptying (20%–40%), gastritis from *H. pylori* (20%–60%), peptic ulcer disease (up to 15% if *H. pylori* is present), and psychosocial factors.[3]

These symptoms or mucosal damage on endoscopy are the diagnostic criteria for GERD. Risk factors include reduced salivary flow, which prolongs acid clearance by damping action of the bicarbonate buffer; delayed gastric emptying; selected medications; and hiatal hernia.

Note that angina from inferior wall coronary ischemia along the diaphragm may present as heartburn. See Table 8-1, Chest Pain, pp. 322–323.

Thirty percent to 90% of patients with asthma and 10% with specialty referral for throat conditions have GERD-like symptoms.

Patients with uncomplicated GERD who do not respond to empiric therapy, patients older than 55 years, and those with "alarm symptoms" warrant endoscopy to detect *esophagitis*, peptic strictures, or *Barrett's esophagus*. In this condition, the squamocolumnar junction is displaced proximally and replaced by intestinal metaplasia, increasing the risk of esophageal adenocarcinoma 30-fold.[9,11-14] Approximately 50% of patients with GERD will have no disease on endoscopy.[15]

Lower Abdominal Pain and Discomfort—Acute and Chronic. Lower abdominal pain and discomfort may be acute or chronic. Asking the patient to point to the pain and characterize all its features, combined with findings on the physical examination, will help you identify possible causes. Some acute pain, especially in the suprapubic area or radiating from the flank, originates in the genitourinary tract (see p. 446).

Acute Lower Abdominal Pain. Patients may complain of *acute pain* localized to the *right lower quadrant*. Find out if it is sharp and continuous, or intermittent and cramping, causing them to double over.

Right lower quadrant pain or pain that migrates from the periumbilical region, combined with abdominal wall rigidity on palpation, is most likely to predict *appendicitis*. In women, consider *pelvic inflammatory disease, ruptured ovarian follicle,* and *ectopic pregnancy.*[16]

Cramping pain radiating to the right or left lower quadrant may be a renal stone.

When patients report acute pain in the *left lower quadrant* or *diffuse abdominal pain,* investigate associated symptoms such as fever and loss of appetite.

Left lower quadrant pain with a palpable mass may be *diverticulitis.* Diffuse abdominal pain with absent bowel sounds and firmness, guarding, or rebound on palpation is seen in *small or large bowel obstruction* (see pp. 472–473).

Chronic Lower Abdominal Pain. If there is *chronic pain* in the quadrants of the lower abdomen, ask about change in bowel habits and alternating diarrhea and constipation.

Change in bowel habits with mass lesion indicates *colon cancer.* Intermittent pain for 12 weeks of the preceding 12 months with relief from defecation, change in frequency of bowel movements, or change in form of stool (loose, watery, pellet-like), without structural or biochemical abnormalities are symptoms of *irritable bowel syndrome.*[17,18]

Gastrointestinal Symptoms Associated With Abdominal Pain. Patients often experience abdominal pain in conjunction with other symptoms. "How is your appetite?" is a good starting question that may lead to other concerns like *indigestion, nausea, vomiting,* and *anorexia. Indigestion* is a general term for distress associated with eating that can have many meanings. Urge your patient to be more specific.

Anorexia, nausea, and vomiting accompany many gastrointestinal disorders; these are all seen in pregnancy, *diabetic ketoacidosis, adrenal insufficiency, hypercalcemia, uremia,* liver disease, emotional states, adverse drug reactions, and other conditions. Induced vomiting without nausea is more indicative of *anorexia/bulimia.*

- *Nausea,* often described as "feeling sick to my stomach," may progress to retching and vomiting. *Retching* describes involuntary spasm of the stomach, diaphragm, and esophagus that precedes and culminates in *vomiting,* the forceful expulsion of gastric contents out of the mouth.

Some patients may not actually vomit but raise esophageal or gastric contents without nausea or retching, called *regurgitation*.

Ask about any vomitus or regurgitated material and inspect it if possible. What color is it? What does the vomitus smell like? How much has there been? You may have to help the patient with the amount: a teaspoon? Two teaspoons? A cupful?

Vomiting and pain indicate *small bowel obstruction*. Fecal odor occurs with *small bowel obstruction* or *gastrocolic fistula*.

Ask specifically if the vomitus contains any blood, and quantify the amount. Gastric juice is clear and mucoid. Small amounts of yellowish or greenish bile are common and have no special significance. Brownish or blackish vomitus with a "coffee grounds" appearance suggests blood altered by gastric acid. Coffee-grounds emesis or red blood is termed *hematemesis*.

Hematemesis may accompany *esophageal* or *gastric varices*, *gastritis*, or *peptic ulcer disease*.

Is there any dehydration or electrolyte imbalance from prolonged vomiting or significant blood loss? Do the patient's symptoms suggest any complications of vomiting, such as aspiration into the lungs, seen in debilitated, obtunded, or elderly patients?

Symptoms of blood loss such as lightheadedness or syncope depend on the rate and volume of bleeding and are rare until blood loss exceeds 500 mL.

- *Anorexia* is loss or lack of appetite. Find out if it arises from intolerance to certain foods or reluctance to eat because of anticipated discomfort. Check for associated symptoms of nausea and vomiting.

Patients may complain of unpleasant *abdominal fullness* after light or moderate meals, or *early satiety*, the inability to eat a full meal. A dietary assessment or recall may be warranted (see Chapter 4, General Survey, Vital Signs, and Pain, pp. 110–111).

Consider *diabetic gastroparesis*, anticholinergic medications, *gastric outlet obstruction*, *gastric cancer*; early satiety in *hepatitis*.

Other Gastrointestinal Symptoms

Dysphagia and/or Odynophagia. Less commonly, patients may report difficulty swallowing from impaired passage of solid foods or liquids from the mouth to the stomach, or *dysphagia*. Food seems to stick, hesitate, or "not go down right," suggesting motility disorders or structural anomalies. The sensation of a lump in the throat or the retrosternal area unassociated with swallowing is not true dysphagia.

For types of dysphagia, see Table 11-2, Dysphagia, p. 474.

Indicators of *oropharyngeal dysphagia* include drooling, nasopharyngeal regurgitation, and cough from aspiration in neuromuscular disorders affecting motility such as stroke or Parkinson's disease; gurgling or regurgitation of undigested food occur in structural conditions like *Zenker's diverticulum*.

Ask the patient to point to where the dysphagia occurs.

Pointing to below the sternoclavicular notch indicates *esophageal dysphagia*.

Pursue which types of foods provoke symptoms: solid foods, or solids and liquids? Establish the timing. When does the dysphagia start? Is it intermittent or persistent? Is it progressing? If so, over what time period? Are there associated symptoms and medical conditions?

If solid foods, consider structural esophageal conditions like *esophageal stricture*, web or *Schatzki's ring*, neoplasm; if solids and liquids, a motility disorder is more likely.

Is there *odynophagia*, or pain on swallowing?

Consider esophageal ulceration from radiation, caustic ingestion, or infection from *Candida, cytomegalovirus, herpes simplex,* or *HIV*. *Odynophagia* can be pill-induced from aspirin or non-steroidal anti-inflammatory agents.

Change in Bowel Function. You will frequently need to assess *bowel function*. Start with open-ended questions: "How are your bowel movements?" "How frequent are they?" "Do you have any difficulties?" "Have you noticed any change?" The range of normal is broad. Current parameters suggest a minimum may be as low as two bowel movements per week.

Some patients may complain of passing excessive gas, or *flatus*, normally about 600 mL/day.

Consider aerophagia, legumes or other gas-producing foods, *intestinal lactase deficiency, or irritable bowel syndrome.*

Diarrhea and Constipation. Patients vary widely in their views of diarrhea and constipation. Increased water content of the stool results in *diarrhea*, or stool volume >200 g in 24 hours. Patients, however, usually focus on the change to loose watery stools or increased frequency.

See Table 11-3, Constipation, p. 475, and Table 11-4, Diarrhea, pp. 476–477.

Ask about the duration. *Acute diarrhea* lasts up to 2 weeks. *Chronic diarrhea* is defined as lasting 4 weeks or more.

Acute diarrhea, especially food-borne, is usually caused by infection;[19,20] chronic diarrhea is typically noninfectious in origin, as in *Crohn's disease* and *ulcerative colitis.*

Ask about the characteristics of the diarrhea, including volume, frequency, and consistency.

Is there mucus, pus, or blood? Is there associated *tenesmus*, a constant urge to defecate, accompanied by pain, cramping, and involuntary straining?

High-volume, frequent watery stools usually are from the small intestine; small-volume stools with tenesmus, or diarrhea with mucus, pus, or blood occur in rectal inflammatory conditions.

Does diarrhea occur at night?

Nocturnal diarrhea usually has pathologic significance.

Are the stools greasy or oily? Frothy? Foul-smelling? Floating on the surface because of excessive gas?

Oily residue, sometimes frothy or floating, occurs with *steatorrhea*, or fatty diarrheal stools, from malabsorption in *celiac sprue, pancreatic insufficiency,* and *small bowel bacterial overgrowth.*

Associated features are important in identifying possible causes. Pursue current medications, including alternative medicines, and especially antibiotics, recent travel, diet patterns, baseline bowel habits, and risk factors for immunocompromise.

Diarrhea is common with use of penicillins and macrolides, magnesium-based antacids, metformin, and herbal and alternative medicines.

Another common symptom is *constipation*. Recent definitions stipulate that constipation should be present for at least 12 weeks of the prior 6 months with at least two of the following conditions: fewer than 3 bowel movements per week; 25% or more defecations with either straining or sensation of incomplete evacuation; lumpy or hard stools; or manual facilitation.[21]

Mechanisms include slow transit and outlet delay from impaired expulsion.

Ask about frequency of bowel movements, passage of hard or painful stools, straining, and a sense of incomplete rectal emptying or pressure.

Check if the patient actually looks at the stool and can describe its color and bulk.

Thin, pencil-like stool occurs in an obstructing "apple-core" lesion of the sigmoid colon.

What remedies has the patient tried? Do medications or stress play a role? Are there associated systemic disorders?

Consider medications such as anticholinergic agents, calcium-channel blockers, iron supplements, and opiates. Constipation also occurs with *diabetes, hypothyroidism, hypercalcemia, multiple sclerosis, Parkinson's disease,* and *systemic sclerosis*.

Occasionally there is no passage of either feces or gas, or *obstipation*.

Obstipation signifies *intestinal obstruction*.

Inquire about the color of stools. Is there *melena*, or black tarry stools, or *hematochezia*, stools that are red or maroon-colored? Pursue such important details as quantity and frequency of any blood.

See Table 11-5, Black and Bloody Stools, p. 478.

Melena may appear with as little as 100 mL of blood from *upper gastrointestinal bleeding;* hematochezia if more than 1,000 mL of blood, usually from *lower gastrointestinal bleeding*.

Is the blood mixed in with stool or on the surface? Does the blood appear as streaks on the toilet paper or is it more copious?

Blood on the surface or toilet paper may occur with *hemorrhoids*.

Jaundice. In some patients, you will be struck by *jaundice* or *icterus*, the yellowish discoloration of the skin and sclerae from increased levels of bilirubin, a bile pigment derived chiefly from the breakdown of hemoglobin. Normally the hepatocytes conjugate, or combine unconjugated bilirubin with other substances, making the bile water soluble, and then excrete it into the bile. The bile passes through the cystic duct into the common bile duct, which also drains the extrahepatic ducts from the liver. More distally, the common bile duct and the pancreatic ducts empty into the duodenum at the ampulla of Vater. Mechanisms of jaundice are listed on next page.

Mechanisms of Jaundice

▶ Increased production of bilirubin
▶ Decreased uptake of bilirubin by the hepatocytes
▶ Decreased ability of the liver to conjugate bilirubin
▶ Decreased excretion of bilirubin into the bile, resulting in absorption of *conjugated* bilirubin back into the blood.

Predominantly unconjugated bilirubin occurs from the first three mechanisms, as in *hemolytic anemia* (increased production) and *Gilbert's syndrome.*

Impaired excretion of conjugated bilirubin is seen in *viral hepatitis, cirrhosis, primary biliary cirrhosis,* and drug-induced cholestasis, as from oral contraceptives, methyl testosterone, and chlorpromazine.

Intrahepatic jaundice can be *hepatocellular,* from damage to the hepatocytes, or *cholestatic,* from impaired excretion as a result of damaged hepatocytes or intrahepatic bile ducts. *Extrahepatic* jaundice arises from obstruction of the extrahepatic bile ducts, most commonly the cystic and common bile ducts.

Gallstones or *pancreatic carcinoma* may obstruct the common bile duct.

As you assess the patient with jaundice, pay special attention to the associated symptoms and the setting in which the illness occurred. What was the *color of the urine* as the patient became ill? When the level of conjugated bilirubin increases in the blood, it may be excreted into the urine, turning the urine a dark yellowish brown or tea color. Unconjugated bilirubin is not water-soluble, so it is not excreted into urine.

Dark urine from bilirubin indicates impaired excretion of bilirubin into the gastrointestinal tract.

Ask also about the *color of the stools.* When excretion of bile into the intestine is completely obstructed, the stools become gray or light colored, or *acholic,* without bile.

Acholic stools may occur briefly in *viral hepatitis;* they are common in obstructive jaundice.

Does the skin itch without other obvious explanation? Is there associated pain? What is its pattern? Has it been recurrent in the past?

Itching occurs in cholestatic or obstructive jaundice; pain may signify a distended liver capsule, *biliary colic,* or *pancreatic cancer.*

Ask about risk factors for liver diseases, such as the following.

Risk Factors for Liver Disease

▶ *Hepatitis:* Travel or meals in areas of poor sanitation, ingestion of contaminated water or foodstuffs (*hepatitis A*); parenteral or mucous membrane exposure to infectious body fluids such as blood, serum, semen, and saliva, especially through sexual contact with an infected partner or use of shared needles for injection drug use (*hepatitis B*); intravenous illicit drug use; or blood transfusion (*hepatitis C*)
▶ *Alcoholic hepatitis* or *alcoholic cirrhosis* (interview the patient carefully about alcohol use)
▶ *Toxic liver damage* from medications, industrial solvents, environmental toxins, or some anesthetic agents
▶ *Gallbladder disease* or *surgery* that may result in extrahepatic biliary obstruction
▶ *Hereditary disorders* in the Family History

THE URINARY TRACT

General questions for a urinary history include: "Do you have any difficulty passing your urine?" "How often do you go?" "Do you have to get up at night? How often?" "How much urine do you pass at a time?" "Is there any pain or burning?" "Do you ever have trouble getting to the toilet in time?" "Do you ever leak any urine? Or wet yourself involuntarily?" Does the patient sense when the bladder is full and when voiding occurs?

Ask women if sudden coughing, sneezing, or laughing makes them lose urine. Roughly half of young women report this experience even before bearing children. Occasional leakage is not necessarily significant. Ask older men, "Do you have trouble starting your stream?" "Do you have to stand close to the toilet to void?" "Is there a change in the force or size of your stream, or straining to void?" "Do you hesitate or stop in the middle of voiding?" "Is there dribbling when you're through?"

Suprapubic Pain. Disorders in the urinary tract may cause pain in either the abdomen or the back. Bladder disorders may cause *suprapubic pain.* In *bladder infection,* pain in the lower abdomen is typically dull and pressure-like. In sudden overdistention of the bladder, pain is often agonizing; in contrast, chronic bladder distention is usually painless.

Dysuria, Urgency, or Frequency. Infection or irritation of either the bladder or urethra often provokes several symptoms. Frequently there is *pain on urination,* usually felt as a burning sensation. Some clinicians refer to this as *dysuria,* whereas others reserve the term *dysuria* for difficulty voiding. Women may report internal urethral discomfort, sometimes described as a pressure, or an external burning from the flow of urine across irritated or inflamed labia. Men typically feel a burning sensation proximal to the glans penis. In contrast, *prostatic pain* is felt in the perineum and occasionally in the rectum.

Other associated symptoms are common. Urinary *urgency* is an unusually intense and immediate desire to void, sometimes leading to involuntary voiding or *urge incontinence.* Urinary *frequency,* or abnormally frequent voiding, may occur. Ask about any related fever or chills, blood in the urine, or any pain in the abdomen, flank, or back (see illustration following). Men with partial obstruction to urinary outflow often report *hesitancy* in starting the urine stream, *straining to void, reduced caliber and force of the urinary stream,* or *dribbling* as voiding is completed.

Polyuria or Nocturia. Three additional terms describe important alterations in the pattern of urination. *Polyuria* refers to a significant increase in 24-hour urine volume, roughly defined as exceeding 3 L. It should be distinguished from urinary frequency, which can involve voiding in high amounts, seen in polyuria, or in small amounts, as in infection. *Nocturia* refers to urinary frequency at night, sometimes defined as awakening the

See Table 11-6, Frequency, Nocturia, and Polyuria, p. 479.

Involuntary voiding or lack of awareness suggests cognitive or neurosensory deficits.

Stress incontinence arises from decreased intraurethral pressure (see pp. 480–481).

These problems are common in men with partial bladder outlet obstruction from *benign prostatic hyperplasia;* also seen with *urethral stricture.*

Pain of sudden overdistention accompanies acute urinary retention.

Painful urination accompanies *cystitis* or *urethritis,* and *urinary tract infections.*[22]

If dysuria, consider bladder stones, foreign bodies, tumors; also *acute prostatitis.* In women, internal burning occurs in *urethritis,* and external burning in *vulvovaginitis.*

Urgency suggests bladder infection or irritation. In men, painful urination without frequency or urgency suggests *urethritis.*

See Table 15-3, Abnormalities of the Prostate, p. 595.

Abnormally high renal production of urine suggests polyuria. Frequency without polyuria during the day or night suggests bladder disorder or impairment to flow at or below the bladder neck.

patient more than once; urine volumes may be large or small. Clarify the patient's daily fluid intake. Note any change in nocturnal voiding patterns and the number of trips to the bathroom.

Urinary Incontinence. Up to 30% of older patients are concerned about *urinary incontinence*, an involuntary loss of urine that may become socially embarrassing or cause problems with hygiene. If the patient reports incontinence, ask when it happens and how often. Find out if the patient is leaking small amounts of urine with increased intra-abdominal pressure from coughing, sneezing, laughing, or lifting. Or following an urge to void, is there an involuntary loss of large amounts of urine? Is there a sensation of bladder fullness, frequent leakage, or voiding of small amounts but difficulty emptying the bladder?

As described earlier, bladder control involves complex neuroregulatory and motor mechanisms (see p. 435). Several central or peripheral nerve lesions may affect normal voiding. Can the patient sense when the bladder is full? And when voiding occurs? Although there are four broad categories of incontinence, a patient may have a combination of causes.

See Table 11-7, Urinary Incontinence, pp. 480–481.

Stress incontinence—when increased abdominal pressure causes bladder pressure to exceed urethral resistance due to poor urethral sphincter tone or poor support of bladder neck; *urge incontinence*—when urgency is followed by immediate involuntary leakage due to uncontrolled detrusor contractions that overcome urethral resistance; *overflow incontinence*—when neurologic disorder or anatomic obstruction from pelvic organs or the prostate limits bladder emptying until the bladder is overdistended.[23,24]

In addition, the patient's functional status may significantly affect voiding behaviors even when the urinary tract is intact. Is the patient mobile? Alert? Able to respond to voiding cues and reach the bathroom? Is alertness or voiding affected by medications?

Functional incontinence may arise from impaired cognition, musculoskeletal problems, or immobility.

Hematuria. Blood in the urine, or *hematuria*, is a major cause for concern. When visible to the naked eye, it is called *gross hematuria*; the urine may appear obviously bloody. Blood may be detected only during microscopic urinalysis, known as *microscopic hematuria*; smaller amounts of blood may tinge the urine with a pinkish or brownish cast. In women, be sure to distinguish menstrual blood from hematuria. If the urine is reddish, ask about medications that might discolor the urine. Test the urine with a dipstick and microscopic examination before you diagnose *hematuria*.

Kidney or Flank Pain; Ureteral Colic. Disorders of the urinary tract may also cause *kidney pain*, often reported as *flank pain* at or below the posterior costal margin near the costovertebral angle. It may radiate anteriorly toward the umbilicus. Kidney pain is a visceral pain usually produced by distention of the renal capsule and typically dull, aching, and steady. *Ureteral pain* is dramatically different. It is usually severe and colicky, originating at the costovertebral angle and radiating around the trunk into the lower quadrant of the abdomen, or possibly into the upper thigh and testicle or labium. Ureteral pain results from sudden distention of the ureter and associated distention of the renal pelvis. Ask about any associated fever, chills, or hematuria.

Kidney pain, fever, and chills occur in *acute pyelonephritis*.

Renal or ureteral colic is caused by sudden obstruction of a ureter, for example, from renal or urinary stones or blood clots.

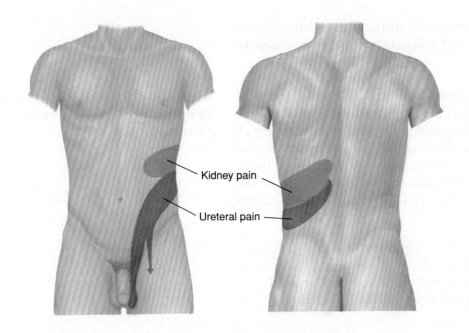

Kidney pain

Ureteral pain

Health Promotion and Counseling: Evidence and Recommendations

Important Topics for Health Promotion and Counseling

- Screening for alcohol abuse
- Risk factors for hepatitis A, B, and C
- Screening for colon cancer

Screening for Alcohol Abuse.   Alert clinicians often notice clues of unhealthy alcohol use from social patterns and behavioral problems that emerge during the history. The patient may report past episodes of pancreatitis, family history of alcoholism, or arrest for intoxicated driving. Examination of the abdomen may reveal such classic findings as hepatosplenomegaly, ascites, or even caput medusa, a collateral pathway of recanalized umbilical veins radiating up the abdomen that decompresses portal vein hypertension.

Current 12-month prevalence of alcohol abuse or dependence is on the rise, affecting 8.5% of the U.S. population, or 15 to 20 million people.[25] Lifetime prevalence is approximately 30%, and in emergency rooms and trauma admissions, prevalence reaches 30% to 40% and 50%, respectively.[26,27] Addictions are increasingly viewed as chronic relapsing behavioral disorders with substance-induced rearrangements of brain neurotransmitters resulting in tolerance, physical dependence, sensitization, craving, and relapse. Alcohol addiction has numerous sequelae and is highly correlated with fatal car accidents,

Other classic findings include spider angiomas, palmar erythema, and peripheral edema.

See Chapter 5, Behavior and Mental Status, p. 150.

See also Chapter 3, Interviewing and the Health History, Alcohol and Illicit Drugs, pp. 88–89.

suicide and other mental health disorders, family disruption, violence, hypertension, cirrhosis hemorrhagic stroke, and malignancies of the upper gastrointestinal tract and liver.

Because early detection of at-risk behaviors may be challenging, learn the basic identifiers for problem drinking. The U.S. Preventive Services Task Force (USPSTF) recommends screening and behavioral counseling for all adults in primary care setting settings, including pregnant women.[28] If your patient drinks alcoholic beverages, begin screening by asking about heavy drinking, then follow up with the well-validated CAGE questions or the Alcohol Use Disorders Identification Test (AUDIT). Keep in mind cutoffs for problem drinking listed below.[29,30]

See Chapter 3, Interviewing and the Health History, for the CAGE questions, p. 88.

Screening for Problem Drinking

Standard Drink Equivalents: 1 standard drink is equivalent to 12 ounces of regular beer or wine cooler, 8 ounces of malt liquor, 5 ounces of wine, or 1.5 ounces of 80-proof spirits

Initial Screening Question: "How many times in the past year have you had 4 or more drinks a day (women), or 5 or more drinks a day (men)?"

Cut Points for Drinks per Day

	Women	Men
	Drinks per day	
Moderate drinking	≤1	≤2
Maximum drinking	≤3	≤4 if **<65 years** (and ≤14 drinks in a week)
		≤3 if **>65 years** (and ≤7 drinks in a week)
Binge drinking*	≥4	≥5

*Brings blood alcohol level to 0.08 g %, usually within 2 hours.

Tailor your recommendations to the severity of the problem, ranging from brief interventions, which are proven to be effective, to long-term rehabilitation. Take advantage of the helpful "Clinician's Guide for Helping Patients Who Drink Too Much."[29]

Risk Factors for Hepatitis A, B, and C. The mainstay for protecting adults against viral hepatitis is adherence to vaccination guidelines for hepatitis A and hepatitis B, the most effective method for preventing infection and transmission. Educating patients about how the hepatitis viruses spread and the benefits of vaccination for groups at risk is also important.

Hepatitis A. Transmission of hepatitis A is fecal/oral. Fecal shedding, followed by poor hand washing, causes contamination of water and foods, leading to infection of household and sexual contacts. Infected children are often asymptomatic, contributing to spread of infection. The Centers for Disease Control and Prevention (CDC) recommends hepatitis A vaccination for all children at age 1 year and for groups at increased risk—travelers to endemic areas, male–male partners, injection and illicit drug users, and persons with chronic liver disease including hepatitis B or C. For immediate protection and prophylaxis for household contacts and travelers, immune serum glob-ulin can be administered within 2 weeks of contact and before travel. Advise washing hands with soap and water before bathroom use, changing diapers, and preparing and eating food.[31]

Hepatitis B. Hepatitis B causes more serious threats to patient health. Approximately 95% of infections in healthy adults are self-limited, with elimi-nation of the virus and development of immunity. Risk of chronic infection is highest when the immune system is immature, occurring in 90% of infected infants and 30% of children infected before age 5 years.[32,33] Fifteen percent to 25% of adults infected after childhood die prematurely from cirrhosis or liver cancer; over 70% are asymptomatic until liver disease is advanced. The CDC recommends screening of all pregnant women and universal vaccination for all infants beginning at birth. For adults, recommendations for vaccination now include high-risk groups, as well as expanded programs in high-risk settings.[34]

Recommendations for Hepatitis B Vaccination: High-Risk Groups and Settings

▶ *Sexual contacts,* including sex partners for those already infected, people with more than one sex partner in the prior 6 months, people seeking eval-uation and treatment for sexually transmitted infections, and men having sex with men

▶ *People with percutaneous or mucosal exposure to blood,* including injection drug users, household contacts of antigen-positive persons, residents and staff of facilities for the developmentally disabled, health care workers, and people on dialysis

▶ *Others,* including travelers to endemic areas, people with chronic liver disease and HIV infection, and people seeking protection from hepatitis B infection

▶ *All adults in high-risk settings,* such as STI clinics, HIV testing and treatment programs, drug-abuse treatment programs and programs for injection drug users, correctional facilities, programs for men having sex with men, chronic hemodialysis facilities and end-stage renal disease programs, and facilities for people with developmental disabilities

▶ *Adults in primary care and specialty settings,* in at-risk groups or requesting the hepatitis B vaccine even without acknowledging a specific risk factor

▶ *Adults in occupational exposure settings,* in occupations involving exposure to blood or other potentially infectious body fluids

Hepatitis C. Hepatitis C is transmitted by repeated percutaneous expo-sure to infected blood and is the most common bloodborne pathogen in the United States, found in approximately 2% of the population.[35–37] However, prevalence reaches 50% to 90% of groups at high risk, namely injection drug users and patients transfused with clotting factors before 1987. Hepatitis C is highly persistent and causes chronic liver disease in 75% of those infected. It accounts for roughly 50% of cirrhosis, end-stage liver disease, and liver cancer. Additional risk factors include history of injection drug use even one time, blood transfusion or organ transplant before 1992, blood transfusion or organ transplant before 1992, hemodialysis, known exposure to the hepatitis C virus from needlesticks or an infected blood or transplant donor, HIV infection, and birth from a hepatitis C–positive mother. Sexual transmission is rare. There is no vaccine, so prevention depends on screening and counseling to avoid risk factors. Response to antiviral therapy is 40% to 80% depending on the viral genotype.

Screening for Colorectal Cancer.   Colorectal cancer is the third most common cancer in both men and women, and it causes almost 10% of deaths from cancer.[38] More than 90% of cases occur after age 50, primarily from neoplastic changes in adenomatous polyps; only about a third of cases have identifiable high-risk factors.[39] Incidence rates are decreasing, except in adults younger than 50 years who fall outside the current age threshold for screening. Overall mortality rates are declining, reflecting improvements in early detection and treatment. However, mortality rates in African Americans are double those of other ethnic groups.

Since population screening rates continue to lag at only 60%, the USPSTF in 2008 conducted a detailed review of newer screening modalities that might expand screening options and availability.[40,41] The USPSTF concluded that several high-sensitivity fecal screening tests are reasonable substitutes for Hemoccult testing, but found insufficient evidence to assess fecal DNA testing or radiation exposure and test performance of computed tomography colonography. The USPSTF established new age cutoffs for screening, summarized below.

Screening for Colorectal Cancer

Assess risk: Begin screening at age 20 years. If high risk, refer for more complex management. If average risk at age 50 (high-risk conditions absent), offer the screening options listed.
- **Common high-risk conditions** (25% of colorectal cancers)
  - Personal history of colorectal cancer or adenoma
  - First-degree relative with colorectal cancer or adenomatous polyps
  - Personal history of breast, ovarian, or endometrial cancer
  - Personal history of ulcerative or Crohn's colitis
- **Hereditary high-risk conditions** (6% of colorectal cancers)
  - Familial adenomatous polyposis
  - Hereditary nonpolyposis colorectal cancer

Screening recommendations—U.S. Preventive Services Task Force 2008
- **Adults age 50 to 75 years—options**
  - High-sensitivity fecal occult blood testing (FOBT) annually
  - Sigmoidoscopy every 5 years with FOBT every 3 years
  - Screening colonoscopy every 10 years
- **Adults age 76 to 85 years**—do not screen routinely, as gain in life-years is small compared to colonoscopy risks, and screening benefits not seen for 7 years; use individual decision making if screening for the first time
- **Adults older than age 85**—do not screen, as "competing causes of mortality preclude a mortality benefit that outweighs harms"

In 2008, the American Cancer Society Colorectal Cancer Advisory Group, consisting of the American Cancer Society, the U.S. Multi-Society Task Force on Colorectal Cancer, and the American College of Radiology, also issued screening guidelines supporting double-contrast barium enema or computed tomography colonography every 5 years and fecal DNA testing.[42]

When adenomas are detected during screening, screening intervals generally narrow to 3 to 5 years. For patients who have first-degree relatives with colorectal cancer or adenomatous polyps, screening often begins at age 40 or 10 years before the youngest case in the affected family.

Screening tests vary in sensitivity and specificity. *Colonoscopy*, which visualizes the entire colon, is considered the highest standard, with a sensitivity and specificity of 90% and 98% when combined with biopsy.[43] In individuals with adenomas, colonoscopy is associated with a 76% to 90% risk reduction for colorectal cancer, particularly for cancer in the left colon and rectum.[44] Colonoscopy misses 10% of adenomas ≥6 mm and 12% of adenomas ≥12 mm. Risk of perforation is 3.8 per 10,000 procedures.[40,41] For *flexible sigmoidoscopy* with biopsy, sensitivity for large distal adenomas or cancer is 88% to 98% and specificity is over 92%. *FOBT* is 50% sensitive as a single test but 90% sensitive when used in annual screening program, with a specificity of 90%. In a recent study, high-sensitivity FOBT and fecal DNA shared a sensitivity of 20% and similar specificities.[45] For best results, high-sensitivity FOBT should involve at-home collection of two stool samples per card from three consecutive bowel movements, or a total of six specimens over a 2- to 3-day period. A single specimen is inadequate due to sensitivity of only 5%.[46] Any positive specimen warrants a follow-up colonoscopy.

Other Interventions for Reducing Risk of Colorectal Cancer. Some evidence suggests that diets high in fat and low in calcium, folate, fiber, and fruits and vegetables increase risk for colorectal cancer; however, results from diet studies are conflicting and further research is needed.[47–49] There is stronger evidence that aspirin, nonsteroidal anti-inflammatory drugs, and postmenopausal estrogen–progesterone therapy reduce the incidence of colorectal cancer and adenomas.[50,51] However, both the National Cancer Institute and the USPSTF recommend against these interventions due to increased risk of gastrointestinal bleeding and of breast cancer, coronary heart disease, and thromboembolic events, respectively.[52]

Techniques of Examination

For a skilled abdominal examination, you need good light and a relaxed and well-draped patient, with exposure of the abdomen from just above the xiphoid process to the symphysis pubis. The groin should be visible. The genitalia should remain draped. The abdominal muscles should be relaxed to enhance all aspects of the examination, but especially palpation.

Tips for Examining the Abdomen

▶ Check if the patient has an empty bladder.

▶ Make the patient comfortable in the supine position, with a pillow under the head and perhaps another under the knees. Slide your hand under the low back to see if the patient is relaxed and lying flat on the table.

▶ Ask the patient to keep the arms at the sides or folded across the chest. When the arms are above the head, the abdominal wall stretches and tightens, making palpation difficult. Move the gown to below the nipple line, and the drape to the level of the symphysis pubis.

▶ Before you begin palpation, ask the patient to point to any areas of pain so that you can examine these areas last.

▶ Warm your hands and stethoscope. To warm your hands, rub them together or place them under hot water. You can also palpate through the patient's gown to absorb warmth from the patient's body before exposing the abdomen.

▶ Approach the patient calmly and avoid quick, unexpected movements. *Watch the patient's face for any signs of pain or discomfort.* Avoid having long fingernails when examining the patient.

▶ Distract the patient, if necessary, with conversation or questions. If the patient is frightened or ticklish, begin palpation with the patient's hand under yours. After a few moments, slip your hand underneath to palpate directly.

An arched back thrusts the abdomen forward and tightens the abdominal muscles.

Visualize each organ in the region you are examining. Stand at the patient's right side and proceed in an orderly fashion with inspection, auscultation, percussion, and palpation. Assess the liver, spleen, kidneys, and aorta.

THE ABDOMEN

Inspection

Starting from your usual standing position at the right side of the bed, inspect the abdomen. As you look at the contour of the abdomen, watch for peristalsis. It is helpful to sit or bend down so that you can view the abdomen tangentially.

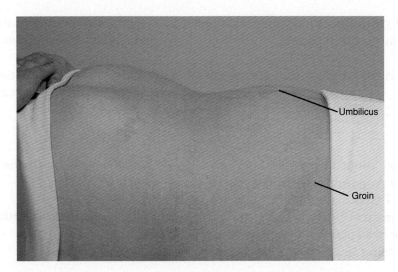

Inspect the surface, contours, and movements of the abdomen, including the following:

- *The skin.* Note:

    Scars. Describe or diagram their location.

    Striae. Old silver striae or stretch marks are normal.

    Dilated veins. A few small veins may be visible normally.

    Rashes or *ecchymoses*

- *The umbilicus.* Observe its contour and location and any inflammation or bulges suggesting a ventral hernia.

- *The contour of the abdomen*

    Is it flat, rounded, protuberant, or scaphoid (markedly concave or hollowed)?

    Do the flanks bulge, or are there any local bulges? Also survey the inguinal and femoral areas.

    Is the abdomen symmetric?

    Are there visible organs or masses? Look for an enlarged liver or spleen that has descended below the rib cage.

Pink–purple striae indicate *Cushing's syndrome*.

Dilated veins can be indicative of *hepatic cirrhosis* or of *inferior vena cava obstruction*.

Ecchymosis of the abdominal wall is seen in intraperitoneal or retroperitoneal hemorrhage.

See Table 11-8, Localized Bulges in the Abdominal Wall, p. 482.

See Table 11-9, Protuberant Abdomens, p. 483.

Observe for bulging flanks of *ascites*; suprapubic bulge of a distended bladder or pregnant uterus; hernias.

Asymmetry suggests an enlarged organ or mass.

Look for the lower abdominal mass of an ovarian or a uterine cancer.

- *Peristalsis.* Observe for several minutes if you suspect intestinal obstruction. Normally, peristalsis may be visible in very thin people.

- *Pulsations.* The normal aortic pulsation is frequently visible in the epigastrium.

Look for the increased peristaltic waves of *intestinal obstruction.*

Look for the increased pulsation of an *aortic aneurysm* or of *increased pulse pressure.*

Auscultation

Auscultation provides important information about bowel motility. *Listen to the abdomen before performing percussion or palpation because these maneuvers may alter the frequency of bowel sounds.* Practice auscultation until you are thoroughly familiar with variations in normal bowel sounds and can detect changes suggestive of inflammation or obstruction. Auscultation may also reveal *bruits,* or vascular sounds resembling heart murmurs, over the aorta or other arteries in the abdomen.

See Table 11-10, Sounds in the Abdomen, p. 484.

Bruits suggest vascular occlusive disease.

Place the diaphragm of your stethoscope gently on the abdomen. Listen for bowel sounds and note their frequency and character. Normal sounds consist of clicks and gurgles, occurring at an estimated frequency of 5 to 34 per minute. Occasionally you may hear *borborygmi,* prolonged gurgles of hyperperistalsis, the familiar "stomach growling." Because bowel sounds are widely transmitted through the abdomen, listening in one spot, such as the right lower quadrant, is usually sufficient.

Bowel sounds may be altered in diarrhea, intestinal obstruction, *paralytic ileus,* and *peritonitis.*

Abdominal Bruits and Friction Rub. If the patient has high blood pressure, listen in the epigastrium and in each upper quadrant for *bruits.* Later in the examination, when the patient sits up, listen also in the costovertebral angles. Epigastric bruits confined to systole are normal.

A bruit in one of these areas that has both systolic and diastolic components strongly suggests *renal artery stenosis* as the cause of hypertension. Four percent to 20% of healthy individuals have abdominal bruits.[53]

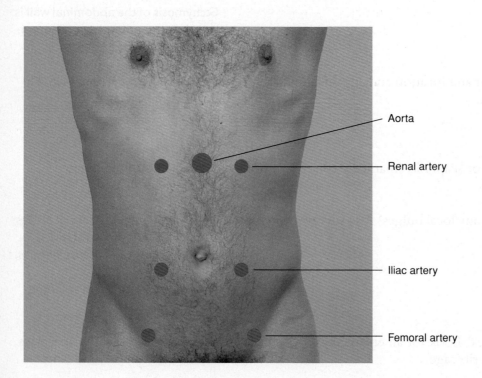

Aorta

Renal artery

Iliac artery

Femoral artery

Listen for bruits over the aorta, the iliac arteries, and the femoral arteries, as illustrated.

Bruits with both systolic and diastolic components suggest the turbulent blood flow from atherosclerotic arterial disease.

Listen over the liver and spleen for *friction rubs.*

Friction rubs are present in hepatoma, gonococcal infection around the liver, splenic infarction, and pancreatic carcinoma.

Percussion

Percussion helps you to assess the amount and distribution of gas in the abdomen, possible masses that are solid or fluid-filled, and the size of the liver and spleen.

Percuss the abdomen lightly in all four quadrants to assess the distribution of *tympany* and *dullness.* Tympany usually predominates because of gas in the gastrointestinal tract, but scattered areas of dullness from fluid and feces are also typical.

A protuberant abdomen that is tympanitic throughout suggests *intestinal obstruction.* See Table 11-9, Protuberant Abdomens, p. 483.

- Note any large dull areas suggesting an underlying mass or enlarged organ. This observation will guide your palpation.

Dull areas can indicate a pregnant uterus, an ovarian tumor, a distended bladder, or a large liver or spleen.

- On each side of a protuberant abdomen, note where abdominal tympany changes to the dullness of solid posterior structures.

Dullness in both flanks prompts further assessment for ascites (see pp. 466–467).

Briefly percuss the lower anterior chest above the costal margins. On the right, you will usually find the dullness of the liver; on the left, the tympany that overlies the gastric air bubble and the splenic flexure of the colon.

In the rare condition of *situs inversus,* organs are reversed—air bubble on the right, liver dullness on the left.

Palpation

Light Palpation. Gentle palpation is especially helpful for eliciting abdominal tenderness, muscular resistance, and some superficial organs and masses. It also serves to reassure and relax the patient.

Keeping your hand and forearm on a horizontal plane, with fingers together and flat on the abdominal wall, palpate the abdomen with a light, gentle, dipping motion. As you move your hand to different quadrants, raise it just off the skin. Gliding smoothly, palpate in all four quadrants.

Identify any superficial organs or masses and any area of tenderness or increased resistance to your hand. If resistance is present, try to distinguish voluntary guarding from involuntary muscular spasm. To do this:

Involuntary rigidity (muscular spasm) typically persists despite these maneuvers, suggesting *peritoneal inflammation.*

- Try all the methods you know to help the patient relax (see p. 452).

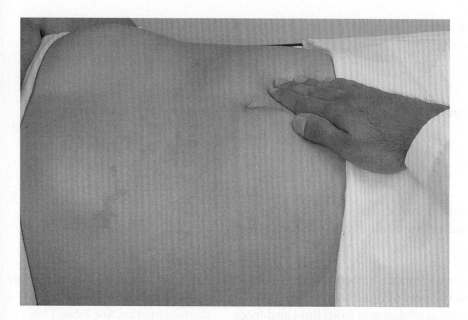

- Feel for relaxation of abdominal muscles that normally accompanies exhalation.

- Ask the patient to mouth-breathe with the jaw dropped open.

Voluntary guarding usually decreases with these maneuvers.

Deep Palpation.   This is usually required to delineate abdominal masses. Again using the palmar surfaces of your fingers, press down in all four quadrants. Identify any masses; note their location, size, shape, consistency, tenderness, pulsations, and any mobility with respiration or pressure from the examining hand. Correlate your palpable findings with their percussion notes.

Abdominal masses may be categorized in several ways: physiologic (pregnant uterus), inflammatory (*diverticulitis* of the colon), vascular (an *abdominal aortic aneurysm*), neoplastic (colon cancer), or obstructive (a distended bladder or dilated loop of bowel).

TWO-HANDED DEEP PALPATION

Assessing Possible Peritonitis. Inflammation of the parietal peritoneum, or peritonitis, signals an *acute abdomen*.[54] Signs of peritonitis include a positive cough test, guarding, rigidity, rebound tenderness, and percussion tenderness.[53] Even before palpation, ask the patient to cough and identify where the cough produces pain. Then palpate gently, starting with one finger then with your hand, to localize the area of pain. As you palpate, check for guarding, rigidity, and rebound tenderness. *Guarding* is a voluntary contraction of the abdominal wall, often accompanied by a grimace that may diminish when the patient is distracted. *Rigidity* is an involuntary reflex contraction of the abdominal wall that persists over several examinations. Assess for rebound tenderness. Ask the patient "Which hurts more, when I press or let go?" Press down with your fingers firmly and slowly, then withdraw your hand quickly. The maneuver is positive if withdrawal produces pain. Percuss gently to check for percussion tenderness.

When positive, these signs roughly double the likelihood of *peritonitis*; rigidity makes peritonitis almost four times more likely.[53] Causes include *appendicitis, cholecystitis,* and a perforation of the bowel wall.

See also Table 11-11, Tender Abdomens, pp. 485–486.

 ## THE LIVER

Because the rib cage shelters most of the liver, direct assessment is difficult. Liver size and shape can be estimated by percussion and palpation. Pressure from your palpating hand helps you to evaluate its surface, consistency, and tenderness.

Percussion

Measure the vertical span of liver dullness in the right midclavicular line. First locate the midclavicular line carefully to avoid inaccurate measurement. Use a light to moderate percussion strike, because examiners with a heavier strike underestimate liver size.[53] Starting at a level below the umbilicus in the right lower quadrant (in an area of tympany, not dullness), percuss upward toward the liver. Identify the *lower border of dullness* in the midclavicular line.

Estimated liver span by percussion is relatively accurate with a 60% to 70% correlation with actual span.

Next, identify the *upper border of liver dullness* in the midclavicular line. Starting at the nipple line, lightly percuss from lung resonance down toward liver dullness. Gently displace a woman's breast as necessary to be sure that you start in a resonant area. The course of percussion is shown on next page.

The span of liver dullness is *increased* when the liver is enlarged.

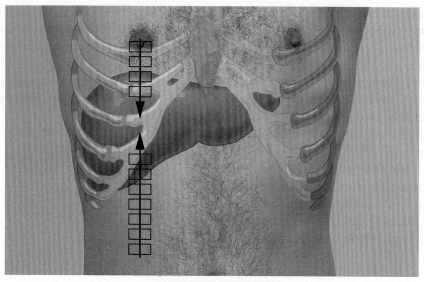

PERCUSSING LIVER SPAN

The span of liver dullness is *decreased* when the liver is small, or when free air is present below the diaphragm, as from a *perforated hollow viscus.* Serial observations may show a decreasing span of dullness with resolution of *hepatitis* or *heart failure* or, less commonly, with progression of *fulminant hepatitis.*

Liver dullness may be displaced downward by the low diaphragm of *chronic obstructive pulmonary disease.* Span, however, remains normal.

Now measure in centimeters the distance between your two points—the vertical span of liver dullness. Normal liver spans, shown below, are generally greater in men than women and in tall people compared to short people. If the liver seems enlarged, outline the lower edge by percussing medially and laterally.

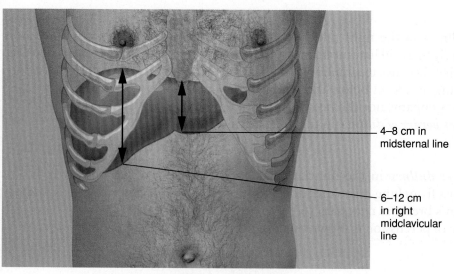

4–8 cm in midsternal line

6–12 cm in right midclavicular line

NORMAL LIVER SPANS

Dullness of a right pleural effusion or consolidated lung, if adjacent to liver dullness, may falsely *increase* the estimate of liver size.

Gas in the colon may produce tympany in the right upper quadrant, obscure liver dullness, and falsely *decrease* the estimate of liver size.

Measurements of liver span by percussion are more accurate when the liver is enlarged with a palpable edge.[55]

Only about half of livers with an edge below the right costal margin are palpable, but when the edge is palpable, the likelihood of hepatomegaly roughly doubles.[53]

Palpation

Place your left hand behind the patient, parallel to and supporting the right 11th and 12th ribs and adjacent soft tissues below. Remind the patient to relax on your hand if necessary. By pressing your left hand upward, the patient's liver may be felt more easily by your other hand.

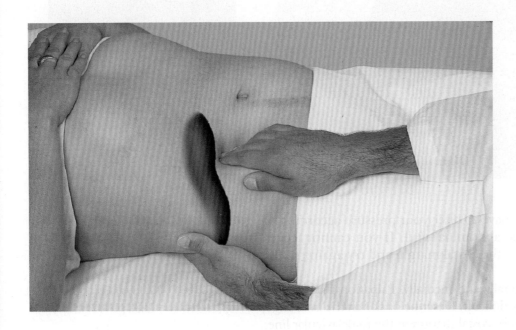

Place your right hand on the patient's right abdomen lateral to the rectus muscle, with your fingertips well below the lower border of liver dullness. Some examiners like to point their fingers up toward the patient's head, whereas others prefer a somewhat more oblique position, as shown on the next page. In either case, press gently in and up.

Ask the patient to take a deep breath. Try to feel the liver edge as it comes down to meet your fingertips. If you feel it, lighten the pressure of your palpating hand slightly so that the liver can slip under your finger pads and you can feel its anterior surface. Note any tenderness. If palpable at all, the normal liver edge is soft, sharp, and regular, with a smooth surface. The normal liver may be slightly tender.

Firmness or hardness of the liver, bluntness or rounding of its edge, and irregularity of its contour suggest an abnormality of the liver.

On inspiration, the liver is palpable about 3 cm below the right costal margin in the midclavicular line. Some people breathe more with the chest than with the diaphragm. It may be helpful to train such a patient to "breathe with the abdomen," thus bringing the liver, as well as the spleen and kidneys, into a palpable position during inspiration.

An obstructed, distended gallbladder may form an oval mass below the edge of the liver and merge with it. The merged area is dull to percussion.

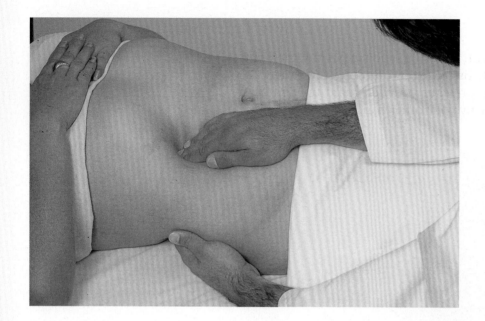

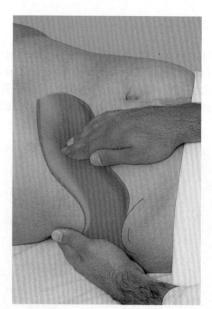

In order to feel the liver, you may have to alter your pressure according to the thickness and resistance of the abdominal wall. If you cannot feel it, move your palpating hand closer to the costal margin and try again.

The edge of an enlarged liver may be missed by starting palpation too high in the abdomen, as shown above.

Try to trace the liver edge both laterally and medially. Palpation through the rectus muscles, however, is especially difficult. Describe or sketch the liver edge, and measure its distance from the right costal margin in the midclavicular line.

See Table 11-12, Liver Enlargement: Apparent and Real, p. 487.

The "hooking technique" may be helpful, especially when the patient is obese. Stand to the right of the patient's chest. Place both hands, side by side, on the right abdomen below the border of liver dullness. Press in with your fingers and up toward the costal margin. Ask the patient to take a deep breath. The liver edge shown below is palpable with the fingerpads of both hands.

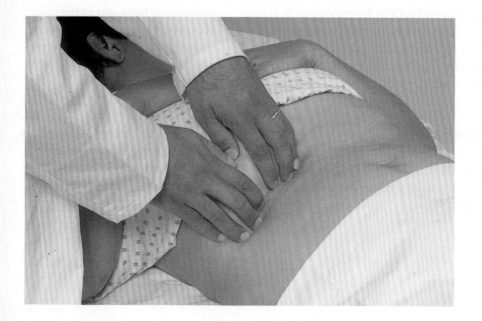

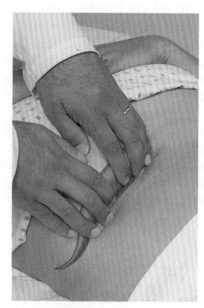

Assessing Percussion Tenderness of a Nonpalpable Liver. Place your left hand flat on the lower right rib cage and gently strike your hand with the ulnar surface of your right fist. Ask the patient to compare the sensation with that produced by a similar strike on the left side.

Tenderness over the liver suggests inflammation, as in *hepatitis*, or congestion, as in *heart failure*.

THE SPLEEN

When a spleen enlarges, it expands anteriorly, downward, and medially, often replacing the tympany of stomach and colon with the dullness of a solid organ. It then becomes palpable below the costal margin. Percussion suggests but does not confirm splenic enlargement. Palpation can confirm the enlargement but often misses large spleens that do not descend below the costal margin.

Percussion

Two techniques may help you to detect *splenomegaly*, an enlarged spleen:

- *Percuss the left lower anterior chest wall* roughly from the border of cardiac dullness at the 6th rib to the anterior axillary line and down to the costal margin, an area termed *Traube's space*. As you percuss along the routes suggested by the arrows in the following figures, note the lateral extent of tympany. Percussion is moderately accurate in detecting splenomegaly (sensitivity, 60%–80%; specificity, 72%–94%).[56]

If percussion dullness is present, palpation correctly detects presence or absence of splenomegaly more than 80% of the time.[56]

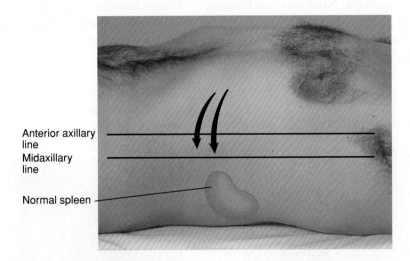

Anterior axillary line
Midaxillary line
Normal spleen

If tympany is prominent, especially laterally, splenomegaly is not likely. The dullness of a normal spleen is usually masked by the dullness of other posterior tissues.

Fluid or solids in the stomach or colon may also cause dullness in Traube's space.

- *Check for a splenic percussion sign*. Percuss the lowest interspace in the left anterior axillary line, as shown next. This area is usually tympanitic. Then ask the patient to take a deep breath, and percuss again. When spleen size is normal, the percussion note usually remains tympanitic.

A change in percussion note from tympany to dullness on inspiration suggests splenic enlargement. This is a *positive splenic percussion sign.*

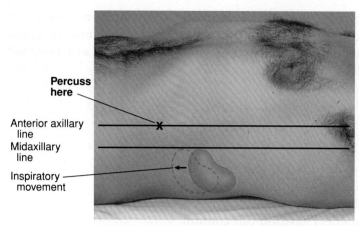

Percuss here

Anterior axillary line

Midaxillary line

Inspiratory movement

NEGATIVE SPLENIC PERCUSSION SIGN

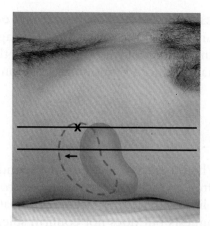

POSITIVE SPLENIC PERCUSSION SIGN

If either or both of these tests is positive, pay extra attention to palpation of the spleen.

The splenic percussion sign may also be positive when spleen size is normal.

Palpation

With your left hand, reach over and around the patient to support and press forward the lower left rib cage and adjacent soft tissue. With your right hand below the left costal margin, press in toward the spleen. Begin palpation low enough so that you are below a possibly enlarged spleen. If your hand is close to the costal margin, it is not sufficiently mobile to reach up under the rib cage. Ask the patient to take a deep breath. Try to feel the tip or edge of the spleen as it comes down to meet your fingertips. Note any tenderness, assess the splenic contour, and measure the distance between the spleen's lowest point and the left costal margin. In approximately 5% of normal adults, the tip of the spleen is palpable. Causes include a low, flat diaphragm, as in chronic obstructive pulmonary disease, and a deep inspiratory descent of the diaphragm.

An enlarged spleen may be missed if the examiner starts too high in the abdomen to feel the lower edge.

Splenomegaly is eight times more likely when the spleen is palpable.[53] Causes include portal hypertension, hematologic malignancies, HIV infection, and splenic infarct or hematoma.

The spleen tip, illustrated below, is just palpable deep to the left costal margin.

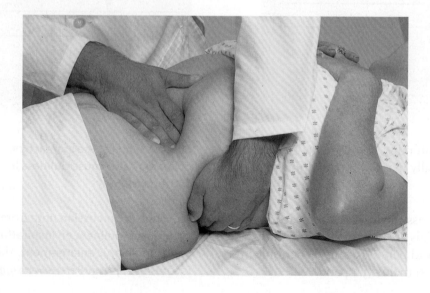

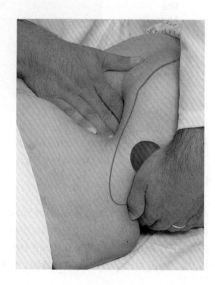

Repeat with the patient lying on the right side with legs somewhat flexed at the hips and knees. In this position, gravity may bring the spleen forward and to the right into a palpable location.

This enlarged spleen is palpable about 2 cm below the left costal margin on deep inspiration.

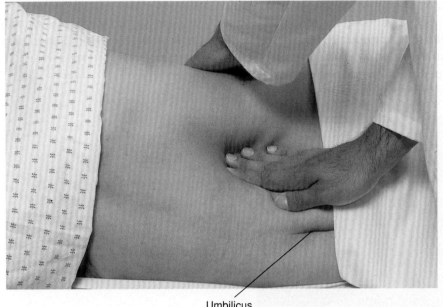

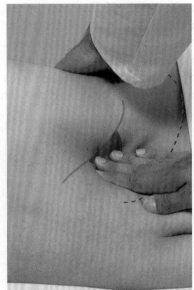

Umbilicus

PALPATING THE SPLEEN—PATIENT LYING ON RIGHT SIDE

THE KIDNEYS

Palpation

Although kidneys are retroperitoneal and not usually palpable, learning the techniques for examination helps you distinguish enlarged kidneys from other enlarged organs and abdominal masses.

Palpation of the Left Kidney. Move to the patient's left side. Place your right hand behind the patient, just below and parallel to the 12th rib, with your fingertips just reaching the costovertebral angle. Lift, trying to displace the kidney anteriorly. Place your left hand gently in the left upper quadrant, lateral and parallel to the rectus muscle. Ask the patient to take a deep breath. At the peak of inspiration, press your left hand firmly and deeply into the left upper quadrant, just below the costal margin. Try to "capture" the kidney between your two hands. Ask the patient to breathe out and then to stop breathing briefly. Slowly release the pressure of your left hand, feeling at the same time for the kidney to slide back into its expiratory position. If the kidney is palpable, describe its size, contour, and any tenderness.

Alternatively, try to feel for the left kidney using a method similar to palpating the spleen. Standing at the patient's right side, with your left hand, reach over and around the patient to lift up beneath the left kidney, and with your right hand, feel deep in the left upper quadrant. Ask the patient to take a deep breath, and feel for a mass. A normal left kidney is rarely palpable.

A left flank mass may represent marked *splenomegaly* or an enlarged left kidney. Suspect *splenomegaly* if a notch is palpated on medial border, the edge extends beyond the midline, percussion is dull, and your fingers can probe deep to the medial and lateral borders but *not* between the mass and the costal margin. Confirm findings with further evaluation.

Attributes indicating an *enlarged kidney* rather than an enlarged spleen include preservation of normal tympany in the left upper quadrant and the ability to probe with your fingers between the mass and the costal margin, but not deep to its medial and lower borders.

Palpation of the Right Kidney. To capture the right kidney, return to the patient's right side. Use your left hand to lift up from the back, and your right hand to feel deep in the right upper quadrant. Proceed as before.

A normal right kidney may be palpable, especially when the patient is thin and the abdominal muscles are relaxed. It may be slightly tender. The patient is usually aware of a capture and release. Occasionally, a right kidney is located more anteriorly and must be distinguished from the liver. The edge of the liver, if palpable, tends to be sharper and extend farther medially and laterally. It cannot be captured. The lower pole of the kidney is rounded.

Causes of kidney enlargement include hydronephrosis, cysts, and tumors. Bilateral enlargement suggests *polycystic kidney disease.*

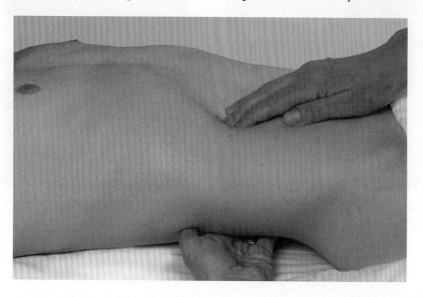

Assessing Percussion Tenderness of the Kidneys. If you find tenderness when examining the abdomen, also check each costovertebral angle. Pressure from your fingertips may be enough to elicit tenderness; if not use fist percussion. Place the ball of one hand in the costovertebral angle and strike it with the ulnar surface of your fist. Use enough force to cause a perceptible but painless jar or thud.

To save the patient from repositioning, integrate this assessment into your examination of the posterior lungs or back.

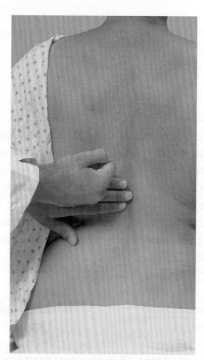

**ASSESSING COSTOVERTEBRAL
ANGLE TENDERNESS**

Pain with pressure or fist percussion suggests *pyelonephritis* but may also have a musculoskeletal cause.

THE BLADDER

The bladder normally cannot be examined unless it is distended above the symphysis pubis. On palpation, the dome of the distended bladder feels smooth and round. Check for tenderness. Use percussion to check for dullness and to determine how high the bladder rises above the symphysis pubis. Bladder volume must be 400 to 600 mL before dullness appears.[53]

Bladder distention from outlet obstruction may be due to *urethral stricture, prostatic hyperplasia;* or from medications and neurologic disorders such as *stroke* or *multiple sclerosis.*

Suprapubic tenderness is common in *bladder infection.*

THE AORTA

Press firmly deep in the upper abdomen, slightly to the left of the midline, and identify the aortic pulsations. In people older than age 50, assess the width of the aorta by pressing deeply in the upper abdomen with one hand on each side of the aorta, as illustrated. In this age group, a normal aorta is not more than 3 cm wide (average, 2.5 cm). This measurement does not include the thickness of the abdominal wall. The ease of feeling aortic pulsations varies greatly with the thickness of the abdominal wall and with the anteroposterior diameter of the abdomen.

Risk factors for abdominal aortic aneurysm (AAA) are age 65 years or older, history of smoking, male gender, and a first-degree relative with a history of AAA repair.[57,58]

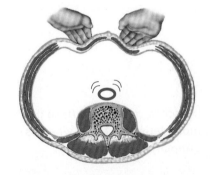 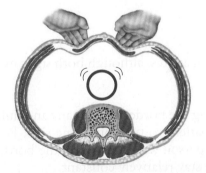

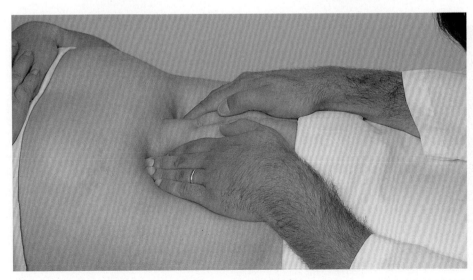

A periumbilical or upper abdominal mass with expansile pulsations that is 3 cm or more wide suggests an AAA. Sensitivity of palpation increases as AAAs enlarge: for widths of 3.0–3.9 cm, 29%; 4.0–4.9 cm, 50%; ≥5.0 cm, 76%.[59,60]

Screening by palpation followed by ultrasound decreases mortality, especially in male smokers 65 years or older. Pain may signal rupture. Rupture is 15 times more likely in AAAs >4 cm than in smaller aneurysms.[60]

SPECIAL TECHNIQUES

Assessment Techniques for:

- Ascites
- Appendicitis
- Acute cholecystitis

- Ventral hernia
- Mass in abdominal wall

Assessing Possible Ascites. A protuberant abdomen with bulging flanks suggests possible ascites. Because ascitic fluid characteristically sinks with gravity, whereas gas-filled loops of bowel rise, percussion gives a dull note in dependent areas of the abdomen. Look for such a pattern by percussing outward in several directions from the central area of tympany. Map the border between tympany and dullness.

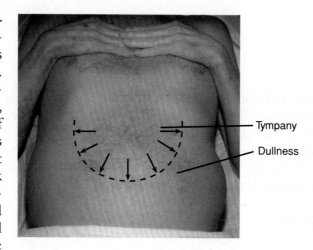

Tympany

Dullness

Ascites occurs in increased hydrostatic pressure in cirrhosis, heart failure, constrictive pericarditis, or inferior vena cava or hepatic vein obstruction. It may signal decreased osmotic pressure in nephrotic syndrome and malnutrition, or ovarian cancer.

Two additional techniques help to confirm ascites, although both signs may be misleading.

- *Test for shifting dullness.* After percussing the border of tympany and dullness with the patient supine, ask the patient to turn onto one side. Percuss and mark the borders again. In a person without ascites, the border between tympany and dullness usually stay relatively constant.

In ascites, dullness shifts to the more dependent side, whereas tympany shifts to the top.

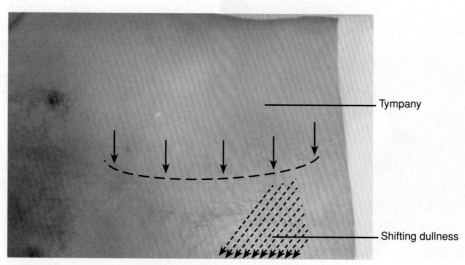

Tympany

Shifting dullness

PATIENT LYING ON RIGHT SIDE

- *Test for a fluid wave.* Ask the patient or an assistant to press the edges of both hands firmly down the midline of the abdomen. This pressure helps to stop the transmission of a wave through fat. While you tap one flank sharply with your fingertips, feel on the opposite flank for an impulse transmitted through the fluid. Unfortunately, this sign is often negative until ascites is obvious, and it is sometimes positive in people without ascites.

An easily palpable impulse suggests ascites. A positive fluid wave, shifting dullness, and peripheral edema make the diagnosis of ascites highly likely with ratios of 3 to 6.[61]

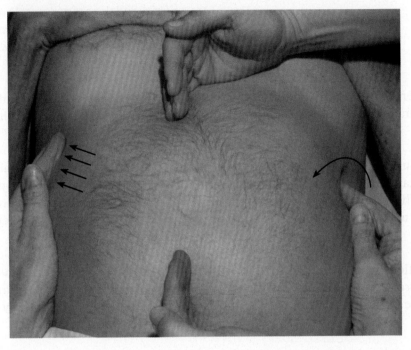

Identifying an Organ or a Mass in an Ascitic Abdomen. Try to *ballotte* the organ or mass, exemplified here by an enlarged liver. Straighten and stiffen the fingers of one hand together, place them on the abdominal surface, and make a brief jabbing movement directly toward the anticipated structure. This quick movement often displaces the fluid so that your fingertips can briefly touch the surface of the structure through the abdominal wall.

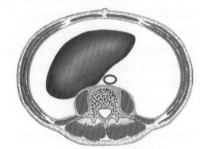
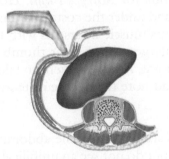

Appendicitis is twice as likely in the presence of guarding, Rosving's sign, and the psoas sign; it is three times more likely if rigidity and McBurney's point tenderness are present.[53]

Assessing Possible Appendicitis. Appendicitis is a common cause of acute abdominal pain. Assess carefully for the peritoneal signs of acute abdomen and the additional signs of McBurney's point tenderness, Rovsing's sign, the psoas sign, and the obturator sign described on the next page.

The pain of *appendicitis* classically begins near the umbilicus, then shifts to the right lower quadrant, where coughing increases it. Older patients report this pattern less frequently than younger ones.[16]

- Ask the patient to point to where the pain began and where it is now. Ask the patient to cough to see where pain occurs.

- Search carefully for an area of local tenderness. Classically "McBurney's point" lies 2 inches from the anterior superior spinous process of ilium on a line drawn from that process to the umbilicus.

Localized tenderness anywhere in the right lower quadrant, even in the right flank, may indicate *appendicitis*.

- Check the tender area for guarding, rigidity, and rebound tenderness.

Early voluntary guarding may be replaced by involuntary muscular rigidity and signs of peritoneal inflammation. There may also be right lower quadrant pain on quick withdrawal or deferred rebound tenderness.

- Check for *Rovsing's sign* and for referred rebound tenderness. Press deeply and evenly in the *left* lower quadrant. Then quickly withdraw your fingers.

Pain in the *right* lower quadrant during *left*-sided pressure is a positive Rovsing's sign.

- Look for a *psoas sign*. Place your hand just above the patient's right knee and ask the patient to raise that thigh against your hand. Alternatively, ask the patient to turn onto the left side. Then extend the patient's right leg at the hip. Flexion of the leg at the hip makes the psoas muscle contract; extension stretches it.

Increased abdominal pain on either maneuver constitutes a *positive psoas sign*, suggesting irritation of the psoas muscle by an inflamed appendix.

- Look for an *obturator sign*. Flex the patient's right thigh at the hip, with the knee bent, and rotate the leg internally at the hip. This maneuver stretches the internal obturator muscle. Internal rotation of the hip is described on p. 649.

Right hypogastric pain constitutes a *positive obturator sign*, from irritation of the obturator muscle by an inflamed appendix.

- *Perform a rectal examination and, in women, a pelvic examination.* These maneuvers may not help you to discriminate between a normal and an inflamed appendix, but they may help to identify an inflamed appendix atypically located within the pelvic cavity or other causes of the abdominal pain.

Right-sided rectal tenderness may also be caused by an inflamed adnexa or an inflamed seminal vesicle.

Assessing Possible Acute Cholecystitis.   When right upper quadrant pain and tenderness suggest acute cholecystitis, look for *Murphy's sign*. Hook your left thumb or the fingers of your right hand under the costal margin at the point where the lateral border of the rectus muscle intersects with the costal margin. Alternatively, if the liver is enlarged, hook your thumb or fingers under the liver edge at a comparable point. Ask the patient to take a deep breath. Watch the patient's breathing and note the degree of tenderness.

A sharp increase in tenderness with a sudden stop in inspiratory effort constitutes a *positive Murphy's sign* of *acute cholecystitis*. Hepatic tenderness may also increase with this maneuver but is usually less well localized.

Assessing Ventral Hernias.   Ventral hernias are hernias in the abdominal wall exclusive of groin hernias. If you suspect but do not see an umbilical or incisional hernia, ask the patient to raise both head and shoulders off the table.

The bulge of a hernia will usually appear with this action.

Inguinal and femoral hernias are discussed in Chapter 13, Male Genitalia and Hernias. They can give rise to important abdominal problems and must not be overlooked.

The cause of intestinal obstruction or peritonitis may be missed by overlooking a strangulated femoral hernia, see pp. 529–530.

Mass in the Abdominal Wall

Distinguishing an Abdominal Mass From a Mass in the Abdominal Wall. An occasional mass is in the abdominal wall rather than inside the abdominal cavity. Ask the patient either to raise the head and shoulders or to strain down, thus tightening the abdominal muscles. Feel for the mass again.

A mass in the abdominal wall remains palpable; an intra-abdominal mass is obscured by muscular contraction.

Recording Your Findings

Note that initially you may use sentences to describe your findings; later you will use phrases. The style below contains phrases appropriate for most write-ups.

Recording the Physical Examination—The Abdomen

"Abdomen is protuberant with active bowel sounds. It is soft and nontender; no palpable masses or hepatosplenomegaly. Liver span is 7 cm in the right midclavicular line; edge is smooth and palpable 1 cm below the right costal margin. Spleen and kidneys not felt. No costovertebral angle (CVA) tenderness."
OR
"Abdomen is flat. No bowel sounds heard. It is firm and boardlike, with increased tenderness, guarding, and rebound in the right midquadrant. Liver percusses to 7 cm in the midclavicular line; edge not felt. Spleen and kidneys not felt. No palpable masses. No CVA tenderness.

Suggests peritonitis from possible *appendicitis* (see pp. 467–468 and pp. 472–473).

Bibliography

Citations

1. Hsaio CJ, Cherry DK, Beatty PC et al. National Ambulatory Medical Care Survey: 2007 Summary—Table 9. National Health Statistics Reports, No 27. November 3, 2010. Available at http://www.cdc.gov/nchs/data/nhsr/nhsr027.pdf. Accessed February 5, 2011.
2. Niska R, Bhulya F, Xu J. National Hospital Ambulatory Medical Care Survey: 2007 emergency Department Summary – Table 10. National Health Statistics Reports, No 26. August 6 2010. Available at http://www.cdc.gov/nchs/data/nhsr/nhsr026.pdf. Accessed February 5, 2011.
3. Talley NJ, Vakil NB, Moayyedi P et al. American Gastroenterological Association technical review on the evaluation of dyspepsia. Gastroenterology 2005;129:1756–1780.
4. Drossman DA. The functional gastrointestinal disorders and the Rome III process. Gastroenterology 2007;130:1377–1390.
5. Ranji SR, Goldman LE, Simel DL et al. Do opiates affect the clinical evaluation of patients with acute abdominal pain? JAMA 2006;296:1764–1774.
6. Whitcomb DC. Acute pancreatitis. N Engl J Med 2006;354: 2142–2150.
7. Guptak WB. In the clinic: acute pancreatitis. Ann Intern Med 2010;153:ITC5-1–ITC5-16.
8. Trowbridge RL, Rutkowshi NK, Shojania KG. Does this patient have acute cholecystitis? JAMA 2003;289:80–86.
9. DeVault KR and Castell DO. Updated guidelines for the diagnosis and treatment of gastroesophageal reflux disease. Am J Gastroenterol 2005;100:190–200.
10. Vaezi MF, Hicks DM, Abelson TI et al. Laryngeal signs and symptoms and gastroesophageal reflux disease (GERD): a critical assessment of cause and effect association. Gastroenterol Hepatol 2003;1:333–344.
11. Talley NJ and Vakil N. Practice guidelines. Guidelines for management of dyspepsia. Am J Gastroenterol 2005;100:2324–2337.
12. Shaheen N and Ransohoff DF. Gastroesophageal reflux, Barrett esophagus, and esophageal cancer. Scientific review. JAMA 2002;287:1972–1981.
13. Wilson JE. In the clinic: gastroesophageal reflux disease. Ann Intern Med 2008;149:ITC2-1–ITC2-16.
14. Wang KK, Sampliner RE. Practice guidelines: updated guidelines 2008 for the diagnosis, surveillance and therapy of Barrett's esophagus. Am J Gastroenterol 2008;103:788–797.
15. Moayyedi P, Talley NJ, Fennerty MB et al. Can the clinical history distinguish between organic and functional dyspepsia? JAMA 2006;295:1566–1576.

16. Paulson EK, Kalady MF, Pappas TN. Suspected appendicitis. N Engl J Med 2003;348:236–242.

17. Mayer EA. Irritable bowel syndrome. N Engl J Med 2008;358:1692–1696.

18. Wilson JE. In the clinic: irritable bowel syndrome. Ann Intern Med 2007;147:ITC7-1–ITC7-16.

19. Theilman NM and Guerrant RL. Acute infectious diarrhea. N Engl J Med 2004;350:38–46.

20. DuPont HL. Bacterial diarrhea. N Engl J Med 2009;361:1560–1569.

21. Longstreth GF, Thompson WG, Chey WD et al. Functional bowel disorders. Gastroenterology 2006;130(5):1480–1491.

22. Drejkonja DM, Johnson JR. Urinary tract infections. Prim Care 2008;35:345–367.

23. Rogers RG. Urinary stress incontinence in women. N Engl J Med 2008;358:1029–1036.

24. Holroyd-Leduc JM, Tannenbaum C, Thorpe KE et al. What type of urinary incontinence does this woman have? JAMA 2008;299:1446–1556.

25. Hasin DS, Stinson FS, Ogburn E et al. Prevalence, correlates, disability, and comorbidity of DSM-IV alcohol abuse and dependence in the United States: results from the National Epidemiologic Survey on Alcohol and Related Conditions. Arch Gen Psychiatry 2007;64:830–842

26. Saitz R. Unhealthy alcohol use. N Engl J Med 2005;352:596–607.

27. Anton RF. Naltrexone for the management of alcohol dependence. N Engl J Med 2008;359:715–772.

28. U.S. Preventive Services Task Force. Screening and Behavioral Counseling Interventions in Primary care to Reduce Alcohol Misuse, in Guide to Clinical Preventive Services 2010-2011. Recommendations of the U.S. Preventive Services Task Force. Available at http://www.ahrq.gov/clinic/pocketgd1011/pocketgd1011.pdf, pp. 131–134. Accessed February 11, 2011.

29. National Institute on Alcohol Abuse and Alcoholism. Helping Patients who Drink Too Much. A Clinician's Guide. Updated January 2007. Available at http://pubs.niaaa.nih.gov/publications/practitioner/cliniciansguide2005/clinicians_guide.htm. Accessed February 11, 2011.

30. Centers for Disease Control and Prevention. Alcohol and public health. Fact sheets. Available at http://www.cdc.gov/alcohol/fact-sheets/alcohol-use.htm. Accessed February 13, 2011.

31. Centers for Disease Control and Prevention. Hepatitis A fact sheet. June 2010. Available at http://www.cdc.gov/hepatitis/A/PDFs/HepAGeneralFactSheet.pdf. Accessed February 11, 2010.

32. Dienstag JL. Hepatitis B virus infection. N Engl J Med 2008;359:1486–1500.

33. Centers for Disease Control and Prevention. Hepatitis B information for health professionals. Available at http://www.cdc.gov/hepatitis/HBV/index.htm. Accessed February 11, 2011.

34. Mast E, Weinbaum CM, Fiore AE et al. Recommendations of the Advisory Committee on Immunization Practices. Part II: Immunization of adults. A comprehensive immunization strategy to eliminate transmission of hepatitis B virus infections. MMWR Morb Mortal Wkly Rep 2006;55(RR16):1–35. Available at http://www.cdc.gov/mmwr/preview/mmwrhtml/rr5516a1.htm?s_cid=rr5516a1_e#box4. Accessed February 11, 2011.

35. Chou R, Clark E, Helfand M. Screening for hepatitis C virus infection. Systematic Evidence Reviews No. 24, Agency for Healthcare Research and Quality. March 2004. Available at http://www.ncbi.nlm.nih.gov/books/NBK43248. Accessed February 11, 2011.

36. Ghany MG, Strader DB, Thomas DL et al. Diagnosis, management, and treatment of hepatitis C: an update. American Association for the Study of Liver Diseases (AASLD) Practice Guidelines. Hepatology 2009;49:1335–1375.

37. Centers for Disease Control and Prevention. Hepatitis C FACs for health professionals. Updated December 2010. Available at http://www.cdc.gov/hepatitis/HCV/HCVfaq.htm. Accessed February 11, 2011.

38. American Cancer Society. Cancer facts and figures 2010. Available at http://www.cancer.org/acs/groups/content/@epidemiologysurveilance/documents/document/acspc-026238.pdf. Accessed February 11, 2011.

39. National Cancer Institute. Colorectal cancer screening. Health professional version. Updated January 28, 2011. Available at http://www.cancer.gov/cancertopics/pdq/screening/colorectal/HealthProfessional/AllPages. Accessed February 12, 2011.

40. U.S. Preventive Services Task Force. Screening for colorectal cancer: U.S. Preventive Services Task Force recommendation statement. Ann Intern Med 2008;148:627–637.

41. Whitlock EP, Lin JS, Liles E et al. Screening for colorectal cancer: A targeted, updated systematic review for the U.S. Preventive Services Task Force. Ann Intern Med 2008;149:638–658.

42. Levin B, Leiberman DA, McFarland B et al. American Cancer Society Colorectal Cancer Advisory Group. Screening and surveillance for the early detection of colorectal cancer and adenomatous polyps, 2008: a joint guideline from the American Cancer Society, the US Multi-Society Task Force on Colorectal Cancer, and the American College of Radiology. CA Cancer J Clin 2008;58:130–160.

43. Weinberg DS. In the clinic. Colorectal cancer screening. Ann Intern Med 2008;148:ITC2-1–ITC2-16.

44. Brenner H, Chang-Claude J, Seiler CM et al. Protection from colorectal cancer after colonoscopy. A population-based, case-control study. Ann Intern Med 2011;154:22–30.

45. Alquist DA, Sargent DJ, Loprinzi CL et al. Stool DNA and occult blood testing for screen detection of colorectal neoplasia. Ann Intern Med 2008;149:441–450.

46. Collins JF, Lieberman DA, Durbin TE et al. Veterans Affairs Cooperative Study #380 Group. Accuracy of screening for rectal occult blood on a single stool sample obtained by digital rectal examination: a comparison with recommended sampling practice. Ann Intern Med 2005;142:81–85.

47. Schatzkin A, Lanza E, Corle D et al. Lack of effect of a low-fat, high-fiber diet on the recurrence of colorectal adenomas. N Engl J Med 2000;342:1149–1155.

48. Alberts DS, Martinez ME, Roe DJ et al. Lack of effect of a high-fiber cereal supplement on the recurrence of colorectal adenomas. N Engl J Med 2000;342:1156–62.

49. Park Y, Leitzmann MF, Subar AF et al. Dairy food, calcium, and risk of cancer in the NIH-AARP Diet and Health Study. Arch Intern Med 2009;169:391–401.

50. Cole BF, Logan RF, Halabi S et al. Aspirin for the chemoprevention of colorectal adenomas: meta-analysis of the randomized trials. J Natl Cancer Inst 2009;101:256–266.

51. National Cancer Institute. Colorectal cancer prevention. Health professional version. Updated August 2010. Available at http://www.cancer.gov/cancertopics/pdq/prevention/colorectal/HealthProfessional. Accessed February 12, 2011.

52. U.S. Preventive Services Task Force. Routine aspirin or nonsteroidal anti-inflammatory drugs for the primary prevention of

colorectal cancer: U.S. Preventive Services Task Force recommendation statement. Ann Intern Med 2007;146:361–364.

53. McGee S. Abdomen, Part 9. Evidence Based Physical Diagnosis, 2nd ed. St. Louis: Saunders, 2007. pp. 346–594.

54. Cope Z. The early diagnosis of the acute abdomen. London: Oxford University Press, 1972.

55. Naylor CD. Physical examination of the liver. JAMA 1994;271:1859–1857.

56. Grover SA, Barkun AN, Sackett DL. Does this patient have splenomegaly? JAMA 1993;270:2218–2221.

57. U.S. Preventive Services Task Force. Screening for abdominal aortic aneurysm: recommendation statement. Ann Intern Med 2005;142:198–202.

58. Birkmeyer JD, Upchurch GR. Evidence-based screening and management of abdominal aortic aneurysm (editorial). Ann Intern Med 2007;146: 749–750.

59. Lederle FA, Simel DL. Does this patient have abdominal aortic aneurysm? JAMA 1999;281(1):77–82.

60. Lederle F. In the clinic. Abdominal aortic aneurysm. Ann Intern Med 2009;150:ITC5-1–ITC5-16.

61. Williams JW, Simel DL. Does this patient have ascites? How to divine fluid in the abdomen. JAMA 1992;267:2645–2648.

62. Brandt LJ, Feuerstadt P, Blaszka MC. Anatomic patterns, patient characteristics, and clinical outcomes in ischemic colitis: a study of 313 cases supported by histology. Am J Gastroenterol 2010;105:2245–2252.

Additional References

Examination of the Abdomen

Barkun AN, Camus M, Green L et al. The bedside assessment of splenic enlargement. Am J Med 1991;91:512–518.

Barkun AN, Camus M, Meagher T et al. Splenic enlargement and Traube's space: how useful is percussion? Am J Med 1989; 87:562–566.

Fink HA, Lederle FA, Roth CS et al. The accuracy of physical examination to detect abdominal aortic aneurysm. Arch Intern Med 2000;160:833–836.

Gu Y, Lim HJ, Moser MA. How useful are bowel sounds in assessing the abdomen? Dig Surg 2010;27:422–426.

Kim LG, Scott AP, Ashton HA et al. A sustained mortality benefit from screening for abdominal aortic aneurysm. Ann Intern Med 2007;52146:699–706.

McGee SR. Percussion and physical diagnosis: separating myth from science. Dis Mon 1995;41:641–688.

Meidl EJ, Ende J. Evaluation of liver size by physical examination. J Gen Intern Med 1993;8:635–637.

Naylor CD. The rational clinical examination. Physical examination of the liver. JAMA 1994;271:1859–1865.

Tamayo SG, Rickman LS, Mathews WC et al. Examiner dependence on physical diagnostic tests for the detection of splenomegaly: a prospective study with multiple observers. J Gen Intern Med 1993;8:69–75.

Turnbull JM. The rational clinical examination. Is listening for abdominal bruits useful in the evaluation of hypertension? JAMA 1995;274:1299–1301.

Yamamoto W, Kono H, Maekawa M et al. The relationship between abdominal pain regions and specific diseases: an epidemiologic approach to clinical practice. J Epidemiol 1997;7:27–32.

Yang JC, Rickman LS, Bosser SK. The clinical diagnosis of splenomegaly. West J Med 1991;155:47–52.

Zoli M, Magalotti D, Grimaldi M et al. Physical examination of the liver: is it still worth it? Am J Gastroenterol 1995;90:1428–1432.

Gastrointestinal and Genitourinary Conditions

American Gastroenterological Association. American Gastroenterological Association Medical Position Statement: guidelines on constipation. Gastroenterology 2000;119:1761–1778.

Bak E, Raman G, Chung M et al. Effectiveness of management strategies for renal artery stenosis: a systematic review. Ann Intern Med 2006;145:901–912.

Bhat S, Coleman HG, Yousef F et al. Risk of malignant progression in Barrett's esophagus patients: results from a large population-based study. J Natl Cancer Inst 2011;103:1049–1057.

Brenner H, Chang-Claude J, Seiler CM et al. Long-term risk of colorectal cancer after negative colonoscopy. J Clin Oncol 2011; 29:3761–367.

Cohen RA, Brown RS. Clinical practice. Microscopic hematuria. N Engl J Med 2003;348:2330–2338.

Feldman M, Friedman LS, Brandt LJ (eds). Sleisenger & Fordtran's Gastrointestinal and Liver Disease: Pathophysiology, Diagnosis, Management, 9th ed. Philadelphia: Saunders Elsevier, 2010.

Ferreira MP, Weems MK. Alcohol consumption by aging adults in the United States: health benefits and detriments. J Am Diet Assoc 2008;108:1668–1676.

Jackson PG, Raiji MT. Evaluation and management of intestinal obstruction. Am Fam Physician 2011;83:159–165.

Jacobs DO. Clinical practice. Diverticulitis. N Engl J Med 2007; 357:2057–2066.

Masson P, Matheson S, Webster AC et al. Meta-analyses in prevention and treatment of urinary tract infections. Infect Dis Clin North Am 2009;23:355–385.

O'Keeffe SA, McNally S, Keogan MT. Investigating painless haematuria. BMJ 2008;337:a260.

Substance Abuse and Mental Health Services Administration. (2010). Alcohol Use, pp. 29–39; see definitions of current, binge, and heavy drinking. In Results from the 2009 National Survey on Drug Use and Health: Volume I. Summary of National Findings (Office of Applied Studies, NSDUH Series H-38A, HHS Publication No. SMA 10-4586 Findings). Rockville, MD. Available at http://oas.samhsa.gov/NSDUH/2k9NSDUH/2k9ResultsP.pdf. Accessed October 22, 2011.

The Bates' suite offers these additional resources to enhance learning and facilitate understanding of this chapter:

- *Bates' Pocket Guide to Physical Examination and History Taking*, 7th edition
- *Bates' Visual Guide to Physical Examination*
- thePoint online resources, for students and instructors: http://thepoint.lww.com

Table 11-1	Abdominal Pain

Problem	Process	Location	Quality
Gastroesophageal reflux disease (GERD)[13,14]	Prolonged exposure of esophagus to gastric acid due to impaired esophageal motility or lower esophageal sphincter action. *Helicobacter pylori* may be present.	Chest or epigastric	Burning (heartburn) Also regurgitation
Peptic Ulcer and Dyspepsia[4,11]	Demonstrated ulcer usually in duodenum or stomach; dyspepsia causes similar symptoms but no ulceration. *H. pylori* infection often present.	Epigastric, may radiate to the back	Variable: gnawing burning, boring, aching, pressing, or hungerlike
Cancer of the Stomach	Predominantly adenocarcinoma (90%–95%)	Increasingly in "cardia" and GE junction; also in distal stomach	Variable
Acute Appendicitis[16]	Acute inflammation of the appendix with distention or obstruction	Poorly localized *periumbilical pain*, followed usually by	Mild but increasing, possibly cramping
		Right lower quadrant pain	Steady and more severe
Acute Cholecystitis[8]	Inflammation of the gallbladder, usually from obstruction of the cystic duct by gallstone	Right upper quadrant or upper abdominal; may radiate to the right scapular area	Steady, aching
Biliary Colic	Sudden obstruction of the cystic duct or common bile duct by a gallstone	Epigastric or right upper quadrant; may radiate to the right scapula and shoulder	Steady, aching; *not* colicky
Acute Pancreatitis[6,7]	Acute inflammation of the pancreas	Epigastric, may radiate to the back or other parts of the abdomen; may be poorly localized	Usually steady
Chronic Pancreatitis	Fibrosis of the pancreas secondary to recurrent inflammation	Epigastric, radiating through to the back	Steady, deep
Cancer of the Pancreas	Predominantly adenocarcinoma (95%)	Epigastric and in either upper quadrant; often radiates to the back	Steady, deep
Acute Diverticulitis	Acute inflammation of a colonic diverticulum, a saclike mucosal outpouching through the colonic muscle	Left lower quadrant	May be cramping at first, but becomes steady
Acute Bowel Obstruction	Obstruction of the bowel lumen, most commonly caused by (1) adhesions or hernias (small bowel), or (2) cancer or diverticulitis (colon)	*Small bowel:* periumbilical or upper abdominal	Cramping
		Colon: lower abdominal or generalized	Cramping
Mesenteric Ischemia[62]	Blood supply to the bowel and mesentery blocked from thrombosis or embolus (acute arterial occlusion), or reduced from hypoperfusion	May be periumbilical at first, then diffuse	Cramping at first, then steady

Timing	Factors That May Aggravate	Factors That May Relieve	Associated Symptoms and Setting
After meals, specifically fatty foods	Lying down, bending over. Physical activity	Antacids; avoiding alcohol, fatty meals, chocolate, selected drugs such as theophylline, calcium channel blockers	Wheezing, chronic cough, shortness of breath, hoarseness, choking sensation, halitosis, sore throat. Increases risk of Barrett's esophagus and esophageal cancer.
Intermittent. Duodenal ulcer is more likely than gastric ulcer or dyspepsia to cause pain that (1) wakes the patient at night, and (2) occurs intermittently over a few weeks, disappears for months, then recurs.	Variable	Food and antacids may bring relief, least commonly in gastric ulcer.	Nausea, vomiting, belching, bloating; heartburn (more common in duodenal ulcer); weight loss (more common in gastric ulcer). Dyspepsia is more common in the young (20–29 years), gastric ulcer in those over 50 years, and duodenal ulcer in those 30–60 years.
The history of pain is typically shorter than in peptic ulcer. Pain is persistent, slowly progressive.	Often food	*Not* relieved by food or antacids	Anorexia, nausea, early satiety, weight loss, and sometimes bleeding. Most common in ages 50–70
Lasts roughly 4–6 hours			
Depends on intervention	Movement or cough	If it subsides temporarily, suspect perforation of the appendix.	Anorexia, nausea, possibly vomiting, which typically follow the onset of pain; low fever
Gradual onset; course longer than in biliary colic	Jarring, deep breathing		Anorexia, nausea, vomiting, fever
Rapid onset over a few minutes, lasts one to several hours and subsides gradually. Often recurrent			Anorexia, nausea, vomiting, restlessness
Acute onset, persistent pain	Lying supine	Leaning forward with trunk flexed	Nausea, vomiting, abdominal distention, fever. Often a history of previous attacks and alcohol abuse or gallstones
Chronic or recurrent course	Alcohol, heavy or fatty meals	Possibly leaning forward with trunk flexed; often intractable	Pancreatic enzyme insufficiency, diarrhea with fatty stools (steatorrhea) and diabetes mellitus.
Persistent pain; relentlessly progressive illness		Possibly leaning forward with trunk flexed; often intractable	Anorexia, nausea, vomiting, weight loss, and jaundice; depression
Often a gradual onset			Fever, constipation. There may be initial brief diarrhea.
Paroxysmal; may decrease as bowel mobility is impaired			Vomiting of bile and mucus (high obstruction) or fecal material (low obstruction). Obstipation develops.
Paroxysmal, though typically milder			Obstipation early. Vomiting late if at all. Prior symptoms of underlying cause.
Usually abrupt in onset, then persistent			Vomiting, diarrhea (sometimes bloody), constipation, shock; older age

Table 11-2   Dysphagia

Process and Problem	Timing	Factors That Aggravate	Factors That Relieve	Associated Symptoms and Conditions
Oropharyngeal Dysphagia, *due to motor disorders affecting the pharyngeal muscles*	Acute or gradual onset and a variable course, depending on the underlying disorder	Attempts to start the swallowing process		Aspiration into the lungs or regurgitation into the nose with attempts to swallow. From stroke, bulbar palsy, or other neuromuscular conditions
Esophageal Dysphagia				
Mechanical Narrowing				
• Mucosal rings and webs	Intermittent	Solid foods	Regurgitation of the bolus of food	Usually none
• Esophageal stricture	Intermittent; may become slowly progressive	Solid foods	Regurgitation of the bolus of food	A long history of heartburn and regurgitation
• Esophageal cancer	May be intermittent at first; progressive over months	Solid foods, with progression to liquids	Regurgitation of the bolus of food	Pain in the chest and back and weight loss, especially late in the course of illness
Motor Disorders				
• Diffuse esophageal spasm	Intermittent	Solids or liquids	Maneuvers described below; sometimes nitroglycerin	Chest pain that mimics angina pectoris or myocardial infarction and lasts minutes to hours; possibly heartburn
• Scleroderma	Intermittent; may progress slowly	Solids or liquids	Repeated swallowing; movements such as straightening the back, raising the arms, or a Valsalva maneuver (straining down against a closed glottis)	Heartburn; other manifestations of scleroderma
• Achalasia	Intermittent; may progress	Solids or liquids		Regurgitation, often at night when lying down, with nocturnal cough; possibly chest pain precipitated by eating

| Table 11-3 | **Constipation** |

Problem	Process	Associated Symptoms and Setting
Life Activities and Habits		
Inadequate Time or Setting for the Defecation Reflex	Ignoring the sensation of a full rectum inhibits the defecation reflex.	Hectic schedules, unfamiliar surroundings, bed rest
False Expectations of Bowel Habits	Expectations of "regularity" or more frequent stools than a person's norm	Beliefs, treatments, and advertisements that promote the use of laxatives
Diet Deficient in Fiber	Decreased fecal bulk	Other factors such as debilitation and constipating drugs may contribute.
Irritable Bowel Syndrome[17,18]	Functional change in frequency or form of bowel movement without known pathology; possibly from change in intestinal bacteria.	Three patterns: diarrhea—predominant, constipation—predominant, or mixed. Symptoms present ≥6 months and abdominal pain for ≥3 months plus at least 2 of 3 features (improvement with defecation; onset with change in stool frequency; onset with change in stool form and appearance)
Mechanical Obstruction		
Cancer of the Rectum or Sigmoid Colon	Progressive narrowing of the bowel lumen from adenocarcinoma	Change in bowel habits; often diarrhea, abdominal pain, bleeding, occult blood in stool. In rectal cancer, tenesmus and pencil-shaped stools. Weight loss.
Fecal Impaction	A large, firm, immovable fecal mass, most often in the rectum	Rectal fullness, abdominal pain, and diarrhea around the impaction; common in debilitated, bedridden, and often elderly patients
Other Obstructing Lesions (such as diverticulitis, volvulus, intussusception, or hernia)	Narrowing or complete obstruction of the bowel	Colicky abdominal pain, abdominal distention, and in intussusception, often "currant jelly" stools (red blood and mucus)
Painful Anal Lesions	Pain may cause spasm of the external sphincter and voluntary inhibition of the defecation reflex.	Anal fissures, painful hemorrhoids, perirectal abscesses
Drugs	A variety of mechanisms	Opiates, anticholinergics, antacids containing calcium or aluminum, and many others
Depression	A disorder of mood. See Table 5-2, Disorders of Mood, p. 167.	Fatigue, anhedonia, sleep disturbance, weight loss
Neurologic Disorders	Interference with the autonomic innervation of the bowel	Spinal cord injuries, multiple sclerosis, Hirschsprung's disease, and other conditions
Metabolic Conditions	Interference with bowel motility	Pregnancy, hypothyroidism, hypercalcemia

Table
11-4 Diarrhea

Problem	Process	Characteristics of Stool
Acute Diarrhea[19] (≤14 days)		
Secretory Infection (non-inflammatory)	Infection by viruses, preformed bacterial toxins (such as *S. aureus*, *B. cereus*, *C. perfringens*, toxigenic *E. coli*, *Vibrio cholerae*), cryptosporidium, *Giardia lamblia*, *rotavirus*	Watery, without blood, pus, or mucus
Inflammatory Infection	Colonization or invasion of intestinal mucosa (nontyphoid *Salmonella*, *Shigella*, *Yersinia*, *Campylobacter*, enteropathic *E. coli*, *Entamoeba histolytica*, *C. difficile*)	Loose to watery, often with blood, pus, or mucus
Drug-Induced Diarrhea	Action of many drugs, such as magnesium-containing antacids, antibiotics, antineoplastic agents, and laxatives	Loose to watery
Chronic Diarrhea (≥30 days)		
Diarrheal Syndrome		
• Irritable bowel syndrome[17,18]	Change in frequency and form of bowel movements without chemical or structural abnormality	Loose; ~50% with mucus; small to moderate volume. Small, hard stools with constipation. May be mixed pattern.
• Cancer of the sigmoid colon	Partial obstruction by a malignant neoplasm	May be blood-streaked
Inflammatory Bowel Disease		
• Ulcerative colitis	Inflammation of the mucosa and submucosa of the rectum and colon with ulceration; typically extends proximally from the rectum	Soft to watery, often containing blood
• Crohn's disease of the small bowel (regional enteritis) or colon (granulomatous colitis)	Chronic transmural inflammation of the bowel wall, in a skip pattern typically involving the terminal ileum and/or proximal colon	Small, soft to loose or watery, usually free of gross blood (enteritis) or with less bleeding than ulcerative colitis (colitis)
Voluminous Diarrhea		
• Malabsorption syndrome	Defective membrane transport or absorption of intestinal epithelium (Crohn's, celiac disease, surgical resection); impaired luminal digestion (pancreatic insufficiency); epithelial defects at brush border (lactose intolerance)	Typically bulky, soft, light yellow to gray, mushy, greasy or oily, and sometimes frothy; particularly foul-smelling; usually floats in toilet
• Osmotic diarrhea		
Lactose intolerance	Deficiency in intestinal lactase	Watery diarrhea of large volume
Abuse of osmotic purgatives	Laxative habit, often surreptitious	Watery diarrhea of large volume
• Secretory diarrhea	Variable: bacterial infection, secreting villous adenoma, fat or bile salt malabsorption, hormone-mediated conditions (gastrin in Zollinger–Ellison syndrome, vasoactive intestinal peptide)	Watery diarrhea of large volume

Timing	Associated Symptoms	Setting, Persons at Risk
Duration of a few days, possibly longer. Lactase deficiency may lead to a longer course.	Nausea, vomiting, periumbilical cramping pain. Temperature normal or slightly elevated	Often travel, a common food source, or an epidemic
An acute illness of varying duration	Lower abdominal cramping pain and often rectal urgency, tenesmus; fever	Travel, contaminated food or water. Frequent anal intercourse.
Acute, recurrent, or chronic	Possibly nausea; usually little if any pain	Prescribed or over-the-counter medications
Worse in the morning; rarely at night.	Crampy lower abdominal pain, abdominal distention, flatulence, nausea. Urgency, pain relieved with defecation.	Young and middle-aged adults, especially women
Variable	Change in usual bowel habits, crampy lower abdominal pain, constipation	Middle-aged and older adults, especially older than 55 years
Onset ranges from insidious to acute. Typically recurrent; may be persistent. May awaken at night.	Milder cramping, lower or generalized abdominal pain, anorexia, weakness; fever if severe. May include episcleritis, uveitis, arthritis, erythema nodosum.	Often young people. Increases risk of colon cancer.
Insidious onset; chronic or recurrent. Diarrhea may wake the patient at night.	Crampy periumbilical or right lower quadrant (enteritis) or diffuse (colitis) pain, with anorexia, low fever, and/or weight loss. Perianal or perirectal abscesses and fistulas. May cause small or large bowel obstruction	Often young people, especially in late teens, but also in middle age. More common in people of Jewish descent. Increases risk of colon cancer
Onset of illness typically insidious	Anorexia, weight loss, fatigue, abdominal distention, often crampy lower abdominal pain. Symptoms of nutritional deficiencies such as bleeding (vitamin K), bone pain and fractures (vitamin D), glossitis (vitamin B), and edema (protein)	Variable, depending on cause
Follows the ingestion of milk and milk products; relieved by fasting	Crampy abdominal pain, abdominal distention, flatulence	In >50% of African Americans, Asians, Native Americans, Hispanics; in 5%–20% of Caucasians
Variable	Often none	Persons with anorexia nervosa or bulimia nervosa
Variable	Weight loss, dehydration, nausea, vomiting, and cramping abdominal pain	Variable depending on cause

Table 11-5	Black and Bloody Stools

Problem	Selected Causes	Associated Symptoms and Setting
Melena Refers to passage of black, tarry (sticky and shiny) stools. Occult blood tests are positive. Involves loss of at least 60 mL of blood into the gastrointestinal tract (less in children), usually from the esophagus, stomach, or duodenum and transit time of 7–14 hours. Less commonly, when transit is slow, blood loss originates in the jejunum, ileum, or ascending colon. In infants, melena may result from swallowing blood during the birth.	Gastritis, GERD, peptic ulcer (gastric or duodenal)	Usually epigastric discomfort from heartburn, dysmotility; if peptic ulcer, pain after meals (delayed, 2–3 hours if duodenal ulcer). May be silent.
	Gastritis or stress ulcers	Recent ingestion of alcohol, aspirin, or other anti-inflammatory drugs; recent bodily trauma, severe burns, surgery, or increased intracranial pressure
	Esophageal or gastric varices	Cirrhosis of the liver or other causes of portal hypertension
	Reflux esophagitis Mallory-Weiss tear in esophageal mucosa due to retching and vomiting	Retching, vomiting, often recent ingestion of alcohol
Black, Nonsticky Stools May result from other causes, with negative occult blood tests. These stools have no pathologic significance.	Ingestion of iron, bismuth salts, licorice, or even chocolate cookies	Asymptomatic
Red Blood in the Stools (hematochezia) Usually originates in the colon, rectum, or anus; much less frequently from the jejunum or ileum. Upper gastrointestinal hemorrhage may also cause red stools; blood loss is then usually large (more than a liter). Rapid transit through the intestinal tract leaves insufficient time for the blood to turn black from oxidation of iron in hemoglobin.	Colon cancer	Often a change in bowel habits, weight loss
	Hyperplasia or adenomatous polyps	Often no other symptoms
	Diverticula of the colon	Often no symptoms unless inflammation causes diverticulitis
	Inflammatory conditions of the colon and rectum	
	• Ulcerative colitis, Crohn's disease	See Table 11-4, Diarrhea, p. 476.
	• Infectious diarrhea	See Table 11-4, Diarrhea, p. 476.
	• Proctitis (various causes including frequent anal intercourse)	Rectal urgency, tenesmus
	Ischemic colitis	Lower abdominal pain, sometimes fever or shock in older adults. Abdomen typically soft to palpation
	Hemorrhoids	Blood on the toilet paper, on the surface of the stool, or dripping into the toilet
	Anal fissure	Blood on the toilet paper or on the surface of the stool; anal pain
Reddish but Nonbloody Stools	Ingestion of beets	Pink urine, which usually precedes the reddish stool; from poor metabolism of betacyanin

Table
11-6 Frequency, Nocturia, and Polyuria

Problem	Mechanisms	Selected Causes	Associated Symptoms
Frequency	Decreased capacity of the bladder		
	• Increased bladder sensitivity to stretch because of inflammation	*Infection*, stones, tumor, or foreign body in the bladder	Burning on urination, urinary urgency, sometimes gross hematuria
	• Decreased elasticity of the bladder wall	Infiltration by scar tissue or tumor	Symptoms of associated inflammation (see above) are common.
	• Decreased cortical inhibition of bladder contractions	Motor disorders of the central nervous system, such as a stroke	Urinary urgency; neurologic symptoms such as weakness and paralysis
	Impaired emptying of the bladder, with residual urine in the bladder		
	• Partial mechanical obstruction of the bladder neck or proximal urethra	Most commonly, benign prostatic hyperplasia; also urethral stricture and other obstructive lesions of the bladder or prostate	Prior obstructive symptoms: hesitancy in starting the urinary stream, straining to void, reduced size and force of the stream, and dribbling during or at the end of urination
	• Loss of peripheral nerve supply to the bladder	Neurologic disease affecting the sacral nerves or nerve roots, e.g., diabetic neuropathy	Weakness or sensory defects
Nocturia *With High Volumes*	Most types of polyuria (see p. 445)		
	Decreased concentrating ability of the kidney with loss of the normal decrease in nocturnal urinary output	Chronic renal insufficiency due to a number of diseases	Possibly other symptoms of renal insufficiency
	Excessive fluid intake before bedtime	Habit, especially involving alcohol and coffee	
	Fluid-retaining, edematous states. Dependent edema accumulates during the day and is excreted when the patient lies down at night.	Heart failure, nephrotic syndrome, hepatic cirrhosis with ascites, chronic venous insufficiency	Edema and other symptoms of the underlying disorder. Urinary output during the day may be reduced as fluid reaccumulates in the body. See Table 12-1, Peripheral Causes of Edema, p. 513.
With Low Volumes	Frequency		
	Voiding while up at night without a real urge, a "pseudofrequency"	Insomnia	Variable
Polyuria	Deficiency of antidiuretic hormone (diabetes insipidus)	A disorder of the posterior pituitary and hypothalamus	Thirst and polydipsia, often severe and persistent; nocturia
	Renal unresponsiveness to antidiuretic hormone (nephrogenic diabetes insipidus)	A number of kidney diseases, including hypercalcemic and hypokalemic nephropathy; drug toxicity, e.g., from lithium	Thirst and polydipsia, often severe and persistent; nocturia
	Solute diuresis		
	• Electrolytes, such as sodium salts	Large saline infusions, potent diuretics, certain kidney diseases	Variable
	• Nonelectrolytes, such as glucose	Uncontrolled diabetes mellitus	Thirst, polydipsia, and nocturia
	Excessive water intake	Primary polydipsia	Polydipsia tends to be episodic. Thirst may not be present. Nocturia is usually absent.

Table	
11-7	**Urinary Incontinence***

Problem	Mechanisms
Stress Incontinence The urethral sphincter is weakened so that transient increases in intra-abdominal pressure raise the bladder pressure to levels that exceed urethral resistance.	In women, often a weakness of the pelvic floor with inadequate muscular support of the bladder and proximal urethra and a change in the angle between the bladder and the urethra (see Chapter 14, p. 562). Causes include childbirth and surgery. Local conditions affecting the internal urethral sphincter, such as postmenopausal atrophy of the mucosa and urethral infection, may also contribute. In men, stress incontinence may follow prostatic surgery.
Urge Incontinence Detrusor contractions are stronger than normal and overcome the normal urethral resistance. The bladder is typically *small*.	Decreased cortical inhibition of detrusor contractions from stroke, brain tumor, dementia, and lesions of the spinal cord above the sacral level Hyperexcitability of sensory pathways, as in bladder infections, tumors, and fecal impaction Deconditioning of voiding reflexes, as in frequent voluntary voiding at low bladder volumes
Overflow Incontinence Detrusor contractions are insufficient to overcome urethral resistance. The bladder is typically *large*, even after an effort to void.	Obstruction of the bladder outlet, as in benign prostatic hyperplasia or tumor Weakness of the detrusor muscle associated with peripheral nerve disease at the sacral level Impaired bladder sensation that interrupts the reflex arc, as from diabetic neuropathy
Functional Incontinence This is a functional inability to get to the toilet in time because of impaired health or environmental conditions.	Problems in mobility resulting from weakness, arthritis, poor vision, or other conditions. Environmental factors such as an unfamiliar setting, distant bathroom facilities, bed rails, or physical restraints
Incontinence Secondary to Medications Drugs may contribute to any type of incontinence listed.	Sedatives, tranquilizers, anticholinergics, sympathetic blockers, and potent diuretics

*Patients may have more than one kind of incontinence.

Symptoms	Physical Signs
Momentary leakage of small amounts of urine with coughing, laughing, and sneezing while the person is in an upright position. A desire to urinate is not associated with pure stress incontinence.	The bladder is not detected on abdominal examination. Stress incontinence may be demonstrable, especially if the patient is examined before voiding and in a standing position. Atrophic vaginitis may be evident.
Involuntary urine loss preceded by an urge to void. The volume tends to be moderate.	The bladder is not detectable on abdominal examination.
Urgency Frequency and nocturia with small to moderate volumes If acute inflammation is present, pain on urination Possibly "pseudo-stress incontinence"—voiding 10–20 seconds after stresses such as a change of position, going up or down stairs, and possibly coughing, laughing, or sneezing	When cortical inhibition is decreased, mental deficits or motor signs of central nervous system disease are often, though not necessarily, present. When sensory pathways are hyperexcitable, signs of local pelvic problems or a fecal impaction may be present.
A continuous dripping or dribbling incontinence Decreased force of the urinary stream Prior symptoms of partial urinary obstruction or other symptoms of peripheral nerve disease may be present.	An enlarged bladder is often found on abdominal examination and may be tender. Other signs include prostatic enlargement, motor signs of peripheral nerve disease, a decrease in sensation (including perineal sensation), and diminished to absent reflexes.
Incontinence on the way to the toilet or only in the early morning	The bladder is not detectable on physical examination. Look for physical or environmental clues to the likely cause.
Variable. A careful history and chart review are important.	Variable

Table
11-8   Localized Bulges in the Abdominal Wall

Localized bulges in the abdominal wall include *ventral hernias* (defects in the wall through which tissue protrudes) and subcutaneous tumors such as *lipomas*. The more common ventral hernias are umbilical, incisional, and epigastric. Hernias and a rectus diastasis usually become more evident when the patient raises head and shoulders from a supine position.

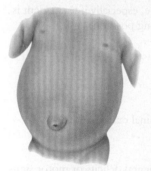

INFANT

Umbilical Hernia
A protrusion through a defective umbilical ring is most common in infants but also occurs in adults. In infants, it usually closes spontaneously within 1 to 2 years.

Diastasis Recti
Separation of the two rectus abdominis muscles, through which abdominal contents form a midline ridge when the patient raises head and shoulders. Often seen in repeated pregnancies, obesity, and chronic lung disease. It has no clinical consequences.

Ridge

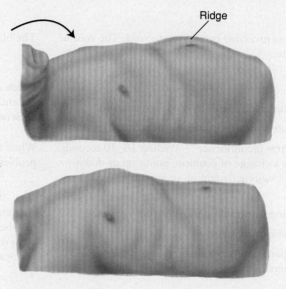

Incisional Hernia
This is a protrusion through an operative scar. Palpate to detect the length and width of the defect in the abdominal wall. A small defect, through which a large hernia has passed, has a greater risk for complications than a large defect.

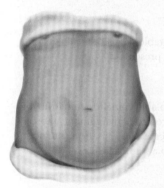

Epigastric Hernia
A small midline protrusion through a defect in the linea alba occurs between the xiphoid process and the umbilicus. With the patient's head and shoulders raised (or with the patient standing), run your fingerpad down the linea alba to feel it.

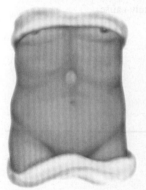

Lipoma
Common, benign, fatty tumors usually in the subcutaneous tissues almost anywhere in the body, including the abdominal wall. Small or large, they are usually soft and often lobulated. Press your finger down on the edge of a lipoma. The tumor typically slips out from under it.

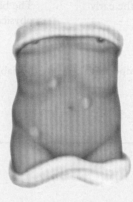

Table
11-9 Protuberant Abdomens

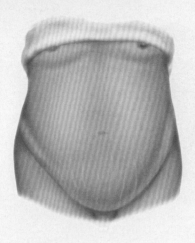

Fat

Fat is the most common cause of a protuberant abdomen. Fat thickens the abdominal wall, the mesentery, and omentum. The umbilicus may appear sunken. A *pannus*, or apron of fatty tissue, may extend below the inguinal ligaments. Lift it to look for inflammation in the skin folds or even for a hidden hernia.

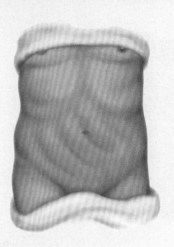

Gas

Gaseous distention may be localized or generalized. It causes a tympanitic percussion note. Increased intestinal gas production from certain foods may cause mild distention. More serious are intestinal obstruction and adynamic (paralytic) ileus. Note the location of the distention. Distention becomes more marked in colonic than in small bowel obstruction.

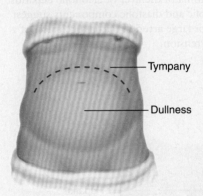

Tympany

Dullness

Tumor

A large, solid tumor, usually rising out of the pelvis, is dull to percussion. Air-filled bowel is displaced to the periphery. Causes include ovarian tumors and uterine myomata. Occasionally a markedly distended bladder may be mistaken for such a tumor.

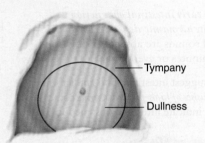

Tympany

Dullness

Pregnancy

Pregnancy is a common cause of a pelvic "mass." Listen for the fetal heart (see pp. 909).

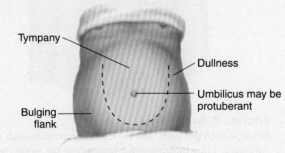

Tympany

Dullness

Bulging flank

Umbilicus may be protuberant

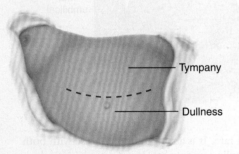

Tympany

Dullness

Ascitic Fluid

Ascitic fluid seeks the lowest point in the abdomen, producing bulging flanks that are dull to percussion. The umbilicus may protrude. Turn the patient onto one side to detect the shift in position of the fluid level (shifting dullness). (See pp. 466–467 for the assessment of ascites.)

Table
11-10   Sounds in the Abdomen

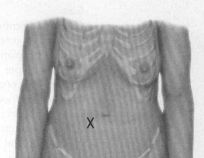

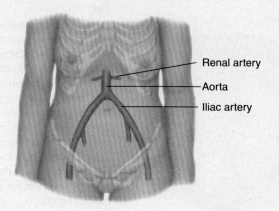

Bowel Sounds

Bowel sounds may be:

- *Increased*, as in diarrhea or *early intestinal obstruction*
- *Decreased*, then absent, as in *adynamic ileus* and *peritonitis*. Before deciding that bowel sounds are absent, sit down and listen where shown for 2 minutes or even longer.

High-pitched tinkling sounds suggest intestinal fluid and air under tension in a dilated bowel. *Rushes of high-pitched sounds* coinciding with an abdominal cramp indicate intestinal obstruction.

Bruits

A *hepatic bruit* suggests carcinoma of the liver or alcoholic hepatitis. *Arterial bruits* with both systolic and diastolic components suggest partial occlusion of the aorta or large arteries. Partial occlusion of a renal artery may explain hypertension.

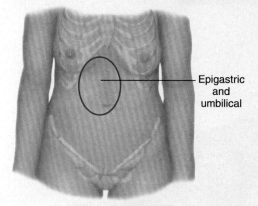

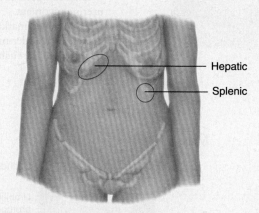

Venous Hum

A venous hum is rare. It is a soft humming noise with both systolic and diastolic components. It indicates increased collateral circulation between portal and systemic venous systems, as in hepatic cirrhosis.

Friction Rubs

Friction rubs are rare. They are grating sounds with respiratory variation. They indicate inflammation of the peritoneal surface of an organ, as in liver cancer, chlamydial or gonococcal perihepatitis, recent liver biopsy, or splenic infarct. When a systolic bruit accompanies a hepatic friction rub, suspect carcinoma of the liver.

Table
11-11   **Tender Abdomens**

Abdominal Wall Tenderness

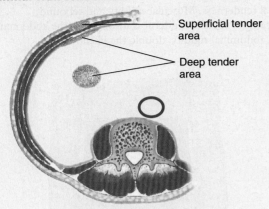

Superficial tender area

Deep tender area

Tenderness may originate in the abdominal wall. When the patient raises the head and shoulders, this tenderness persists, whereas tenderness from a deeper lesion (protected by the tightened muscles) decreases.

Visceral Tenderness

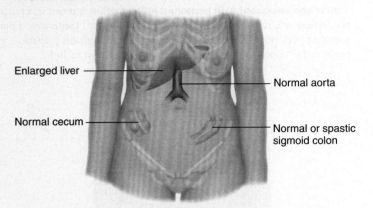

Enlarged liver

Normal aorta

Normal cecum

Normal or spastic sigmoid colon

The structures shown may be tender to deep palpation. Usually the discomfort is dull with no muscular rigidity or rebound tenderness. A reassuring explanation to the patient may prove quite helpful.

Tenderness From Disease in the Chest and Pelvis

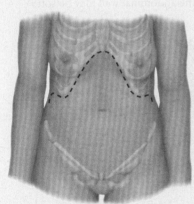

Unilateral or bilateral, upper or lower abdomen

Acute Pleurisy

Abdominal pain and tenderness may result from acute pleural inflammation. When unilateral, it may mimic acute cholecystitis or appendicitis. Rebound tenderness and rigidity are less common; chest signs are usually present.

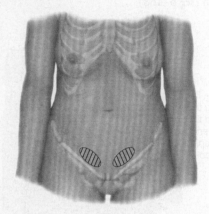

Acute Salpingitis

Frequently bilateral, the tenderness of acute salpingitis (inflammation of the fallopian tubes) is usually maximal just above the inguinal ligaments. Rebound tenderness and rigidity may be present. On pelvic examination, motion of the uterus causes pain.

(table continues on page 486)

Table
11-11 Tender Abdomens (*continued*)

Tenderness of Peritoneal Inflammation

Tenderness associated with peritoneal inflammation is more severe than visceral tenderness. Muscular rigidity and rebound tenderness are frequently but not necessarily present. Generalized peritonitis causes exquisite tenderness throughout the abdomen, together with boardlike muscular rigidity. These signs on palpation, especially abdominal rigidity, double the likelihood of peritonitis.[53] Local causes of peritoneal inflammation include:

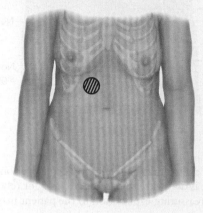

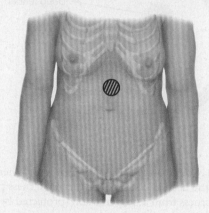

Acute Cholecystitis[8]

Signs are maximal in the right upper quadrant. Check for Murphy's sign (see p. 468).

Acute Pancreatitis

In acute pancreatitis, epigastric tenderness and rebound tenderness are usually present, but the abdominal wall may be soft.

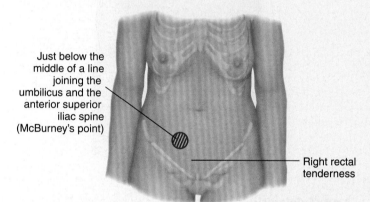

Just below the middle of a line joining the umbilicus and the anterior superior iliac spine (McBurney's point)

Right rectal tenderness

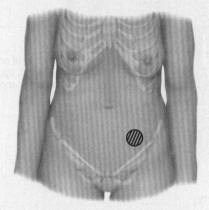

Acute Appendicitis[16]

Right lower quadrant signs are typical of acute appendicitis but may be absent early in the course (McBurney's point). The typical area of tenderness is illustrated. Explore other portions of the right lower quadrant as well as the right flank.

Acute Diverticulitis

Acute diverticulitis most often involves the sigmoid colon and then resembles a left-sided appendicitis.

Table

11-12   **Liver Enlargement: Apparent and Real**

A palpable liver does not necessarily indicate hepatomegaly (an enlarged liver), but more often results from a change in consistency—from the normal softness to an abnormal firmness or hardness, as in cirrhosis. Clinical estimates of liver size should be based on both percussion and palpation, although even these techniques are far from perfect.[53]

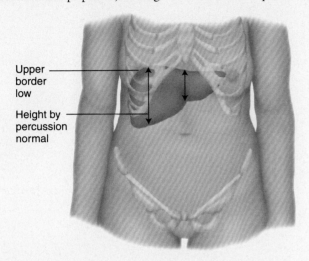

Upper border low

Height by percussion normal

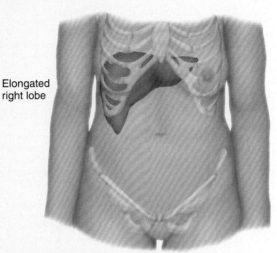

Elongated right lobe

Downward Displacement of the Liver by a Low Diaphragm

This finding is common when the diaphragm is low (e.g., in COPD). The liver edge may be palpable well below the costal margin. Percussion, however, reveals a low upper edge, and the vertical span of the liver is normal.

Normal Variations in Liver Shape

In some people, especially those with a lanky build, the liver tends to be elongated so that its right lobe is easily palpable as it projects downward toward the iliac crest. Such an elongation, sometimes called *Riedel's lobe*, represents a variation in shape, not an increase in liver volume or size. Examiners can only estimate the upper and lower borders of an organ with three dimensions and differing shapes. Some error is unavoidable.

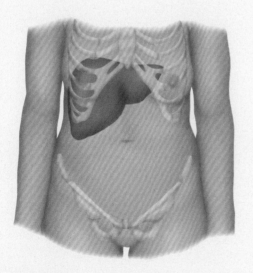

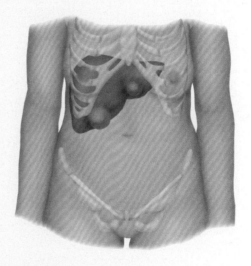

Smooth Large Liver

Cirrhosis may produce an enlarged liver with a firm, *nontender* edge. The cirrhotic liver may also be scarred and contracted. Many other diseases may produce similar findings such as hemochromatosis, amyloidosis, and lymphoma. An enlarged liver with a smooth, *tender* edge suggests inflammation, as in hepatitis, or venous congestion, as in right-sided heart failure.

Irregular Large Liver

An enlarged liver that is firm or hard and has an irregular edge or surface suggests *hepatocellular carcinoma*. There may be one or more nodules. The liver may or may not be tender.

The Peripheral Vascular System

Careful assessment of the peripheral vascular system is essential for detection of *peripheral arterial disease (PAD)*, found in roughly 8 million Americans, approximately 12% of the population, but "silent" in roughly half of those affected.[1,2] Prevalence increases with age, from 7% in adults ages 60 to 69 to 23% in adults 80 years of age and older.[3] Detection is doubly important because PAD is both a marker for cardiovascular morbidity and mortality, and a harbinger of functional decline. Risk of death from myocardial infarction and stroke triples in adults with PAD. Improved screening and prevention is the focus of two major reports from an interdisciplinary task force of the American College of Cardiology and the American Heart Association in 2005 and 2010, referenced throughout this chapter.[1,4]

Thromboembolic disorders of the *peripheral venous system* are also common, seen in an estimated 1% of adults above age 60.[5] Roughly one-third of patients present with pulmonary thromboembolism, and two-thirds with deep venous thrombosis (DVT), often in hospital settings.[6] Recent reports show that superficial venous thrombosis may also accompany DVT and increase risk of pulmonary thromboembolism.[7]

Anatomy and Physiology

ARTERIES

Arteries contain three concentric layers of tissue: the *intima*, the *media*, and the *adventitia*. The *internal elastic membrane* borders the intima and the media; the *external elastic membrane* separates the media from the adventitia.

Injury to vascular endothelial cells provokes thrombus formation, atheromas, and the vascular lesions of hypertension.[8]

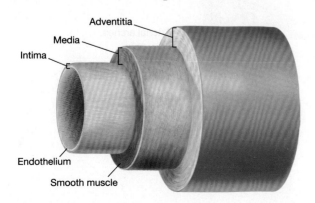

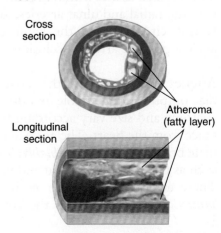

Surrounding the lumen of all blood vessels is the *intima*, a single continuous lining of endothelial cells with remarkable metabolic properties.[8] Intact endothelium synthesizes regulators of thrombosis such as prostacyclin, plasminogen activator, and heparinlike molecules. It produces prothrombotic molecules such as Von Willebrand factor and plasminogen activator inhibitor. It modulates blood flow and vascular reactivity through synthesis of vasoconstrictors like endothelin and angiotensin-converting enzyme, and vasodilators such as nitric oxide and prostacyclin. The intimal endothelium also regulates immune and inflammatory reactions through elaboration of interleukins, adhesion molecules, and histocompatibility antigens.

The *media* is composed of smooth muscle cells that dilate and constrict to accommodate blood pressure and flow. Its inner and outer boundaries consist of elastic fibers, or *elastin*, and are called *internal and external elastic laminae*, or membranes. Small arterioles called the *vasa vasorum* perfuse the media. The outer layer of the artery is the *adventitia*, connective tissue containing nerve fibers and the vasa vasorum.

Arterial pulses are palpable in arteries lying close to the body surface. In the arms, note pulsations in:

- The *brachial artery* at the bend of the elbow just medial to the biceps tendon

- The *radial artery* on the lateral flexor surface

- The *ulnar artery* on the medial flexor surface, although overlying tissues may obscure the ulnar artery

Two vascular arches within the hand interconnect the radial and ulnar arteries, doubly protecting circulation to the hand and fingers against possible arterial occlusion.

Arteries must respond to the variations in cardiac output during systole and diastole. Their anatomy and size vary according to their distance from the heart. The aorta and its immediate branches are *large or highly elastic arteries* such as the common carotid and iliac arteries. These arteries course into *medium-sized or muscular arteries* such as the coronary and

An *atheroma* begins in the intima as lipid-filled foam cells and then becomes fatty streaks. *Complex atheromas* are thickened asymmetric plaques that narrow the lumen, reducing blood flow, and weaken the underlying media. They have a soft lipid core and a fibrous cap of smooth muscle cells and a collagen-rich matrix. Plaque rupture may precede thrombosis.[8,9]

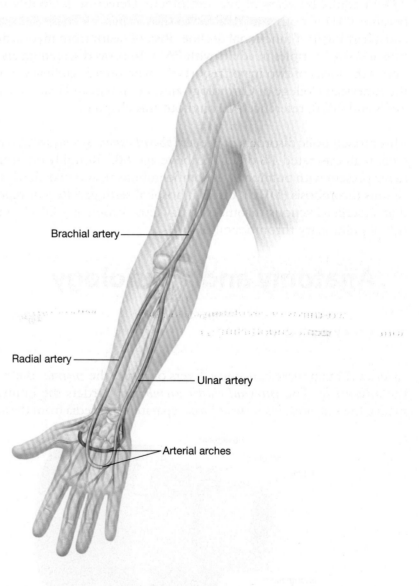

Brachial artery

Radial artery

Ulnar artery

Arterial arches

renal arteries. The elastic recoil and smooth muscle contraction and relaxation in the media of large and medium-sized arteries produce arterial pulsatile flow. Medium-sized arteries divide into *small arteries* less than 2 mm in diameter and even smaller *arterioles* with diameters from 20 to 100 micrometers. Resistance to blood flow occurs primarily in the arterioles. Recall that resistance is inversely proportional to the fourth power of the vessel diameter, known as the law of LaPlace. From the arterioles, blood flows into the vast network of *capillaries*, each the diameter of a single red blood cell, only 7 to 8 microns (μm) across. Capillaries have an endothelial cell lining but no media, facilitating rapid diffusion of oxygen and carbon dioxide.

In the legs, locate pulsations in:

- The *femoral artery* just below the inguinal ligament, midway between the anterior superior iliac spine and the symphysis pubis

- The *popliteal artery*, an extension of the femoral artery that passes medially behind the femur, palpable just behind the knee. The popliteal artery divides into the two arteries perfusing the lower leg and foot, listed below

- The *dorsalis pedis artery* on the dorsum of the foot just lateral to the extensor tendon of the big toe

- The *posterior tibial artery* behind the medial malleolus of the ankle. An interconnecting arch between its two chief arterial branches protects circulation to the foot.

VEINS

Unlike arteries, veins are thin-walled and highly distensible, with a capacity for up to two-thirds of circulating blood flow. The *venous intima* consists of nonthrombogenic endothelium. Protruding into the lumen are valves that promote unidirectional venous return to the heart. The *media* contains circumferential rings of elastic tissue and smooth muscle that change vein caliber in response to even minor changes in venous pressure.[8,10]

Veins from the arms, upper trunk, and head and neck drain into the *superior vena cava*, which empties into the right atrium. Veins from the legs and lower trunk drain upward into the *inferior vena cava*. Because of their weaker wall structure, the leg veins are susceptible to irregular dilatation, compression, ulceration, and invasion by tumors, and warrant special attention.

Deep and Superficial Venous System (Legs). The *deep veins* of the legs carry approximately 90% of venous return from the lower extremities. They are well supported by surrounding tissues.

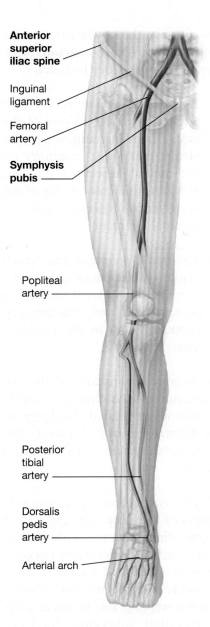

Anterior superior iliac spine

Inguinal ligament

Femoral artery

Symphysis pubis

Popliteal artery

Posterior tibial artery

Dorsalis pedis artery

Arterial arch

In contrast, the *superficial veins* are subcutaneous, with relatively poor tissue support. They include:

- The *great saphenous vein*, which originates on the dorsum of the foot, passes just anterior to the medial malleolus, continues up the medial aspect of the leg, and joins the femoral vein of the deep venous system below the inguinal ligament

- The *small saphenous vein*, which begins on the lateral side of the foot, passes upward along the posterior calf, and joins the deep venous system in the popliteal fossa

Anastomotic veins connect the two saphenous veins that are readily visible when dilated. Bridging or *perforating veins* connect the superficial system with the deep system.

When competent, the one-way valves of the deep, superficial, and perforating veins propel blood toward the heart, preventing pooling, venous stasis, and backward flow. Contraction of the calf muscles during walking also serves as a venous pump, squeezing blood upward against gravity.

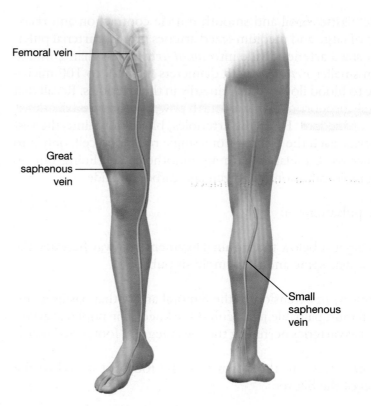

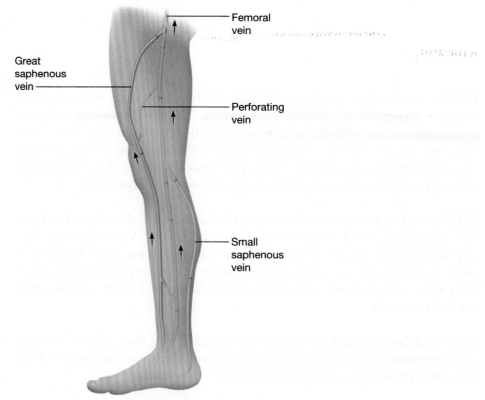

THE LYMPHATIC SYSTEM AND LYMPH NODES

The lymphatic system is an extensive vascular network that drains lymph fluid from body tissues and returns it to the venous circulation. The system starts peripherally as blind lymphatic capillaries, continues centrally as thin vascular channels, then as collecting ducts, and empties into the major veins at the neck. Lymph fluid transported through these channels is filtered through lymph nodes interposed along the way.

Lymph nodes are round, oval, or bean-shaped structures that vary in size according to their location. Some lymph nodes, such as the preauricular nodes, if palpable at all, are typically very small. The inguinal nodes, by contrast, are relatively larger—often 1 cm in diameter and occasionally even 2 cm in an adult.

In addition to its vascular functions, the lymphatic system plays an important role in the body's immune system. Cells within the lymph nodes engulf cellular debris and bacteria and produce antibodies.

Only the superficial lymph nodes are accessible to physical examination. These include the cervical nodes (p. 249), the axillary nodes (p. 407), and nodes in the arms and legs.

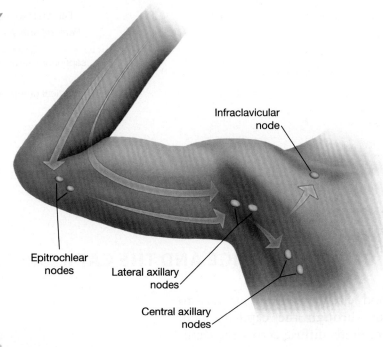

Recall that the axillary lymph nodes drain most of the arm. Lymphatics from the ulnar surface of the forearm and hand, the little and ring fingers, and the adjacent surface of the middle finger, however, drain first into the *epitrochlear nodes*. These are located on the medial surface of the arm approximately 3 cm above the elbow. Lymphatics from the rest of the arm drain mostly into the axillary nodes. A few may go directly to the infraclavicular nodes.

The lymphatics of the lower limb, following the venous supply, consist of both deep and superficial systems. Only the superficial nodes are palpable. The *superficial inguinal nodes* include two groups. The *horizontal group* lies in a chain high in the anterior thigh below the inguinal ligament. It drains the superficial portions of the lower abdomen and buttock, the external genitalia (but not the testes), the anal canal and perianal area, and the lower vagina.

The *vertical group* clusters near the upper part of the saphenous vein and drains a corresponding region of the leg. By contrast, lymphatics from the portion of leg drained by the small saphenous vein (the heel and outer aspect of the foot) join the deep system at the level of the popliteal space. Lesions in this space are not usually associated with palpable inguinal lymph nodes.

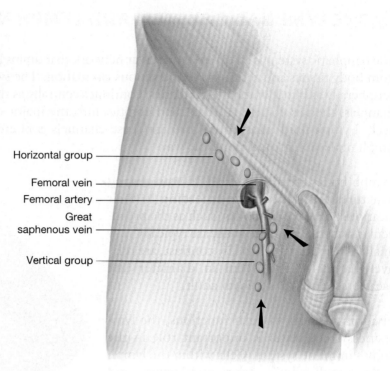

Horizontal group

Femoral vein

Femoral artery

Great saphenous vein

Vertical group

FLUID EXCHANGE AND THE CAPILLARY BED

Blood circulates from arteries to veins through the capillary bed. Here fluids diffuse across the capillary membrane, maintaining a dynamic equilibrium between the vascular and interstitial spaces. Blood pressure (*hydrostatic pressure*) within the capillary bed, especially near the arteriolar end, forces fluid out into the tissue spaces. This movement is aided by the relatively weak osmotic attraction of proteins within the tissues (*interstitial colloid oncotic pressure*) and is opposed by the hydrostatic pressure of the tissues.

As blood continues through the capillary bed toward the venous end, its hydrostatic pressure falls, and another force gains dominance. This is the *colloid oncotic pressure of plasma proteins*, which pulls fluid back into the vascular tree. Net flow of fluid, which was directed outward on the

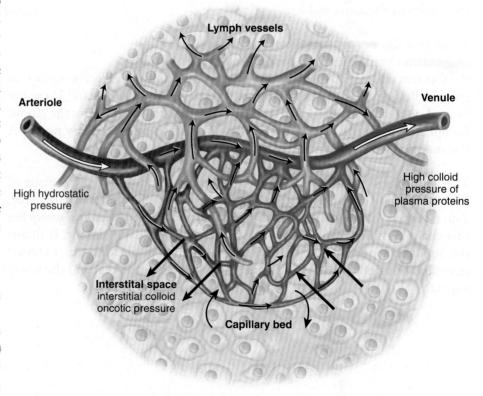

Lymph vessels

Arteriole

Venule

High hydrostatic pressure

High colloid pressure of plasma proteins

Interstital space interstitial colloid oncotic pressure

Capillary bed

arteriolar side of the capillary bed, reverses and turns inward on the venous side. Lymphatic capillaries, which also play an important role in this equilibrium, remove excessive fluid, including protein, from the interstitial space.

Lymphatic dysfunction or disturbances in hydrostatic or osmotic forces can all disrupt this equilibrium, resulting in an accumulation of interstitial fluid termed edema. See Table 12-1, Some Peripheral Causes of Edema, p. 513.

The Health History

Common or Concerning Symptoms

▶ Abdominal, flank, or back pain
▶ Pain in the arms or legs
▶ Intermittent claudication
▶ Cold, numbness, pallor in the legs; hair loss
▶ Swelling in calves, legs, or feet
▶ Color change in fingertips or toes in cold weather
▶ Swelling with redness or tenderness

As defined in the 2005 guidelines from the American College of Cardiology and the American Heart Association, *peripheral arterial disease* (PAD) refers to stenotic, occlusive, and aneurysmal disease of the aorta, its visceral arterial branches, and the arteries of the lower extremities, exclusive of the coronary arteries.[4] Be aware that pain in the extremities may arise from the skin, peripheral vascular system, musculoskeletal system, or nervous system. It also may be referred, like the pain of myocardial infarction that radiates to the left arm.

See Table 12-2, Painful Peripheral Vascular Disorders and Their Mimics, pp. 514–515.

Ask about abdominal, flank, or back pain, especially in older smokers. Is there unusual constipation or distention? Check for urinary retention, difficulty voiding, or renal colic.

An expanding hematoma from abdominal aortic aneurysm (AAA) may cause symptoms by compressing the bowel, aortic branch arteries, or the ureters.[11]

Ask about any pain or cramping in the legs during exertion that is relieved by rest within 10 minutes, termed *intermittent claudication*.

Symptomatic limb ischemia with exertion is present in *atherosclerotic PAD*. Pain with walking or prolonged standing, radiating from the spinal area into the buttocks, thighs, lower legs, or feet, is present in *neurogenic claudication*, with a likelihood ratio (LR) of 7.4 for *spinal stenosis* if the pain is relieved by sitting and a LR over 6 if the pain is relieved by bending forward or if bilateral buttock or leg pain is present.[12]

Ask also about *coldness, numbness,* or *pallor* in the legs or *feet* or *loss of hair* over the anterior tibial surfaces.

Hair loss over the anterior tibiae occurs with decreased arterial perfusion. "Dry" or brown–black ulcers from *gangrene* may ensue.

Because most patients with PAD report minimal symptoms, ask specifically about the PAD warning signs that follow, particularly in patients 50 years or older and those with risk factors, especially smoking, but also diabetes, hypertension, elevated cholesterol, African-American ethnicity or coronary artery disease (see pp. 352–353). When symptoms or risk factors described below are present, careful examination and testing of the ankle–brachial index are warranted (see also p. 516).

Only 10% to 30% of patients have the classic triad of leg pain with exertion that stops with rest.[13,14] The low symptom rate may reflect functional declines in walking, even though PAD is present or progressing.[15]

Peripheral Arterial Disease "Warning Signs"

▶ Fatigue, aching, numbness, or pain that limits walking or exertion in the legs; if present, identify the location. Ask also about erectile dysfunction.

▶ Any poorly healing or nonhealing wounds of the legs or feet

▶ Any pain present when at rest in the lower leg or foot and changes when standing or supine

▶ Abdominal pain after meals and associated "food fear" and weight loss

▶ Any first-degree relatives with an abdominal aortic aneurysm

Symptom location suggests the site of arterial ischemia:
• buttock, hip: *aortoiliac*
• erectile dysfunction: *iliac–pudendal*
• thigh: *common femoral* or *aortoiliac*
• upper calf: *superficial femoral*
• lower calf: *popliteal*
• foot: *tibial* or *peroneal*

Abdominal pain, "food fear," and weight loss suggest intestinal ischemia of the *celiac* or *superior* or *inferior mesenteric arteries.*

Prevalence of abdominal aortic aneurysms in first-degree relatives is 15% to 28%.[4]

Health Promotion and Counseling: Evidence and Recommendations

Important Topics for Health Promotion and Counseling

▶ Screening for peripheral arterial disease; the ankle–brachial index (ABI)
▶ Screening for renal artery disease
▶ Screening for abdominal aortic aneurysm

Screening for Peripheral Arterial Disease: The Ankle–Brachial Index.
PAD is a common manifestation of atherosclerosis, affecting from 12% to 29% of community populations.[13,16] Prevalence increases with age and the presence

of cardiovascular risk factors. PAD and cardiovascular disease co-occur in 16% of patients.[13] Despite widespread prevalence, PAD is commonly missed in office practices.[13,17] Although the U.S. Preventive Services Task Force does not advocate screening, the American College of Cardiology/American Heart Association guidelines support "case-finding" in those at risk, as detailed below.

Risk Factors for Lower-Extremity Peripheral Arterial Disease

▶ Age 50 years, or younger if diabetes or atherosclerosis risk factor of smoking, dyslipidemia, hypertension, or hyperhomocysteinemia
▶ Age 50 to 69 years and history of smoking or diabetes
▶ Age 70 years or older
▶ Leg symptoms with exertion or ischemic rest pain
▶ Abnormal lower extremity pulses
▶ Known atherosclerotic coronary, carotid, or renal artery disease

Source: Hirsch AT, Haskal ZJ, Hertzer NR, et al. ACC/AHA 2005 guidelines for the management of patients with peripheral arterial disease. J Am Coll Cardiol 2005;47:1239–1312.

Learn to assess PAD by using the ankle–brachial index (ABI). The ABI is reliable, reproducible, and easy to perform in the office, with a sensitivity and specificity of 95% and 99%, respectively.[14] Clinicians or office staff can easily measure systolic blood pressure in the arms and in the pedal pulses, using Doppler ultrasound. These values can be entered into calculators available at selected Web sites (see American College of Physicians, at http://cpsc.acponline.org/enhancements/232abiCalc.html).

See Table 12-3, Using the Ankle–Brachial Index, p. 516.

For patients with PAD and claudication, the 2010 guidelines of the American College of Cardiology and the American Heart Association strongly recommend *supervised exercise*, shown by numerous studies to be highly effective in increasing walking capability.[1,18,19] Even though calf muscles are weaker in patients with PAD, supervised treadmill exercise is superior to lower extremity resistance training for improving 6-minute walk performance.[20–22] Gait speed is emerging as a predictor of survival in older adults.[23] Patients with ABIs in the lowest categories have a 20% to 25% annual mortality risk.[13] Those with higher daily physical activity lower both their risk of mortality and of cardiovascular events.[24]

Other interventions that reduce onset and progression of PAD include tobacco cessation, treatment of hyperlipidemia, optimal control of diabetes and hypertension, use of antiplatelet agents, meticulous foot care and well-fitting shoes, and if needed, surgical revascularization.

Screening for Renal Artery Disease. Atherosclerotic renal artery disease affects 7% of adults 65 years or older, increasing to 22% to 55% of those with PAD and 30% of those with documented coronary disease.[4,25] Fibromuscular dysplasia also causes stenotic lesions, usually in women under age 40, but is less common.[26] The American College of Cardiology and the

American Heart Association recommend diagnostic studies for renal artery disease, usually beginning with Doppler measurement of renal artery velocity, for patients with the conditions below.

Conditions Suspicious for Renal Artery Disease

▶ Hypertension if age ≤30 years
▶ Severe hypertension if age ≥55 years
▶ Accelerated, resistant, or malignant hypertension
▶ New worsening of renal function or worsening after use of an angiotensin-converting enzyme inhibitor or an angiotensin-receptor blocking agent
▶ An unexplained small kidney
▶ Sudden unexplained pulmonary edema, especially in the setting of worsening renal function

See Chapter 9, p. 354, for guidelines for assessing blood pressure. The frequency of hypertension arising from renal artery stenosis is unknown.

Screening for Abdominal Aortic Aneurysm (AAA). Early detection of AAA, the leading cause of sudden death, is critical for survival.[11,27] AAA is defined as an infrarenal aortic diameter ≥3 cm, and is found in over 50% of older male smokers. Rupture and mortality increases dramatically when the aortic diameter exceeds 5.5 cm. Risk factors are smoking, age 65 years or older, family history, coronary artery disease, PAD, hypertension, and hyperlipidemia. Because symptoms are uncommon and screening reduces mortality by 40%, the U.S. Preventive Services Task Force recommends one-time screening by ultrasound in men between the ages of 65 and 75 years with a history of having ever smoked, defined as smoking more than 100 cigarettes in a lifetime.[28] Ultrasound is 95% sensitive and 100% specific for diagnosis of AAA. Palpation is also useful when the aortic diameter reaches ≥4 cm.[11] Due to lower prevalence, data on the benefits of screening nonsmokers and women are inconclusive.

Techniques of Examination

Important Areas of Examination

The Arms	The Abdomen	The Legs
▶ Size, symmetry, skin color	▶ Aortic width	▶ Size, symmetry, skin color
▶ Radial pulse, brachial pulse	▶ Pulsatile mass	▶ Femoral pulse and inguinal lymph nodes
▶ Epitrochlear lymph nodes		▶ Popliteal, dorsalis pedis, and posterior tibial pulses
		▶ Peripheral edema

The American College of Cardiology and the American Heart Association have urged clinicians to intensify their focus when examining the peripheral vascular system.[4] Recall that peripheral arterial disease is often asymptomatic and underdiagnosed, leading to significant morbidity and mortality. As you learn and practice the techniques of the vascular examination, observe the 2005 recommendations for examining the peripheral arterial system. Review the techniques for assessing blood pressure, the carotid artery, the aorta, and the renal and femoral arteries on the pages indicated below.

Summary: Key Components of the Peripheral Arterial Examination

▶ Measure blood pressure in both arms (see Chapter 4, pp. 121–123).
▶ Palpate carotid upstroke, auscultate for bruits (see Chapter 9, pp. 367–368).
▶ Auscultate for aortic, renal, and femoral bruits; palpate aorta and determine maximal diameter (see Chapter 11, pp. 454–455, 465).
▶ Palpate brachial, radial, ulnar, femoral, popliteal, dorsalis pedis, and posterior arteries.
▶ Inspect ankles and feet for color, temperature, skin integrity; note any ulcerations; check for hair loss, trophic skin changes, hypertrophic nails.

Source: Hirsch AT, Haskal ZJ, Hertzer NR, et al. ACC/AHA 2005 guidelines for the management of patients with peripheral arterial disease. J Am Coll Cardiol 2005;47:1239–1312.

Asymmetric blood pressures as seen in *coarctation of the aorta* and *dissecting aortic aneurysm*.

ARMS

Inspect both arms from the fingertips to the shoulders. Note:

● Their size, symmetry, and any swelling

Lymphedema of the arm and hand may follow axillary node dissection and radiation therapy.

● The venous pattern

Prominent veins in an edematous arm suggest venous obstruction.

● The color of the skin and nail beds and the texture of the skin

Palpate the radial pulse with the pads of your fingers on the flexor surface of the wrist laterally. Partially flexing the patient's wrist may help you feel this pulse. Compare the pulses in both arms.

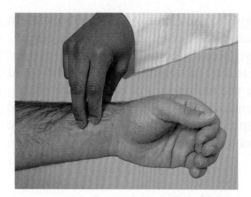

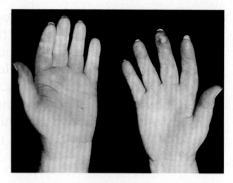

In *Raynaud's disease*, wrist pulses are typically normal, but spasm of more distal arteries causes episodes of sharply demarcated pallor of the fingers (see Table 12-2, Painful Peripheral Vascular Disorders and Their Mimics, pp. 514–515).

There are several systems for grading the amplitude of the arterial pulses. One system uses a scale of 0 to 3, as below.[4] Use the scale adopted by your institution.

Note that if an artery is widely dilated, it is *aneurysmal*.

Recommended Grading of Pulses

3+	Bounding
2+	Brisk, expected (normal)
1+	Diminished, weaker than expected
0	Absent, unable to palpate

Bounding carotid, radial, and femoral pulses are present in *aortic insufficiency*; asymmetric diminished pulses occur in *arterial occlusion* from atherosclerosis or embolism.

If you suspect arterial insufficiency, feel for the *brachial pulse*. Flex the patient's elbow slightly, and palpate the artery just medial to the biceps tendon at the antecubital crease. The brachial artery can also be felt higher in the arm in the groove between the biceps and triceps muscles.

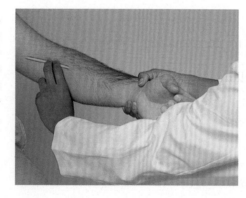

Feel for one or more *epitrochlear nodes*. With the patient's elbow flexed to about 90 degrees and the forearm supported by your hand, reach around behind the arm and feel in the groove between the biceps and triceps muscles, about 3 cm above the medial epicondyle. If a node is present, note its size, consistency, and tenderness.

Epitrochlear nodes are difficult or impossible to identify in most normally healthy people.

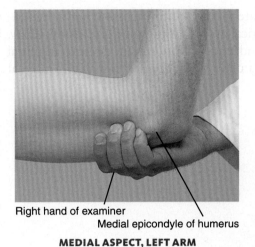

Right hand of examiner

Medial epicondyle of humerus

MEDIAL ASPECT, LEFT ARM

An enlarged epitrochlear node may arise from local or distal infection, or may be associated with generalized lymphadenopathy.

ABDOMEN

For techniques of examination of the abdominal aorta, see Chapter 11, Abdomen, pp. 454–455, 465. In brief, listen for aortic, renal, and femoral bruits. Palpate and estimate the width of the abdominal aorta in the epigastric area by measuring the aortic width between two fingers, especially in older adults due to higher risk of AAA. Assess for a pulsatile mass.

The sensitivity of aortic palpation for AAA ≥4 cm is 60%. Sensitivity for a pulsatile mass, detected in only 50% of diagnosed ruptures, is 40% to 60%. Note that an inguinal mass suspicious for an incarcerated hernia is often diagnosed as AAA at surgery.[11]

 LEGS

The patient should be lying down and draped so that the external genitalia are covered and the legs fully exposed. A good examination is impossible through stockings or socks.

Inspection.   Examine both legs from the groin and buttocks to the feet. Note:

● Their size, symmetry, and any swelling

● The venous pattern and any venous enlargement

● Any pigmentation, rashes, scars, or ulcers

● The color and texture of the skin, the color of the nail beds, and the distribution of hair on the lower legs, feet, and toes

See Table 12-4, Chronic Insufficiency of Arteries and Veins, p. 517.

See Table 12-5, Common Ulcers of the Ankles and Feet, p. 518.

Warmth and redness over calf signal cellulitis.

The Inguinal Lymph Nodes. Palpate the *superficial inguinal nodes*, including both the horizontal and the vertical groups. Note their size, consistency, and discreteness, and note any tenderness. Nontender, discrete inguinal nodes up to 1 cm or even 2 cm in diameter are frequently palpable in normal people.

Lymphadenopathy refers to enlargement of the nodes, with or without tenderness. Distinguish between local and generalized lymphadenopathy, respectively, by finding either a causative lesion in the drainage area, or enlarged nodes in at least two other noncontiguous lymph node regions.

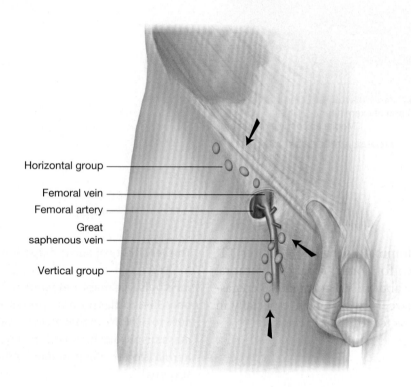

Horizontal group

Femoral vein

Femoral artery

Great saphenous vein

Vertical group

The Peripheral Arteries. *Palpate the pulses* to assess the arterial circulation.

- *The femoral pulse.* Press deeply, below the inguinal ligament and about midway between the anterior superior iliac spine and the symphysis pubis. As in deep abdominal palpation, the use of two hands, one on top of the other, may be helpful, especially in obese patients.

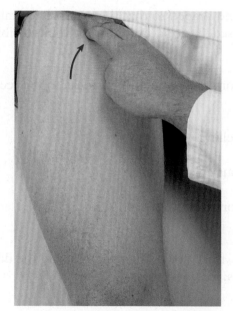

A diminished or absent pulse makes partial or complete proximal occlusion 10 times more likely.[29] If the occlusion is at the aortic or iliac level, all pulses distal to the occlusion are typically affected. Chronic arterial occlusion, usually from atherosclerosis, causes *intermittent claudication*, p. 514, postural color changes, and trophic changes in the skin, pp. 508–509.

An exaggerated, widened femoral pulse suggests a *femoral aneurysm*, a pathologic dilatation of the artery.

- *The popliteal pulse.* The patient's knee should be somewhat flexed, with the leg relaxed. Place the fingertips of both hands so that they just meet in the midline behind the knee and press them deeply into the popliteal fossa. The popliteal pulse is often more difficult to find than other pulses. It is deeper and feels more diffuse.

An exaggerated, widened popliteal pulse suggests an aneurysm of the popliteal artery. Popliteal and femoral aneurysms are not common. They are usually caused by atherosclerosis and occur primarily in men older than 50 years.

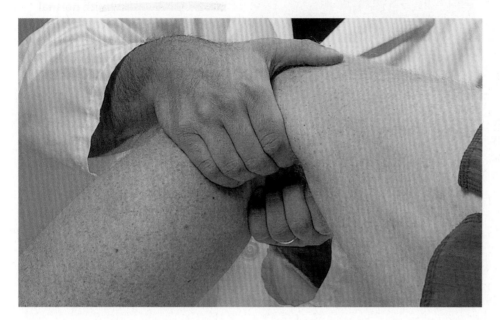

If you cannot feel the popliteal pulse with this approach, try with the patient prone. Flex the patient's knee to about 90 degrees, let the lower leg relax against your shoulder or upper arm, and press your two thumbs deeply into the popliteal fossa.

Atherosclerosis (arteriosclerosis obliterans) most commonly obstructs arterial circulation in the thigh. The femoral pulse is normal, the popliteal decreased or absent.

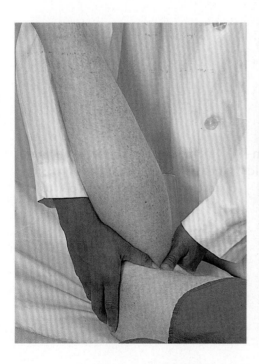

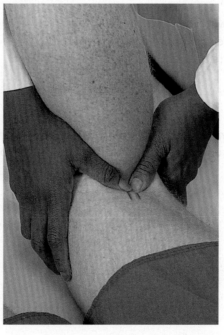

- *The dorsalis pedis pulse.* Feel the dorsum of the foot (not the ankle) just lateral to the extensor tendon of the great toe. If you cannot feel a pulse, explore the dorsum of the foot more laterally.

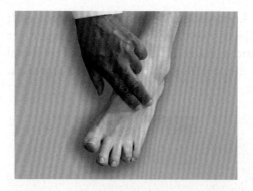

The dorsalis pedis artery may be congenitally absent or may branch higher in the ankle. Search for a pulse more laterally.

Absent pedal pulses with normal femoral and popliteal pulses make atherosclerotic disease in the lower popliteal artery or its branches 14 times more likely, seen in *diabetes mellitus*.[29]

- *The posterior tibial pulse.* Curve your fingers behind and slightly below the medial malleolus of the ankle. This pulse may be hard to feel in a fat or edematous ankle.

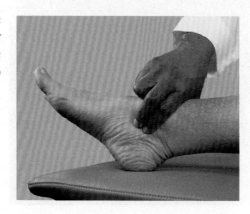

Sudden arterial occlusion from embolism or thrombosis causes pain and numbness or tingling. The limb distal to the occlusion becomes cold, pale, and pulseless. Emergency treatment is required.

Tips for Palpating Difficult Pulses

1. Position your body and examining hand comfortably; awkward positions decrease your tactile sensitivity.
2. Place your hand properly and linger there, varying the pressure of your fingers to pick up a weak pulsation. If unsuccessful, explore the area deliberately.
3. Do not confuse the patient's pulse with your own pulsating fingertips. If you are unsure, count your own heart rate and compare it with the patient's. The rates are usually different. Your carotid pulse is convenient for this comparison.

Note the temperature of the feet and legs with the backs of your fingers. Compare one side with the other. Bilateral coldness is most often caused by a cold environment or anxiety.

Coldness, especially when unilateral or associated with other signs, suggests inadequate arterial perfusion.

The Peripheral Veins. *Look for edema.* Compare one foot and leg with the other, noting their relative size and the prominence of veins, tendons, and bones.

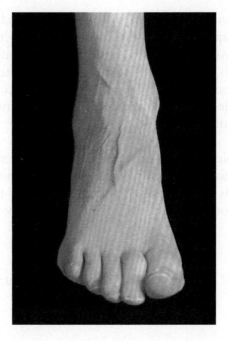

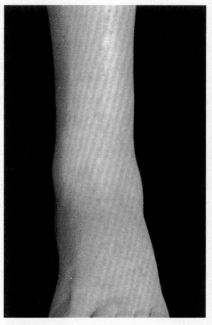

Edema causes swelling that may obscure the veins, tendons, and bony prominences.

Check for pitting edema. Press firmly but gently with your thumb for at least 2 seconds (1) over the dorsum of each foot, (2) behind each medial malleolus, and (3) over the shins. Look for *pitting*—a depression caused by pressure from your thumb. Normally there is none. The severity of edema is graded on a four-point scale, from slight to very marked.

See Table 12-1, Some Peripheral Causes of Edema, p. 513.

Shown below is 3+ pitting edema.

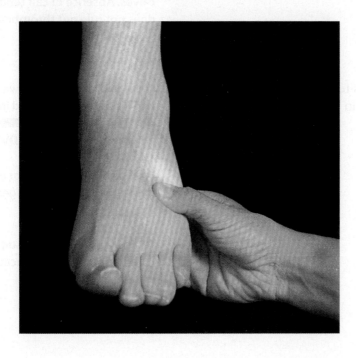

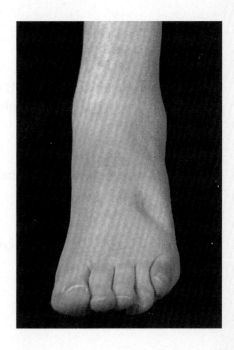

If you detect unilateral edema, *measure the legs* to identify the edema and to follow its course. With a flexible tape, measure (1) the forefoot, (2) the smallest possible circumference above the ankle, (3) the largest circumference at the calf, and (4) the midthigh, a measured distance above the patella with the knee extended. Compare one side with the other. A difference of more than 1 cm just above the ankle or 2 cm at the calf is unusual in normally healthy people and suggests edema.

Calf asymmetry increases the likelihood of DVT. Also consider muscle tear or trauma, Baker's cyst (posterior knee) and muscular atrophy.

If edema is present, look for possible causes in the peripheral vascular system. These include recent deep venous thrombosis, chronic venous insufficiency from previous deep venous thrombosis or incompetence of the venous valves, and lymphedema. Note the extent of the swelling. How far up the leg does it go?

In DVT, the location of edema suggests the location of the occlusion: the popliteal vein when the lower leg or the ankle is swollen; the iliofemoral veins when the entire leg is swollen.

Is the swelling unilateral or bilateral? Are the veins unusually prominent?

Venous distention suggests a venous cause of edema. Bilateral edema is present in *heart failure, cirrhosis, and nephrotic syndrome*.

Try to identify any venous tenderness that may accompany deep venous thrombosis. Palpate the groin just medial to the femoral pulse for tenderness of the femoral vein. Next, with the patient's leg flexed at the knee and relaxed, palpate the calf. With your fingerpads, gently compress the calf muscles against the tibia, and search for any tenderness or cords. DVT, however, may have no demonstrable signs, and diagnosis often depends on clinical suspicion and other testing.

A painful, pale swollen leg, together with tenderness in the groin over the femoral vein, suggests deep *iliofemoral thrombosis*. Risk of pulmonary embolism in proximal vein thrombosis is 50%.[5] Only half of patients with DVT in the calf have tenderness and cords deep in the calves. Absence of calf tenderness does not rule out thrombosis.

Note the *color of the skin*.

- Is there a local area of redness? If so, note its temperature, and gently try to feel the firm cord of a thrombosed vein in the area. The calf is most often involved.

Local swelling, redness, warmth, and a subcutaneous cord in *superficial thrombophlebitis* is an emerging risk factor for DVT.[7]

- Are there brownish areas near the ankles?

Brownish discoloration or ulcers just above the malleolus suggest *chronic venous insufficiency*.

- Note any ulcers in the skin. Where are they?

Thickened brawny skin suggests lymphedema and advanced venous insufficiency.

Ask the patient to stand, and *inspect the saphenous system for varicosities*. The standing posture allows any varicosities to fill with blood and makes them visible. You can easily miss them when the patient is in a supine position. Feel for any varicosities, noting any signs of thrombophlebitis.

Varicose veins are dilated and tortuous. Their walls may feel somewhat thickened. Many varicose veins can be seen in the leg on p. 509.

SPECIAL TECHNIQUES

Evaluating the Arterial Supply to the Hand. If you suspect arterial insufficiency in the arm or hand, try to feel the *ulnar pulse* as well as the radial and brachial pulses. Feel for it deeply on the flexor surface of the wrist medially. Partially flexing the patient's wrist may help you. The pulse of a normal ulnar artery, however, may not be palpable.

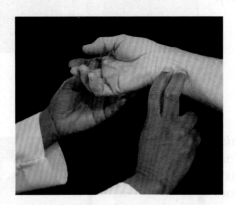

Arterial occlusive disease is much less common in the arms than in the legs. Absent or diminished pulses at the wrist are found in acute embolic occlusion and in *Buerger's disease,* or *thromboangiitis obliterans.*

The *Allen test* gives further information. This test is also useful to ensure the patency of the ulnar artery before puncturing the radial artery for blood samples. The patient should rest with hands in lap, palms up.

Ask the patient to make a tight fist with one hand; then compress both radial and ulnar arteries firmly between your thumbs and fingers.

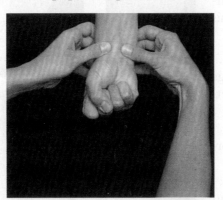

Next, ask the patient to open the hand into a relaxed, slightly flexed position. The palm is pale.

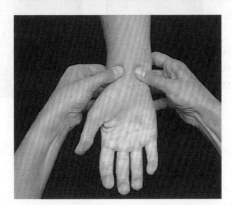

Extending the hand fully may cause pallor and a falsely positive test.

Release your pressure over the ulnar artery. If the ulnar artery is patent, the palm flushes within about 3 to 5 seconds.

Patency of the radial artery may be tested by releasing the radial artery while still compressing the ulnar artery.

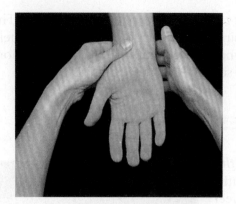
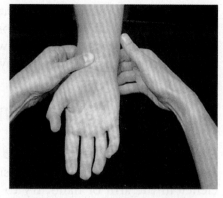

Persisting pallor indicates occlusion of the ulnar artery or its distal branches.

Marked pallor on elevation suggests *arterial insufficiency*.

Postural Color Changes of Chronic Arterial Insufficiency. If pain or diminished pulses suggest arterial insufficiency, look for postural color changes. Raise both legs to about 60 degrees until maximal pallor of the feet develops, usually within a minute. In light-skinned persons, either maintenance of normal color, as seen in this right foot, or slight pallor is normal.

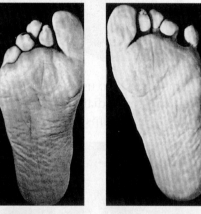

Then ask the patient to sit up with legs dangling down. Compare both feet, noting the time required for:

- Return of pinkness to the skin, normally about 10 seconds or less

- Filling of the veins of the feet and ankles, normally about 15 seconds

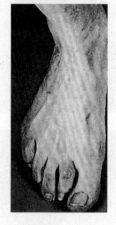
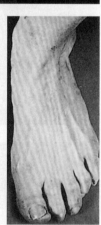

This right foot has normal color and the veins on the foot have filled. These normal responses suggest an adequate circulation.

The left foot is still pale, and the veins are just starting to fill, signs of arterial insufficiency.

Source of foot photos: Kappert A, Winsor T. Diagnosis of Peripheral Vascular Disease. Philadelphia: FA Davis, 1972.

Look for any unusual *rubor* (dusky redness) to replace the pallor of the dependent foot. Rubor may take a minute or more to appear.

Normal responses accompanied by diminished arterial pulses suggest that good collateral circulation has developed around an arterial occlusion.

Color changes may be difficult to see in darker-skinned persons. Inspect the soles of the feet for these changes, and use tangential lighting to see the veins.

Persisting rubor on dependency suggests arterial insufficiency (see p. 518). When veins are incompetent, dependent rubor and the timing of color return and venous filling are not reliable tests of arterial insufficiency.

Mapping Varicose Veins. Mapping can show which veins are insufficient, and their origin. You can map out the course and connections of varicose veins by transmitting pressure waves along the blood-filled veins. With the patient standing, place your palpating fingers gently on a vein and, with your other hand below it, compress the vein sharply. Feel for a pressure wave transmitted to the fingers of your upper hand. A palpable pressure wave indicates that the two parts of the vein are connected.

A wave may also be transmitted downward, but not as easily.

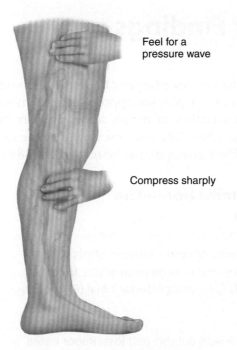

Feel for a pressure wave

Compress sharply

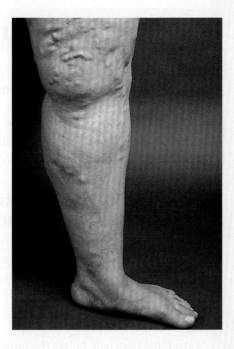

Evaluating the Competency of Venous Valves. By the *retrograde filling (Trendelenburg) test*, you can assess the valvular competency in both the communicating veins and the saphenous system. Start with the patient supine. Elevate one leg to about 90 degrees to empty it of venous blood.

Next, occlude the great saphenous vein in the upper thigh by manual compression, using enough pressure to occlude this vein but not the deeper vessels. Ask the patient to stand. While you keep the vein occluded, watch for venous filling in the leg. Normally the saphenous vein fills from below, taking about 35 seconds as blood flows through the capillary bed into the venous system.

Rapid filling of the superficial veins while the saphenous vein is occluded indicates incompetent valves in the communicating veins. Blood flows quickly in a retrograde direction from the deep to the saphenous system.

After the patient stands for 20 seconds, release the compression and look for sudden additional venous filling. Normally there is none; competent valves in the saphenous vein block retrograde flow. Slow venous filling continues.

Sudden additional filling of superficial veins after release of compression indicates incompetent valves in the saphenous vein.

When both steps of this test are normal, the response is termed negative–negative. Negative–positive and positive–negative responses may also occur.

When both steps are abnormal, the test is positive–positive.

Recording Your Findings

Note that initially you may use sentences to describe your findings; later you will use phrases. The style below contains phrases appropriate for most write-ups. Recall that the written description of lymph nodes appears in Chapter 7, The Head and Neck (see p. 256). Likewise, assessment of the carotid pulse is recorded in Chapter 9, The Cardiovascular System (see p. 385).

Recording the Physical Examination—The Peripheral Vascular System

"Extremities are warm and without edema. No varicosities or stasis changes. Calves are supple and nontender. No femoral or abdominal bruits. Brachial, radial, femoral, popliteal, dorsalis pedis (DP), and posterior tibial (PT) pulses are 2+ and symmetric."

OR

"Extremities are pale below the midcalf, with notable hair loss. Rubor noted when legs dependent but no edema or ulceration. Bilateral femoral bruits; no abdominal bruits heard. Brachial and radial pulses 2+; femoral, popliteal, DP and PT pulses 1+." (Alternatively, pulses can be recorded as below.)

Suggests atherosclerotic *peripheral arterial disease*

	Radial	Brachial	Femoral	Popliteal	Dorsalis Pedis	Posterior Tibial
RT	2+	2+	1+	1+	1+	1+
LT	2+	2+	1+	1+	1+	1+

Bibliography

Citations

1. Olin JW, Allie DE, Belkin M et al. ACCF/AHA/ACR/SCAI/SIR/SVM/SVN/SVS 2010 performance measures for adults with peripheral artery disease: a report of the American College of Cardiology Foundation/American Heart Association Task Force on performance measures, the American College of Radiology, the Society for Cardiac Angiography and Interventions, the Society for Interventional Radiology, the Society for Vascular Medicine, the Society for Vascular Nursing, and the Society for Vascular Surgery (Writing Committee to Develop Clinical Performance Measures for Peripheral Artery Disease). Circulation 2010;122:2583–2618.
2. Allison MA, Ho E, Denenberg JO, et al. Ethnic-specific prevalence of peripheral arterial disease in the United States. Am J Prev Med 2007;32:328–333.
3. Ostchega Y, Paulose-Ram R, Dillon CF et al. Prevalence of peripheral arterial disease and risk factors in persons aged 60 or older: data from the National Health and Nutrition Examination Survey 1999–2004. J am Geriatir Soc 2007;55:583–589.

4. Hirsch AT, Haskal ZJ, Hertzer NR et al. ACC/AHA 2005 Practice Guidelines for the management of patients with peripheral arterial disease (lower extremity, renal, mesenteric, and abdominal aortic): a collaborative report from the American Association for Vascular Surgery/Society for Vascular Surgery, Society for Cardiovascular Angiography and Interventions, Society for Vascular Medicine and Biology, Society of Interventional Radiology, and the ACC/AHA Task Force on Practice Guidelines (Writing Committee to Develop Guidelines for the Management of Patients With Peripheral Arterial Disease): endorsed by the American Association of Cardiovascular and Pulmonary Rehabilitation; National Heart, Lung, and Blood Institute; Society for Vascular Nursing; TransAtlantic Inter-Society Consensus; and Vascular Disease Foundation. J Am Coll Cardiol 2005;47:1239–1312.

5. Bates SM, Ginsberg JS. Treatment of deep-vein thrombosis. N Engl J Med 2004;351:268–277.

6. Goodacre S. In the clinic: Deep venous thrombosis. Ann Intern Med 2008;149:ITC3-1–ITC3-16.

7. Decousus H, Quere I, Presles E et al. Superficial venous thromboembolism and venous thromboembolism. A large, prospective epidemiologic study. Ann Intern Med 2010;152:218–244.

8. Schoen FJ. Blood vessels. In Kumar VK, Fausto N, Abbas AK (eds.) Robbins and Cotran Pathologic Basis of Disease, 8th ed. Philadelphia: Elsevier, 2010.

9. Hansson GK. Inflammation, atherosclerosis, and coronary artery disease. N Engl J Med 2005;351:1685–1698.

10. Lam FY, Griswold ME, Moneta GL. Venous and lymphatic disease. In Brunicardi C, Anderson DA, Billiard TR, et al (eds.). Schwartz's Principles of surgery, 9th ed. New York: McGraw Hill, 2010.

11. Lederle FA. In the clinic. Abdominal aortic aneurysm. Ann Intern Med 2009;150:ITC5-1–ITC5-16.

12. Suri P, Rainville J, Kalichman L et al. Does this older adult with lower extremity pain have the clinical syndrome of lumbar spinal stenosis? JAMA 2010;304:2628–2636.

13. Hirsch AT, Criqui MH, Treat-Jacobsen D et al. Peripheral arterial disease detection, awareness, and treatment in primary care. JAMA 2001;286:1317–1324.

14. McDermott MM, Greenland P, Liu K et al. The ankle-brachial index is associated with leg function and physical activity: the walking and leg circulation study. Ann Intern Med 2002;136:873–883.

15. McDermott MM, Liu K, Greenland P et al. Functional decline in peripheral arterial disease—associations with the ankle brachial index and leg symptoms. JAMA 2004;292:453–461.

16. Newman AB. Peripheral arterial disease: insights from population studies of older adults. J Am Geriatr Soc 2000;48:1157–1162.

17. Wilson J, Laine C, Goldman D. In the clinic: peripheral arterial disease. Ann Intern Med 2007;146:ITC3-1–ITC3-16.

18. Nicolaï SPA, Teijink JAW, Prins MH et al. Multicenter randomized clinical trial of supervised exercise therapy with or without feedback versus walking advice for intermittent claudication. J Vasc Surg 2010;52:348–355.

19. McDermott MM, Liu K, Ferrucci L et al. Physical performance in peripheral arterial disease: a slower rate of decline in patients who walk more. Ann Intern Med 2006;144:10–20.

20. McDermott MM, Guralnik JM, Ferruci L et al. Asymptomatic peripheral arterial disease is associated with more adverse lower extremity characteristics than intermittent claudication. Circulation 2008;117:2484–2491.

21. Koutakis P, Johanning JM, Haynatzki GR et al. Abnormal joint powers before and after the onset of claudication symptoms. J Vasc Surg 2010;52:340–347.

22. McDermott MM, Ades P, Guralnik JM et al. Treadmill exercise and resistance training in patients with peripheral arterial disease with and without intermittent claudication: a randomized controlled trial. JAMA 2009;301:165–174.

23. Studeski S, Perera S, Patel K et al. Gait speed and survival in older adults. JAMA 2011;305:50–58.

24. Garg PK, Tian L, Criqui MH et al. Physical activity during daily life and mortality in patients with peripheral arterial disease. Circulation 2006;1114:242–248.

25. Balk E, Raman G, Chung M et al. Effectiveness of management strategies for renal artery stenosis: a systematic review. Ann Intern Med 2006;146:901–912.

26. Dworkin LD, Cooper CJ. Renal-artery stenosis. N Engl J Med 2009;361:1972–1978.

27. Lederle FA, Simel DL. The rational clinical examination. Does this patient have abdominal aortic aneurysm? JAMA 1999;281:77–82.

28. U.S. Preventive Services Task Force. Screening for abdominal aortic aneurysm: recommendation statement. Ann Intern Med 2005;142:198–202.

29. McGee S. Part 10, Extremities, in Evidence Based Physical Diagnosis, 2nd ed. St Louis: Elsevier, 2007. pp. 597–622.

30. De Araujo T, Valencia J, Federman D et al. Managing the patient with venous ulcers. Ann Intern Med 2003;138:326–334.

Additional References

Aslam F, Haque A, Foody J, Lee LV. Peripheral arterial disease: current perspectives and new trends in management. South Med J 2009;102:1141–1149.

Boin F, Wigley FM. Understanding, assessing and treating Raynaud's phenomenon. Curr Opin Rheumatol 2005;17:752–760.

Boulton AJM, Kirsner RS, Vileikyte L. Neuropathic diabetic foot ulcers. N Engl J Med 2004;351:48–55.

Colman RW, Marder VJ, Clowes AW (eds). Hemostasis and Thrombosis: Basic Principles and Clinical Practice, 5th ed. Philadelphia: Lippincott Williams & Wilkins, 2006.

Creager M, Dzau VJ, Loscalzo J. Vascular Medicine: A Companion to Braunwald's Heart Disease. Philadelphia: Saunders Elsevier, 2006.

Hill J, Treasure T; National Clinical Guideline Centre for Acute and Chronic Conditions. Reducing the risk of venous thromboembolism in patients admitted to hospital: summary of NICE guidance. BMJ. 2010;Jan 27;340:c95.

Khan NA, Rahim Sa, Anand SS et al. Does the clinical examination predict lower extremity peripheral arterial disease? JAMA 2006; 295:536–546.

Klein LW. Atherosclerosis regression, vascular remodeling, and plaque stabilization. J Am Coll Cardiol 2007;49:271–273.

O'Rourke MF, Hashimoto J. Mechanical factors in arterial aging: a clinical perspective. J Am Coll Cardiol 2007;50:1–13.

Qaseem A, Snow V, Barry P et al. Current diagnosis of venous thromboembolism in primary care: a clinical practice guideline from the American Academy of Family Physicians and the American College of Physicians. Ann Intern Med 2007;146:454–458.

Warren AG, Brorson H, Borud LJ et al. Lymphedema: a comprehensive review. Ann Plast Surg 2007;59:464–472.

Wells PS, Owen C, Doucette S et al. Does this patient have deep vein thrombosis? JAMA 2006;295:199–207.

Wigley FM. Vascular disease in scleroderma. Clin Rev Allergy Immunol 2009;36:150–175.

The Bates' suite offers these additional resources to enhance learning and facilitate understanding of this chapter:

- *Bates' Pocket Guide to Physical Examination and History Taking,* 7th edition
- *Bates' Visual Guide to Physical Examination*
- thePoint online resources, for students and instructors: http://thepoint.lww.com

Table
12-1
Some Peripheral Causes of Edema

Approximately one-third of total body water is extracellular, or outside the body's cells. Approximately 25% of extracellular fluid is plasma; the remainder is interstitial fluid. At the arteriolar end of the capillaries, *hydrostatic pressure* in the blood vessels and *colloid oncotic pressure* in the interstitium cause fluid to move into the tissues; at the venous end of the capillaries and in the lymphatics, hydrostatic pressure in the interstitium and the colloid oncotic pressure of plasma proteins cause fluid to return to the vascular compartment. Several clinical conditions disrupt this balance, resulting in *edema*, or a clinically evident accumulation of interstitial fluid. Not depicted below is *capillary leak syndrome*, in which protein leaks into the interstitial space, seen in burns, angioedema, snake bites, and allergic reactions.

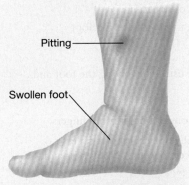

Pitting Edema

Edema is soft, bilateral, with pitting after 1 to 2 seconds of thumb pressure on the anterior tibiae and feet. There is no skin thickening, ulceration, or pigmentation. Pitting edema results from several conditions: when legs are dependent from prolonged standing or sitting, which leads to increased hydrostatic pressure in the veins and capillaries; heart failure leading to decreased cardiac output; nephrotic syndrome, cirrhosis, or malnutrition leading to low albumin and decreased intravascular colloid oncotic pressure; and selected medications. Pitting reflects the viscosity of the edema fluid, usually low in protein concentration.[29]

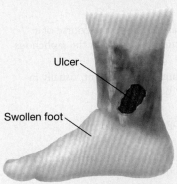

Chronic Venous Insufficiency

Edema is soft, with pitting on pressure, and occasionally bilateral. Look for brawny changes and skin thickening, especially near the ankle. Ulceration, brownish pigmentation, and edema in the feet are common. Arises from chronic obstruction and from incompetent valves in the deep venous system.

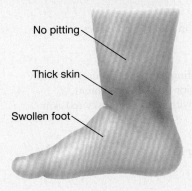

Lymphedema

Edema is soft in the early stages, then becomes indurated, hard, and nonpitting. Skin is markedly thickened; ulceration is rare. There is no pigmentation. Edema is found in the feet and toes, often bilaterally. Lymphedema develops when lymph channels are obstructed by tumor, fibrosis, or inflammation, and in cases of axillary node dissection and radiation.

Table	
12-2	**Painful Peripheral Vascular Disorders and Their Mimics**

Problem	Process	Location of Pain
Arterial Disorders **Atherosclerosis (arteriosclerosis obliterans)**		
• Intermittent claudication	Episodic muscular ischemia induced by exercise, due to atherosclerosis of large or medium-sized arteries	Usually calf muscles, but also may be in the buttock, hip, thigh, or foot, depending on the level of obstruction
• Rest pain	Ischemia even at rest	Distal pain, in the toes or forefoot
Acute Arterial Occlusion	Embolism or thrombosis, possibly superimposed on arteriosclerosis obliterans	Distal pain, usually involving the foot and leg
Raynaud's Disease and Phenomenon	*Raynaud's disease:* Episodic spasm of the small arteries and arterioles; no vascular occlusion *Raynaud's phenomenon:* Syndrome secondary to other conditions such as collagen vascular disease, arterial occlusion, trauma, drugs	Distal portions of one or more fingers. Pain is usually not prominent unless fingertip ulcers develop. Numbness and tingling are common.
Venous Disorders		
Superficial Thrombophlebitis	Clot formation and acute inflammation in a superficial vein	Pain in a local area along the course of a superficial vein, most often in the saphenous system
Deep Venous Thrombosis (DVT)	Clot formation in a deep vein	Tight, bursting pain, if present, usually in the calf; may be painless.
Chronic Venous Insufficiency (deep)	Chronic venous engorgement secondary to venous occlusion or incompetency of venous valves	Diffuse aching of the leg(s)
Thromboangiitis Obliterans (Buerger's Disease)	Inflammatory and thrombotic occlusions of small arteries and also of veins, occurring in smokers	• Intermittent claudication, particularly in the arch of the foot • Rest pain in the fingers or toes
Compartment Syndrome	Pressure builds from trauma or bleeding into one of the four major muscle compartments between the knee and ankle. Each compartment is enclosed by fascia and thus cannot expand to accommodate increasing pressure.	Tight, bursting pain in calf muscles, usually in the anterior tibial compartment, sometimes with overlying dusky red skin.
Acute Lymphangitis	Acute bacterial infection (usually streptococcal) spreading up the lymphatic channels from a portal of entry such as an injured area or an ulcer	An arm or a leg
Mimics*		
Acute Cellulitis	Acute bacterial infection of the skin and subcutaneous tissues	Arms, legs, or elsewhere
Erythema Nodosum	Raised tender bilateral subcutaneous lesions seen in systemic conditions such as pregnancy, sarcoidosis, tuberculosis, streptococcal infections, inflammatory bowel disease	Anterior surfaces of both lower legs

*Mistaken primarily for acute superficial thrombophlebitis.

Timing	Factors That Aggravate	Factors That Relieve	Associated Manifestations
Fairly brief; pain usually forces the patient to rest.	Exercise such as walking	Rest usually stops the pain in 1–3 min.	Local fatigue, numbness, diminished pulses, often signs of arterial insufficiency (see p. 518)
Persistent, often worse at night	Elevation of the feet, as in bed	Sitting with legs dependent	Numbness, tingling, trophic signs and color changes of arterial insufficiency (see p. 518)
Sudden onset; associated symptoms may occur without pain.			Coldness, numbness, weakness, absent distal pulses
Relatively brief (minutes) but recurrent	Exposure to cold, emotional upset	Warm environment	Color changes in the distal fingers: severe pallor (essential for the diagnosis) followed by cyanosis and then redness
An acute episode lasting days or longer			Local redness, swelling, tenderness, a palpable cord, possibly fever
Often hard to determine because of lack of symptoms	Walking	Elevation speeds relief	Possible swelling of the foot and calf, local calf tenderness. Prior history of DVT
Chronic, increasing as the day wears on	Prolonged standing	Elevation of the leg(s)	Chronic edema, pigmentation, possibly ulceration (see p. 518)
• Fairly brief but recurrent	• Exercise	• Rest	Distal coldness, sweating, numbness, and cyanosis; ulceration and gangrene at the tips of fingers or toes; migratory thrombophlebitis
• Chronic, persistent, may be worse at night		• Permanent cessation of smoking helps both kinds of pain (but patients seldom stop)	
Several hours if *acute* (pressure must be relieved to overt necrosis). During exercise if *chronic*.	*Acute:* anabolic steroids; surgical complication; crush injury. *Chronic:* occurs with exercise	*Acute:* surgical incision to relieve pressure. *Chronic:* avoiding exercise; ice elevation	Tingling, burning sensations in calf; muscles may feel tight, full, numbness, paralysis if unrelieved
An acute episode lasting days or longer			Red streak(s) on the skin, with tenderness, enlarged, tender lymph nodes, and fever
An acute episode lasting days or longer			A local area of diffuse swelling, redness, and tenderness with enlarged, tender lymph nodes and fever; no palpable cord
Pain associated with a series of lesions over several weeks			Lesions recur in crops; often malaise, joint pains, and fever

Table
12-3   Using the Ankle–Brachial Index

Instructions for Measuring the Ankle–Brachial Index (ABI)

1. Patient should rest supine in a warm room for at least 10 minutes before testing.

2. Place blood pressure cuffs on both arms and ankles as illustrated, then apply ultrasound gel over brachial, dorsalis pedis, and posterior tibial arteries.

3. Measure systolic pressures in the arms
   - Use vascular Doppler to locate brachial pulse
   - Inflate cuff 20 mm Hg above last audible pulse
   - Deflate cuff slowly and record pressure at which pulse becomes audible
   - Obtain 2 measures in each arm and record the average as the brachial pressure in that arm

4. Measure systolic pressures in ankles
   - Use vascular Doppler to locate dorsalis pedis pulse
   - Inflate cuff 20 mm Hg above last audible pulse
   - Deflate cuff slowly and record pressure at which pulse becomes audible
   - Obtain 2 measures in each ankle and record the average as the dorsalis pedis pressure in that leg
   - Repeat above steps for posterior tibial arteries

5. Calculate ABI

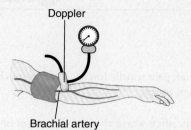

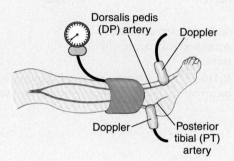

$$\text{Right ABI} = \frac{\text{highest right average ankle pressure (DP or PT)}}{\text{highest average arm pressure (right or left)}}$$

$$\text{Left ABI} = \frac{\text{highest left average ankle pressure (DP or PT)}}{\text{highest average arm pressure (right or left)}}$$

Site	1st reading	2nd reading	Average	Site	1st reading	2nd reading	Average
Left brachial				Right brachial			
Left dorsalis pedis				Right dorsalis pedis			
Left posterior tibial				Right posterior tibial			

Ankle–Brachial Index Calculator

$$A - BI = S_A \div S_B$$

Enter values for systolic pressure at:

The ankle: ☐ mm/Hg

The brachial artery: ☐ mm/Hg

Ankle–brachial index: ☐

Interpretation of Ankle–Brachial Index

>0.90 (with a range of 0.90 to 1.30) = Normal lower extremity blood flow
<0.89 to >0.60 = Mild PAD
<0.59 to >0.40 = Moderate PAD
<0.39 = Severe PAD

Sources: *Ankle–Brachial Calculator*—American College of Physicians. Available at http//cpsc.acponline.org/enhancements/232abiCalc.html. Accessed January 30, 2010 . Wilson JF, Laine C, Goldman D. In the clinic: peripheral arterial disease. Ann Int Med 2007;146:ITC 3-1.

Table	
12-4	**Chronic Insufficiency of Arteries and Veins**

Chronic Arterial Insufficiency (Advanced)

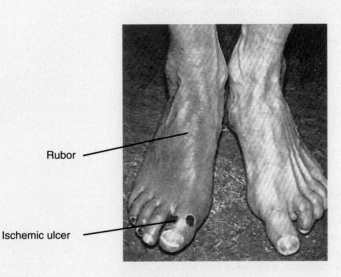

Rubor

Ischemic ulcer

Chronic Venous Insufficiency (Advanced)

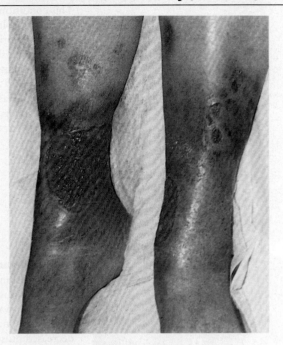

	Chronic Arterial Insufficiency (Advanced)	Chronic Venous Insufficiency (Advanced)
Pain	Intermittent claudication, progressing to pain at rest	Often painful
Mechanism	Tissue ischemia	Venous hypertension
Pulses	Decreased or absent	Normal, though may be difficult to feel through edema
Color	Pale, especially on elevation; dusky red on dependency	Normal, or cyanotic on dependency Petechiae and then brown pigmentation appear with chronicity.
Temperature	Cool	Normal
Edema	Absent or mild; may develop as the patient tries to relieve rest pain by lowering the leg	Present, often marked
Skin Changes	Trophic changes: thin, shiny, atrophic skin; loss of hair over the foot and toes; nails thickened and ridged	Often brown pigmentation around the ankle, stasis dermatitis, and possible thickening of the skin and narrowing of the leg as scarring develops
Ulceration	If present, involves toes or points of trauma on feet	If present, develops at sides of ankle, especially medially
Gangrene	May develop	Does not develop

Sources of photos: *Arterial Insufficiency*—Kappert A, Winsor T. Diagnosis of Peripheral Vascular Disease. Philadelphia, FA Davis, 1972; *Venous Insufficiency*—Marks R: Skin Disease in Old Age. Philadelphia, JB Lippincott, 1987.

Table 12-5   Common Ulcers of the Ankles and Feet

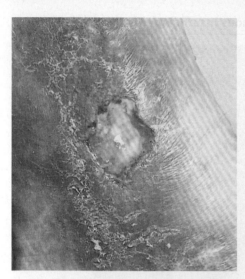

Chronic Venous Insufficiency

This condition usually appears over the medial and sometimes the lateral malleolus. The ulcer contains small, painful granulation tissue and fibrin; necrosis or exposed tendons are rare. Borders are irregular, flat, or slightly steep. Pain affects quality of life in 75% of patients. Associated findings include edema, reddish pigmentation and purpura, venous varicosities, the eczematous changes of stasis dermatitis (redness, scaling, and pruritus), and at times cyanosis of the foot when dependent. Gangrene is rare.[30]

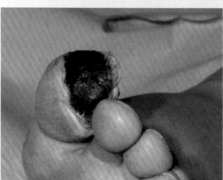

Arterial Insufficiency

This condition occurs in the toes, feet, or possibly areas of trauma (e.g., the shins). Surrounding skin shows no callus or excess pigment, although it may be atrophic. Pain often is severe unless neuropathy masks it. Gangrene may be associated, along with decreased pulses, trophic changes, foot pallor on elevation, and dusky rubor on dependency.

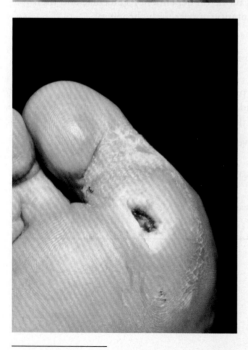

Neuropathic Ulcer

This condition develops in pressure points of areas with diminished sensation; seen in diabetic neuropathy, neurologic disorders, and Hansen disease. Surrounding skin is calloused. There is no pain, so the ulcer may go unnoticed. In uncomplicated cases, there is no gangrene. Associated signs include decreased sensation and absent ankle jerks.

Source of photos: Marks R. Skin Disease in Old Age. Philadelphia: JB Lippincott, 1987.

Male Genitalia and Hernias

Anatomy and Physiology

Review the anatomy of the male genitalia. The *shaft of the penis* is formed by three columns of vascular erectile tissue: the *corpus spongiosum*, containing the urethra, and two *corpora cavernosa*. The corpus spongiosum forms the bulb of the penis, ending in the cone-shaped *glans* with its expanded base, or *corona*. In uncircumcised men, the glans is covered by a loose, hoodlike

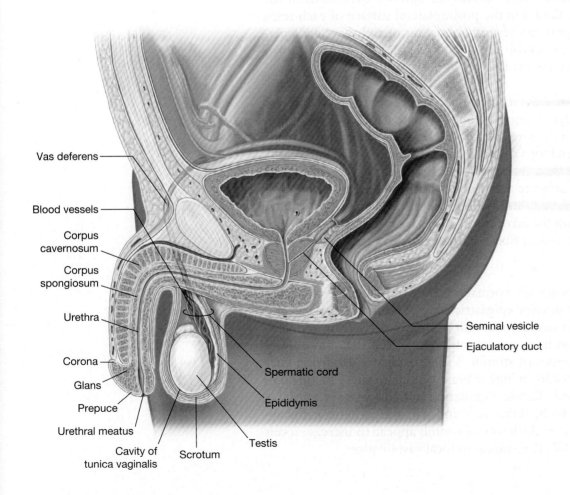

Vas deferens

Blood vessels

Corpus cavernosum

Corpus spongiosum

Urethra

Corona

Glans

Prepuce

Urethral meatus

Cavity of tunica vaginalis

Scrotum

Testis

Epididymis

Spermatic cord

Ejaculatory duct

Seminal vesicle

fold of skin called the *prepuce* or *foreskin* where *smegma*, or secretions of the glans, may collect. The urethra is located ventrally in the shaft of the penis; urethral abnormalities may sometimes be felt there. The urethra opens into the vertical, slitlike *urethral meatus*, located somewhat ventrally at the tip of the glans.

The testes contain interstitial tissue and seminiferous tubules. Gonadotropin-releasing hormone (GRH) from the hypothalamus stimulates pituitary secretion of luteinizing hormone (LH) and follicle-stimulating hormone (FSH). LH acts on the interstitial Leydig cells to promote synthesis of testosterone, which is converted by the enzyme 5α reductase to 5α dihydrotestosterone. It is 5α dihydrotestosterone that triggers pubertal growth of the male genitalia, prostate, seminal vesicles, and secondary sex characteristics such as facial and body hair, musculoskeletal growth, and enlargement of the larynx with its associated low-pitched voice. Testosterone is also converted to small amounts of estradiol by the enzyme CYP 19 aromatase. FSH regulates sperm production in the germ cells and Sertoli cells of the tubules.

Surrounding or appended to the testes are several structures. The *scrotum* is a loose, wrinkled pouch divided into two compartments, each containing a testis or testicle. Covering the testis, except posteriorly, is the serous membrane of the *tunica vaginalis*, which cloaks the anterior two-thirds of the testis and can accumulate fluid. On the posterolateral surface of each testis is the softer, comma-shaped *epididymis*, consisting of tightly coiled spermatic ducts that provide a reservoir for storage, maturation, and transport of sperm from the testis to the *vas deferens*.

During ejaculation, the *vas deferens*, a cordlike structure, transports sperm from the tail of the epididymis along a somewhat circular route to the urethra. The *vas* ascends from the scrotal sac into the pelvic cavity through the external inguinal ring, then loops over the ureter to the prostate behind the bladder. There it merges with the *seminal vesicle* to form the *ejaculatory duct*, which traverses the prostate and empties into the urethra. Secretions from the *vasa deferentia*, the seminal vesicles, and the prostate all contribute to the seminal fluid. Within the scrotum, each vas is closely associated with blood vessels, nerves, and muscle fibers. These structures make up the *spermatic cord*.

Male sexual function depends on normal levels of testosterone, adequate arterial blood flow to the inferior epigastric artery and its cremasteric and pubic branches, and intact neural innervation from α-adrenergic and cholinergic pathways. Erection from venous engorgement of the corpora cavernosa results from two types of stimuli. Visual, auditory, or erotic cues trigger sympathetic outflow from higher brain centers to the T11 through L2 levels of the spinal cord. Tactile stimulation initiates sensory impulses from the genitalia to S_2 to S_4 reflex arcs and parasympathetic pathways through the pudendal nerve. Both sets of stimuli appear to increase levels of nitric oxide and cyclic GMP, resulting in local vasodilation.

Lymphatics.   Lymphatics from the penile and scrotal surfaces drain into the inguinal nodes. *When you find an inflammatory or possibly malignant lesion* on these surfaces, *assess the inguinal nodes especially carefully* for enlargement or tenderness. The lymphatics of the testes drain into the abdomen, where enlarged nodes are clinically undetectable. See p. 493 for further discussion of the inguinal nodes.

Anatomy of the Groin.   Because hernias are relatively common, it is important to understand the anatomy of the groin. The basic landmarks are the anterior superior iliac spine, the pubic tubercle, and the inguinal ligament that runs between them. Find these on yourself or a colleague.

The *inguinal canal*, which lies above and approximately parallel to the inguinal ligament, forms a tunnel for the vas deferens as it passes through the abdominal muscles. The exterior opening of the tunnel, the *external inguinal ring*, is a triangular, slitlike structure palpable just above and lateral to the pubic tubercle. The internal opening of the canal, the *internal inguinal ring*, is approximately 1 cm above the midpoint of the inguinal ligament. Neither canal nor internal ring is palpable through the abdominal wall. When loops of bowel force their way through weak areas of the inguinal canal, they produce *inguinal hernias,* as illustrated on p. 538.

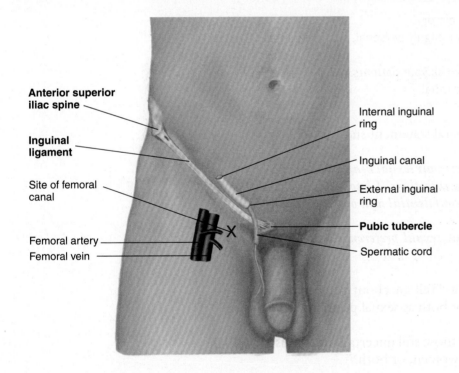

Anterior superior iliac spine

Inguinal ligament

Site of femoral canal

Femoral artery

Femoral vein

Internal inguinal ring

Inguinal canal

External inguinal ring

Pubic tubercle

Spermatic cord

Indirect inguinal hernias develop at the internal inguinal ring, where the spermatic cord exits the abdomen. *Direct inguinal hernias* arise more medially from weakness in the floor of the inguinal canal and are associated with straining and heavy lifting.

Another route for a herniating mass is the *femoral canal*, below the inguinal ligament. Although you cannot see it, you can estimate its location by placing your right index finger, from below, on the right femoral artery. Your middle finger will then overlie the femoral vein; your ring finger, the femoral canal. Femoral hernias protrude here.

Femoral hernias are more likely to present as emergencies with bowel incarceration or strangulation.

The Health History

Common or Concerning Symptoms

▶ Sexual orientation and sexual response
▶ Penile discharge or lesions
▶ Scrotal pain, swelling, or lesions
▶ Sexually transmitted infections (STIs) and diseases (STDs)

Sexual Orientation and Sexual Response

Sexual Orientation.   Discussing gender identity and sexual function touches a vital and multifaceted core of your patients' lives. Reflect on any biases you may have so they do not interfere with your professional responses to patient disclosures and concerns. A neutral nonjudgmental approach, supporting the patient's gender and sexual identity, is critical for ensuring your patient's health and well-being. To put your patients at ease as you explore the sexual history, adopt the tips below.

See also Chapter 3, The Sexual History, pp. 86–87.

Tips for Taking the Sexual History

▶ Explain why you are taking the sexual history.
▶ Note that you realize this information is highly personal, and encourage the patient to be open and direct.
▶ Relate that you gather this history from all your patients.
▶ Affirm that your conversation is confidential.

For example, you can begin with a general statement such as:

"To provide good care, I need to review your sexual health and see if you are at risk for any sexually transmitted infections. I know this is a sensitive area. Any information you share is confidential and only between us."

Continue with neutral questions about *sexual preference* and *gender and sexual identity* such as:

● "What is your relationship status?" or "Tell me about your sexual preference. Do you prefer men, women, or both as sexual partners?"

● Furthermore, to open discussion for those still uncertain or confused, ask "Are you sexually attracted to men, women, or both?"

Gay, Lesbian, Bisexual, and Transgender Health Care.   Two recent surveys suggest that 7% to 8% of men and 4% to 7% of women report they are gay, lesbian, or bisexual.[1,2] During clinical encounters, these patients often experience significant anxiety related to fears of being accepted; they may be uncomfortable disclosing their sexual behaviors and still fluctuating in their sexual identity. When they experience bias or discrimination, they are unlikely to reveal their sexual identity or concerns.[3] Gay, lesbian, transgender, and bisexual patients have higher rates of depression, anxiety, drug use, sexual victimization, and risk of infection with HIV and sexually transmitted infections (STIs; also referred to as sexually transmitted diseases [STDs]).[4–6] Furthermore, reports indicated that clinicians are often unprepared to respond to questions about fertility and transgender issues like hormonal therapy and surgery. Expand your knowledge and clinical skills about gay, lesbian, and transgender health from the many resources available.[6–10]

Sexual Response. Continue with questions about *sexual response*. "How is sexual function for you?" "How is your current relationship?" "Are you satisfied with your relationship and your sexual activity?" "What about your ability to perform sexually?" If the patient expresses relational or sexual concerns, explore both their psychological and physiologic dimensions. Ask about the meaning of the relationship in the patient's life. Also ask about any changes in desire or frequency of sexual activity. What is the patient's view of the cause, what responses has he tried, and what are his hopes?

Direct questions help you to assess each phase of the sexual response. To assess *libido*, or desire, ask "Have you maintained interest in sex?" For the *arousal phase*, ask "Can you achieve and maintain an erection?" Explore the timing, severity, setting, and any other factors that may be contributing to problems. Have any changes in the relationship with his partner or in his life circumstances coincided with onset of a problem? Are there circumstances when erection is normal? On awakening in the early morning or during the night? With other partners? With masturbation?

Lack of libido may arise from psychogenic causes such as depression, endocrine dysfunction, or side effects of medications.

Erectile dysfunction may be from psychogenic causes, especially if early morning erection is preserved; it may also reflect decreased testosterone, decreased blood flow in the hypogastric arterial system, impaired neural innervation, and diabetes.[11]

Other questions relate to the phase of *orgasm* and *ejaculation* of semen. If ejaculation is premature, or early and out of control, ask "About how long does intercourse last?" "Do you climax too soon?" "Do you feel you have control over climaxing?" "Do you think your partner would like intercourse to last longer?" For reduced or absent ejaculation, "Do you find that you cannot have an orgasm even though you can have an erection?" Try to determine whether the problem involves the pleasurable sensation of orgasm, the ejaculation of seminal fluid, or both. Review the frequency and setting of the problem, medications, surgery, and neurologic symptoms.

Premature ejaculation is common, especially in young men. Less common is reduced or absent ejaculation affecting middle-aged or older men. Possible causes are medications, surgery, neurologic deficits, or lack of androgen. Lack of orgasm with ejaculation is usually psychogenic.

Penile Discharge or Lesions, Scrotal Swelling or Pain, and STIs. Ask about any discharge from the penis, dripping, or staining of underwear. If penile discharge is present, clarify the amount, color, and any fever, chills, rash, or associated symptoms.

Look for yellow penile discharge in *gonorrhea;* white discharge in *non-gonococcal urethritis* from *Chlamydia*. See Table 13-1, Sexually Transmitted Infections of the Male Genitalia (p. 534).

Rash, tenosynovitis, monoarticular arthritis, even meningitis, not always with urogenital symptoms, occur in *disseminated gonorrhea*.

Inquire about sores or growths on the penis. Ask about *swelling or pain in the scrotum.*

Look for ulcer in syphilitic *chancre, herpes;* warts from *human papillomavirus (HPV);* swelling in *mumps orchitis,* scrotal edema, testicular cancer; pain in *testicular torsion, epididymitis, orchitis.*

See Table 13-2, Abnormalities of the Penis and Scrotum, p. 535, and Table 13-3, Abnormalities of the Testis, p. 536.

Review any previous genital symptoms or past history of infection from herpes, gonorrhea, or syphilis. Men with multiple or same sex partners, illicit drug use, or prior history of STIs are at increased risk of HIV infection and other new STIs.

Because STIs may involve other parts of the body, additional questions are often indicated. An introductory explanation may be useful. "Sexually transmitted infections can involve any body opening where you have sex. It's important for you to tell me which openings you use." And further, as needed, "Do you have oral sex? Anal sex?" If the patient's answers are affirmative, ask about symptoms such as sore throat, diarrhea, rectal bleeding, and anal itching or pain.

Infections from oral–penile transmission include *gonorrhea, chlamydia, syphilis,* and *herpes.* Symptomatic or asymptomatic proctitis may follow anal intercourse.

Because many infected individuals do not have symptoms or risk factors, ask all patients, "Do you have any concerns about the HIV infection?" and discuss the need for *universal testing for HIV.*[12–14]

Health Promotion and Counseling: Evidence and Recommendations

Important Topics for Health Promotion and Counseling

▶ Prevention of STIs and HIV
▶ Screening for testicular cancer and testicular self-examination

Prevention of STIs and HIV Infection.   The case for aggressive clinician education, early detection during history taking and physical examination, and treatment for STIs and HIV is compelling. The growing burden of STIs affects the health of all segments of the population, but especially adolescents and young adults. The Institute of Medicine has documented that U.S. rates of STIs are the highest in the industrialized world.[15] In 2009, the Centers for Disease Control and Prevention (CDC) estimated 19 million new STIs each year, with almost half in the age group 15 to 24 years.[16] Of the 1.5 million new cases reported in 2009, approximately 80% were infections from chlamydia, 19% from gonorrhea, and 1% from syphilis. The CDC notes that these figures underestimate the "true national burden" of STIs; many cases are unreported, and viral infections such as human papillomavirus and genital herpes are not subject to requirements for mandatory reporting. Only half of people at risk receive recommended screening services.

The *HIV and AIDS* population continues to grow. More than 1.1 million Americans are currently infected with HIV, with approximately 56,000 new infections annually.[17] At highest risk are African American men and men having sex with men. In 2008, more than 50% of new infections occurred in African American men and approximately 55% occurred in the male-to-male transmission group. An estimated 20% of infected individuals are unaware of their infected status, increasing the spread of disease, and over 30% of diagnoses are "late," defined as an AIDS diagnosis made 12 months or less from an initial HIV diagnosis. The Centers for Disease Control and Prevention continues to urge *universal testing from ages 18 to 64, regardless of risk*; currently only 45% of adults in this age spectrum have been tested. Groups at high risk should be tested annually—men with male sex partners, individuals with multiple partners, past or present injection drug users, sex workers' individuals with past or present partners who have a history of STIs, HIV infection, injection drug use, or bisexual practice, and recipients of blood transfusions between 1978 and 1985.[13] The presence of any STI, including hepatitis B and chancroid, warrants testing for coinfection with HIV. Advances in treatment now mean that an HIV-positive person diagnosed at age 25 who receives high-quality care can live an additional 39 years.

Clinicians must master the skills of eliciting the sexual history and asking frank but tactful questions about sexual practices. Key information includes the patient's sexual orientation, the number of partners in the past month, and any history of past STIs (see also pp. 86–87). Careful screening for alcohol and drug use, especially injection drugs, is also important. Counseling should be interactive and combine information about general risk reduction with personalized messages for reducing risk in the patient's individual situation. Adopting this approach, termed *client-centered counseling*, especially by trained clinicians, has been shown to lower high-risk behaviors.[18] Explore available resources to improve your effectiveness in this critical area.[19,20]

As you counsel patients, encourage men to seek prompt attention for any genital lesions or penile discharge. Address preventive behaviors such as using condoms, limiting the number of sexual partners, and establishing regular health care for treatment of STIs and HIV. *Correct use of male condoms* is highly effective in preventing the transmission of HIV, HPV, and other STIs.[18,21] Key instructions should include: using a new condom with each sex act, applying the condom before any sexual contact occurs, adding only water-based lubricants, and holding the condom during withdrawal to keep it from slipping off. Recommend *HPV vaccination* with Gardasil for boys and men ages 9 through 26 for prevention of genital warts.[22–25] (See also Chapter 14, p. 550.)

Screening for Testicular Cancer and Testicular Self-Examination.

Testicular cancer is rare, but it is the most common cancer in men ages 15 to 34, and four times more common in white men compared to black men. Risk factors are family history and a history of cryptorchidism, which increases risk two- to eightfold and is present in 7% to 10% of men with testicular cancer.[26] Evidence to guide recommendations for screening is scant, and in 2010 the U.S. Preventive Services Task Force was unable to find any studies that directly addressed the benefits or harms of screening.[27] As advised by the American Cancer Society, encourage men, especially those between the ages of 15 and 34, to perform monthly *testicular self-examinations* and seek clinician assessment for any of the following: any painless lump, swelling, or enlargement in either testicle; pain or discomfort in a testicle or the scrotum; a feeling of heaviness or a sudden fluid collection in the scrotum; or a dull ache in the lower abdomen or the groin.[28] See p. 531 for patient instructions for self-examination.

Techniques of Examination

Many students feel uneasy about examining a man's genitalia. "How will the patient react?" "Will he have an erection?" "Will he let me examine him?" It is reassuring to explain each step of the examination so that the patient knows what to expect. Request an assistant to accompany you. Occasionally, male patients have erections during the examination. If this happens, explain that this is a normal response, finish your examination, and proceed with an unruffled demeanor. If the man refuses to be examined, you should respect his wishes.

A good genital examination can be done with the patient either standing or supine. To check for hernias or varicoceles, however, the patient should stand, and you should sit comfortably on a chair or stool. A gown conveniently covers the patient's chest and abdomen. *Wear gloves* throughout the examination. Expose the genitalia and inguinal areas. For younger patients, review the sexual maturity ratings on p. 866.

THE PENIS

Inspection

Inspect the penis, including:

- The *skin*

- The *prepuce* (foreskin). If present, retract the prepuce or ask the patient to retract it. This step is essential for the detection of chancres and carcinomas. Smegma, a cheesy, whitish material, may accumulate normally under the foreskin.

- The *glans*. Look for any ulcers, scars, nodules, or signs of inflammation.

Check the skin around the base of the penis for excoriations or inflammation. Look for nits or lice at the bases of the pubic hairs.

Note the location of the urethral meatus.

Compress the glans gently between your index finger above and your thumb below. This maneuver should open the urethral meatus and allow you to inspect it for discharge. Normally there is none.

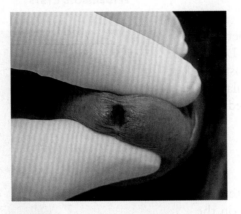

If the patient has reported a discharge that you are unable to see, ask him to strip, or milk, the shaft of the penis from its base to the glans. Alternatively, do it yourself. This maneuver may expel some discharge from the urethral meatus for appropriate examination. Have a glass slide and culture materials ready.

Palpation

Palpate any abnormality of the penis, noting any tenderness or induration. Palpate the shaft of the penis between your thumb and first two fingers, noting any induration. Palpation of the shaft may be omitted in a young, asymptomatic male patient.

If you retract the foreskin, replace it before proceeding on to examine the scrotum.

See Table 13-2, Abnormalities of the Penis and Scrotum, p. 535.

Phimosis is a tight prepuce that cannot be retracted over the glans. *Paraphimosis* is a tight prepuce that, once retracted, cannot be returned. Edema ensues.

Balanitis is inflammation of the glans; *balanoposthitis* is inflammation of the glans and prepuce.

Pubic or genital excoriations suggest lice (crabs) or, sometimes, scabies.

Hypospadias is a congenital, ventral displacement of the meatus on the penis (p. 535).

Profuse yellow discharge occurs in *gonococcal urethritis*; scanty white or clear discharge in *nongonococcal urethritis*. Definitive diagnosis requires Gram stain and culture.

Induration along the ventral surface of the penis suggests a *urethral stricture* or possibly a *carcinoma*. Tenderness in the indurated area suggests periurethral inflammation secondary to a urethral stricture.

THE SCROTUM AND ITS CONTENTS

Inspection

Inspect the scrotum, including:

- The *skin*. Lift up the scrotum so that you can see its posterior surface.

- The *scrotal contours*. Note any swelling, lumps, or veins.

There may be dome-shaped white or yellow papules or nodules formed by occluded follicles filled with keratin debris of desquamated follicular epithelium. Such *epidermoid cysts* are common, frequently multiple, and benign.

See Table 13-2, Abnormalities of the Penis and Scrotum, p. 535.

Rashes, epidermoid cysts, rarely skin cancer may be observed.

A poorly developed scrotum on one or both sides suggests *cryptorchidism* (an undescended testicle). Common scrotal swellings include indirect *inguinal hernias, hydroceles, scrotal edema,* and, rarely, testicular carcinoma.

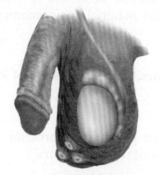

EPIDERMOID CYSTS

Palpation

Palpate each testis and epididymis between your thumb and first two fingers. Locate the epididymis on the superior posterior surface of each testicle. It feels nodular and cordlike and should not be confused with an abnormal lump.

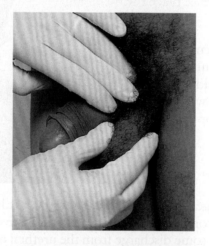

Note size, shape, consistency, and tenderness; feel for any nodules. Pressure on the testis normally produces a deep visceral pain.

Palpate each spermatic cord, including the vas deferens, between your thumb and fingers, from the epididymis to the superficial inguinal ring.

Note any nodules or swellings.

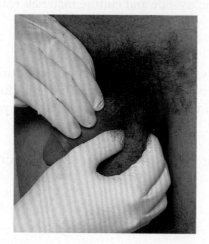

See Table 13-3, Abnormalities of the Testis, p. 536, and Table 13-4, Abnormalities of the Epididymis and Spermatic Cord, p. 537.

Tender, painful scrotal swelling is present in *acute epididymitis, acute orchitis, torsion of the spermatic cord,* or a *strangulated inguinal hernia.*

Any painless nodule in the testis must raise the possibility of *testicular cancer,* a potentially curable cancer with a peak incidence between the ages of 15 and 34 years.

Multiple tortuous veins in this area, usually on the left, may be palpable and even visible, indicating a *varicocele,* p. 537.

The vas deferens, if chronically infected, may feel thickened or beaded. A cystic structure in the spermatic cord suggests a *hydrocele of the cord.*

Swelling in the scrotum other than the testicles can be evaluated by transillumination. After darkening the room, shine the beam of a strong flashlight from behind the scrotum through the mass. Look for transmission of the light as a red glow.

Swellings containing serous fluid, such as *hydroceles,* light up with a red glow, or transilluminate. Those containing blood or tissue, such as a normal testis, a tumor, or most hernias, do not.

HERNIAS

Inspection

Sitting comfortably in front of the patient, with the patient standing and an assistant present, *inspect the inguinal regions and genitalia* for bulging areas and asymmetry. As you observe, ask the patient to strain and bear down (the Valsalva maneuver) to increase intra-abdominal pressure, making it easier to detect any hernias.

A bulge that appears with straining suggests a *hernia.*

Palpation

Palpate for an inguinal hernia, using the techniques below. Continue to face the patient, who should still be standing.

See Table 13-5, Course, Presentation, and Differentiation of Hernias in the Groin, p. 538.

- To examine for right inguinal hernias, place the tip of your right index finger close to the inferior margin of the scrotal sac, then move your finger upward along the inguinal canal, invaginating the scrotum.

- Follow the spermatic cord upward to the inguinal ligament. Find the triangular slitlike opening of the *external inguinal ring* just above and lateral to the pubic tubercle. Palpate the external inguinal ring and its floor. Ask the patient to bear down. Search for any bulges or masses against the side or pulp of the index finger above the inguinal ligament near the pubic tubercle.

A bulge near the external inguinal ring suggests a *direct inguinal hernia.* A bulge near the internal inguinal ring suggests an *indirect inguinal hernia.* Experts note that distinguishing the type of hernia is difficult, with sensitivity and specificity of 75% and 95%. Detecting either type of mass warrants surgical evaluation.[29,30]

- The external ring may be large enough for you to gently palpate obliquely along the inguinal canal toward the *internal inguinal ring.* Ask the patient to bear down. Check for a bulge that slides down the inguinal canal and taps against the fingertip.

- To examine for left inguinal hernias, use the same techniques with the left index finger.

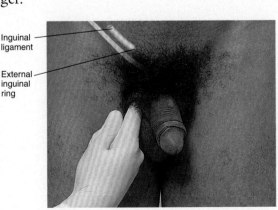

Inguinal ligament

External inguinal ring

Palpate for a femoral hernia by placing your fingers on the anterior thigh in the region of the femoral canal. Ask the patient to strain down again or cough. Note any swelling or tenderness.

Evaluating a Possible Scrotal Hernia.   If you find a large scrotal mass and suspect that it may be a hernia, ask the patient to lie down. The mass may return to the abdomen by itself. If so, it is a hernia. If not:

● Can you get your fingers above the mass in the scrotum?

If you can, suspect a *hydrocele*.

● Listen to the mass with a stethoscope for bowel sounds.

Bowel sounds may be heard over a hernia, but not over a hydrocele.

If the findings suggest a hernia, gently try to reduce it (return it to the abdominal cavity) by sustained pressure with your fingers. Do not attempt this maneuver if the mass is tender or the patient reports nausea and vomiting.

A hernia is *incarcerated* when its contents cannot be returned to the abdominal cavity. A hernia is *strangulated* when the blood supply to the entrapped contents is compromised. Suspect strangulation in the presence of tenderness, nausea, and vomiting, and consider surgical intervention. See Table 13-5, Course, Presentation, and Differentiation of Hernias in the Groin, p. 538.

History may be helpful here. The patient can usually tell you what happens to his swelling on lying down and may be able to demonstrate how he reduces it himself.

SPECIAL TECHNIQUES

The Testicular Self-Examination

The incidence of testicular cancer is low, about 4 per 100,000 men, but it is the most common cancer of young men between ages 15 and 34. Although the testicular self-examination (TSE) has not been formally endorsed as a screen for testicular carcinoma, teach your patient the TSE to enhance health awareness and self-care. When detected early, testicular carcinoma has an excellent prognosis. Risk factors include cryptorchidism, which confers a high risk for testicular carcinoma in the undescended testicle; a history of carcinoma in the contralateral testicle; mumps orchitis; an inguinal hernia; and a hydrocele in childhood.

Patient Instructions for the Testicular Self-Examination

This examination is best performed after a warm bath or shower. The heat relaxes the scrotum and makes it easier to find anything unusual.

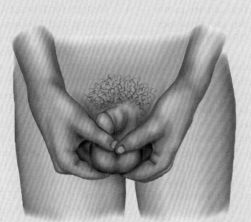

▶ Standing in front of a mirror, check for any swelling on the skin of the scrotum.

▶ With the penis out of the way, examine each testicle separately.

▶ Cup the testicle between your thumb and fingers with both hands and roll it gently between the fingers. One testicle may be larger than the other; that is normal, but be concerned about any lump or area of pain.

▶ Find the epididymis. This is a soft, tubelike structure at the back of the testicle that collects and carries sperm, and is not an abnormal lump.

▶ If you find any lump, don't wait. See your doctor. The lump may just be an infection, but if it is cancer, it will spread unless stopped by treatment.

Source: Medline Plus. U.S. National Library of Medicine and National Institutes of Health. Medical Encyclopedia—Testicular self-examination. Available at www.nlm.nih.gov/medlineplus/ency/article/003909.htm. Accessed December 19, 2010.

Recording Your Findings

Note that initially you may use sentences to describe your findings; later you will use phrases. The style below contains phrases appropriate for most write-ups.

Recording the Physical Examination—Male Genitalia and Hernias

"Circumcised male. No penile discharge or lesions. No scrotal swelling or discoloration. Testes descended bilaterally, smooth, without masses. Epididymis nontender. No inguinal or femoral hernias."

OR

"Uncircumcised male; prepuce easily retractible. No penile discharge or lesions. No scrotal swelling or discoloration. Testes descended bilaterally; right testicle smooth; 1 × 1 cm firm nodule on left lateral testicle. It is fixed and nontender. Epididymis nontender. No inguinal or femoral hernias."

Suspicious for *testicular carcinoma*, the most common form of cancer in men between the ages of 15 and 34.

Bibliography

Citations

1. Hebernick D, Reece M, Schick V et al. Sexual activity in the United States: results from a national probability sample of men and women ages 14–94. J Sex Medicine 2010;7(Suppl 5): 255–265.

2. Gates GJ. Same sex couples and the gay, lesbian, and bisexual population: new estimates from the American Community Survey. October 2006. Available at http://www.law.ucla. edu/williamsinstitute/publications/SameSexCouplesandG-LBpopACS.pdf. Accessed December 19, 2010.

3. Polek CA, Hardie TL, Crowley EM. Lesbians' disclosure of sexual orientation and satisfaction with care. J Transcult Nurs 2008;19:243–249.

4. Conron KJ, Mimiaga MJ, Landers SJ. A population-based study of sexual orientation identity and gender differences in adult health. Am J Public Health 2010;100:1953–1960.

5. McLaughlin KA, Hatzenbuehler ML, Keyes KM. Responses to discrimination and psychiatric disorders among black, Hispanic, female, and lesbian, gay, and bisexual individuals. Am J Public Health 2010;100:1477–1484.

6. Centers for Disease Control and Prevention. Lesbian, gay, bisexual, and transgender health. Updated November 2, 2010. Available at http://www.cdc.gov/lgbthealth/index.htm. Accessed December 18, 2010.

7. Kelley L, Chou CL, Dibble SL et al. A critical intervention in lesbian, gay, bisexual, and transgender health: knowledge and attitude outcomes among second-year medical students. Teach Learn Med 2008;20:248–253.

8. National Coalition for LGTB Health. Available at http://lgbthealth.webolutionary.com/home. Accessed December 18, 2010.

9. Mayer KH, Bradford JB, Makadon HJ et al. Sexual and gender minority health: what we know and what needs to be done. Am J Public Health 2008;98:989–995.

10. Wolitsky RJ, Stall R, Valdiserri RO, eds. Unequal Opportunity: Health Disparities Affecting Gay and Bisexual Men in the United States. New York: Oxford University Press, 2008.

11. McVary KT. Clinical practice: erectile dysfunction. N Engl J Med 2007;357:2472–2481.

12. Workowsi KA, Levine WC, Wasserheit JN. U.S. Centers for Disease Control and Prevention guidelines for the treatment of sexually transmitted diseases: an opportunity to unify clinical and public health practice. Ann Intern Med 2002;137:255–262.

13. USPSTF. Screening for HIV. April 2007. Available at http://www.uspreventiveservicestaskforce.org/uspstf05/hiv/hivrs.htm#clinical. Accessed October 18, 2010.

14. Qaseem A, Snow V, Shekelle P et al. Clinical guidelines: screening for HIV in health care settings: a guidance statement from the American College of Physicians and HIV Medicine Association. Ann Intern Med 2009;150:125–131.

15. Institute of Medicine. Committee on Prevention and Control of Sexually Transmitted Diseases. The Hidden Epidemic: Confronting Sexually Transmitted Diseases. Washington, DC: National Academy Press, 1997. pp. 1–432.

16. Centers for Disease Control and Prevention. Trends in sexually transmitted diseases in the United States: 2009 national data for gonorrhea, chlamydia, and syphilis. Updated November 22, 2010. Available at http://www.cdc.gov/std/stats09/trends.htm Accessed December 28, 2010.

17. Centers for Disease Control and Prevention. Vital Signs: HIV testing and diagnosis among adults—United States, 2001–2009. Morbidity and Mortality Weekly Report 2010;59(47): 1550–1555. Available at http://www.cdc.gov/mmwr/preview/mmwrhtml/mm5947a3.htm?s_cid=mm5947a3_w. Accessed December 19, 2010.

18. Workowski KA, Berman S. Sexually transmitted diseases treatment guidelines, 2010. Centers for Disease Control and Prevention. Morbidity and Mortality Weekly Report 2010;59(RR12):1–110. Available at http://www.cdc.gov/mmwr/preview/mmwrhtml/rr5912a1.htm. Accessed December 31, 2010.

19. Centers for Disease Control and Prevention. National Network of STD/HIV Prevention Training Centers. Available at http://depts.washington.edu/nnptc. Accessed December 31, 2010.

20. DEBI. Diffusion of effective behavioral interventions. Available at http://effectiveinterventions.org/en/home.aspx. Accessed December 31, 2010.

21. Centers for Disease Control and Prevention. Male latex condoms and sexually transmitted diseases. Condoms and STDs: fact sheet for public health personnel. Available at http://www.cdc.gov/condomeffectiveness/latex.htm. Accessed December 31, 2010.

22. Advisory Committee on Immunization Practices, Centers for Disease Control. Morbidity and Mortality Weekly Report. Quadrivalent Human Papillomavirus Vaccine. Recommendations of the Advisory Committee on Immunization Practices. March 12, 2007/56 (Early Release). pp. 1–54. Available at http://www.cdc.gov/mmwr/preview/mmwrhtml/rr56e312a1.htm. Accessed December 4, 2010.

23. Garland SM, Hernandez-Avila M, Wheller CM et al. Quadrivalent vaccine against human papillomavirus to prevent anogenital diseases. N Engl J Med 2007;356:1928–1943.

24. Centers for Disease Control and Prevention. Vaccine Information Statement (Interim)-Human Papillomavirus (HPV) Gardasil. March 30, 2010. Available at http://www.cdc.gov/vaccines/pubs/vis/downloads/vis-hpv-gardasil.pdf. Accessed December 4, 2010.

25. Winer RL, Hughes JP, Feng Q et al. Condom use and the risk of genital human papillomavirus infection in young women. NEJM 2006;354:2645–2654.

26. National Cancer Institute. Testicular cancer screening. Health professional version. Updated July 23, 2010. Available at http://www.cancer.gov/cancertopics/pdq/screening/testicular/healthprofessional/allpages. Accessed December 19, 2010.

27. Lin K, Sharangpani R. Screening for testicular cancer: an evidence review for the U. S. Preventive Services task force. Ann Intern Med 2010;153:396–399.

28. American Cancer Society. Testicular cancer. Updated July 20, 2010. Available at http://www.cancer.org/acs/groups/cid/documents/webcontent/003142–pdf.pdf. Accessed December 19, 2010.

29. Van den Berg JC, de Valois JC, Go PM et al. Detection of groin hernia with physical examination, ultrasound, and MRI compared with laparoscopic findings. Invest Radiol 1999;34:739–74.

30. Sayad P, Abdo Z, Cacchione R et al. Incidence of incipient contralateral hernia during laparoscopic hernia repair. Surg Endosc 2000;14:543–545.

Additional References

Bosl GJ, Bajorin DF, Sheinfeld J et al. Cancer of the testis. In: DeVita VT, Lawrence TS, Rosenberg SA, eds. Cancer: Principles and Practice of Oncology, 9th ed. Philadelphia: Wolters Kluwer Health/Lippincott Williams & Wilkins. pp. 1463–1485, 2011.

Centers for Disease Control and Prevention. Clinical prevention guidance. In: Sexually transmitted diseases treatment guidelines, 2010. MMWR Recomm Rep 2010;59(RR-12):2–8. Available at http://www.guideline.gov/content.aspx?id=25577&search=sexually+transmitted+disease. Accessed November 4, 2011.

DeBusk RF. Sexual activity in patients with angina. JAMA 2003; 290:3129–3132.

Gupta R, Warren T, Wald A. Genital herpes. Lancet 2007; 370(9605):2127–2137.

Handsfield HH. Color Atlas and Synopsis of Sexually Transmitted Diseases, 3rd ed. New York: McGraw-Hill Medical, 2011.

Kaufman DS, Saksena MA, Young RH et al. Case records of the Massachusetts General Hospital. Case 6-2007. A 28-year-old man with a mass in the testis. N Engl J Med 2007;356:842–849.

Kiowski W, Brunner H, Schalcher C. Sex, the heart, and heart failure. Semin Cardiothorac Vasc Anesth 2006;10:256–258.

Markland AD, Vaughan CP, Johnson TM 2nd et al. Incontinence. Med Clin North Am 2011;95:539–554.

Pettersson A, Richiardi L, Nordenskjold A et al. Age at surgery for undescended testis and risk of testicular cancer. N Engl J Med 2007;356:1835–1841.

Qaseem A, Snow V, Denberg TD et al. Clinical guidelines: hormonal testing and pharmacologic treatment of erectile dysfunction: a clinical practice guideline from the American College of Physicians. Ann Intern Med 2009;151:639–649.

Sherman V, Macho JR, Brunicardi C. Ch 37, Inguinal hernias. In Brunicardi FC, Andersen DK, Billiar TR et al (eds). Schwartz's Principles of Surgery, 9th ed. New York: McGraw-Hill, 2010.

U. S. Preventive Services Task Force. Screening for genital herpes. March 2005. Available at http://www.ahrq.gov/clinic/uspstf/uspsherp.htm. Accessed November 4, 2011.

Wein AJ, Kavoussi LR Campbell MF et al (eds). Campbell-Walsh Urology. Philadelphia: Elsevier Saunders, 2012.

The Bates' suite offers these additional resources to enhance learning and facilitate understanding of this chapter:

• *Bates' Pocket Guide to Physical Examination and History Taking*, 7th edition
• *Bates' Visual Guide to Physical Examination*
• thePoint online resources, for students and instructors: http://thePoint.lww.com

Table
13-1   **Sexually Transmitted Infections of Male Genitalia**

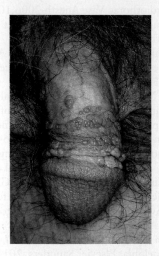

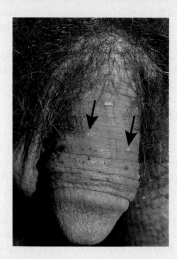

Genital Warts (condylomata acuminata)

- *Appearance:* Single or multiple papules or plaques of variable shapes; may be round, acuminate (or pointed), or thin and slender. May be raised, flat, or cauliflowerlike (verrucous).
- *Causative organism: Human papillomavirus (HPV),* usually from subtypes 6, 11; carcinogenic subtypes rare, approximately 5% to 10% of all anogenital warts. *Incubation:* weeks to months; infected contact may have no visible warts.
- Can arise on penis, scrotum, groin, thighs, anus; usually asymptomatic, occasionally cause itching and pain.
- May disappear without treatment.

Genital Herpes Simplex

- *Appearance:* Small scattered or grouped vesicles, 1 to 3 mm in size, on glans or shaft of penis. Appear as erosions if vesicular membrane breaks.
- *Causative organism:* Usually *Herpes simplex virus 2* (90%), a double-stranded DNA virus. *Incubation:* 2 to 7 days after exposure.
- Primary episode may be asymptomatic; recurrence usually less painful, of shorter duration.
- Associated with fever, malaise, headache, arthralgias; local pain and edema, lymphadenopathy.
- Need to distinguish from genital herpes zoster (usually in older patients with dermatomal distribution); candidiasis.

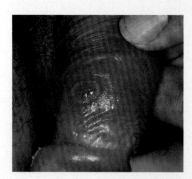

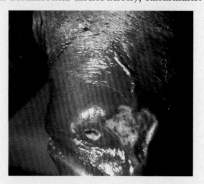

Primary Syphilis

- *Appearance:* Small red papule that becomes a *chancre,* or *painless* erosion up to 2 cm in diameter. Base of chancre is clean, red, smooth, and glistening; borders are raised and indurated. Chancre heals within 3 to 8 weeks.
- *Causative organism: Treponema pallidum,* a spirochete. *Incubation:* 9 to 90 days after exposure.
- May develop inguinal lymphadenopathy within 7 days; lymph nodes are rubbery, nontender, mobile.
- 20% to 30% of patients develop secondary syphilis while chancre still present (suggests coinfection with HIV).
- Distinguish from: genital herpes simplex; chancroid; granuloma inguinale from *Klebsiella granulomatis* (rare in the United States; 4 variants, so difficult to identify).

Chancroid

- *Appearance:* Red papule or pustule initially, then forms a *painful* deep ulcer with ragged nonindurated margins; contains necrotic exudate, has a friable base.
- *Causative organism: Haemophilus ducreyi,* an anaerobic bacillus. *Incubation:* 3 to 7 days after exposure.
- Painful inguinal adenopathy; suppurative buboes in 25% of patients.
- Need to distinguish from: primary syphilis; genital herpes simplex; lymphomogranuloma venereum, granuloma inguinale from *Klebsiella granulomatis* (both rare in the United States).

Table
13-2   Abnormalities of the Penis and Scrotum

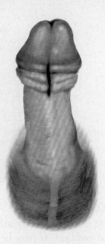

Hypospadias

A congenital displacement of the urethral meatus to the inferior surface of the penis. A groove extends from the actual urethral meatus to its normal location on the tip of the glans.

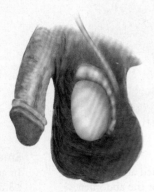

Scrotal Edema

Pitting edema may make the scrotal skin taut; seen in heart failure or nephrotic syndrome.

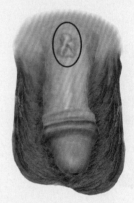

Peyronie's Disease

Palpable, nontender, hard plaques are found just beneath the skin, usually along the dorsum of the penis. The patient complains of crooked, painful erections.

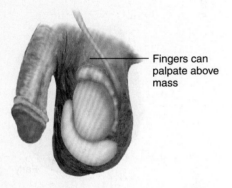

Fingers can palpate above mass

Hydrocele

A nontender, fluid-filled mass within the tunica vaginalis. It transilluminates, and the examining fingers can get above the mass within the scrotum.

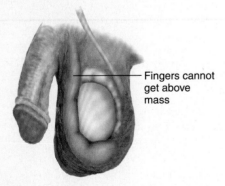

Fingers cannot get above mass

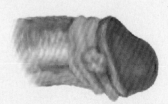

Carcinoma of the Penis

An indurated nodule or ulcer that is usually nontender. Limited almost completely to men who are not circumcised, it may be masked by the prepuce. Any persistent penile sore is suspicious.

Scrotal Hernia

Usually an *indirect inguinal hernia*, that comes through the external inguinal ring, so the examining fingers cannot get above it within the scrotum.

Table
13-3
Abnormalities of the Testis

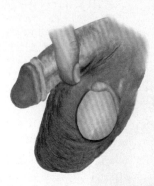

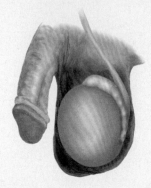

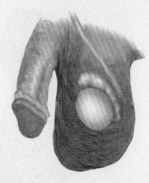

Cryptorchidism

The testis is atrophied and may lie in the inguinal canal or the abdomen, resulting in an unfilled scrotum. As above, there is no palpable left testis or epididymis. Cryptorchidism markedly raises the risk for testicular cancer.

Small Testis

In adults, testicular length is usually ≤3.5 cm. Small, firm testes in *Klinefelter's syndrome*, usually ≤2 cm. Small, soft testes suggesting atrophy are seen in cirrhosis, myotonic dystrophy, use of estrogens, and hypopituitarism; may also follow orchitis.

Acute Orchitis

The testis is acutely inflamed, painful, tender, and swollen. It may be difficult to distinguish from the epididymis. The scrotum may be reddened. Seen in mumps and other viral infections; usually unilateral.

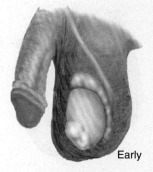

Early

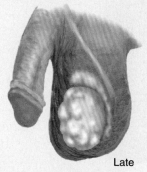

Late

Tumor of the Testis

Usually appears as a painless nodule. Any nodule within the testis warrants investigation for malignancy.

As a testicular neoplasm grows and spreads, it may seem to replace the entire organ. The testicle characteristically feels heavier than normal.

Table 13-4
Abnormalities of the Epididymis and Spermatic Cord

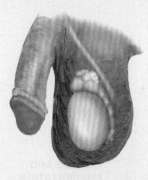

Spermatocele and Cyst of the Epididymis

A painless, movable cystic mass just above the testis suggests a spermatocele or an epididymal cyst. Both transilluminate. The former contains sperm, and the latter does not, but they are clinically indistinguishable.

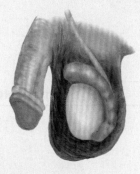

Acute Epididymitis

An acutely inflamed epididymis is tender and swollen and may be difficult to distinguish from the testis. The scrotum may be reddened and the vas deferens inflamed. It occurs chiefly in adults, most commonly with *Chlamydia* infection. Coexisting urinary tract infection or prostatitis supports the diagnosis.

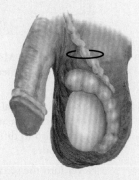

Tuberculous Epididymitis

The chronic inflammation of tuberculosis produces a firm enlargement of the epididymis, which is sometimes tender, with thickening or beading of the vas deferens.

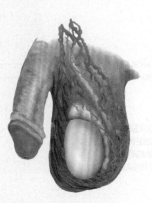

Varicocele of the Spermatic Cord

Varicocele refers to varicose veins of the spermatic cord, usually found on the left. It feels like a soft "bag of worms" separate from the testis, and slowly collapses when the scrotum is elevated in the supine patient. Infertility may be associated.

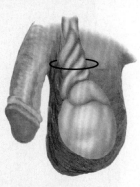

Torsion of the Spermatic Cord

Torsion, or twisting, of the testicle on its spermatic cord produces an acutely painful, tender, and swollen organ that is retracted upward in the scrotum. The scrotum becomes red and edematous. There is no associated urinary infection. Torsion, most common in adolescents, is a surgical emergency because of obstructed circulation.

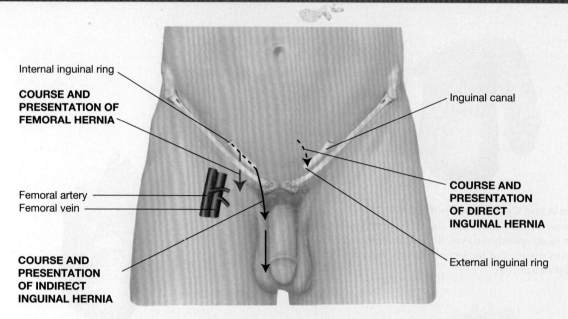

Inguinal Hernias

	Indirect	Direct	Femoral Hernias
Frequency, Age, and Sex	Most common, all ages, both sexes. Often in children; may be in adults	Less common. Usually in men older than 40; rare in women	Least common. More common in women than in men
Point of Origin	Above inguinal ligament, near its midpoint (the internal inguinal ring)	Above inguinal ligament, close to the pubic tubercle (near the external inguinal ring)	Below the inguinal ligament; appears more lateral than an inguinal hernia. Can be hard to differentiate from lymph nodes
Course	Often into the scrotum	Rarely into the scrotum	Never into the scrotum
(Examining finger in inguinal canal during straining)	The hernia comes down the inguinal canal and touches the fingertip.	The hernia bulges anteriorly and pushes the side of the finger forward.	The inguinal canal is empty.

Female Genitalia

Anatomy and Physiology

Review the anatomy of the external female genitalia, or *vulva*, including the *mons pubis*, a hair-covered fat pad overlying the symphysis pubis; the *labia majora*, rounded folds of adipose tissue; the *labia minora*, thinner pinkish-red folds that extend anteriorly to form the *prepuce*; and the *clitoris*. The *vestibule* is the boat-shaped fossa between the labia minora. In its posterior portion lies the vaginal opening, the *introitus*, which in virgins may be hidden by the *hymen*. The term *perineum* refers to the tissue between the introitus and the anus.

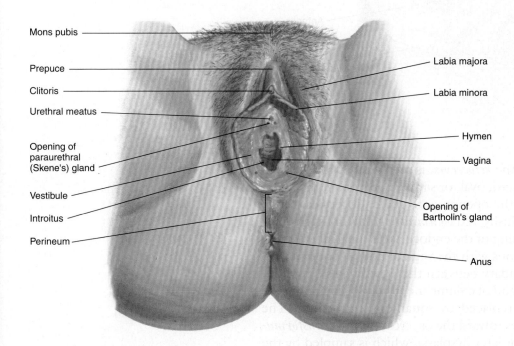

The *urethral meatus* opens into the vestibule between the clitoris and the vagina. Just posterior to it on either side lie the openings of the *paraurethral* (Skene's) *glands*.

The openings of *Bartholin's glands* are located posteriorly on either side of the vaginal opening but are not usually visible. Bartholin's glands themselves are situated more deeply.

The *vagina* is a musculomembranous tube extending upward and posteriorly between the urethra and the rectum. Its upper third lies at a horizontal plane and terminates in the cup-shaped *fornix*. The vaginal mucosa lies in transverse folds, or rugae.

The vagina lies almost at a right angle to the *uterus*, a flattened fibromuscular structure shaped like an inverted pear. The uterus has two parts: the body, or *corpus*, and the cervix, both joined at the *isthmus*. The convex upper surface of the body is termed the uterine *fundus*. The distal cervix protrudes into the vagina, dividing the upper vagina into three recesses, the *anterior*, *posterior*, and *lateral fornices*.

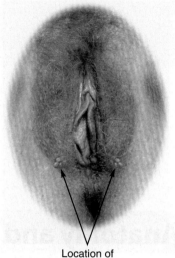

Location of
Bartholin's glands

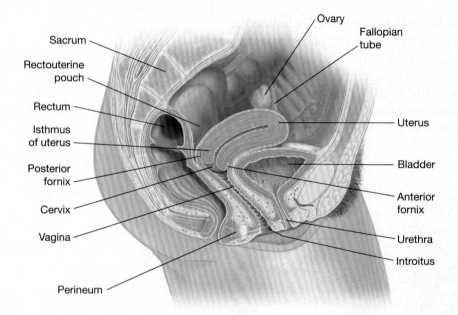

Sacrum

Rectouterine
pouch

Rectum

Isthmus
of uterus

Posterior
fornix

Cervix

Vagina

Perineum

Ovary

Fallopian
tube

Uterus

Bladder

Anterior
fornix

Urethra

Introitus

The vaginal surface of the cervix, the *ectocervix*, is seen easily with the help of a speculum. At its center is a round, oval, or slitlike depression, the *external os* of the cervix, which marks the opening into the endocervical canal. The ectocervix is covered by the plushy, red *columnar epithelium* surrounding the os, which resembles the lining of the endocervical canal, and a shiny pink *squamous epithelium* continuous with the vaginal lining. The *squamocolumnar junction* forms the boundary between these two types of epithelium. During puberty, the broad band of columnar epithelium encircling the os, called *ectropion*, is gradually replaced by squamous epithelium. The squamocolumnar junction migrates toward the os, creating the *transformation zone*. This is the area at risk for later dysplasia, which is sampled by the Papanicolaou, or Pap, smear.

A *fallopian tube* with a fanlike tip extends from each side of the uterus toward the ovary. The two ovaries are almond-shaped structures that vary considerably in size but average approximately $3.5 \times 2 \times 1.5$ cm from adulthood through menopause. The ovaries are palpable on pelvic examination in roughly half of women during the reproductive years. Normally, fallopian tubes cannot be felt. The term *adnexa*, a plural Latin word meaning appendages, refers to the ovaries, tubes, and supporting tissues.

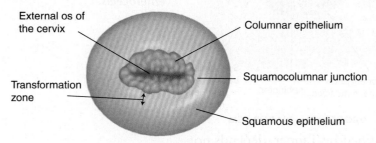

External os of the cervix

Columnar epithelium

Transformation zone

Squamocolumnar junction

Squamous epithelium

CERVICAL EPITHELIA AND TRANSFORMATION ZONE

The ovaries have two primary functions: the production of ova and the secretion of hormones, including estrogen, progesterone, and testosterone. Increased hormonal secretions during puberty stimulate the growth of the uterus and its endometrial lining, enlargement of the vagina, and thickening of the vaginal epithelium. They also stimulate the development of secondary sex characteristics, including the breasts and pubic hair.

The parietal peritoneum extends downward behind the uterus into a cul-de-sac called the *rectouterine pouch* (pouch of Douglas). You can just reach this area on rectovaginal examination.

The pelvic organs are supported by a sling of tissues composed of muscle, ligaments, and endopelvic fascia. The anatomy and innervation of these support structures are complex, but link to several common symptoms and conditions.[1,2] In brief, the pelvis contains two basins, as illustrated. The abdominal viscera reside in the broad major basin, which narrows to the inferior inlet of the basin of the minor pelvis. The *levator ani* and the *coccygeus muscles* attach to the inner surface of the minor pelvis and form the *pelvic*

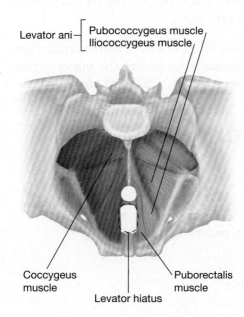

Levator ani — Pubococcygeus muscle
Iliococcygeus muscle

Coccygeus muscle

Levator hiatus

Puborectalis muscle

Weakness of the levator ani may cause sagging of the pelvic floor, widening the urogenital hiatus, and prolapse the pelvic organs.

diaphragm. The urethra, vagina, and anorectum pass through the keylike opening in the center of the pelvic diaphragm, the *urogenital (levator) hiatus.*

Below the pelvic diaphragm is the second supporting structure, the *urogenital diaphragm.* This diaphragm includes: the *ischiocavernosus and bulbocavernosus muscles,* which provide structural support for the distal urethra; the *perineal body* and *perineal membrane* anteriorly, just below the vagina and the uterus; and the *anal sphincter* posteriorly. These two diaphragms constitute the *pelvic floor.*

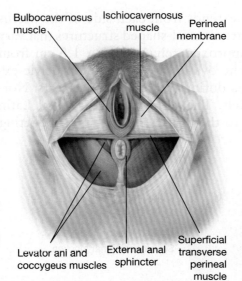

Bulbocavernosus muscle | Ischiocavernosus muscle | Perineal membrane

Levator ani and coccygeus muscles | External anal sphincter | Superficial transverse perineal muscle

UROGENITAL DIAPHRAGM

Loss of urethral support contributes to *stress incontinence.* Weakness of the perineal body from childbirth predisposes to *rectoceles* and *enteroceles.*

Assessment of sexual maturity in girls, as classified by Tanner, depends not on internal examination, but on the growth of pubic hair and the development of breasts. Tanner's stages, or sexual maturity ratings, as they relate to pubic hair and breasts are shown in Chapter 18, Assessing Children: Infancy Through Adolescence, pp. 864–867.

In most women, pubic hair spreads downward in a triangular pattern, pointing toward the vagina. In 10% of women, it may form an inverted triangle, pointing toward the umbilicus. This growth is usually not completed until the middle 20s or later.

Just before menarche, there is a physiologic increase in vaginal secretions—a normal change that sometimes worries a girl or her mother. As menses become established, increased secretions or *leukorrhea* coincide with ovulation. They also accompany sexual arousal. These normal discharges must be differentiated from those of infectious processes.

Lymphatics. Lymph from the vulva and lower vagina drains into the inguinal nodes. Lymph from the internal genitalia, including the upper vagina, flows into the pelvic and abdominal lymph nodes, which are not palpable.

The Health History

Common Concerns

> Menarche, menstruation, menopause, postmenopausal bleeding
> Pregnancy
> Vulvovaginal symptoms
> Sexual orientation and sexual response
> Pelvic pain—acute and chronic
> Sexually transmitted infections (STIs)

Menarche, Menstruation, Menopause.   Learn to recognize patterns of menstrual flow, using the terms below.

The Menstrual History—Helpful Definitions

▶ *Menarche*—age at onset of menses
▶ *Menopause*—absence of menses for 12 consecutive months, usually occurring between 48 and 55 years
▶ *Postmenopausal bleeding*—bleeding occurring 6 months or more after cessation of menses
▶ *Amenorrhea*—absence of menses
▶ *Dysmenorrhea*—pain with menses, often with bearing down, aching, or cramping sensation in the lower abdomen or pelvis
▶ *Premenstrual syndrome (PMS)*—a cluster of emotional, behavioral, and physical symptoms occurring 5 days before menses for three consecutive cycles
▶ *Abnormal uterine bleeding*—bleeding between menses; includes infrequent, excessive, prolonged, or postmenopausal bleeding

Questions about *menarche, menstruation,* and *menopause* often give you an opportunity to explore the patient's concerns and attitude about her body. When talking with an adolescent girl, for example, opening questions might include: "How did you first learn about monthly periods? How did you feel when they started? Many girls worry when their periods aren't regular or come late. Has anything like that bothered you?" You can explain that girls in the United States usually begin to menstruate between the ages of 9 and 16 years, and often it takes 1 year or more before periods settle into a reasonable, regular pattern. Age at menarche is variable, depending on genetic endowment, socioeconomic status, and nutrition. The interval between periods ranges roughly from 24 to 32 days; flow lasts from 3 to 7 days.

For the menstrual history, ask the patient how old she was when her menstrual periods began, or age at *menarche.* When did her *last menstrual period* (*LMP*) start, and, if possible, the one before that, termed *prior menstrual period,* or *PMP.* How often does she have periods, as measured by the interval between the first days of successive periods? How regular or irregular are they? How long do they last? How heavy is the flow? What color is it? Flow can be assessed roughly by the number of pads or tampons used daily. Because women vary in their practices for sanitary measures, however, ask the patient whether she usually soaks a pad or tampon, spots it lightly, etc. Further, does she use more than one at a time? Does she have any bleeding between periods? Any bleeding after intercourse?

Ask a middle-aged or older woman if she has stopped menstruating. When? Did any symptoms accompany her transition to menopause? Has she had any bleeding since?

The dates of previous periods can signal possible pregnancy or menstrual irregularities.

Unlike the normal dark red menstrual discharge, excessive flow tends to be bright red and may include "clots" (not true fibrin clots).

Up to 50% of women report *dysmenorrhea*, or pain with menses. Ask if the patient has any discomfort or pain before or during her periods. If so, what is it like, how long does it last, and does it interfere with usual activities? Are there other associated symptoms? Dysmenorrhea may be *primary*, without an organic cause, or *secondary*, with an organic cause.

Premenstrual syndrome (PMS) includes emotional and behavioral symptoms such as depression, angry outbursts, irritability, anxiety, confusion, crying spells, sleep disturbance, poor concentration, and social withdrawal.[3] Ask about signs such as bloating and weight gain, swelling of the hands and feet, and generalized aches and pains. Criteria for diagnosis are symptoms and signs in the 5 days prior to menses for at least three consecutive cycles; cessation of symptoms and signs within 4 days after onset of menses; and interference with daily activities.

Amenorrhea refers to the absence of periods. Absence of ever initiating periods is called *primary amenorrhea*; cessation of periods after they have been established is *secondary amenorrhea*. Pregnancy, lactation, and menopause are physiologic forms of the secondary type.

Ask about any abnormal bleeding. The term *abnormal uterine bleeding* encompasses several patterns.

Patterns of Abnormal Bleeding

▶ *Polymenorrhea*, or less than 21-day intervals between menses
▶ *Oligomenorrhea*, or infrequent bleeding
▶ *Menorrhagia*, or excessive flow
▶ *Metrorrhagia*, or intermenstrual bleeding
▶ Postcoital bleeding

Menopause typically occurs between the ages of 48 and 55, peaking at a median age of 51. It is defined retrospectively as cessation of menses for 12 months, progressing through several stages of erratic cyclical bleeding. These stages of variable cycle length, often with vasomotor symptoms like hot flashes, flushing, and sweating, represent *perimenopause*. The ovaries stop producing estradiol or progesterone and estrogen levels drop significantly, although some testosterone synthesis persists.[4,5] Pituitary secretion of luteinizing hormone and follicle-stimulating hormone levels gradually becomes markedly elevated. Low levels of estradiol remain detectable due to conversion of adrenal steroids in peripheral fat tissue.

Primary dysmenorrhea results from increased prostaglandin production during the luteal phase of the menstrual cycle, when estrogen and progesterone levels decline.

Causes of *secondary dysmenorrhea* include endometriosis, adenomyosis (endometriosis in the muscular layers of the uterus), pelvic inflammatory disease, and endometrial polyps.

Other causes of *secondary amenorrhea* include low body weight from any cause, including malnutrition and anorexia nervosa, stress, chronic illness, and hypothalamic–pituitary–ovarian dysfunction.

Causes vary by age group and include pregnancy, cervical or vaginal infection or cancer, cervical or endometrial polyps or hyperplasia, fibroids, bleeding disorders, and hormonal contraception or replacement therapy. *Postcoital bleeding* suggests cervical polyps or cancer, or, in an older woman, atrophic vaginitis.

Women may ask about alternative compounds and botanicals for relief of menopause-related symptoms. Most have not been well studied or proven to be beneficial. Estrogen replacement relieves symptoms but increases other health hazards (see p. 553).[6] Only a few medications have been shown to affect symptoms.[7]

During the menopausal transition, women may experience mood shifts, change in self-concept, hot flashes from vasomotor changes, accelerated bone loss, increases in total and LDL cholesterol, and vulvovaginal atrophy accompanied by symptoms such as vaginal drying, dysuria, and, at times, dyspareunia. Studies suggest that only vasomotor symptoms, vaginal symptoms, and trouble sleeping are consistently linked to menopause. Urinary symptoms may occur in the absence of infection, due to atrophy of the urethra and urinary trigone.

Often you will ask, "How do (did) you feel about not having your periods anymore? Has it affected your life in any way?" Ask about any bleeding after menopause.

Causes of *postmenopausal bleeding* include endometrial cancer, hormone replacement therapy, and uterine and cervical polyps.

Pregnancy. Questions relating to pregnancy include "Have you ever been pregnant? How many times? ... How many living children do you have? ... Have you ever had a miscarriage or an abortion? How many times?" Ask about any difficulties during pregnancy and the timing and circumstances of any abortion, whether spontaneous or induced. How did the woman experience these losses? Obstetricians commonly record the pregnancy history using the "gravida para" system.

The Gravida Para Notation

▶ G = gravida, or total number of pregnancies
▶ P = para, or outcomes of pregnancies. After P, you will often see the notations F (full-term), P (premature), A (abortion), and L (living child).

Inquire about methods of contraception used by the patient and her partner. Is the patient satisfied with the method chosen? Are there any questions about the options available?

If amenorrhea suggests a *current pregnancy*, inquire about the history of intercourse and *common early symptoms:* tenderness, tingling, or increased size of the breasts; urinary frequency; nausea and vomiting; easy fatigability; and feelings that the baby is moving, usually noted at about 20 weeks. Be sensitive to the patient's feelings about these topics; explore them when the patient has special concerns. (See also Chapter 19, The Pregnant Woman, p. 893.)

Amenorrhea followed by heavy bleeding suggests a *threatened abortion* or *dysfunctional uterine bleeding* related to lack of ovulation.

Vulvovaginal Symptoms. The most common vulvovaginal symptoms are *vaginal discharge* and local *itching.* Follow your usual approach. If the patient reports a discharge, inquire about its amount, color, consistency, and odor. Ask about any local *sores* or *lumps* in the vulvar area. Are they painful or not? Because patients vary in their understanding of anatomical terms, be prepared to try alternative phrasing such as "Any itching (or other symptoms) near your vagina? ... between your legs? ... where you urinate?"

See Table 14-1, Lesions of the Vulva, p. 568; and Table 14-2, Vaginal Discharge, p. 569.

Sexual Orientation and Sexual Response

Sexual Orientation.   Patients immediately sense your receptiveness to their concerns in this sensitive and vital area of their health. Using neutral and nonjudgmental questions, ask "What is your relationship status?" or "Tell me about your sexual preference, if it is men, women, or both?" For those who are uncertain, ask about their feelings of sexual attraction. About 4% to 7% of women report they are lesbian or bisexual; some may be transgender. They may be anxious or fearful during clinical encounters. Probe existing resources to learn about their health issues. An informed and neutral manner will help your patients to express their concerns more openly.[8–15]

Sexual Response.   Start with general questions such as "How is sex for you?" Or "Are you having any problems with sex?" You can also ask, "Are you satisfied with your sex life as it is now? Has there been any significant change in the last few years? Are you satisfied with your ability to perform sexually? How satisfied do you think your partner is? Do you feel that your partner is satisfied with the frequency of sexual activity?"

If the patient has concerns about sexual activity, ask her to tell you about it. Direct questions help you assess each phase of the sexual response: desire, arousal, and orgasm. "Do you have an interest in (appetite for) sex?" inquires about the desire phase. For the orgasmic phase, "Are you able to reach climax (reach an orgasm or 'come')?" "Is it important for you to reach climax?" For arousal, "Do you get sexually aroused? Do you lubricate easily (get wet or slippery)? Do you stay too dry?"

Ask also about *dyspareunia,* or pain with intercourse. If present, try to localize the symptom. Is it near the outside, occurring at the start of intercourse, or does she feel it farther in, when her partner is pushing deeper? *Vaginismus* refers to an involuntary spasm of the muscles surrounding the vaginal orifice that makes penetration during intercourse painful or impossible.

In addition to ascertaining the nature of a sexual problem, ask about its onset, severity (persistent or sporadic), setting, and factors, if any, that make it better or worse. What does the patient think is the cause of the problem, what has she tried to do about it, and what does she hope for? The setting of sexual dysfunction is an important but complicated topic, involving the patient's general health; medications and drugs, including use of alcohol; her partner's and her own knowledge of sexual practices and techniques; her attitudes, values, and fears; the relationship and communication between partners; and the setting in which sexual activity takes place.

See also The Sexual History in Chapter 3, pp. 86–87, and Tips for Taking a Sexual History and the discussion on gay, lesbian, and transgender health in Chapter 13, p. 522.

Sexual dysfunction is classified by the phase of sexual response. A woman may lack desire; she may fail to become aroused and attain adequate vaginal lubrication; or, despite adequate arousal, she may be unable to reach orgasm. Causes include lack of estrogen, medical illness, and psychiatric conditions.

Superficial pain suggests local inflammation, atrophic vaginitis, or inadequate lubrication; deeper pain may be from pelvic disorders or pressure on a normal ovary. The cause of *vaginismus* may be physical or psychological.

More commonly, however, a sexual problem is related to situational or psychosocial factors.

Pelvic Pain—Acute and Chronic.   Many women volunteer a history of pelvic pain. *Acute pelvic pain* in menstruating girls and women warrants immediate attention. The differential diagnosis is broad but includes such life-threatening conditions as *ectopic pregnancy*, *ovarian torsion*, and *appendicitis*. As you gather the history of the onset, timing, features of the pain, and associated symptoms, you will need to consider infectious, gastrointestinal, and urinary causes. Be sure to ask about sexually transmitted infections, recent insertion of an intra-uterine device (IUD), and any symptoms in the sexual partner. A careful pelvic examination, with attention to vital signs, and testing for pregnancy will help you narrow your diagnosis and guide further testing.

The most common cause of acute pelvic pain is *pelvic inflammatory disease (PID)*, followed by *ruptured ovarian cyst*, and *appendicitis*.[16] STIs and recent IUD insertion are red flags for PID. Always rule out *ectopic pregnancy* first with serum or urine testing.

Also consider *mittelschmerz*, or pain from ovulation at midcycle, *ruptured ovarian cyst*, and *tubo-ovarian abscess*.

Chronic pelvic pain refers to pain that lasts more than six months and does not respond to treatment.[17] It accounts for approximately 10% of ambulatory referrals to gynecologists and approximately 20% of hysterectomies.[18,19] Determining the cause may take time since gynecologic, urologic, gastrointestinal, and musculoskeletal conditions all need to be considered. The Pelvic Pain Assessment Form of the International Pelvic Pain Society, which includes screening questions for depression and physical and sexual abuse, as well as a pain map that women complete, may be helpful.[20] Asking the woman to keep a daily pain journal may also be useful.

Endometriosis, from retrograde menstrual flow and extension of the uterine lining outside the uterus, affects 50% to 60% of women and girls with pelvic pain.[21] Other causes include *adenosis* and *fibroids*, from tumors in the uterine wall or submucosal or subserosal surfaces arising from the smooth muscle cells of the myometrium. Chronic pelvic pain is a red flag for a history of *sexual abuse*. Also consider *pelvic floor spasm* from myofascial pain with trigger points on examination (see p. 562).

Sexually Transmitted Infections (STIs).   Local symptoms or findings on physical examination may raise the possibility of *sexually transmitted infections* (also referred to as *sexually transmitted diseases [STDs]*). After establishing the usual attributes of any symptoms, identify sexual orientation (male, female, or both). Inquire about sexual contacts and establish the number of sexual partners in the prior month. Ask if the patient has concerns about HIV infection, desires HIV testing, or has current or past partners at risk. Also ask about oral and anal sex and, if indicated, about symptoms involving the mouth, throat, anus, and rectum. Review the past history of venereal disease. "Have you ever had herpes? ... any other problems such as gonorrhea? ... syphilis? ... pelvic infections?" Continue with the more general questions suggested on pp. 86–87.

Health Promotion and Counseling: Evidence and Recommendations

Important Topics for Health Promotion and Counseling

▶ Cervical cancer screening: Pap smear and HPV infection
▶ Ovarian cancer: symptoms and risk factors
▶ Sexually transmitted infections and HIV
▶ Options for family planning
▶ Menopause and hormone replacement therapy

Cervical Cancer Screening: The Pap Smear and Human Papillomavirus (HPV) Infection. Widespread screening by *Papanicolaou (Pap) smear* has contributed to a significant decline in the incidence of and mortality from cervical cancer. The U.S. Preventive Services Task Force notes that "the goal of cytologic screening is to sample the transformation zone, the area where physiologic transformation from columnar endocervical epithelium to squamous (ectocervical) epithelium takes place and where dysplasia and cancer arise."[22] There are two primary types of cervical cancer. Approximately 80% to 90% are squamous cell carcinomas; the remaining 10% to 20% are adenocarcinomas in glandular cells.

Risk factors for cervical cancer are both viral and behavioral. Genital HPV infection is the most common STI in the United States.[23] Approximately 15% of the population, or 20 million Americans, are currently infected, including 50% to 80% of sexually active teenage girls and young women.[24] Over 90% of genital HPV infections are cleared by the immune system in 1 to 2 years. HPV infection with high-risk, or oncogenic, subtypes is found in virtually all cervical cancers. The most important risk factor for cervical cancer is *persistent infection with high-risk HPV subtypes*, especially HPV 16 or HPV 18. These two subtypes alone cause roughly 70% of cervical cancers, usually over the course of many years.[23,25] Even the 10% of women with persistent infection rarely progress to cervical cancer if they get regular screening that promotes early detection and treatment. Genital infection with low-risk subtypes, such as HPV 6 and HPV 11, is associated with genital warts.

Two notable risk factors for cervical cancer include *failure to undergo screening*, which accounts for roughly half of women diagnosed with cervical cancer, and *multiple sexual partners*. Other risk factors include smoking, immunosuppression from any cause including HIV infection, long-term use of oral contraception, coinfection with *Chlamydia*, parity, prior cervical cancer, and genetic polymorphisms affecting the entry of HPV DNA into cervical cells.[22]

New Pap Smear Screening Guidelines. The American College of Obstetricians and Gynecologists (ACOG) issued new guidelines in March 2012 recommending increasing the screening intervals for women ages 21 to 65 and ending screening at age 65. These recommendations reflect scientific advances in understanding how persistent HPV infection leads to cervical cancer. The ACOG guidelines have been widely adopted, and conform closely to those of the American Cancer Society and the U.S. Preventive Services Task Force.[22,26] These guidelines underscore the importance of carefully reviewing each woman's Pap smear history. Further, for clinicians to safely extend screening intervals, women need to know their recent Pap smear results, particularly if they change from one clinician to another.

Cervical Cancer Screening Guidelines: ACOG 2009[27]

First screen	Begin screening at age 21. *Rationale:* high rates of clearance of HPV infection; low incidence of cervical cancer; avoids unnecessary procedures that could affect cervical competence and childbearing.
Women ages 21–29	Screen every 3 years with cytology. Can use either liquid-based or conventional cytology. *Rationale:* detection rates comparable to annual screening.
Women ages 30–65	Screen every 3 years with cytology if three consecutive negative screening tests, no history of invasive carcinoma from CIN 2 or CIN 3, and no risk factors such as HIV infection, immunocompromise, or exposure in utero to diethylstilbestrol (DES) or with cytology and HPV testing every 5 years. *Rationale:* low risk of cervical cancer if three prior screening tests documented as negative, especially if co-testing with both cytology and high-risk HPV DNA is negative.
Women with hysterectomy	Discontinue screening *if hysterectomy for benign indications* and no prior history of high-grade CIN. *Rationale:* very low risk of vaginal cancer. *If hysterectomy for CIN2, CIN3, or cancer and cervix removed,* continue annual screening for 20 years after postsurveillance period. *Rationale:* risk still present for persistent or recurrent disease.
Women ages ≥65	Discontinue screening if three or more negative cytology tests in a row and no abnormal test results in the past 20 years. *Rationale:* low risk of cervical cancer because cervical cancer develops slowly and risk factors decrease with age.

Take the time to understand how Pap smear results are reported. Current classification and management guidelines are based on the Bethesda System of the National Cancer Institute, revised in 2001.[28,29] The principal categories are provided below. Management depends on the cervical cancer risk and often involves repeat cytology, colposcopy, and DNA testing for HPV.

Conventional Pap smears have a sensitivity and specificity for detecting cervical cancer of 30% to 87% and 86% to 100%, respectively. For liquid-based cytology these figures are 61% to 95% and 78% to 82%.[23]

Classification of Pap Smear Cytology: The Bethesda System (2001)

▸ *Negative for intraepithelial lesion or malignancy:* No cellular evidence of neoplasia is present, although other organisms like *Trichomonas, Candida,* or *Actinomyces* may be reported in this category. Shifts in flora consistent with bacterial vaginosis or cellular changes from herpes simplex may also be reported.

▸ *Epithelial cell abnormalities:* These include precancerous or cancerous lesions:

  ▸ *Squamous cells,* including *atypical squamous cells* (ASC), which may be of undetermined significance (ASC-US); *low-grade squamous intraepithelial lesions* (LSIL), including mild dysplasia; *high-grade squamous intraepithelial lesions* (HSIL), including moderate and severe dysplasia with features suspicious for invasion; and invasive *squamous cell carcinoma.*

  ▸ *Glandular cells,* including *atypical endocervical cells* or *atypical endometrial cells,* specified or not otherwise specified (NOS); *atypical endocervical cells* or *atypical glandular cells, favor neoplastic; endocervical adenocarcinoma in situ;* and *adenocarcinoma*

▸ *Other malignant neoplasms,* such as sarcomas or lymphomas, both rare

The HPV Vaccine. In 2007, the Centers for Disease Control and Prevention[23,30] recommended routine vaccination of *girls before their first sexual contact* places them at risk for exposure to HPV, usually at ages 11 or 12 but possibly starting at age 9. The quadrivalent vaccine Gardasil, given in a three-dose series, targets HPV 16, 18, 6, and 11 and prevents most cases of cervical cancer.[31] The vaccine also reduces risk of anogenital warts, invasive anogenital cancers, and vulvar and vaginal cancers.[31,32]

American adolescents initiate sexual activity early: 8% before age 13; 33% by ninth grade, and 66% by the end of high school.[33] *Catch-up vaccination* is recommended for girls and women ages 13 to 26 if they have not had all three doses. The vaccine is still highly effective for girls and women who are already sexually active.[24]

Vaccinated women should still get pelvic examinations and Pap smear screening to assess infection or cervical cellular changes from other oncogenic HPV subtypes. Consistent use of condoms does not eliminate risk of cervical HPV infection.[34]

Gardasil vaccination is also recommended for *boys and men ages 9 through 26,* ideally before their first sexual contact, since it prevents genital warts. The bivalent vaccine, which targets only HPV 16 and 18, is not recommended for boys and men.

Ovarian Cancer: Symptoms and Risk Factors. Many women remain fearful of ovarian cancer. Although ovarian cancer is relatively rare, it is the fifth leading cause of cancer-related death for women.[35] Two-thirds of women affected are over age 55; most are diagnosed when the disease is already metastatic to the peritoneal cavity or other organs. Five-year survival in these women is only 25%, compared to 80% to 90% for those with early stage disease.[36] Currently there are no effective screening tests, so clinicians face the challenge of improving identification of symptoms. In women over 50, *three symptoms* merit special attention: abdominal distention, abdominal bloating, and urinary frequency, however these are usually reported within 3 months of diagnosis, and frequently occur in other conditions.[36]

Risk factors for ovarian cancer include family history and presence of the BRCA1 or BRCA2 gene mutation. Risk is tripled if there is a first-degree relative with breast or ovarian cancer. Carriers of BRCA1 and BRCA2 have a lifetime risk of 39% to 46% and 12% to 20%, respectively.[35] Over 90% of ovarian cancers appear to be random. Risk is decreased by use of oral contraceptives, pregnancy, and a history of breast-feeding.

Women frequently ask about *CA-125* testing. The CA-125 level is neither sensitive nor specific.[35] Although CA-125 is elevated in more than 80% of women with ovarian cancer and helps predict relapse after treatment, it is also elevated in many other conditions and cancers, including pregnancy, endometriosis, uterine fibroids, pelvic inflammatory disease, benign cysts, and pancreatic, beast, lung, gastric, and colon cancer. Current investigations of combined screening with CA-125, transvaginal ultrasound, and selected tumor markers have not demonstrated benefits that improve survival.

STIs and HIV Infection. U.S. rates of STIs are the highest in the industrialized world. *Chlamydia trachomatis* is the most commonly reported STI in the United States and the most common STI in women.[37,38] Most women are asymptomatic and infection remains undiagnosed. If untreated, 40% of women will develop pelvic inflammatory disease (PID) and 20% will become infertile. Prevalence is highest in women ages 15 to 19, closely followed by women ages 20 to 24. African American women and American Indian/Alaskan natives are at highest risk for infection. As with other STIs, risk factors are: age less than 24 and sexually active; prior infection with *Chlamydia* or other STIs, new or multiple partners, inconsistent condom use, and occupational sex work. Detection, groups most affected, and consequences of underdiagnosis and treatment are similar for *gonorrhea*. Infection with *syphilis* is less common, but increasing in women.[39,40]

To improve detection and treatment, the CDC and the U.S. Preventive Services Task Force strongly recommend:

- Annual screening for cervical *Chlamydia* in all sexually active and pregnant women age 26 and younger and in older women at increased risk

- Screening these groups for *Chlamydia* whenever Pap smears are done, or using nucleic acid amplification urine tests for *Chlamydia* and *gonorrhea*, which are equally sensitive and less invasive

- Routine screening for *syphilis* of all sexually active women at increased risk and of all pregnant women

- Routine screening for *gonorrhea* of sexually active women and pregnant women who are at increased risk

In the United States, *HIV and AIDS infection* rates are increasing fastest in women, who now account for 25% of all cases.[41] Transmission in women is primarily heterosexual. Among infected women, 60% are African American, 20% are Latina, and 17% are Caucasian. Heterosexual transmission is more likely in the following settings: infected partner with high viral load of HIV-1; cervical ectopy; sex during menstruation; and male partner without circumcision. Recurrent vulvocandidiasis, concurrent STIs, abnormal Pap smears (occurring in 40% of HIV-positive women), and HPV infections are warnings for testing for HIV. In 2006, the CDC published new guidelines recommending *universal HIV testing for everyone in the age range of 13 to 64*, because many infections occur in people without known risk factors.[42] This recommendation was affirmed by the U.S. Preventive Services Task Force in its updated recommendations of 2007.[43] Of the estimated 1 million persons living in the United States with HIV/AIDS, roughly 25% have undiagnosed disease and are unaware of their infection, and 10% to 25% of people testing positive do not report high-risk behaviors.[44]

As with men, clinicians should assess risk factors for STIs and HIV infection by taking a careful sexual history and counseling patients about spread of disease and how to reduce high-risk practices. Key to effective clinician counseling are respect, compassion, a nonjudgmental attitude, and use of open-ended and understandable questions such as "Tell me about any new sex partners" and "Have you ever had anal sex, meaning 'penis in rectum/anus sex'?" The CDC recommends interactive client-centered counseling, tailored to the person's specific risk factors and situation. Training in prevention counseling improves effectiveness. You can begin at the excellent Web sites recommended by the CDC such as http://effectiveinterventions.org or http://depts.washington.edu/nnptc/.

See Chapter 3, Interviewing and the Health History, pp. 86–87, on eliciting the sexual history, and Chapter 13, Male Genitalia and Hernias, pp. 524–526, on risk factors for HIV infection.

Options for Family Planning. More than half of U.S. pregnancies are unintended.[45] Among pregnancies in teens ages 18 years and younger, this number climbs to over 65%.[46] It is important to counsel girls and women about the timing of ovulation in the menstrual cycle and how to plan or prevent pregnancy. Clinicians should be familiar with the numerous options for contraception and their effectiveness. These include natural methods (periodic abstinence, withdrawal, lactation); barrier methods (condom, diaphragm, cervical cap); implantable methods (intrauterine device, subdermal implant); pharmacologic interventions (spermicide, birth control pill, subdermal implant of levonorgestrel, estrogen/progesterone injectables and patch, vaginal ring); and surgery (tubal ligation; transcervical sterilization). Take the time to understand the patient or couple's concerns and preferences, and respect these preferences whenever possible. Continued use of a preferred method is superior to a more effective method that is abandoned. For teenagers, a confidential setting eases discussion of topics that may seem private and difficult to explore.

Menopause and Hormone Replacement Therapy (HRT). For many women, menopause is a profound transition, evoking a gamut of responses and a series of physiologic changes ranging from mood shifts to hot flashes to vaginal drying and bone loss. Be informed about the *risks and benefits of hormone replacement therapy* with estrogen and progesterone, a topic women ask about frequently. Three major randomized trials since 1998, all with disease-event outcomes, have shown that HRT poses increased risk of stroke and pulmonary embolism, and no benefit or increased risk of coronary events.[47–50] The coronary risk may diminish 3 years after stopping HRT.[51] Two of the three trials reported a 25% increase in risk of breast cancer. [47,48,51] A recent follow-up study of postmenopausal women taking combined estrogen and progesterone in the Women's Health Initiative (WHI) series showed a 25% increased risk of invasive breast cancer, an increased risk of breast cancers presenting with positive lymph nodes, and increased breast cancer mortality.[52] The WHI Memory Study found a twofold increase in risk of dementia in older users of HRT.[53] These risks arise primarily from estrogen effects. Although risks of hip fracture and colon cancer decline, ACOG, the North American Menopause Society, and the U.S. Preventive Services Task Force advise using HRT only for menopausal symptoms and at minimal doses, for the shortest acceptable duration, usually in the range of 1 to 2 years.[6,54–56]

Techniques of Examination

Important Areas of Examination

External Examination	Internal Examination
▶ Mons pubis	▶ Vagina, vaginal walls
▶ Labia majora and minora	▶ Cervix
▶ Urethral meatus, clitoris	▶ Uterus, ovaries
▶ Vaginal introitus	▶ Pelvic muscles
▶ Perineum	▶ Rectovaginal wall

Approach to the Pelvic Examination. Many students feel uneasy or uncomfortable when doing their first pelvic examinations. At the same time, patients have their own concerns. Some women have had painful, embarrassing, or even demeaning experiences during previous examinations; others may be facing a pelvic examination for the first time. Some fear what the clinician may find, and how findings may affect their lives. Asking the patient's permission to perform the examination shows courtesy and respect.

If a Pap smear is to be collected using the glass-slide technique, time the examination so that it does not occur during menses, because blood can interfere with interpretation.

In liquid-based cytology, blood cells can be filtered out.[57]

A woman having her first pelvic examination may not know what to expect. Using three-dimensional models, showing her the equipment, letting her handle the speculum, and explaining each step in advance can help her to learn about her body and be more comfortable. A careful, gentle technique is especially important for minimizing any pain or discomfort.

The woman's response to the pelvic examination may reveal clues about her feelings about the examination and her sexuality. If she pulls away, adducts her thighs, or reacts negatively to the examination, you can gently comment, "I notice you are having some trouble relaxing. Is it just being here, or are you troubled by the examination? . . . Is anything worrying you?" Behaviors that seem to present an obstacle may lead you to a better understanding of your patient's concerns. Adverse reactions may signal prior physical or sexual abuse and should be explored.[58]

Indications for a pelvic examination during adolescence include menstrual abnormalities such as amenorrhea, excessive bleeding, or dysmenorrhea; unexplained abdominal pain; vaginal discharge; the prescription of contraceptives; bacteriologic and cytologic studies in a sexually active girl; and the patient's own desire for assessment.

See Chapter 18, Assessing Children: Infancy Through Adolescence.

Tips for the Successful Pelvic Examination

The Patient	The Examiner
▸ Avoids intercourse, douching, or use of vaginal suppositories for 24 to 48 hours before examination	▸ Obtains permission; selects chaperone
▸ Empties bladder before examination	▸ Explains each step of the examination in advance
▸ Lies supine, with head and shoulders elevated, arms at sides or folded across chest to enhance eye contact and reduce tightening of abdominal muscles	▸ Drapes patient from midabdomen to knees; depresses drape between knees to provide eye contact with patient
	▸ Avoids unexpected or sudden movements
	▸ Chooses a speculum that is the correct size
	▸ Warms speculum with tap water
	▸ Monitors comfort of the examination by watching the patient's face
	▸ Uses excellent but gentle technique, especially when inserting the speculum (see next page)

Helping the patient to relax is essential for an adequate examination. Adopting the tips recommended helps ensure the patient's comfort. Be sure always to *wear gloves*, both during the examination and when handling equipment and specimens. Plan ahead, so that any needed equipment and culture media are readily at hand.

Note that male examiners should be accompanied by female chaperones. Female examiners should also be assisted if the patient is physically or emotionally disturbed, or to otherwise facilitate the examination.

Rape Victims. Cases of *rape* merit special evaluation, and usually require gynecologic consultation and documentation. Often there is a special rape kit, provided in many emergency departments, that must be used to ensure a chain of custody for evidence. Specimens must be labeled carefully with name, date, and time. Additional information may be needed for further legal investigation.

Choosing Equipment. You should have within reach a good light, a vaginal speculum of appropriate size, water-soluble lubricant, and equipment for taking Pap smears, bacteriologic cultures and DNA probes, or other diagnostic testing materials, such as potassium hydroxide and normal saline. Review the supplies and procedures of your own facility before taking cultures and other samples.

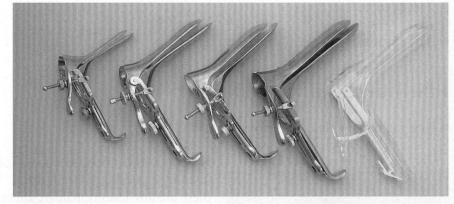

Specula are made of metal or plastic and come in two basic shapes, named for Pedersen and Graves. Both are available in small, medium, and large sizes. The medium Pedersen speculum is usually most comfortable for sexually active women. The narrow-bladed Pedersen speculum is best for the patient with a relatively small introitus, such as a virgin or an elderly woman. The Graves specula are best suited for parous women with vaginal prolapse.

Before using a speculum, be sure you know how to open and close its blades, lock the blades in an open position, and release them again. Although the instructions in this chapter refer to a metal speculum, you can easily adapt them to a plastic speculum by handling it before use.

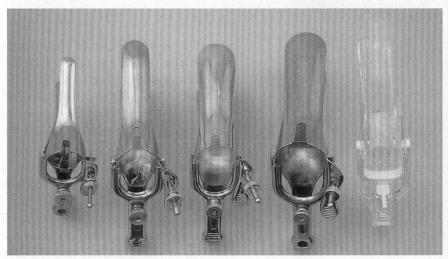

Plastic specula typically make a loud click or may pinch when locked or released. Forewarn the patient to avoid unnecessary surprise.

SPECULA, FROM LEFT TO RIGHT: SMALL METAL PEDERSEN, MEDIUM METAL PEDERSEN, MEDIUM METAL GRAVES, LARGE METAL GRAVES, AND LARGE PLASTIC PEDERSEN

Positioning the Patient. Drape the patient appropriately and then assist her into the lithotomy position. Help her to place first one heel and then the other into the stirrups. She may be more comfortable with shoes on than with bare feet. Then ask her to slide all the way down the examining table until her buttocks extend slightly beyond the edge. Her thighs should be flexed, abducted, and externally rotated at the hips. Support her head with a pillow.

EXTERNAL EXAMINATION

Assess the Sexual Maturity of an Adolescent Patient. You can assess pubic hair during either the abdominal or the pelvic examination. Note its character and distribution, and rate it according to Tanner's stages, described on p. 867.

Delayed puberty is often familial or related to chronic illness. It may also arise from abnormal function of the hypothalamus, anterior pituitary gland, or ovaries.

Examine the External Genitalia. Seat yourself comfortably and warn the patient that you will be touching her genital area. Inspect the mons pubis, labia, and perineum. Separate the labia and inspect:

Excoriations or itchy, small, red maculopapules suggest *pediculosis pubis* (lice or "crabs"). Look for nits or lice at the bases of the pubic hairs.

- The labia minora

- The clitoris

Enlarged clitoris is seen in masculinizing conditions.

- The urethral meatus

Observe for *urethral caruncle, prolapse of the urethral mucosa* (p. 570); tenderness in interstitial cystitis

- The vaginal opening, or introitus

Note any inflammation, ulceration, discharge, swelling, or nodules. If there are any lesions, palpate them.

For descriptions of *Herpes simplex, Behçet's disease, syphilitic chancre,* and *epidermoid cyst,* see Table 14-1, Lesions of the Vulva, p. 568.

If there is a history or an appearance of labial swelling, check *Bartholin's glands.* Insert your index finger into the vagina near the posterior end of the introitus. Place your thumb outside the posterior part of the labium majus. Palpate each side in turn, at approximately the "4-o'clock" and "8-o'clock" positions, between your finger and thumb, checking for swelling or tenderness. Note any discharge exuding from the duct opening of the gland. If any is present, culture it.

A *Bartholin's gland* may become acutely or chronically infected and then produce a swelling. See Table 14-3, Bulges and Swelling of the Vulva, Vagina, and Urethra, p. 570.

PALPATING BARTHOLIN'S GLAND

INTERNAL EXAMINATION

Insert the Speculum. Select a speculum of appropriate size and shape, and moisten it with warm, but not hot, water. (Lubricants or gels may interfere with cytologic studies and bacterial or viral cultures.) *Let the patient know when you are about to insert the speculum and apply downward pressure.* You can enlarge the vaginal introitus by lubricating one finger with water and applying downward pressure at its lower margin. Check the location of the cervix to help angle the speculum more accurately. Enlarging the introitus greatly eases insertion of the speculum and the patient's comfort. With your other hand (usually the left), introduce the closed speculum past your fingers at a somewhat downward slope. Be careful not to pull on the pubic hair or pinch the labia with the speculum. Separating the labia majora with your other hand can help to avoid this.

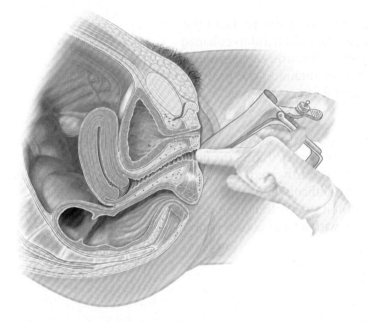

The Small Introitus

Many virginal vaginal orifices admit a single examining finger. Modify your technique so as to use your index finger only. A small Pedersen speculum may make inspection possible. When the vaginal orifice is even smaller, an adequate bimanual examination can be performed by placing one finger in the rectum rather than in the vagina, but warn the patient first!

Similar techniques may be indicated in elderly women if the introitus has become atrophied and tight.

An *imperforate hymen* occasionally delays menarche. Be sure to check for this possibility when menarche seems unduly late in relation to the development of a girl's breasts and pubic hair.

Two methods help you to avoid placing pressure on the sensitive urethra. (1) When inserting the speculum, hold it at an angle (see photo), and then

(2) slide the speculum inward along the posterior wall of the vagina, applying downward pressure to keep the vaginal introitus relaxed.

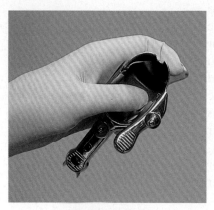

ENTRY ANGLE

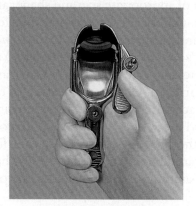

ANGLE AT FULL INSERTION

After the speculum has entered the vagina, remove your fingers from the introitus. You may wish to switch the speculum to the right hand to enhance maneuverability of the speculum and subsequent collection of specimens. Rotate the speculum into a horizontal position, maintaining the pressure posteriorly, and insert it to its full length. Be careful not to open the blades of the speculum prematurely.

Inspect the Cervix. Open the speculum carefully. Rotate and adjust the speculum until it cups the cervix and brings it into full view. Position the light until you can see the cervix well. When the uterus is retroverted, the cervix points more anteriorly than illustrated. If you have difficulty finding the cervix, withdraw the speculum slightly and reposition it on a different slope. If discharge obscures your view, wipe it away gently with a large cotton swab.

See retroversion of the uterus, p. 573.

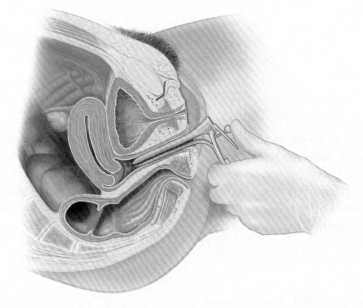

See Table 14-4, Variations in the Cervical Surface, p. 571; Table 14-5, Shapes of the Cervical Os, p. 572; and Table 14-6, Abnormalities of the Cervix, p. 572.

Note the color of the cervix, its position, the characteristics of its surface, and any ulcerations, nodules, masses, bleeding, or discharge. Inspect the cervical os for discharge.

Look for lateral displacement of the cervix in *endometriosis* involving the uterosacral ligaments.

Maintain the open position of the speculum by tightening the thumb-screw.

A yellowish discharge on the endo-cervical swab suggests mucopuru-lent cervicitis, commonly caused by *Chlamydia trachomatis, Neisseria gonorrhoeae,* or *herpes simplex* (p. 572). Raised, friable, or lobed wartlike lesions occur in *condylomata* or *cervical cancer.*

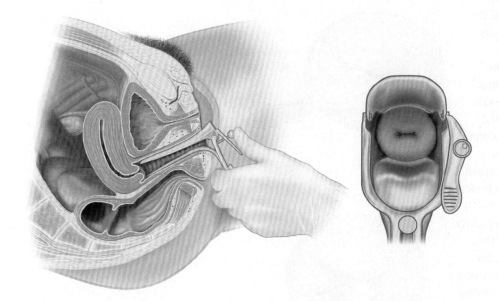

Obtain Specimens for Cervical Cytology (Pap Smears).

Obtain one specimen from the endocervix and another from the ectocer-vix, or a combination specimen using the cervical brush ("broom"). For best results the patient should not be menstruating. She should avoid intercourse and use of douches, tampons, contraceptive foams or creams, or vaginal suppositories for 48 hours before the examination. For sexually active women age 26 or younger, and for other asymptomatic women at increased risk for infection, plan to culture the cervix routinely for *Chlamydia trachomatis.*[37]

Chlamydial infection is linked to urethritis, cervicitis, pelvic inflam-matory disease, ectopic pregnancy, infertility, and chronic pelvic pain. Risk factors include age younger than 26, multiple partners, and prior history of STIs.

Obtaining the Pap Smear: Options for Specimen Collection

Cervical Broom
Many clinicians use a plastic brush tipped with a broomlike fringe for collection of a single specimen containing both squamous and columnar epithelial cells. Rotate the tip of the brush in the cervical os, in a full clock-wise direction, then place the sample directly into preservative so that the labora-tory can prepare the slide (liquid-based cytology).

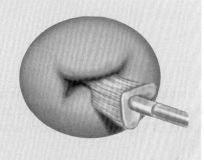

Use of the cervical broom and liquid-based cytology is increas-ingly common, and can also be used to test for *Chlamydia* and *gonorrhea.*

   Alternatively, stroke each side of the brush on the glass slide. Promptly place the slide in solution or spray with a fixative as described below.

(continued)

Obtaining the Pap Smear: Options for Specimen Collection (*continued*)

Cervical Scrape and Endocervical Brush
Cervical Scrape. Place the longer end of the scraper in the cervical os. Press, turn, and scrape in a full circle, making sure to include the *transformation zone* and the *squamocolumnar junction.* Smear the specimen on a glass slide. Set the slide in a safe spot that is easy to reach. Note that first doing the cervical scrape reduces obscuring the cells with blood, which sometimes appears after use of the endocervical brush.

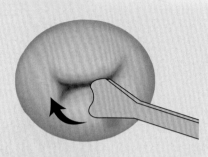

    Endocervical Brush. Take the endocervical brush and place it in the cervical os. Roll it between your thumb and index finger, clockwise and counterclockwise. Remove the brush and pick up the slide you have set aside. Smear the slide with the brush, using a gentle painting motion to avoid destroying any cells. Place the slide into an ether–alcohol solution at once, or spray it promptly with a special fixative.

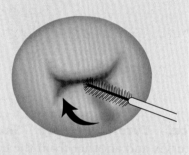

    Note that for pregnant women, a cotton-tipped applicator, moistened with saline, is advised in place of the endocervical brush.

Inspect the Vagina. Withdraw the speculum slowly while observing the vagina. As the speculum clears the cervix, release the thumbscrew and maintain the open position of the speculum with your thumb. During withdrawal, inspect the vaginal mucosa, noting its color and any inflammation, discharge, ulcers, or masses.

See Table 14-2, Vaginal Discharge, p. 569.

Vaginitis with discharge can result from *Candida, Trichomonas vaginalis,* bacterial vaginosis. Diagnosis depends on laboratory tests because sensitivity and specificity of discharge characteristics are low.[59–61] *Vaginal cancer* is rare; DES exposure in utero and HPV infection are risk factors.

Check for bulging in the vaginal wall. You may wish remove either the upper or lower blade of the speculum (or use a single blade speculum) and ask the woman to bear down to assess the location of vaginal wall relaxation or the degree of uterine prolapse.

Close the speculum as it emerges from the introitus, avoiding both excessive stretching or pinching of the mucosa.

Use of the lower blade as a retractor during bearing down helps expose anterior vaginal wall defects such as *cystoceles*; likewise use of the upper blade helps expose *rectoceles*. The standardized Pelvic Organ Quantification (POP-Q) system and diagram is widely used.[62] See Table 14-3, Bulges and Swelling of the Vulva, Vagina, and Urethra, p. 570.

Perform a Bimanual Examination. Lubricate the index and middle fingers of one of your gloved hands, and *from a standing position*, insert them into the vagina, again exerting pressure primarily posteriorly. Your thumb should be abducted, your ring and little fingers flexed into your palm. Pressing inward on the perineum with your flexed fingers causes little if any discomfort and allows you to position your palpating fingers correctly. Note any nodularity or tenderness in the vaginal wall, including the region of the urethra and the bladder anteriorly.

Stool in the rectum may simulate a rectovaginal mass, but unlike a malignant mass, it can usually be dented by digital pressure. Rectovaginal examination confirms the distinction.

Palpate the cervix, noting its position, shape, consistency, regularity, mobility, and tenderness. Normally the cervix can be moved somewhat without pain. Feel the fornices around the cervix.

Cervical motion tenderness and/or adnexal tenderness suggest *pelvic inflammatory disease*, ectopic pregnancy, and appendicitis.

Palpate the uterus. Place your other hand on the abdomen about midway between the umbilicus and the symphysis pubis. While you elevate the cervix and uterus with your pelvic hand, press your abdominal hand in and down, trying to grasp the uterus between your two hands. Note its size, shape, consistency, and mobility, and identify any tenderness or masses.

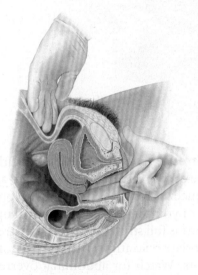

See Table 14-7, Positions of the Uterus, p. 573, and Table 14-8, Abnormalities of the Uterus, p. 574.

Uterine enlargement suggests pregnancy, uterine myomas (fibroids), or malignancy.

Now slide the fingers of your pelvic hand into the anterior fornix and palpate the body of the uterus between your hands. In this position, your pelvic fingers can feel the anterior surface of the uterus, and your abdominal hand can feel part of the posterior surface.

Nodules on the uterine surfaces suggest *myomas* (see p. 574).

If you cannot feel the uterus with either of these maneuvers, it may be tipped posteriorly (retrodisplaced). Slide your pelvic fingers into the posterior fornix and feel for the uterus butting against your fingertips. An obese or poorly relaxed abdominal wall may also prevent you from feeling the uterus even when it is located anteriorly.

See *retroversion* and *retroflexion of the uterus* (p. 573).

Palpate each ovary. Place your abdominal hand on the right lower quadrant, and your pelvic hand in the right lateral fornix. Press your abdominal hand in and down, trying to push the adnexal structures toward your pelvic hand. Try to identify the right ovary or any adjacent adnexal masses. By moving your hands slightly, slide the adnexal structures between your fingers, if possible, and note their size, shape, consistency, mobility, and tenderness. Repeat the procedure on the left side.

Three to 5 years after menopause, ovaries are atrophic and usually nonpalpable. In postmenopausal women, investigate a palpable ovary for possible *ovarian cyst* or *ovarian cancer*. Pelvic pain, bloating, increased abdominal size, and urinary tract symptoms are more common in women with ovarian cancer.[35]

Normal ovaries are somewhat tender. They are usually palpable in slender, relaxed women but are difficult or impossible to feel in women who are obese or tense.

Adnexal masses can also arise from a *tubo-ovarian abscess, salpingitis* or inflammation of the fallopian tubes from PID, or ectopic pregnancy. Distinguish such a mass from a uterine myoma. See Table 14-9, Adnexal Masses, p. 575.

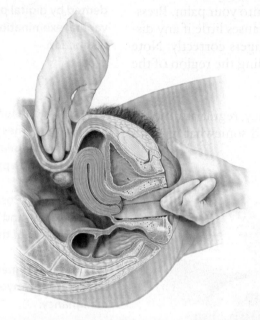

Assess the Pelvic Floor Muscles for Strength and Tenderness. Withdraw your examining fingers just clear of the cervix, and then spread them against the vaginal walls. Ask the patient to squeeze around your fingers as long and as hard as she can. Snug compression of your fingers, moving them upward and inward, that lasts 3 or more seconds is full strength. Check for strength, tenderness during contraction, appropriate relaxation after contraction, and endurance in all four vaginal quadrants. Watch for abdominal overrecruitment or tightening of the adductor or gluteal muscles.

In patients with pelvic pain or vaginal wall tenderness, palpate the external pelvic floor muscles in a clockwise rotation to identify trigger points.[64]

Muscle weakness from aging, vaginal deliveries, neurologic conditions can occur; it may be associated with *stress incontinence*. Overrecruitment with tightening, vaginal wall tenderness, and referred pain may be found in pelvic pain from *pelvic floor spasm, interstitial cystitis, vulvodynia,* and *urethral spasm.*[63]

Trigger point tenderness in pelvic floor muscles can be seen in *pelvic floor spasm.*

Symphysis pubis

Ischiocavernosus muscle

Bulbocavernousus muscle

Superficial transverse perineal muscle

Perineal body

Levator ani muscles

12
1
2
3
4
5
6
7
8
9
10
11

Do a Rectovaginal Examination if Indicated. The rectovaginal examination has three primary purposes: to palpate a retroverted uterus, the uterosacral ligaments, cul-de-sac, and adnexa; to screen for colorectal cancer in women 50 years or older; and to assess pelvic pathology.[57,65]

After withdrawing your fingers from the bimanual examination, change your gloves and lubricate your fingers as needed (see note below on lubricants). Slowly reintroduce your index finger into the vagina and your middle finger into the rectum. Ask the patient to strain down as you do this to relax her anal sphincter. Mention that this may stimulate an urge to move her bowels, but this will not occur. Apply pressure against the anterior and lateral walls with the examining fingers, and downward pressure with the hand on the abdomen.

Nodularity, and thickening of the uterosacral ligaments occur in endometriosis; also pain with uterine movement.

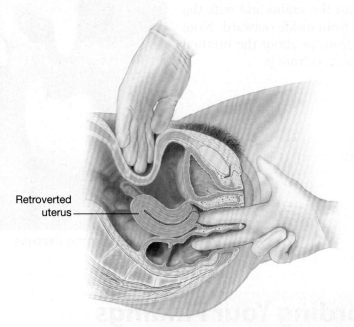

Retroverted uterus

Check the rectal vault for masses. If a Hemoccult test is planned, you should change gloves to avoid contaminating fecal material with any blood provoked by the Pap smear. After the examination, wipe off the external genitalia and rectum, or offer the patient some tissue so she can do it herself.

See Chapter 15, The Anus, Rectum, and Prostate, pp. 589, 593–594.

Using Lubricants

If you use a tube of lubricant during a pelvic or rectal examination, you may inadvertently contaminate it by touching the tube with your gloved fingers after touching the patient. To avoid this problem, let the lubricant drop onto your gloved fingers without allowing contact between the tube and the gloves. If you or your assistant should inadvertently contaminate the tube, discard it. Small disposable tubes for use with one patient circumvent this problem.

HERNIAS

Hernias of the groin occur in women as well as in men, but they are much less common. The examination techniques are basically the same as for men (see pp. 529–530). A woman should also stand up to be examined. To feel an indirect inguinal hernia, however, palpate in the labia majora and upward to just lateral to the pubic tubercles.

An indirect inguinal hernia is the most common hernia in women. A femoral hernia ranks next in frequency.

SPECIAL TECHNIQUES

If you suspect urethritis or inflammation of the paraurethral glands, insert your index finger into the vagina and milk the urethra gently from inside outward. Note any discharge from or about the urethral meatus. If present, culture it.

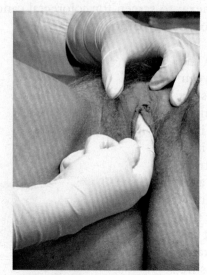

MILKING THE URETHRA

Urethritis may arise from infection with *Chlamydia trachomatis* or *Neisseria gonorrhoeae*.

Recording Your Findings

Note that initially you may use sentences to describe your findings; later you will use phrases. The style below contains phrases appropriate for most write-ups.

Recording the Pelvic Examination—Female Genitalia

"No inguinal adenopathy. External genitalia without erythema, lesions, or masses. Vaginal mucosa pink. Cervix parous, pink, and without discharge. Uterus anterior, midline, smooth, and not enlarged. No adnexal tenderness. Pap smear obtained. Rectovaginal wall intact. Rectal vault without masses. Stool brown and Hemoccult negative."

OR

"Bilateral shotty inguinal adenopathy. External genitalia without erythema or lesions. Vaginal mucosa and cervix coated with thin white homogeneous discharge with mild fishy odor. After swabbing cervix, no discharge visible in cervical os. Uterus midline; no adnexal masses. Rectal vault without masses. Stool brown and Hemoccult negative."

Suggests bacterial vaginosis

Bibliography

Citations

1. Herschorn S. Female pelvic floor anatomy: the pelvic floor, supporting structures, and pelvic organs. Rev Urol 2004;6 (Suppl 5):S2–S10.

2. Ashton-Miller, Howard D, Delancey JOL. The functional anatomy of the female pelvic floor and stress continence control system. Scand J Urol Suppl 2001;207:S1–S12.

3. American College of Obstetricians and Gynecologists. Premenstrual syndrome. March 2010. Available at http://www.acog.org/publications/patient_education/bp057.cfm. Accessed November 14, 2010.

4. Grady D. Management of menopausal symptoms. N Engl J Med 2006;355:2238–2247.

5. Col NF, Fairfield KM, Ewan-Whyte C et al. In the clinic. Menopause. Ann Int Med 2009;150: ITC4–ITC 11.

6. North American Menopause Society. Estrogen and progestogen use in postmenopausal women: 2010 position statement of the North American menopause society. Menopause 2010; 17:242–255.

7. Newton KM, Reed SD, LaCroix AZ et al. Treatment of vasomotor symptoms of menopause with black cohosh, multibotanicals, soy, hormone therapy, or placebo: a randomized trial. Ann Intern Med 145:869–879, 2006.

8. Bjorkman M, Malterud K. Lesbian women's experiences with health care: a qualitative study. Scand J Prim Health Care 2009;27:238–243.

9. Polek CA, Hardie TL, Crowley EM. Lesbians' disclosure of sexual orientation and satisfaction with care. J Transcult Nurs 2008;19:243–249.

10. Seaver MR, Freund KM, Wright LM et al. Healthcare preferences among lesbians: a focus group analysis. J Womens Health 2008;17:215–225.

11. Hebernick D, Reece M, Schick V et al. Sexual activity in the United States: results from a national probability sample of men and women ages 14–94. J Sex Medicine 2010;7(Suppl 5): 255–265.

12. Gates GJ. Same sex couples and the gay, lesbian, and bisexual population: new estimates from the American Community Survey. October 2006. Available at http://www.law.ucla.edu/williamsinstitute/publications/SameSexCouplesandGLBpopACS.pdf. Accessed December 19, 2010.

13. Conron KJ, Mimiaga MJ, Landers SJ. A population-based study of sexual orientation identity and gender differences in adult health. Am J Public Health 2010;100:19531960.

14. McLaughlin KA, Hatzenbuehler ML, Keyes KM. Responses to discrimination and psychiatric disorders among black, Hispanic, female, and lesbian, gay, and bisexual individuals. Am J Public Health 2010;100:1477–1484.

15. Centers for Disease Control and Prevention. Lesbian, gay, bisexual, and transgender health. Updated November 2, 2010. Available at http://www.cdc.gov/lgbthealth/index.htm. Accessed December 18, 2010.

16. Kruzka PS and Kruszka SJ. Evaluation of acute pelvic pain in women. Am Fam Physician 2010;82:141–147.

17. Guidice LC. Endometriosis. N Engl J Med 2010;362:2389–2398.

18. American College of Obstetricians and Gynecologists. Pelvic Pain. ACOG Education Pamphlet APO99. January 2006. Available at http://www.acog.org/publications/patient_education/bp099.cfm. Accessed October 23, 2010.

19. Reiter RC. A profile of women with chronic pelvic pain. Clin Obstet Gynec 1990;33:130–136.

20. Farquhar CM and Steiner CA. Hysterectomy rates in the United States 1990–1997. Obstet Gynecol 2002;99: 229–234.

21. International Pelvic Pain Society. Pelvic Pain Assessment Form. Available at http://www.pelvicpain.org/pdf/History_and_Physical_Form/IPPS-H&PformR-MSW.pdf. Accessed October 23, 2010.

22. U.S. Preventive Services Task Force. Screening for Cervical Cancer. April 2012. Available at http://www.uspreventiveservices-taskforce.org/uspstf/uspscerv.htm. Accessed August 22, 2012.

23. Centers for Disease Control and Prevention. Human Papillomavirus: HPV Information for Clinicians. April 2007. Available at http://www.cdc.gov/std/hpv/common-clinicians/ClinicianBro-br.pdf. Accessed December 4, 2010.

24. Goldstein MA, Goodman A, del Carmen MG et al. Case 10–2009: a 23-year-old woman with an abnormal Papanicolaou smear. N Engl J Med 2009;360:1337–1344.

25. Huh WK. Human papillomavirus infection: a concise review of natural history. Obstet Gynecol 2009;114:139–143.

26. The American Congress of Obstetricians and Gynecologists. New Cervical Cancer Screening Recommendations from the U.S. Preventive Services Task Force and the American Cancer Society/American Society for Colposcopy and Cervical Pathology/American Society for Clinical Pathology, Available at http://www.acog.org/About_ACOG/Announcements/New_Cervical_Cancer_Screening_Recommendations. Accessed August 22, 2012.

27. American College of Obstetricians and Gynecologists Committee on Practice Bulletins–Gynecology. ACOG Practice Bulletin no. 109: Cervical cytology screening. Obstet Gynecol 2009;114:1409–1420.

28. Solomon D, Davey D, Kurman R et al. The 2001 Bethesda system: terminology for reporting results of cervical cytology. JAMA 2004;291:2990–2993.

29. Wright TC, Cox JT, Massad JS. 2001 consensus guidelines for the management of women with cervical cytologic abnormalities. JAMA 2002;287:2120–2119.

30. Advisory Committee on Immunization Practices, Centers for Disease Control. Morbidity and Mortality Weekly Report. Quadrivalent Human Papillomavirus Vaccine. Recommendations of the Advisory Committee on Immunization Practices. March 12 2007/56 (Early Release). Pp. 1–54. Available at http://www.cdc.gov/mmwr/preview/mmwrhtml/rr56e312a1.htm. Accessed December 4, 2010.

31. Centers for Disease Control and Prevention. Vaccine Information Statement (Interim)-Human Papillomavirus (HPV) Gardasil. March 30, 2010. Available at http://www.cdc.gov/vaccines/pubs/vis/downloads/vis-hpv-gardasil.pdf. Accessed December 4, 2010.

32. Garland SM, Hernandez-Avila M, Wheller CM et al. Quadrivalent vaccine against human papillomavirus to prevent anogenital diseases. N Engl J Med 2007;356:1928–1943.

33. Steinbrook R. The potential of human papilloma virus vaccines: perspective. N Engl J Med 2007;354:1109–1112.

34. Winer RL, Hughes JP, Feng Q et al. Condom use and the risk of genital human papillomavirus infection in young women. N Engl J Med 2006;354:2645–2654.

35. Clarke-Pearson DL. Screening for ovarian cancer. N Engl J Med 2009;316:170–177.

36. Hamilton W, Peters TJ, Bankhead C et al. Risk of ovarian cancer in women with symptoms in primary care: population based case-control study. BMJ 2009;339:b2998–b3005.

37. Centers for Disease Control and Prevention, Division of STD Prevention, National Center for HIV/AIDS, Viral Hepatitis, STD, and TB Prevention. Sexually Transmitted Diseases in the United States, 2008. National Surveillance Data for Chlamydia, Gonorrhea, and Syphilis. Available at http://www.cdc.gov/std/stats08/trends.htm. Accessed October 18, 2010.

38. U. S. Preventive Services Task Force. Screening for Chlamydial infection. June 2007. Available at http://www.uspreventiveservicestaskforce.org/uspstf07/chlamydia/chlamydiars.htm#clinical. Accessed October 16, 2010.

39. U. S. Preventive Services Task Force. Screening for gonorrhea. May 2005. Available at http://www.uspreventiveservicestaskforce.org/uspstf/uspsgono.htm. Accessed October 18, 2010.

40. U. S. Preventive Services Task Force. Screening for syphilis infection. July 2004. Available at http://www.uspreventiveservicestaskforce.org/uspstf/uspssyph.htm. Accessed October 18, 2010.

41. Centers for Disease Control and Prevention. Diagnoses of HIV infection and AIDS in the United States and Dependent Areas, 2008. See also Commentary. Available at http://www.cdc.gov/hiv/surveillance/resources/reports/2008report/index.htm. Accessed October 18, 2010.

42. Workowsi KA, Levine WC, Wasserheit JN. U.S. Centers for Disease Control and Prevention guidelines for the treatment of sexually transmitted diseases: an opportunity to unify clinical and public health practice. Ann Intern Med 2002;137:255–262.

43. U. S. Preventive Services Task Force. Screening for HIV. April 2007. Available at http://www.uspreventiveservicestaskforce.org/uspstf05/hiv/hivrs.htm#clinical. Accessed October 18, 2010.

44. Qaseem A, Snow V, Shekelle P et al. Clinical guidelines: screening for HIV in health care settings: a guidance statement from the American College of Physicians and HIV Medicine Association. Ann Intern Med 2009;150:125–131.

45. Centers for Disease Control and Prevention. Teen Pregnancy. September 20 2010. Available at http://www.cdc.gov/Teen-Pregnancy, Accessed October 18, 2010.

46. Centers for Disease Control and Prevention. Unintended pregnancy prevention: contraception. Updated August 5, 2009. Available at http://www.cdc.gov/reproductivehealth/UnintendedPregnancy/Contraception.htm. Accessed October 18, 2010.

47. Hulley S, Grady D, Busht et al, for the Heart and Estrogen/Progestin Replacement Study Research Group. Randomized trial of estrogen plus progestin for secondary prevention of coronary heart disease in postmenopausal women. JAMA 1998;280:605–613.

48. Writing Group for the Women's Health Initiative Investigators. Risks and benefits of estrogen plus progestin in healthy postmenopausal women. JAMA 2002;288:321–333

49. Womens' Health Initiative Steering Committee. Effects of conjugated equine estrogen in postmenopausal women with hysterectomy. JAMA 2004;291:1701–1712.

50. Hulley SB, Grady D. The HWI estrogen alone trial—do things look any better? (editorial) JAMA 2004;291:1769–1779.

51. Women's Health Initiative Investigators. Health risks and benefits 3 years after stopping randomized treatment with estrogen and progestin. JAMA 2008;299:1036–1045.

52. Chlebowski RT, Garnet LA, Gass M et al. Estrogen plus progestin and breast cancer incidence and mortality in postmenopausal women. JAMA 2010;304:1684–1692.

53. Women's Health Initiative Memory Study Investigators. Estrogen plus progestin and the incidence of dementia and mild cognitive impairment in post-menopausal women: the Women's Health Initiative Memory Study: a randomized controlled trial. JAMA 2003;289:2651–2662.

54. American College of Obstetricians and Gynecologists. Hormone therapy. December 2007. Available at http://www.acog.org/publications/patient_education/bp066.cfm. Accessed October 22, 2010.

55. American College of Obstetricians and Gynecologists. The college responds to new report from the Women's Health Initiative regarding estrogen plus progestin hormone therapy and breast cancer. October 2010. Available at http://www.acog.org/from_home/misc/20101021WHIResponse.cfm. Accessed October 22, 2010

56. U.S. Preventive Services Task Force. Hormone Replacement Therapy for the Prevention of Chronic Conditions in Post-menopausal Women. May 2005. Available at http://www.uspreventiveservicestaskforce.org/uspstf/uspspmho.htm. Accessed October 22, 2010

57. Edelman A, Anderson J, Lai S et al. Pelvic examination. N Engl J Med 2007;356:e26–28.

58. Weitlauf JC, Frayne SM, Finney JW et al. Sexual violence, post-traumatic stress disorder, and the pelvic examination: how do beliefs about the safety, necessity, and utility of the examination influence patient experiences? J Women's Health 2010; 19:1271–1280.

59. Wilson JF. In the clinic: vaginitis and cervicitis. Ann Intern Med 2009;151:ITC3-1-ITC3-16.

60. Eckhert LO. Acute vulvovaginitis. N Engl J Med 2006;355:1244–1252.

61. Anderson MR, Klink K, Cohrssen A. Evaluation of vaginal complaints. JAMA 2004;291:1368–1370.

62. Bump RC, Mattiasson A, Bo K et al. The standardization of terminology of female pelvic organ prolapse and pelvic floor dysfunction. Am J Obstet Gynecol 1996;175:10–17.

63. Wieslander CK. Clinical approach and office evaluation of the patient with pelvic floor dysfunction. Obstet Gynecol Clin North Am 2009;36:445–462.

64. Steege JF, Metzger DA, Levy BS. Chronic Pelvic Pain: An Integrated Approach. Philadelphia: Saunders, 1998.

65. Padilla LA, Radosevich DM, Milad MPl. Accuracy of the pelvic examination in detecting adnexal masses. Obstet Gynelcol 2000;96:593–598.

66. Ehrmann DA. Polycystic ovary syndrome. N Engl J Med 2005;352:1223–1236.

67. Barnhart KT. Ectopic pregnancy. N Engl J Med 2009;361:379–387.

BIBLIOGRAPHY

Additional References

Azziz R, Carmina E, Dewailly D et al. The Androgen Excess and PCOS Society criteria for the polycystic ovary syndrome: the complete task force report. Fertil Steril 2009;91:456–488.

Berek J, Novak E (eds). Berek & Novak's Gynecology, 15th ed. Philadelphia: Wolters Kluwer Health/Lippincott Williams & Wilkins, 2012.

Collaborative Group on Epidemiological Studies of Ovarian Cancer, Beral V, Doll R et al. Ovarian cancer and oral contraceptives: collaborative reanalysis of data from 45 epidemiological studies including 23,257 women with ovarian cancer and 87,303 controls. Lancet 2008;371(9609):303–314.

Freeman EW, Sammel MD, Lin H et al. Duration of menopausal hot flushes and associated risk factors. Obstet Gynecol 2011; 117:1095–1194.

Gibbs RS, Danforth DN (eds). Danforth's obstetrics and gynecology, 10th ed. Philadelphia: Wolters Kluwer/Lippincott Williams & Wilkins, 2008.

Gupta R, Warren T, Wald A. Genital herpes. Lancet 2007; 370(9605):2127–2137.

Holroyd-Leduc JM, Tannenbaum C, Thorpe KE et al. What type of urinary incontinence does this woman have? JAMA 2008; 299:1446–1456.

Lee SC, Kaunitz AM, Sanchez-Ramos L et al. The oncogenic potential of endometrial polyps: A systematic review and meta-analysis. Obstet Gynecol 2010;116:1197–1205.

Lowe NK, Neal JL, Ryan-Wenger NA. Accuracy of the clinical diagnosis of vaginitis compared with a DNA probe laboratory standard. Obstet Gynecol 2009;113:89–95.

Mac Bride MB, Rhodes DJ, Shuster LT. Vulvovaginal atrophy. Mayo Clin Proc 2010;85:87–94.

Meyers DS, Halvorson H, Luckhaupt S. Screening for chlamydial infection: an evidence update for the U.S. Preventive Services Task Force. Ann Intern Med 2007;147:135–42.

Nelson HD. Menopause. Lancet 2008;371(9614):760–770.

Newton KM, Reed SD, LaCroix AZ et al. Treatment of vasomotor symptoms of menopause with black cohosh, multibotanicals, soy, hormone therapy, or placebo: a randomized trial. Ann Intern Med 2006;145:869–879.

Nygaard I, Barber MD. Prevalence of symptomatic pelvic floor disorders in US women. JAMA 2008;300:1311–1316.

Rebbeck TR, Kauff ND, Domchek SM. Meta-analysis of risk reduction estimates associated with risk-reducing salpingo-oophorectomy in BRCA1 or BRCA2 mutation carriers. J Natl Cancer Inst 2009;101:80–87.

Sirovich BE, Welch HG. Cervical cancer screening among women without a cervix. JAMA 2004;291:2990–2993.

Utz AL, Schaefer PW, Snuderl M. Case records of the Massachusetts General Hospital. Case 20-2010. A 32-year-old woman with oligomenorrhea and infertility. N Engl J Med 2010; 363:178–186.

Wooster R, Weber BL. Breast and ovarian cancer. N Engl J Med 2003;348:2339–2347.

Workowski KA, Berman S. Sexually transmitted diseases treatment guidelines, 2010. Centers for Disease Control and Prevention. Morbidity and Mortality Weekly Report 2010;59(RR12):1-110, December 17 2010. Available at http://www.cdc.gov/mmwr/preview/mmwrhtml/rr5912a1.htm. Accessed December 31, 2010.

> **The Bates' suite offers these additional resources to enhance learning and facilitate understanding of this chapter:**
>
> - *Bates' Pocket Guide to Physical Examination and History Taking*, 7th edition
> - *Bates' Visual Guide to Physical Examination*
> - thePoint online resources, for students and instructors: http://thepoint.lww.com

Table
14-1   Lesions of the Vulva

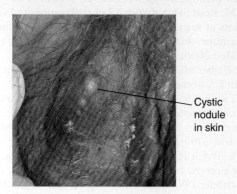

Epidermoid Cyst

A small, firm, round cystic nodule in the labia suggests an epidermoid cyst. These are yellowish in color. Look for the dark punctum marking the blocked opening of the gland.

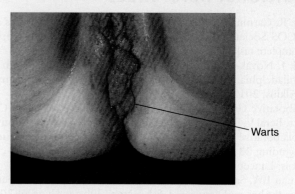

Venereal Wart (*Condyloma Acuminatum*)

Warty lesions on the labia and within the vestibule suggest condyloma acuminatum. These result from infection with *human papillomavirus.*

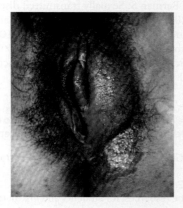

Syphilitic Chancre

A firm, painless ulcer suggests the chancre of primary syphilis. Because most chancres in women develop internally, they often go undetected.

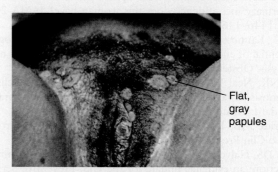

Secondary Syphilis (*Condyloma Latum*)

Slightly raised, round or oval, flat-topped papules covered by a gray exudate suggest condylomata lata. These constitute one manifestation of secondary syphilis and are contagious.

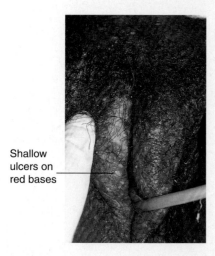

Genital Herpes

Shallow, small, painful ulcers on red bases suggest a herpes infection. Initial infection may be extensive, as shown. Recurrent infections usually are confined to a small local patch.

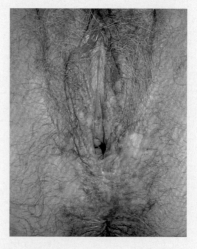

Carcinoma of the Vulva

An ulcerated or raised red vulvar lesion in an elderly woman may indicate vulvar carcinoma.

| Table | | |
| 14-2 | **Vaginal Discharge** | 569 |

Vaginal discharge from vaginitis must be distinguished from a physiologic discharge. The latter is clear or white and may contain white clumps of epithelial cells; it is not malodorous. It is also important to distinguish vaginal from cervical discharges. Use a large cotton swab to wipe off the cervix. If no cervical discharge is present in the os, suspect a vaginal origin and consider the causes below. Remember that diagnosis of cervicitis or vaginitis hinges on careful collection and analysis of the appropriate laboratory specimens.[60,61]

	Trichomonal Vaginitis	Candidal Vaginitis	Bacterial Vaginosis
Cause	*Trichomonas vaginalis*, a protozoan; often but not always acquired sexually	*Candida albicans*, a yeast (normal overgrowth of vaginal flora); many factors predispose, including antibiotic therapy	Bacterial overgrowth probably from anaerobic bacteria; may be transmitted sexually
Discharge	Yellowish green or gray, possibly frothy; often profuse and pooled in the vaginal fornix; may be malodorous	White and curdy; may be thin but typically thick; not as profuse as in trichomonal infection; not malodorous	Gray or white, thin, homogeneous, malodorous; coats the vaginal walls; usually not profuse, may be minimal
Other Symptoms	Pruritus (though not usually as severe as with *Candida* infection); pain on urination (from skin inflammation or possibly urethritis); dyspareunia	Pruritus; vaginal soreness; pain on urination (from skin inflammation); dyspareunia	Unpleasant fishy or musty genital odor
Vulva and Vaginal Mucosa	Vestibule and labia minora may be reddened. Vaginal mucosa may be diffusively reddened, with small red granular spots or petechiae in the posterior fornix. In mild cases, the mucosa looks normal.	The vulva and even the surrounding skin are often inflamed and sometimes swollen to a variable extent. Vaginal mucosa often reddened, with white, often tenacious patches of discharge. The mucosa may bleed when these patches are scraped off. In mild cases, the mucosa looks normal.	Vulva usually normal. Vaginal mucosa usually normal
Laboratory Evaluation	Scan saline wet mount for trichomonads	Scan potassium hydroxide (KOH) preparation for branching hyphae of *Candida*.	Scan saline wet mount for *clue cells* (epithelial cells with stippled borders); sniff for fishy odor after applying KOH ("whiff test"); vaginal secretions with pH >4.5

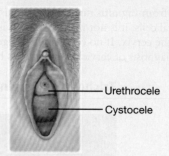

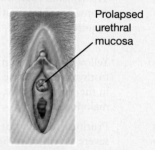

Urethrocele
Cystocele

Cystocele

A cystocele is a bulge of the upper two-thirds of the anterior vaginal wall, together with the bladder above it. It results from weakened supporting tissues.

Cystourethrocele

When the entire anterior vaginal wall, together with the bladder and urethra, is involved in the bulge, a cystourethrocele is present. A groove sometimes defines the border between urethrocele and cystocele, but is not always present.

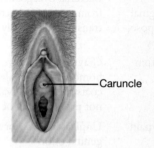

Caruncle

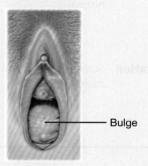

Prolapsed urethral mucosa

Urethral Caruncle

A urethral caruncle is a small, red, benign tumor visible at the posterior part of the urethral meatus. It occurs chiefly in postmenopausal women and usually causes no symptoms. Occasionally, a carcinoma of the urethra is mistaken for a caruncle. To check, palpate the urethra through the vagina for thickening, nodularity, or tenderness, and feel for inguinal lymphadenopathy.

Prolapse of the Urethral Mucosa

Prolapsed urethral mucosa forms a swollen red ring around the urethral meatus. It usually occurs before menarche or after menopause. Identify the urethral meatus at the center of the swelling to make this diagnosis.

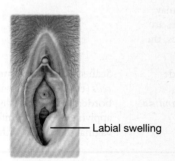

Labial swelling

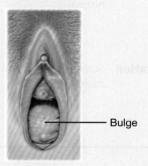

Bulge

Bartholin's Gland Infection

Causes of a Bartholin's gland infection include trauma, gonococci anaerobes like bacteroides and peptostreptococci, and *Chlamydia trachomatis.* Acutely, it appears as a tense, hot, very tender abscess. Look for pus coming out of the duct or erythema around the duct opening. Chronically, a nontender cyst is felt. It may be large or small.

Rectocele

A rectocele is a herniation of the rectum into the posterior wall of the vagina, resulting from a weakness or defect in the endopelvic fascia.

Table
14-4   Variations in the Cervical Surface

Two kinds of epithelia cover the cervix: (1) shiny pink *squamous epithelium*, which resembles the vaginal epithelium, and (2) deep red, plushy *columnar epithelium*, which is continuous with the endocervical lining. These meet at the *squamocolumnar junction*. When this junction is at or inside the cervical os, only squamous epithelium is seen. A ring of columnar epithelium is often visible to a varying extent around the os—the result of a normal process that accompanies fetal development, menarche, and the first pregnancy.*

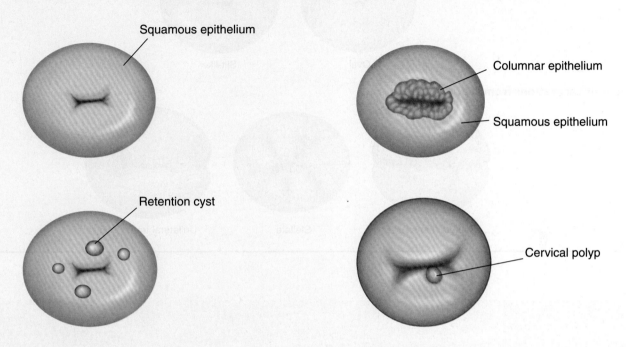

With increasing estrogen stimulation during adolescence, all or part of this columnar epithelium is transformed into squamous epithelium by a process termed *metaplasia*. This change may block the secretions of columnar epithelium and cause *retention cysts*, also called *nabothian cysts*. These appear as translucent nodules on the cervical surface and have no pathologic significance.

A cervical polyp usually arises from the endocervical canal, becoming visible when it protrudes through the cervical os. It is bright red, soft, and rather fragile. When only the tip is seen, it cannot be differentiated clinically from a polyp originating in the endometrium. Polyps are benign but may bleed.

*Terminology is in flux. Other terms for the columnar epithelium visible on the ectocervix are *ectropion*, *ectopy*, and *eversion*.

Table 14-5	Shapes of the Cervical Os

Normal

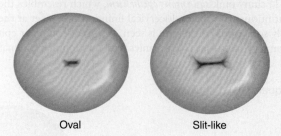

Oval   Slit-like

Types of Lacerations from Delivery

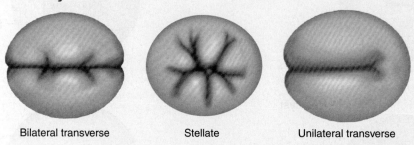

Bilateral transverse   Stellate   Unilateral transverse

Table 14-6	Abnormalities of the Cervix

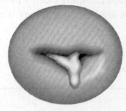

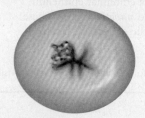

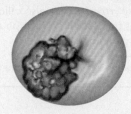

Mucopurulent Cervicitis

Mucopurulent cervicitis produces purulent yellow drainage from the cervical os, usually from *Chlamydia trachomatis*, *Neisseria gonorrhoeae*, or herpes infection. These infections are sexually transmitted and may occur without symptoms or signs.

Carcinoma of the Cervix

Carcinoma of the cervix begins in an area of metaplasia. In its earliest stages, it cannot be distinguished from a normal cervix. In later stages, an extensive, irregular, cauliflowerlike growth may develop. Early frequent intercourse, multiple partners, smoking, and infection with human papillomavirus increase the risk for cervical cancer.

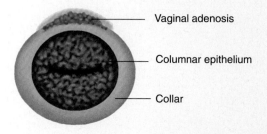

Vaginal adenosis

Columnar epithelium

Collar

Fetal Exposure to Diethylstilbestrol (DES)

Daughters of women who took DES during pregnancy are at greatly increased risk for several abnormalities, including (1) columnar epithelium that covers most or all of the cervix, (2) vaginal adenosis, i.e., extension of this epithelium to the vaginal wall, and (3) a circular collar or ridge of tissue, of varying shapes, between the cervix and vagina. Much less common is an otherwise rare carcinoma of the upper vagina.

Table
14-7   Positions of the Uterus

Retroversion and retroflexion are usually normal variants.

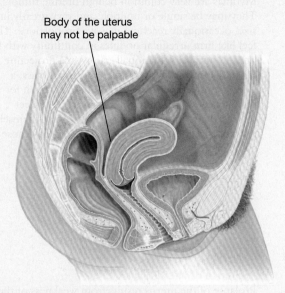

Body of the uterus
may not be palpable

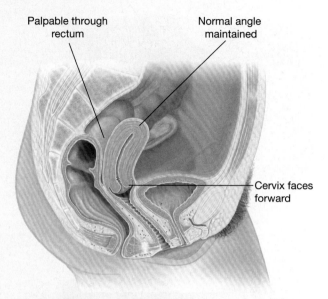

Palpable through
rectum

Normal angle
maintained

Cervix faces
forward

Retroversion of the Uterus

Retroversion of the uterus refers to a tilting backward of the entire uterus, including both body and cervix. It is a common variant occurring in approximately 20% of women. Early clues on pelvic examination are a cervix that faces forward and a uterine body that cannot be felt by the abdominal hand. In *moderate retroversion*, the body may not be palpable with either hand. In *marked retroversion*, the body can be felt posteriorly, either through the posterior fornix or through the rectum. A retroverted uterus is usually both mobile and asymptomatic. Occasionally, such a uterus is fixed and immobile, held in place by conditions such as endometriosis or pelvic inflammatory disease.

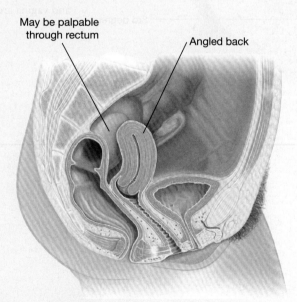

May be palpable
through rectum

Angled back

Retroflexion of the Uterus

Retroflexion of the uterus refers to a backward angulation of the body of the uterus in relation to the cervix. The cervix maintains its usual position. The body of the uterus is often palpable through the posterior fornix or through the rectum.

Table 14-8   Abnormalities of the Uterus

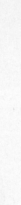
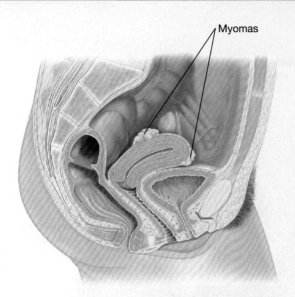

Myomas

Myomas of the Uterus (Fibroids)

Myomas are very common benign uterine tumors. They may be single or multiple and vary greatly in size, occasionally reaching massive proportions. They feel like firm, irregular nodules in continuity with the uterine surface. Occasionally, a myoma projecting laterally can be confused with an ovarian mass; a nodule projecting posteriorly can be mistaken for a retroflexed uterus. Submucous myomas project toward the endometrial cavity and are not themselves palpable, although they may be suspected because of an enlarged uterus.

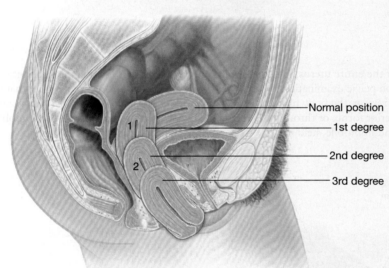

Normal position
1st degree
2nd degree
3rd degree

Prolapse of the Uterus

Prolapse of the uterus results from weakness of the supporting structures of the pelvic floor and is often associated with a cystocele and rectocele. In progressive stages, the uterus becomes retroverted and descends down the vaginal canal to the outside:

- In *first-degree prolapse*, the cervix is still well within the vagina.
- In *second-degree prolapse*, it is at the introitus.
- In *third-degree prolapse* (procidentia), the cervix and vagina are outside the introitus.

Table
14-9   Adnexal Masses

Adnexal masses most commonly result from disorders of the fallopian tubes or ovaries. Three examples—often hard to differentiate—are described. In addition, inflammatory disease of the bowel (such as diverticulitis), carcinoma of the colon, and a pedunculated myoma of the uterus may simulate an adnexal mass.

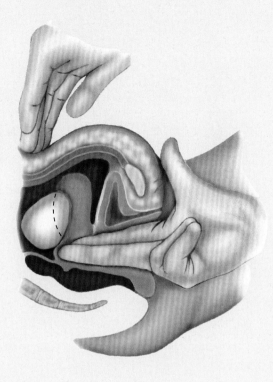

Ovarian Cysts and Ovarian Cancer

Ovarian cysts and tumors may be detected as adnexal masses on one or both sides. Later, they may extend out of the pelvis. Cysts tend to be smooth and compressible, tumors more solid and often nodular. Uncomplicated cysts are not usually tender.

Small (≤6 cm in diameter), mobile, cystic masses in a young woman are usually benign and often disappear after the next menstrual period. Diagnosis of *polycystic ovary syndrome* rests on exclusion of several endocrine disorders and 2 of the 3 features listed: absent or irregular menses; hyperandrogenism (hirsutism, acne, alopecia, elevated serum testosterone); and confirmation of polycystic ovaries on ultrasound. Obesity and absence of lactation outside pregnancy or childbirth are additional predictors.[66]

Ovarian cancer is relatively rare and usually presents at an advanced stage. Symptoms include pelvic pain, bloating, increased abdominal size, and urinary tract symptoms[35]; often there is a palpable ovarian mass. Currently there are no reliable screening tests. A strong family history of breast or ovarian cancer is an important risk factor but occurs in only 5% of cases.

Ruptured Tubal Pregnancy

A ruptured tubal pregnancy spills blood into the peritoneal cavity, causing severe abdominal pain and tenderness. Guarding and rebound tenderness are sometimes associated. A unilateral adnexal mass may be palpable, but tenderness often prevents its detection. Faintness, syncope, nausea, vomiting, tachycardia, and shock may be present, reflecting the hemorrhage. There may be a prior history of amenorrhea or other symptoms of a pregnancy.[67]

Pelvic Inflammatory Disease

Pelvic inflammatory disease (PID) is most often a result of sexually transmitted infection of the fallopian tubes (salpingitis) or of the tubes and ovaries (salpingo-oophoritis). It is caused by *Neisseria gonorrhoeae, Chlamydia trachomatis,* and other organisms. *Acute* disease is associated with very tender, bilateral adnexal masses, although pain and muscle spasm usually make it impossible to delineate them. Movement of the cervix produces pain. If not treated, a *tubo-ovarian abscess* or infertility may ensue.

Infection of the fallopian tubes and ovaries may also follow delivery of a baby or gynecologic surgery.

The Anus, Rectum, and Prostate

Anatomy and Physiology

The gastrointestinal tract terminates in a short segment, the *anal canal*. The external margin of the anal canal is poorly demarcated, but the moist, hairless appearance of its skin usually distinguishes it from the surrounding perianal skin. The muscle actions of the voluntary *external anal sphincter* and involuntary *internal anal sphincter* normally hold the anal canal closed. The internal anal sphincter is an extension of the muscular coat of the rectal wall.

Note carefully the angle of the anal canal, on a line roughly between the anus and umbilicus. Unlike the rectum above it, the canal is liberally supplied by somatic sensory nerves, and a poorly directed finger or instrument will produce pain.

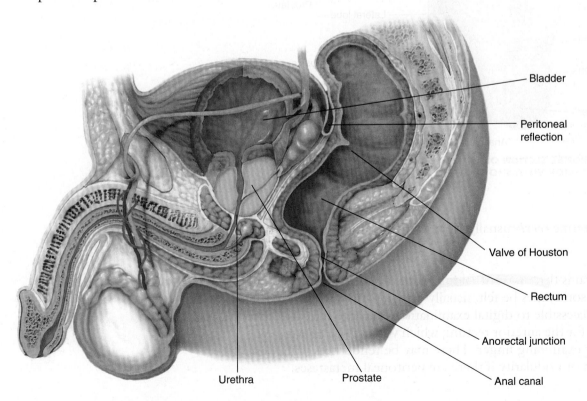

- Bladder
- Peritoneal reflection
- Valve of Houston
- Rectum
- Anorectal junction
- Anal canal
- Urethra
- Prostate

A serrated line marking the change from skin to mucous membrane demarcates the anal canal from the rectum. This anorectal junction, often called the *pectinate* or *dentate line*, is also the boundary between somatic and visceral nerve supplies. It is easily visible on proctoscopic examination, but is not palpable.

Above the anorectal junction, the rectum balloons out and turns posteriorly into the hollow of the coccyx and the sacrum. In the male, the three lobes of the *prostate gland* surround the urethra. The prostate gland is small during childhood, but between puberty and approximately 20 years, it increases roughly fivefold in size. Prostate volume further expands as the gland becomes hyperplastic (see p. 595). The two lateral lobes lie against the anterior rectal wall, where they are palpable as a rounded, heart-shaped structure approximately 2.5 cm long. They are separated by a shallow *median sulcus* or groove, also palpable. Note that the third, or median, lobe is anterior to the urethra and cannot be examined. The *seminal vesicles*, shaped like rabbit ears above the prostate, are also not normally palpable.

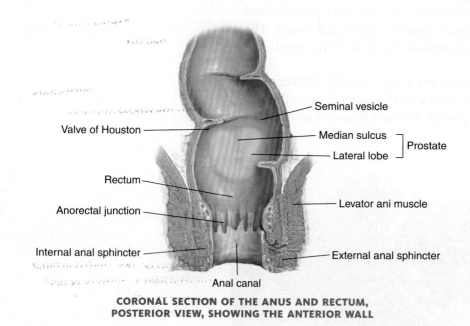

Valve of Houston

Seminal vesicle

Median sulcus
Lateral lobe ⎫ Prostate ⎬
⎭

Rectum

Anorectal junction

Levator ani muscle

Internal anal sphincter

External anal sphincter

Anal canal

CORONAL SECTION OF THE ANUS AND RECTUM, POSTERIOR VIEW, SHOWING THE ANTERIOR WALL

In the female, the uterine *cervix* usually is palpable through the anterior wall of the rectum.

The rectal wall contains three inward foldings, called *valves of Houston*. The lowest of these can sometimes be felt, usually on the patient's left. Most of the rectum that is accessible to digital examination does not have a peritoneal surface, except for the anterior rectum, which you may be able to reach with the tip of your examining finger. There may be tenderness from peritoneal inflammation or nodularity if there are peritoneal metastases.

The Health History

Common or Concerning Symptoms

▶ Change in bowel habits
▶ Blood in the stool
▶ Pain with defecation; rectal bleeding or tenderness
▶ Anal warts or fissures
▶ Weak stream of urine
▶ Burning with urination

Other chapters have addressed many of the symptoms related to the anorectal area and the prostate. For example, you will need to ask if there has been any change in the pattern of bowel function or the size or caliber of the stools, diarrhea or constipation, and abnormal color of the stools. Review the health history on pp. 442–443 regarding these symptoms, as well as queries about *blood in the stool*, ranging from black stools, suggesting *melena*, to the red blood of *hematochezia*, to *bright-red blood per rectum*. Also ask about the presence of mucus.

See Table 11-3, Constipation, p. 475, and Table 11-5, Black and Bloody Stools, p. 478.

Change in bowel pattern, especially stools of thin pencil-like shape, may warn of *colon cancer*. Blood in the stool may be from polyps or cancer, or from gastrointestinal bleeding or local hemorrhoids; mucus may accompany *villous adenoma*.

Be sure to ask about any personal or family history of colonic polyps or colorectal cancer. Is there any history of inflammatory bowel disease?

Positive answers to these questions indicate increased risk for colorectal cancer and a need for further testing and surveillance (see Screening Recommendations, Chapter 11, pp. 450–451).

Is there any pain on defecation? Any itching? Any extreme tenderness in the anus or rectum? Is there any mucopurulent discharge or bleeding? Any ulcerations? Does the patient have anal intercourse?

Proctitis may be indicated by itching, anorectal pain, tenesmus, or discharge or bleeding from infection or *rectal abscess*. Causes include *gonorrhea, chlamydia, lymphogranuloma venereum*, receptive anal intercourse, ulcerations of *herpes simplex*, chancre of *primary syphilis* (see Table 13-1, Sexually Transmitted Infections of Male Genitalia, p. 534). Itching in younger patients may be from pinworms.

Is there any history of anal warts or anal fissures?

Genital warts may occur from *human papillomavirus, condylomata lata* in secondary syphilis. Anal fissures can be found in *proctitis, Crohn's disease.*

In men, review the pattern of urination (see pp. 445–446). Does the patient have any difficulty starting or holding back the urine stream? Is the flow weak? What about frequent urination, especially at night? Or pain or burning as urine is passed? Any blood in the urine or semen or pain with ejaculation? Is there frequent pain or stiffness in the lower back, hips, or upper thighs?

Also in men, is there any feeling of discomfort or heaviness in the prostate area at the base of the penis? Any associated malaise, fever, or chills?

These symptoms suggest urethral obstruction as in *benign prostatic hyperplasia (BPH)* or *prostate cancer*, especially in men older than 70 years.[1-3] The AUA Symptom Index helps quantify BPH severity and need for referral. See Table 15-1, BPH Symptom Score Index: American Urological Association (AUA), p. 592.

These symptoms suggest possible *prostatitis*.

Health Promotion and Counseling: Evidence and Recommendations

Important Topics for Health Promotion and Counseling

▶ Screening for prostate cancer
▶ Screening for colorectal cancer
▶ Counseling for sexually transmitted infections

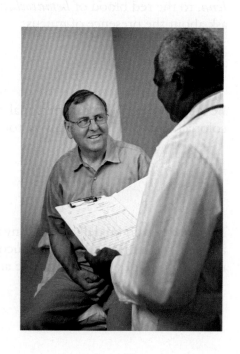

Screening for Prostate Cancer

Risk Factors for Prostate Cancer. Prostate cancer is the leading cancer diagnosed in U.S. men and the second leading cause of death in men, after lung cancer.[4] Although lifetime risk of diagnosis is high, approximately 17%, biologic risk and mortality are only 3%. Approximately 60% of cancers are "organ-confined" at diagnosis, and are slow to invade beyond the prostate capsule.[5] Age, ethnicity, and family history are the primary risk factors.

● *Age.* After age 50 years, the risk of prostate cancer increases sharply with each advancing decade. For white men, the probability of diagnosis rises from 2.1% from ages 50 to 59, to 8% after age 70. For African American men, the increase in probability of diagnosis is even higher, rising from 3.8% to 11.2%.[5]

● *Ethnicity.* For undetermined reasons, incidence rates are significantly higher in African American men than in Caucasian men: 232 cases per 100,000 compared with 146 cases per 100,000, even after adjustments for access to care. Prostate cancer occurs at an earlier age and more advanced stage in African American men. In African American men with <12 years of education, the risk of death from prostate cancer doubles compared to white men.

- **Family history.** Recall that family history is a strong risk factor as you interview your patients. Men with one affected first-degree relative, namely a father or brother, are two to three times more likely to have prostate cancer. Risk of diagnosis in men with two or more affected relatives increases three- to fivefold. Genetics also play a role, especially men with the BRCA2 mutation. Presence of autosomal dominant and X-linked alleles also increase risk and are under investigation.[5,6]

- **Diet.** A series of studies suggests an association between prostate cancer and the high intake of saturated fat from diary and animal sources, but evidence is inconclusive. A recent study showed no evidence of decreased risk from selenium or vitamin E.[7]

The Complexities of Screening. Screening for prostate cancer is fraught with dilemmas. The most common methods for screening, the *prostate-specific antigen (PSA)* test and the *digital rectal exam (DRE)*, are far from ideal. The literature on the characteristics of these tests is reviewed below, followed by sections on current screening recommendations and shared decision making.

- **PSA.** PSA is a glycoprotein produced by prostate epithelial cells. It is a biomarker for early detection of prostate cancer, but it has a number of limitations as a screening test.

  - PSA can be elevated in a number of benign conditions such as hyperplasia, prostatitis, ejaculation, and urinary retention, causing *false positives*. Many men who do not have prostate cancer will test positive and go on to biopsy to determine diagnosis. Some men with prostate cancer will not have an elevated PSA, causing *false negatives.*

  - Cancer can be found at virtually all levels of PSA, so setting cutpoints for intervention is problematic. In the Prostate Cancer Prevention Trial, cancer was found in 10% of men with PSA levels of 0.6 to 1.0 ng/mL, in 24% with levels 2.1 to 3.0, and in 27% with levels 3.1 to 4.0.[8] The common cutpoint for proceeding to biopsy is 4.0 ng/mL. Most men with prostate cancer on biopsy have asymptomatic nonpalpable tumors. Lowering the cutpoint raises the risk of increasing diagnosis and intervention in cancers that may be indolent.

  - PSA does not distinguish small volume indolent cancers from aggressive life-threatening disease. In a number of studies, early diagnosis has not been shown to reduce mortality. PSA screening extends *lead time*, or the time that screening alone advances diagnosis, by 5 to 7 years. Screening also increases *overdiagnosis*, or diagnosis in men who would not have clinical symptoms during their lifetime, by an estimated 23% to 43%.[9] PSA screening can lead to harm from *overtreatment*, as many overdiagnosed patients receive curative surgery or radiation for cancers that may be indolent. The U.S. Preventive Services Task Force (USPSTF) and the National Cancer Institute have determined that "20% to 70% of men who had no problems before radical prostatectomy or external-beam radiation therapy will have reduced sexual function and/or urinary problems."[5]

A number of modifications of PSA screening have been investigated, including use of age-specific cutpoints, PSA density, PSA velocity, and PSA doubling time, but to date these strategies have not been shown to improve health outcomes.[10]

- **DRE.** The DRE has a low sensitivity of 59%, with a specificity of 94%.[11] It detects tumors on the posterior and lateral aspects of the gland but misses the 25% to 35% of tumors arising in other areas. Suspicious findings of nodules, asymmetry, and induration should be pursued. In the past, key organizations have recommended combining PSA with DRE to achieve small gains in detection, but as shown below, recommendations to use DRE for screening are becoming less common.

- *Use of PSA and DRE in recent studies.* The difficulties of using PSA and DRE for screening are illustrated by two large randomized controlled trials published in 2009: the U.S. Prostate, Lung, Colorectal, and Ovarian (PLCO) Cancer Screening Trial of 76,693 men and the Prostate-Cancer Mortality in a Randomized European Study (ERSPC) of 182,000 men.[12-14] It was hoped that these studies would clarify screening guidelines, but the results were conflicting: The PLCO study reported no benefit from screening in reducing mortality; the ERSPC study showed a 20% reduction in mortality in men ages 55 to 69 years at the time of randomization, but at the cost of a overdiagnosis and a 76% false-positive rate on biopsy. In the PLCO study, men were offered either annual PSA testing for 6 years and DRE for 4 years or usual care. PSA ≥4.0 ng/mL was considered positive for prostate cancer. Problems with this study included high levels of prescreening and "contamination" from PSA testing in the control group, improvements in treatment that may have reduced the benefit of screening overall, and closing the study at 7 years, a follow-up interval that may have been too short to show the benefits of screening. The ERSPC study recruited patients from seven different centers with slightly different age criteria and screening intervals. The screening group was usually offered PSA screening once every 4 years; this was not offered to the control group. Average follow-up was 8.8 years. Six of the centers used a PSA cutoff for biopsy of 3.0 ng/mL; one used 4.0 ng/mL. Differences in diagnosis and treatment between the screening and control groups were not delineated.

A 2010 meta-analysis of six randomized controlled studies totaling 387,286 participants also showed that screening leads to early diagnosis, especially of early-stage cancers, but has no significant effect on prostate cancer mortality or overall mortality.[15] The authors point out that all six trials had one or more significant limitations in study methodology, ranging from inadequate concealment of randomization before or after recruitment, termed allocation concealment, to short length of follow-up.

Screening Guidelines From Major Organizations. The perplexing current state of evidence and the variations in screening guidelines across key expert groups put the onus on clinicians to thoroughly understand screening issues and communicate effectively and collaboratively when counseling patients.

Most major medical organizations recommend discussion of the risks and benefits of PSA testing and *individualized screening decisions* beginning at age 50. In 2008, the USPSTF stated that "current evidence is insufficient to assess the balance of benefits and harms of screening for prostate cancer in men younger than age 75 years."[16,17] In men 75 years of age and older, the USPSTF found the incremental benefits of treatment detected by screening as "small to none." The *American Cancer Society (ACS)* guidelines in 2010 recommend informed decision making about screening beginning at age 50 for men at average risk, at age 45 for men at high risk from a single affected first-degree relative, and at age 40 for men at very high risk from two or more affected relatives.[18] For those men choosing screening, the ACS recommends PSA testing with optional DRE every 2 years, if the PSA is <2.5 ng/mL, and annually if the PSA is ≥2.5 mg/dL. The ACS states that asymptomatic men with less than a 10-year life expectancy should not be offered screening; this encompasses about half of men at age 75 due to significant comorbidities. To help men make informed decisions, the ACS urges clinicians to offer a number of decision aids, detailed below. The *American Urological Association* recommends a baseline PSA and DRE at age 40 for asymptomatic men with more than a 10-year life expectancy and "for well-informed men who wish to pursue early diagnosis," then continued surveillance.[19]

Other experts have adopted risk stratification to reduce unnecessary treatment. One study targeted chemoprevention with 5α reductase inhibitors to high-risk men with at least one negative biopsy; however, risk of later high-grade cancers was not notably affected.[20,21] Another study determined that men with a PSA ≤1 ng/mL at age 60 are unlikely to develop life-threatening cancers; 90% of deaths from prostate cancer occurred in men with a PSA above 2 at age 60.[22]

Chemoprevention. Use of chemoprevention remains an area of active research and entails complex decision making for clinicians and patients. Testosterone is converted to the principal intracellular androgen, dihydrotestosterone, by 5α reductase isoenzymes type 1 and type 2. Finasteride inhibits the type 2 isoenzyme and dutasteride inhibits both type 1 and type 2. These agents appear to shrink or inhibit growth of existing cancers rather than prevent them. Although these agents appear to reduce cancer detected on random biopsies, it is unclear whether they reduce clinically significant, or high-grade, cancers.[20,21,23] They clearly ameliorate BPH symptoms and suppress PSA during treatment, so it is important to multiply the PSA by 2.0 to 2.5, depending on how many years the patient has been treated, to recalculate thresholds for biopsy.

Counseling Men About Prostate Cancer

The Challenges of Communicating Screening Benefits and Risks. Clinicians face a number of challenges when promoting informed patient screening decisions: complex and conflicting evidence, time pressures that make lengthy discussions difficult, and patient understanding of statistics and testing. One promising strategy is the *Ask-Tell-Ask* approach, derived from motivational interviewing and readiness models of behavior change.[24–26] Clinicians are urged to first *Ask*, to assess the patient's desire for information, for example, "Have you thought about whether you want to be screened for prostate cancer?" An "anchor point" question such as "Patients vary in how much they would like to hear before making a decision. What would help you make this decision?" gives patients permission express a range of responses and suggests there is "no right answer." The next step in this model is *Tell*, filling in the information requested by the patient, keeping the patient's educational level in mind and using appropriate decision aids. Finally, *Ask* if the patient is ready to make a decision, for example, "Does screening sound like something you want to do?" If the patient is unsure, clinicians are encouraged to make a patient-centered recommendation based on concerns and values the patient has already shared. (See also Chapter 2, Clinical Reasoning, Assessment and Plan, and the Patient Record, pp. 25–53.)

Resources for Prostate Cancer Information. Encourage men to take advantage of the many resources available to help them make decisions about prostate cancer screening.

Decision Aids for Prostate Cancer Screening

Testing for Prostate Cancer (American Cancer Society):
www.cancer.org/acs/groups/content/@nho/documents/document/acspc-024618.pdf

PSA Testing (Foundation for Informed Decision Making):
www.healthcrossroads.com/example/crossroad.aspx?contentGUID=fc326615-5b29-47f1-87c3-9a3e2d946919

Prostate Cancer Screening: A Decision Guide (Centers for Disease Control and Prevention). See also Web sites for African Americans and Hispanic Americans:
www.cdc.gov/cancer/prostate/pdf/prosguide.pdf
www.cdc.gov/cancer/prostate/pdf/aaprosguide.pdf
www.cdc.gov/cancer/prostate/pdf/prostate_cancer_spanish.pdf

Prostate Cancer Screening: Should you get a PSA test? (Mayo Clinic):
www.mayoclinic.com/health/prostate-cancer/HQ01273

PROSDEX: A PSA Decision Aid (University of Cardiff):
www.prosdex.com/index_content.htm

Source: American Cancer Society. Cancer facts and figures 2010—prostate cancer, p 29. Available at http://www.cancer.org/acs/groups/content/@epidemiologysurveilance/documents/document/acspc-026238.pdf All Web sites accessed December 12, 2010.

Screening for Colorectal Cancer.   In 2008, both the USPSTF and the ACS Colorectal Cancer Advisory Group, consisting of the ACS, the U.S. Multi-Society Task Force on Colorectal Cancer, and the American College of Radiology, updated screening guidelines for colorectal cancer (CRC).[27-29] These guidelines are reviewed in Chapter 11, The Abdomen, on pp. 450. An abbreviated summary is provided below.

- Identify patients at average or increased risk, ideally by age 20 years, but earlier if there are high-risk factors such as inflammatory bowel disease or a family history of an inherited polyposis syndrome (see p. 450).

- *Offer patients at average risk a range of screening options beginning at age 50 years:* annual screening with high-sensitivity fecal occult blood tests (FOBTs); sigmoidoscopy every 5 years, with high-sensitivity FOBT every 3 years; or screening colonoscopy every 10 years.[27] The ACS Colorectal Cancer Advisory Group also endorses the options of double-contrast barium enema or computed tomography colonography every 5 years.[29]

- Patients at increased risk should undergo colonoscopy every 3 to 5 years.

For best results, high-sensitivity FOBT should involve at-home collection of six samples over a 2- to 3-day period. The single sample test collected during DRE is considered inadequate due to low sensitivity.[30] Note that DRE is not a recommended screening method because it covers only 7 cm to 8 cm of the rectum.

Counseling for Sexually Transmitted Infections (STIs).   Anal intercourse places men and women at risk for perianal and rectal abrasions and transmission of HIV and other STIs. Protective measures include abstinence from high-risk behaviors (see pp. 524–526), use of condoms, and good hygiene.

Techniques of Examination

For many patients and examiners, the rectal examination is the least popular segment of the physical examination. It may cause discomfort for the patient, but it is rarely painful. You may choose to omit the rectal examination in adolescents who have no relevant complaints. In middle-aged or older adults, it is useful for screening and assessing symptoms. Aim for a calm demeanor, an explanation to the patient of what he or she may feel, gentleness, and slow movement of your finger.

MALE

Choose one of several suitable patient positions for conducting the examination. Often, the clinician asks the patient to stand and lean forward with his upper body resting across the examining table and hips flexed. For most purposes, the side-lying position, depicted below, is satisfactory and allows good visualization of the perianal and sacrococcygeal areas.

No matter how you position the patient, your examining finger cannot reach the full length of the rectum. If a rectosigmoid cancer is suspected or screening is warranted, consider sigmoidoscopy or colonoscopy.

Ask the patient to lie on his left side with his buttocks close to the edge of the examining table near you. Flexing the patient's hips and knees, especially in the upper leg, stabilizes his position and improves visibility. Drape the patient appropriately and adjust the light for the best view. Glove your hands and spread the buttocks apart.

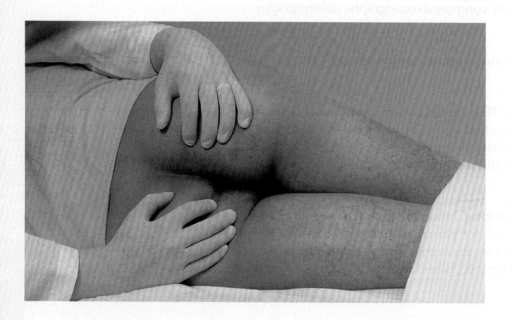

- *Inspect the sacrococcygeal and perianal areas* for lumps, ulcers, inflammation, rashes, or excoriations. Adult perianal skin is normally more pigmented and somewhat coarser than the skin over the buttocks. Palpate any abnormal areas, noting lumps or tenderness.

- *Examine the anus and rectum.* Lubricate your gloved index finger, explain to the patient what you are going to do, and tell him that the examination may trigger an urge to move his bowels but that this will not occur. Ask him to strain down. Inspect the anus, noting any lesions.

Anal and perianal lesions include hemorrhoids, venereal warts, herpes, syphilitic chancre, and carcinoma. A linear crack or tear suggests *anal fissure* from large, hard stools, inflammatory bowel disease, or STIs. Consider *pruritus ani* if there is swollen, thickened, fissured perianal skin with excoriations.

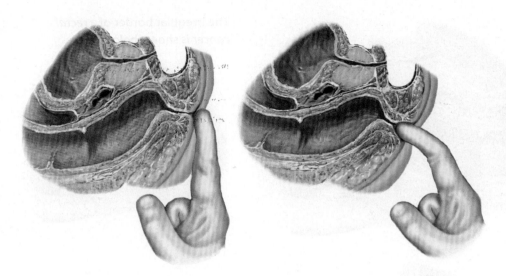

Tender, purulent, reddened mass with fever or chills accompanies an *anal abscess*. Abscesses tunneling to the skin surface from the anus or rectum may form a clogged or draining *anorectal fistula*. Fistulas may ooze blood, pus, or feculent mucus. Consider anoscopy or sigmoidoscopy for better visualization.

As the patient strains, place the pad of your gloved and lubricated index finger over the anus.

As the sphincter relaxes, gently insert your fingertip into the anal canal in the direction pointing toward the umbilicus. If you feel the sphincter tighten, pause and reassure the patient. When, in a moment, the sphincter relaxes, proceed.

Occasionally, severe tenderness prevents entry and internal examination. Do not try to force it. Instead, place your fingers on both sides of the anus, gently spread the orifice, and ask the patient to strain down. Look for a lesion, such as an anal fissure, that might explain the tenderness.

If you can proceed without undue discomfort to the patient, note:

- The sphincter tone of the anus. Normally, the muscles of the anal sphincter close snugly around your finger. Initial resting tone reflects the integrity of the internal anal sphincter. To check external sphincter tone, ask the patient to bear down and squeeze the rectal muscles.

- Tenderness, if any

- Induration

- Irregularities or nodules

Insert your finger into the rectum as far as possible. Rotate your hand clockwise to palpate as much of the rectal surface as possible on the patient's right side, then counterclockwise to palpate the surface posteriorly and on the patient's left side.

Sphincter tightness may occur with anxiety, inflammation, or scarring; laxity occurs in neurologic diseases, such as S2-4 cord lesions.

Induration may be caused by inflammation, scarring, or malignancy.

See Table 15-2, Abnormalities of the Anus, Surrounding Skin, and Rectum, pp. 593–594.

Note any nodules, irregularities, or induration. To bring a possible lesion into reach, take your finger off the rectal surface, ask the patient to strain down, and palpate again.

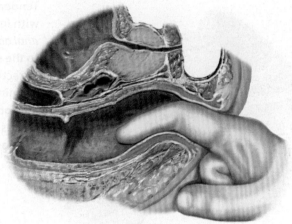

The irregular border of a *rectal cancer* is shown below.

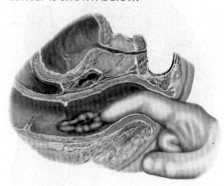

Then rotate your hand further counterclockwise so that your finger can examine the *posterior surface of the prostate gland*. By turning your body somewhat away from the patient, you can feel this area more easily. Tell the patient that examining his prostate gland may prompt an urge to urinate.

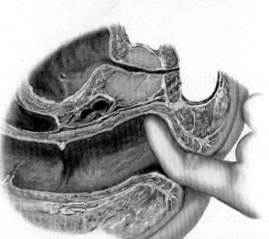

Sweep your finger carefully over the prostate gland, identifying its lateral lobes and the median sulcus between them. Note the size, shape, and consistency of the prostate, and identify any nodules or tenderness. The normal prostate is rubbery and nontender.

See Table 15-3, Abnormalities of the Prostate, p. 595.

If possible, *extend your finger above the prostate* to the region of the seminal vesicles and the peritoneal cavity and sweep the anterior wall. Note any nodules or tenderness.

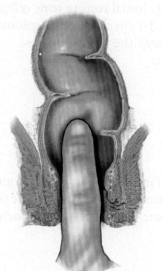

Findings include a rectal "shelf" of peritoneal metastases (see p. 594) or the tenderness of peritoneal inflammation.

Gently withdraw your finger, and wipe the anus or give the patient tissues. Note the color of any fecal matter on your glove, and test it for occult blood.

A single fecal occult blood test is not an adequate screen for *colon cancer*.[30] (See p. 585.)

PALPATING THE PROSTATE

FEMALE

The rectum is usually examined after the female genitalia while the woman is in the lithotomy position. This position allows you to conduct the bimanual examination and delineate a possible adnexal or pelvic mass. It allows you to test the integrity of the rectovaginal wall and may help you to palpate a cancer high in the rectum.

If you need to examine only the rectum, the lateral position is satisfactory and affords a much better view to the perianal and sacrococcygeal areas. Use the same techniques for examination that you use for men. Note that the cervix is readily palpated through the anterior wall. Sometimes a retroverted uterus is also palpable. Do not mistake either of these, or a vaginal tampon, for a tumor.

Recording Your Findings

Note that initially you may use sentences to describe your findings; later you will use phrases. The style below contains phrases appropriate for most write-ups.

Recording the Physical Examination—The Anus, Rectum, and Prostate

"No perirectal lesions or fissures. External sphincter tone intact. Rectal vault without masses. Prostate smooth and nontender with palpable median sulcus. (Or in a female, uterine cervix nontender.) Stool brown and Hemoccult negative."
OR
"Perirectal area inflamed; no ulcerations, warts, or discharge. Unable to examine external sphincter, rectal vault, or prostate because of spasm of external sphincter and marked inflammation and tenderness of anal canal."
OR

Raises concern of proctitis from infectious cause

"No perirectal lesions or fissures. External sphincter tone intact. Rectal vault without masses. Left lateral prostate lobe with 1- × 1-cm firm, hard nodule; right lateral lobe smooth; median sulcus obscured. Stool brown and Hemoccult negative."

Raises concern of prostate cancer

Bibliography

Citations

1. Barry MJ, Fowler FJ, O'Leary M et al. The American Urological Association symptom index for benign prostatic hyperplasia. J Urol 1992;148:1549–1557.

2. American Urological Association. Management of BPH. 2003, updated 2006. Available at http://www.auanet.org/content/guidelines-and-quality-care/clinical-guidelines.cfm?sub=bph. Accessed December 5, 2010.

3. Edwards JL. Diagnosis and management of benign prostatic hyperplasia. Am Fam Physician 2008;77:1403–1410.

4. American Cancer Society. Cancer facts and figures 2010 - prostate cancer (pp. 23–37). Available at http://www.cancer.org/acs/groups/content/@epidemiologysurveilance/documents/document/acspc-026238.pdf. Accessed December 5, 2010.

5. National Cancer Institute. Prostate cancer screening. Health professional version. Updated December 3, 2010. Available at http://www.cancer.gov/cancertopics/pdq/screening/prostate/healthprofessional/allpages. Accessed December 10, 2010.

6. Johns LE, Houlston RS. A systematic review and meta-analysis of familial prostate cancer risk. BJU Int 2003;91:789–794.

7. Lippman SM, Klein EA, Goodman PJ et al. Effect of selenium and vitamin E on risk of prostate cancer and other cancers: the Selenium and Vitamin E Cancer Prevention Trial (SELECT). JAMA 2009;301:39–51.

8. Thompson IM, Pauler DK, Goodman PJ et al. Prevalence of prostate cancer among men with a prostate-specific antigen level ≤ 4.0 ng per milliliter. N Engl J Med 2004;350:2239–2246.

9. Draisma G. Etzioni R et al. Lead time and overdiagnosis in prostate-specific antigen screening: importance of methods and context. J Natl Cancer Inst 2009;101:374–383.

10. U.S. Preventive Services Task Force. Screening for Prostate Cancer: U.S. Preventive Services Task Force Recommendation Statement. August 2008. Available at http://www.uspreventiveservicestaskforce.org/uspstf08/prostate/prostaters.htm. Accessed December 5, 2010.

11. Hoogendam A, Buntinx F, de Vet HC. The diagnostic value of digital rectal examination in primary care screening for prostate cancer: a meta-analysis. Fam Pract 1999;6:621–626.

12. Andriole GL, Crawford ED, Grubb RL et al. Mortality results from a randomized prostate-cancer screening trial. N Engl J Med 2009;360:1310–1319.

13. Schroder FH, Hugosson J, Roobol MJ et al. Screening and prostate-cancer mortality in a randomized European study. N Engl J Med 2009;360:1320–1328.

14. Barry MJ. Screening for prostate cancer—a controversy that refuses to die. (editorial) N Engl J Med 2009;360:1351–1354.

15. Djulbegovic M, Beyth RJ, Neuberger MM et al. Screening for prostate cancer: systematic review and meta-analysis of randomized controlled trials. BMJ 2010;341:c4543.

16. U.S. Preventive Services Task Force. Screening for prostate cancer: U.S. Preventive Services Task Force recommendation statement. Ann Intern Med 2008;149:185–191.

17. Lin K, Lipsitz R, Miller R et al. Benefits and harms of prostate-specific antigen screening for prostate cancer: an evidence update for the U. S. Preventive Services Task Force. Ann Intern Med 2008;149:192–199.

18. American Cancer Society. American Cancer Society recommendation for early detection of prostate cancer. Updated December 1 2010. Available at http://www.cancer.org/Cancer/ProstateCancer/MoreInformation/ProstateCancerEarlyDetection/prostate-cancer-early-detection-acs-recommendations. Accessed December 11, 2010.

19. American Urological Association. Prostate specific antigen best practice statement: 2009 update. Available at http://www.auanet.org/content/media/psa09.pdf. Accessed December 5, 2010.

20. Andriole GL, Bostwick DG, Brawley OW et al. Effect of dutasteride on the risk of prostate cancer. N Engl J Med 2010;362:1192–1202.

21. Walsh PC. Chemoprevention of prostate cancer (editorial). N Engl J Med 2010;362:1237–1238.

22. Vickers AJ, Cronin AM, Björk T et al. Prostate specific antigen concentration at age 60 and death or metastasis from prostate cancer: case-control study. BMJ 2010;341:c4521.

23. Thompson IM, Goodman PJ, Tangen CM et al. The influence of finasteride on the development of prostate cancer. N Engl J Med 2003;349:215–224.

24. Gaster B, Edwards K, Trinidad SB et al. Patient-centered discussions about prostate cancer screening: a real-world approach. Ann Intern Med 2010;153:661–665.

25. Hettema J, Steele J et al. Motivational interviewing. Ann Rev Clin Psychol 2005;1:91–111.

26. Kemp EC, Floyd MR et al. Patients prefer the method of "tell-back-collaborative inquiry" to assess understanding of medical information. J Am Board Fam Med 2008;21:24–30.

27. U.S. Preventive Services Task Force. Screening for colorectal cancer: U.S. Preventive Services Task Force recommendation statement. Ann Intern Med 2008;148:627–637.

28. Whitlock EP, Lin JS, Liles E et al. Screening for colorectal cancer: a targeted, updated systematic review for the U.S. Preventive Services Task Force. Ann Intern Med 2008;149:638–658.

29. Levin B, Leiberman DA, McFarland B et al. American Cancer Society Colorectal Cancer Advisory Group. Screening and surveillance for the early detection of colorectal cancer and adenomatous polyps, 2008: a joint guideline from the American Cancer Society, the US Multi-Society Task Force on Colorectal Cancer, and the American College of Radiology. CA Cancer J Clin 2008;58:130–160.

30. Collins JF, Lieberman DA, Durbin TE et al. Veterans Affairs Cooperative Study #380 Group. Accuracy of screening for rectal occult blood on a single stool sample obtained by digital rectal examination: a comparison with recommended sampling practice. Ann Intern Med 2005;142:81–85.

Additional References

Dube C, Rostum A, Lewin G et al. The use of aspirin for primary prevention of colorectal cancer: a systematic review prepared for the U.S. Preventive Services Task Force. Ann Intern Med 2007;146:365–375.

Hugosson J, Carlsson S, Aus G et al. Mortality results from the Goteborg randomised population-based prostate-cancer screening trial. Lancet Oncol 2010;11:725–732.

Hull TL. Ch 122, Diseases of the Anorectum. In Feldman M, Friedman LS, Brandt LJ (eds). *Sleisenger & Fordtran's Gastrointestinal and Liver Disease: Pathophysiology, Diagnosis, Management*, 2-volume set, 9th ed. Philadelphia: Saunders/Elsevier, 2010.

Ilic D, O'Connor D, Green S et al. Screening for prostate cancer. Cochrane Database Syst Rev 3:CD004720, 2006.

National Cancer Institute. Colorectal screening. Health professional version. Available at http://www.cancer.gov/cancertopics/pdq/screening/colorectal/healthprofessional/allpages. Accessed December 12, 2010.

National Cancer Institute. Colorectal cancer prevention. Health professional version. Available at http://www.cancer.org/acs/groups/content/@epidemiologysurveilance/documents/document/acspc-026238.pdf. Accessed December 12, 2010.

Philip J, Dutta RS, Ballal M et al. Is a digital rectal examination necessary in the diagnosis and clinical staging of early prostate cancer? BJU Int 2005;95:969–971.

Shteynshlyuger A, Andriole GL. Prostate cancer: to screen or not to screen? Urol Clin North Am 2010;37:1–9.

U.S. Preventive Services Task Force. Screening for Prostate Cancer: U.S. Preventive Services Task Force Recommendation Statement DRAFT: Summary of Recommendation and Evidence. October 2011. Available at http://www.uspreventiveservicestaskforce.org/draftrec3.htm. Accessed November 6, 2011.

The Bates' suite offers these additional resources to enhance learning and facilitate understanding of this chapter:

• *Bates' Pocket Guide to Physical Examination and History Taking*, 7th edition
• *Bates' Visual Guide to Physical Examination*
• thePoint online resources, for students and instructors: http://thepoint.lww.com

Score or ask the patient to score each of the questions below. Higher scores (maximum 35) indicate more severe symptoms; scores ≤7 are considered mild and generally do not warrant treatment.

PART A	Not at All	Less Than 1 Time in 5	Less Than Half the Time	About Half the Time	More Than Half the Time	Almost Always	Total Points for Each Row
1. Incomplete emptying: Over the past month, how often have you had a sensation of not emptying your bladder completely after you finished urinating?	0	1	2	3	4	5	
2. Frequency: Over the past month, how often have you had to urinate again <2 hours after you finished urinating?	0	1	2	3	4	5	
3. Intermittency: Over the past month, how often have you stopped and started again several times when you urinated?	0	1	2	3	4	5	
4. Urgency: Over the past month, how often have you found it difficult to postpone urination?	0	1	2	3	4	5	
5. Weak stream: Over the past month, how often have you had a weak urinary stream?	0	1	2	3	4	5	
6. Straining: Over the past month, how often have you had to push or strain to begin urination?	0	1	2	3	4	5	
PART B	**None**	**1 Time**	**2 Times**	**3 Times**	**4 Times**	**5 Times**	**Points for Part B**
7. Nocturia: Over the past month, how many times did you most typically get up to urinate from the time you went to bed at night until the time you got up in the morning?	0	1	2	3	4	5	

TOTAL PARTS A and B (maximum 35) _____

Adapted from: Madsen FA, Bruskewitz RC. Clinical manifestations of benign prostatic hyperplasia. Urol Clin North Am 1995:22:291–298.

Table
15-2
Abnormalities of the Anus, Surrounding Skin, and Rectum

Pilonidal Cyst and Sinus

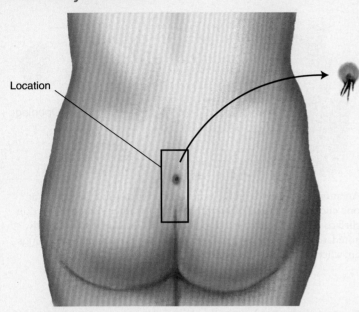

Location

A pilonidal cyst is a fairly common, probably congenital, abnormality located in the midline superficial to the coccyx or the lower sacrum. Look for the opening of a sinus tract. This opening may exhibit a small tuft of hair surrounded by a halo of erythema. Although pilonidal cysts are generally asymptomatic, except perhaps for slight drainage, abscess formation and secondary sinus tracts may complicate the picture.

External Hemorrhoids (*Thrombosed*)

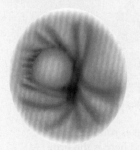

External hemorrhoids are dilated hemorrhoidal veins that originate below the pectinate line and are covered with skin. They seldom produce symptoms unless thrombosis occurs. This causes acute local pain that increases with defecation and sitting. A tender, swollen, bluish, ovoid mass is visible at the anal margin.

Internal Hemorrhoids (*Prolapsed*)

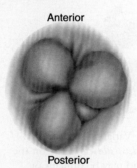

Anterior

Posterior

Internal hemorrhoids are enlargements of the normal vascular cushions located above the pectinate line. They are not usually palpable. Sometimes, especially during defecation, internal hemorrhoids may cause bright-red bleeding. They may also prolapse through the anal canal and appear as reddish, moist, protruding masses, typically located in one or more of the positions illustrated.

Prolapse of the Rectum

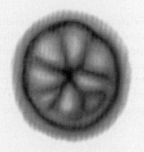

On straining for a bowel movement, the rectal mucosa, with or without its muscular wall, may prolapse through the anus, appearing as a doughnut or rosette of red tissue. A prolapse involving only mucosa is relatively small and shows radiating folds, as illustrated. When the entire bowel wall is involved, the prolapse is larger and covered by concentrically circular folds.

(table continues on page 594)

Anal Fissure

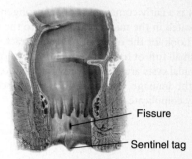

Fissure

Sentinel tag

An anal fissure is a very painful oval ulceration of the anal canal, found most commonly in the midline posteriorly, less commonly in the midline anteriorly. Its long axis lies longitudinally. There may be a swollen "sentinel" skin tag just below it. Gentle separation of the anal margins may reveal the lower edge of the fissure. The sphincter is spastic; the examination is painful. Local anesthesia may be required.

Anorectal Fistula

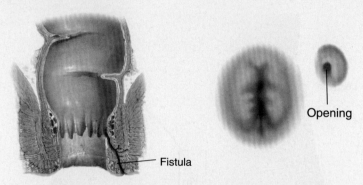

Opening

Fistula

An anorectal fistula is an inflammatory tract or tube that opens at one end into the anus or rectum and at the other end onto the skin surface (as shown here) or into another viscus. An abscess usually antedates such a fistula. Look for the fistulous opening or openings anywhere in the skin around the anus.

Polyps of the Rectum

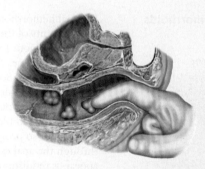

Polyps of the rectum are fairly common. Variable in size and number, they can develop on a stalk (*pedunculated*) or lie on the mucosal surface (*sessile*). They are soft and may be difficult or impossible to feel even when in reach of the examining finger. Proctoscopy and biopsy are needed for differentiation of benign from malignant lesions.

Cancer of the Rectum

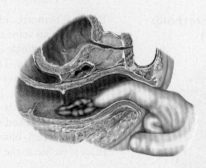

Asymptomatic carcinoma of the rectum makes routine rectal examination important for adults. Illustrated here is the firm, nodular, rolled edge of an ulcerated cancer.

Rectal Shelf

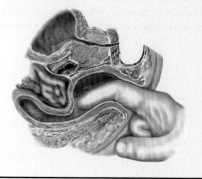

Widespread peritoneal metastases from any source may develop in the area of the peritoneal reflection anterior to the rectum. A firm to hard nodular rectal "shelf" may be just palpable with the tip of the examining finger. In a woman, this shelf of metastatic tissue develops in the rectouterine pouch, behind the cervix and the uterus.

Table
15-3   **Abnormalities of the Prostate**

Normal Prostate Gland

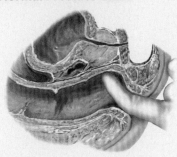

As palpated through the anterior rectal wall, the normal prostate is a rounded, heart-shaped structure approximately 2.5 cm long. The median sulcus can be felt between the two lateral lobes. Only the posterior surface of the prostate is palpable. Anterior lesions, including those that may obstruct the urethra, are not detectable by physical examination.

Prostatitis

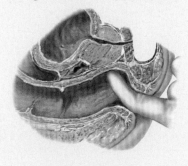

Acute bacterial prostatitis, illustrated here, presents with fever and urinary tract symptoms such as frequency, urgency, dysuria, incomplete voiding, and sometimes low back pain. The gland feels tender, swollen, "boggy," and warm. Examine it gently. More than 80% of infections are caused by gram-negative aerobes such as *E. coli*, *Enterococcus*, and *Proteus*. In men younger than 35, consider sexual transmission of *Neisseria gonorrhea* and *Chlamydia trachomatis*.

Chronic bacterial prostatitis is associated with recurrent urinary tract infections, usually from the same organism. Men may be asymptomatic or have symptoms of dysuria or mild pelvic pain. The prostate gland may feel normal, without tenderness or swelling. Cultures of prostatic fluid usually show infection with *E. coli*.

It may be challenging to distinguish these conditions from the more common *chronic pelvic pain syndrome*, seen in up to 80% of symptomatic men who report obstructive or irritative symptoms on voiding but show no evidence of prostate or urinary tract infection. Physical examination findings are not predictable, but examination is needed to assess any prostate induration or asymmetry suggestive of carcinoma.

Benign Prostatic Hyperplasia

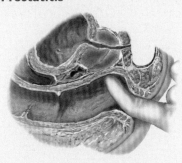

Benign prostatic hyperplasia is a nonmalignant enlargement of the prostate gland that increases with age, present in more than 50% of men by 50 years. Symptoms arise both from smooth-muscle contraction in the prostate and bladder neck and from compression of the urethra. They may be irritative (urgency, frequency, nocturia), obstructive (decreased stream, incomplete emptying, straining), or both, and are seen in more than one-third of men by 65 years. The affected gland may be normal in size, or may feel symmetrically enlarged, smooth, and firm, though slightly elastic; there may be obliteration of the median sulcus and more notable protrusion into the rectal lumen.

Cancer of the Prostate

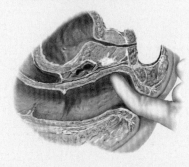

Cancer of the prostate is suggested by an area of hardness in the gland. A distinct hard nodule that alters the contour of the gland may or may not be palpable. As the cancer enlarges, it feels irregular and may extend beyond the confines of the gland. The median sulcus may be obscured. Hard areas in the prostate are not always malignant. They may also result from prostatic stones, chronic inflammation, and other conditions.

The Musculoskeletal System

Musculoskeletal disorders are the leading cause of medical-office visits in the United States. These disorders total 91 million visits, or 7.9% of all ambulatory care visits, making competent office examinations ever more important. Three of the top ten ambulatory diagnoses are musculoskeletal.[1] Arthritis alone affects one in five Americans, or 19% of the population, and is the leading cause of disability, costing more than $128 billion a year; back and spine problems rank second, affecting almost 17% of Americans.[2,3] Low back pain, the fifth most frequent reason for office visits, represents a continuing clinical challenge; 85% of low back pain cases are "nonspecific," yet this category is one of the most common and expensive causes of work-related disability.[4,5]

Estimated Prevalence and Average Age at Onset for Common Musculoskeletal Conditions in the U.S.

Condition	Prevalence	
Low back pain	26 million	
Osteoarthritis	17 million	
Fibromyalgia	3.7 million	
RA	2.1 million	
Gout	2.1 million	Women / Men
Carpal tunnel	2.0 million	
PMR	450K	
Ankylosing spondylitis	300K	
SLE	239K	
Psoriatic arthritis	160K–275K	
Scleroderma	≤34K	
Myositis	≤25K	DM / DM/PM

Age at onset, years (0–80)

Prevalences for most conditions vary between the sexes. Osteoarthritis, for example, is more common in women, especially in the knee.

RA, rheumatoid arthritis; PMR, polymyalgia rheumatica; SLE, systemic lupus erythematosus; DM, dermatomyositis; PM, polymyositis.

Source: Cush JJ, Lipsky PE. Approach to articular and musculoskeletal disorders. In: Kasper DL, Braunwald E, Fauci AS, et al., eds. Harrison's Principles of Internal Medicine, 16th ed. New York: McGraw-Hill, 2005 (Data 1998).

Each of the major joints has a unique profile of anatomy and directional movement. In this chapter the Anatomy and Physiology section and Techniques for Examination *are combined*, to help students apply their knowledge of the anatomy and function of each joint to the specific examination techniques needed. These sections follow a head-to-toe sequence, beginning with the jaw and joints of the upper extremities. Sharpen your skills as you inspect the surface structures and contours of each joint learn to visualize the joint's underlying anatomy. Visualization helps trigger the examination techniques and maneuvers you will need to perform. In a sense, for joints anatomy is destiny...

Chapter Organization

> ▶ **Joint Structure and Function**
> ▶ **The Health History**
> ▶ **Health Promotion and Counseling**
> ▶ **Examination of Specific Joints: Anatomy and Physiology and Related Examination Techniques**
>> ▶ The chapter follows a "head-to-toe" sequence: *temporomandibular joint, shoulder, elbow, wrist and hand, spine, hip, knee and lower leg, ankle and foot.*
>
> ▶ For each joint, there are subsections on *Joint Overview, Bony Structures and Joints, Muscle Groups and Additional Structures,* and *Examination Techniques.*
>> ▶ *Joint Overview* presents the distinguishing anatomical and functional characteristics of each joint.
>> ▶ *Techniques of Examination* presents the fundamental steps for examining that joint—*inspection, palpation* of bony and soft-tissue structures, assessment of *range of motion* (the arc of measurable joint movement in a single plane), and *maneuvers* to test the joint's function and stability.

OVERVIEW: JOINT STRUCTURE AND FUNCTION

It is helpful to begin by reviewing some anatomical terminology.

- *Articular structures* include the joint capsule and articular cartilage, the synovium and synovial fluid, intra-articular ligaments, and juxta-articular bone. Articular cartilage is comprised of a collagen matrix containing charged ions and water, allowing the cartilage to change shape in response to pressure or load, acting as a cushion for underlying bone. Synovial fluid provides nutrition to the adjacent relatively avascular articular cartilage.

Articular disease typically involves swelling and tenderness of the entire joint and limits both active and passive range of motion due either to stiffness or to pain.

- *Extra-articular structures* include periarticular ligaments, tendons, bursae, muscle, fascia, bone, nerve, and overlying skin.

Extra-articular disease typically involves selected regions of the joint and types of movement.

  - *Ligaments* are ropelike bundles of collagen fibrils that connect bone to bone.

- *Tendons* are collagen fibers connecting muscle to bone.

- *Bursae* are pouches of synovial fluid that cushion the movement of tendons and muscles over bone or other joint structures.

To understand joint function, study the various types of joints and how they articulate, or interconnect, and the role of bursae in easing joint movement.

Types of Joint Articulation

There are three primary types of joint articulation—synovial, cartilaginous, and fibrous—allowing varying degrees of movement.

Joints

Type of Joint	Extent of Movement	Example
Synovial	Freely movable	Knee, shoulder
Cartilaginous	Slightly movable	Vertebral bodies of the spine
Fibrous	Immovable	Skull sutures

Synovial Joints. The bones do not touch each other, and the joint articulations are *freely movable* within the limits surrounding ligaments. The bones are covered by *articular cartilage* and separated by a *synovial cavity* that cushions joint movement. A *synovial membrane* lines the synovial cavity and secretes a small amount of viscous lubricating fluid, the *synovial fluid*. The membrane is attached at the margins of the articular cartilage and pouched or folded to accommodate joint movement. Surrounding the joint is a fibrous *joint capsule,* which is strengthened by ligaments extending from bone to bone.

Cartilaginous Joints. These joints, such as those between vertebrae and the symphysis pubis, are slightly movable. Fibrocartilaginous discs separate the bony surfaces. At the center of each disc is the *nucleus pulposus,* somewhat gelatinous fibrocartilaginous material that serves as a cushion or shock absorber between bony surfaces.

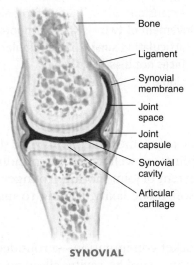

SYNOVIAL

CARTILAGINOUS

Fibrous Joints. In these joints, such as the sutures of the skull, intervening layers of fibrous tissue or cartilage hold the bones together. The bones are almost in direct contact, which allows *no appreciable movement.*

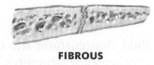

FIBROUS

Structure of Synovial Joints

As you learn about the examination of the musculoskeletal system, think about how the anatomy of the joint relates to its movement.

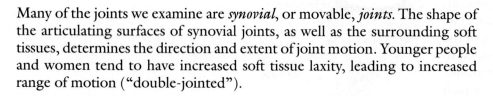

Synovial Joints

Type of Joint	Articular Shape	Movement	Example
Spheroidal (ball and socket)	Convex surface in concave cavity	Wide-ranging flexion, extension, abduction, adduction, rotation, circumduction	Shoulder, hip
Hinge	Flat, planar	Motion in one plane; flexion, extension	Interphalangeal joints of hand and foot; elbow
Condylar	Convex or concave	Movement of two articulating surfaces not dissociable	Knee; temporomandibular joint

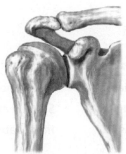

SPHEROIDAL JOINT (BALL AND SOCKET)

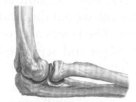

HINGE JOINT

Many of the joints we examine are *synovial*, or movable, *joints*. The shape of the articulating surfaces of synovial joints, as well as the surrounding soft tissues, determines the direction and extent of joint motion. Younger people and women tend to have increased soft tissue laxity, leading to increased range of motion ("double-jointed").

- *Spheroidal joints* have a ball-and-socket configuration—a rounded, convex surface articulating with a concave cuplike cavity, allowing a wide range of rotatory movement, as in the shoulder and hip.

- *Hinge joints* are flat, planar, or slightly curved, allowing only a gliding motion in a single plane, as in flexion and extension of the digits.

- In *condylar joints*, such as the knee, the articulating surfaces are convex or concave. These joints allow flexion, extension, rotation, and motion in the coronal plane.

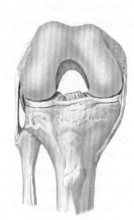

CONDYLAR JOINT

Bursae.   Easing joint action are *bursae*, roughly disc-shaped synovial sacs that allow adjacent muscles or muscles and tendons to glide over each other during movement. They lie between the skin and the convex surface of a bone or joint (as in the prepatellar bursa of the knee, p. 652) or in areas where tendons or muscles rub against bone, ligaments, or other tendons or muscles (as in the subacromial bursa of the shoulder, pp. 617–618).

Knowledge of the underlying joint anatomy and movement will help you assess joints subjected to trauma. Your knowledge of the soft-tissue structures, ligaments, tendons, and bursae will help you evaluate the changes of overuse and arthritis.

The Health History

Common or Concerning Symptoms

▶ Low back pain
▶ Neck pain
▶ Monoarticular or polyarticular joint pain
▶ Inflammatory or infectious joint pain
▶ Joint pain with systemic features such as fever, chills, rash, anorexia, weight loss, weakness
▶ Joint pain with symptoms from other organ systems

Joint pain is one of the leading complaints of patients seeking health care. In addition to obtaining the seven features of any joint pain, adopt the three tips below to guide your subsequent examination and diagnosis:

See Chapter 3, Interviewing and the Health History, for the seven features of pain, pp. 70–71.

Tips for Assessing Joint Pain

▶ Ask the patient to *"point to the pain."* This may save considerable time because the patient's verbal description may be imprecise.
▶ Clarify and record when the pain started and the *mechanism of injury*, particularly if there is a history of trauma.
▶ Determine whether the pain is *localized or diffuse, acute or chronic, inflammatory or noninflammatory*.

Low Back Pain.   You may wish to begin with "Any pains in your back?" because two-thirds of adults have low back pain at least once during their lifetime, usually between the ages of 30 and 50 years. Low back pain is the second most common reason for office visits. Using open-ended questions, get a clear picture of the problem, especially location or radiation of the pain or any history of trauma.

See Table 16-1, Low Back Pain, p. 668.

Approximately 85% of patients have *idiopathic low back pain* (this term is preferred to "sprain" or "strain") usually from musculoligamentous injuries and age-related degenerative processes of the intervertebral discs and facet joints.[5]

Determine if the pain is *on the midline*, over the vertebrae, or *off the midline*.

For *midline back pain*, assess for musculoligamentous injury, disc herniation, vertebral collapse, spinal cord metastases, and, rarely, *epidural abscess*. For *pain off the midline*, assess for muscle strain, sacroiliitis, trochanteric bursitis, sciatica, and hip arthritis; also for renal conditions like pyelonephritis or stones.

Is there radiation into the buttock or lower extremity? Is there any associated numbness or paresthesias?

Sciatica is radicular gluteal and posterior leg pain in the S1 distribution that increases with cough or Valsalva (see pp. 732–733 for related neurologic findings). Leg pain that resolves with rest and/or lumbar forward flexion occurs in *spinal stenosis*.

What about associated bladder or bowel dysfunction?

Consider *cauda equina syndrome* from S2–4 midline disc or tumor if there is bowel or bladder dysfunction (usually urinary retention with overflow incontinence), especially if there is saddle anesthesia or perineal numbness.[5]

Elicit any *key warning signs, or "red flags," for serious underlying systemic disease:* age older than 50 years, history of cancer, unexplained weight loss, pain lasting more than 1 month or not responding to treatment, pain at night or present at rest, history of intravenous drug use, or presence of infection.

In cases of low back pain plus another indicator, there is a 10% probability of serious systemic disease.[6,7]

Neck Pain.   Neck pain is also common. Although neck pain is usually self-limited, it is important to ask about radiation into the arm, especially the shoulder. Be sure to elicit symptoms related to the "red flags" listed earlier. Persistent pain after blunt trauma or a motor vehicle collision warrants further evaluation.[8]

See Table 16-2, Pains in the Neck, p. 669.

Radicular pain arises from spinal nerve compression, most commonly C7 followed by C6. Unlike low back pain, it is usually caused by foraminal impingement from degenerative joint changes (70% to 75%) rather than disc herniation (20% to 25%).[9,10]

Monoarticular or Polyarticular Joint Pain.   To pursue other musculoskeletal disorders, ask "Do you have any pains in your joints?" Joint pain may be localized, diffuse, or systemic. Ask the patient to point to the pain.

- If the joint pain is localized and involves only one joint, it is *monoarticular*. Pain originating in the small joints of the hands and feet is more sharply localized than pain from larger joints. Pain from the hip joint is especially deceptive. Although typically in the groin or buttock, it is sometimes felt in the anterior thigh or partly or solely in the knee.

Pain in one joint suggests injury, monoarticular arthritis, possible tendinitis, or bursitis. Lateral hip pain near the greater trochanter suggests *trochanteric bursitis*.

- Patients may report joint pain that is *polyarticular*, involving several joints. If polyarticular, what is the *pattern of involvement* . . . migrating from joint to joint or steadily spreading from one joint to multiple joints? Is the involvement symmetric, affecting similar joints on both sides of the body?

- Joint pain may also be *extra-articular*, involving bones, muscles, and tissues around the joint such as the tendons, bursae, or even overlying skin. Generalized "aches and pains" are called *myalgias* if in muscles, and *arthralgias* if there is pain but no evidence of arthritis.

Timing. Assess the chronicity, quality, and severity of the joint symptoms. *Timing* is especially important. Did the pain or discomfort develop rapidly over the course of a few hours or insidiously over weeks or even months? Has the pain progressed slowly or fluctuated, with periods of improvement and worsening? How long has the pain lasted? What is it like over the course of a day? . . . In the morning? . . . As the day wears on?

If more rapid in onset, how did the pain arise? Was there an acute injury or overuse from repetitive motion of the same part of the body? If the pain comes from trauma, what was the *mechanism of injury* or the series of events that caused the joint pain? Furthermore, what aggravates or relieves the pain? What are the effects of exercise, rest, and treatment?

Inflammation. Try to determine whether the problem is *inflammatory* or *noninflammatory*. Is there *tenderness, warmth,* or *redness?* These features are best assessed on examination, but patients can sometimes guide you to points of tenderness. Ask about systemic symptoms such as fever or chills.

Swelling and Stiffness. Additional symptoms can help you decide if the pain is *articular* in origin, such as *swelling, stiffness,* or *decreased range of motion.* Localize any *swelling* as accurately as possible. If *stiffness* is present, it may be difficult to assess because people use the term differently. Musculoskeletal stiffness refers to a perceived tightness or resistance to movement, the opposite of feeling limber. It is often associated with discomfort or pain. If the patient does not report stiffness spontaneously, ask about it and try to calculate its duration. Find out when the patient gets up in the morning and when the joints feel the most limber. Healthy people experience stiffness and muscular soreness after unusually strenuous muscular exertion, usually peaking within 2 days.

To assess *limitations of motion,* ask about changes in level of activity because of problems with the involved joint. When relevant, inquire specifically about the patient's ability to walk, stand, lean over, sit, sit up, rise from a sitting position, climb, pinch, grasp, turn a page, open a door handle or jar, and about daily activities such as combing hair, brushing teeth, eating, dressing, and bathing.

Migratory pattern of spread is seen in *rheumatic fever* or *gonococcal arthritis;* progressive additive pattern with symmetric involvement, in *rheumatoid arthritis*. Inflammatory arthritides are more common in women.

Extra-articular pain occurs in inflammation of bursae (*bursitis*), tendons (*tendinitis*), or tendon sheaths (*tenosynovitis*); also in *sprains* from stretching or tearing of ligaments.

Severe pain of rapid onset in a red, swollen joint suggests *acute septic arthritis* or *gout.*[11,12] In children, consider *osteomyelitis* in bone contiguous to a joint.

See Table 16-3, Patterns of Pain In and Around the Joints, pp. 670–671.

Fever, chills, warmth, redness are seen in *septic arthritis;* also consider *gout* or possible *rheumatic fever.*

Pain, swelling, loss of active and passive motion, or "locking" suggest *articular joint pain;* loss of active but not passive motion and tenderness outside the joint are seen in *nonarticular pain.*

Stiffness and limited motion after inactivity, sometimes called *gelling,* occurs in degenerative joint disease but usually lasts only a few minutes; stiffness lasting 30 minutes or more is present in *rheumatoid arthritis* and other inflammatory arthritides. Stiffness also occurs in *fibromyalgia* and *polymyalgia rheumatica (PMR).*[13,14]

Systemic Features. Some joint problems have *systemic* features such as fever, chills, rash, anorexia, weight loss, and weakness.

Generalized symptoms are common in *rheumatoid arthritis, systemic lupus erythematosus (SLE), PMR,* and other inflammatory arthritides. High fever and chills suggest an infectious cause.

Note that other joint disorders may be linked to *organ systems outside the musculoskeletal system.* Symptoms elsewhere in the body can give important clues to these conditions. Ask about any family history of joint or muscle disorders. Be alert to the symptoms and disorders below.

Leukemia can infiltrate the synovium; chemotherapy can also cause joint pain.

Joint Pain and Systemic Disorders

▸ *Skin conditions*
  ▸ A butterfly rash on the cheeks
  ▸ The scaly rash and pitted nails of psoriasis
  ▸ A few papules, pustules, or vesicles on reddened bases, located on the distal extremities
  ▸ An expanding erythematous patch early in an illness
  ▸ Hives
  ▸ Erosions or scaling on the penis and crusted, scaling papules on the soles and palms
  ▸ The maculopapular rash of rubella
  ▸ Clubbing of the fingernails (see p. 202)
▸ Red, burning, and itchy eyes (*conjunctivitis*)
▸ Preceding *sore throat*

▸ *Diarrhea, abdominal pain, cramping*

▸ Symptoms of *urethritis*

▸ Mental status change, facial or other weakness, stiff neck

Systemic lupus erythematosus

Psoriatic arthritis

Gonococcal arthritis

Lyme disease

Serum sickness, drug reaction

Reiter's syndrome, which includes arthritis, urethritis, and uveitis

Arthritis of *rubella*

Hypertrophic osteoarthropathy

Reiter's syndrome, Behçet's syndrome[15]

Acute rheumatic fever or *gonococcal arthritis*

Arthritis with *ulcerative colitis, regional enteritis, scleroderma*

Reiter's syndrome or possibly *gonococcal arthritis*

Lyme disease with central nervous system involvement

Health Promotion and Counseling: Evidence and Recommendations

Important Topics for Health Promotion and Counseling

▸ Nutrition, weight, and physical activity
▸ Profiling low back pain
▸ Osteoporosis: screening and prevention
▸ Preventing falls

Maintaining the integrity of the musculoskeletal system brings many habits of a healthy lifestyle into play—nutrition, fitness, optimal weight, and preventing injury from collisions, falls, or sports. Each joint has its own specific vulnerabilities to trauma and wear. Proper lifting, avoiding falls, household safety measures, and a balanced exercise program are key ingredients to protecting and preserving well-functioning joints and muscles, and help delay the incursions of arthritis, chronic back pain, and osteoporosis, all important targets for Healthy People 2020.[3]

Nutrition, Weight, and Physical Activity. The habits of a healthy lifestyle convey direct benefits to the skeleton and muscles. Good nutrition supplies the calcium needed for bone mineralization and bone density. Weight appropriate to height and body frame reduces excess mechanical stress on weight-bearing joints like the hips and knees. Exercise helps to maintain bone mass (especially weight-bearing), improve mood and outlook, and manage stress.

See Chapter 4, Beginning the Physical Examination: General Survey, Vital Signs, and Pain, pp. 105–140, for further discussion of nutrition and weight.

The goals for Healthy People 2020 reflect the ever-increasing importance of physical activity for all Americans.[3] Currently, only 20% of adults engage in meaningful physical activity each week; avoiding inactivity is paramount. Physical activity reduces risk of osteoporosis, obesity, cardiovascular disease, hypertension, type 2 diabetes, breast and colon cancer, falls, and depression. For substantial health benefits, Healthy People 2020 endorses the first set of national guidelines ever published, *Physical Activity Guidelines for Americans*, released in 2008.[16]

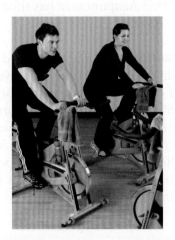

Physical Activity Guidelines for Americans 2008

▶ At least 2 hours and 30 minutes a week of moderate-intensity, or 1 hour and 15 minutes a week of vigorous-intensity, *aerobic physical activity*, or a combination that is equivalent

▶ Moderate- or high-intensity *muscle-strengthening activity* that involves all major muscle groups on 2 or more days a week

The report includes guidelines for helping the many who are currently sedentary to gradually build up their activity level, starting with 10 minutes of exercise a day.

Profiling Low Back Pain. From 60% to 80% of the U.S. population experiences low back pain at least once in a lifetime. Roughly 90% of acute episodes resolve within 4 to 6 weeks. However, 25% of patients have a recurrence within the next year, and 7% develop chronic low back pain, costing over $90 billion annually for medical care and lost worker productivity.[17–20]

See Table 16-1, Low Back Pain, p. 668, for serious causes of low back pain, including back pain with sciatica, *compression fracture, malignancy, ankylosing spondylitis,* and infection including *osteomyelitis.*

Symptom severity and imaging findings correlate poorly with functional outcome, giving rise to many studies that have explored predictors of outcome and the utility of therapeutic and workplace interventions. Although optimal weight, physical fitness, workplace interventions, and low back supports during lifting and physical work have other health benefits, they have not been shown to prevent low back pain.[21,22] One of the most important outcome predictors is *depression*, which doubles the incidence of new low back pain in asymptomatic patients.[23] *Other predictors of chronic back pain* persisting to 1 year include: maladaptive pain-coping behaviors related to fear of movements that could make pain worse, leading to avoidance of work, movement, or other activities; high somatization scores; poor general health; high levels of baseline functional impairment; and prior history of chronic or low back pain.[24] Current evidence supports active exercise with minimal bed rest or delay of back-specific exercises while pain is acute, cognitive-behavioral counseling, occupational interventions targeting graded exercise with early return to modified work, and treatment of depression and psychiatric comorbidities.[22,24–26] Acupuncture has shown promise, but with mixed results.[27,28]

Osteoporosis: Screening and Prevention. Like arthritis and back pain, osteoporosis is a major threat to health in America, affecting over 5 million people over age 50 years.[18,29,30] Half of all postmenopausal women sustain an osteoporosis-related fracture; 25% develop vertebral deformities; and 15% suffer from hip fracture with ensuing chronic pain, disability, and increased mortality. Men are also at risk; one in four over age 50 years has an osteoporosis-related fracture. The population with osteopenia is even larger, affecting over 34 million people, including 12 million men. More than half of fragility fractures occur in this group.[31]

Risk Factors for Osteoporosis and Fracture

- Prior fragility fracture
- Postmenopausal status in women
- Age ≥50 years
- Weight ≤70 kg or 154 lbs
- Low dietary calcium
- Vitamin D deficiency
- Tobacco and alcohol use
- Family history of fracture in a first-degree relative
- Use of corticosteroids
- Medical conditions such as thyrotoxicosis, celiac sprue, chronic renal disease, organ transplantation, diabetes, HIV, primary or secondary hypogonadism, multiple myeloma, and anorexia nervosa
- Medications such as aromatase inhibitors for breast cancer, methotrexate, selected antiseizure medications, immunosuppressive agents, and antigonadal therapy
- Inflammatory disorders of the musculoskeletal, pulmonary, or gastrointestinal systems, including rheumatoid arthritis

Screening Recommendations 2011.   As of 2011, the U.S. Preventive Services Task Force (USPSTF) recommends osteoporosis screening for women 65 years of age and older and for younger women whose fracture risk equals or exceeds that of a 65-year-old white woman with no additional risk factors.[29] The USPSTF finds that evidence about risks and benefits for men is insufficient for recommending routine screening. Screen your patients for the many risk factors listed on the preceding page, and proceed to further assessment.

Assessing Fracture Risk.   The USPSTF defines osteoporosis as "a systemic skeletal condition characterized by low bone mass and microarchitectural deterioration of bone tissue that increases bone fragility and risk for fractures."[32] The USPSTF supports use of the FRAX calculator developed by the World Health Organization for assessing risk, available at the Web site. The FRAX calculator generates fracture risk based on age, body mass index, parental fracture history, use of glucocorticoids, presence of rheumatoid arthritis or secondary osteoporosis, and tobacco and alcohol use. It has been validated for black, Hispanic, and Asian women in the United States and has calculators that are continent- and country-specific.

Prior low-impact fracture from standing height or less is the greatest risk factor for subsequent fracture.

The Web site for the FRAX Calculator for Assessing Fracture Risk for the United States is http://www.shef.ac.uk/FRAX/tool.jsp?country=9

The Task Force recommends a *10-year fracture risk threshold of 9.3% for osteoporotic fracture* to determine need for bone density screening and therapeutic interventions. The FRAX calculator also provides 10-year risk of hip fracture.

Measuring Bone Density.   Bone strength depends on bone quality, bone density, and overall bone size. Since there is no direct measure of bone strength, bone mineral density, which provides roughly 70% of bone strength, is used as a reasonable surrogate. DXA (or DEXA, dual energy x-ray absorptiometry) scanning is the optimal standard for measuring bone density, diagnosing osteoporosis, and guiding treatment decisions. DXA measurement of bone density at the femoral neck is considered the best predictor of hip fracture.

The World Health Organization scoring criteria for *T-scores* and *Z-scores*, measured in standard deviations, are used worldwide. A 10% drop in bone density, equivalent to 1.0 standard deviation, portends a 20% increase in risk for fracture.

World Health Organization Bone Density Criteria

▸ **Osteoporosis**   T score < −2.5 (>2.5 standard deviations below the mean for young adult white women)

▸ **Osteopenia**   T score −2.5 to 1.5 (1.0 to 2.5 standard deviations below the mean for young adult white women)

Peak bone mass is reached by age 30. Bone loss due to age-related declines in estrogen and testosterone is initially rapid, then becomes slow and continuous. *Osteoporosis is also common in hepatic and renal disease.*

Bone densitometry scoring also includes Z-scores for age-matched controls. These are useful when screening young people, since they are more closely matched in age, height, and weight.

Calcium and Vitamin D.   *Calcium* is the most abundant mineral in the body, and is essential for bone health, muscle function, nerve transmission, vascular function, and intracellular signaling and hormonal secretion.[33] Serum calcium is tightly regulated; less that 1% of total body calcium supports these metabolic functions. The remaining 99% of the body calcium supply is stored in teeth and in bones, where calcium deposits are subject to constant remodeling from deposition and resorption that determines bone quality and strength.

Humans acquire *vitamin D* from sunlight, food, and dietary supplements.[34,35] Vitamin D from the skin and diet is metabolized in the liver to 25-hydroxyvitamin D, which determines the patient's vitamin D level. Without vitamin D, only 10% to 15% of dietary calcium is absorbed. Parathyroid hormone (PTH) enhances renal tubular absorption of calcium and stimulates conversion of 25-hydroxyvitamin D in the kidneys to 1,25-dihydroxyvitamin D, its active form. PTH also activates osteoblasts, which lay down new bone matrix, and indirectly stimulates osteoclasts, which dissolve bone matrix, causing osteopenia, osteoporosis, increased risk of fracture, and muscle weakness.

In 2010, the Institute of Medicine issued new recommendations for intake of calcium and vitamin D in the amounts listed below, recognizing their key role in reducing risk of osteoporosis and fractures.[36–38] The Institute report concludes that serum 25-hydroxyvitamin D levels of 20 ng/mL are sufficient to maintain bone health and warns that levels of above 50 ng/mL may have adverse effects. The Institute of Medicine states that evidence supporting the extraskeletal benefits of vitamin D relating to cancer and immune disorders is insufficient for establishing nutritional requirements.

Studies published since 2010 have questioned the use of calcium supplements for managing osteoporosis due to modest increases in risk of cardiovascular events, especially myocardial infarction.[39,40] Supplements in the absence of dietary deficiencies may not be advisable, pending further investigation. There have been no reports of harm associated with calcium intake from dietary sources.

Recommended Dietary Intakes of Calcium and Vitamin D for Adults (Institute of Medicine 2010)

Age Group	Calcium (elemental) mg/day	Vitamin D IU/day
19–50	1,000	600
50–71		
Women	1,200	600
Men	1,000	600
71 and above	1,200	800

Source: Ross AC, Manson JE, Abrams SA et al. The 2011 report on dietary reference intakes for calcium and vitamin D from the Institute of Medicine: what clinicians need to know. J Endocrinol Metab 2011;96:53–58.

In the U.S., women over age 50 and men over age 70 fall below the recommended dietary guidelines, so advise supplements for these groups.[33] There are two main forms of calcium supplements, calcium carbonate and calcium citrate. Supplements contain variable amounts of elemental calcium. Patients can read these amounts on the Supplemental Facts panel. Calcium carbonate is less expensive and should be consumed with food. Calcium citrate is absorbed more easily in individuals with reduced levels of stomach acid and can be taken with or without food. How much calcium is absorbed depends on the total amount consumed at one time and falls at higher doses; for best absorption, counsel patients to take doses of 500 mg at two separate times.

Antiresorptive and Anabolic Agents. The therapeutic uses of these agents for treating osteoporosis are summarized briefly here.[35] Antiresorptive agents inhibit osteoclast activity and slow bone remodeling, allowing better mineralization of bone matrix and stabilization of the trabecular microarchitecture. These agents include bisphosphonates, selective estrogen-receptor modulators (SERMs), calcitonin, and postmenopausal estrogen (now contraindicated due to associated risks of breast cancer and vascular thrombosis).[41] Bisphosphonates have also created controversy related to very low associated risks of osteonecrosis of the jaw and atypical femur fractures.[42–44]

Anabolic agents such as parathyroid hormone stimulate bone formation by acting primarily on osteoblasts but require subcutaneous administration and monitoring for hypercalcemia. They are reserved for moderate to severe cases of osteopenia and patients whose bone density has not improved on bisphosphonates.

Preventing Falls. More than one in three adults over age 65 years falls each year, exacting a heavy toll in morbidity and mortality.[45] Falls are the leading cause of nonfatal injuries and prompt a dramatic rise in death rates after age 65 years, increasing from 7 per 100,000 in the general population, to 13 per 100,000 for adults age 65 to 74 years, to more than 174 per 100,000 after age 85.[46] Among older adults, falls are the number one cause of fractures, hospital admissions for trauma, and loss of independence. One-third of patients with fractures are admitted to nursing homes. Risk factors are both cognitive and physiologic and include unstable gait, unbalanced posture, loss of strength, cognitive loss, deficits in vision and proprioception, and osteoporosis. Poor lighting, stairs, chairs at awkward heights, slippery or irregular surfaces, and ill-fitting shoes are environmental hazards that can usually be corrected. Work with your patients and their families to modify such risks whenever possible. Arrange for home health assessments to target needed home safety measures. Above all, counsel all older adults about falls prevention and encourage them to pursue exercise programs that improve their strength and balance.[47]

Sports injuries, especially of the anterior cruciate ligament (ACL), are a significant source of musculoskeletal disorders.

See Table 4-5, Nutrition Counseling: Sources of Nutrients, p. 139, for food sources of calcium and vitamin D.

See Chapter 14, Female Genitalia, p. 553, for discussion of hormone replacement therapy.

See also Chapter 20, Assessing Older Adults, for further discussion of Assessing and Preventing Falls, pp. 943–944.

Once injured, articular cartilage is replaced by less resilient fibrocartilage, increasing risk of pain and osteoarthritis.

Rates of ACL tears are substantially higher in women, possibly related to increased ligamentous laxity related to estrogen cycling, or to differing anatomy and neuromuscular control. ACL injury prevention programs are now common.

Examination of Specific Joints: Anatomy and Physiology and Techniques of Examination

Important Areas of Examination for Each of the Major Joints

> ▶ Inspection for joint symmetry, alignment, bony deformities, and swelling
> ▶ Inspection and palpation of surrounding tissues for skin changes, nodules, muscle atrophy, tenderness
> ▶ Range of motion and maneuvers to test joint function and stability, and integrity of ligaments, tendons, bursae, especially if pain or trauma
> ▶ Assessment of inflammation, especially swelling, warmth, redness

During the interview, you have evaluated the patient's ability to carry out normal activities of daily living. Keep these abilities in mind during your physical examination.

During the general survey, you have assessed the patient's general appearance, body proportions, and ease of movement. Now visualize the underlying anatomy of the joints and recall the key elements of the history, for example, the mechanism of injury if there is trauma, or the time course of symptoms and limitations in function in arthritis.

Your examination should be systematic. It should include inspection, palpation of bony structures and related joint and soft-tissue structures, assessment of range of motion, and *special maneuvers* to test specific movements. Recall that the anatomical shape of each joint determines its range of motion. There are two phases to *range of motion*: *active* (by the patient) and *passive* (by the examiner).

If patients have painful joints, move them gently, or let them move more comfortably by themselves, showing you how they manage. If the joint has been injured, consider an x-ray before attempting movement.

Tips for Successful Examination of the Musculoskeletal System

▶ During inspection, look for *symmetry* of involvement. Is there a symmetric change in joints on both sides of the body, or is the change only in one or two joints?

Note any *joint deformities* or *malalignment of bones or joints*.

▶ Use inspection and palpation to assess the *surrounding tissues*, noting skin changes, subcutaneous nodules, and muscle atrophy. Note any *crepitus*, an audible or palpable crunching during movement of tendons or ligaments over bone or areas of cartilage loss. This may occur in joints without pain but is more significant when associated with symptoms or signs.

▶ Test range of motion and maneuvers (described for each joint) to demonstrate *limitations in range of motion* or joint instability from excess mobility of joint ligaments, called *ligamentous laxity*.

▶ Finally, test *muscle strength* to aid in the assessment of joint function (for these techniques, see Chapter 17, pp. 710–715).

Signs of Inflammation and Arthritis (first recorded by Celsus in the first century A.D.) Watch for:

▶ *Swelling.* Palpable swelling may involve: (1) the synovial membrane, which can feel boggy or doughy; (2) effusion from excess synovial fluid within the joint space; or (3) soft-tissue structures such as bursae, tendons, and tendon sheaths.

▶ *Warmth.* Use the backs of your fingers to compare the involved joint with its unaffected contralateral joint, or with nearby tissues if both joints are involved.

▶ *Tenderness.* Try to identify the specific anatomical structure that is tender. Trauma may also cause tenderness.

▶ *Redness.* Redness of the overlying skin is the *least* common sign of inflammation near the joints and is usually seen in more superficial joints like fingers, toes, and knees.

Acute involvement of only one joint suggests trauma, septic arthritis, or gout. *Rheumatoid arthritis* is typically polyarticular and symmetrical.[12,48]

Seen in *Dupuytren's contracture* (p. 676), bowlegs (*genu varum*) or knock-knees (*genu valgum*).

Look for subcutaneous nodules in *rheumatoid arthritis* or *rheumatic fever*; effusions in trauma; crepitus over inflamed joints (in *osteoarthritis*), or over the inflamed tendon sheaths of *tenosynovitis*.

Decreased range of motion is present in arthritis, inflammation of tissues around a joint, fibrosis in or around a joint, or bony fixation (*ankylosis*). Ligamentous laxity of the ACL occurs in knee trauma; muscle atrophy or weakness is seen in *rheumatoid arthritis*.

Palpable bogginess or doughiness of the synovial membrane indicates *synovitis*, which is often accompanied by effusion. Palpable joint fluid is present in effusion, tenderness over the tendon sheaths in *tendinitis*.

Increased warmth is seen in arthritis, tendinitis, bursitis, *osteomyelitis*.

Diffuse tenderness and warmth over a thickened synovium suggest arthritis or infection; focal tenderness suggests injury.

Redness over a tender joint suggests septic or gouty arthritis, or possibly *rheumatoid arthritis*.

The detail needed for examination of the musculoskeletal system varies widely. This section presents examination techniques for both comprehensive and targeted assessment of joint function. Patients with extensive or severe musculoskeletal problems will require more time.

To help organize your approach to the musculoskeletal examination, study the following flowchart on musculoskeletal complaints.

See also Chapter 1, Overview: Physical Examination and History Taking, pp. 3–24, and Chapter 4, Beginning the Examination: General Survey, Vital Signs, and Pain, p. 116, for briefer examination techniques for those without musculoskeletal symptoms.

Approach to Musculoskeletal Complaints

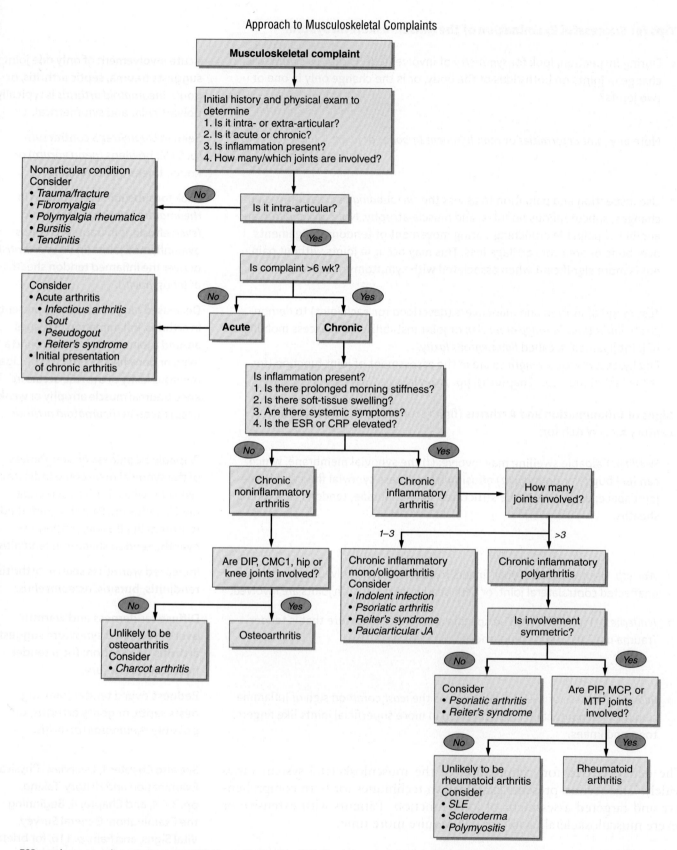

ESR, erythrocyte sedimentation rate; CRP, C-reactive protein; DIP, distal interphalangeal; CMC, carpometacarpal; PIP, proximal interphalangeal; MCP, metacarpophalangeal; MTP, metatarsophalangeal; PMR, polymyalgia rheumatica; SLE, systemic lupus erythematosus; JA, juvenile arthritis.

Adapted from: Kasper DL, Braunwald E, Fauci AS, et al., eds. Harrison's Principles of Internal Medicine, 16th ed. New York: McGraw-Hill, 2005.

TEMPOROMANDIBULAR JOINT (TMJ)

Overview, Bony Structures, and Joints

The temporomandibular joint (TMJ) is the most active joint in the body, opening and closing up to 2,000 times a day. It is formed by the fossa and articular tubercle of the temporal bone and the condyle of the mandible. It lies midway between the external acoustic meatus and the zygomatic arch.

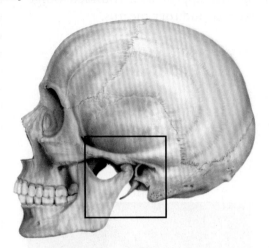

A fibrocartilaginous disc cushions the action of the condyle of the mandible against the synovial membrane and capsule of the articulating surfaces of the temporal bone. Hence, it is a condylar synovial joint.

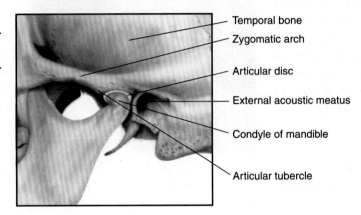

- Temporal bone
- Zygomatic arch
- Articular disc
- External acoustic meatus
- Condyle of mandible
- Articular tubercle

Muscle Groups and Additional Structures

The principal muscles opening the mouth are the *external pterygoids*. Closing the mouth are the muscles innervated by Cranial Nerve V, the trigeminal nerve—the *masseter*, the *temporalis*, and the *internal pterygoids* (see p. 685).

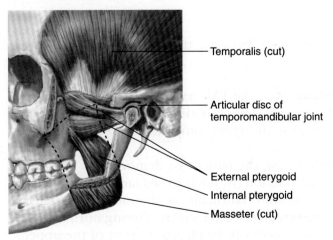

- Temporalis (cut)
- Articular disc of temporomandibular joint
- External pterygoid
- Internal pterygoid
- Masseter (cut)

Techniques of Examination

Inspection and Palpation. Inspect the face for symmetry. Inspect the TMJ for swelling or redness. Swelling may appear as a rounded bulge approximately 0.5 cm anterior to the external auditory meatus.

Facial asymmetry is seen in *TMJ syndrome*. Typical features are unilateral chronic pain with chewing, jaw clenching, or teeth grinding, often associated with stress; patients may also present with headache. Pain with chewing also occurs in *trigeminal neuralgia, temporal arteritis*.

Swelling, tenderness, and decreased range of motion are present in inflammation or arthritis.

To locate and palpate the joint, place the tips of your index fingers just in front of the tragus of each ear and ask the patient to open his or her mouth. The fingertips should drop into the joint spaces as the mouth opens. Check for smooth range of motion; note any swelling or tenderness. Snapping or clicking may be felt or heard in normal people.

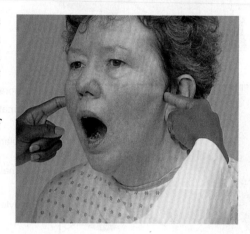

Dislocation of the TMJ may be seen in trauma.

Palpable crepitus or clicking is present in poor occlusion, meniscus injury, or synovial swelling from trauma.

Palpate the muscles of mastication:

- The *masseters*, externally at the angle of the mandible

- The *temporal muscles*, externally during clenching and relaxation of the jaw

- The *pterygoid muscles*, internally between the tonsillar pillars at the mandible

Pain and tenderness occur on palpation in *TMJ syndrome*.

Range of Motion and Maneuvers. The TMJ has glide and hinge motions in its upper and lower portions, respectively. Grinding or chewing consists primarily of gliding movements in the upper compartments.

Range of motion is threefold: ask the patient to demonstrate opening and closing, protrusion and retraction (by jutting the mandible forward), and lateral, or side-to-side, motion. Normally, as the mouth is opened wide, three fingers can be inserted between incisors. During normal protrusion of the jaw, the bottom teeth can be placed in front of the upper teeth.

THE SHOULDER

Overview

The glenohumeral joint of the shoulder is distinguished by wide-ranging movement in all directions. This joint is largely uninhibited by bony structures. The humeral head contacts less than one third of the surface area of the glenoid fossa and virtually dangles from the scapula, attached by the joint capsule, the intra-articular capsular ligaments, the glenoid labrum, and a meshwork of muscles and tendons.

The shoulder derives its mobility from a complex interconnected structure of four joints, three large bones, and three principal muscle groups, often referred to as the *shoulder girdle*. These structures are viewed as *dynamic stabilizers*, or those capable of movement, or *static stabilizers*, those incapable of movement.

- *Dynamic stabilizers:* the SITS muscles of the rotator cuff (supraspinatus, infraspinatus, teres minor, and subscapularis), which move the humerus and compress and stabilize the humeral head within the glenoid cavity.

- *Static stabilizers:* the bony structures of the shoulder girdle, the labrum, the articular capsule, and the glenohumeral ligaments. The *labrum* is a fibrocartilaginous ring that surrounds the glenoid and deepens its socket, providing greater stability to the humeral head. The joint capsule is strengthened by tendons of the rotator cuff and glenohumeral ligaments, adding to joint stability.

This meshwork of muscles can make distinguishing shoulder from neck disorders difficult.

Bony Structures

The bony structures of the shoulder include the humerus, the clavicle, and the scapula. The scapula is anchored to the axial skeleton only by the sternoclavicular joint and inserting muscles, often called the *scapulothoracic articulation* because it is not a true joint.

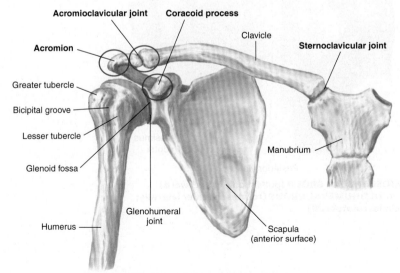

IMPORTANT BONES OF THE SHOULDER

Identify the *manubrium*, the *sternoclavicular joint*, and the *clavicle*. Also identify the *tip of the acromion*, the *greater tubercle of the humerus*, and the *coracoid process*, which are important features of shoulder anatomy.

Joints

Three different joints articulate at the shoulder:

- The *glenohumeral joint*. In this joint, the head of the humerus articulates with the shallow glenoid fossa of the scapula. This joint is deeply situated and not normally palpable. It is a ball-and-socket joint, allowing the arm its wide arc of movement—flexion, extension, abduction (movement away from the trunk), adduction (movement toward the trunk), rotation, and circumduction.

- The *sternoclavicular joint*. The convex medial end of the clavicle articulates with the concave hollow in the upper sternum.

- The *acromioclavicular joint*. The lateral end of the clavicle articulates with the acromion process of the scapula.

Muscle Groups

Three groups of muscles attach at the shoulder:

The Scapulohumeral Group. This group extends from the scapula to the humerus and includes the muscles inserting directly on the humerus, known as *"SITS muscles"* of the *rotator cuff*:

- *Supraspinatus*—runs above the glenohumeral joint; inserts on the greater tubercle

- *Infraspinatus* and *teres minor*—cross the glenohumeral joint posteriorly; insert on the greater tubercle

- *Subscapularis* (not illustrated)—originates on the anterior surface of the scapula and crosses the joint anteriorly; inserts on the lesser tubercle

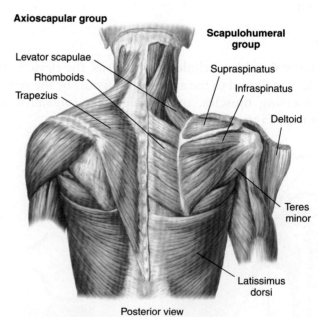

Axioscapular group

Scapulohumeral group

Levator scapulae
Rhomboids
Trapezius

Supraspinatus
Infraspinatus
Deltoid
Teres minor
Latissimus dorsi

Posterior view

AXIOSCAPULAR GROUP (pulls shoulder backward)
SCAPULOHUMERAL GROUP (rotates shoulder laterally; includes rotator cuff)

The scapulohumeral group rotates the shoulder laterally (the *rotator cuff*) and depresses and rotates the head of the humerus. See pp. 624–625 for discussion of rotator cuff injuries.

The Axioscapular Group. This group attaches the trunk to the scapula and includes the trapezius, rhomboids, serratus anterior, and levator scapulae. These muscles rotate the scapula.

The Axiohumeral Group. This group attaches the trunk to the humerus and includes the pectoralis major and minor and the latissimus dorsi. These muscles produce internal rotation of the shoulder.

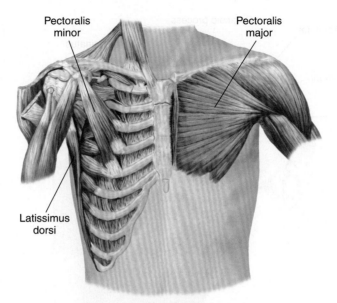

Pectoralis minor

Pectoralis major

Latissimus dorsi

Anterior view

AXIOHUMERAL GROUP (rotates shoulder internally)

The biceps and triceps, which connect the scapula to the bones of the forearm, are also involved in shoulder movement, especially forward flexion (biceps) and extension (triceps).

Additional Structures

Also important to shoulder movement are the *articular capsule and bursae*. Surrounding the glenohumeral joint is a fibrous articular capsule formed by the tendon insertions of the rotator cuff and other capsular structures. The loose fit of the capsule allows the shoulder bones to separate, and contributes to the shoulder's wide range of movement. The capsule is lined by a synovial membrane with two outpouchings—the *subscapular bursa* and the *synovial sheath of the tendon of the long head of the biceps*.

To locate the biceps tendon, rotate your arm externally and find the tendinous cord that runs just medial to the greater tubercle. Roll it under your fingers. This is the tendon of the long head of the biceps. It runs in the bicipital groove between the greater and lesser tubercles.

The principal bursa of the shoulder is the *subacromial bursa*, positioned between the acromion and the head of the humerus and overlying the supraspinatus tendon. Abduction of the shoulder compresses this bursa. Normally, the supraspinatus tendon and the subacromial bursa are not palpable. However, if the bursal surfaces are inflamed (*subacromial bursitis*), there may be tenderness just below the tip of the acromion, pain with abduction and rotation, and loss of smooth movement.

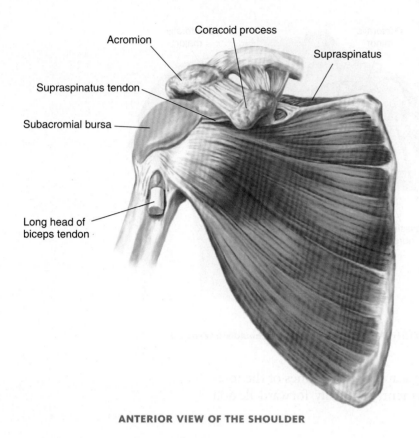

ANTERIOR VIEW OF THE SHOULDER

Techniques of Examination

Inspection. Observe the shoulder and shoulder girdle anteriorly, and inspect the scapulae and related muscles posteriorly.

Note any swelling, deformity, muscle atrophy or fasciculations (fine tremors of the muscles), or abnormal positioning.

Look for swelling of the joint capsule anteriorly or a bulge in the subacromial bursa under the deltoid muscle. Survey the entire upper extremity for color change, skin alteration, or unusual bony contours.

Palpation. Begin by palpating the bony structures of the shoulder, and then palpate any area of pain.

● Beginning medially, at the *sternoclavicular joint,* trace the clavicle laterally with your fingers.

Scoliosis may cause elevation of one shoulder. With *anterior dislocation of the shoulder*, the rounded lateral aspect of the shoulder appears flattened.[49,50]

Atrophy of the supraspinatus and infraspinatus with increased prominence of scapular spine can appear within 2 to 3 weeks of a *rotator cuff tear*.

A significant amount of synovial fluid is needed before the glenohumeral joint capsule appears distended. Swelling of the acromioclavicular joint is easier to identify since it is more superficial.

See Table 16-4, Painful Shoulders, pp. 672–673.

- From behind, follow the bony spine of the scapula laterally and upward until it becomes the acromion (**A**), the summit of the shoulder. Its upper surface is rough and slightly convex. Identify the anterior tip of the acromion.

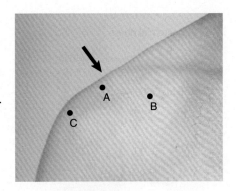

- With your index finger on top of the acromion, just behind its tip, press medially with your thumb to find the slightly elevated ridge that marks the distal end of the clavicle at the *acromioclavicular joint* (shown by the arrow). Move your thumb medially and down a short step to the next bony prominence, the *coracoid process* (**B**) of the scapula.

- With your thumb on the coracoid process, allow your fingers to fall on and grasp the lateral aspect of the humerus to palpate the *greater tubercle* (**C**), where the SITS muscles insert.

- Next, to palpate the *biceps tendon* in the intertubercular groove, keep your thumb on the coracoid process and your fingers on the lateral aspect of the humerus. Remove your index finger and place it halfway between the coracoid process and the greater tubercle on the anterior surface of the arm. As you check for tendon tenderness, rolling the tendon under the fingertips may be helpful. You can also rotate the glenohumeral joint externally, locate the muscle distally near the elbow, and track the muscle and its tendon proximally into the intertubercular groove.

See also Bicipital Tendinitis in Table 16-4, Painful Shoulders, pp. 672–673.

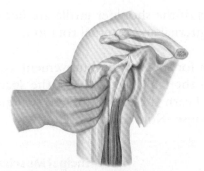

PALPATION OF THE BICIPITAL GROOVE AND TENDON

- To examine the *subacromial* and *subdeltoid bursae* and the *SITS muscles*, first passively extend the humerus by lifting the elbow posteriorly. This rotates these structures so that they are anterior to the acromion. Palpate carefully over the subacromial and subdeltoid bursae. The underlying palpable SITS muscles are:

  - Supraspinatus—directly under the acromion

  - Infraspinatus—posterior to supraspinatus

  - Teres minor—posterior and inferior to the supraspinatus

  - Subscapularis—inserts anteriorly and is not palpable

Localized tenderness arises from *subacromial* or *subdeltoid bursitis*, degenerative changes, or calcific deposits in the rotator cuff.

Swelling suggests a *bursal tear* that communicates with the articular cavity.

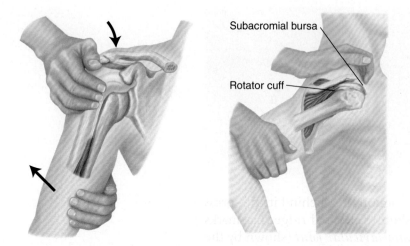

Subacromial bursa

Rotator cuff

Tenderness over the SITS muscle insertions and inability to abduct the arm above shoulder level are seen in sprains, tears, and tendon rupture of the rotator cuff, most commonly the *supraspinatus*. See Table 16-4, Painful Shoulders, pp. 672–673.

- The fibrous articular capsule and the broad, flat tendons of the rotator cuff are so closely associated that they must be examined simultaneously. Swelling in the capsule and synovial membrane is often best detected by looking down on the shoulder from above. Palpate the capsule and synovial membrane beneath the anterior and posterior acromion to check for injury or arthritis.

Tenderness and effusion suggest synovitis of the glenohumeral joint. If the margins of the capsule and synovial membrane are palpable, a moderate to large effusion is present; if synovitis is minimal, it cannot be detected on palpation.

Range of Motion and Maneuvers

Range of Motion.   The six motions of the shoulder girdle are flexion, extension, abduction, adduction, and internal and external rotation.

Standing in front of the patient, watch for smooth fluid movement as the patient performs the motions listed in the table below. Note the specific muscles responsible for each motion. Learn the clear simple instructions that prompt the requested patient response. Note muscle strength.

Restricted range of motion occurs in *bursitis, capsulitis, rotator cuff tears* or *sprains*, and *tendinitis*.

Shoulder Movement	Principal Muscles Affecting Movement	Patient Instructions
Flexion 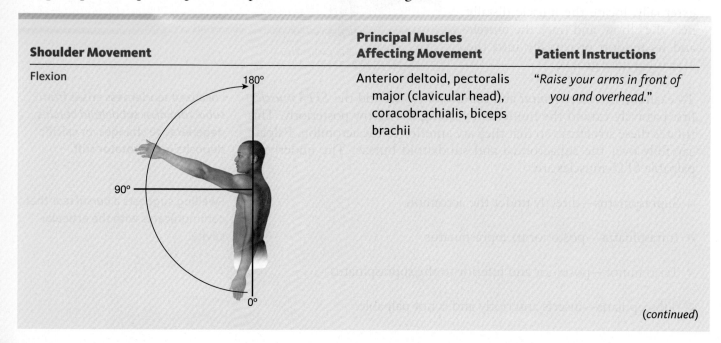	Anterior deltoid, pectoralis major (clavicular head), coracobrachialis, biceps brachii	*"Raise your arms in front of you and overhead."*

(continued)

Shoulder Movement	Principal Muscles Affecting Movement	Patient Instructions
Extension 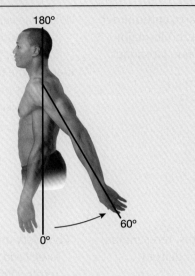	Latissimus dorsi, teres major, posterior deltoid, triceps brachii (long head)	"*Raise your arms behind you.*"
Abduction 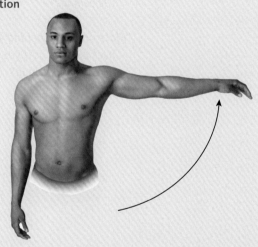	Supraspinatus, middle deltoid, serratus anterior (via upward rotation of the scapula)	"*Raise your arms out to the side and overhead.*" Note that to test *pure gleno-humeral motion,* the patient should raise the arms to shoulder level at 90 degrees, with palms facing down. To test *scapulothoracic motion,* the patient should turn the palms up and raise the arms an additional 60 degrees. The final 30-degrees tests combined glenohumeral and scapulothoracic motion.
Adduction 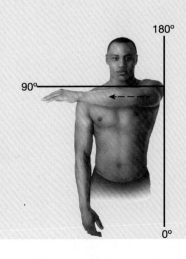	Pectoralis major, coracobrachialis, latissimus dorsi, teres major, subscapularis	"*Cross your arm in front of your body.*"

(continued)

Shoulder Movement	Principal Muscles Affecting Movement	Patient Instructions
Internal Rotation	Subscapularis, anterior deltoid, pectoralis major, teres major, latissimus dorsi	*"Place one hand behind your back and touch your shoulder blade."* Identify the highest midline spinous process the patient is able to reach.
External Rotation	Infraspinatus, teres minor, posterior deltoid	*"Raise your arm to shoulder level; bend your elbow and rotate your forearm toward the ceiling."* or *"Place one hand behind your neck or head as if you are brushing your hair."*

90°

Maneuvers. The examination of the shoulder often requires selective evaluation of specific motions and structures. There are more than 20 different maneuvers for testing shoulder function, but not all are well studied.[51] Common recommended maneuvers, with evidence when available, are described on pp. 623–625. Using these maneuvers takes practice and supervision, but you will find them helpful in identifying shoulder pathology.

Note that the most common cause of shoulder pain involves the rotator cuff. Compression of the rotator cuff muscles and tendons between the head of the humerus and the acromion causes "impingement signs" or pain during maneuvers such as Neer's, Hawkin's, and the drop-arm tests, described below. However, the best predictors of rotator cuff tear are supraspinatus weakness on abduction, infraspinatus weakness during external rotation, and a positive impingement sign.[51–53]

An age of 60 years or older and a positive drop-arm test are the findings most likely to identify a degenerative rotator cuff tear, with likelihood ratios (LRs) of 3.2 and 5.0, respectively. The combined findings of supraspinatus weakness, infraspinatus weakness, and a positive impingement sign increase the likelihood ratio of a tear to 48.0; when all three are absent, the LR falls to 0.02, virtually ruling out the diagnosis.[51,53]

Maneuvers for Examining the Shoulder

Structure	Technique
Acromioclavicular Joint	Palpate and compare both joints for swelling or tenderness. Adduct the patient's arm across the chest, sometimes called the *"crossover test."*

(continued)

See Table 16-4, Painful Shoulders, pp. 672–673. Localized tenderness or pain with *adduction* suggests inflammation or arthritis of the acromioclavicular joint, but sensitivity and specificity of tenderness is approximately 95% and 10%; and of pain with adduction, approximately 80% and 50%.[51]

Maneuvers for Examining the Shoulder (continued)

Structure	Technique	
Overall Shoulder Rotation	Ask the patient to touch the opposite scapula using the two motions shown below (the *Apley scratch* test).	Difficulty with these motions suggests a *rotator cuff disorder* or *adhesive capsulitis*.

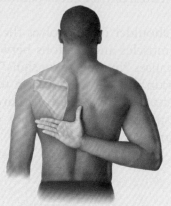

Tests abduction and external rotation.	Tests adduction and internal rotation.

Rotator Cuff	Test *Neer's impingement sign.* Press on the scapula to prevent scapular motion with one hand, and raise the patient's arm with the other. This compresses the greater tuberosity of the humerus against the acromion.	Pain during this maneuver is a *positive test,* indicating possible inflammation or *rotator cuff tear.*

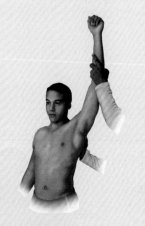

	Test *Hawkin's impingement sign.* Flex the patient's shoulder and elbow to 90 degrees with the palm facing down. Then, with one hand on the forearm and one on the arm, rotate the arm internally. This compresses the greater tuberosity against the cor- acoacromial ligament.	Pain during this maneuver is a *positive test,* indicating possible inflammation or *rotator cuff tear.*

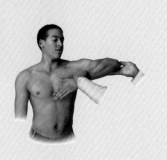

(continued)

Maneuvers for Examining the Shoulder (*continued*)

Structure	Technique	
	Test *supraspinatus strength* (sometimes called the "empty can test"). Elevate the arms to 90 degrees and internally rotate the arms with the thumbs pointing down, as if emptying a can. Ask the patient to resist as you place downward pressure on the arms. 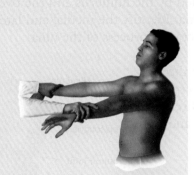	Weakness during this maneuver is a *positive test,* indicating possible *rotator cuff tear.*
	Test *infraspinatus strength.* Ask the patient to place arms at the side and flex the elbows to 90 degrees with the thumbs turned up. Provide resistance as the patient presses the forearms outward. 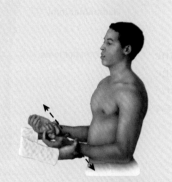	Weakness during this maneuver is a *positive test,* indicating possible *rotator cuff tear* or *bicipital tendinitis.*
	Test *forearm supination.* Flex the patient's forearm to 90 degrees at the elbow and pronate the patient's wrist. Provide resistance when the patient supinates the forearm. 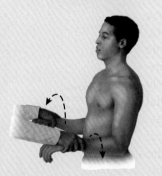	Pain during this maneuver is a *positive test,* indicating inflammation of the long head of the biceps tendon and possible *rotator cuff tear.*
	Test the *"drop-arm" sign.* Ask the patient to fully abduct the arm to shoulder level (or up to 90 degrees) and lower it slowly. Note that abduction above shoulder level, from 90 degrees to 120 degrees, reflects action of the deltoid muscle. 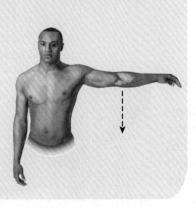	If the patient cannot hold the arm fully abducted at shoulder level or cannot control lowering the arm, the test is *positive,* indicating a *rotator cuff tear* (LR, 5.0).[51]

■ THE ELBOW

Overview, Bony Structures, and Joints

The elbow helps position the hand in space and stabilizes the lever action of the forearm. The elbow joint is formed by the humerus and the two bones of the forearm, the radius and the ulna. Identify the medial and lateral epicondyles of the humerus and the olecranon process of the ulna.

These bones have three articulations: the *humeroulnar joint*, the *radiohumeral joint*, and the *radioulnar joint*. All three share a large common articular cavity and an extensive synovial lining.

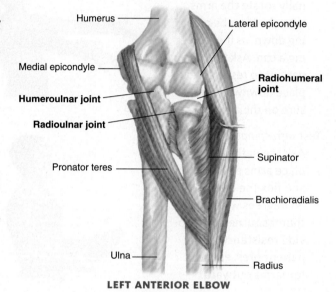

LEFT ANTERIOR ELBOW

Muscle Groups and Additional Structures

Muscles traversing the elbow include the *biceps* and *brachioradialis* (flexion), the *brachialis*, the *triceps* (extension), the *pronator teres* (pronation), and the *supinator* (supination).

Note the location of the *olecranon bursa* between the olecranon process and the skin. The bursa is not normally palpable but swells and becomes tender when inflamed. The *ulnar nerve* runs posteriorly in the ulnar groove between the medial epicondyle and the olecranon process. The radial nerve is adjacent to the lateral epicondyle. On the ventral forearm, the *median nerve* is just medial to the brachial artery in the antecubital fossa.

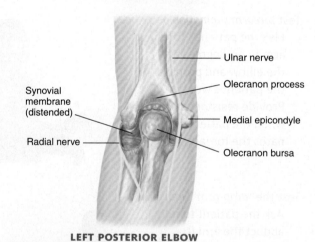

LEFT POSTERIOR ELBOW

Techniques of Examination

Inspection. Support the patient's forearm with your opposite hand so that the elbow is flexed to about 70 degrees. Identify the medial and lateral epicondyles and the olecranon process of the ulna. Inspect the contours of the elbow, including the extensor surface of the ulna and the olecranon process. Note any nodules or swelling.

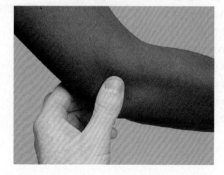

See Table 16-5, Swollen or Tender Elbows, p. 674.

Swelling over the olecranon process is found in *olecranon bursitis* (see p. 674); inflammation or synovial fluid occurs in arthritis.

Palpation. Palpate the olecranon process and press over the epicondyles for tenderness or effusion. Note any displacement of the olecranon.

Note any displacement of the olecranon process.

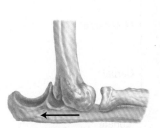

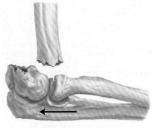

POSTERIOR DISLOCATION OF THE ELBOW

SUPRACONDYLAR FRACTURE OF THE ELBOW

Palpate the grooves between the epicondyles and the olecranon process, where the synovium is most easily examined. Normally you cannot palpate either the synovium or the olecranon bursa.

The sensitive ulnar nerve can be felt posteriorly between the olecranon process and the medial epicondyle.

Range of Motion and Maneuvers. Range of motion includes flexion and extension at the elbow and pronation and supination of the forearm. In the following table, note the specific muscles responsible for each motion and the instructions that prompt the requested patient response.

Elbow Movement	Primary Muscles Affecting Movement	Patient Instructions
Flexion	Biceps brachii, brachialis, brachioradialis	*"Bend your elbow."*
Extension	Triceps brachii, anconeus	*"Straighten your elbow."*
Supination	Biceps brachii, supinator	*"Turn your palms up, as if carrying a bowl of soup."*
Pronation	Pronator teres, pronator quadratus	*"Turn your palms down."*

THE WRIST AND HANDS

Overview

The wrist and hands form a complex unit of small highly active joints used almost continuously during waking hours. There is little protection from overlying soft tissue, increasing vulnerability to trauma and disability.

Tenderness distal to the epicondyle is common in *lateral epicondylitis* (tennis elbow) and less common in *medial epicondylitis* (pitcher's or golfer's elbow).

The olecranon is displaced posteriorly in *posterior dislocation of the elbow* and *supracondylar fracture*.

After injury, preservation of active range of motion and full elbow extension makes fracture highly unlikely. When intact, these actions have a sensitivity of 100% and specificity of 50% to >97% for absence of fracture.[54,55]

Full elbow extension also makes intra-articular effusion or hemarthrosis unlikely.

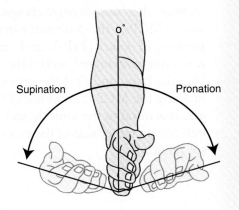

Bony Structures

The wrist includes the distal radius and ulna and eight small carpal bones. At the wrist, identify the bony tips of the radius and the ulna.

The carpal bones lie distal to the wrist joint. Identify the carpal bones, each of the five metacarpals, and the proximal, middle, and distal phalanges. Note that the thumb has only two phalanges.

Joints

The numerous joints of the wrist and hand make the hands unusually dextrous.

- *Wrist joints.* The wrist joints include the *radiocarpal* or *wrist joint*, the *distal radioulnar joint*, and the *intercarpal joints*. The joint capsule, articular disc, and synovial membrane of the wrist join the radius to the ulna and to the proximal carpal bones. On the dorsum of the wrist, locate the groove of the *radiocarpal joint*. This joint provides most of the flexion and extension at the wrist because the ulna does not articulate directly with the carpal bones.

- *Hand joints.* The joints of the hand include the *metacarpophalangeal joints* (MCPs), the *proximal interphalangeal joints* (PIPs), and the *distal interphalangeal joints* (DIPs). Flex the hand and find the groove marking the MCP joint of each finger. It is distal to the knuckle and is best felt on either side of the extensor tendon.

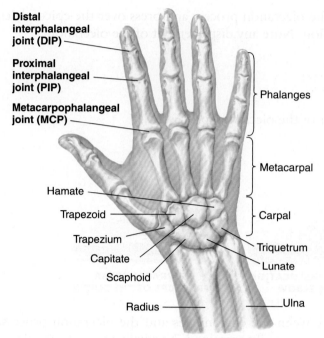

Distal interphalangeal joint (DIP)
Proximal interphalangeal joint (PIP)
Metacarpophalangeal joint (MCP)
Phalanges
Metacarpal
Hamate
Trapezoid
Trapezium
Capitate
Scaphoid
Carpal
Triquetrum
Lunate
Radius
Ulna

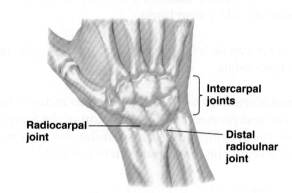

Intercarpal joints
Radiocarpal joint
Distal radioulnar joint

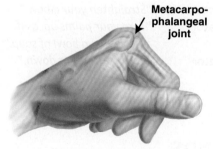

Metacarpophalangeal joint

Degenerative changes at the first carpometacarpal joint of the thumb are more common in women.

Muscle Groups

Wrist flexion arises from the two carpal muscles, located on the radial and ulnar surfaces. Two radial and one ulnar muscle provide wrist extension. Supination and pronation result from muscle contraction in the forearm.

The thumb is powered by three muscles that form the thenar eminence and provide flexion, abduction, and opposition. The muscles of extension are at the base of the thumb along the radial margin. Movement in the digits depends on action of the flexor and extensor tendons of muscles in the forearm and wrist.

The intrinsic muscles of the hand attaching to the metacarpal bones are involved in flexion (*lumbricals*), abduction (*dorsal interossei*), and adduction (*palmar interossei*) of the fingers.

Additional Structures

Soft-tissue structures, especially tendons and tendon sheaths, are especially important to movement of the wrist and hand. Six extensor tendons and two flexor tendons pass across the wrist and hand to insert on the fingers. Through much of their course these tendons travel in tunnel-like sheaths, generally palpable only when swollen or inflamed.

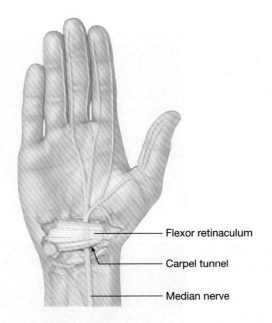

Flexor retinaculum

Carpel tunnel

Median nerve

Be familiar with the structures in the *carpal tunnel*, a channel beneath the palmar surface of the wrist and proximal hand. The channel contains the sheath and flexor tendons of the forearm muscles and the *median nerve*.

Holding the tendons and tendon sheath in place is a transverse ligament, the *flexor retinaculum*. The median nerve lies between the flexor retinaculum and the tendon sheath. The median nerve provides sensation to the palm and the palmar surface of most of the thumb, the second and third digits, and half of the fourth digit. It also innervates the thumb muscles of flexion, abduction, and opposition.

Techniques of Examination

Inspection. Observe the position of the hands in motion to see if movements are smooth and natural. When the fingers are relaxed they should be slightly flexed; the fingernail edges should be in parallel.

Guarded movement suggests injury. Abnormal finger alignment is seen in flexor tendon damage.

Inspect the palmar and dorsal surfaces of the wrist and hand carefully for swelling over the joints.

Note any deformities of the wrist, hand, or finger bones, as well as any angulation.

Observe the contours of the palm, namely the thenar and hypothenar eminences.

Note any thickening of the flexor tendons or flexion contractures in the fingers.

Palpation. At the wrist, palpate the distal radius and ulna on the lateral and medial surfaces. Palpate the groove of each wrist joint with your thumbs on the dorsum of the wrist, your fingers beneath it. Note any swelling, bogginess, or tenderness.

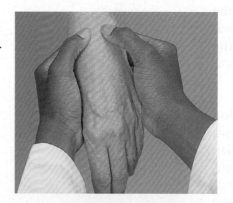

Palpate the radial styloid bone and the *anatomical snuffbox,* a hollowed depression just distal to the radial styloid process formed by the abductor and extensor muscles of the thumb. The "snuffbox" becomes more visible with lateral extension of the thumb away from the hand (abduction).

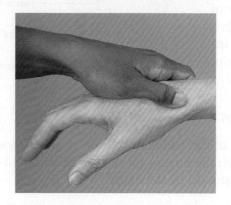

Diffuse swelling is common in arthritis or infection; local swelling suggests a ganglion. See Table 16-6, Arthritis in the Hands, p. 675, and Table 16-7, Swellings and Deformities of the Hands, p. 676.

In *osteoarthritis,* look for Heberden's nodes at the DIP joints and Bouchard's nodes at the PIP joints. In *rheumatoid arthritis,* there is symmetric deformity in the PIP, MCP, and wrist joints, and ulnar deviation.

Thenar atrophy occurs in median nerve compression from *carpal tunnel syndrome;* hypothenar atrophy in *ulnar nerve compression.*

Flexion contractures in the ring, fifth, and third fingers, or *Dupuytren's contractures,* arise from thickening of the palmar fascia (see p. 676).

Tenderness over the distal radius occurs in *Colles' fracture* from a fall, especially in patients with osteoporosis. Any tenderness or bony step-offs are suspicious for fracture.

Swelling and/or tenderness suggests *rheumatoid arthritis* if bilateral and of several weeks' duration.

Tenderness over the extensor and abductor tendons of the thumb at the radial styloid suggests *de Quervain's tenosynovitis* and *gonococcal tenosynovitis.* See Table 16-8, Tendon Sheath, Palmar Space, and Finger Infections, p. 677.

Tenderness over the "snuffbox" suggests *scaphoid fracture,* the most common injury of the carpal bones. Poor blood supply puts the scaphoid bone at risk for *avascular necrosis.*

Palpate the eight carpal bones lying distal to the wrist joint, and then each of the five metacarpals and the proximal, middle, and distal phalanges.

Palpate any other area where you suspect an abnormality.

Compress the MCP joints by squeezing the hand from each side between the thumb and fingers. Alternatively, use your thumb to palpate each MCP joint just distal to and on each side of the knuckle as your index finger feels the head of the metacarpal in the palm. Note any swelling, bogginess, or tenderness.

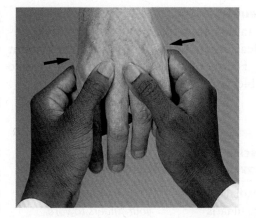

Synovitis in the MCPs is painful with this pressure—a point to remember when shaking hands.

The MCPs are often boggy or tender in *rheumatoid arthritis*, but are rarely involved in osteoarthritis. Pain with compression also occurs in *posttraumatic arthritis*.

Now examine the fingers and thumb. Palpate the medial and lateral aspects of each PIP joint between your thumb and index finger, again checking for swelling, bogginess, bony enlargement, or tenderness.

PIP changes are seen in *rheumatoid arthritis*; Bouchard's nodes in *osteoarthritis*. Pain at the base of the thumb occurs in *carpometacarpal arthritis*.

Hard dorsolateral nodules on the DIP joints, or *Heberden's nodes*, are common in osteoarthritis; DIP joints are involved in *psoriatic arthritis*.

Using the same techniques, examine the DIP joints.

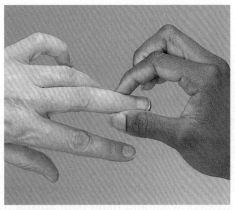

HEBERDEN'S NODES

In any area of swelling or inflammation, palpate along the tendons inserting on the thumb and fingers.

Tenderness and swelling are seen in in *tenosynovitis*, or inflammation of the tendon sheaths. *De Quervain's tenosynovitis* involves the extensor and abductor tendons of the thumb as they cross the radial styloid. See Table 16-8, Tendon Sheath, Palmar Space, and Finger Infections, p. 677.

Wrists: Range of Motion and Maneuvers

Range of Motion. Refer to the table below for specific muscles responsible for each movement and use clear instructions that prompt the patient to properly follow your directions. For techniques of testing wrist muscle strength, turn to Chapter 17, The Nervous System, pp. 711–712.

Conditions that impair range of motion include *arthritis, tenosynovitis,* and *Dupuytren's contracture.* See Table 16-7, Swellings and Deformities of the Hands, p. 676.

Wrist Movement	Primary Muscles Affecting Movement	Patient Instructions
Flexion	Flexor carpi radialis, flexor carpi ulnaris	*"With palms down, point your fingers toward the floor."*
Extension	Extensor carpi ulnaris, extensor carpi radialis longus, extensor carpi radialis brevis	*"With palms down, point your your fingers toward the ceiling."*
Adduction (radial deviation)	Flexor carpi ulnaris	*"With palms down, bring your fingers toward the midline."*
Abduction (ulnar deviation)	Flexor carpi radialis	*"With palms down, bring your fingers away from the midline."*

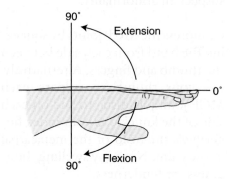

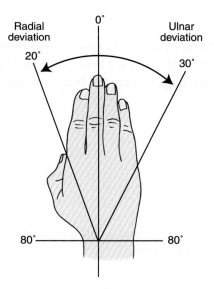

Maneuvers. Several maneuvers useful for assessing common office complaints relating to the wrist are listed on the next page. For complaints of dropping objects, inability to twist lids off jars, aching at the wrist or even the forearm, and numbness of the first three digits, learn these tests for assessing *carpal tunnel syndrome.* Note the distribution of the median, radial, and ulnar nerve innervations of the wrist and hand on the next page. Remember to assess more proximal causes of wrist and hand pain arising in the cervical cord and nerve roots.

Onset of *carpal tunnel syndrome* is often related to repetitive motion with wrists flexed (as in keyboard use or mail-sorting), pregnancy, rheumatoid arthritis, diabetes, or hypothyroidism.

Thenar atrophy may also be present.

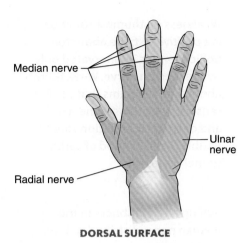

DORSAL SURFACE

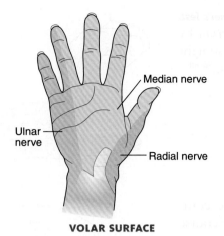

VOLAR SURFACE

Decreased sensation in the median nerve distribution characterizes *carpal tunnel syndrome.*

You can test sensation as follows:

- Pulp of the index finger—median nerve

- Pulp of the fifth finger—ulnar nerve

- Dorsal web space of the thumb and index finger—radial nerve

Hand Grip. Test *hand grip strength* by asking the patient to grasp your second and third fingers. This tests function of wrist joints, the finger flexors, and the intrinsic muscles and joints of the hand.

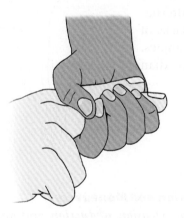

Decreased grip strength is a *positive test* for weakness of the finger flexors and/or intrinsic muscles of the hand. It may also result from pain from degenerative joint changes.

Wrist pain and grip weakness occur in *de Quervain's tenosynovitis.* There is decreased grip strength in *arthritis, carpal tunnel syndrome,* epicondylitis, and *cervical radiculopathy.*

Thumb Movement. Test the thumb function if there is wrist pain by asking the patient to grasp the thumb against the palm and then move the wrist toward the midline in ulnar deviation (commonly called *Finkelstein's test*).

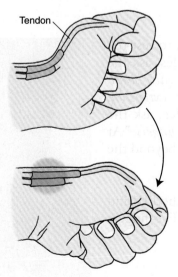

Tendon

Pain during this maneuver identifies *de Quervain's tenosynovitis* from inflammation of the abductor pollicis longus and extensor pollicis brevis tendons and tendon sheaths. This condition, like *carpal tunnel syndrome,* is more common in women.

Carpal Tunnel—Thumb Abduction, Tinel's Test, and Phalen's Test. Test *thumb abduction* by asking the patient to raise the thumb straight up as you apply downward resistance.[56–58]

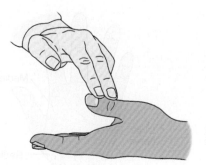

Weakness on thumb abduction is a *positive test*; the abductor pollicis longus is innervated only by the median nerve. Weak thumb abduction, diagrams that confirm sensory symptoms in the hand, and decreased sensation roughly double the likelihood of carpal tunnel disease.[56]

Test *Tinel's sign* for median nerve compression by tapping lightly over the course of the median nerve in the carpal tunnel as shown.

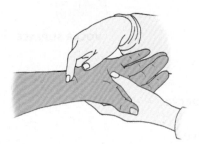

Aching and numbness in the median nerve distribution is a *positive test*.

Test *Phalen's sign* for median nerve compression by asking the patient to hold the wrists in flexion for 60 seconds. Alternatively, ask the patient to press the backs of both hands together to form right angles. These maneuvers compress the median nerve.

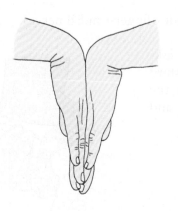

Numbness and tingling in the median nerve distribution within 60 seconds is a *positive test*.

Tinel's and Phalen's signs do not reliably predict positive electrodiagnosis of carpal tunnel disease.[56]

Fingers and Thumbs: Range of Motion and Maneuvers

Range of Motion. Assess *flexion, extension, abduction,* and *adduction* of the fingers.

- *Flexion and extension.* For *flexion*, to test the lumbricals and finger flexor muscles, ask the patient to *"Make a tight fist with each hand, thumb across the knuckles."* For *extension*, to test the finger extensor muscles, ask the patient to *"Extend and spread the fingers."* At the MCPs, the fingers may extend beyond the neutral position.

  Test the flexion and extension of the PIP and DIP joints (lumbrical muscles). The fingers should open and close easily.

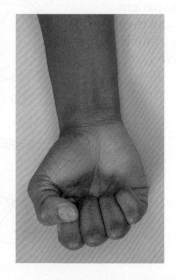

- *Abduction and adduction.* Ask the patient to spread the fingers apart (abduction from dorsal interossei) and back together (adduction from palmar interossei). Check for smooth, coordinated movement.

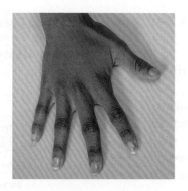

Look for impaired hand movement in arthritis, trigger finger, and Dupuytren's contracture.

Thumbs. At the *thumb,* assess *flexion, extension, abduction, adduction,* and *opposition.* Each of these movements is powered by a related muscle of the thumb.

Ask the patient to move the thumb across the palm and touch the base of the fifth finger to test *flexion,* and then to move the thumb back across the palm and away from the fingers to test *extension.*

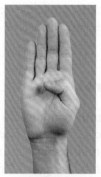
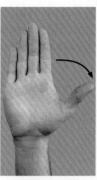

FLEXION   **EXTENSION**

Next, ask the patient to place the fingers and thumb in the neutral position with the palm up, then have the patient move the thumb anteriorly away from the palm to assess abduction and back down for adduction. To test opposition, or movements of the thumb across the palm, ask the patient to touch the thumb to each of the other fingertips.

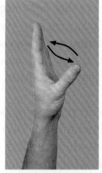
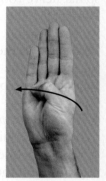

ABDUCTION   **OPPOSITION**
AND ADDUCTION

A full examination of the wrist and hand involves detailed testing of muscle strength and sensation, found in Chapter 17, The Nervous System, pp. 710–713.

THE SPINE

Overview

The vertebral column, or spine, is the central supporting structure of the trunk and back. The *concave curves* of the cervical and lumbar spine and the *convex curves* of the thoracic and sacrococcygeal spine help distribute upper body weight to the pelvis and lower extremities and cushion the concussive impact of walking or running.

The complex mechanics of the back reflect the coordinated action of:

- The vertebrae and intervertebral discs

- An interconnecting system of ligaments between anterior vertebrae and posterior vertebrae, ligaments between the spinous processes, and ligaments between the lamina of two adjacent vertebrae

- Large superficial muscles, deeper intrinsic muscles, and muscles of the abdominal wall

Bony Structures

The vertebral column contains 24 vertebrae stacked on the sacrum and coccyx. A typical vertebra contains sites for joint articulations, weight bearing, and muscle attachments, as well as foramina for the spinal nerve roots and peripheral nerves. Anteriorly, the *vertebral body* supports weight bearing. The posterior *vertebral arch* encloses the spinal cord. Review the location of the vertebral processes and foramina, with particular attention to:

- The *spinous process* projecting posteriorly in the midline and the two transverse processes at the junction of the *pedicle* and the *lamina*. Muscles attach at these processes.

- The *articular processes*—two on each side of the vertebra, one facing up and one facing down, at the junction of the pedicles and laminae, often called *articular facets*.

- The *vertebral foramen*, which encloses the spinal cord, the *intervertebral foramen*, formed by the inferior and superior articulating process of adjacent vertebrae, creating a channel for the spinal nerve roots; and in the cervical vertebrae, the *transverse foramen* for the vertebral artery.

Representative Cervical and Lumbar Vertebrae

C4–5 Coronal and Lateral Views

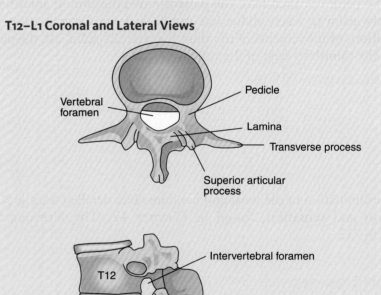

T12–L1 Coronal and Lateral Views

The proximity of the spinal cord and spinal nerve roots to their bony vertebral casing and the intervertebral discs makes them especially vulnerable to disc herniation, impingement from degenerative changes in the vertebrae and facets, and trauma.

Joints

The spine has slightly movable cartilaginous joints between the vertebral bodies and between the articular facets. Between the vertebral bodies are the *intervertebral discs,* each consisting of a soft mucoid central core, the *nucleus pulposus,* rimmed by the tough fibrous tissue of the *annulus fibrosis.* The intervertebral discs cushion movement between vertebrae and allow the vertebral column to curve, flex, and bend. The flexibility of the spine is largely determined by the angle of the articular facet joints relative to the plane of the vertebral body, and varies at different levels of the spine. Note that the vertebral column angles sharply posterior at the *lumbosacral junction* and becomes immovable. The mechanical stress at this angulation contributes to the risk for disc herniation and subluxation, or slippage (*spondylolisthesis*), of L5 on S1.

Muscle Groups

The *trapezius* and *latissimus dorsi* form the large outer layer of muscles attaching to each side of the spine. They overlie two deeper muscle layers—a layer attaching to the head, neck, and spinous processes (*splenius capitis, splenius cervicis,* and *sacrospinalis*) and a layer of smaller intrinsic muscles between vertebrae. Muscles attaching to the anterior surface of the vertebrae, including the *psoas* muscle and muscles of the abdominal wall, assist with flexion.

Muscles moving the neck and lower vertebral column are summarized in the table on p. 639.

Techniques of Examination

Inspection. Begin by observing the patient's posture when entering the room, including the position of both the neck and trunk.

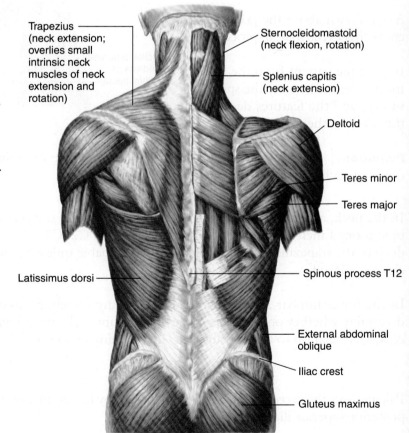

Trapezius (neck extension; overlies small intrinsic neck muscles of neck extension and rotation)

Sternocleidomastoid (neck flexion, rotation)

Splenius capitis (neck extension)

Deltoid

Teres minor

Teres major

Spinous process T12

Latissimus dorsi

External abdominal oblique

Iliac crest

Gluteus maximus

Assess the patient for erect position of the head, neck, and back; for smooth, coordinated neck movement; and for ease of gait.

Neck stiffness signals arthritis, muscle strain, or other underlying pathology that should be pursued. Headache may be present.

Drape or gown the patient to expose the entire back for complete inspection. If possible, the patient should be upright in the natural standing position, with feet together and arms hanging at the sides. The head should be midline in the same plane as the sacrum, and the shoulders and pelvis should be level.

Viewing the patient from behind, identify the following:

- Spinous processes, usually more prominent at C7 and T1 and more evident on forward flexion

- Paravertebral muscles on either side of the midline

- Iliac crests

- Posterior superior iliac spines, usually marked by skin dimples.

A line drawn above the posterior iliac crests crosses the spinous process of L4.

Inspect the patient from the side and from behind. Evaluate the spinal curvatures and the features described in the table on the next page.

Lateral deviation and rotation of the head suggest *torticollis*, from contraction of the sternocleidomastoid muscle.

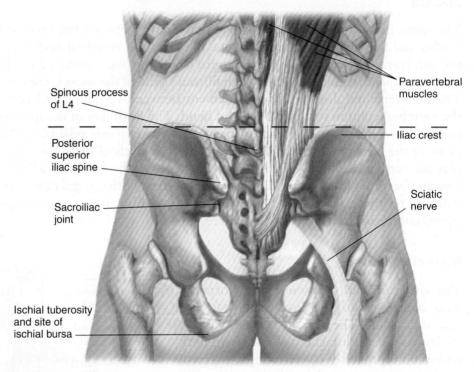

Spinous process of L4

Posterior superior iliac spine

Sacroiliac joint

Ischial tuberosity and site of ischial bursa

Paravertebral muscles

Iliac crest

Sciatic nerve

Palpation. From a sitting or standing position, palpate the spinous processes of each vertebra with your thumb.

In the neck, also palpate the *facet joints* that lie between the cervical vertebrae about 1 inch lateral to the spinous processes of C2–C7. These joints lie deep to the trapezius muscle and may not be palpable unless the neck muscles are relaxed.

In the lower lumbar area, check carefully for any vertebral "step-offs" to determine whether one spinous process seems unusually prominent (or recessed) in relation to the one above it. Identify any tenderness.

Palpate over the *sacroiliac joint,* often identified by the dimple overlying the posterior superior iliac spine.

You may wish to percuss the spine for tenderness by thumping, but not too roughly, with the ulnar surface of your fist.

Tenderness suggests fracture or dislocation if preceded by trauma, underlying infection, or arthritis.

Tenderness occurs in arthritis, especially at the facet joints between C5 and C6

Step-offs occur in *spondylolisthesis,* or forward slippage of one vertebra, which may compress the spinal cord. Vertebral tenderness is suspicious for fracture or infection.

Tenderness over the sacroiliac joint is common in sacroiliitis. *Ankylosing spondylitis* may produce sacroiliac tenderness.[59]

Pain on percussion may arise from *osteoporosis, infection,* or *malignancy.*

Inspection of the Spine

View of Patient	Focus of Inspection		
From the side	Cervical, thoracic, and lumbar curves	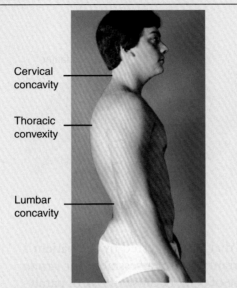 Cervical concavity — Thoracic convexity — Lumbar concavity —	Increased *thoracic kyphosis* occurs with aging. In children, a correctable structural deformity should be pursued.
From behind	Upright spinal column (an imaginary line should fall from C7 through the gluteal cleft) Alignment of the shoulders, the iliac crests, and the skin creases below the buttocks (gluteal folds)	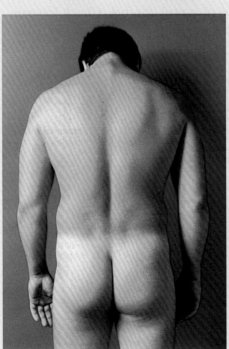	In *scoliosis,* there is lateral and rotatory curvature of the spine to bring the head back to midline. Scoliosis often becomes evident during adolescence, before symptoms appear. *Unequal shoulder heights* occur in: scoliosis; Sprengel's deformity of the scapula, from the attachment of an extra bone or band between the upper scapula and C7; "winging" of the scapula, from loss of innervation of the serratus anterior muscle by the long thoracic nerve; and contralateral weakness of the trapezius. *Unequal heights of the iliac crests,* or *pelvic tilt,* suggest unequal lengths of the legs and disappear when a block is placed under the shorter limb. Scoliosis and hip abduction or adduction may also cause a pelvic tilt. "Listing" of the trunk to one side is seen with a herniated lumbar disc.
	Skin markings, tags, or masses		Birthmarks, port-wine stains, hairy patches, and lipomas often overlie bony defects such as *spina bifida.* Café-au-lait spots (discolored patches of skin), skin tags, and fibrous tumors are common in *neurofibromatosis.*

Inspect and palpate the *paravertebral muscles* for tenderness and spasm. Muscles in spasm feel firm and knotted and may be visible.

Spasm occurs in degenerative and inflammatory processes of muscles, overuse, prolonged contraction from abnormal posture, or anxiety.

With the patient's hip flexed and the patient lying on the opposite side, palpate the *sciatic nerve*, the largest nerve in the body, consisting of nerve roots from L4, L5, S1, S2, and S3. The nerve lies midway between the greater trochanter and the ischial tuberosity as it leaves the pelvis through the sciatic notch.

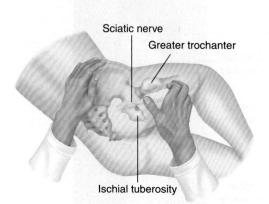

Sciatic nerve
Greater trochanter
Ischial tuberosity

Sciatic nerve tenderness suggests a herniated disc or mass lesion impinging on the contributing nerve roots. This nerve is difficult to palpate in most patients.

Palpate for tenderness in any other areas that are suggested by the patient's symptoms. Recall that low back pain warrants careful assessment for *cauda equina compression*, the most serious cause of pain, because of risk of paralysis of the affected limb or loss of bladder or bowel control. Check for pain radiation into the buttock, perineum, or legs.

Herniated intervertebral discs, most common at L5–S1 or L4–L5, may produce tenderness of the spinous processes, the intervertebral joints, the paravertebral muscles, the sacrosciatic notch, and the sciatic nerve.

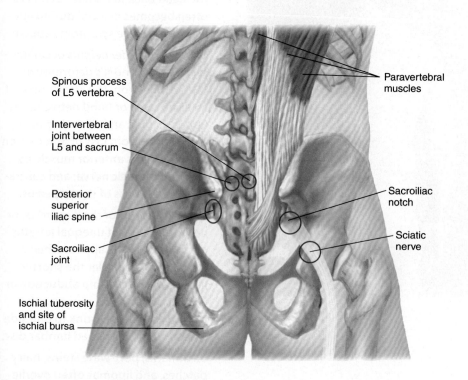

Spinous process of L5 vertebra

Intervertebral joint between L5 and sacrum

Posterior superior iliac spine

Sacroiliac joint

Ischial tuberosity and site of ischial bursa

Paravertebral muscles

Sacroiliac notch

Sciatic nerve

Rheumatoid arthritis may also cause tenderness of the intervertebral joints.

Remember that tenderness in the costovertebral angles may signify kidney infection rather than a musculoskeletal problem.

See Table 16-1, Low Back Pain, p. 668.

Range of Motion and Maneuvers

Range of Motion: Neck. The neck is the most mobile portion of the spine, remarkable for its seven fragile vertebrae supporting the 10- to 15-pound head. *Flexion* and *extension* occur primarily between the skull and C1, the atlas; *rotation* at C1–C2, the axis; and *lateral bending* at C2–C7.

Limitations in range of motion can arise from stiffness from arthritis, pain from trauma, overuse, or muscle spasm such as *torticollis*.

In the table below, note the specific muscles responsible for each motion and the instructions that prompt the requested patient response.

Neck Movement	Primary Muscles Affecting Movement	Patient Instructions
Flexion	Sternocleidomastoid, scalene, prevertebral muscles	*"Bring your chin to your chest."*
Extension	Splenius capitis and cervicis, small intrinsic neck muscles	*"Look up at the ceiling."*
Rotation	Sternocleidomastoid, small intrinsic neck muscles	*"Look over one shoulder, and then the other."*
Lateral Bending	Scalenes and small intrinsic neck muscles	*"Bring your ear to your shoulder."*

Tenderness, loss of sensation, or weakness warrant careful neurologic testing of the neck and upper extremities.

Range of Motion: Spinal Column. Now assess range of motion in the spinal column. In the table below, note the specific muscles responsible for each motion and the instructions that prompt the requested patient response.

Back Movement	Primary Muscles Affecting Movement	Patient Instructions
Flexion	Psoas major, psoas minor, quadratus lumborum; abdominal muscles attaching to the anterior vertebrae, such as the internal and external obliques and rectus abdominis	*"Bend forward and try to touch your toes."* Note the smoothness and symmetry of movement, the range of motion, and the curve in the lumbar area. As flexion proceeds, the lumbar concavity should flatten out.
Extension	Deep intrinsic muscles of the back, such as the erector spinae and transversospinalis groups	*"Bend back as far as possible."* Support the patient by placing your hand on the posterior superior iliac spine, with your fingers pointing toward the midline.

(continued)

It is important to assess any complaints or findings of neck, shoulder, or arm pain, numbness, or weakness for possible cervical cord or nerve root compression. See Table 16-2, Pains in the Neck, p. 669.

Tenderness at C1–C2 in *rheumatoid arthritis* suggests possible risk for subluxation and high cervical cord compression and needs prompt additional assessment.

Deformity of the thorax on forward bending, especially differences in height of the scapulae, suggests *scoliosis.*

Persistence of lumbar lordosis suggests muscle spasm or *ankylosing spondylitis.*

Decreased *spinal mobility* is common in *osteoarthritis* and *ankylosing spondylitis,* among other conditions.[59–61]

Back Movement	Primary Muscles Affecting Movement	Patient Instructions
Rotation	Abdominal muscles, intrinsic muscles of the back	*"Rotate from side to side."* Stabilize the patient's pelvis by placing one hand on the patient's hip and the other on the opposite shoulder. Then rotate the trunk by pulling the shoulder anteriorly and then the hip posteriorly. Repeat these maneuvers for the opposite side.
Lateral Bending	Abdominal muscles, intrinsic muscles of the back	*"Bend to the side from the waist."* Stabilize the patient's pelvis by placing your hand on the patient's hip. Repeat for the opposite side.

As with the neck, pain or tenderness with these maneuvers, particularly with radiation into the leg, warrants careful neurologic testing of the lower extremities.

Underlying cord or nerve root compression should be considered. Note that arthritis, tumor, or infection in the hip, rectum, or pelvis may cause symptoms in the lumbar spine. See Table 16-1, Low Back Pain, p. 668.

See Chapter 17, The Nervous System, for the Straight Leg Raise Test, pp. 732–733.

THE HIP

Overview

The hip joint is deeply embedded in the pelvis and is notable for its strength, stability, and wide range of motion. The stability of the hip joint, essential for weight bearing, arises from the deep fit of the head of the femur into the acetabulum, its strong fibrous articular capsule, and the powerful muscles crossing the joint and inserting below the femoral head, providing leverage for movement of the femur.

Bony Structures and Joints

The hip joint lies below the middle third of the inguinal ligament but in a deeper plane. It is a ball-and-socket joint; note how the rounded head of the femur articulates with the cuplike cavity of the acetabulum. Because of its overlying muscles and depth, it is not readily palpable. Review the bones of the pelvis—the *acetabulum*, the *ilium*, and the *ischium*—and the connection inferiorly at the *symphysis pubis* and posteriorly with the sacroiliac bone.

On the *anterior surface of the hip,* locate the following bony structures:

- The iliac crest at the level of L4

- The iliac tubercle

- The anterior superior iliac spine

- The greater trochanter

- The pubic tubercle

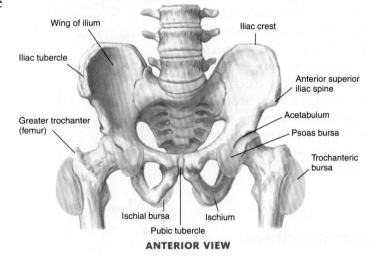

ANTERIOR VIEW

On the *posterior surface of the hip,* locate the following:

- The posterior superior iliac spine

- The greater trochanter

- The ischial tuberosity

- The sacroiliac joint

Note that an imaginary line between the posterior superior iliac spines crosses the joint at S2.

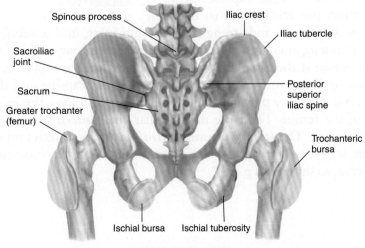

POSTERIOR VIEW

Muscle Groups

Four powerful muscle groups move the hip. Picture these groups as you examine patients, and remember that, to move the femur or any bone in a given direction, the muscle must cross the joint line.

The *flexor group* lies anteriorly and flexes the thigh. The primary hip flexor is the *iliopsoas,* extending from above the iliac crest to the lesser trochanter. The *extensor group* lies posteriorly and extends the thigh. The *gluteus maximus* is the primary extensor of the hip. It forms a band crossing from its origin along the medial pelvis to its insertion below the trochanter.

The *adductor group* is medial and swings the thigh toward the body. The muscles in this group arise from the rami of the pubis and ischium and insert on the posteromedial aspect of the femur. The *abductor group* is lateral, extending from the iliac crest to the greater trochanter, and moves the thigh away from the body. This group includes the *gluteus medius* and *minimus.* These muscles help stabilize the pelvis during the stance phase of gait.

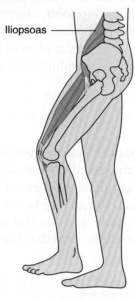
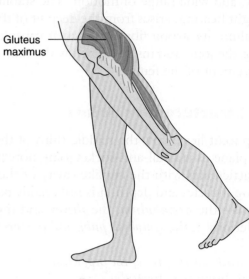

Iliopsoas

Gluteus maximus

Flexor Group

Extensor Group

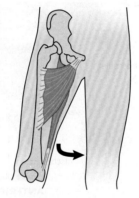
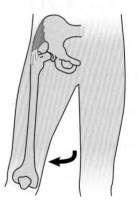

Adductor Group

Abductor Group

Additional Structures

A strong, dense articular capsule, extending from the acetabulum to the femoral neck, encases and strengthens the hip joint, and is reinforced by three overlying ligaments and lined with synovial membrane. There are three principal bursae at the hip. Anterior to the joint is the *psoas* (also termed *iliopectineal* or *iliopsoas) bursa,* overlying the articular capsule and the psoas muscle. Find the bony prominence lateral to the hip joint—the *greater trochanter* of the femur. The large multilocular *trochanteric bursa* lies on its posterior surface. The *ischial* (or *ischiogluteal) bursa,* not always present, lies under the *ischial tuberosity,* on which a person sits. Note its proximity to the sciatic nerve, as shown on p. 647.

Techniques of Examination

Inspection.   Inspection of the hip begins with careful observation of the patient's gait on entering the room. Observe the two phases of gait:

- *Stance*—when the foot is on the ground and bears weight (60% of the walking cycle)

Most hip problems appear during the weight-bearing stance phase.

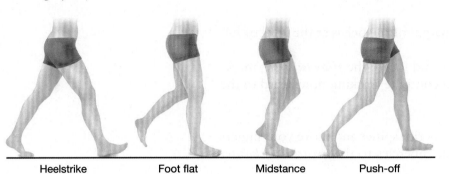

Heelstrike   Foot flat   Midstance   Push-off

THE STANCE PHASE OF GAIT

- *Swing*—when the foot moves forward and does not bear weight (40% of the cycle)

Observe the gait for the width of the base, the shift of the pelvis, and flexion of the knee. The width of the base should be 2 to 4 inches from heel to heel. Normal gait has a smooth, continuous rhythm, achieved in part by contraction of the abductors of the weight-bearing limb. Abductor contraction stabilizes the pelvis and helps maintain balance, raising the opposite hip. The knee should be flexed throughout the stance phase, except when the heel strikes the ground to counteract motion at the ankle.

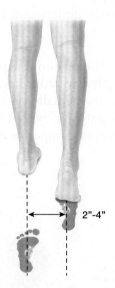

2"-4"

A wide base suggests cerebellar disease or foot problems.

Hip dislocation, arthritis, leg length discrepancy, or abductor weakness can cause the pelvis to drop on the opposite side, producing a waddling gait.

Lack of knee flexion, which makes the leg functionally longer, interrupts the smooth pattern of gait with circumduction of the extremity, or swinging the leg out to the side.

Observe the lumbar portion of the spine for the amount of lordosis and, with the patient supine, assess the length of the legs for symmetry. (To measure leg length, see Special Techniques, p. 662).

Loss of lordosis may reflect *paravertebral spasm*; excess lordosis suggests a *flexion deformity* of the hip.

Changes in apparent leg length are seen in abduction or adduction deformities and scoliosis. Leg shortening and external rotation suggest *hip fracture*.

Inspect the anterior and posterior surfaces of the hip for any areas of muscle atrophy or bruising. The joint is too deeply situated to detect swelling.

Palpation

Bony Landmarks.   Palpate the surface landmarks of the hip, identified on p. 643. On the anterior aspect of the hips, these can be located as follows:

- Identify the *iliac crest* at the upper margin of the pelvis at the level of L4.

- Follow the downward anterior curve and locate the *iliac tubercle*, marking the widest point of the crest, and continue tracking downward to the *anterior–superior iliac spine*.

- Place your thumbs on the anterior–superior spines and move your fingers downward and laterally from the iliac tubercles to the *greater trochanter* of the femur.

- Then move your thumbs medially and obliquely to the *pubic tubercle*, which lies at the same level as the greater trochanter.

On the *posterior aspect* of the hips, find the bony landmarks below.

- Palpate the *posterior–superior iliac spine* directly underneath the visible dimples just above the buttocks.

- Placing your left thumb and index finger over the posterior superior iliac spine, next locate the *greater trochanter* laterally with your fingers at the level of the gluteal fold, and place your thumb medially on the *ischial tuberosity*. The *sacroiliac joint* is not always palpable but may be tender. Note that an imaginary line along the posterior–superior iliac spines crosses the joint at S2.

Sacroiliac joint tenderness suggests *sacroiliitis*.

Inguinal Structures.   With the patient supine, ask the patient to place the heel of the leg being examined on the opposite knee. Then palpate along the inguinal ligament, which extends from the anterior–superior iliac spine to the pubic tubercle. The femoral nerve, artery, and vein bisect the overlying inguinal ligament; lymph nodes lie medially. The mnemonic **NAVEL** may help you remember the lateral-to-medial sequence of **N**erve–**A**rtery–**V**ein–Empty space–**L**ymph node.

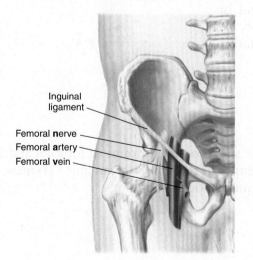

Inguinal ligament

Femoral nerve
Femoral artery
Femoral vein

Bulges along the ligament suggest an *inguinal hernia* or, on occasion, an *aneurysm*.

Enlarged lymph nodes suggest infection in the lower extremity or pelvis.

Tenderness in the groin area may be from *synovitis* of the hip joint, *arthritis, bursitis*, or possibly *psoas abscess*.

Bursae. If the hip is painful, palpate the (psoas) bursa, below the inguinal ligament but on a deeper plane.

With the patient resting on one side and the hip flexed and internally rotated, palpate the *trochanteric bursa* lying over the greater trochanter. Normally, the *ischiogluteal bursa,* over the ischial tuberosity, is not palpable unless inflamed.

Focal tenderness over the trochanter confirms *trochanteric bursitis.* Tenderness over the posterolateral surface of the greater trochanter occurs in localized tendinitis or muscle spasm from referred hip pain, and iliotibial band tendinitis.

Look for tenderness in *ischiogluteal bursitis* or "weaver's bottom"; because of the adjacent sciatic nerve, this may mimic sciatica.

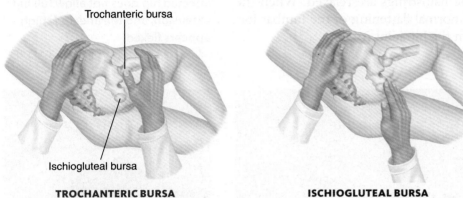

Trochanteric bursa

Ischiogluteal bursa

TROCHANTERIC BURSA   **ISCHIOGLUTEAL BURSA**

Range of Motion and Maneuvers

Range of Motion. Assess hip range of motion, referring to the table below for specific muscles responsible for each movement. Review the instructions to the patient.

Hip Movement	Primary Muscles Affecting Movement	Patient Instructions
Flexion	Iliopsoas	*"Bend your knee to your chest and pull it against your abdomen."*
Extension (actually hyperextension)	Gluteus maximus	*"Lie face down, then bend your knee and lift it up."* Or *"Lying flat, move your lower leg away from the midline and down over the side of the table."*
Abduction	Gluteus medius and minimus	*"Lying flat, move your lower leg away from the midline."*
Adduction	Adductor brevis, adductor longus, adductor magnus, pectineus, gracilis	*"Lying flat, bend your knee and move your lower leg toward the midline."*
External Rotation	Internal and external obturators, quadratus femoris, superior and inferior gemelli	*"Lying flat, bend your knee and turn your lower leg and foot across the midline."*
Internal Rotation	Iliopsoas	*"Lying flat, bend your knee and turn your lower leg and foot away from the midline."*

Maneuvers. Often the examiner must assist the patient with movements of the hip, so further detail is provided below for knee flexion, abduction, adduction, and external and internal rotation.

● *Flexion.* With the patient supine, place your hand under the patient's lumbar spine. Ask the patient to bend each knee in turn up to the chest and pull it firmly against the abdomen. Note that the hip can flex further when the knee is flexed because the hamstrings are relaxed. When the back touches your hand, indicating normal flattening of the lumbar lordosis, further flexion must arise from the hip joint itself.

In *flexion deformity of the hip,* as the opposite hip is flexed (with the thigh against the chest), the affected hip does not allow full hip extension, and the affected thigh appears flexed.

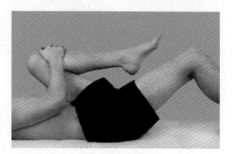

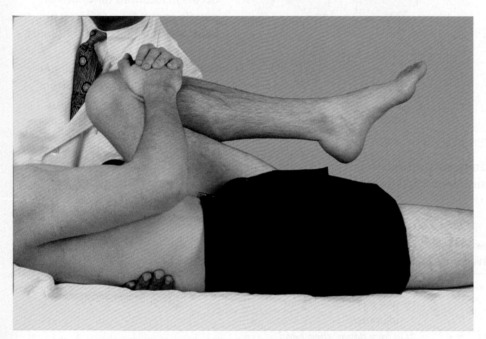

HIP FLEXION AND FLATTENING OF LUMBAR LORDOSIS

As the thigh is held against the abdomen, observe the degree of flexion at the hip and knee. Normally, the anterior portion of the thigh can almost touch the chest wall. Note whether the opposite thigh remains fully extended, resting on the table.

Flexion deformity may be masked by an increase, rather than flattening, in lumbar lordosis and an anterior pelvic tilt.

● *Extension.* With the patient lying face down, extend the thigh toward you in a posterior direction. Alternatively, carefully position the supine patient near the edge of the table and extend the leg posteriorly.

● *Abduction.* Stabilize the pelvis by pressing down on the opposite anterior–superior iliac spine with one hand. With the other hand, grasp the ankle and abduct the extended leg until you feel the iliac spine move. This movement marks the limit of hip abduction.

Restricted abduction is common in hip *osteoarthritis.*

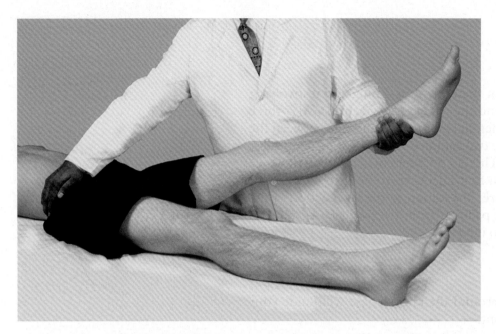

- *Adduction*. With the patient supine, stabilize the pelvis, hold one ankle, and move the leg medially across the body and over the opposite extremity.

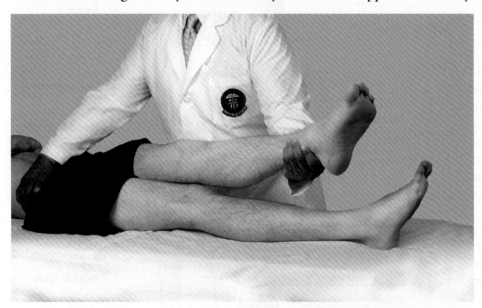

- *External and internal rotation.* Flex the leg to 90 degrees at hip and knee, stabilize the thigh with one hand, grasp the ankle with the other, and swing the lower leg—medially for external rotation at the hip, and laterally for internal rotation. Although confusing at first, it is the motion of the head of the femur in the acetabulum that identifies these movements.

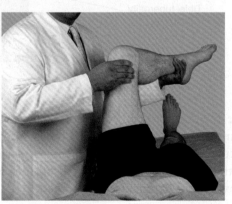

Restrictions of internal and external rotation are sensitive indicators of hip disease such as arthritis.[62,63]

THE KNEE

Overview

The knee joint is the largest joint in the body. It is a hinge joint involving three bones: the femur, the tibia, and the patella (or knee cap), with three articular surfaces, two between the femur and the tibia and one between the femur and the patella. Note how the two rounded condyles of the femur rest on the relatively flat tibial plateau. There is no inherent stability in the knee joint itself, making it dependent on four ligaments to hold its articulating femur and tibia in place. This feature, in addition to the lever action of the femur on the tibia and the lack of padding from overlying fat or muscle, makes the knee highly vulnerable to injury.

Bony Structures

Learn the bony landmarks in and around the knee. These will guide your examination of this complicated joint.

- On the *medial surface,* identify the *adductor tubercle,* the *medial epicondyle* of the femur, and the *medial condyle* of the tibia.

- On the *anterior surface,* identify the patella, which rests on the anterior articulating surface of the femur midway between the epicondyles, embedded in the tendon of the quadriceps muscle. This tendon continues below the knee joint as the *patellar tendon,* which inserts distally on the *tibial tuberosity.*

- On the *lateral surface,* find the *lateral epicondyle* of the femur, the *lateral condyle* of the tibia, and the head of the *fibula.*

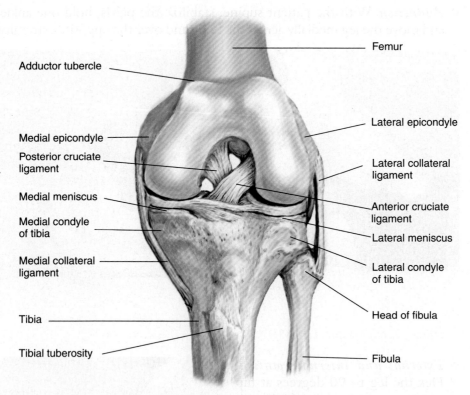

Adductor tubercle

Medial epicondyle

Posterior cruciate ligament

Medial meniscus

Medial condyle of tibia

Medial collateral ligament

Tibia

Tibial tuberosity

Femur

Lateral epicondyle

Lateral collateral ligament

Anterior cruciate ligament

Lateral meniscus

Lateral condyle of tibia

Head of fibula

Fibula

ANTERIOR ASPECT OF THE KNEE

Joints

Two condylar *tibiofemoral joints* are formed by the convex curves of the medial and lateral condyles of the femur as they articulate with the concave condyles of the tibia. The third articular surface is the *patellofemoral joint.* The patella slides on the groove of the anterior aspect of the distal femur, called the *trochlear groove,* during flexion and extension of the knee.

Problems with patellar tracking, for example in patients with shallower grooves, especially women, can lead to arthritis, anterior knee pain, and patellar dislocation.

Muscle Groups

Powerful muscles move and support the knee. The *quadriceps femoris* extends the knee, covering the anterior, medial, and lateral aspects of the thigh. The *hamstring muscles* lie on the posterior aspect of the thigh and flex the knee.

In women, quadriceps contraction tends to have a more lateral pull (Q angle) that alters patellar tracking, contributing to anterior knee pain.

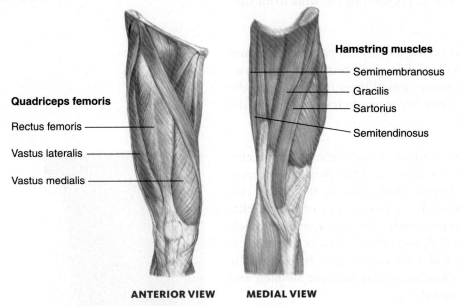

Quadriceps femoris

Rectus femoris

Vastus lateralis

Vastus medialis

Hamstring muscles

Semimembranosus

Gracilis

Sartorius

Semitendinosus

ANTERIOR VIEW   **MEDIAL VIEW**

Additional Structures

The menisci and two important pairs of ligaments, the collaterals and the cruciates, are crucial to stability of the knee. Identify these structures on the illustrations on p. 650 and below.

- The *medial and lateral menisci* cushion the action of the femur on the tibia. These crescent-shaped fibrocartilaginous discs add a cup-like surface to the otherwise flat tibial plateau.

- The *medial collateral ligament (MCL),* not easily palpable, is a broad, flat ligament connecting the medial femoral epicondyle to the medial condyle of the tibia. The medial portion of the MCL also attaches to the medial meniscus.

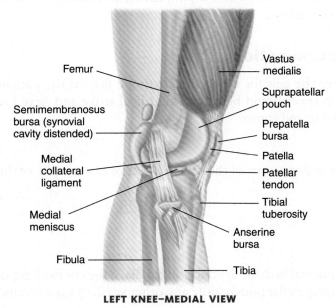

Femur

Semimembranosus bursa (synovial cavity distended)

Medial collateral ligament

Medial meniscus

Fibula

Vastus medialis

Suprapatellar pouch

Prepatella bursa

Patella

Patellar tendon

Tibial tuberosity

Anserine bursa

Tibia

LEFT KNEE—MEDIAL VIEW

- The *lateral collateral ligament (LCL)* connects the lateral femoral epicondyle and the head of the fibula. The MCL and LCL provide medial and lateral stability to the knee joint.

- The *anterior cruciate ligament (ACL)* crosses obliquely from the anterior medial tibia to the lateral femoral condyle, preventing the tibia from sliding forward on the femur.

- The *posterior cruciate ligament (PCL)* crosses from the *posterior* tibia and lateral meniscus to the medial femoral condyle, preventing the tibia from slipping backward on the femur. Because these ligaments lie within the knee joint, they are not palpable. They are nonetheless crucial to the anteroposterior stability of the knee.

Observe the concavities that are usually evident at each side of the patella, the "negative infrapatellar space," and also above it. Occupying these areas is the synovial cavity of the knee, the largest joint cavity in the body. This cavity includes an extension 6 cm above the upper border of the patella, lying upward and deep to the quadriceps muscle, the *suprapatellar pouch.* The joint cavity covers the anterior, medial, and lateral surfaces of the knee, as well as the condyles of the femur and tibia posteriorly. Although the synovium is not normally detectable, these areas may become swollen and tender when the joint is inflamed or injured.

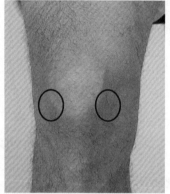

NOTE THE NEGATIVE INFRAPATELLAR SPACES MEDIAL AND LATERAL TO THE PATELLA

Several bursae lie near the knee. The *prepatellar bursa* lies between the patella and the overlying skin. The *anserine bursa* lies 1 to 2 inches below the knee joint on the medial surface, proximal and medial to the attachments of the medial hamstring muscles on the proximal tibia. It cannot be palpated due to these overlying tendons. Now identify the large *semimembranosus bursa* that communicates with the joint cavity, also on the posterior and medial surfaces of the knee.

Techniques of Examination

Inspection.   Observe the gait for a smooth, rhythmic flow as the patient enters the room. The knee should be extended at heel strike and flexed at all other phases of swing and stance.

Stumbling or "giving way" of the knee during heel strike suggests *quadriceps weakness* or abnormal patellar tracking.

Check the alignment and contours of the knees. Observe any atrophy of the quadriceps muscles.

Bowlegs (*genu varum*) and knock-knees (*genu valgum*) are common; flexion contracture (inability to extend fully) is seen in limb paralysis or hamstring tightness.

Look for loss of the normal hollows around the patella, a sign of swelling in the knee joint and suprapatellar pouch; note any other swelling in or around the knee.

Swelling over the patella suggests *prepatellar bursitis.* Swelling over the tibial tubercle suggests *infrapatellar* or, if more medial, *anserine bursitis.*

Palpation. Ask the patient to sit on the edge of the examining table with the knees in flexion. In this position, bony landmarks are more visible, and the muscles, tendons, and ligaments are more relaxed, making them easier to palpate.

Pay special attention to any areas of tenderness. Pain is a common complaint in knee problems, and localizing the structure causing pain is important for accurate evaluation.

The Tibiofemoral Joint. Palpate the *tibiofemoral joint.* Facing the knee, place your thumbs in the soft-tissue depressions on either side of the *patellar tendon.* Identify the groove of the tibiofemoral joint. Note that the inferior pole of the patella lies at the tibiofemoral joint line. As you press your thumbs downward, you can feel the edge of the tibial plateau. Follow it medially, then laterally, until you are stopped by the converging femur and tibia. By moving your thumbs upward toward the midline to the top of the patella, you can follow the articulating surface of the femur and identify the margins of the joint.

Note any irregular bony ridges along the joint margins.

Osteoarthritis **is likely when there are tender bony ridges along the joint margins, genu varum deformity, and stiffness lasting 30 minutes or less (likelihood ratios: 11.8, 3.4, and 3.0).[51,64–66] Crepitus may also be present.**

Palpate the *medial meniscus* by pressing on the medial soft-tissue depression along the upper edge of the tibial plateau. It is easier to palpate the medial meniscus if the tibia is slightly internally rotated. Place the knee in slight flexion and palpate the *lateral meniscus* along the lateral joint line.

A medial meniscus tear with point tenderness is more common after trauma.[67,68]

Assess *the medial and lateral joint compartments* of the tibiofemoral joint with the knee flexed on the examining table to approximately 90 degrees. Pay special attention to any areas of pain or tenderness.

- *Medial compartment.* Medially, move your thumbs upward to palpate the *medial femoral condyle.* The *adductor tubercle* is posterior to the medial femoral condyle. Move your thumbs downward to palpate the *medial tibial plateau.*

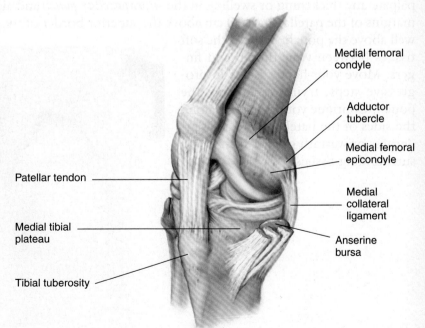

Medial femoral condyle

Adductor tubercle

Medial femoral epicondyle

Medial collateral ligament

Anserine bursa

Patellar tendon

Medial tibial plateau

Tibial tuberosity

Also medially, palpate along the joint line and identify the *medial collateral ligament*, which connects the medial epicondyle of the femur to the medial condyle and superior medial surface of the tibia. Palpate along this broad, flat ligament from its origin to insertion.

MCL tenderness after injury is suspicious for an MCL tear; LCL injuries are less frequent.

- *Lateral compartment.* Lateral to the patellar tendon, move your thumbs upward to palpate the *lateral femoral condyle* and downward to palpate the *lateral tibial plateau.* When the knee is flexed, the femoral epicondyles are lateral to the femoral condyles.

Also on the lateral surface, ask the patient to cross one leg so the ankle rests on the opposite knee and find the *lateral collateral ligament,* a firm cord that runs from the lateral femoral epicondyle to the head of the fibula.

Assess the *patellofemoral compartment.* Now locate the *patella* and trace the *patellar tendon* distally until you palpate the *tibial tuberosity.* Ask the patient to extend the knee to make sure the patellar tendon is intact.

Tenderness over the tendon or inability to extend the knee suggests a partial or complete tear of the patellar tendon.

With the patient supine and the knee extended, compress the patella against the underlying femur, and gently move it medially and laterally, assessing for crepitus and pain. Ask the patient to tighten the quadriceps as the patella moves distally in the trochlear groove. Check for a smooth sliding motion (the *patellofemoral grinding test*).

Pain and crepitus suggest roughening of the patellar undersurface that articulates with the femur. Similar pain may occur with climbing or going down stairs, or getting up from a chair.

Pain with compression and with patellar movement during quadriceps contraction suggests *chondromalacia,* or degenerative patella (the *patellofemoral syndrome*).

The Suprapatellar Pouch, Prepatellar Bursa, and Anserine Bursa. Try to palpate any thickening or swelling in the *suprapatellar pouch* and along the margins of the patella. Start 10 cm above the superior border of the patella, well above the pouch, and feel the soft tissues between your thumb and fingers. Move your hand distally in progressive steps, trying to identify the pouch. Continue your palpation along the sides of the patella. Note any tenderness or warmth greater than in the surrounding tissues.

Swelling above and adjacent to the patella suggests synovial thickening or effusion in the knee joint.

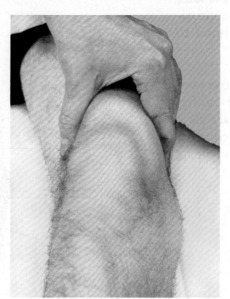

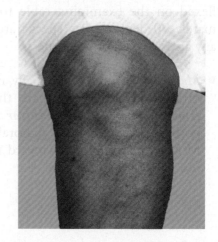

Thickening, bogginess, or warmth in these areas indicates synovitis or nontender effusions from osteoarthritis.

Check three other bursae for bogginess or swelling. Palpate the *prepatellar bursa*. Palpate over the *anserine bursa* on the posteromedial side of the knee between the medial collateral ligament and the tendons inserting on the medial tibial and plateau. On the posterior surface, with the leg extended, check the medial aspect of the popliteal fossa.

Prepatellar bursitis ("housemaid's knee") arises from excessive kneeling; *anserine bursitis* from running, valgus knee deformity, fibromyalgias, osteoarthritis; a *popliteal* or *"baker's" cyst* from distention of the gastrocnemius semimembranosus bursa from underlying arthritis or trauma.

Palpation Tests for Effusion in the Knee Joint. Learn to apply three tests for detecting fluid in the knee joint: the bulge sign, the balloon sign, and balloting the patella.

- The *bulge sign (for minor effusions)*. With the knee extended, place the left hand above the knee and apply pressure on the suprapatellar pouch, displacing or "milking" fluid downward. Stroke downward on the medial aspect of the knee and apply pressure to force fluid into the lateral area. Tap the knee just behind the lateral margin of the patella with the right hand.

A fluid wave or bulge on the medial side between the patella and the femur is considered a positive bulge sign consistent with an effusion.

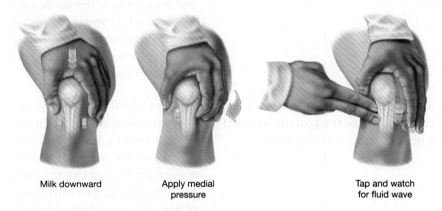

Milk downward   Apply medial   Tap and watch
                pressure   for fluid wave

- The *balloon sign (for major effusions)*. Place the thumb and index finger of your right hand on each side of the patella; with the left hand, compress the suprapatellar pouch against the femur. Feel for fluid entering (or ballooning into) the spaces next to the patella under your right thumb and index finger.

When the knee joint contains a large effusion, suprapatellar compression ejects fluid into the spaces adjacent to the patella. A palpable fluid wave signifies a positive "balloon sign." A returning fluid wave into the suprapatellar pouch confirms an effusion.

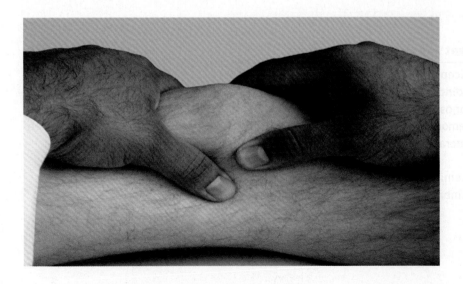

- *Ballotting the patella*. To assess large effusions, you can also compress the suprapatellar pouch and "ballotte" or push the patella sharply against the femur. Watch for fluid returning to the suprapatellar pouch.

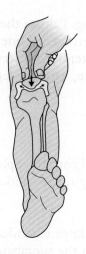

Palpable fluid returning into the pouch further confirms the presence of a large effusion.

A palpable patellar click with compression may also occur, but yields more false positives.

Gastrocnemius and Soleus Muscles, Achilles Tendon. Palpate the gastrocnemius and soleus muscles on the posterior surface of the lower leg. Their common tendon, the Achilles, is palpable from about the lower third of the calf to its insertion on the calcaneus.

A defect in the muscles with tenderness and swelling suggests a *ruptured Achilles tendon;* tenderness and thickening of the tendon above the calcaneus, sometimes with a protuberant posterolateral bony process of the calcaneus, suggests *Achilles tendinitis.*

To test the integrity of the *Achilles tendon,* place the patient prone with the knee and ankle flexed at 90 degrees, or alternatively, ask the patient to kneel on a chair. Squeeze the calf and watch for plantar flexion at the ankle.

Absence of plantar flexion is a positive test indicating rupture of the Achilles tendon. Sudden severe pain "like a gunshot wound," an ecchymosis from the calf into the heel, and a flat-footed gait with absence of "toe-off" may also be present.

Range of Motion and Maneuvers

Range of Motion. Now assess knee range of motion, referring to the table below for specific muscles responsible for each movement and for instructions to the patient.

Knee Movement	Primary Muscles Affecting Movement	Patient Instructions	
Flexion	Hamstring group: biceps femoris, semitendinosus, and semimembranosus	"Bend or flex your knee." Or "Squat down to the floor."	
Extension	Quadriceps: rectus femoris, vastus medialis, lateralis, and intermedius	"Straighten your leg." Or "After you squat down to the floor, stand up."	Crepitus with flexion and extension suggests osteoarthritis.
Internal Rotation	Sartorius, gracilis, semitendinosus, semimembranosus	"While sitting, swing your lower leg toward the midline."	
External Rotation	Biceps femoris	"While sitting, swing your lower leg away from the midline."	

Maneuvers. You will often need to test ligamentous stability and integrity of the menisci, particularly when there is a history of trauma or palpable tenderness.[67,68] Always examine both knees and compare findings.

Maneuvers for Examining the Knee

Structure	Maneuver
Medial meniscus and lateral meniscus 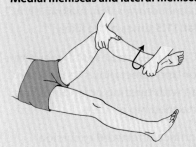	**McMurray Test.** With the patient supine, grasp the heel and flex the knee. Cup your other hand over the knee joint with fingers and thumb along the medial joint line. From the heel, externally rotate the lower, then push on the lateral side to apply a valgus stress on the medial side of the joint. At the same time, slowly extend the lower leg in external rotation. The same maneuver with internal rotation of the foot stresses the lateral meniscus. If a click is felt or heard at the joint line during flexion and extension of the knee, or if tenderness is noted along the joint line, further assess the meniscus for a posterior tear.
Medial collateral ligament (MCL) 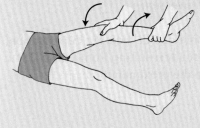	**Abduction (or Valgus) Stress Test.** With the patient supine and the knee slightly flexed, move the thigh about 30 degrees laterally to the side of the table. Place one hand against the lateral knee to stabilize the femur and the other hand around the medial ankle. Push medially against the knee and pull laterally at the ankle to open the knee joint on the medial side (*valgus stress*).
Lateral collateral ligament (LCL) 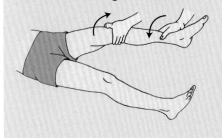	**Adduction (or Varus) Stress Test.** With the thigh and knee in the same position, change your position so you can place one hand against the medial surface of the knee and the other around the lateral ankle. Push laterally against the knee and pull medially at the ankle to open the knee joint on the lateral side (*varus stress*). *(continued)*

A click or pop along the medial joint with valgus stress, external rotation, and leg extension suggests a probable *tear of the posterior portion of the medial meniscus*. The tear may displace meniscal tissue, causing "locking" on full knee extension.

A McMurray sign and locking make a medial meniscus tear 8.2 and 3.2 times more likely.[51]

Pain or a gap in the medial joint line points to ligamentous laxity and a partial tear of the *medial collateral ligament*. Most injuries are on the medial side.

Pain or a gap in the lateral joint line points to ligamentous laxity and a partial tear of the *lateral collateral ligament*.

Maneuvers for Examining the Knee (continued)

Structure	Maneuver	
Anterior cruciate ligament (ACL) 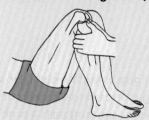	**Anterior Drawer Sign.** With the patient supine, hips flexed and knees flexed to 90 degrees and feet flat on the table, cup your hands around the knee with the thumbs on the medial and lateral joint line and the fingers on the medial and lateral insertions of the hamstrings. Draw the tibia forward and observe if it slides forward (like a drawer) from under the femur. Compare the degree of forward movement with that of the opposite knee.	A few degrees of forward movement are normal if equally present on the opposite side. A forward jerk showing the contours of the upper tibia is a *positive anterior drawer sign,* making an ACL tear 11.5 times more likely.[51]
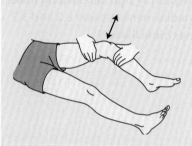	**Lachman Test.** Place the knee in 15 degrees of flexion and external rotation. Grasp the distal femur on the lateral side with one hand and the proximal tibia on the medial side with the other. With the thumb of the tibial hand on the joint line, simultaneously pull the tibia forward and the femur back. Estimate the degree of forward excursion.	ACL injuries occur with hyperextension and direct blows to the knee and with twisting or landing on an extended hip or knee. Significant forward excursion indicates an *ACL tear* (likelihood increases by 17.0 if *positive test*).[51]
Posterior cruciate ligament (PCL) 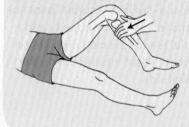	**Posterior Drawer Sign.** Position the patient and place your hands in the positions described for the anterior drawer test. Push the tibia posteriorly and observe the degree of backward movement in the femur.	If the PCL is injured, the proximal tibia falls back, a *positive posterior drawer sign.* Isolated *PCL tears* are less common, usually resulting from a direct blow to the proximal tibia.

THE ANKLE AND FOOT

Overview

The total weight of the body is transmitted through the ankle to the foot. The ankle and foot must balance the body and absorb the impact of the heel strike and gait. Despite thick padding along the toes, sole, and heel and stabilizing ligaments at the ankles, the ankle and foot are frequent sites of sprain and bony injury.

Bony Structures and Joints

The ankle is a hinge joint formed by the *tibia*, the *fibula*, and the *talus*. The tibia and fibula act as a mortise, stabilizing the joint while bracing the talus like an inverted cup.

The principal joints of the ankle are the *tibiotalar joint*, between the tibia and the talus, and the *subtalar (talocalcaneal) joint*.

Note the principal landmarks of the ankle: the *medial malleolus,* the bony prominence at the distal end of the tibia, and the *lateral malleolus,* at the distal end of the fibula. Lodged under the talus and jutting posteriorly is the *calcaneus,* or heel bone.

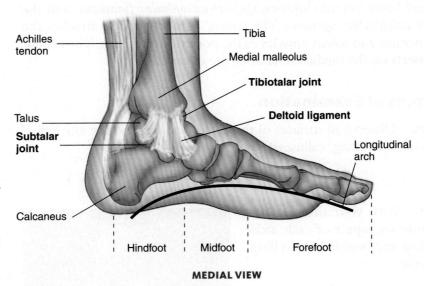

MEDIAL VIEW

An imaginary line, the *longitudinal arch,* spans the foot, extending from the calcaneus of the hind foot along the tarsal bones of the midfoot (see cuneiform, navicular, and cuboid bones in the illustration below) to the forefoot metatarsals and toes. The *heads of the metatarsals* are palpable in the ball of the foot. In the forefoot, identify the *metatarsophalangeal joints,* proximal to the webs of the toes, and the *proximal and distal interphalangeal joints* of the toes.

Muscle Groups and Additional Structures

Movement at the ankle (tibiotalar) joint is limited to dorsiflexion and plantar flexion. *Plantar flexion* is powered by the gastrocnemius, the posterior tibial muscle, and the toe flexors. Their tendons run behind the malleoli. The *dorsiflexors* include the anterior tibial muscle and the toe extensors. They lie prominently on the anterior surface, or dorsum, of the ankle, anterior to the malleoli.

Ligaments extend from each malleolus onto the foot.

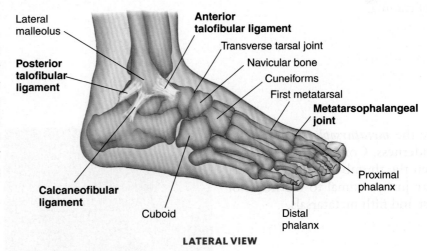

LATERAL VIEW

- Medially, the triangle-shaped *deltoid ligament* fans out from the inferior surface of the medial malleolus to the talus and proximal tarsal bones, protecting against stress from eversion (heel bows outward).

- Laterally, the three ligaments are less substantial, with higher risk for injury: the *anterior talofibular ligament*, most at risk in injury from inversion (heel bows inward) injuries; the *calcaneofibular ligament*; and the *posterior talofibular ligament*. The strong Achilles tendon attaches the gastrocnemius and soleus muscles to the posterior calcaneus. The plantar fascia inserts on the medial tubercle of the calcaneus.

Techniques of Examination

Inspection.   Observe all surfaces of the ankles and feet, noting any deformities, nodules, swelling, calluses, or corns.

See Table 16-9, Abnormalities of the Feet (p. 678) and Table 16-10, Abnormalities of the Toes and Soles (p. 679).

Palpation.   With your thumbs, palpate the anterior aspect of each *ankle joint*, noting any bogginess, swelling, or tenderness.

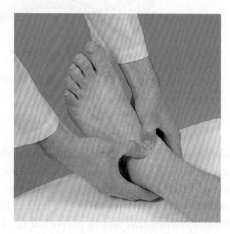

Localized tenderness is often present in arthritis, ligamentous injury, or infection of the ankle.

Feel along the *Achilles tendon* for nodules and tenderness.

Check for rheumatoid nodules and tenderness, commonly found in Achilles tendinitis, bursitis, or partial tear from trauma.

Palpate the heel, especially the posterior and inferior calcaneus, and the plantar fascia for tenderness.

Bone spurs may be present on the calcaneus. Focal heel tenderness on palpation of the plantar fascia suggests *plantar fasciitis,* seen in prolonged standing or heel-strike exercise and also in *rheumatoid arthritis, gout.*[69–71]

Palpate for tenderness over the medial and lateral malleolus, especially in cases of trauma.

Tenderness along the posterior medial malleolus suggests *posterior tibial tendinitis* and causes flat feet.

Palpate the *metatarsophalangeal joints* for tenderness. Compress the forefoot between the thumb and fingers. Exert pressure just proximal to the heads of the first and fifth metatarsals.

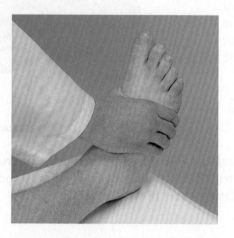

After trauma, inability to bear weight after four steps and tenderness over the posterior aspects of either malleolus, especially the medial malleolus, is suspicious for ankle fracture (known as the Ottawa ankle rule).[72,73]

Tenderness on compression is an early sign of *rheumatoid arthritis.* Acute inflammation of the first metatarsophalangeal joint suggests *gout.*

Palpate the heads of the five metatarsals and the grooves between them with your thumb and index finger. Place your thumb on the dorsum of the foot and your index finger on the plantar surface.

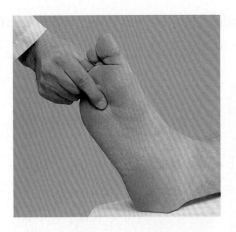

Pain and tenderness, called *metatarsalgia*, occurs in trauma, arthritis, vascular compromise.

Tenderness over the third and fourth metatarsal heads on the plantar surface signals *Morton's neuroma* (see p. 678).

Forefoot abnormalities like hallux valgus, metatarsalgia, and *Morton's neuroma* are more common in women who wear high-heeled shoes with narrow toe boxes.

Range of Motion and Maneuvers

Range of Motion. Assess flexion and extension at the tibiotalar (ankle) joint. In the foot, assess inversion and eversion at the subtalar and transverse tarsal joints.

Ankle and Foot Movement	Primary Muscles Affecting Movement	Patient Instructions
Ankle Flexion (plantar flexion)	Gastrocnemius, soleus, plantaris, tibialis posterior	*"Point your foot toward the floor."*
Ankle Extension (dorsiflexion)	Tibialis anterior, extensor digitorum longus, and extensor hallucis longus	*"Point your foot toward the ceiling."*
Inversion	Tibialis posterior and anterior	*"Bend your heel inward."*
Eversion	Peroneus longus and brevis	*"Bend your heel outward."*

Maneuvers

- *The Ankle (Tibiotalar) Joint.* Dorsiflex and plantar flex the foot at the ankle.

Pain during movements of the ankle and the foot helps to localize possible arthritis.

- *The Subtalar (Talocalcaneal) Joint.* Stabilize the ankle with one hand, grasp the heel with the other, and invert and evert the foot by turning the heel inward then outward.

An arthritic joint is frequently painful when moved in any direction, whereas a ligamentous sprain produces maximal pain when the ligament is stretched. For example, in a common form of sprained ankle, inversion and plantar flexion of the foot cause pain, whereas eversion and plantar flexion are relatively pain free.

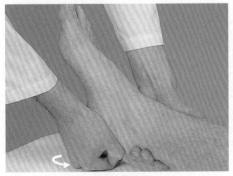

INVERSION

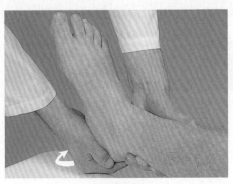

EVERSION

- *The Transverse Tarsal Joint.* Stabilize the heel and invert and evert the forefoot.

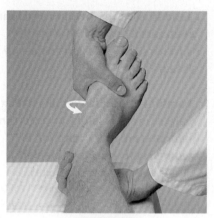
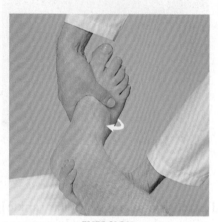

INVERSION   **EVERSION**

- *The Metatarsophalangeal Joints.* Move the proximal phalanx of each toe up and down.

Pain suggests acute synovitis. Instability occurs in chronic synovitis and claw-toe deformity.

 SPECIAL TECHNIQUES

Measuring the Length of Legs. If you suspect that the patient's legs are unequal in length, measure them. Get the patient relaxed in the supine position and symmetrically aligned with legs extended. With a tape, measure the distance between the anterior superior iliac spine and the medial malleolus. The tape should cross the knee on its medial side.

Unequal leg length suggests scoliosis.

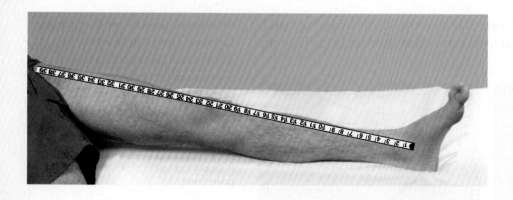

Describing Limited Motion of a Joint. Measurement of motion can be described in degrees. Pocket goniometers are available for this purpose. In the two examples shown below, the red lines indicate the range of the patient's movement, and the black lines suggest the normal range.

Observations may be described in several ways. The numbers in parentheses show abbreviated descriptions.

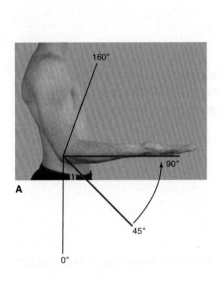

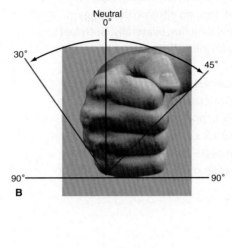

A. The elbow flexes from 45 degrees to 90 degrees (45° → 90°),

-or-

The elbow has a flexion deformity of 45 degrees and can be flexed farther to 90 degrees (45° → 90°).

B. Supination at elbow = 30 degrees (0° → 30°)
Pronation at elbow = 45 degrees (0° → 45°)

Recording Your Findings

The examples on the next page contain phrases appropriate for most write-ups. Note that use of the anatomical terms specific to the structure and function of individual joint problems makes your write-up of musculoskeletal findings more meaningful and informative.

Recording the Examination—The Musculoskeletal System

"Full range of motion in all joints of the upper and lower extremities. No evidence of swelling or deformity."

OR

"Full range of motion in all joints. Hand with degenerative changes of Heberden's nodes at the distal interphalangeal joints, Bouchard's nodes at proximal interphalangeal joints. Mild pain with flexion, extension, and rotation of both hips. Full range of motion in the knees, with moderate crepitus; no effusion but boggy synovium and osteophytes along the tibiofemoral joint line bilaterally. Both feet with hallux valgus at the first metatarsophalangeal joints."

Suggests *osteoarthritis*

OR

"Right knee with moderate effusion and tenderness over medial meniscus along the joint line. Moderate laxity of anterior cruciate ligament (ACL) on Lachman test; posterior cruciate ligament (PCL) and medial and lateral collateral ligaments (MCL, LCL) intact—no posterior drawer sign or tenderness with varus or valgus stress. Patellar tendon intact—patient able to extend lower extremity. All other joints with good range of motion, no other deformity or swelling."

Suggests *partial tear of medial meniscus and ACL,* possibly from sports injury or trauma

Bibliography

Citations

1. Schappert SM, Rechtsteiner EA. Ambulatory medical care utilization estimates for 2007. National Center for Health Statistics. Vital Health Stat 2011;13(169):1–45. Available at http://www.cdc.gov/nchs/data/series/sr_13/sr13_169.pdf. Accessed May 21, 2011.
2. Brault MW, Hootman J, Helmick CG et al. Prevalence and most common causes of disability among adults, United States, 2005. MMWR 2009;58:421–426.
3. U.S. Department of Health and Human Services. Healthy People 2020. Physical Activity, Objectives. Available at http://www.healthypeople.gov/2020/topicsobjectives2020/objectiveslist.aspx?topicid=33. Accessed May 27, 2011.
4. Deyo RA, Mirza SK, Martin BI. Back pain prevalence and visit rates: estimates from U.S. national surveys, 2002. Spine 2006;31:2724–2727.
5. Deyo RA, Weinstein JN. Primary care. Low back pain. N Engl J Med 2001;344:363–370.
6. Deyo RA. Diagnostic evaluation of LBP. Reaching a specific diagnosis is often impossible. Arch Int Med 2002;162:1444–1447.
7. Lurie JD, Gerber PD, Sox HC. A pain in the back. N Engl J Med 2000;343:723–726.
8. Hoffman JR, Mower WR, Wolfson AB et al. Validity of a set of clinical criteria to rule out injury to the cervical spine in patients with blunt trauma. N Engl J Med 2000;343:94–99.
9. Devereaux MW. Neck and low back pain. Med Clin North Am 2003;87:643–662.
10. Carette S, Fehlings MG. Cervical radiculopathy. N Engl J Med 2005;353:392–399.
11. Margaretten ME, Kohlwes J, Moore D et al. Does this adult patient have septic arthritis? JAMA 2007;297:1478–1488.
12. Huizinga TQJ, Pincus T. In the clinic. Rheumatoid arthritis. Ann Intern Med 2010;153:ITC1-1–ITC1-16.
13. Abeles AM, Pillinger MH, Abeles M. Narrative review: the pathophysiology of fibromyalgia. Ann Intern Med 2007;146:726–734.
14. Salvarani C, Cantini F, Hunder GG. Polymyalgia rheumatica and giant-cell arteritis. Lancet 2008;372:234–245.
15. Sakane T, Takleno M, Suzuke N et al. Behçet's disease. N Engl J Med 1999;341:1284–1291.
16. U.S. Department of Health and Human Services. 2008 Guidelines for Physical Activity. Available at http://www.health.gov/PAGuidelines/guidelines/default.aspx. Accessed May 27 2011.
17. Stanton TR, Henschke N, Maher CG et al. After an episode of acute low back pain, recurrence is unpredictable and not as common as previously thought. Spine 2008;33;2923–2928.
18. U.S. Department of Health and Human Services. Healthy People 2020. Arthritis, Osteoporosis, and Chronic Low Back Pain—Overview. Available at http://www.healthypeople.gov/2020/topicsobjectives2020/overview.aspx?topicid=3. Accessed May 28, 2011.
19. Luo X, Pietrobon R, Sun SX et al. Estimates and patterns of direct health care expenditures among individuals with back pain in the United States. Spine 2004;29:79–86.
20. Martin BI, Deyo RA, Mirza SK et al. Expenditures and health status among adults with back and neck problems. JAMA 2008;299:656–664.

21. U.S. Preventive Services Task Force. Primary care interventions to prevent low back pain in adults: recommendation statement. Rockville MD, Agency for Healthcare Research and Quality, February 2004. Available at http://www.uspreventiveservicestaskforce.org/3rduspstf/lowback/lowbackrs.htm. Accessed May 28, 2011.

22. Wilson JE. In the clinic. Low back pain. Ann Intern Med 2008;148:ITC5-1–ITC5-16.

23. Jarvik JG, Hollinworth W, Heagerty FJ et al. Three-year incidence of low back pain in an initially asymptomatic cohort: clinical and imaging risk factors. Spine 2005;30:1541–1548.

24. Chou R, Shekelle P. Will this patient develop persistent disabling low back pain? JAMA 2010;303:1295–1302.

25. Lamb SE, Hansen Z, Lall R et al. Group cognitive behavioral treatment for low-back pain in primary care: a randomized controlled trial and cost-effectiveness analysis. Lancet 2010; 375:916–923.

26. Staal JB, Hlobil H, Twoisk JWR et al. Graded activity for low back pain in occupational health care. Ann Intern Med 2004;140:77–84.

27. Berman BM, Langevin HH, Witt CM et al. Acupuncture for chronic low back pain. N Engl J Med 2010;363:454–461

28. Cherkin DC, Sherman KJ, Avins Al et al. A randomized trial comparing acupuncture, simulated acupuncture, and usual care for chronic low back pain. Arch Intern Med 2009;169:858–866.

29. U.S. Preventive Services Task Force. Screening for osteoporosis. Recommendation statement. January 2011. Available at http://www.uspreventiveservicestaskforce.org/uspstf10/osteoporosis/osteors.htm. Accessed July 8, 2012.

30. Centers for Disease Control and Prevention. Key statistics from NHANES 2005–2006 – osteopenia. Available at http://wwwn.cdc.gov/nchs/nhanes/bibliography/key_statistics.aspx. Accessed May 29, 2011.

31. Raisz LG. Screening for osteoporosis. N Engl J Med 2005; 353:164–171.

32. Nelson HD, Haney EM, Chou R et al. Screening for osteoporosis: systematic review to update the 2002 U.S. Preventive Services Task Force Recommendation. Evidence Synthesis No. 77. AHRQ Publication No. 2010;10–05145-EF-1. Rockville, MD: Agency for Healthcare Research and Quality, July 2010.

33. Office of Dietary Supplements, National Institute of Health. Dietary Supplement Fact Sheet – Calcium. Available at http://ods.od.nih.gov/factsheets/calcium/#en1. Accessed May 30, 2011.

34. Holnick MF. Vitamin D deficiency. N Engl J Med 2007;357: 266–281.

35. Rosen CJ. Vitamin D insufficiency. N Engl J Med 2011; 364:248–254.

36. Ross AC, Manson JE, Abrams SA et al. The 2011 report on dietary reference intakes for calcium and vitamin D from the Institute of Medicine: what clinicians need to know. J Endocrinol Metab 2011;96:53–58.

37. Institute of Medicine. 2011 Dietary reference intakes for calcium and vitamin D. Washington, DC: The National Academies Press, 2011.

38. Holick MF, Binkley NC, Bischoff-Ferrari HA et al. Evaluation, treatment, and prevention of vitamin D deficiency: an Endocrine Society Clinical Practice Guideline. J Clin Endo Metab 2011;96:1911–1930.

39. Bolland MJ, Avenell A, Baron JA et al. Effect of calcium supplements on risk of myocardial infarction and cardiovascular events: meta-analysis. BMJ 2010;341:c3691.

40. Bolland MJ, Grey A, Avenell A et al. Calcium supplements with or without vitamin D and risk of cardiovascular events: reanalysis of the Women's Health Initiative limited access dataset and meta-analysis. BMJ 2011;342:d2040.

41. North American Menopause Society. Estrogen and progestogen use in postmenopausal women: 2010 position statement of the North American Menopause Society. Menopause 2010;17:242–255.

42. Barasch A, Cunha-Cruz J, Curro FA et al. Risk factors for osteonecrosis of the jaws: a case-control study from the CONDOR Dental PBRN. J Dent Res 2011;90:439–444.

43. Fellows JL, Rindal DB, Barasch A et al. ONJ in two dental practice-based research network regions. J Dent Res 2011;90: 433–438.

44. Park-Wyllie LY, Mamdani MM, Juurlink DN et al. Bisphosphonate use and the risk of subtrochanteric or femoral shaft fractures in older women. JAMA 2011;305:783–789.

45. National Institute on Aging. NIH SeniorHealth. Falls and Older Adults. Available at http://nihseniorhealth.gov/falls/aboutfalls/01.html. Accessed May 28 2011.

46. National Center for Injury Prevention and Control, Centers for Disease Prevention and Control. 2007, United States-Unintentional Fall Deaths and Rates per 100,000. Available at http://webappa.cdc.gov/cgi-bin/broker.exe. Accessed May 28, 2011.

47. U.S. Preventive Services Task Force. Interventions to Prevent Falls in Older Adults, Topic Page. February 2011. Available at http://www.uspreventiveservicestaskforce.org/uspstf/uspsfalls.htm. Accessed May 29, 2011.

48. Aletaha D, Neogi T, Silman AJ et al. 2010 Rheumatoid arthritis classification criteria: an American College of Rheumatology/European League Against Rheumatism collaborative initiative. Arthritis Rheum 2010;62:2569–2591.

49. Liume JJ, Verhagen AP, Meidema HS et al. Does this patient have an instability of the shoulder or a labrum lesion? The rational clinical examination. JAMA 2004;292:1989–1999.

50. Woodward TW, Best TM. The painful shoulder. Part II. Acute and chronic disorders. Am Fam Physician 2000;61:3291–3300.

51. McGee S. Ch. 53, Examination of the musculoskeletal system—the shoulder. In Evidence-based Physical Diagnosis, 2nd ed. St. Louis: Saunders, 2007.

52. Matsen FA. Rotator cuff failure. N Engl J Med 2008;358:2138–2147.

53. Murrell GA, Walton. Diagnosis of rotator cuff tears. Lancet 2001;357:769–770.

54. Appleboam A, Reuben AD, Benger JR et al. Elbow extension test to rule out elbow fracture: multicentre prospective validation and observational study of diagnostic accuracy in adults and children. BMJ 2008;337:2428–2433.

55. Darracq MA, Vinson DR, Panacek EA. Preservation of active range of motion after acute elbow trauma predicts absence of elbow fracture. Am J Emerg Med 2008;26:779–782.

56. D'Arcy CA, McGee S. Does this patient have carpal tunnel syndrome? The rational clinical examination. JAMA 2000;283: 3110–3117.

57. Sarwark JF (ed). Hand and Wrist, in Essentials of Musculoskeletal Care, 4th ed. Rosemont, IL: American Academy of Orthopedic Surgeons, 2010.

58. Katz JN, Simmons BP. Carpal tunnel syndrome. N Engl J Med 2002;346:1807–1811.

59. Braun J, Sieper J. Ankylosing spondylitis. Lancet 2007;369: 1379–1390.

60. Haywood KL, Garratt AM, Jordan K et al. Spinal mobility in ankylosing spondylitis: reliability, validity and responsiveness. Rheumatology 2004;43:750–757.

61. Laine C, Goldman DR, Wilson JE. In the clinic. Osteoarthritis. Ann Intern Med 2007;147:ITC8-1–ITC8-16.

62. Lane NE. Osteoarthritis of the hip. N Engl J Med 2007;357: 1413–1421.

63. Steultjens MPM, Dekker J, van Baar ME et al. Range of joint motion and disability in patients with osteoarthritis of the knee or hip. Rheumatology 2000;39:955–961.

64. Altman R, Asch E, Bloch D et al. Development of criteria for the classification and reporting of osteoarthritis. Classification of osteoarthritis of the knee. Arthritis Rheum 1986;29:1039–1049.

65. Cibere J, Bellamy N, Thorne A et al. Reliability of the knee examination in osteoarthritis. Arthritis Rheum 2004;50:458–468.

66. Felson DT. Osteoarthritis of the knee. N Engl J Med 2006;354: 841–848.

67. Solomon DH, Simel DL, Bates DW, et al. Does this patient have a torn meniscus or ligament of the knee? Value of the physical examination. The rational physical examination. JAMA 2001;286:1610–1620.

68. Jackson JL, O'Malley PG, Kroenke K. Evaluation of acute knee pain in primary care. Ann Intern Med 139:575–588, 2003.

69. Clemow C, Pope B, Woodall HE. Tools to speed your heel pain diagnosis. J Fam Pract 2008;57:714–723.

70. Cole C, Seto C, Gazewood J. Plantar fasciitis: evidence based review of diagnosis and therapy. Am Fam Phys 2005;72:2237–2242.

71. Buchbinder R. Plantar fasciitis. N Engl J Med 2004;350: 2159–2166.

72. Seah R, Mani-Babu S. Managing ankle sprains in primary care: what is best practice? A systematic review of the last 10 years of evidence. Br Med Bull 2011;97:105–135.

73. Stiell IG, Greenberg GH, McKnight RD et al. Decision rules for the use of radiography in acute ankle injuries: refinement and prospective validation. JAMA 1993;269:1127–1132.

74. Chou R, Qaseem A, Sonow V et al. Diagnosis and treatment of low back pain: a joint clinical practice guideline from the American College of Physicians and the American Pain Society. Ann Intern Med 2007;147:478–491.

75. McGee S. Ch. 60, Disorders of the nerve roots, plexi, and peripheral nerves, in Evidence-based Physical Diagnosis, 2nd ed. St. Louis: Saunders, 2007.

76. Suri P, Rainville J, Kalichman L et al. Does this older adult with lower extremity pain have the clinical syndrome of lumbar spinal stenosis? JAMA 2010;304:2628–2636.

77. Katz JN, Harris MB. Lumbar spinal stenosis. N Engl J Med 2008;358:818–825.

78. Palumbo A, Anderson K. Multiple myeloma. N Engl J Med 2011;364:1046–1060.

79. Davis BT, Pasternak MS. Case 19–2007: a 19-year-old college student with fever and joint pain. N Engl J Med 2007;356: 2631–2637.

80. Wilson JE. In the clinic. Gout. Ann Intern Med 2010;152: ITC1–ITC16.

81. Dore RK. The gout diagnosis. Cleve Clin J Med 2008;75:S17–S21.

Additional References

Bialosky JE, Bishop MD, Cleland JA. Individual expectation: an overlooked, but pertinent, factor in the treatment of individuals experiencing musculoskeletal pain. Phys Ther 2010;90:1345–1355.

Burbank KM, Stevenson JH, Czarnecki GR et al. Chronic shoulder pain: part I. Evaluation and diagnosis. Am Fam Physician 2008;77:453–460.

Carragee EJ, Alamin TF, Miller JL et al. Discographic, MRI and psychosocial determinants of low back pain disability and remission: a prospective study in subjects with benign persistent back pain. Spine J 2005;5:23–35.

Chou R, Huffman AH. Nonpharmacologic therapies for acute and chronic low back pain: a review of the evidence for an American Pain Society/American College of Physicians Clinical Practice Guideline. Ann Intern Med 2007;147:492–504.

Darouiche RO. Spinal epidural abscess. N Engl J Med 2006;355: 2012–2020.

Escalante Y, Saavedra JM, García-Hermoso A et al. Physical exercise and reduction of pain in adults with lower limb osteoarthritis: a systematic review. J Back Musculoskelet Rehabil 2010;23:175–186.

Firestein GS, Kelley WN. Kelley's Textbook of Rheumatology, 9th ed. Philadelphia: Saunders/Elsevier, 2013.

Goldenberg DL, Burckhardt C, Crofford L. Management of fibromyalgia syndrome. JAMA 2004;292:2388–2395.

Hegedus EJ, Cook C, Hasselblad V. Physical examination tests for assessing a torn meniscus in the knee: a systematic review with meta-analysis. J Orthop Sports Phys Ther 2007;37:541–550.

Hoppenfeld S, Hutton R. Physical Examination of the Spine and Extremities. New York: Appleton-Century-Crofts, 1976.

Hunter DJ. In the clinic. Osteoarthritis. Ann Intern Med 2007;147(3):ITC8-1–ITC8-16.

Ma L, Cranney A, Holroyd-Leduc JM. Acute monoarthritis: what is the cause of my patient's painful swollen joint? CMAJ 2009;180:59–65.

Main C, Wood P, Hollis S et al. The distress and risk assessment method (DRAM): a simple patient classification to identify distress and evaluate the risk of a poor outcome. Spine 1992;17:42–52.

Porcheret M, Jordan K, Croft P. Treatment of knee pain in older adults in primary care: development of an evidence-based model of care. Rheumatology 2007;46:638–648.

Peul WC, van Houwelingen HC, van den Hout WB et al. Surgery versus prolonged conservative treatment for sciatica. N Engl J Med 2007;356:2245–2256.

Roddy E, Zhang W, Doherty M, Arden NK et al. Evidence-based recommendations for the role of exercise in the management of osteoarthritis of the hip or knee–the MOVE consensus. Rheumatology (Oxford) 2005;44:67–73.

Sarwark JF, American Academy of Orthopaedic Surgeons, American Academy of Pediatrics. Essentials of Musculoskeletal Care,

4th ed. Rosemont, IL: American Academy of Orthopedic Surgeons, 2010.

Sawitzke AD, Shi H, Finco MF, et al. Clinical efficacy and safety of glucosamine, chondroitin sulphate, their combination, celecoxib or placebo taken to treat osteoarthritis of the knee: 2-year results from GAIT. Ann Rheum Dis 2010;69:1459–1464.

Scholten RJ, Opstelten W, van der Plas CG. Accuracy of physical diagnostic tests for assessing ruptures of the anterior cruciate ligament: a meta-analysis. J Fam Pract 2003;52:689–694.

U.S. Preventive Services Task Force. Behavioral counseling in primary care to promote physical activity: recommendations and rationale. Rockville, MD: Agency for Healthcare Research and Quality, July 2002. Available at http://www.uspreventiveservicestaskforce.org/3rduspstf/physactivity/physactrr.htm. Accessed May 27, 2010.

Van Nies JA, de Jong Z, Vand der Helm-van Mil Ah et al. Improved treatment strategies reduce the increased mortality risk in early RA patients. Rheumatology 2010;49:2210–2216.

Vignon E, Valat JP, Rossignol M et al. Osteoarthritis of the knee and hip and activity: a systematic international review and synthesis (OASIS). Joint Bone Spine 2006;73:442–455.

Vrooman PCAJ, de Krom MCTFM, Knotternus JA. Predicting the outcome of sciatica at short- term follow-up. Br J Gen Pract 2002;52:119–123.

Wang C, Schmid CH, Hibberd PL et al. Tai Chi is effective in treating knee osteoarthritis: a randomized controlled trial. Arthritis Rheum 2009;61:1545–1553.

Wang C, Schmid CH, Rones R. A randomized trial of Tai Chi for fibromyalgia. N Engl J Med 2010;363:743–754.

Witt JC, Stevens JC. Neurologic disorders masquerading as carpal tunnel syndrome: 12 cases of failed carpal tunnel release. Mayo Clin Proc 2000;75:409–413.

Wolfe F, Smythe HA, Yunus MB et al. The American College of Rheumatology 1990 Criteria for the Classification of Fibromyalgia. Report of the Multicenter Criteria Committee. Arthritis Rheum 1990;33:160–172.

Zimmerli W. Clinical practice. Vertebral osteomyelitis. N Engl J Med 2010;362:1022–1029.

The Bates' suite offers these additional resources to enhance learning and facilitate understanding of this chapter:

- *Bates' Pocket Guide to Physical Examination and History Taking*, 7th edition
- *Bates' Visual Guide to Physical Examination*
- thePoint online resources, for students and instructors: http://thepoint.lww.com

Table 16-1 Low Back Pain

Patterns	Possible Causes	Physical Signs
Mechanical Low Back Pain[5,74] Aching pain in the lumbosacral area; may radiate into lower leg, especially along L5 (lateral leg) or S1 (posterior leg) dermatomes. Refers to anatomic or functional abnormality in absence of neoplastic, infectious, or inflammatory disease. Usually acute (<3 months), idiopathic, benign, and self-limiting; represents 97% of symptomatic low back pain. Commonly work related and occurring in patients 30 to 50 years. Risk factors include heavy lifting, poor conditioning, obesity.	Often arises from muscle and ligament injuries (~70%) or age-related intervertebral disc or facet disease (~4%). Causes also include herniated disc (~4%), spinal stenosis (~3%), compression fractures (~4%), and spondylolisthesis (2%).	Paraspinal muscle or facet tenderness, pain with back movement, loss of normal lumbar lordosis, but no motor or sensory loss or reflex abnormalities. In osteoporosis, check for thoracic kyphosis, percussion tenderness over a spinous process, or fractures in the thoracic spine or hip.
Sciatica (Radicular Low Back Pain)[5,22,75] Shooting pain below the knee, commonly into the lateral leg (L5) or posterior calf (S1); typically accompanies low back pain. Patients report associated paresthesias and weakness. Bending, sneezing, coughing, straining during bowel movements often worsen pain.[1]	Sciatic pain very sensitive, ~95%, and specific, ~88%, for disc herniation. Usually from herniated intervertebral disc with compression or traction of nerve root(s) in people 50 years or older. Involves L5 and S1 roots in ~95% of disc herniations. Root or spinal cord compression from neoplastic conditions in fewer than 1% of cases. Tumor or midline disc herniation in bowel or bladder dysfunction, leg weakness from cauda equina syndrome (S2–4).	Disc herniation most likely if calf wasting, weak ankle dorsiflexion, absent ankle jerk, positive crossed straight-leg raise (pain in affected leg when healthy leg tested); negative straight-leg raise makes diagnosis highly unlikely. Ipsilateral straight-leg raise sensitive, about 65% to 98%, but not specific, about 10% to 60%.
Lumbar Spinal Stenosis[76,77] "Pseudoclaudication" pain in the back or legs with walking that improves with rest, lumbar flexion (which decompresses spinal cord), or both. Pain vague but usually bilateral, with paresthesias in one or both legs.	Arises from hypertrophic degenerative disease of one or more vertebral facets and thickening of the ligamentum flavum, causing narrowing of the spinal canal centrally or in lateral recesses. More common after age 60 years.	Posture may be flexed forward, with lower extremity weakness and hyporeflexia. Thigh pain after 30 seconds of lumbar extension. Straight-leg raise usually negative.
Chronic Back Stiffness[59,60]	*Ankylosing spondylitis*, an inflammatory polyarthritis, most common in men younger than 40 years. *Diffuse idiopathic hyperostosis (DISH)* affects men more than women, usually 50 years or older	
Nocturnal Back Pain, Unrelieved by Rest[5,78]	Consider *metastatic malignancy* to the spine from cancer of the prostate, breast, lung, thyroid, and kidney, and multiple myeloma.	Loss of the normal lumbar lordosis, muscle spasm, limited anterior and lateral flexion. Improves with exercise. Lateral immobility of the spine, especially in thoracic area.
Pain Referred from the Abdomen or Pelvis Usually a deep, aching pain; the level varies with the source. Accounts for ~2% of low back pain.	Peptic ulcer, pancreatitis, pancreatic cancer, chronic prostatitis, endometriosis, dissecting aortic aneurysm, retroperitoneal tumor, and other causes.	Variable with the source. Local vertebral tenderness may be present. Spinal movements are not painful and range of motion is not affected. Look for signs of the primary disorder.

Table
16-2   Pains in the Neck

Patterns	Possible Causes	Physical Signs
Mechanical Neck Pain Aching pain in the cervical paraspinal muscles and ligaments with associated muscle spasm and stiffness and tightness in the upper back and shoulder, lasting up to 6 weeks. No associated radiation, paresthesias, or weakness. Headache may be present.	Mechanism poorly understood, possibly sustained muscle contraction. Associated with poor posture, stress, poor sleep, poor head position during activities such as computer use, watching television, and driving.	Local muscle tenderness, pain on movement. No neurologic deficits. Possible trigger points in *fibromyalgia*. *Torticollis* if prolonged abnormal neck posture and muscle spasm.
Mechanical Neck Pain—Whiplash[9] Mechanical neck pain with aching paracervical pain and stiffness, often beginning the day after injury. Occipital headache, dizziness, malaise, and fatigue may be present. Chronic whiplash syndrome if symptoms last more than 6 months; occurs in 20% to 40% of injuries.	Musculoligamentous sprain or strain from forced hyperflexion–hyperextension injury to the neck, as in rear-end collisions.	Localized paracervical tenderness, decreased neck range of motion, perceived weakness of the upper extremities. Causes of cervical cord compression such as fracture, herniation, head injury, or altered consciousness are excluded.
Cervical Radiculopathy—from nerve root compression[9,10] Sharp burning or tingling pain in the neck and one arm, with associated paresthesias and weakness. Sensory symptoms often in myotomal pattern, deep in muscle, rather than dermatomal pattern.	Dysfunction of cervical spinal nerve, nerve roots, or both from foraminal encroachment of the spinal nerve (~75%), herniated cervical disc (~25%). Rarely from tumor, syrinx, or multiple sclerosis. Mechanisms may involve hypoxia of the nerve root and dorsal ganglion, release of inflammatory mediators.	C7 nerve root affected most often (45%–60%), with weakness in triceps and finger flexors and extensors. C6 nerve root involvement also common, with weakness in biceps, brachioradialis, wrist extensors.
Cervical Myelopathy—from cervical cord compression[9] Neck pain with bilateral weakness and paresthesias in both upper and lower extremities, often with urinary frequency. Hand clumsiness, palmar paresthesias, and gait changes may be subtle. Neck flexion often exacerbates symptoms.	Usually from cervical *spondylosis,* defined as cervical degenerative disc disease from spurs, protrusion of ligamentum flavum, and/or disc herniation (~80%); also from cervical stenosis from osteophytes, ossification of ligamentum flavum. Large central or paracentral disc herniation may also compress cord.	Hyperreflexia; clonus at the wrist, knee, or ankle; extensor plantar reflexes (positive Babinski signs); and gait disturbances. May also see *Lhermitte's sign:* neck flexion with resulting sensation of electrical shock radiating down the spine. Confirmation of cervical myelopathy warrants neck immobilization and neurosurgical evaluation.

Table	
16-3	**Patterns of Pain In and Around the Joints**

Problem	Process	Common Locations	Pattern of Spread	Onset	Progression and Duration
Rheumatoid Arthritis[12,48,79]	Chronic inflammation of *synovial membranes* with secondary erosion of adjacent cartilage and bone, and damage to ligaments and tendons	Hands (proximal interphalangeal and metacarpophalangeal joints), feet (metatarsopha-langeal joints), wrists, knees, elbows, ankles	Symmetrically additive: progresses to other joints while persisting in the initial ones	Usually insidious	Often chronic, with remissions and exacerbations
Osteoarthritis (*degenerative joint disease*)[22]	Degeneration and progressive loss of *cartilage* within the joints, damage to underlying bone, and formation of new bone at the margins of the cartilage	Knees, hips, hands (distal, sometimes proximal interphalangeal joints), cervical and lumbar spine, and wrists (first carpometacarpal joint); also joints previously injured or diseased	Additive; however, only one joint may be involved.	Usually insidious	Slowly progressive, with temporary exacerbations after periods of overuse
Gouty Arthritis[80,81]					
Acute Gout	An inflammatory reaction to microcrystals of monosodium urate	Base of the big toe (the first metatarso-phalangeal joint), the instep or dorsa of feet, the ankles, knees, and elbows	Early attacks usually confined to one joint	Sudden; often at night; often after injury, surgery, fasting, or excessive food or alcohol intake	Occasional isolated attacks lasting days up to 2 weeks; they may get more frequent and severe, with persisting symptoms
Chronic Tophaceous Gout	Multiple local accumulations of sodium urate in the joints and other tissues (*tophi*), with or without inflammation	Feet, ankles, wrists, fingers, and elbows	Additive, not so symmetric as rheumatoid arthritis	Gradual development of chronicity with repeated attacks	Chronic symptoms with acute exacerbations
Polymyalgia Rheumatica[14]	A disease of unclear etiology in people older than 50, especially women; overlaps with giant cell arteritis	Muscles of the hip and shoulder girdles and neck; symmetric		Insidious or abrupt, even appearing overnight	Chronic but ultimately self-limiting
Fibromyalgia Syndrome[13]	Widespread musculoskeletal pain and tender points. Mechanism may involve aberrant pain signaling and amplification	"All over," but especially in the neck, shoulders, hands, low back, and knees	Shifts unpredictably or worsens in response to immobility, excessive use, or exposure to cold	Variable	Chronic, with "ups and downs"

Swelling	Redness, Warmth, and Tenderness	Stiffness	Limitation of Motion	Generalized Symptoms
Frequent swelling of synovial tissue in joints or tendon sheaths; also subcutaneous nodules	Tender, often warm, but seldom red	Prominent, often for an hour or more in the mornings, also after inactivity	Often develops	Weakness, fatigue, weight loss, and low fever are common.
Small effusions in the joints may be present, especially in the knees; also bony enlargement	Possibly tender, seldom warm, and rarely red	Frequent but brief (usually 5–10 min), in the morning and after inactivity	Often develops	Usually absent
Present, within and around the involved joint	Exquisitely tender, hot, and red	Not evident	Motion is limited primarily by pain.	Fever may be present. Consider also septic arthritis.
Present as tophi in joints, bursae, and subcutaneous tissues. Check ears and extensor surfaces for tophi.	Tenderness, warmth, and redness may be present during exacerbations.	Present	Present	Possibly fever; patient may also develop symptoms of renal failure and renal stones.
Swelling and edema may be present over dorsum of hands, wrists, feet	Muscles often tender, but not warm or red	Prominent, especially in the morning	Pain restricts movement, especially in shoulders	Malaise, depression, anorexia, weight loss, and fever, but no true weakness
None	Multiple specific and symmetric tender "trigger points," often not recognized until the examination	Present, especially in the morning	Absent, though stiffness is greater at the extremes of movement	A disturbance of sleep, usually associated with morning fatigue; overlaps with depression

Table
16-4 Painful Shoulders
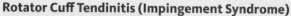

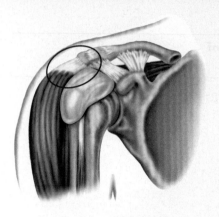

Rotator Cuff Tendinitis (Impingement Syndrome)

Repeated shoulder motion, for example, from throwing or swimming, can cause edema and hemorrhage followed by inflammation, most commonly involving the supraspinatus tendon. Acute, recurrent, or chronic pain may result, often aggravated by activity. Patients report sharp catches of pain, grating, and weakness when lifting the arm overhead. When the supraspinatus tendon is involved, tenderness is maximal just below the tip of the acromion. In older adults, bone spurs on the undersurface of the acromion may contribute to symptoms.

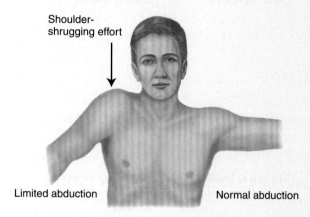

Shoulder-shrugging effort

Limited abduction   Normal abduction

Rotator Cuff Tears

The rotator cuff muscles and tendons compress the humeral head into the concave glenoid fossa and strengthen arm movement—the subscapularis in internal rotation, the supraspinatus in elevation, and the infraspinatus and teres minor in external rotation.[52] Injury from a fall, trauma, or repeated impingement against the acromion and the coracoacromial ligament may cause a partial or full-thickness tear of the rotator cuff, the most common clinical problem of the shoulder, especially in older patients. Patients complain of chronic shoulder pain, night pain, or catching and grating when raising the arm overhead. Weakness or tears of the tendons usually start in the supraspinatus tendon and progress posteriorly and anteriorly. Look for atrophy of the deltoid, supraspinatus, or infraspinatus muscles. Palpate anteriorly over the anterior greater tuberosity of the humerus to check for a defect in muscle attachment and below the acromion for crepitus during arm rotation. In a complete tear, active abduction and forward flexion at the glenohumeral joint are severely impaired, producing a characteristic shrug of the shoulder and a positive "drop arm" test (see p. 625).

Calcific Tendinitis

Calcific tendinitis is a degenerative process in the tendon associated with the deposition of calcium salts that usually involves the supraspinatus tendon. Acute, disabling attacks of shoulder pain may occur, usually in patients older than age 30, more often in women. The arm is held close to the side, and all motions are severely limited by pain. Tenderness is maximal below the tip of the acromion. The subacromial bursa, which overlies the supraspinatus tendon, may be inflamed. Chronic, less severe pain may also occur.

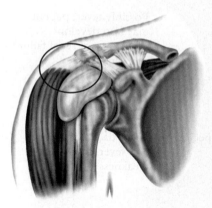

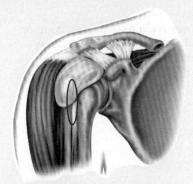

Bicipital Tendinitis

Inflammation of the long head of the biceps tendon and tendon sheath causes anterior shoulder pain resembling and often coexisting with rotator cuff tendinitis. Both conditions may involve impingement injury. Tenderness is maximal in the bicipital groove. Externally rotate and abduct the arm to separate this area from the subacromial tenderness of supraspinatus tendinitis. With the patient's arm at the side, elbow flexed to 90 degrees, ask the patient to supinate the forearm against your resistance. Increased pain in the bicipital groove confirms this condition. Pain during resisted forward flexion of the shoulder with the elbow extended is also indicative.

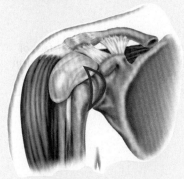

Adhesive Capsulitis (Frozen Shoulder)

Adhesive capsulitis refers to fibrosis of the glenohumeral joint capsule, manifested by diffuse, dull, aching pain in the shoulder and progressive restriction of active and passive range of motion, especially in external rotation, with localized tenderness. The condition is usually unilateral and occurs in people aged 40 to 60. There is often an antecedent disorder of the shoulder or another condition (such as myocardial infarction) that has decreased shoulder movements. The disorder may take 6 months to 2 years to resolve. Stretching exercises may help.

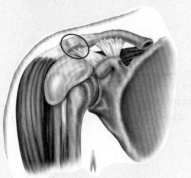

Acromioclavicular Arthritis

Acromioclavicular arthritis is relatively common, usually arising from prior direct injury to the shoulder girdle with resulting degenerative changes. Tenderness is localized over the acromioclavicular joint. Patients report pain with movements of the scapula and arm abduction.

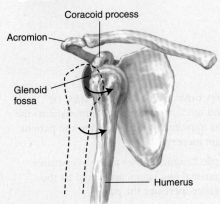

Coracoid process

Acromion

Glenoid fossa

Humerus

Anterior Dislocation of the Humerus[49-51]

Shoulder instability from anterior subluxation or dislocation of the humerus usually results from a fall or forceful throwing motion, then can become common unless treated or the precipitating motion is avoided. The shoulder seems to "slip out of the joint" when the arm is abducted and externally rotated, causing a *positive apprehension sign* for anterior instability when the examiner places the arm in this position. Any shoulder movement may cause pain, and patients hold the arm in a neutral position. The rounded lateral aspect of the shoulder appears flattened. Dislocations may also be inferior, posterior (relatively rare), and multidirectional.

Table 16-5 Swollen or Tender Elbows

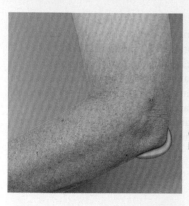

Olecranon bursitis

Olecranon Bursitis

Swelling and inflammation of the olecranon bursa may result from trauma, gout, or rheumatoid arthritis. The swelling is superficial to the olecranon process and may reach 6 cm in diameter. Consider aspiration for both diagnosis and symptomatic relief.

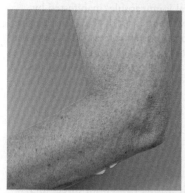

Rheumatoid nodules

Rheumatoid Nodules

Subcutaneous nodules may develop at pressure points along the extensor surface of the ulna in patients with rheumatoid arthritis or acute rheumatic fever. They are firm and nontender. They are not attached to the overlying skin but may be attached to the underlying periosteum. They can develop in the area of the olecranon bursa, but often occur more distally.

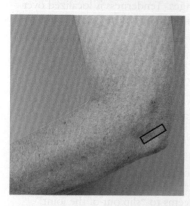

Arthritis

Arthritis of the Elbow

Synovial inflammation or fluid is felt best in the grooves between the olecranon process and the epicondyles on either side. Palpate for a boggy, soft, or fluctuant swelling and for tenderness. Causes include rheumatoid arthritis, gout and pseudogout, osteoarthritis, and trauma. Patients report pain, stiffness, and restricted motion.

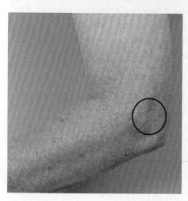

Epicondylitis

Epicondylitis

Lateral epicondylitis (tennis elbow) follows repetitive extension of the wrist or pronation–supination of the forearm. Pain and tenderness develop 1 cm distal to the lateral epicondyle and possibly in the extensor muscles close to it. When the patient tries to extend the wrist against resistance, pain increases.

Medial epicondylitis (pitcher's, golfer's, or Little League elbow) follows repetitive wrist flexion, as in throwing. Tenderness is maximal just lateral and distal to the medial epicondyle. Wrist flexion against resistance increases the pain.

Table
16-6 **Arthritis in the Hands**

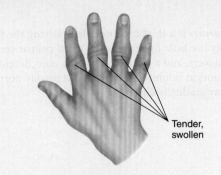

Tender,
swollen

Acute Rheumatoid Arthritis

Tender, painful, stiff joints in *rheumatoid arthritis*, usually with *symmetric* involvement on both sides of the body. The proximal interphalangeal, metacarpophalangeal, and wrist joints are the most frequently affected. Note the fusiform or spindle-shaped swelling of the proximal interphalangeal joints in acute disease.

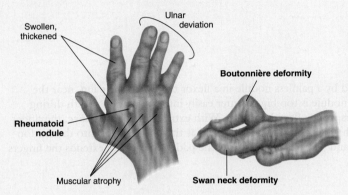

Ulnar
deviation

Swollen,
thickened

Boutonnière deformity

Rheumatoid
nodule

Muscular atrophy

Swan neck deformity

Chronic Rheumatoid Arthritis

In chronic disease, note the swelling and thickening of the metacarpophalangeal and proximal interphalangeal joints. Range of motion becomes limited, and fingers may deviate toward the ulnar side. The interosseous muscles atrophy. The fingers may show *"swan neck"* deformities (hyperextension of the proximal interphalangeal joints with fixed flexion of the distal interphalangeal joints). Less common is a *boutonnière deformity* (persistent flexion of the proximal interphalangeal joint with hyperextension of the distal interphalangeal joint). Rheumatoid nodules are seen in the acute or the chronic stage.

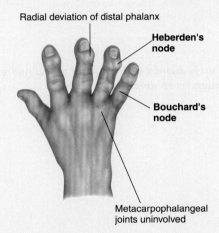

Radial deviation of distal phalanx

Heberden's
node

Bouchard's
node

Metacarpophalangeal
joints uninvolved

Osteoarthritis *(Degenerative Joint Disease)*

Heberden's nodes on the dorsolateral aspects of the distal interphalangeal joints from bony overgrowth of osteoarthritis. Usually hard and painless, they affect the middle-aged or elderly; often associated with arthritic changes in other joints. Flexion and deviation deformities may develop. *Bouchard's nodes* on the proximal interphalangeal joints are less common. The metacarpophalangeal joints are spared.

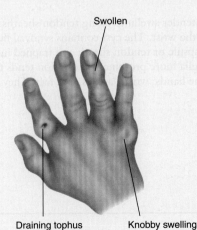

Swollen

Draining tophus   Knobby swelling

Chronic Tophaceous Gout

The deformities of long-standing chronic tophaceous gout can mimic rheumatoid arthritis and osteoarthritis. Joint involvement is usually not as symmetric as in rheumatoid arthritis. Acute inflammation may be present. Knobby swellings around the joints ulcerate and discharge white chalklike urates.

Table	
16-7	**Swellings and Deformities of the Hands**

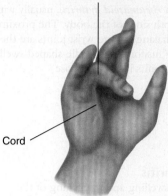

Flexion contraction

Cord

Dupuytren's Contracture

The first sign of a *Dupuytren's contracture* is a thickened nodule overlying the flexor tendon of the ring finger and possibly the little finger near the distal palmar crease. Subsequently, the skin in this area puckers, and a thickened fibrotic cord develops between palm and finger. Finger extension is limited, but flexion is usually normal. Flexion contracture of the fingers may gradually ensue.

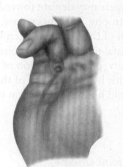

Trigger Finger

Trigger finger is caused by a painless nodule in a flexor tendon in the palm, near the metacarpal head. The nodule is too big to enter easily into the tendon sheath during extension of the fingers from a flexed position. With extra effort or assistance, the finger extends and flexes with a palpable and audible snap as the nodule pops into the tendon sheath. Watch, listen, and palpate the nodule as the patient flexes and extends the fingers.

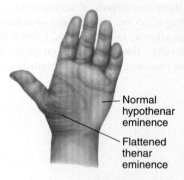

Normal hypothenar eminence

Flattened thenar eminence

Thenar Atrophy

Thenar atrophy suggests a *median nerve disorder* such as *carpal tunnel syndrome* (see p. 634). Hypothenar atrophy suggests an *ulnar nerve disorder.*

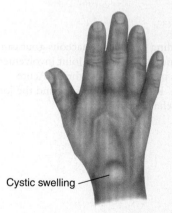

Cystic swelling

Ganglion

Ganglia are cystic, round, usually nontender swellings along tendon sheaths or joint capsules, frequently at the dorsum of the wrist. The cyst contains synovial fluid arising from erosion or tearing of the joint capsule or tendon sheath and trapped in the cystic cavity. Flexion of the wrist makes ganglia more prominent; extension tends to obscure them. Ganglia may also develop on the hands, wrists, ankles, and feet. They can disappear spontaneously.

Table	
16-8	**Tendon Sheath, Palmar Space, and Finger Infections**

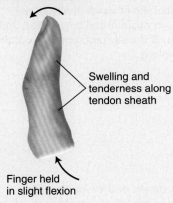

Pain on extension

Swelling and tenderness along tendon sheath

Finger held in slight flexion

Acute Tenosynovitis

Infection of the flexor tendon sheaths, *acute tenosynovitis*, may follow local injury. Unlike arthritis, tenderness and swelling develop not in the joint but along the course of the tendon sheath, from the distal phalanx to the level of the metacarpophalangeal joint. The finger is held in slight flexion; finger extension is very painful.

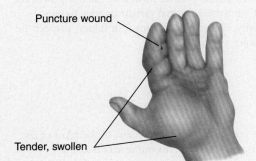

Puncture wound

Tender, swollen

Acute Tenosynovitis and Thenar Space Involvement

If the infection progresses, it may extend from the tendon sheath into the adjacent fascial spaces within the palm. Infections of the index finger and thenar space are illustrated. Early diagnosis and treatment are important.

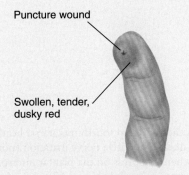

Puncture wound

Swollen, tender, dusky red

Felon

Injury to the fingertip may result in infection of the enclosed fascial spaces of the finger pad, usually from *Staphylococcus aureus*. Severe pain, localized tenderness, swelling, and dusky redness are characteristic. Early diagnosis and treatment, usually incision and drainage, are important. If vesicles are present, consider *herpetic whitlow* instead, usually seen in health care workers exposed to *herpes simplex virus* in human saliva.

Table
16-9
Abnormalities of the Feet

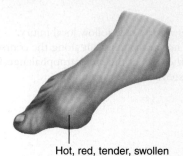

Hot, red, tender, swollen

Acute Gouty Arthritis

The metatarsophalangeal joint of the great toe is the initial site of attack in 50% of the episodes of *acute gouty arthritis*. It is characterized by a very painful and tender, hot, dusky red swelling that extends beyond the margin of the joint. It is easily mistaken for a cellulitis. The ankle, tarsal joints, and knee are also commonly involved.

Medial border becomes convex

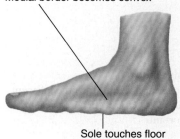

Sole touches floor

Flat Feet

Signs of *flat feet* may be apparent only when the patient stands, or they may become permanent. The longitudinal arch flattens so that the sole approaches or touches the floor. The normal concavity on the medial side of the foot becomes convex. Tenderness may be present from the medial malleolus down along the medial-plantar surface of the foot. Swelling may develop anterior to the malleoli. "Flat foot" may be a normal variant or arise from posterior tibial tendon dysfunction, seen in obesity, diabetes, and prior foot injury. Inspect the shoes for excess wear on the inner sides of the soles and heels.

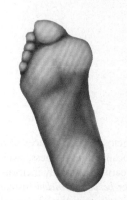

Hallux Valgus

In *hallux valgus,* there is lateral deviation of the great toe and enlargement of the head of the first metatarsal on its medial side, forming a bursa or bunion. This bursa may become inflamed. Women are 10 times more likely to be affected than men.

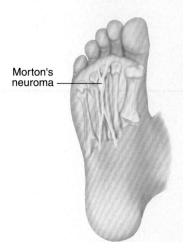

Morton's neuroma

Morton's Neuroma

Look for tenderness over the plantar surface between the third and fourth metatarsal heads, from perineural fibrosis of the common digital nerve due to repetitive nerve irritation (not a true neuroma). Check for pain radiating to the toes when you press on the plantar interspace and squeeze the metatarsals with your other hand. Symptoms include hyperesthesia, numbness, aching, and burning from the metatarsal heads into the third and fourth toes.

Table
16-10   **Abnormalities of the Toes and Soles**

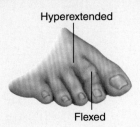

Red, tender

Granulation tissue

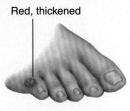

Hyperextended

Flexed

Red, thickened

Ingrown Toenail

The sharp edge of a toenail may dig into and injure the lateral nail fold, resulting in inflammation and infection. A tender, reddened, overhanging nail fold, sometimes with granulation tissue and purulent discharge, results. The great toe is most often affected.

Hammer Toe

Most commonly involving the second toe, a hammer toe is characterized by hyperextension at the metatarsophalangeal joint with flexion at the proximal interphalangeal joint. A corn frequently develops at the pressure point over the proximal interphalangeal joint.

Corn

A corn is a painful conical thickening of skin that results from recurrent pressure on normally thin skin. The apex of the cone points inward and causes pain. Corns characteristically occur over bony prominences such as the fifth toe. When located in moist areas such as pressure points between the fourth and fifth toes, they are called soft corns.

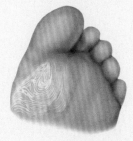

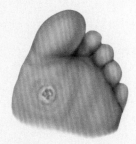

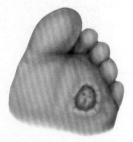

Callus

Like a corn, a callus is an area of greatly thickened skin that develops in a region of recurrent pressure. Unlike a corn, a callus involves skin that is normally thick, such as the sole, and is usually painless. If a callus is painful, suspect an underlying plantar wart.

Plantar Wart

A plantar wart is a hyperkeratotic lesion caused by *human papillomavirus,* located on the sole of the foot. It may look like a callus. Look for the characteristic small dark spots that give a stippled appearance to a wart. Normal skin lines stop at the wart's edge. It is tender if pinched side to side, whereas a callus is tender to direct pressure.

Neuropathic Ulcer

When pain sensation is diminished or absent, as in diabetic neuropathy, neuropathic ulcers may develop at pressure points on the feet. Although often deep, infected, and indolent, they are painless. Underlying osteomyelitis and amputation may ensue. Early detection of loss of sensation using a nylon filament is the standard of care in diabetes.

The Nervous System

Assessment of the nervous system calls for mastery of the complex skills of examination and clinical reasoning, and a commitment to lifelong learning. The nervous system examination begins with formal assessment of mental status to test cognition and memory, described in Chapter 5. Continue with the examination of the cranial nerves, the motor system, the sensory system, and the reflexes, which is the focus of this chapter. As you acquire the techniques for these increasingly important components of physical examination, especially for our aging population, make the discipline of neurologists your creed—always think through the three guiding questions below that organize your findings. Test your conclusions against the findings of your teachers, colleagues, and neurologists to refine your expertise.

See Chapter 5, Behavior and Mental Status, pp. 141–169, for the principles and techniques of the mental status examination.

Guiding Questions for Examination of the Nervous System

▶ Is the mental status intact?
▶ Are your findings symmetric? Do right-sided findings match left-sided findings?
▶ Where is the lesion? If findings are asymmetric or abnormal, is the lesion in the *central nervous system*, involving the brain, brainstem, or spinal cord, or in the *peripheral nervous system*, involving the 12 pairs of cranial nerves or the peripheral nerves?

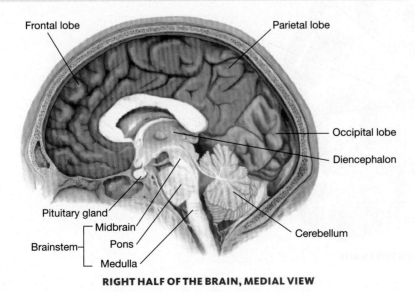

Frontal lobe
Parietal lobe
Occipital lobe
Diencephalon
Pituitary gland
Midbrain
Pons
Brainstem
Medulla
Cerebellum

RIGHT HALF OF THE BRAIN, MEDIAL VIEW

Anatomy and Physiology

CENTRAL NERVOUS SYSTEM

The Brain

The brain has four regions: the cerebrum, the diencephalon, the brainstem, and the cerebellum. Each cerebral hemisphere is subdivided into frontal, parietal, temporal, and occipital lobes.

The brain is a vast network of interconnecting *neurons* (nerve cells), consisting of cell bodies and their *axons*—single long fibers that conduct impulses to other parts of the nervous system.

Brain tissue may be gray or white. *Gray matter* consists of aggregations of neuronal cell bodies. It rims the surfaces of the cerebral hemispheres, forming the cerebral cortex. *White matter* consists of neuronal axons that are coated with myelin. The myelin sheaths, which create the white color, allow nerve impulses to travel more rapidly.

Deep in the brain lie additional clusters of gray matter. These include the *basal ganglia*, which affect movement, and the thalamus and the hypothalamus, structures in the diencephalon. The *thalamus* processes sensory impulses and relays them to the cerebral cortex. The *hypothalamus* maintains homeostasis and regulates temperature, heart rate, and blood pressure. The hypothalamus affects the endocrine system and governs emotional behaviors such as anger and sexual drive. Hormones secreted in the hypothalamus act directly on the pituitary gland.

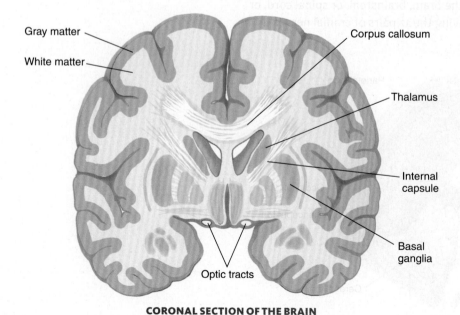

Gray matter

White matter

Corpus callosum

Thalamus

Internal capsule

Basal ganglia

Optic tracts

CORONAL SECTION OF THE BRAIN

The *internal capsule* is a white-matter structure where myelinated fibers converge from all parts of the cerebral cortex and descend into the brainstem. The *brainstem*, which connects the upper part of the brain with the spinal cord, has three sections: the midbrain, the pons, and the medulla.

Consciousness relies on the interaction between intact cerebral hemispheres and a structure in the diencephalon and upper brainstem, the *reticular activating (arousal) system*.

The *cerebellum*, which lies at the base of the brain, coordinates all movement and helps maintain the body upright in space.

The Spinal Cord

Below the medulla, the central nervous system extends into the elongated *spinal cord*, encased within the bony vertebral column and terminating at the first or second lumbar vertebra. The cord provides a series of segmental relays with the periphery, serving as a conduit for information flow to and from the brain. The motor and sensory nerve pathways relay neural signals that enter and exit the cord through posterior and anterior nerve roots and the spinal and peripheral nerves.

The spinal cord is divided into segments: cervical, from C1 to C8; thoracic, from T1 to T12; lumbar, from L1 to L5; sacral, from S1 to S5; and coccygeal. The spinal cord is thickest in the cervical segment, which contains nerve tracts to both the upper and lower extremities.

Note that the spinal cord is not as long as the vertebral canal. The lumbar and sacral roots travel the longest intraspinal distance and fan out like a horse's tail at L1–2, giving rise to the term *cauda equina*. To avoid injury to the spinal cord, most lumbar punctures are performed at the L3–4 or L4–5 vertebral interspaces.[1,2]

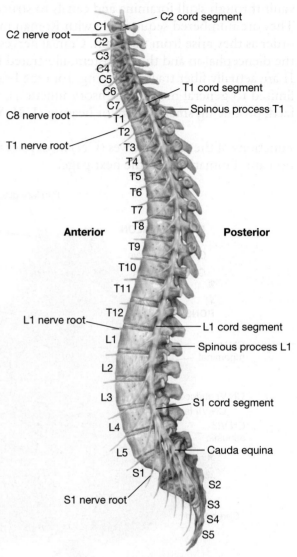

THE SPINAL CORD, LATERAL VIEW

PERIPHERAL NERVOUS SYSTEM

The *peripheral nervous system* consists of both cranial nerves and peripheral nerves that project to the heart, visceral organs, skin, and limbs. It controls the *somatic nervous system*, which regulates muscle movements and response to the sensations of touch and pain, and the *autonomic nervous system* that connects to internal organs and generates autonomic reflex responses. The autonomic nervous system consists of the *sympathetic nervous system*, which "mobilizes organs and their functions during times of stress and arousal, and the *parasympathetic nervous system*, which conserves energy and resources during times of rest and relaxation."[3]

The Cranial Nerves

Twelve pairs of special nerves called *cranial nerves* emerge from the cranial vault through skull foramina and canals to structures in the head and neck. They are numbered sequentially with Roman numerals in rostral to caudal order as they arise from the brain. Cranial nerves III through XII arise from the diencephalon and the brainstem, illustrated below. Cranial nerves I and II are actually fiber tracts emerging from the brain. Some cranial nerves are limited to general motor or sensory functions, whereas others are specialized, producing smell, vision, or hearing (I, II, VIII).

Functions of the cranial nerves (CN) most relevant to the physical examination are summarized on the next page.

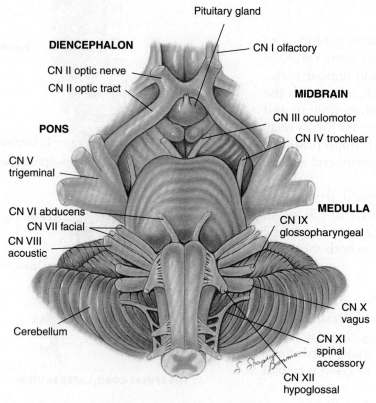

Pituitary gland

DIENCEPHALON

CN I olfactory

CN II optic nerve

CN II optic tract

MIDBRAIN

CN III oculomotor

CN IV trochlear

PONS

CN V trigeminal

CN VI abducens

CN VII facial

CN VIII acoustic

MEDULLA

CN IX glossopharyngeal

CN X vagus

CN XI spinal accessory

CN XII hypoglossal

Cerebellum

INFERIOR SURFACE OF THE BRAIN

The Peripheral Nerves

The peripheral nervous system includes spinal and peripheral nerves that carry impulses to and from the cord. Thirty-one pairs of nerves attach to the spinal cord: 8 cervical, 12 thoracic, 5 lumbar, 5 sacral, and 1 coccygeal. Each nerve has an anterior (ventral) root containing motor fibers, and a posterior (dorsal) root containing sensory fibers. The anterior and posterior roots merge to form a short *spinal nerve,* <5 mm long. Spinal nerve fibers commingle with similar fibers from other levels in plexuses outside the cord, from which *peripheral nerves* emerge. Most peripheral nerves contain both *sensory* (afferent) and *motor* (efferent) fibers.

Cranial Nerves

No.	Name	Function
I	**Olfactory**	Sense of smell
II	**Optic**	Vision
III	**Oculomotor**	Pupillary constriction, opening the eye (lid elevation), and most extraocular movements
IV	**Trochlear**	Downward, internal rotation of the eye
V	**Trigeminal**	*Motor*—temporal and masseter muscles (jaw clenching), lateral pterygoids (lateral jaw movement)
		Sensory—facial. The nerve has three divisions: (1) ophthalmic, (2) maxillary, and (3) mandibular.

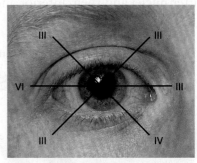

RIGHT EYE (CN III, IV, VI)

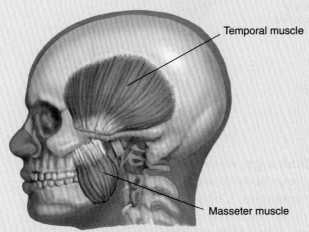

Temporal muscle

Masseter muscle

CN V—MOTOR

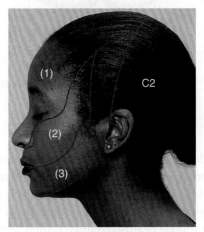

(1)

(2)

(3)

C2

CN V—SENSORY

No.	Name	Function
VI	**Abducens**	Lateral deviation of the eye
VII	**Facial**	*Motor*—facial movements, including those of facial expression, closing the eye, and closing the mouth
		Sensory—taste for salty, sweet, sour, and bitter substances on the anterior two-thirds of the tongue
VIII	**Acoustic**	Hearing (cochlear division) and balance (vestibular division)
IX	**Glossopharyngeal**	*Motor*—pharynx
		Sensory—posterior portions of the eardrum and ear canal, the pharynx, and the posterior tongue, including taste (salty, sweet, sour, bitter)
X	**Vagus**	*Motor*—palate, pharynx, and larynx
		Sensory—pharynx and larynx
XI	**Spinal accessory**	*Motor*—the sternomastoid and upper portion of the trapezius
XII	**Hypoglossal**	*Motor*—tongue

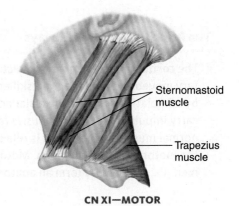

Sternomastoid muscle

Trapezius muscle

CN XI—MOTOR

Like the brain, the spinal cord contains both gray matter and white matter. The gray matter consists of aggregations of nerve cell nuclei and dendrites that are surrounded by white tracts of nerve fibers connecting the brain to the peripheral nervous system. Note the butterfly appearance of the gray-matter nuclei and their anterior and posterior horns.

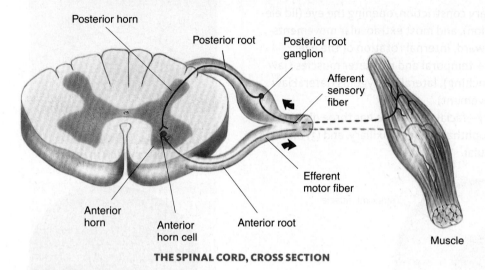

THE SPINAL CORD, CROSS SECTION

MOTOR PATHWAYS

Motor pathways are complex avenues that extend from *upper motor neurons* through long white matter tracts to synapses with *lower motor neurons,* and continue to the periphery through peripheral nerve structures. Upper motor neurons, or nerve cell bodies, lie in the motor strip of the cerebral cortex and in several brainstem nuclei; their axons synapse with motor nuclei in the brainstem (for cranial nerves) and in the spinal cord (for peripheral nerves). Lower motor neurons have cell bodies in the spinal cord, termed anterior horn cells; their axons transmit impulses through the anterior roots and spinal nerves into peripheral nerves, terminating at the neuromuscular junction.

Three kinds of motor pathways impinge on the anterior horn cells: the corticospinal tract, the basal ganglia system, and the cerebellar system. Additional pathways originating in the brainstem mediate flexor and extensor tone in limb movement and posture, most notably in coma (see Table 17-14, p. 762).

The Principal Motor Pathways

▶ The **corticospinal (pyramidal) tract**. The corticospinal tracts mediate voluntary movement and integrate skilled, complicated, or delicate movements by stimulating selected muscular actions and inhibiting others. They also carry impulses that inhibit *muscle tone,* the slight tension maintained by normal muscle even when it is relaxed. The corticospinal tracts originate in the motor cortex of the brain. Motor fibers travel down into the lower medulla, where they form an anatomical structure resembling a pyramid.

(continued)

The Principal Motor Pathways (*continued*)

There, most of these fibers cross to the opposite or *contralateral* side of the medulla, continue downward, and synapse with anterior horn cells or with intermediate neurons. Tracts synapsing in the brainstem with motor nuclei of the cranial nerves are termed *corticobulbar*.

▶ The *basal ganglia system*. This exceedingly complex system includes motor pathways between the cerebral cortex, basal ganglia, brainstem, and spinal cord. It helps to maintain muscle tone and to control body movements, especially gross automatic movements such as walking.

▶ The *cerebellar system*. The cerebellum receives both sensory and motor input and coordinates motor activity, maintains equilibrium, and helps to control posture.

All of these higher motor pathways affect movement only through the lower motor neuron systems, sometimes called the "final common pathway." Any movement, whether initiated voluntarily in the cortex, "automatically" in the basal ganglia, or reflexly in the sensory receptors, must ultimately be translated into action via the anterior horn cells. A lesion in any of these areas will affect movement or reflex activity.

When the corticospinal tract is damaged or destroyed, its functions are reduced or lost below the level of injury. *When upper motor neuron systems are damaged above the crossover of its tracts in the medulla, motor impairment develops on the opposite or contralateral side. In damage below the crossover, motor impairment occurs on the same or ipsilateral side of the body.* The affected limb becomes weak or paralyzed, and skilled, complicated, or delicate movements are performed poorly when compared with gross movements.

In upper motor neuron lesions, muscle tone is increased and deep tendon reflexes are exaggerated. Damage to the lower motor neuron systems causes ipsilateral weakness and paralysis, but in this case, muscle tone and reflexes are decreased or absent.

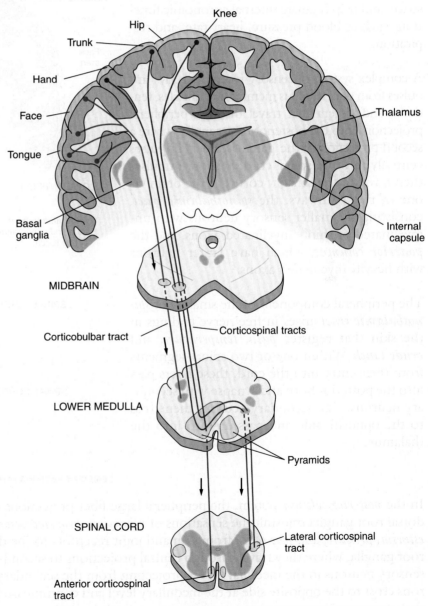

MOTOR PATHWAYS: CORTICOSPINAL AND CORTICOBULBAR TRACTS

Disease of the basal ganglia system or cerebellar system does not cause paralysis, but can be disabling. Damage to the basal ganglia system produces changes in muscle tone (most often an increase), disturbances in posture and gait, a slowness or lack of spontaneous and automatic movements termed *bradykinesia*, and various involuntary movements. Cerebellar damage impairs coordination, gait, and equilibrium, and decreases muscle tone.

SENSORY PATHWAYS

Sensory impulses not only participate in reflex activity, as previously described, but also give rise to conscious sensation, calibrate body position in space, and help regulate internal autonomic functions such as blood pressure, heart rate, and respiration.

A complex system of sensory receptors relays impulses from skin, mucous membranes, muscles, tendons, and viscera that travel through peripheral projections into the posterior root ganglia, where a second projection of the ganglia directs impulses centrally into the spinal cord. Sensory impulses then travel to the sensory cortex of the brain via one of two pathways: the *spinothalamic tract*, consisting of smaller sensory neurons with unmyelinated or thinly myelinated axons, and the *posterior columns*, which have larger neurons with heavily myelinated axons.[4]

The peripheral component of the small fiber *spinothalamic tract* arises in free nerve endings in the skin that register *pain, temperature,* and *crude touch*. Within one or two spinal segments from their entry into the cord, these fibers pass into the posterior horn and synapse with secondary neurons. The secondary neurons then cross to the opposite side and pass upward into the thalamus.

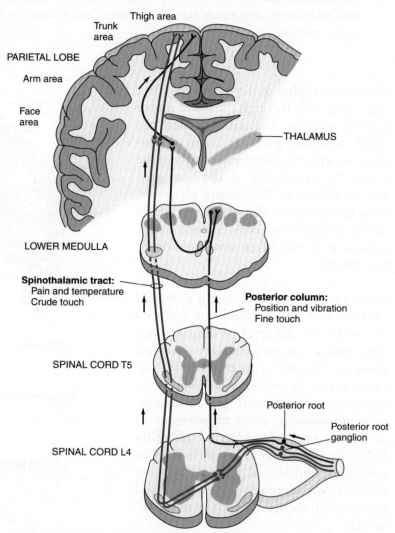

SENSORY PATHWAYS: SPINOTHALAMIC TRACT AND POSTERIOR COLUMNS

In the *posterior column* system, the peripheral large fiber projections of the dorsal root ganglia transmit the sensations of *vibration, proprioception, kinesthesia, pressure,* and *fine touch* from skin and joint receptors to the dorsal-root ganglia, where they travel through central projections to second-order sensory neurons in the medulla. Fibers projecting from the secondary neurons cross to the opposite side at the medullary level and continue on to the thalamus.

Diabetic patients with small fiber neuropathy report sharp, burning, or shooting foot pain, whereas those with large fiber neuropathy experience numbness and tingling or even no sensation at all.[5]

At the *thalamic level*, the general quality of sensation is perceived (e.g., pain, cold, pleasant, unpleasant), but fine distinctions are not made. For full perception, a third group of sensory neurons sends impulses from the thalamus to the *sensory cortex* of the brain. Here, stimuli are localized and higher-order discriminations are made.

Lesions at different points in the sensory pathways produce different kinds of sensory loss. Patterns of sensory loss, together with their associated motor findings, help you to identify where the causative lesions might be. A lesion in the sensory cortex may not impair the perception of pain, touch, and position, for example, but does impair finer discrimination. A person so affected cannot appreciate the size, shape, or texture of an object by feeling it and, therefore, cannot identify it. Loss of position and vibration sense, with preservation of other sensations, points to disease of the posterior columns, whereas loss of all sensations from the waist down, together with paralysis and hyperactive reflexes in the legs, indicates transection of the spinal cord. Crude and light touch are often preserved despite partial damage to the cord, because impulses originating on one side of the body travel up both sides of the cord.

See Table 17-1, Disorders of the Central and Peripheral Nervous Systems, pp. 744–745.

Dermatomes.   A *dermatome* is the band of skin innervated by the sensory root of a single spinal nerve. Knowledge and testing of dermatomes help localize a lesion to a specific spinal cord segment.

See the dermatome "maps" on pp. 723 and 724.

SPINAL REFLEXES: THE DEEP TENDON RESPONSE

The deep tendon or muscle stretch reflexes are relayed over structures of both the central and peripheral nervous systems. Recall that a *reflex* is an involuntary stereotypical response that may involve as few as two neurons, one afferent (sensory) and one efferent (motor), across a single synapse. The deep tendon reflexes in the arms and legs are such monosynaptic reflexes. They illustrate the simplest unit of sensory and motor function. Other reflexes are polysynaptic, involving interneurons interposed between sensory and motor neurons.

To elicit a deep tendon reflex, briskly tap the tendon of a partially stretched muscle. For the reflex to occur, all components of the reflex arc must be intact: sensory nerve fibers, spinal cord synapse, motor nerve fibers, neuromuscular junction, and muscle fibers. Tapping the tendon activates special sensory fibers in the partially stretched muscle, triggering a sensory impulse that travels to the spinal cord via a peripheral nerve. The stimulated sensory fiber synapses directly with the anterior horn cell innervating the same muscle. When the impulse crosses the neuromuscular junction, the muscle suddenly contracts, completing the reflex arc.

Because each deep tendon reflex involves specific spinal segments, together with their sensory and motor fibers, an abnormal reflex can help you locate a pathologic lesion. Learn the segmental levels of the deep tendon reflexes. You can remember them easily by their numerical sequence in ascending order from ankle to triceps: S1–L2, L3, L4–C5, C6, C7.

Deep Tendon Reflexes

Ankle reflex	Sacral 1 primarily
Knee reflex	Lumbar 2, 3, 4
Supinator (brachioradialis) reflex	Cervical 5, 6
Biceps reflex	Cervical 5, 6
Triceps reflex	Cervical 6, 7

Reflexes may be initiated by stimulating skin as well as muscle. Stroking the skin of the abdomen, for example, produces a localized muscular twitch. Superficial (cutaneous) reflexes and their corresponding spinal segments include the following:

Cutaneous Stimulation Reflexes

Abdominal reflexes—upper	Thoracic 8, 9, 10
—lower	Thoracic 10, 11, 12
Plantar responses	Lumbar 5, Sacral 1
Anal reflex	Sacral 2, 3, 4

The Health History

Common or Concerning Symptoms

▶ Headache
▶ Dizziness or vertigo
▶ Generalized, proximal, or distal weakness
▶ Numbness, abnormal or loss of sensations
▶ Loss of consciousness, syncope, or near-syncope
▶ Seizures
▶ Tremors or involuntary movements

Two of the most common symptoms in neurologic disorders are *headache* and *dizziness*. Review the discussions of these symptoms in Chapter 7, Head and Neck.

See Chapter 7, Head and Neck, pp. 205–291.

Headache. Headaches have many causes, ranging from benign to life threatening, and always warrant careful assessment. Headaches from neurologic causes such as subarachnoid hemorrhage, meningitis, or mass lesions are especially ominous. The wise clinician pursues the complaint of headache with attention to the history and a careful neurologic examination.

See Table 7-1, Primary Headaches, p. 259, and Table 7-2, Secondary Headaches, pp. 260–261.

Primary headaches include migraine, tension, cluster, and chronic daily headaches; *secondary headaches* arise from underlying structural, systemic, or infectious causes and may be life threatening.[6–9]

Always assess the severity of the headache and its location, duration, and any associated symptoms such as double vision, visual changes, weakness, or loss of sensation. Is the headache exacerbated by coughing, sneezing, or sudden head movements, which can increase intracranial pressure? Is there fever, stiff neck, or a parameningeal focus like ear, sinus, or throat infection that may signal meningitis?

Subarachnoid hemorrhage often presents as "the worst headache of my life."[10–12] Severe headache and stiff neck accompany *meningitis*.[13,14] Dull headache increased by coughing and sneezing, especially in the same location, occurs in mass lesions from *brain tumors* or *abscess*.

An atypical presentation of the patient's usual migraine may be suspicious for stroke, especially in women using hormonal contraceptives.[15–18]

Migraine headache is often preceded by an aura or prodrome. Migraine is highly likely if three of the five "POUND" features are present: **P**ulsatile or throbbing; **O**ne-day duration, or lasts 4 to 72 hours if untreated; **U**nilateral; **N**ausea or vomiting; **D**isabling or intensity causing interruption of daily activity.[19–22]

Always look for unusual headache warning signs, such as sudden onset "like a thunderclap," onset after age 50 years, and associated symptoms such as fever and stiff neck. Examine for papilledema and focal neurologic signs.

See table on "Headache Warning Signs" on p. 206 in Chapter 7.

Dizziness or Vertigo. As you learned in Chapter 7, Head and Neck, *dizziness* and *light-headedness* are common, somewhat vague, complaints that prompt a more specific history and a careful neurologic examination focusing on the presence of nystagmus and focal neurologic signs. Especially in older patients, be sure to ask about medications.

Feeling light-headed, weak in the legs, or about to faint points to *presyncope* from arrhythmia, orthostatic hypotension, vasovagal stimulation, or side effects from blood pressure and other medications.

Does the patient feel faint or ready to fall or pass out (*presyncope*)? Or unsteady and off balance (*disequilibrium* or *ataxia*)? Or is there *true vertigo*, a spinning sensation within the patient or of the surroundings. If there is true vertigo, establish the time course of symptoms, which is helpful for distinguishing types of peripheral vestibular disorders.

Vertigo often reflects vestibular disease, usually from peripheral causes in the inner ear such as *benign positional vertigo, labyrinthitis,* and *Ménière's disease.*

See Table 7-4, Dizziness and Vertigo, p. 263, for distinguishing symptoms and time course.

If there are localizing symptoms or signs like double vision (*diplopia*), difficulty forming words (*dysarthria*), or problems with gait or balance (*ataxia*), investigate the central causes of vertigo.

Ataxia, diplopia, and dysarthria are suspicious for vertebrobasilar *transient ischemic attack* or *stroke*.[23–26] Also consider *posterior fossa tumor* and *vertebrobasilar* or *hemicranial migraine*.[27]

See Table 17-2 , Types of Stroke, pp. 746–747.

Weakness. Weakness is another common symptom with many causes and which bears careful investigation. Elicit a full history to clarify what the patient means—fatigue, apathy, drowsiness, or actual loss of strength. In true motor weakness, the cause may involve a nerve, the neuromuscular junction, or a muscle. Time course and location are especially important. Is the onset sudden, gradual or subacute, or chronic, over a long period of time?

Abrupt onset of motor and sensory deficits occurs in *transient ischemic attack* and *stroke*.[23–26,28] Progressive subacute onset of distal lower extremity weakness suggests *Guillain–Barré syndrome.* Chronic, more gradual, onset of weakness in the lower extremities can be seen in metastatic cord lesions and lumbar disc disease.

What areas of the body are involved? Is the weakness generalized, or focal to the face or a limb? Does it involve one side of the body or both sides? What movements are affected? As you listen to the patient's story, identity the patterns below:

Focal or asymmetric weakness has many causes, both central (ischemic, thrombotic, or mass lesions) and peripheral, which range from nerve injury to the neuromuscular junction disorders, to *myopathies,* or intrinsic muscle diseases.

Proximal—in the shoulder or hip girdle, for example

Distal—in the hands or feet

Symmetric—in the same areas on both sides of the body

Asymmetric—types of weakness include focal, in a portion of the face or extremity; monoparesis, in an extremity; paraparesis, in both extremities; and hemiparesis, in one side of the body

To identify *proximal weakness,* ask about difficulty with movements such as combing hair, reaching up to a shelf, getting up out of a chair, or climbing a high step. Does the weakness get worse with repetition and improve after rest? Are there associated sensory or other symptoms?

Proximal limb weakness, usually symmetric and without sensory loss, occurs in myopathies from alcohol, drugs like glucocorticoids, and inflammatory muscle disorders like *myositis* and *dermatomyositis.* In the neuromuscular junction disorder *myasthenia gravis,* there is proximal typically asymmetric weakness that gets worse with effort (fatigability), often with associated *bulbar symptoms* such as diplopia, ptosis, dysarthria, and dysphagia.[29]

To identify *distal weakness,* ask about hand movements when opening a jar or can or using scissors or a screwdriver, or problems such as tripping when walking.

Bilateral predominantly distal weakness suggests a *polyneuropathy,* as in diabetes.

Loss of Sensation. In a patient who reports numbness, ask the patient to be more precise. Is there tingling like "pins and needles," altered sensations called paresthesias, distorted sensations or dysesthesias, or is sensation completely absent?

Sensory changes may arise at several levels: local nerve compression or "entrapment," seen in hand numbness in distributions specific to the median, ulnar, or radial nerve; nerve root compression with dermatomal sensory loss from vertebral bone spurs or herniated discs; or central lesions from *stroke* or *multiple sclerosis*.

In dysesthesias, light touch or pinprick, for example, may cause a burning or irritating sensation.

Burning pain occurs in painful *sensory neuropathies* from conditions like diabetes.[30]

Establish the pattern of sensory loss. Is there a stocking-glove distribution? Are sensory deficits patchy, nondermatomal, and occurring in more than one limb?

A pattern of stocking, then glove, sensory loss occurs in *polyneuropathies*, especially from diabetes; multiple patchy areas of sensory loss in different limbs suggest *mononeuritis multiplex*, seen in diabetes and rheumatoid arthritis.

Transient Loss of Consciousness (Syncope or Fainting). Patient reports of fainting or "passing out" are common and warrant a meticulous history to guide management and assess for possible hospital admission.[31] Begin by finding out exactly what the patient means. Did the patient hear external noise or voices throughout the episode, feel light-headed or weak, but fail to actually lose consciousness, consistent with near syncope or presyncope? Or did the patient actually experience complete loss of consciousness, a case of true syncope, defined as a sudden but temporary loss of consciousness and postural tone from transient global hypoperfusion to the brain?

See Table 17-3, Syncope and Similar Disorders, pp. 748–749.

Causes include seizures, "neurocardiogenic" or *vasovagal syncope, orthostatic hypotension*, and cardiac disease including arrhythmias, especially ventricular tachycardia and bradyarrhythmias. Stroke or subarachnoid hemorrhage are unlikely to cause syncope unless there are focal findings and damage to both hemispheres.

Elicit a complete description of the event. What was the patient doing when the episode occurred? Was the patient standing, sitting, or lying down? Were there any triggers or warning symptoms? How long did the episode last? Could voices still be heard? Importantly, were onset and offset slow or fast? Were there any palpitations? Is there a history of heart disease, which has a sensitivity and specificity for a cardiac cause of over 85%?[32]

Ask if anyone observed the episode, and consider the possibility of a seizure based on the features described in the following section.

In *vasovagal syncope*, a common cause of syncope, look for a prodrome of nausea, diaphoresis, and pallor triggered by a fearful or unpleasant event, then vagally mediated hypotension, often with slow onset and offset. In syncope from arrhythmias, onset and offset are often sudden, reflecting loss and recovery of cerebral perfusion.

Seizures. Patients may recount spells or faints that raise suspicion of seizure, a sudden excessive electrical discharge from cortical neurons. Seizures may be symptomatic, with an identifiable cause, or idiopathic. A careful history is important to rule out other causes of loss of consciousness and acute symptomatic seizures that have discernible explanations.

If there is more than one seizure, consider epilepsy, defined as two or more seizures that are not provoked by other illnesses or circumstances.[34] The incidence of epilepsy in the United States is 3%; in over 60% to 70% of affected patients, no cause is identified.

Epilepsy does not always involve loss of consciousness, depending on the type. It is usually classified as generalized or partial, based on the where in the cortex seizure activity is initiated. If available, ask a witness what the patient looked like before, during, and after the episode. Was there any seizurelike movement of the arms or legs? Any incontinence of the bladder or bowel? What about any drowsiness or impaired memory after the event?

Ask about age at onset, frequency, change in frequency or symptom pattern, and use of medications, alcohol, or illicit drugs. Check for any history of head injury.

Tremors. Tremor, "a rhythmic oscillatory movement of a body part resulting from the contraction of opposing muscle groups," is the most common movement disorder.[35] It may be an isolated finding or part of a neurologic disorder. Ask about any tremor, shaking, or body movements that the patient seems unable to control. Does the tremor occur at rest? Does it get worse with voluntary intentional movement or with sustained postures?

Distinct from these symptoms is restless legs syndrome, present in 6% to 12% of the U.S. population, often with an unpleasant sensation in the legs, especially at night, that gets worse during rest and improves with activity.

See Table 17-4, Seizure Disorders, pp. 750–751.

Common causes of *acute symptomatic seizures* include head trauma; alcohol, cocaine, and other drugs; withdrawal from alcohol, benzodiazepines, and barbiturates; metabolic insults from low or high glucose or low calcium or sodium; acute stroke; and meningitis or encephalitis.[33]

Tonic–clonic motor activity, bladder or bowel incontinence, and *postictal state* characterize generalized seizures. Unlike syncope, tongue biting or bruising of limbs may occur.

Epilepsy is more common in infants and older adults. The baseline neurologic examination is frequently normal.

Generalized epilepsy syndromes usually begin in childhood or adolescence; adult seizures are usually partial.

See Table 17-5, Tremors and Involuntary Movements, pp. 752–753.

Low-frequency unilateral resting tremor, rigidity, and bradykinesia typify *Parkinson disease*.[36–38] *Essential tremors* are high-frequency, bilateral, upper extremity tremors that occur with both limb movement and sustained posture; head, voice, and leg tremor may also be present.[35]

Reversible causes include pregnancy, renal disease, and iron deficiency.[39]

Health Promotion and Counseling: Evidence and Recommendations

Important Topics for Health Promotion and Counseling

▶ Preventing stroke or transient ischemic attack (TIA)
▶ Reducing risk of peripheral neuropathy
▶ Preventing the "three D's": delirium, dementia, and depression

Preventing Stroke and Transient Ischemic Attack (TIA). Stroke from cerebrovascular disease is the third leading cause of death in the United States and the leading cause of long-term disability in the workforce and general population.[40] *Stroke* is a sudden neurologic deficit caused by cerebrovascular ischemia (87%) or hemorrhage (13%). *Hemorrhagic strokes* may be intracerebral (10% of all strokes) or subarachnoid (3% of all strokes).

See Table 17-2, Types of Stroke, pp. 746–747.

New definitions of ischemic stroke and TIA, established in 2009, are important for clinical assessment and stroke prevention; of note, diagnoses are no longer time-based. Pointing to scientific advances in imaging, the American Heart Association (AHA) and the American Stroke Association (ASA) issued tissue-based definitions that encourage early neurodiagnostic imaging and risk stratification for TIA.[41]

● *Ischemic stroke* is "an infarction of central nervous system tissue" that may be symptomatic or silent. "Symptomatic ischemic strokes are manifest by clinical signs of focal or global cerebral, spinal, or retinal dysfunction caused by central nervous system infarction. A silent stroke is a documented central nervous system infarction that was asymptomatic."

● *TIA* is now defined as "a transient episode of neurological dysfunction caused by focal brain, spinal cord, or retinal ischemia, without acute infarction." The 2009 guidelines recommend neurodiagnostic imaging within 24 hours of symptom onset and routine noninvasive imaging of the carotid and intracranial vessels.

The AHA/ASA report cites the well-validated ABCD2 scoring system for early prediction of stroke 2, 7, and 90 days after TIA: **A**ge >60 years; initial **B**lood pressure >140/90; **C**linical features of focal weakness or impaired speech without focal weakness; **D**uration up to or more than 60 minutes; and **D**iabetes.[42]

TIAs are a major risk factor for subsequent stroke: 5% of patients have a stroke within 2 days and 10% within 90 days. Stroke risk is highest in those with age greater than 60 years, diabetes, focal symptoms of weakness or impaired speech, and a TIA lasting more than 10 minutes. An additional 15% of patients with TIA have other adverse outcomes within 90 days, including death in over 2% and a recurrent TIA in over 12%.[40,43]

Stroke at a Glance

Key Facts for Prevention and Patient Education

▶ Stroke affects 7,000,000 Americans at a cost of $40 billion annually.

▶ Stroke prevalence and mortality are disproportionately higher in *African Americans*, compared to whites:

  ▶ *Prevalence, black vs. white men:* 4.5% vs. 2.4%; black vs. white women 4.4% vs. 3.3%

  ▶ *Mortality per 100,000, black vs. white men*—67 vs. 40; black vs. white women—55 vs. 40

▶ The prevalence of silent stroke increases progressively from 11% between ages 55 and 64 to 43% after age 85.

▶ Individuals with TIA have a 1-year mortality of ~12%, and a 10-year risk of stroke and death from cardiovascular disease of 19% and 43%.

▶ *Women* ages 45 to 54 are twice as likely as men to report previous stroke. Midlife risk factors now include autoimmune collagen vascular disease and history of preeclampsia, gestational diabetes, and pregnancy-induced hypertension.

▶ Public awareness of stroke warning signs is improving, but only 17% of the U. S. population are aware of correct warning signs and would call 911 if they thought someone was having a stroke.

▶ Stroke outcomes markedly improve if therapy is given within 3 hours of onset of symptoms; however, the median emergency room arrival time from symptom onset is 3 to 6 hours.

▶ Physician awareness of warning signs, risk factors, and prevention remains insufficient.

Source: Roger VL, Go AS, Lloyd-Jones DM, et al. Heart disease and stroke statistics–2011 update: a report from the American Heart Association. *Circulation* 2001;123:e18–e209. Rosamond W, Flegal K, Friday G, et al. Heart disease and stroke statistics—2007 update: a report from the American Heart Association Statistics Committee and Stroke Statistics Subcommittee. Circulation 2007;115:e69–e171.

Cardiovascular disease, including stroke, is the greatest contributor to the 6-year disparity in life expectancy for African Americans compared to whites.[44] Other contributing factors include a higher prevalence of hypertension, diabetes, left ventricular hypertrophy, and income and insurance gaps.[45–47]

See Chapter 9, Cardiovascular System, for discussion of the AHA/ASA 2011 guidelines for preventing cardiovascular disease in women that address the increased risk of midlife stroke and death from coronary heart disease, pp. 350–351.[48–50]

See also table on American Heart Association Cardiovascular Risk Categories for Women 2011, p. 351. Note that preeclampsia increases risk of hypertension 3- to 6-fold and risk of diabetes 3- to 4-fold, both stroke risk factors.[41]

Symptoms and signs of stroke depend on the vascular territory affected in the brain. The most common cause of ischemic symptoms is occlusion of the *middle cerebral artery,* which causes visual field cuts and contralateral hemiparesis and sensory deficits. Occlusion of the left middle cerebral artery often produces *aphasia*; and occlusion of the right middle cerebral artery, *neglect* or *inattention* to the opposite side of the body.

See Table 17-2, Types of Stroke, pp. 746–747.

See p. 154 in Chapter 5 and Table 17-6, Disorders of Speech, p. 754, for discussion of *aphasia.*

Stroke Warning Signs. The AHA and the ASA urge patients to seek immediate care for any of the warning signs below. You should teach these to your patients.

AHA/ASA Stroke Attack Warning Signs

▶ Sudden numbness or weakness of the face, arm, or leg

▶ Sudden confusion, trouble speaking or understanding

▶ Sudden trouble seeing in one or both eyes

▶ Sudden trouble walking, dizziness, or loss of balance or coordination

▶ Sudden severe headache

Stroke Risk Factors—Primary Prevention.   Recognizing that stroke and coronary heart disease share common cardiovascular risk factors and threats to health, in 2010, Healthy People 2020 and the AHA presented a new concept of "cardiovascular health" that encompasses seven health behaviors and health factors, and a new set of combined impact goals for the coming decade:

By 2020, to improve the cardiovascular health of all Americans by 20%, while reducing deaths from cardiovascular disease and stroke by 20%.[51,52]

For primary prevention, target both modifiable and disease-specific risk factors, detailed in the table to follow. Modifiable risk factors for *ischemic stroke* are hypertension, smoking, hyperlipidemia, diabetes, excess weight, lack of exercise, and heavy alcohol use. Careful management of the disease-specific risk factors, namely atrial fibrillation and carotid artery disease, also reduce risk of stroke.[53] Learn the indications for using aspirin in healthy and diabetic individuals.[54–56]

For prevention of *hemorrhagic stroke*, optimal blood pressure control is essential. The additional risk factors for the most common cause of hemorrhagic stroke, ruptured aneurysms in the circle of Willis, are familiar— smoking and alcohol use, as well as family history in a first-degree relative.

See Chapter 9, Cardiovascular System, for discussion of the new, more aggressive, guidelines for cardiovascular screening and the table on cardiovascular health behaviors and health factors, pp. 352–354.

Stroke Risk Factors—Primary Prevention for Ischemic Stoke

Behavioral Risk Factors

▶ **Hypertension** Hypertension is the leading risk factor for both ischemic and hemorrhagic stroke. Individuals with blood pressure <120/80 have roughly half the lifetime risk of stroke compared to those with hypertension. Optimal blood pressure control in African Americans and older adults leads to significant reduction in stroke risk.

▶ **Smoking** Smoking doubles the risk of ischemic stroke and triples the risk of subarachnoid hemorrhage. It takes 5 years for ex-smokers to drop to the same risk level as nonsmokers.

▶ **Dyslipidemia** Growing evidence from cardiovascular studies using statin agents shows that reducing dyslipidemia reduces stroke risk by up to 20%.

▶ **Diabetes** Stroke risk doubles in individuals with impaired glucose tolerance and triples in those with diabetes. Reasonable goals are blood pressure <130/80 and HgA1C of 7%. Statin therapy is also beneficial if LDL is ≥ 160.

▶ **Weight** Obesity doubles risk of stroke.

▶ **Exercise** As with coronary heart disease, hypertension, and diabetes, moderate exercise like brisk walking for 150 minutes a week or 30 minutes on most days improves cardiovascular health.

(continued)

Stroke Risk Factors—Primary Prevention for Ischemic Stoke *(continued)*

▷ **Alcohol use**   Heavy alcohol use has a direct dose-dependent effect on the risk of hemorrhagic stroke and appears to increase risk of ischemic stroke through the interaction of its effects on hypertension, hypercoagulable states, cardiac arrhythmias, and reductions in cerebral blood flow.

Disease-Specific Risk Factors

▷ **Atrial fibrillation**   Valvular (rheumatic) and nonvalvular atrial fibrillation increases risk of stroke 5- and 17-fold, respectively, compared to controls. Risk for ischemic stroke with warfarin therapy and aspirin therapy are ~68% and ~20%, but individual risk levels are variable. When considering antithrombotic therapy, experts recommend individual risk stratification into high-, moderate-, and low-risk groups to balance risk of stroke against risk of bleeding. CHADS2 is a commonly used scoring system based on **C**ongestive heart failure, **H**ypertension, **A**ge >75 years, **D**iabetes, and prior **S**troke/TIA. Patients with atrial fibrillation at highest risk are those with additional stroke risk factors: prior TIA or stroke, hypertension, diabetes, poor left ventricular function, rheumatic mitral valve disease, and women over age 75.

▷ **Carotid artery disease**   The prevalence of atherosclerotic carotid artery disease of the extracranial carotid arteries in the U.S. population over age 65 is 1%. Medical therapy in individuals with asymptomatic carotid artery stenosis of 60% to 70% has improved, with an annual stroke rate of 1% annually. Experts recommend risk factor reduction and medical therapy, reserving endarterectomy and stenting for highly selected individuals. In 2007, the U.S. Preventive Services Task Force recommended against screening the general population due to lack of evidence that use of duplex ultrasonography reduces stroke.

Sources: Roger VL, Go AS, Lloyd-Jones DM, et al. Heart disease and stroke statistics–2011 update: a report from the American Heart Association. Circulation 2011;123:e18–e209; Goldstein LB, Bushnell CD, Adams RJ, et al. Guidelines for the primary prevention of stroke. A guideline for healthcare professionals from the American Heart Association/American Stroke Association. Stroke 2001;42:517–584; Straus SE, Majumdar SR, McAlister FA. New evidence for stroke prevention. Scientific review. JAMA 2002;288:1388–1395; Wolff T, Guirgulis-Blake J, Miller T, et al. Screening for carotid artery stenosis: an update of the evidence for the U.S. Preventive Services Task Force. Ann Intern Med 2007;147:860–870.

TIA and Stroke—Secondary Prevention. For the patient who has already suffered TIA or stroke, focus on identifying causes, reducing cardiovascular risk factors, and minimizing risk of recurrence. Note that "stroke in a young person" often involves unusual causes such as collagen vascular disease, Takayasu's arteritis, cervical or cerebral artery dissection, or cocaine and illicit drug use.[57] As you gain clinical experience, you will turn to the literature on management, treatment, and rehabilitation in this group of patients.[24,58–60] Learn the indications for secondary prevention with aspirin or anticoagulants.[54,56,61,62]

History, onset, medications review, and careful neurologic examination for level of consciousness and focal findings are essential for diagnosis, followed by neuroimaging to distinguish ischemic from hemorrhagic stroke.

Categories of ischemic stroke include large artery atherosclerotic infarction whether extracranial, intracranial, artery-to-artery embolic, or thrombotic in situ; cardiac embolism; small vessel lacunar disease; unusual causes such as dissection, hypercoagulable states, and paradoxical embolisms through the foramen ovale; and cryptogenic (cause undetermined).[63]

Reducing Risk of Diabetic Peripheral Neuropathy. Diabetes causes several types of peripheral neuropathy. The most common is *distal symmetric sensorimotor polyneuropathy*, which is slowly progressive and asymptomatic in up to 50% of patients, increasing risk of foot injury and amputation.[64] Those with symptoms report burning electrical pain in the lower extremities, usually at night. Diabetic patients and clinicians should examine the diabetic's feet frequently. Clinicians should promote optimal glycemic control and monitor vibration perception with a 128-Hz tuning fork and plantar pressure sensation with a 5.07 Semmes-Weinstein monofilament.[5] Maintaining HgA1C at $\leq 7.4\%$ reduces the odds of onset of neuropathy by 60%.[65] Other diabetic neuropathies are *autonomic dysfunction, mononeuritis multiplex,* and *diabetic amyotrophy*, which can cause thigh pain and proximal lower extremity weakness, initially unilateral.

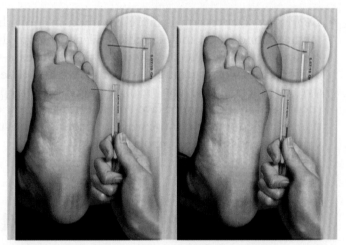

PRESS THE PERPENDICULAR MONOFILAMENT AGAINST THE SKIN AT THE GREAT TOE AND METATARSALS UNTIL IT BENDS. THIS TEST IS POSITIVE IF THE PATIENT CANNOT FEEL THE MONOFILAMENT.

Preventing the "Three D's": Delirium, Dementia, and Depression. Delirium and dementia are increasingly common in clinical practice, with subtle presentations that call for early detection as you assess cognition and mental status. Depression may compound the difficulties of diagnosis. Review the discussion of these disorders in Chapter 20, Assessing the Older Adult, and Chapter 5, Mental Status and Behavior. Brief summaries are provided here:

See Chapter 20, Assessing Older Adults, pp. 939–940, and Table 20-4, Delirium and Dementia, p. 964.

See also Chapter 5, Behavior and Mental Status, pp. 141–169.

- *Delirium.* Delirium, a multifactorial syndrome, is an acute confusional state marked by sudden onset, fluctuating course, inattention, and, at times, changes in level of consciousness. Prevalence is 30% in hospitalized adults age 70 years and older. A useful schema distinguishes predisposing from precipitating factors. Since over 50% of cases are undetected, and delirium is highly associated with poor patient outcomes, screening with the Confusional Assessment Method (CAM) algorithm is recommended.[66] In a recent review of 11 instruments, the CAM had the best supportive data for bedside use and takes only 5 minutes.[67] In 2011, the National Institutes of Health (NIH) issued clinical excellence guidelines for prevention that feature successful multicomponent interventions by interdisciplinary teams that target key clinical precipitants.[68]

● *Dementia.* Dementia is increasingly prevalent, affecting up to 5 million Americans, but underdiagnosed in primary care offices.[69,70] Assessing dementia is complex, and involves teasing out distinguishing age-related changes in cognition from mild cognitive impairment and Alzheimer disease.[71] A 2011 NIH review states that "currently, firm conclusions cannot be drawn about the association of any modifiable risk factor with cognitive decline or Alzheimer disease."[72] Although research on the role of antihypertensive medication, omega-3 fatty acids, physical activity, and cognitive exercise is promising, "highly reliable consensus-based diagnostic criteria for cognitive decline, mild cognitive impairment, and Alzheimer disease are lacking, and available criteria have not been uniformly applied," including for use of pharmaceutical agents.[72,73]

The Mini-Mental State Examination, which takes 7 to 10 minutes to administer, is the best studied, and at a cutpoint of 23 to 24, has a median likelihood ratio of 6.3 for a positive test and 0.19 for a negative test.[69]

See also discussion of the Mini-Cog on p. 940 and the Mini-Cog screening tool in Table 20-5, Screening for Dementia: The Mini-Cog, on p. 965.

● *Depression.* Depression is more common in individuals with significant medical conditions, including several neurologic disorders—dementia, epilepsy, multiple sclerosis, and Parkinson disease—and is also underdiagnosed. Two screening questions have a 90% sensitivity for depressive disorders: Have you been feeling down, depressed, or hopeless (depressed mood)? and, Have you felt little interest or pleasure in doing things (anhedonia)? In those who are depressed, be sure to assess suicidality and the possibility of bipolar disorder.

Techniques of Examination

Important Areas of Examination

▶ Mental status—see Chapter 5, Behavior and Mental Status
▶ Cranial nerves I through XII
▶ Motor system: muscle bulk, tone, and strength; coordination, gait, and stance
▶ Sensory system: pain and temperature, position and vibration, light touch, discrimination
▶ Deep tendon, abdominal, and plantar reflexes

Return to the three important questions that govern the neurologic examination:

● Is the mental status intact?

● Are right-sided and left-sided findings symmetric?

● If the findings are asymmetric or otherwise abnormal, does the causative lesion lie in the *central nervous system* or the *peripheral nervous system*?

In this section, you will learn the techniques for a practical and reasonably comprehensive examination of the nervous system, in accordance with recommendations of the American Academy of Neurology.[74-76] It is important to master the techniques for a thorough examination, which at first may seem both numerous and difficult. With supervision, practice, and dedication, you will come to feel comfortable evaluating neurologic symptoms and disease. Be an active learner; seek feedback from your instructors and consulting neurologists to make sure you are using skilled and proper technique. Take advantage of teaching videos available through the Web sites of the American Academy of Neurology and Wayne State University.[77,78]

The amount of detail in an appropriate neurologic examination varies widely. As you gain experience, you will find that in healthy people your examination will be relatively brief. When you detect abnormal findings, your examination will become more comprehensive. Be aware that neurologists may use many other techniques in specific situations.

For efficiency, you should integrate the neurologic assessment with other parts of your examination. Survey the patient's mental status and speech during the interview, for example, even though you may do further testing during your neurologic evaluation. Assess some of the cranial nerves as you examine the head and neck, and inspect the arms and legs for neurologic abnormalities while you also observe the peripheral vascular and musculoskeletal systems. Chapter 1 provides an outline for this kind of integrated approach. Think about and describe your findings, however, in terms of the nervous system as a whole.

See the Screening Neurologic Examination recommended by the American Academy of Neurology below.

See Chapter 1, Overview Examination and History Taking table on "The Physical Examination: Suggested Sequence," p. 17.

See also the American Academy of Neurology videotape of an even briefer screening examination for patients with no neurologic symptoms, limited to pupils, extraocular movements, facial symmetry, gait, and tandem walk, available at http://www.aan.com/globals/axon/assets/5456.mov.[79]

Guidelines for a Screening Neurologic Examination From the American Academy of Neurology

Students should be able to perform a brief screening neurologic examination that is sufficient to detect significant neurologic disease even in patients with no neurologic complaints. Although the exact sequence of such screening may vary, it should contain at least some assessment of mental status, cranial nerves, strength, gait and coordination, sensation, and reflexes. One example of a screening examination is given here.

Mental Status—level of alertness, appropriateness of responses, orientation to date and place

Cranial Nerves
- Visual acuity
- Pupillary light reflex
- Eye movements
- Hearing
- Facial strength—smile, eye closure

Motor System
- Strength—shoulder abduction, elbow extension, wrist extension, finger abduction, hip flexion, knee flexion, ankle dorsiflexion
- Gait—casual, tandem
- Coordination—fine finger movements, finger-to-nose

(continued)

Guidelines for a Screening Neurologic Examination From the American Academy of Neurology (*continued*)

Sensory System—one modality at toes—can be light touch, pain/temperature, or proprioception

Reflexes

▶ Deep tendon reflexes—biceps, patellar, Achilles

▶ Plantar responses

Note: If there is reason to suspect neurologic disease based on the patient's history or the results of any components of the screening examination, a more complete neurologic examination is necessary.

Source: Adapted from the American Academy of Neurology. Available at http://www.aan.com/globals/axon/assets/2770.pdf. Accessed January 2, 2008.

Whether you conduct a comprehensive or screening examination, organize your thinking into five categories: (1) mental status, speech, and language; (2) cranial nerves; (3) the motor system; (4) the sensory system; and (5) reflexes. If your findings are abnormal, begin to group them into patterns of central or peripheral disorders.

THE CRANIAL NERVES

Overview. The examination of the cranial nerves (abbreviated as CN) can be summarized as follows.

Summary: Cranial Nerves I–XII

I	Smell
II	Visual acuity, visual fields, and ocular fundi
II, III	Pupillary reactions
III, IV, VI	Extraocular movements
V	Corneal reflexes, facial sensation, and jaw movements
VII	Facial movements
VIII	Hearing
IX, X	Swallowing and rise of the palate, gag reflex
V, VII, X, XII	Voice and speech
XI	Shoulder and neck movements
XII	Tongue symmetry and position

Cranial Nerve I—Olfactory. Test the *sense of smell* by presenting the patient with familiar nonirritating odors. First, be sure that each nasal passage is open by compressing one side of the nose and asking the patient to sniff through the other. The patient should then close both eyes. Occlude one nostril and test smell in the other with such substances as cloves,

Loss of smell occurs in sinus conditions, head trauma, smoking, aging, and the use of cocaine and in *Parkinson disease.*

coffee, soap, or vanilla. Avoid noxious triggers like ammonia that might stimulate CN V. Ask if the patient smells anything and, if so, what. Test the other side. A person normally perceives odor on each side and can often identify it.

Cranial Nerve II—Optic. Test visual acuity.

See Chapter 7, Head and Neck, for more detailed discussion of examination techniques for Visual Acuity and Visual Fields, pp. 221–223, Pupils, pp. 225–226, and optic fundi, including use of the ophthalmoscope, pp. 228–232.

Inspect the optic fundi with your ophthalmoscope, paying special attention to the optic discs.

Inspect each disc carefully for bulging and blurred margins (*papilledema*); pallor (*optic atrophy*); and cup enlargement (*glaucoma*).

Test the visual fields by confrontation. Occasionally, in stroke patients for example, patients will complain of partial loss of vision, and testing of both eyes reveals a *visual field defect*, or abnormality in peripheral vision, such as *homonymous hemianopsia*. Testing one eye would not confirm the finding.

See Table 7-6, Visual Field Defects, p. 265. Look for prechiasmal, or anterior, defects seen in *glaucoma, retinal emboli, optic neuritis* (visual acuity poor); bitemporal hemianopsias from defects at the optic chiasm, usually from *pituitary tumor*; homonymous hemianopsias or quadrantanopsia in postchiasmal lesions, usually in the *parietal lobe*, with associated findings of stroke (visual acuity normal).[80]

Cranial Nerves II and III—Optic and Oculomotor. Inspect the size and shape of the pupils, and compare one side with the other. *Anisocoria*, or a difference of >0.4 mm in the diameter of one pupil compared to the other, is seen in up to 38% of healthy individuals. Test the *pupillary reactions to light*.

See Table 7-10, Pupillary Abnormalities, p. 269. If the large pupil reacts poorly to light or anisocoria worsens in light, the large pupil has abnormal pupillary constriction, seen in *CN III palsy*. If ptosis and ophthalmoplegia also present, consider *intracranial aneurysm* if patient awake, and *transtentorial herniation* if patient comatose.

Also check the *near response* (p. 220), which tests pupillary constriction (pupillary constrictor muscle), convergence (medial rectus muscles), and accommodation of the lens (ciliary muscle).

If both pupils react to light and anisocoria worsens in darkness, the small pupil has abnormal pupillary dilation, seen in *Horner's syndrome* and *simple anisocoria*.[80]

Cranial Nerves III, IV, and VI—Oculomotor, Trochlear, and Abducens. Test the *extraocular movements* in the six cardinal directions of gaze, and look for loss of conjugate movements in any of the six directions, which causes *diplopia*. Ask the patient which direction makes the diplopia worse and inspect the eye closely for asymmetric deviation of movement. Determine if the diplopia is *monocular* or *binocular* by asking the patient to cover one eye, or perform the cover–uncover test.

See Chapter 7, Head and Neck (pp. 226–228) for a more detailed discussion of techniques for testing extraocular movements.

See Table 7-11, Dysconjugate Gaze, p. 270. Monocular diplopia is seen in local problems with glasses or contact lenses, cataracts, astigmatism, or ptosis. Binocular diplopia occurs in *CN III, IV, VI neuropathy* (40% of patients), eye muscle disease from *myasthenia gravis, trauma, thyroid ophthalmopathy, and internuclear ophthalmoplegia.*[80]

Check convergence of the eyes.

Identify any *nystagmus*, an involuntary jerking movement of the eyes with quick and slow components. Note the direction of gaze in which it appears, the plane of the nystagmus (horizontal, vertical, rotary, or mixed), and the direction of the quick and slow components. *Nystagmus is named for the direction of the quick component.* Ask the patient to fix his or her vision on a distant object and observe if the nystagmus increases or decreases.

See Table 17-7, Nystagmus, pp. 755–756. Nystagmus is seen in *cerebellar disease*, especially with gait ataxia and dysarthria (increases with retinal fixation), and *vestibular disorders* (decreases with retinal fixation); and in *internuclear ophthalmoplegia.*

Look for *ptosis* (drooping of the upper eyelids). A slight difference in the width of the palpebral fissures may be a normal variation in approximately one-third of all people.

Ptosis suggests *3rd nerve palsy* (CN III), *Horner's syndrome* (ptosis, meiosis, anhidrosis), or *myasthenia gravis.*

Cranial Nerve V—Trigeminal

Motor. While palpating the temporal and masseter muscles in turn, ask the patient to clench the teeth. Note the strength of muscle contraction. Ask the patient to move the jaw side to side.

Difficulty clenching the jaw or moving it to the opposite side occurs in masseter and lateral pterygoid weakness, respectively.

Look for unilateral weakness in CN V pontine lesions; bilateral weakness in bilateral hemispheric disease.

Central nervous system patterns from stroke include ipsilateral facial and body sensory loss from contralateral cortical or thalamic lesion; ipsilateral face but contralateral body sensory loss in brainstem lesions.

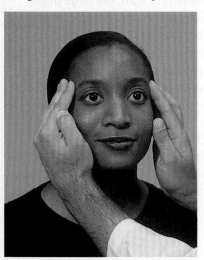

PALPATING TEMPORAL MUSCLES

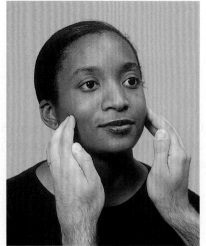

PALPATING MASSETER MUSCLES

Sensory. After explaining what you plan to do, test the forehead, cheeks, and jaw on each side for *pain sensation*. Suggested areas are indicated by the circles. The patient's eyes should be closed. Use a suitable sharp object, occasionally substituting the blunt end for the point as a stimulus. Ask the patient to report whether it is "sharp" or "dull" and to compare sides.

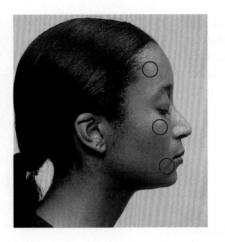

Isolated facial sensory loss occurs in peripheral nerve disorders like *trigeminal neuralgia.*

To avoid transmitting infection, use a new object for each patient. You can create a sharp wood splinter by breaking or twisting a cotton swab. The cotton end of the swab can also be used as a dull stimulus.

If you find an abnormality, confirm it by testing *temperature sensation.* Two test tubes, filled with hot and ice-cold water, are the traditional stimuli. A tuning fork may also be used. It usually feels cool. If you are near running water, the fork is easily made colder or warm. Dry it before use. Touch the skin and ask the patient to identify "hot" or "cold."

Then test for *light touch*, using a fine wisp of cotton. Ask the patient to respond whenever you touch the skin.

Corneal Reflex. Test the *corneal reflex.* Ask the patient to look up and away from you. Approaching from the other side, out of the patient's line of vision, and avoiding the eyelashes, touch the cornea (not just the conjunctiva) lightly with a fine wisp of cotton. If the patient is apprehensive, however, first touching the conjunctiva may allay fear.

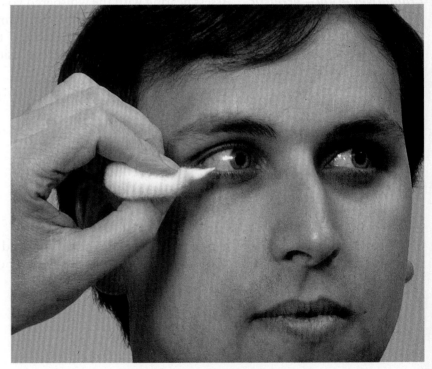

Look for blinking of the eyes, the normal reaction to this stimulus. The sensory limb of this reflex is carried in CN V, and the motor response, in CN VII. Use of contact lenses frequently diminishes or abolishes this reflex.

Blinking is absent in lesions of CN V or VII. Absent blinking and sensorineural hearing loss occur in *acoustic neuroma.*

Cranial Nerve VII—Facial. Inspect the face, both at rest and during conversation with the patient. Note any asymmetry (e.g., of the nasolabial folds), and observe any tics or other abnormal movements.

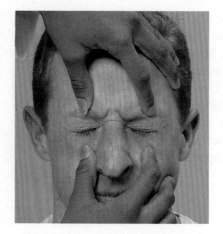

Ask the patient to:

1. Raise both eyebrows.

2. Frown.

3. Close both eyes tightly so that you cannot open them. Test muscular strength by trying to open them, as illustrated.

4. Show both upper and lower teeth.

5. Smile.

6. Puff out both cheeks.

Flattening of the nasolabial fold and drooping of the lower eyelid suggest facial weakness.

A peripheral injury to CN VII, also seen in *Bell's palsy*, affects both the upper and lower face; a central lesion affects mainly the lower face. Loss of taste, hyperacusis, and increased or decreased tearing also occur in *Bell's palsy*.[81] See Table 17-8, Types of Facial Paralysis, p. 757.

In unilateral facial paralysis, the mouth droops on the paralyzed side when the patient smiles or grimaces.

Cranial Nerve VIII—Acoustic. Assess hearing with the whispered voice test. If hearing loss is present, determine if the loss is *conductive*, from impaired "air through ear" transmission, or *sensorineural*, from damage to the cochlear branch of CN VIII. Test for *air and bone conduction*, using the Rinne test, and *lateralization*, using the Weber test.

The whispered voice test is both sensitive (>90%) and specific (>80%) when assessing presence or absence of hearing loss.[80]

See techniques for Weber and Rinne tests on pp. 237–238 and Table 7-21, Patterns of Hearing Loss, p. 281.

Excess cerumen, otosclerosis, and *otitis media* cause conductive hearing loss; *presbyacusis* from aging commonly reflects sensorineural hearing loss.

Specific tests of the vestibular function of CN VIII are rarely included in the typical neurologic examination. Consult textbooks of neurology or otolaryngology as the need arises.

Vertigo with hearing loss and nystagmus typifies *Ménière's disease.* See Table 7-4, Dizziness and Vertigo, p. 263, and Table 17-7, Nystagmus, pp. 755–756. For caloric stimulation testing of comatose patients, see pp. 736–737.

Cranial Nerves IX and X—Glossopharyngeal and Vagus. Listen to the patient's *voice*. Is it hoarse, or does it have a nasal quality?

Hoarseness occurs in vocal cord paralysis; nasal voice in paralysis of the palate.

Is there difficulty in swallowing?

Difficulty swallowing suggests pharyngeal or palatal weakness.

Ask the patient to say "ah" or to yawn as you watch the *movements of the soft palate and the pharynx*. The soft palate normally rises symmetrically, the uvula remains in the midline, and each side of the posterior pharynx moves medially, like a curtain. The slightly curved uvula seen occasionally as a normal variation should not be mistaken for a uvula deviated by a lesion of CN X.

The palate fails to rise with a bilateral lesion of CN X. In unilateral paralysis, one side of the palate fails to rise and, together with the uvula, is pulled toward the normal side (see p. 247 in Chapter 7).

Warn the patient that you are going to test the *gag reflex*, which consists of elevation of the tongue and soft palate and constriction of the pharyngeal muscles. Stimulate the back of the throat lightly on each side in turn and note the gag reflex. Many normally healthy people have a diminished gag reflex.

Unilateral absence of this reflex suggests a lesion of CN IX, and perhaps CN X.

Cranial Nerve XI—Spinal Accessory.   From behind, look for atrophy or fasciculations in the trapezius muscles, and compare one side with the other. Fasciculations are fine flickering irregular movements in small groups of muscle fibers. Ask the patient to shrug both shoulders upward against your hands. Note the strength and contraction of the trapezii.

Trapezius weakness with atrophy and fasciculations indicates a peripheral nerve disorder. In trapezius muscle paralysis, the shoulder droops, and the scapula is displaced downward and laterally.

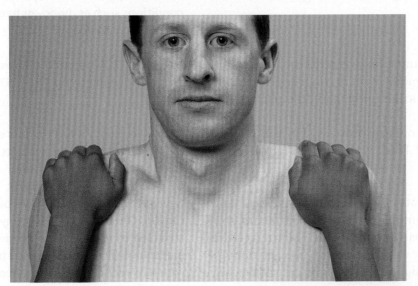

Ask the patient to turn his or her head to each side against your hand. Observe the contraction of the opposite sternomastoid and note the force of the movement against your hand.

A supine patient with bilateral weakness of the sternomastoids has difficulty raising the head off the pillow.

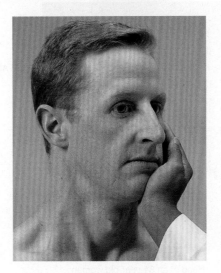

Cranial Nerve XII—Hypoglossal.   Listen to the articulation of the patient's words. This depends on CN V, VII, and X, as well as XII. Inspect the patient's tongue as it lies on the floor of the mouth. Look for any atrophy or fasciculations. Some coarser restless movements are often seen in a normal tongue. Then, with the patient's tongue protruded, look for

For poor articulation, or *dysarthria*, see Table 17-6, Disorders of Speech (p. 754). Tongue atrophy and fasciculations occur in *amyotrophic lateral sclerosis*, and *polio*.

asymmetry, atrophy, or deviation from the midline. Ask the patient to move the tongue from side to side, and note the symmetry of the movement. In ambiguous cases, ask the patient to push the tongue against the inside of each cheek in turn as you palpate externally for strength.

In a unilateral cortical lesion, the protruded tongue deviates transiently in a direction away from the side of the cortical lesion, toward the side of weakness.

THE MOTOR SYSTEM

As you assess the motor system, focus on body position, involuntary movements, characteristics of the muscles (bulk, tone, and strength), and coordination. These components are described below in sequence. You may either use this sequence or check each component in the arms, legs, and trunk in turn. If you see an abnormality, identify the muscle(s) involved. Determine whether the abnormality is central or peripheral in origin, and begin to learn which nerves innervate the affected muscles.

Body Position. Observe the patient's body position during movement and at rest.

Abnormal positions alert you to conditions such as mono- or hemiparesis from stroke.

Involuntary Movements. Watch for involuntary movements such as tremors, tics, or fasciculations. Note their location, quality, rate, rhythm, and amplitude, and their relation to posture, activity, fatigue, emotion, and other factors.

See Table 17-5, Tremors and Involuntary Movements, pp. 752–753.

Muscle Bulk. Inspect the size and contours of muscles. Do the muscles look flat or concave, suggesting atrophy? If so, is the process unilateral or bilateral? Is it proximal or distal?

When looking for atrophy, pay particular attention to the hands, shoulders, and thighs. The thenar and hypothenar eminences should be full and convex, and the spaces between the metacarpals, where the dorsal interosseous muscles lie, should be full or only slightly depressed. However, atrophy of hand muscles may occur with normal aging, as shown on the right below.

Muscular *atrophy* refers to a loss of muscle bulk, or wasting. It results from diseases of the peripheral nervous system such as diabetic neuropathy, as well as diseases of the muscles themselves. *Hypertrophy* is an increase in bulk with proportionate strength, whereas increased bulk with diminished strength is called *pseudohypertrophy*, seen in the *Duchenne form of muscular dystrophy*.

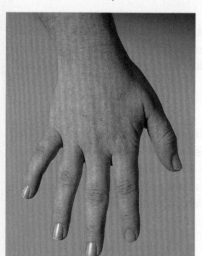

Hand of a 44-year-old woman

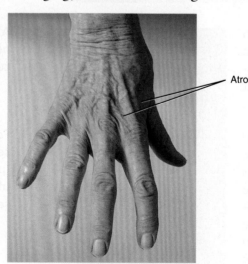

Hand of an 84-year-old woman

Atrophy

Flattening of the thenar and hypothenar eminences and furrowing between the metacarpals suggest atrophy. Localized atrophy of the thenar and hypothenar eminences occurs in median and ulnar nerve damage, respectively.

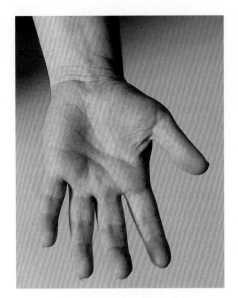
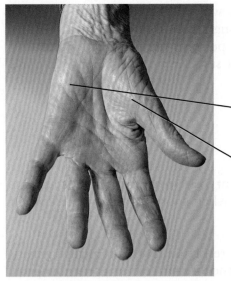

Hypothenar eminence

Flattening of the thenar
eminence due to mild atrophy

Hand of a 44-year-old woman

Hand of an 84-year-old woman

Other causes of muscular atrophy
include motor neuron diseases,
disease affecting the peripheral
motor system projecting from the
spinal cord, and protein–calorie
malnutrition.

Be alert for fasciculations in atrophic muscles. If absent, tap on the muscle
with a reflex hammer to try to stimulate them.

Fasciculations with atrophy and
muscle weakness suggest disease
of the peripheral motor unit.

Muscle Tone.   When a normal muscle with an intact nerve supply is relaxed
voluntarily, it maintains a slight residual tension known as *muscle tone*. This
can be assessed best by feeling the muscle's resistance to passive stretch.
Persuade the patient to relax. Take one hand with yours and, while supporting the elbow, flex and extend the patient's fingers, wrist, and elbow, and
put the shoulder through a moderate range of motion. With practice, these
actions can be combined into a single smooth movement. On each side,
note muscle tone—the resistance offered to your movements. Tense patients
may show increased resistance. With repeated practice, you will learn the feel
of normal resistance.

Decreased resistance suggests
disease of the peripheral nervous
system, cerebellar disease, or the
acute stages of spinal cord injury.
See Table 17-9, Disorders of Muscle
Tone, p. 758.

If you suspect decreased resistance, hold the forearm and shake the hand
loosely back and forth. Normally the hand moves back and forth freely but
is not completely floppy.

Marked floppiness indicates muscle
hypotonia or *flaccidity*, usually from
a disorder of the peripheral motor
system.

If resistance is increased, determine whether it varies as you move the limb
or whether it persists throughout the range of movement and in both directions, as for example, during both flexion and extension. Feel for any jerki-
ness in the resistance.

To assess muscle tone in the legs, support the patient's thigh with one hand,
grasp the foot with the other, and flex and extend the patient's knee and
ankle on each side. Note the resistance to your movements.

Spasticity is velocity-dependent
increased tone that worsens at
the extremes of range. Spasticity,
seen in central corticospinal tract
diseases, is rate-dependent, increasing with rapid movement. *Rigidity*
is increased resistance throughout
the range of movement and in both
directions; it is not rate-dependent.

Muscle Strength. Normal people vary widely in their strength, and your standard of normal, while admittedly rough, should allow for such variables as age, sex, and muscular training. A person's dominant side is usually slightly stronger than the nondominant side. Keep this difference in mind when you compare sides.

Test muscle strength by asking the patient to actively resist your movement. Remember that a muscle is strongest when shortest, and weakest when longest.

If the muscles are too weak to overcome resistance, test them against gravity alone or with gravity eliminated. When the forearm rests in a pronated position, for example, dorsiflexion at the wrist can be tested against gravity alone. When the forearm is midway between pronation and supination, extension at the wrist can be tested with gravity eliminated. Finally, if the patient fails to move the body part, watch or feel for weak muscular contraction.

Impaired strength is called weakness, or *paresis*. Absence of strength is called paralysis, or plegia. *Hemiparesis* refers to weakness of one-half of the body; *hemiplegia* to paralysis of one-half of the body. *Paraplegia* means paralysis of the legs; *quadriplegia* means paralysis of all four limbs.

See Table 17-1, Disorders of the Central and Peripheral Nervous Systems, pp. 744–745.

Scale for Grading Muscle Strength

Muscle strength is graded on a 0 to 5 scale:
0—No muscular contraction detected
1—A barely detectable flicker or trace of contraction
2—Active movement of the body part with gravity eliminated
3—Active movement against gravity
4—Active movement against gravity and some resistance
5—Active movement against full resistance without evident fatigue. This is normal muscle strength.

Source: Medical Research Council. Aids to the examination of the peripheral nervous system. London: Bailliere Tindall, 1986.

More experienced clinicians make further distinctions by using plus or minus signs toward the stronger end of this scale. Thus 4+ indicates good but not full strength, while 5–; means a trace of weakness.

Methods for testing the major muscle groups are described in the following text. The spinal root innervations and the muscles affected are shown in parentheses. To localize lesions in the spinal cord or the peripheral nervous system more precisely, additional testing may be necessary. For these specialized methods, refer to texts of neurology.

Test flexion (C5, C6—biceps) *and extension* (C6, C7, C8—triceps) *at the elbow* by having the patient pull and push against your hand.

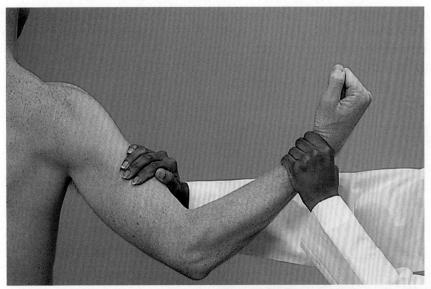

FLEXION AT ELBOW

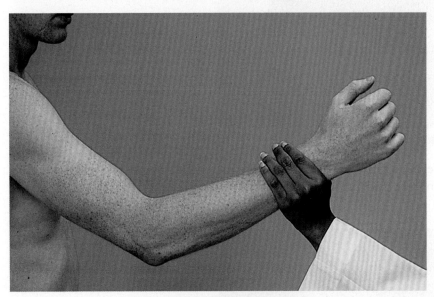

EXTENSION AT ELBOW

Test extension at the wrist (C6, C7, C8, radial nerve—extensor carpi radialis longus and brevis) by asking the patient to make a fist and resist your pulling it down.

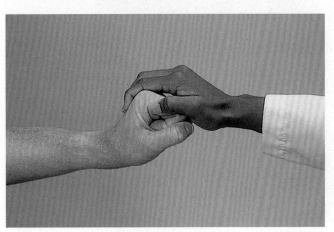

EXTENSION AT WRIST

Weakness of extension is seen in peripheral nerve disease, from radial nerve damage, and in central nervous system disease, producing hemiplegia, seen in *stroke* or *multiple sclerosis*.

Test the grip (C7, C8, T1). Ask the patient to squeeze two of your fingers as hard as possible and not let them go. (To avoid getting hurt by hard squeezes, place your own middle finger on top of your index finger.) You should normally have difficulty removing your fingers from the patient's grip. Testing both grips simultaneously with arms extended or in the lap facilitates comparison.

A weak grip is seen in cervical radiculopathy, *de Quervain's tenosynovitis*, *carpal tunnel syndrome*, arthritis, and epicondylitis.

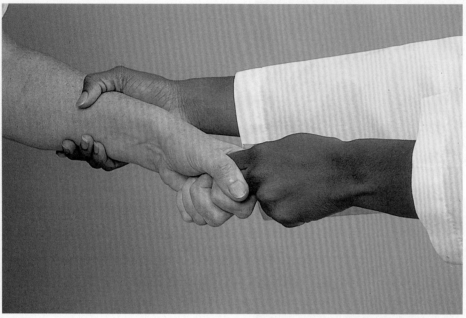

TEST OF GRIP

Test finger abduction (C8, T1, ulnar nerve). Position the patient's hand with palm down and fingers spread. Instructing the patient not to let you move the fingers, try to force them together.

Weak finger abduction occurs in ulnar nerve disorders.

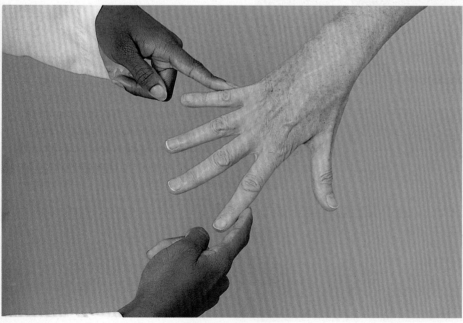

FINGER ABDUCTION

Test opposition of the thumb (C8, T1, median nerve). The patient should try to touch the tip of the little finger with the thumb, against your resistance.

Look for weak opposition of the thumb in median nerve disorders such as *carpal tunnel syndrome* (see p. 634 in Chapter 16).

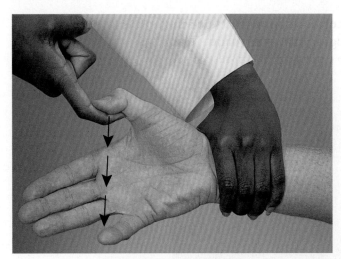

OPPOSITION OF THE THUMB

You may already have assessed *muscle strength of the trunk* during other segments of the examination, namely:

● Flexion, extension, and lateral bending of the spine, and

● Thoracic expansion and diaphragmatic excursion during respiration.

Test flexion at the hip (L2, L3, L4—iliopsoas) by placing your hand on the patient's thigh and asking the patient to raise the leg against your hand.

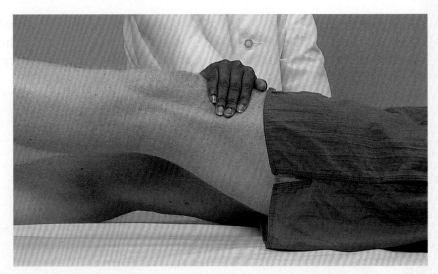

FLEXION OF THE HIP

Test adduction at the hips (L2, L3, L4—adductors). Place your hands firmly on the bed between the patient's knees. Ask the patient to bring both legs together.

Symmetric weakness of the proximal muscles suggests a *myopathy*; symmetric weakness of distal muscles suggests a *polyneuropathy*, or disorder of peripheral nerves.

Test abduction at the hips (L4, L5, S1—gluteus medius and minimus). Place your hands firmly on the bed outside the patient's knees. Ask the patient to spread both legs against your hands.

Test extension at the hips (S1—gluteus maximus). Have the patient push the posterior thigh down against your hand.

Test extension at the knee (L2, L3, L4—quadriceps). Support the knee in flexion and ask the patient to straighten the leg against your hand. The quadriceps is the strongest muscle in the body, so expect a forceful response.

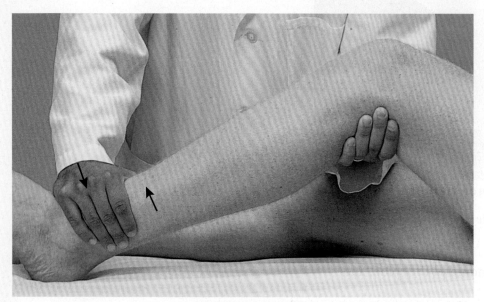

EXTENSION AT THE KNEE

Test flexion at the knee (L4, L5, S1, S2—hamstrings) as shown below. Place the patient's leg so that the knee is flexed with the foot resting on the bed. Tell the patient to keep the foot down as you try to straighten the leg.

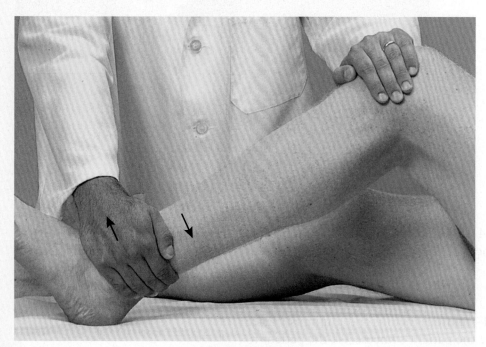

FLEXION AT THE KNEE

Test dorsiflexion (mainly L4, L5—tibialis anterior) and *plantar flexion* (mainly S1—gastrocnemius, soleus) at the ankle by asking the patient to pull up and push down against your hand.

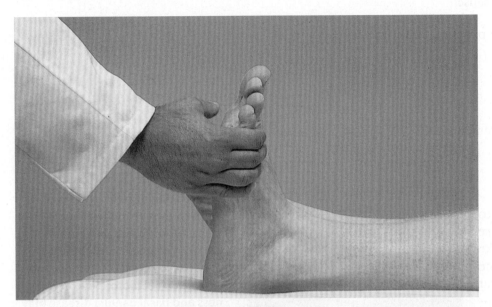

DORSIFLEXION AT THE ANKLE

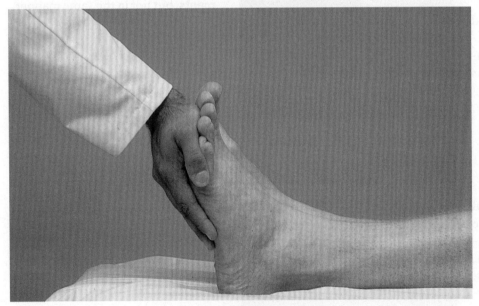

PLANTAR FLEXION AT THE ANKLE

Coordination. Coordination of muscle movement requires that four areas of the nervous system function in an integrated way:

● The motor system, for muscle strength

● The cerebellar system (also part of the motor system), for rhythmic movement and steady posture

In cerebellar disease, look for nystagmus, dysarthria, hypotonia, and ataxia.

- The vestibular system, for balance and for coordinating eye, head, and body movements

- The sensory system, for position sense

To assess coordination, observe the patient's performance in:

- Rapid alternating movements

- Point-to-point movements

- Gait and other related body movements

- Standing in specified ways

Rapid Alternating Movements

Arms. Show the patient how to strike one hand on the thigh, raise the hand, turn it over, and then strike the back of the hand down on the same place. Urge the patient to repeat these alternating movements as rapidly as possible.

Observe the speed, rhythm, and smoothness of the movements. Repeat with the other hand. The nondominant hand often performs somewhat less well.

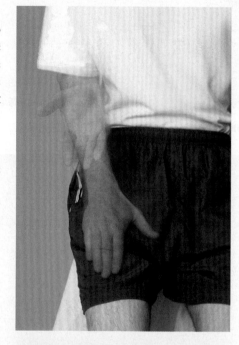

In cerebellar disease, one movement cannot be followed quickly by its opposite and movements are slow, irregular, and clumsy. This abnormality is called *dysdiadochokinesis.* Upper motor neuron weakness and basal ganglia disease may also impair rapid alternating movements, but not in the same manner.

Show the patient how to tap the distal joint of the thumb with the tip of the index finger, again as rapidly as possible. Again, observe the speed, rhythm, and smoothness of the movements. The nondominant side often performs less well.

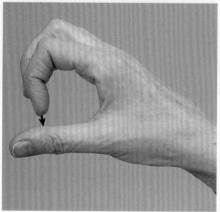

Legs. Ask the patient to tap your hand as quickly as possible with the ball of each foot in turn. Note any slowness or awkwardness. The feet normally perform less well than the hands.

Dysdiadochokinesis occurs in cerebellar disease.

Point-to-Point Movements

Arms—Finger-to-Nose Test. Ask the patient to touch your index finger and then his or her nose alternately several times. Move your finger about so that the patient has to alter directions and extend the arm fully to reach it. Observe the accuracy and smoothness of movements, and watch for any tremor. Normally the patient's movements are smooth and accurate.

In cerebellar disease, movements are clumsy, unsteady, and inappropriately varying in their speed, force, and direction. The finger may initially overshoot its mark, but finally reaches it fairly well, termed *dysmetria*. An *intention tremor* may appear toward the end of the movement. See Table 17-5, Tremors and Involuntary Movements, p. 752.

Now hold your finger in one place so that the patient can touch it with one arm and finger outstretched. Ask the patient to raise the arm overhead and lower it again to touch your finger. After several repeats, ask the patient to close both eyes and try several more times. Repeat on the other side. Normally a person can touch the examiner's finger successfully with eyes open or closed. These maneuvers test position sense and the functions of both the labyrinth and the cerebellum.

Cerebellar disease causes incoordination that worsens with eyes closed. If present, this suggests loss of position sense. Repetitive and consistent deviation to one side, referred to as *past pointing*, worse with the eyes closed, suggests cerebellar or vestibular disease.

Legs—Heel-to-Shin Test. Ask the patient to place one heel on the opposite knee, and then run it down the shin to the big toe. Note the smoothness and accuracy of the movements. Repetition with the patient's eyes closed tests for position sense. Repeat on the other side.

In cerebellar disease, the heel may overshoot the knee and then oscillate from side to side down the shin. When position sense is lost, the heel is lifted too high and the patient tries to look. With eyes closed, performance is poor.

Gait. Ask the patient to:

Abnormalities of gait increase risk of falls.

- *Walk across the room* or down the hall, then turn, and come back. Observe posture, balance, swinging of the arms, and movements of the legs. Normally balance is easy, the arms swing at the sides, and turns are accomplished smoothly.

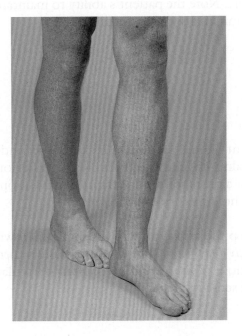

A gait that lacks coordination, with reeling and instability, is called *ataxic*. Ataxia may be due to cerebellar disease, loss of position sense, or intoxication. See Table 17-10, Abnormalities of Gait and Posture, p. 759.

- *Walk heel-to-toe* in a straight line—a pattern called *tandem walking*.

Tandem walking may reveal an ataxia not previously obvious.

- *Walk on the toes*, then *on the heels*—sensitive tests, respectively, for plantar flexion and dorsiflexion of the ankles, as well as for balance.

Walking on toes and heels may reveal distal muscular weakness in the legs. Inability to heel-walk is a sensitive test for corticospinal tract damage.

- *Hop in place* on each foot in turn (if the patient is not too ill). Hopping involves the proximal muscles of the legs as well as the distal ones and requires both good position sense and normal cerebellar function.

Difficulty with hopping may be due to weakness, lack of position sense, or cerebellar dysfunction.

- *Do a shallow knee bend,* first on one leg, then on the other. Support the patient's elbow if you think the patient is in danger of falling.

Difficulty in doing a shallow knee bend suggests proximal weakness (extensors of the hip), weakness of the quadriceps (the extensor of the knee), or both.

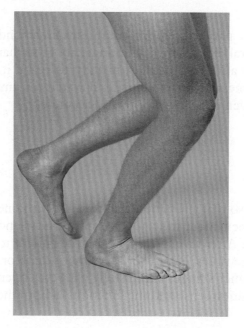

- *Rising from a sitting position* without arm support and *stepping up* on a sturdy stool are more suitable tests than hopping or knee bends when patients are old or less robust.

Proximal muscle weakness involving the pelvic girdle and legs causes difficulty with both of these activities.

Stance.   The following two tests can often be performed concurrently. They differ only in the patient's arm position and in what you are assessing. In each case, stand close enough to the patient to prevent a fall.

The Romberg Test.   This is mainly a test of position sense. The patient should first stand with feet together and eyes open and then close both eyes for 30 to 60 seconds without support. Note the patient's ability to maintain an upright posture. Normally only minimal swaying occurs.

In ataxia from dorsal column disease and loss of position sense, vision compensates for the sensory loss. The patient stands fairly well with eyes open but loses balance when they are closed, a *positive Romberg sign.* In *cerebellar ataxia,* the patient has difficulty standing with feet together whether the eyes are open or closed.

Test for Pronator Drift.   The patient should stand for 20 to 30 seconds with both arms straight forward, palms up, and with eyes closed. A person who cannot stand may be tested for a pronator drift in the sitting position. In either case, a normal person can hold this arm position well.

Now, instructing the patient to keep the arms up and eyes shut, as shown on the next page, *tap the arms briskly downward.* The arms normally return smoothly to the horizontal position. This response requires muscular strength, coordination, and a good sense of position.

Pronator drift is the pronation of one forearm. It is both sensitive and specific for a corticospinal tract lesion originating in the contralateral hemisphere. Downward drift of the arm with flexion of fingers and elbow may also occur.[82]

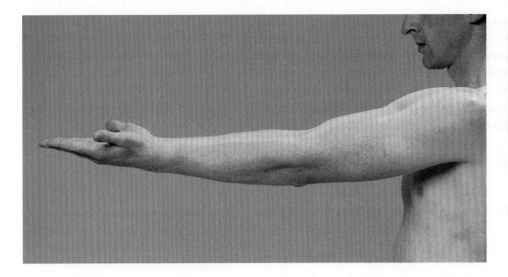

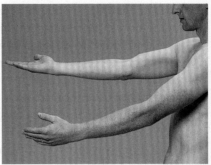

A sideward or upward drift, sometimes with searching, writhing movements of the hands, suggests loss of position sense; the patient may not recognize the displacement and, if told to correct it, does so poorly. In cerebellar incoordination, the arm returns to its original position but overshoots and bounces.

THE SENSORY SYSTEM

To evaluate the sensory system, you will test several kinds of sensation:

- Pain and temperature (spinothalamic tracts)

- Position and vibration (posterior columns)

- Light touch (both of these pathways)

- Discriminative sensations, which depend on some of the above sensations but also involve the cortex

Familiarize yourself with each kind of test so that you can use it as indicated. When you detect abnormal findings, correlate them with motor and reflex activity. Assess the patient carefully as you consider the following questions: Is the underlying lesion central or peripheral? Is the sensory loss bilateral or unilateral? Does it have a pattern suggesting a dermatomal distribution, a polyneuropathy, or a spinal cord syndrome with a loss of pain and temperature sensation but intact touch and vibration? To advance in physical diagnosis of nervous system disorders, you will need to work with specialists to refine your examination and learn the complex presentations of many sensory syndromes.

See Table 17-1, Disorders of the Central and Peripheral Nervous Systems, pp. 744–745.

See textbooks in Additional References, pp. 742–743, for discussion of *spinal cord syndromes* with crossed sensory findings, both ipsilateral and contralateral to the cord injury.

Patterns of Testing. Because sensory testing quickly fatigues many patients, producing unreliable results, conduct the examination as efficiently as possible. Pay special attention to those areas where there are symptoms such as numbness or pain, where there are motor or reflex abnormalities that suggest a lesion of the spinal cord or peripheral nervous system, and where there are trophic changes, such as absent or excessive sweating, atrophic skin, or cutaneous ulceration. Repeat testing at another time is often required to confirm abnormalities.

Meticulous sensory mapping helps to establish the level of a spinal cord lesion and to determine whether a more peripheral lesion is in a nerve root, a major peripheral nerve, or one of its branches.

The following patterns of testing help you to identify sensory deficits accurately and efficiently.

- *Compare symmetric areas* on the two sides of the body, including the arms, legs, and trunk.

A hemisensory loss pattern suggests a lesion in the opposite cerebral hemisphere; a sensory level suggests a spinal cord lesion.

- When testing pain, temperature, and touch sensation, also *compare the distal with the proximal areas* of the extremities. Further, scatter the stimuli so as to sample most of the dermatomes and major peripheral nerves (see pp. 723–724). One suggested pattern includes both shoulders (C4), the inner and outer aspects of the forearms (C6 and T1), the thumbs and little fingers (C6 and C8), the fronts of both thighs (L2), the medial and lateral aspects of both calves (L4 and L5), the little toes (S1), and the medial aspect of each buttock (S3).

Symmetric distal sensory loss suggests a *polyneuropathy*. You may miss this finding unless you compare distal and proximal sensation.

- When testing vibration and position sensation, first test the fingers and toes. If these are normal, you may safely assume that more proximal areas will also be normal.

- *Vary the pace of your testing.* This is important so that the patient does not merely respond to your repetitive rhythm.

- When you detect an area of sensory loss or hypersensitivity, *map out its boundaries* in detail. Stimulate first at a point of reduced sensation, and move by progressive steps until the patient detects the change. An example is shown here.

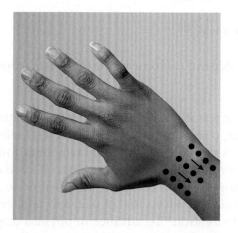

Here all sensation in the hand is lost. Repetitive testing in a proximal direction reveals a gradual change to normal sensation at the wrist. This pattern fits neither a peripheral nerve nor a dermatome (see pp. 723–724). If bilateral, it suggests the "glove and stocking" sensory loss of a *polyneuropathy*, often seen in *alcoholism* and *diabetes*.

By identifying the distribution of sensory abnormalities and the kinds of sensations affected, you can infer where the causative lesion might be. A motor deficit or reflex abnormality also helps in this localizing process.

Before each of the following tests, show the patient what you plan to do and what responses you want. Unless otherwise specified, the patient's eyes should be closed during actual testing.

Pain. Use a sharp safety pin, a broken cotton swab, or other suitable tool. Occasionally, substitute the blunt end for the point. Ask the patient, "Is this sharp or dull?" or, when making comparisons, "Does this feel the same as this?" Apply the lightest pressure needed for the stimulus to feel sharp, and try not to draw blood.

To prevent transmitting a blood-borne infection, *discard the pin or other device safely. Do not reuse it on another person.*

Temperature. Temperature testing is often omitted if pain sensation is normal, but include it if there are sensory deficits. Use two test tubes, filled with hot and cold water, or a tuning fork heated or cooled by water. Touch the skin and ask the patient to identify "hot" or "cold."

Light Touch. With a fine wisp of cotton, touch the skin lightly, avoiding pressure. Ask the patient to respond whenever a touch is felt, and to compare one area with another. Calloused skin is normally relatively insensitive and should be avoided.

Vibration. Use a relatively low-pitched tuning fork of 128 Hz. Tap it on the heel of your hand and place it firmly over a distal interphalangeal joint of the patient's finger, then over the interphalangeal joint of the big toe. Ask what the patient feels. If you are uncertain whether it is pressure or vibration, ask the patient to tell you when the vibration stops, and then touch the fork to stop it. If vibration sense is impaired, proceed to more proximal bony prominences (e.g., wrist, elbow, medial malleolus, patella, anterior superior iliac spine, spinous processes, and clavicles).

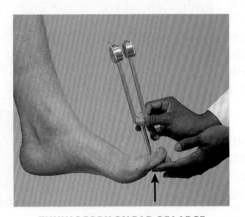

TUNING FORK ON PAD OF LARGE TOE, NOT BONE

Proprioception (Position). Grasp the patient's big toe, *holding it by its sides* between your thumb and index finger, and then pull it away from the other toes. This prevents extraneous tactile stimuli from affecting position testing. Demonstrate "up" and "down" as you move the patient's toe clearly upward and downward. Then, with the patient's eyes closed, ask for a response of "up" or "down" when moving the large toe in a small arc.

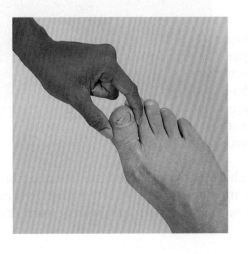

Analgesia refers to absence of pain sensation, *hypalgesia* to decreased sensitivity to pain, and *hyperalgesia* to increased sensitivity.

Anesthesia is absence of touch sensation, *hypesthesia* is decreased sensitivity, and *hyperesthesia* is increased sensitivity.

Vibration sense is often the first sensation to be lost in a peripheral neuropathy and increases the likelihood of peripheral neuropathy 16-fold.[5] Common causes include *diabetes* and *alcoholism*. Vibration sense is also lost in posterior column disease, for example, *tertiary syphilis* or *vitamin B₁₂ deficiency.*

Testing vibration sense in the trunk may be useful in estimating the level of a cord lesion.

Loss of position sense, like loss of vibration sense, is seen in *tabes dorsalis, multiple sclerosis,* or *B₁₂ deficiency* from posterior column disease, and in peripheral neuropathy from diabetes.

Repeat several times on each side, avoiding simple alternation of the stimuli. If position sense is impaired, move proximally to test it at the ankle joint. In a similar fashion, test position in the fingers, moving proximally, if indicated, to the metacarpophalangeal joints, wrist, and elbow.

Discriminative Sensations. Several additional techniques test the ability of the sensory cortex to correlate, analyze, and interpret sensations. Because discriminative sensations depend on touch and position sense, they are useful only when these sensations are either intact or only slightly impaired.

Screen a patient with *stereognosis*, and proceed to other methods if indicated. The patient's eyes should be closed during all these tests.

When touch and position sense are normal or only slightly impaired, a disproportionate decrease in, or loss of, discriminative sensations suggests disease of the sensory cortex. Stereognosis, number identification, and two-point discrimination are also impaired in posterior column disease.

- *Stereognosis.* Stereognosis refers to the ability to identify an object by feeling it. Place in the patient's hand a familiar object such as a coin, paper clip, key, pencil, or cotton ball, and ask the patient to tell you what it is. Normally a patient will manipulate it skillfully and identify it correctly within 5 seconds. Asking the patient to distinguish "heads" from "tails" on a coin is a sensitive test of stereognosis.

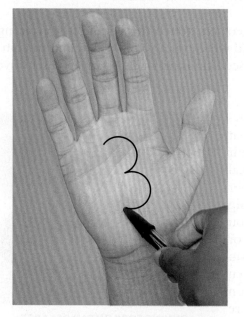

Astereognosis refers to the inability to recognize objects placed in the hand.

- *Number identification (graphesthesia).* When motor impairment, arthritis, or other conditions prevent the patient from manipulating an object well enough to identify it, test the ability to identify numbers. With the blunt end of a pen or pencil, draw a large number in the patient's palm. A normal person can identify most such numbers.

The inability to recognize numbers, or *graphesthesia*, suggests a lesion in the sensory cortex.

- *Two-point discrimination.* Using the two ends of an opened paper clip, or the sides of two pins, touch a finger pad in two places simultaneously. Alternate the double stimulus irregularly with a one-point touch. Be careful not to cause pain.

Find the minimal distance at which the patient can discriminate one from two points (normally <5 mm on the finger pads). This test may be used on other parts of the body, but normal distances vary widely from one body region to another.

Lesions of the sensory cortex increase the distance between two recognizable points.

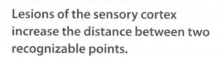

- *Point localization.* Briefly touch a point on the patient's skin. Then ask the patient to open both eyes and point to the place touched. Normally a person can do so accurately. This test, together with the test for extinction, is especially useful on the trunk and the legs.

- *Extinction.* Simultaneously stimulate corresponding areas on both sides of the body. Ask where the patient feels your touch. Normally both stimuli are felt.

Dermatomes. Knowledge of dermatomes helps you localize neurologic lesions to a specific level of the spinal cord, particularly in spinal cord injury. *A dermatome is the band of skin innervated by the sensory root of a single spinal nerve.* Dermatome patterns are mapped in the next two figures, using the

Lesions of the sensory cortex impair the ability to localize points accurately.

With lesions of the sensory cortex, only one stimulus may be recognized. The stimulus on the side opposite the damaged cortex is extinguished.

In spinal cord injury, the sensory level may be several segments *lower* than the spinal lesion, for reasons that are not well understood. Tapping for the level of vertebral pain may be helpful.[80]

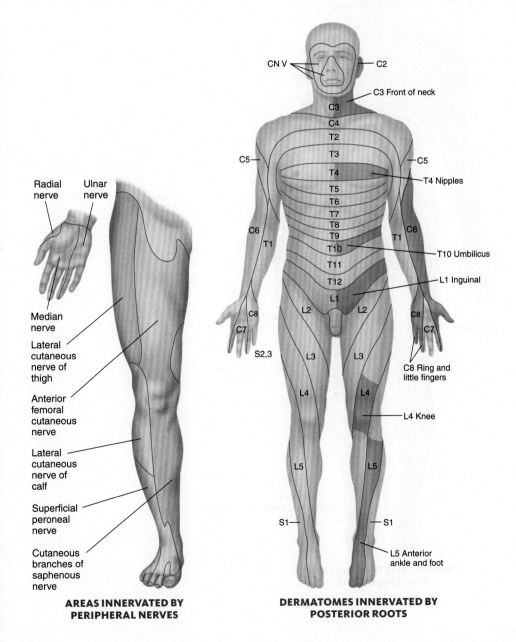

AREAS INNERVATED BY PERIPHERAL NERVES

DERMATOMES INNERVATED BY POSTERIOR ROOTS

international standard recommended by the American Spinal Injury Association.[83] Dermatome levels are more variable than these diagrams suggest. They overlap at their upper and lower margins and also slightly across the midline.

Do not try to memorize all the dermatomes. Instead, focus on learning the dermatomes shaded in green. The distribution of selected areas innervated by peripheral nerves is shown in the figures on the left.

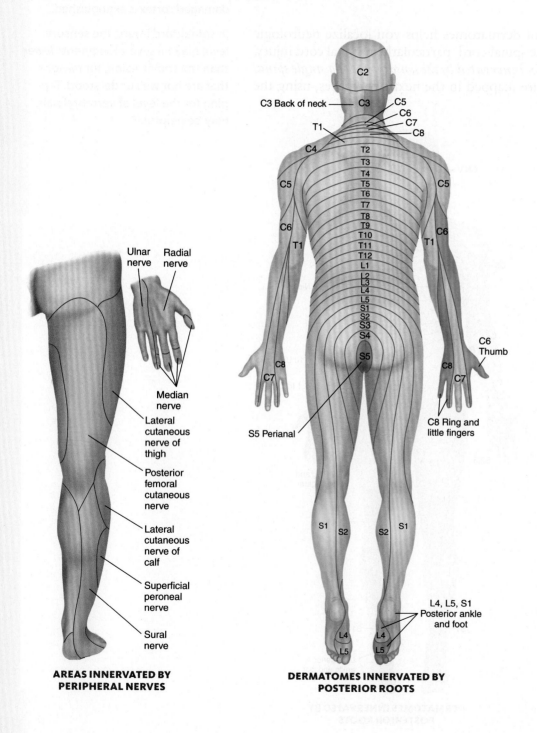

**AREAS INNERVATED BY
PERIPHERAL NERVES**

**DERMATOMES INNERVATED BY
POSTERIOR ROOTS**

DEEP TENDON REFLEXES

Eliciting the *deep tendon reflexes* involves a series of examiner skills. Be sure to select a properly weighted reflex hammer. Learn when to use either the pointed or the flat end of the hammer. For example, the pointed end is useful for striking small areas, such as your finger as it overlies the biceps tendon. Test the reflexes as follows:

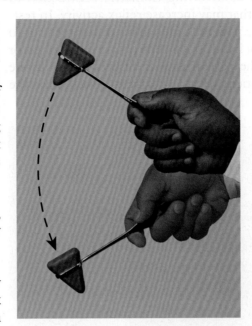

- Encourage the patient to relax, then position the limbs properly and symmetrically.

- Hold the reflex hammer loosely between your thumb and index finger so that it swings freely in an arc within the limits set by your palm and other fingers.

- With your wrist relaxed, strike the tendon briskly using a rapid wrist movement. Your strike should be quick and direct, not glancing.

- Note the speed, force, and amplitude of the reflex response and grade the response using the scale below. Always compare the response of one side with the other. Reflexes are usually graded on a 0 to 4+ scale.[84]

Hyperactive reflexes (hyperreflexia) are seen in central nervous system lesions along the descending corticospinal tract. Look for associated upper motor neuron findings of weakness, spasticity, or a positive Babinski sign.

Hypoactive or *absent reflexes (hyporeflexia)* are seen in diseases of spinal nerve roots, spinal nerves, plexuses, or peripheral nerves. Look for associated findings of lower motor unit disease, namely weakness, atrophy, and fasciculations.[80]

Scale for Grading Reflexes

4+	Very brisk, hyperactive, with *clonus* (rhythmic oscillations between flexion and extension)
3+	Brisker than average; possibly but not necessarily indicative of disease
2+	Average; normal
1+	Somewhat diminished; low normal
0	No response

Reflex response depends partly on the force of your stimulus. Use no more force than you need to provoke a definite response. Differences between sides are usually easier to assess than symmetric changes. Symmetrically diminished or even absent reflexes may be found in normal people.

Reinforcement.   If the patient's reflexes are symmetrically diminished or absent, use *reinforcement*, a technique involving isometric contraction of other muscles for up to 10 seconds that may increase reflex activity. In testing arm reflexes, for example, ask the patient to clench his or her teeth or to squeeze one thigh with the opposite hand. If leg reflexes are diminished or absent, reinforce them by asking the patient to lock fingers and pull one hand against the other. Tell the patient to pull just before you strike the tendon.

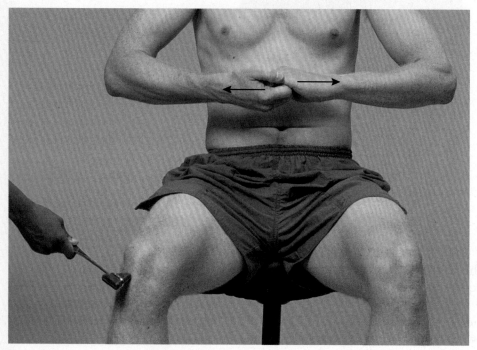

REINFORCEMENT OF KNEE REFLEX

The Biceps Reflex (C5, C6).   The patient's arm should be partially flexed at the elbow with palm down. Place your thumb or finger firmly on the biceps tendon. Strike with the reflex hammer so that the blow is aimed directly through your digit toward the biceps tendon.

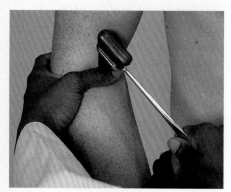

PATIENT SITTING

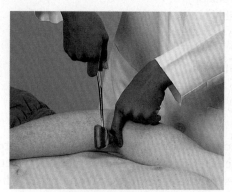

PATIENT LYING DOWN

Observe flexion at the elbow, and watch for and feel the contraction of the biceps muscle.

The Triceps Reflex (C6, C7). The patient may be sitting or supine. Flex the patient's arm at the elbow, with palm toward the body, and pull it slightly across the chest. Strike the triceps tendon above the elbow. Use a direct blow from directly behind it. Watch for contraction of the triceps muscle and extension at the elbow.

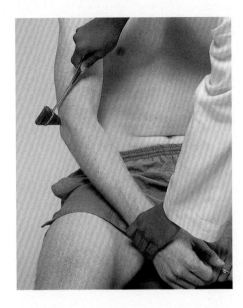
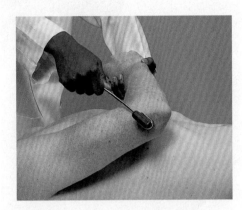

If you have difficulty getting the patient to relax, try supporting the upper arm as illustrated on the right. Ask the patient to let the arm go limp, as if it were "hung up to dry." Then strike the triceps tendon.

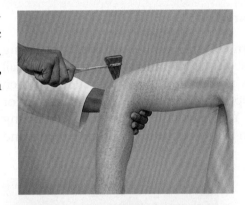

The Supinator or Brachioradialis Reflex (C5, C6). The patient's hand should rest on the abdomen or the lap, with the forearm partly pronated. Strike the radius with the point or flat edge of the reflex hammer, about 1 to 2 inches above the wrist. Watch for flexion and supination of the forearm.

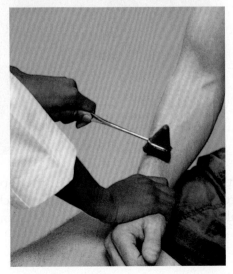

The Knee Reflex (L2, L3, L4). The patient may be either sitting or lying down as long as the knee is flexed. Briskly tap the patellar tendon just below the patella. Note contraction of the quadriceps with extension at the knee. A hand on the patient's anterior thigh lets you feel this reflex.

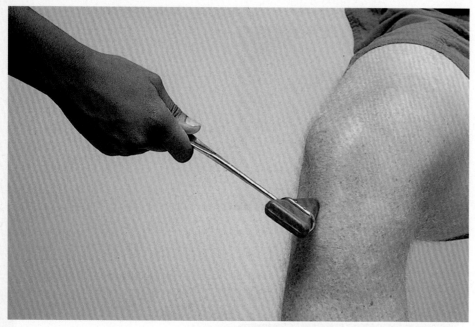

PATIENT SITTING

Two methods are useful when examining the supine patient. Supporting both knees at once, as shown below on the left, allows you to assess small differences between knee reflexes by repeatedly testing one reflex and then the other. Sometimes, however, supporting both legs is uncomfortable for both the examiner and the patient. You may wish to rest your supporting arm under the patient's leg, as shown below on the right. Some patients find it easier to relax with this method.

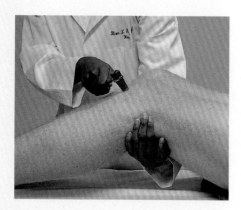 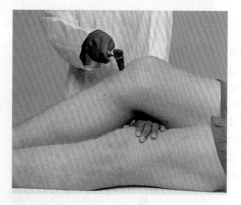

The Ankle Reflex (primarily S1). If the patient is sitting, dorsiflex the foot at the ankle. Persuade the patient to relax. Strike the Achilles tendon. Watch and feel for plantar flexion at the ankle. Note also the speed of relaxation after muscular contraction.

The slowed relaxation phase of reflexes in *hypothyroidism* is often easily seen and felt in the ankle reflex.

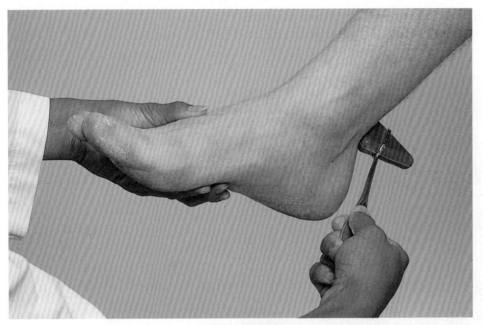

PATIENT SITTING

When the patient is lying down, flex one leg at both hip and knee and rotate it externally so that the lower leg rests across the opposite shin. Then dorsiflex the foot at the ankle and strike the Achilles tendon.

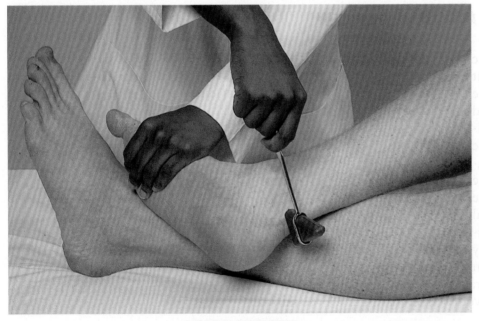

PATIENT LYING DOWN

Clonus. If the reflexes seem hyperactive, test for *ankle clonus.* Support the knee in a partly flexed position. With your other hand, dorsiflex and plantar flex the foot a few times while encouraging the patient to relax, and then sharply dorsiflex the foot and maintain it in dorsiflexion. Look and feel for rhythmic oscillations between dorsiflexion and plantar flexion. In most normal people, the ankle does not react to this stimulus. A few clonic beats may be seen and felt, especially when the patient is tense or has exercised.

Sustained clonus indicates central nervous system disease. The ankle plantar flexes and dorsiflexes repetitively and rhythmically. When clonus is present, the reflex is graded 4+ (see p. 725).

Clonus may also be elicited at other joints. A sharp downward displacement of the patella, for example, may elicit patellar clonus in the extended knee.

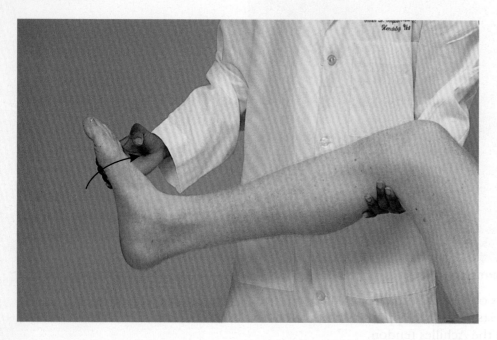

CUTANEOUS STIMULATION REFLEXES

The Abdominal Reflexes. Test the abdominal reflexes by lightly but briskly stroking each side of the abdomen, above (T8, T9, T10) and below (T10, T11, T12) the umbilicus, in the directions illustrated. Use a key, the wooden end of a cotton-tipped applicator, or a tongue blade twisted and split longitudinally. Note the contraction of the abdominal muscles and deviation of the umbilicus toward the stimulus. Obesity may mask an abdominal reflex. In this situation, use your finger to retract the patient's umbilicus away from the side to be stimulated. Feel with your retracting finger for the muscular contraction.

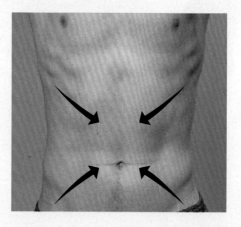

Abdominal reflexes may be absent in both central and peripheral nerve disorders.

The Plantar Response (L5, S1). With an object such as a key or the wooden end of an applicator stick, stroke the lateral aspect of the sole from the heel to the ball of the foot, curving medially across the ball. Use the lightest stimulus that will provoke a response, but be increasingly firm if necessary. Note movement of the big toe, normally plantar flexion.

Dorsiflexion of the big toe is a *positive Babinski response* from a central nervous system lesion in the corticospinal tract; it is also seen in unconscious states from drug or alcohol intoxication or in the postictal period following a seizure.

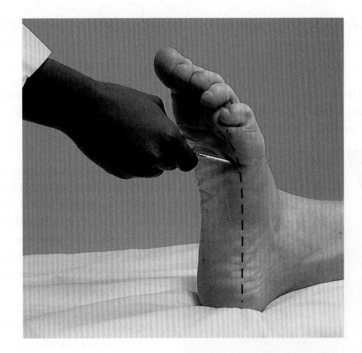

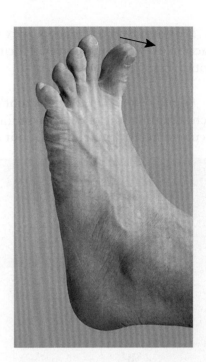

Some patients withdraw from this stimulus by flexing the hip and the knee. Hold the ankle, if necessary, to complete your observation. It is sometimes difficult to distinguish withdrawal from a Babinski response.

A marked Babinski response is occasionally accompanied by reflex flexion at hip and knee.

The Anal Reflex. Using a dull object, such as a cotton swab, stroke outward in the four quadrants from the anus. Watch for reflex contraction of the anal musculature.

Loss of the anal reflex suggests a lesion in the S2–3–4 reflex arc, is seen in cauda equina lesions.

SPECIAL TECHNIQUES

Meningeal Signs. Testing for these signs is important if you suspect meningeal inflammation from meningitis or subarachnoid hemorrhage.

Neck Mobility/Nuchal Rigidity. First, make sure there is no injury to the cervical vertebrae or cervical cord. In trauma settings, this may require evaluation by x-ray. Then, with the patient supine, place your hands behind the patient's head and flex the neck forward, until the chin touches the chest if possible. Normally the neck is supple, and the patient can easily bend the head and neck forward.

Inflammation in the subarachnoid space causes resistance to movement that stretches the spinal nerves (neck flexion), the femoral nerve (Brudzinski's sign), or the sciatic nerve (Kernig's sign).

Neck stiffness with resistance to flexion is found in 57% to 92% of patients with *acute bacterial meningitis* and 21% to 86% with *subarachnoid hemorrhage*.[80] It is most reliably present in patients with severe meningeal inflammation, but in suspected or moderate cases, sensitivity is low and specificity data is limited.[85]

Brudzinski's Sign. As you flex the neck, watch the hips and knees in reaction to your maneuver. Normally they should remain relaxed and motionless.

Flexion of both the hips and knees is a *positive Brudzinski's sign*.

Kernig's Sign. Flex the patient's leg at both the hip and the knee, and then straighten the knee. Discomfort behind the knee during full extension occurs in many normal people, but should not produce pain.

Pain and increased resistance to extending the knee are a *positive Kernig's sign*.

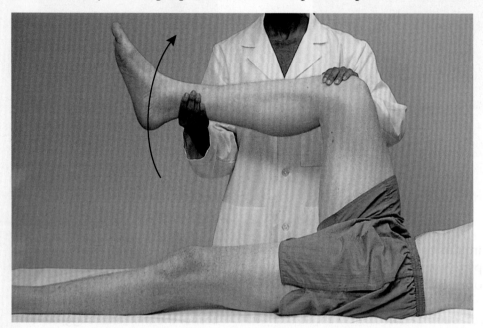

The mechanism of this sign is similar to the positive straight-leg-raise test, described on p. 733. Compression of a lumbar or sacral nerve root or the sciatic nerve causes radicular or sciatic pain radiating into the leg when the nerves are stretched as the leg is extended.

The frequency of Brudzinski's and Kernig's signs in patients with meningitis has a reported range of 5% to 60%; sensitivity is low at approximately 5% and specificity data is limited.[80,85]

Lumbosacral Radiculopathy: Straight-Leg Raise. If the patient has low back pain with nerve pain that radiates down the leg, commonly called *sciatica* if in the S_1 distribution, test straight-leg raising on each side in turn. Place the patient in the supine position. Raise the patient's relaxed and straightened leg,

See Table 16-1, Low Back Pain, p. 668.

Compression of the spinal nerve root as it passes through the vertebral foramen causes a painful *radiculopathy* with associated muscle weakness and dermatomal sensory loss, usually from a herniated disc. More than 95% of disc herniations occur at L5–S1, where the spine angles sharply posterior. Look for confirming ipsilateral calf wasting and weak ankle dorsiflexion, which make the diagnosis of sciatica five times more likely.[80]

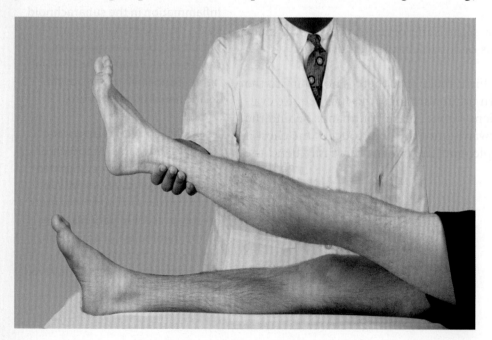

flexing the leg at the hip, then dorsiflex the foot. Some examiners first raise the patient's leg with the knee flexed, then extend the leg.

Assess the degree of elevation at which pain occurs, the quality and distribution of the pain, and the effects of dorsiflexion. Tightness or discomfort in the buttocks or hamstrings is common during these maneuvers; do not interpret this as "radiating pain" or a positive test.

Pain radiating into the ipsilateral leg is a *positive straight-leg test* for *lumbosacral radiculopathy*. Foot dorsiflexion can further increase leg pain in *lumbosacral radiculopathy, sciatic neuropathy,* or both. Increased pain when the contralateral healthy leg is raised is a *positive crossed straight-leg-raising sign*. These maneuvers stretch the affected nerve roots and sciatic nerve.

In addition, be sure to examine motor and sensory function and reflexes at the lumbosacral levels.

Sensitivity and specificity of positive ipsilateral straight-leg raise for lumbosacral radiculopathy in patients with sciatica is roughly 95% and 25%; of crossed straight-leg raise, 40% and 90%.

Asterixis. Asterixis helps identify metabolic encephalopathy in patients whose mental functions are impaired. Asterixis is caused by abnormal function of the diencephalic motor centers that regulate agonist and antagonist muscle tone and maintain posture.[86]

Sudden, brief, nonrhythmic flexion of the hands and fingers indicates asterixis, seen in liver disease, uremia, and hypercapnia.

Ask the patient to "stop traffic" by extending both arms, with hands cocked up and fingers spread. Watch for 1 to 2 minutes, coaxing the patient as necessary to maintain this position.

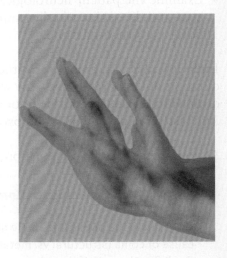

Winging of the Scapula. When the shoulder muscles seem weak or atrophic, look for winging. Ask the patient to extend both arms and push against your hand or against a wall. Observe the scapulae. Normally they lie close to the thorax.

In winging, shown next, the medial border of the scapula juts backward. It suggests weakness of the serratus anterior muscle, seen in *muscular dystrophy* or injury to the long thoracic nerve.

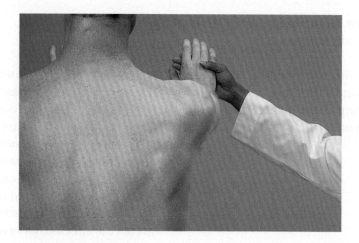

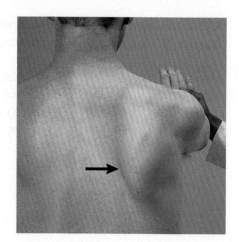

In very thin but normal people, the scapulae may appear "winged" even when the musculature is intact.

The Stuporous or Comatose Patient. Coma signals a potentially life-threatening event affecting the two hemispheres, the brainstem, or both.[87,88] The usual sequence of history, physical examination, and laboratory evaluation does not apply. Instead, you must:

- First assess the ABCs (airway, breathing, and circulation)

- Establish the patient's level of consciousness

- Examine the patient neurologically. Look for focal or asymmetric findings, and determine whether impaired consciousness arises from a metabolic or a structural cause.

Interview relatives, friends, or witnesses to establish the speed of onset and duration of unconsciousness, any warning symptoms, precipitating factors, or previous episodes, and the prior appearance and behavior of the patient. Any history of past medical and psychiatric illnesses is also useful.

As you proceed to the examination, remember two cardinal DON'Ts:

"Don'ts" When Assessing the Comatose Patient

▷ *Don't* dilate the pupils, the single most important clue to the underlying cause of coma (structural vs. metabolic), and
▷ *Don't* flex the neck if there is any question of trauma to the head or neck. Immobilize the cervical spine and get an x-ray first to rule out fractures of the cervical vertebrae that could compress and damage the spinal cord.

Airway, Breathing, and Circulation. Quickly check the patient's color and pattern of breathing. Inspect the posterior pharynx and listen over the

See Table 17-11, Metabolic and Structural Coma, p. 760.

Be familiar with the Glasgow Coma Scale.[89] See Table 17-12, Glasgow Coma Scale, p. 760.

Five clinical signs strongly predict death or poor outcome, with likelihood ratios of 5 to 12: at 24 hours—absent corneal response, absent pupillary response, absent withdrawal response to pain, no motor response; at 72 hours—no motor response.[90]

trachea for stridor to make sure the airway is clear. If respirations are slowed or shallow, or if the airway is obstructed by secretions, consider intubating the patient as soon as possible while stabilizing the cervical spine.

Assess the remaining vital signs: pulse, blood pressure, and *rectal* temperature. If hypotension or hemorrhage is present, establish intravenous access and begin intravenous fluids. (Further emergency management and laboratory studies are beyond the scope of this text.)

Level of Consciousness. Level of consciousness primarily reflects the patient's capacity for arousal, or wakefulness. It is determined by the level of activity that the patient can be aroused to perform in response to escalating stimuli from the examiner.

Five clinical levels of consciousness are described in the table below, together with related techniques for examination. Increase your stimuli in a stepwise manner, depending on the patient's response.

When you examine patients with an altered level of consciousness, describe and record exactly what you see and hear. Imprecise use of terms such as lethargy, obtundation, stupor, or coma may mislead other examiners.

Level of Consciousness (Arousal): Techniques and Patient Response

Level	Technique	
Alertness	Speak to the patient in a normal tone of voice. An alert patient opens the eyes, looks at you, and responds fully and appropriately to stimuli (arousal intact).	
Lethargy	Speak to the patient in a loud voice. For example, call the patient's name or ask "How are you?"	A lethargic patient appears drowsy but opens the eyes and looks at you, responds to questions, and then falls asleep.
Obtundation	Shake the patient gently as if awakening a sleeper.	An obtunded patient opens the eyes and looks at you but responds slowly and is somewhat confused. Alertness and interest in the environment are decreased.
Stupor	Apply a painful stimulus. For example, pinch a tendon, rub the sternum, or roll a pencil across a nail bed. (No stronger stimuli needed!)	A stuporous patient arouses from sleep only after painful stimuli. Verbal responses are slow or even absent. The patient lapses into an unresponsive state when the stimulus ceases. There is minimal awareness of self or the environment.
Coma	Apply repeated painful stimuli.	A comatose patient remains unarousable with eyes closed. There is no evident response to inner need or external stimuli.

Neurologic Evaluation

Respirations. Observe the rate, rhythm, and pattern of respirations. Because neural structures that govern breathing in the cortex and brainstem overlap those that govern consciousness, abnormalities of respiration often occur in coma.

See Table 17-11, Metabolic and Structural Coma, p. 760, and Table 4-7, Abnormalities in Rate and Rhythm of Breathing, p. 140.

Pupils. Observe the size and equality of the pupils and test their reaction to light. The presence or absence of the light reaction is one of the most important signs distinguishing structural from metabolic causes of coma. The light reaction often remains intact in metabolic coma.

See Table 17-13, Pupils in Comatose Patients, p. 761.

Structural lesions from stroke, abscess, or tumor mass may lead to asymmetrical pupils and loss of light reaction.

Ocular Movement. Observe the position of the eyes and eyelids at rest. Check for horizontal deviation of the eyes to one side (*gaze preference*). When the oculomotor pathways are intact, the eyes look straight ahead.

In structural hemispheric lesions, the eyes "look at the lesion" in the affected hemisphere.

In irritative lesions from epilepsy or early cerebral hemorrhage, the eyes "look away" from the affected hemisphere.

Oculocephalic Reflex (Doll's Eye Movements). This reflex helps to assess brainstem function in a comatose patient. Holding the upper eyelids open so that you can see the eyes, turn the head quickly, first to one side and then to the other. Make sure the patient has no neck injury before performing this test.

In a comatose patient with absence of doll's eye movements, shown below, the ability to move both eyes to one side is lost, suggesting a lesion of the midbrain or pons.

In a comatose patient with an intact brainstem, as the head is turned, the eyes move toward the opposite side (the doll's eye movements). In the adjacent photo, for example, the patient's head has been turned to the right; her eyes have moved to the left. Her eyes still seem to gaze at the camera. The doll's eye movements are intact.

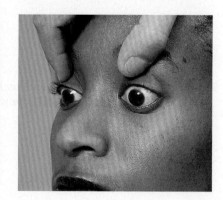

Oculovestibular Reflex (With Caloric Stimulation). If the oculocephalic reflex is absent and you seek further assessment of brainstem function, test the oculovestibular reflex. Note that this test is almost never performed in an awake patient.

Make sure the eardrums are intact and the canals clear. You must elevate the patient's head to 30 degrees to perform the test accurately. Place a kidney basin under the ear to catch any overflowing water. With a large syringe, inject ice water through a small catheter that is lying in (but not plugging) the ear canal. Watch for deviation of the eyes in the horizontal plane. You may need to use up to 120 mL of ice water to elicit a response. In the co-matose patient with an *intact brainstem*, the eyes drift *toward* the irrigated ear. Repeat on the opposite side, waiting 3 to 5 minutes if necessary for the first response to disappear.

No response to stimulation suggests brainstem injury.

Posture and Muscle Tone.   Observe the patient's posture. If there is no spon-taneous movement, you may need to apply a painful stimulus (see p. 735). Classify the resulting pattern of movement as:

See Table 17-14, Abnormal Postures in Comatose Patients, p. 762. Two stereotypic responses predominate: *decorticate rigidity* and *decerebrate rigidity.*

- *Normal–avoidant*—the patient pushes the stimulus away or withdraws.

- *Stereotypic*—the stimulus evokes abnormal postural responses of the trunk and extremities.

- *Flaccid paralysis or no response*

No response on one side suggests a corticospinal tract lesion.

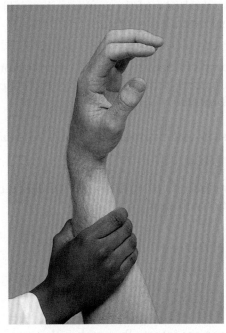

Test muscle tone by grasping each forearm near the wrist and raising it to a vertical position. Note the position of the hand, which is usually only slightly flexed at the wrist.

The hemiplegia of sudden cerebral accidents is usually flaccid at first. The limp hand drops to form a right angle with the wrist.

Then lower the arm to about 12 or 18 inches off the bed and drop it. Watch how it falls. A normal arm drops somewhat slowly.

A flaccid arm drops rapidly, like a flail.

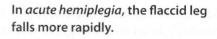
Support the patient's flexed knees. Then extend one leg at a time at the knee and let it fall (see below). Compare the speed with which each leg falls.

In *acute hemiplegia*, the flaccid leg falls more rapidly.

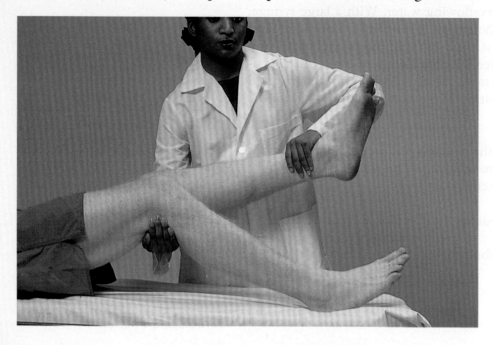

Flex both legs so that the heels rest on the bed and then release them. The normal leg returns slowly to its original extended position.

In acute hemiplegia, the flaccid leg falls rapidly into extension, with external rotation at the hip.

Further Examination.   As you complete the neurologic examination, check for facial asymmetry and asymmetries in motor, sensory, and reflex function. Test for meningeal signs if indicated.

Meningeal signs suggest *meningitis, subarachnoid hemorrhage.*[11]

As you proceed to the general physical examination, check for unusual odors.

Consider alcohol, liver failure, or uremia.

Look for abnormalities of the skin, including color, moisture, evidence of bleeding disorders, needle marks, and other lesions.

Note any jaundice, cyanosis, or the cherry red color of carbon monoxide poisoning.

Examine the scalp and skull for signs of trauma.

Look for bruises, lacerations, or swelling.

Examine the fundi carefully.

Examine closely for papilledema and hypertensive retinopathy.

Check to make sure the corneal reflexes are intact. Remember that use of contact lenses may abolish these reflexes.

Corneal reflex loss occurs in coma and lesions affecting CN V or CN VII.

Inspect the ears and nose, and examine the mouth and throat.

Blood or cerebrospinal fluid in the nose or the ears suggests a skull fracture; otitis media suggests a possible brain abscess.

Be sure to evaluate the heart, lungs, and abdomen.

Tongue injury suggests a seizure.

Recording Your Findings

Note that initially you may use sentences to describe your findings; later you will use phrases. The style below contains phrases appropriate for most write-ups. Note the five components of the examination and write-up of the nervous system.

Recording the Examination—The Nervous System

"**Mental Status:** Alert, relaxed, and cooperative. Thought process coherent. Oriented to person, place, and time. Detailed cognitive testing deferred. **Cranial Nerves:** I—not tested; II through XII intact. **Motor:** Good muscle bulk and tone. Strength 5/5 throughout. Cerebellar—Rapid alternating movements (RAMs), finger-to-nose (F→N), heel-to-shin (H→S) intact. Gait with normal base. Romberg—maintains balance with eyes closed. No pronator drift. **Sensory:** Pinprick, light touch, position, and vibration intact. **Reflexes:** 2+ and symmetric with plantar reflexes downgoing."

OR

"**Mental Status:** The patient is alert and tries to answer questions but has difficulty finding words. **Cranial Nerves:** I—not tested; II—visual acuity intact; visual fields full; III, IV, VI—extraocular movements intact; V motor—temporal and masseter strength intact, sensory corneal reflexes present; VII motor—prominent right facial droop and flattening of right nasolabial fold, left facial movements intact, sensory—taste not tested; VIII—hearing intact bilaterally to whispered voice; IX, X—gag intact; XI—strength of sternomastoid and trapezius muscles 5/5; XII—tongue midline. **Motor:** strength in right biceps, triceps, iliopsoas, gluteals, quadriceps, hamstring, and ankle flexor and extensor muscles 3/5 with good bulk but increased tone and spasticity; strength in comparable muscle groups on the left 5/5 with good bulk and tone. Gait—unable to test. Cerebellar—unable to test on right due to right arm and leg weakness; RAMs, F→N, H→S intact on left. Romberg—unable to test due to right leg weakness. Right pronator drift present. **Sensory:** decreased sensation to pinprick over right face, arm, and leg; intact on the left. Stereognosis and two-point discrimination not tested. **Reflexes** (can record in two ways):

	Biceps	Triceps	Brach	Knee	Ankle	Plantar
RT	4+	4+	4+	4+	4+	↑
LT	2+	2+	2+	2+	1+	↓

OR

Suggests left hemispheric CVA in distribution of the left middle cerebral artery, with right-sided hemiparesis.

Bibliography

Citations

1. Straus SE, Thorpe KE, Holroyd-Leduc J. How do I perform a lumbar puncture and analyze the results to diagnose bacterial meningitis? JAMA 2006;296:2012–2022.
2. Ellenby MS, Tegtmeyer K, Lai S et al. Lumbar puncture. N Engl J Med 2006;355:e12.
3. National Institute of Neurologic Disorders and Stroke, National Institutes of Health. Spinal cord injury: hope through research. Updated June 22, 2011. Available at http://www.ninds.nih.gov/disorders/sci/detail_sci.htm. Accessed July 2, 2011.
4. Chad DA, Stone JH, Gupta R. Case 14-2011: a woman with asymmetric sensory loss and paresthesias. N Engl J Med 2011; 364:1856–1865.
5. Kanji JN, Anglin RE, Hunt DL et al. Does this patient with diabetes have large-fiber peripheral neuropathy? JAMA 2010;303:1526–1532.
6. Taylor FR. Diagnosis and classification of headache. Prim Care 2004;31:243–259.
7. Lipton RB, Bigal ME, Steiner TJ et al. Classification of primary headaches. Neurology 2004;63:427–435.
8. Headache Classification Subcommittee of the International Headache Society. The International Classification of Headache Disorders: 2nd edition. Cephalalgia 2004;24 (Suppl 1): 9–160.
9. Olesen J, Steiner T, Bousser MG et al. Proposals for new standardized general diagnostic criteria for the secondary headaches. Cephalalgia 2009;29:1331–1336.
10. Schwedt TJ, Matharu MS, Dodick DW. Thunderclap headache. Lancet Neurol 2006;5:621–631.
11. Suarez JI, Tarr RW, Selman WR. Aneurysmal subarachnoid hemorrhage. N Engl J Med 2006;354: 387–396.
12. Brisman JL, Song JK, Newell DW. Cerebral aneurysms. N Engl J Med 2006;355:928–939.
13. Logan SA, MacMahon E. Viral meningitis. BMJ 2008; 336(7634):36–40.
14. Van de Beek D, de Gans J, Spanjaard L et al. Clinical features and prognostic factors in adults with bacterial meningitis. N Engl J Med 2004;351:1849–1859.
15. Lipton RB, Bigal ME, Diamond M et al. Migraine prevalence, disease burden, and the need for preventative therapy. Neurology 2007;68:343–349.
16. Spector JT, Kahn SR, Jones MR et al. Migraine headache and ischemic stroke risk: an updated meta-analysis. Am J Med 2010;123:612–624.
17. Chang CL, Donaghy M, Poulter N. Migraine and stroke in young women: case-control study. The World Health Organisation Collaborative Study of Cardiovascular Disease and Steroid Hormone Contraception. BMJ 1999;318(7175):13–18.
18. Kurth T, Slomke MA, Kase CS et al. Migraine, headache, and the risk of stroke in women: a prospective study. Neurology 2005;64:1020–1026.
19. Wilson JF, Migraine. Ann Intern Med 2007;144:ITC-1–ITC-16.
20. Detsky ME, McDonald DR, Baerlocher MO et al. Does this patient with headache have a migraine or need neuroimaging? JAMA 2006;296:1274–1283.
21. American Academy of Neurology. AAN encounter kit for headache. Available at http://www.aan.com/go/practice/quality/headache. Accessed July 4, 2011.
22. Lipton RB, Dodick D, Sadovsky R et al. A self-administered screener for migraine in primary care: The ID Migraine™ validation study. Neurology 2003;61:375–382.
23. Cuccharia G, Kasner SE. In the clinic. Transient ischemic attack. Ann Intern Med 2011;154:ITC-1–ITC-16.
24. van der Worp HB, van Gijn J. Acute ischemic stroke. New Engl J Med 2007;357:572–579.
25. Runchey S, McGee S. Does this patient have a hemorrhagic stroke? Clinical findings distinguishing hemorrhagic stroke from ischemic stroke. JAMA 2010;303:2280–2286.
26. Savitz SI, Caplan LR. Vertebrobasilar disease. N Engl J Med 2005; 352:2618–2626.
27. Chan Y. Differential diagnosis of dizziness. Curr Opin Otolaryngol Head Neck Surg 2009;17:200–203.
28. Goldstein LB, Simel DL. Is this patient having a stroke? JAMA 2005;293:2391–2402.
29. Scherer K, Bedlack RS, Simel DL. Does this patient have myasthenia gravis? JAMA 2005;293(15):1906–1914.
30. Mendell JR, Sahenk Z. Painful sensory neuropathy. N Engl J Med 2003;348(13):1243–1255.
31. Parry SW, Tan MP. An approach to the evaluation and management of syncope in adults. BMJ 2010;340:c880.
32. Chen LY, Benditt DG, Shen WK. Management of syncope in adults: an update. Mayo Clin Proc 2008;83:1280–1293. Available at http://www.mayoclinicproceedings.com/content/83/11/1280.full.pdf.
33. American College of Physicians. Epilepsy syndromes and their diagnosis. In Neurology, Medical Knowledge Self-Assessment Program (MKSAP) 15. Philadelphia: American College of Physicians, 2006. pp. 74–83.
34. French JA, Pedley TA. Initial management of epilepsy. New Engl J Med 2008;359:166–176.
35. Benito-Leon J, Louis ED. Clinical update: diagnosis and treatment of essential tremor. Lancet 2007;369(9568):1152–1154.
36. Rao G, Fisch L, Srinivasan S et al. Does this patient have Parkinson disease? JAMA 2003;289:347–353.
37. Jankovic J. Parkinson's disease: clinical features and diagnosis. J Neurol Neurosurg Psychiatry 2008;79:368–376.
38. LeWitt PA. Levodopa for the treatment of Parkinson's disease. N Engl J Med 2008;359:2468–2476.
39. Hening WZ. Current guidelines and standards of practice for restless legs syndrome. Am J Med 2007;120(1 Suppl 1):S22–S27.
40. Roger VL, Go AS, Lloyd-Jones DM et al. Heart disease and stroke statistics–2011 update: a report from the American Heart Association. Circulation 2011;123:e18–e209. Available at http://circ.ahajournals.org/cgi/reprint/CIR.0b013e3182009701. Accessed July 6, 2011.
41. Easton JD, Saver JL, Albers GW et al. Definition and evaluation of transient ischemic attack: a scientific statement for healthcare professionals from the American Heart Association/American Stroke Association Stroke Council; Council on Cardiovascular Radiology and Intervention; Council on Cardiovascular Nursing; and the Interdisciplinary Council on Peripheral Vascular Disease. Stroke 2009;40: 2276–2293.
42. Johnston SC, Rothwell PM, Nguyen-Huynh MN et al. Validation and refinement of scores to predict very early stroke risk

after transient ischaemic attack. Lancet 2007;369(9558):283–292.

43. Johnston SC, Gress DR, Browner WS et al. Short-term prognosis after emergency department diagnosis of TIA. JAMA 2000;284:2901–2906.

44. Cruz-Flores S, Rabinstein A, Biller J et al. Racial-ethnic disparities in stroke care: the American experience. A statement for healthcare professionals from the American Heart Association/American Stroke Association. Stroke 2011;42:2091–2166. Available at http://stroke.ahajournals.org/content/42/7/2091.full.pdf. Accessed July 7, 2011.

45. Fowler-Brown A, Corbie-Smith G, Garrett J et al. Risk of cardiovascular events and death: does insurance matter? J Gen Intern Med 2007;22:502–507.

46. Shen JJ, Washington EL. Disparities in outcomes among patients with stroke associated with insurance status. Stroke 2007;38:1010–1016.

47. Kleindorfer DO, Lindsell C, Broderick JP et al. Impact of socioeconomic status on stroke incidence: a population-based study. Ann Neurol 2006;60:480–484.

48. Mosca L, Benjamin EJ, Berra K et al. Effectiveness-based guidelines for the prevention of cardiovascular disease in women—2011 update: a guideline from the American Heart Association. Circulation 2011;123: [e-pub ahead of print]. Available at http://dx.doi.org/10.1161/CIR.0b013e31820faaf8.

49. Towfighi A, Markovic D, Ovbiagele B. Persistent sex disparity in midlife stroke prevalence in the United States. Cerebrovasc Dis 2011;31:322–328.

50. Towfighi A, Saver JL, Engelhardt R et al. A midlife stroke surge among women in the United States. Neurology 2007;69:1898–1904.

51. Healthy People 2020. 2020 topics and objectives – heart disease and stroke. Available at http://www.healthypeople.gov/2020/topicsobjectives2020/objectiveslist.aspx?topicId=21. Accessed July 8, 2011.

52. Lloyd-Jones DM, Hong Y, Labarthe D et al; on behalf of the American Heart Association Strategic Planning Task Force and Statistics Committee. Defining and setting national goals for cardiovascular health promotion and disease reduction: the American Heart Association's Strategic Impact Goal through 2020 and beyond. Circulation 2010;121:586–613. Available at http://circ.ahajournals.org/content/121/4/586.full.pdf.

53. Goldstein LB, Bushnell CD, Adams RJ et al on behalf of the American Heart Association Stroke Council, Council on Cardiovascular Nursing Council on Epidemiology and Prevention Council for High Blood Pressure Research, Council on Peripheral Vascular Disease, and Interdisciplinary Council on Quality of Care and Outcomes Research. Guidelines for the primary prevention of stroke. A guideline for healthcare professionals from the American Heart Association/American Stroke Association. Stroke 2011;42:517–584. Available at http://stroke.ahajournals.org/content/42/2/517.full.pdf. Accessed July 7, 2011.

54. U.S. Preventive Services Task Force. Aspirin for the primary prevention of cardiovascular disease: a U.S. Preventive Services Task Force recommendation statement. Ann Intern Med 2009;150:396–404.

55. Wolff T, Miller T, Ko S. Aspirin for the primary prevention of cardiovascular events: An update of the evidence for the U.S. Preventive Services Task Force. Ann Intern Med 2009;150:396–404.

56. Pignone M, Alberts MJ, Colwell JA et al. Aspirin for primary prevention of cardiovascular events in people with diabetes: a position statement of the American Diabetes Association, a scientific statement of the American Heart Association, and an expert consensus document of the American College of Cardiology Foundation. Circulation 2010;121:2694–2701.

57. Larrue V, Berhoune N, Massabuau P et al. Etiologic investigation of ischemic stroke in young adults. Neurology 2011;76:1983–1988.

58. Adams HP Jr, del Zoppo G, Alberts MJ et al. Guidelines for the early management of adults with ischemic stroke: a guideline from the American Heart Association/American Stroke Association Stroke Council, Clinical Cardiology Council, Cardiovascular Radiology and Intervention Council, and the Atherosclerotic Peripheral Vascular Disease and Quality of Care Outcomes in Research Interdisciplinary Working Groups. Stroke 2007;38:1655–1711.

59. Brott TG, Halperin JL, Abbara S et al. 2011 ASA/ACCF/AHA/AANN/AANS/ACR/ASNR/CNS/SAIP/SCAI/SIR/SNIS/SVM/SVS guideline on the management of patients with extracranial carotid and vertebral artery disease: executive summary: a report of the American College of Cardiology Foundation/ American Heart Association Task Force on Practice Guidelines, and the American Stroke Association, American Association of Neuroscience Nurses, American Association of Neurological Surgeons, American College of Radiology, American Society of Neuroradiology, Congress of Neurological Surgeons, Society of Atherosclerosis Imaging and Prevention, Society for Cardiovascular Angiography and Interventions, Society of Interventional Radiology, Society of NeuroInterventional Surgery, Society for Vascular Medicine, and Society for Vascular Surgery. J Am Coll Cardiol 2011;57:1002–1044.

60. Wechsler LR. Intravenous thrombolytic therapy for acute ischemic stroke. N Engl J Med 2011;364:2138–2146.

61. Antithrombotic Trialists' Collaboration. Aspirin in the primary and secondary prevention of vascular disease: collaborative meta-analysis of individual participant data from randomized trials. Lancet 2009;373(9678):1849–1860.

62. Wolff T, Guirgulis-Blake J, Miller T et al. Screening for carotid artery stenosis: an update of the evidence for the U.S. Preventive Services Task Force. Ann Intern Med 2007;147:860–870.

63. American College of Physicians. Stroke. In Neurology, Medical Knowledge Self-Assessment Program (MKSAP) 15. Philadelphia: American College of Physicians, 2006. pp. 3–19.

64. Boulton AJ, Vinik AT, Arezzo JC et al. Diabetic neuropathies. A statement by the American Diabetes Association. Diabetes Care 2005;28:956–962.

65. Martin CL, Albers J, Herman WH et al. Neuropathy among the Diabetes Control and Complications Trial Cohort 8 years after trial completion. Diabetes Care 2006;29:340–344.

66. Marcantonio ER. In the clinic: delirium. Ann Intern Med 2011;154:ITC6-1– ITC6–16.

67. Wong CL, Holroyd-Leduc J, Simel DL et al. Does this patient have delirium? Value of bedside instruments. JAMA 2010;304:779–786.

68. O'Mahony R, Murthy L, Akunne A et al. Synopsis of the National Institute for Health and clinical excellence guideline for prevention of delirium. Ann Intern Med 2011;154:746–751.

69. Holsinger T, Deveau J, Boustani M et al. Does this patient have dementia? JAMA 2007;297:2391–2404.

70. Blass DM, Rabins DV. In the clinic: dementia. Ann Intern Med 2008;148:ITC4-1–ITC4–16.

71. Petersen RC. Mild cognitive impairment. N Engl J Med 2011; 364:2227–2234.

72. Daviglus ML, Bell CC, Berrettini W et al. National Institutes of Health state-of-the-science conference statement: preventing Alzheimer disease and cognitive decline. Ann Intern Med 2010;153:176–181.

73. Plassman BL. Williams JW, Burke JR et al. Systematic review: factors associated with risk for and possible prevention of cognitive decline in later life. Ann Intern Med 2010;153:182–193.

74. American Academy of Neurology. Neurology clerkship core curriculum guidelines. Available at http://www.aan.com/globals/axon/assets/2770.pdf. Accessed July 14, 2011.

75. Gelb DJ, Gunderson CH, Henry KA et al. The neurology clerkship core curriculum. Neurology 2002;58:849–852.

76. Moore FGA, Chalk C. The essential neurologic examination. Neurology 2009;72:2020–2023.

77. Scherokman B, Selwa L, Alguire PC. Approach to common neurological symptoms in internal medicine. Internal medicine curriculum in neurology. American Academy of Neurology and American College of Physicians. Available at http://www.aan.com/go/education/curricula/internal/toc. Accessed July 14, 2011.

78. Wayne State University, Pearson JC. Neurology Teaching Videos. See 6870 videos of examination techniques. Available at http://www.ntv.wright.edu. Accessed July 14, 2011.

79. Scherokman B, Alguire PC. Video: general screening examination for patients with no neurologic symptoms. American Academy of Neurology – Internal Medicine Curriculum in Neurology. Available at http://www.aan.com/globals/axon/assets/5456.mov. Accessed July 14, 2011.

80. McGee S. Evidence-Based Physical Diagnosis, 2nd ed. St. Louis: Saunders, 2005.

81. Gilden DH. Bell's palsy. N Engl J Med 2004;351:1323–1331.

82. Teitelbaum JS, Eliasziw M, Garner M. Tests of motor function in patients suspected of having mild unilateral cerebral lesions Can J Neurol Sci 2002;29:337–344.

83. Maynard FM, Bracken MB, Creasey G et al. International standards for neurological and functional classification of spinal cord injury. Spinal Cord 1997;35(5):266–274. See also American Spinal Cord Injury Association dermatome diagram available at http://www.asia-spinalinjury.org/publications/59544_sc_Exam_Sheet_r4.pdf. Accessed July 14, 2011.

84. Hallett M. NINDS myotatic reflex scale. Neurology 1993;43: 2723.

85. Thomas KE, Hasbun R, Jekel J et al. the diagnostic accuracy of Kernig's sign, Brudzinski's sign, and nuchal rigidity in adults with suspected meningitis. Clin Infect Dis 2002; 35:46–52.

86. Mendizabal M, Silva MO. Asterixis. N Engl J Med 2010;363:9.

87. Bateman DE. Neurological assessment of coma. J Neurolol Neurosurg Psychiatry 2001;71(Suppl 1):i13–17.

88. Laureys S, Owen AM, Schiff ND. Brain function in coma, vegetative state, and related disorders. Lancet Neurol 2004;3:537–546.

89. Teasdale G, Jennett B. Assessment of coma and impaired consciousness. A practical scale. Lancet 1974;304:7872):81–84.

90. Booth CM, Boone RH, Tomlinson G et al. Is this patient dead, vegetative, or severely neurologically impaired? Assessing outcome for comatose survivors of cardiac arrest. JAMA 2004;291:870–879.

91. Freeman R. Neurogenic orthostatic hypotension. N Engl J Med 2008;3548:615–628.

92. Gupta V, Lipsitz LA. Orthostatic hypotension in the elderly: diagnosis and treatment. Am J Med 2007;120:841–847.

Additional References

Adams SM, Knowles PD. Evaluation of a first seizure. Am Fam Physician 2007;75:1342–1347.

Aids to the Examination of the Peripheral Nervous System: Medical Research Council Memorandum No. 45. London: Her Majesty's Stationery Office, 1976.

Ay H, Gungor L, Arsaya EM et al. A score to predict early risk of recurrence after ischemic stroke. Neurology 2010;74:128–135. Epub 2009 Dec 16.

Berg AT, Berkovic, SF, Brodie MJ et al. Revised terminology and concepts for organization of seizures and epilepsies: Report of the ILAE Commission on Classification and Terminology, 2005–2009. Epilepsia 2010;51:676–685.

Boyer EW, Shannon M. The serotonin syndrome. N Engl J Med 2005;352:1112–1120.

Bril V, England J, Franklin GM et al. Evidence-based guideline: treatment of painful diabetic neuropathy: report of the American Academy of Neurology, the American Association of Neuromuscular and Electrodiagnostic Medicine, and the American Academy of Physical Medicine and Rehabilitation. Neurology 2011;76:1758–1765.

Brouwer MC, Tunkel AR, van de Beek D. Epidemiology, diagnosis, and antimicrobial treatment of acute bacterial meningitis. Clin Microbiol Rev 2010;23:467–492.

Campbell WW, DeJong RN, Haerer AF. DeJong's The Neurologic Examination, 6th ed. Philadelphia, Lippincott Williams & Wilkins, 2005.

Chandana SR, Movva S, Arora M et al. Primary brain tumors in adults. Am Fam Physician 2008;77:1423–1430.

Cucchiara B, Kasner SE. In the clinic. Transient ischemic attack. Ann Int Med 2011;154:ITC1–ITC16.

Darouiche RO. Spinal epidural abscess and subdural empyema. Handb Clin Neurol 2010;96:91–99.

Detsky ME, McDonald DR, Baerlocher MO et al. Does this patient with headache have a migraine or need neuroimaging? JAMA 2006;296:1272–1283.

Fraser GA, Chalk C. The essential neurologic examination. Neurology 2009;72:2020–2023.

Freeman R. Clinical practice. Neurogenic orthostatic hypotension. N Engl J Med 2008;358:615–624.

Gardner P. Prevention of meningococcal disease. N Engl J Med 2006;355:1466–1473.

Gilman S, Manter JT, Gatz AJ et al. Manter and Gatz's Essentials of Clinical Neuroanatomy and Neurophysiology, 10th ed. Philadelphia: FA Davis, 2003.

Grubb BP. Neurocardiogenic syncope. N Engl J Med 2004;352(10): 1004–1010.

Haanpaa ML, Backonja M, Bennett MI et al. Assessment of neuropathic pain in primary care. Am J Med 2009;122:S13–S21.

BIBLIOGRAPHY

Heaton RK, Clifford DB, Franklin DR et al. HIV-associated neurocognitive disorders persist in the era of potent antiretroviral therapy. CHARTER study. Neurology 2010;75:2087–2096.

Katz JN, Harris MB. Lumbar spinal stenosis. N Engl J Med 2008; 358:818–825.

Kim LG, Johnson TL, Marson AG et al. Prediction of risk of seizure recurrence after a single seizure and early epilepsy: further results from the MESS trial. Lancet Neurol 2006;5:317–322.

Magnetic Resonance Angiography in Relatives of Patients with Subarachnoid Hemorrhage Study Group. Risks and benefits of screening for intracranial aneurysms in first-degree relatives of patients with sporadic subarachnoid hemorrhage. N Engl J Med 1999;341:1344–1350.

McGee S. Evidence-Based Physical Diagnosis, 2nd ed. St. Louis: Saunders, 2005. See especially Ch 54, Visual field defects, pp. 663–670; Ch 19, The pupils, pp. 203–233; Ch 55, Nerves of the eye muscles (III, IV, and VI): approach to diplopia, pp. 671–689; Ch 61, Coordination and cerebellar testing, pp. 793–800; Ch 56, Miscellaneous Cranial Nerves, pp. 690–706; Ch 21, Hearing, pp. 242–249; Ch 5, Stance and gait, pp. 57–74; Ch 58, Examination of the sensory system, pp. 736–753; Ch 59, Examination of the reflexes, pp. 754–771; Ch 60, Disorders of the nerve roots, plexi, and peripheral nerves, pp. 772–792; and Ch 23, Meninges, pp. 277–282.

National Institutes of Health–National Institute of Neurological Disorders and Stroke. NIH Stroke Scale. Revised October 1 2003. Available at http://www.ninds.nih.gov/doctors/NIH_Stroke_Scale.pdf. Accessed November 26, 2011.

Pascuzzi RM. Peripheral neuropathy. Med Clin North Am 2009;93:317–342, vii–viii.

Pickett CA, Jackson JL, Hemann BA et al. Carotid bruits and cerebrovascular disease risk – a meta-analysis. Stroke 2010;41:2295–2302.

Posner JB, Saper CB, Schiff ND, Plum F. The diagnosis of stupor and coma. Contemporary Neurology Series 71, 4th ed. New York: Oxford University Press, 2007.

Renoux C, Dell'Aniello S, Garbe E et al. Transdermal and oral hormone replacement therapy and the risk of stroke: a nested case-control study. BMJ 2010;340:c2519.

Romero-Ortuno R, Cogan L, Foran T et al. Continuous noninvasive orthostatic blood pressure measurements and their relationship with orthostatic intolerance, falls, and frailty in older people. J Am Geriatr Soc 2011;59:655–665.

Ropper AH, Samuels M. Adams and Victor's Principles of Neurology, 9th ed. New York: McGraw-Hill, 2009.

Ropper AH, Gorson KC. Concussion. N Engl J Med 2007;356:166–172.

Rosamond W, Flegal K, Friday G et al. Heart disease and stroke statistics–2007 update: a report from the American Heart Association Statistics Committee and Stroke Statistics Subcommittee. Circulation 2007;115:e69–e171.

Rosenberg RN. Atlas of Clinical Neurology, 3rd ed. Philadelphia: Springer, 2009.

Rowland LP, Pedley TA, Kneass W. Merritt's Neurology. Philadelphia: Wolters Kluwer/Lippincott Williams & Wilkins, 2010.

Saltzman CL, Rashid R, Hayes A et al. 4.5 Gram monofilament sensation beneath both first metatarsal heads indicates protective foot sensation in diabetic patients. J Bone Joint Surg 2004;86:717–723.

Straus SE, Majumdar SR, McAlister FA. New evidence for stroke prevention. Scientific review. JAMA 2002;288:1388–1395.

Sun BC, Derose SF, Liang L et al. Predictors of 30-day serious events in older patients with syncope. Ann Emerg Med 2009;54:760–768.

Suri P, Rainville, Kalichman L et al. Does this older adult with lower extremity pain have the clinical syndrome of lumbar spinal stenosis? JAMA 2010;304:2628–2636.

Task Force for the Diagnosis and Management of Syncope, developed in collaboration with European Society of Cardiology; European Heart Rhythm Association; Heart Failure Association; Heart Rhythm Society, Moya A, Sutton R, Ammirati F et al. Guidelines for the diagnosis and management of syncope (version 2009). Eur Heart J 2009;30:2631–2671. Available at http://eurheartj.oxfordjournals.org/content/30/21/2631.full.pdf+html. Accessed November 26, 2011.

van Gijn J, Kerr RS, Rinkel GJ. Subarachnoid haemorrhage. Lancet 2007;369(9558):306–318.

Velickovic M, Gracies JM. Movement disorders: keys to identifying and treating tremor. Geriatrics 2002;57:32–39.

Witt JC, Stevens JC. Neurologic disorders masquerading as carpal tunnel syndrome: 12 cases of failed carpal tunnel release. Mayo Clin Proc 2000;75:409–413.

Yew KS, Cheng E. Acute stroke diagnosis. Am Fam Physician 2009; 80:33–40.

The Bates' suite offers these additional resources to enhance learning and facilitate understanding of this chapter:

- *Bates' Pocket Guide to Physical Examination and History Taking,* 7th edition
- Bates' *Visual Guide to Physical Examination*
- thePoint online resources, for students and instructors: http://thepoint.lww.com

Table 17-1

Disorders of the Central and Peripheral Nervous Systems

Central Nervous System Disorders

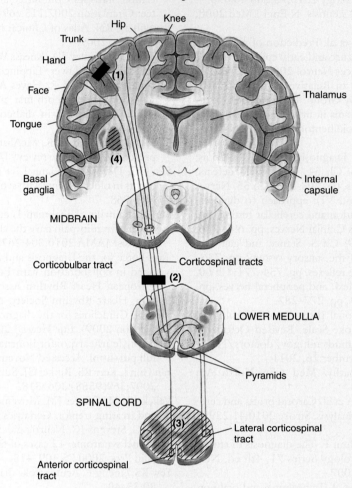

Typical Findings

Location of Lesion	Motor	Sensory	Deep Tendon Reflexes	Examples of Cause
Cerebral Cortex (1)	Chronic contralateral corticospinal-type weakness and spasticity. Flexion is stronger than extension in the arm, plantar flexion is stronger than dorsiflexion in the foot, and the leg is externally rotated at the hip.	Contralateral sensory loss in the limbs and trunk on the same side as the motor deficits	↑	Cortical stroke
Brainstem (2)	Weakness and spasticity as above, plus cranial nerve deficits such as diplopia (from weakness of the extraocular muscles) and dysarthria	Variable; no typical sensory findings	↑	Brainstem stroke, acoustic neuroma
Spinal Cord (3)	Weakness and spasticity as above, but often affecting both sides (when cord damage is bilateral), causing paraplegia or quadriplegia depending on the level of injury	Dermatomal sensory deficit on the trunk bilaterally at the level of the lesion, and sensory loss from tract damage below the level of the lesion	↑	Trauma, causing cord compression

Typical Findings

Location of Lesion	Motor	Sensory	Deep Tendon Reflexes	Examples of Cause
Subcortical Gray Matter: Basal Ganglia (4)	Slowness of movement (bradykinesia), rigidity, and tremor	Sensation not affected	Normal or ↓	Parkinsonism
Cerebellar (not illustrated)	Hypotonia, ataxia, and other abnormal movements, including nystagmus, dysdiadochokinesis, and dysmetria	Sensation not affected	Normal or ↓	Cerebellar stroke, brain tumor

Peripheral Nervous System Disorders

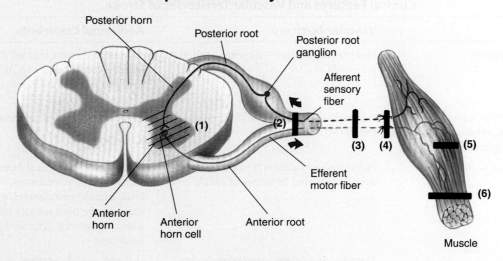

Typical Findings

Location of Lesion	Motor	Sensory	Deep Tendon Reflexes	Examples of Cause
Anterior Horn Cell (1)	Weakness and atrophy in a segmental or focal pattern; fasciculations	Sensation intact	↓	Polio, amyotrophic lateral sclerosis
Spinal Roots and Nerves (2)	Weakness and atrophy in a root-innervated pattern; sometimes with fasciculations	Corresponding dermatomal sensory deficits	↓	Herniated cervical or lumbar disc
Peripheral Nerve—Mono-neuropathy (3)	Weakness and atrophy in a peripheral nerve distribution; sometimes with fasciculations	Sensory loss in the pattern of that nerve	↓	Trauma
Peripheral Nerve—Polyneuropathy (4)	Weakness and atrophy more distal than proximal; sometimes with fasciculations	Sensory deficits, commonly in stocking-glove distribution	↓	Peripheral polyneuropathy of alcoholism, diabetes
Neuromuscular Junction (5)	Fatigability more than weakness	Sensation intact	Normal	Myasthenia gravis
Muscle (6)	Weakness usually more proximal than distal; fasciculations rare	Sensation intact	Normal or ↓	Muscular dystrophy

Table
17-2   **Types of Stroke**

Assessing patients with stroke involves three fundamental questions, based on a careful history and detailed physical examination: *What brain area and related vascular territory explain the patient's findings? Is the stroke ischemic or hemorrhagic? If ischemic, is the mechanism thrombus or embolus?* Stroke is a medical emergency, and timing is of the essence. Answers to these questions are critical to patient outcomes and use of antithrombotic therapies.

In *acute ischemic stroke*, ischemic brain injury begins with a central core of very low perfusion and often irreversible cell death. This core is surrounded by an *ischemic penumbra* of metabolically disturbed cells that are still potentially viable, depending on restoration of blood flow and duration of ischemia. Because most irreversible damage occurs in the first 3 to 6 hours after onset of symptoms, therapies targeted to the 3-hour window achieve the best outcomes, with recovery in up to 50% of patients in some studies.

Clinician performance in diagnosing stroke improves with training.[58] Understanding the pathophysiology of stroke takes dedication, expert supervision to improve techniques of neurologic examination, and perseverance. *This brief overview is intended to prompt further study and practice.* Accuracy in clinical examination is achievable, and more important than ever in determining patient therapy.[25,28,60] Turn to pp. 695–698 and review the discussion of *stroke risk factors–primary and secondary prevention*.

Clinical Features and Vascular Territories of Stroke

Clinical Finding	Vascular Territory	Additional Comments
Contralateral leg weakness	*Anterior circulation*—anterior cerebral artery (ACA)	Includes stem of Circle of Willis connecting internal carotid artery to ACA, and the segment distal to ACA and its anterior choroidal branch
Contralateral face, arm > leg weakness, sensory loss, field cut, aphasia (left MCA) or neglect, apraxia (right MCA)	*Anterior circulation*—middle cerebral artery (MCA)	Largest vascular bed for stroke
Contralateral motor or sensory deficit without cortical signs	*Subcortical circulation**—lenticulostriate deep penetrating branches of MCA	Small vessel subcortical *lacunar infarcts* in internal capsule, thalamus, or brainstem. Four common syndromes: pure motor hemiparesis; pure sensory hemianesthesia; ataxic hemiparesis; clumsy hand—dysarthria syndrome
Contralateral field cut	*Posterior circulation*—posterior cerebral artery (PCA)	Includes paired vertebral and basilar artery, paired posterior cerebral arteries. Bilateral PCA infarction causes cortical blindness but preserved pupillary light reaction.
Dysphagia, dysarthria, tongue/palate deviation and/or ataxia with crossed sensory/motor deficits (= ipsilateral face with contralateral body)	*Posterior circulation*—brainstem, vertebral, or basilar artery branches	
Oculomotor deficits and/or ataxia with crossed sensory/motor deficits	*Posterior circulation*—basilar artery	Complete basilar artery occlusion—"locked-in syndrome" with intact consciousness but with inability to speak and quadriplegia

*Learn to differentiate cortical from subcortical involvement. *Subcortical or lacunar syndromes* do not affect higher cognitive function, language, or visual fields.

Source: Adapted from American College of Physicians. Stroke, in Neurology. Medical Knowledge Self-Assessment Program (MKSAP) 14. Philadelphia: American College of Physicians, 2006. pp. 52–68.

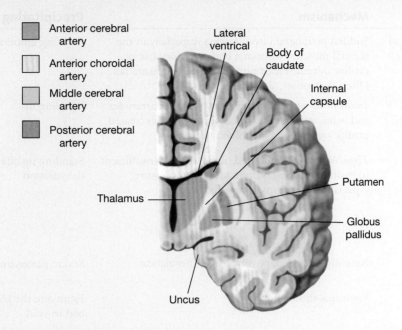

Anterior cerebral artery

Anterior choroidal artery

Middle cerebral artery

Posterior cerebral artery

Lateral ventrical

Body of caudate

Internal capsule

Putamen

Globus pallidus

Uncus

Thalamus

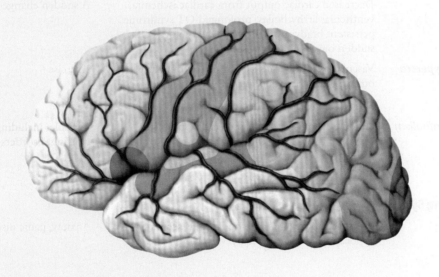

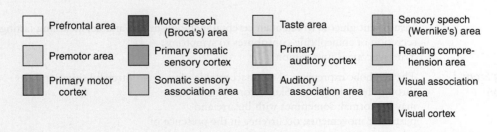

Prefrontal area

Premotor area

Primary motor cortex

Motor speech (Broca's) area

Primary somatic sensory cortex

Somatic sensory association area

Taste area

Primary auditory cortex

Auditory association area

Sensory speech (Wernike's) area

Reading comprehension area

Visual association area

Visual cortex

Table
17-3   Syncope and Similar Disorders

Problem	Mechanism	Precipitating Factors
Vasodepressor or Vasovagal Syncope (*the common faint*)	Sudden peripheral vasodilatation, especially in the skeletal muscles, without a compensatory rise in cardiac output. Heart rate then blood pressure fall. Often slow onset, slow offset.	A strong emotion such as fear or pain
Orthostatic (Postural) Hypotension[91,92] (*orthostatic*)	*Inadequate vasoconstrictor reflexes* in both arterioles and veins, with resultant venous pooling, decreased cardiac output, and low blood pressure	Standing up
	Hypovolemia, a diminished blood volume insufficient to maintain cardiac output and blood pressure, especially in the upright position	Standing up after hemorrhage or dehydration
Cough Syncope	Neurally mediated, possible vagal stimulation	Severe paroxysm of coughing
Micturition Syncope	Vasovagal stimulation	Emptying the bladder after getting out of bed to void
Cardiovascular Disorders[31,32]		
Arrhythmias	Decreased cardiac output from cardiac ischemia, ventricular arrhythmias, prolonged QT syndrome, persistent bradycardia, infrafascicular block. Often sudden onset; sudden offset.	A sudden change in rhythm
Aortic Stenosis and Hypertrophic Cardiomyopathy	Vascular resistance falls with exercise, but cardiac output cannot rise due to outflow obstruction.	Exercise
Myocardial Infarction	Sudden arrhythmia or decreased cardiac output	Variable
Massive Pulmonary Embolism	Sudden hypoxia or decreased cardiac output	Variable, including prolonged bed rest and clotting disorders
Disorders Resembling Syncope		
Hypocapnia due to Hyperventilation	Constriction of cerebral blood vessels secondary to hypocapnia induced by hyperventilation	Anxiety, panic disorder
Hypoglycemia	Insufficient glucose to maintain cerebral metabolism; secretion of epinephrine contributes to symptoms. True syncope is uncommon.	Variable, including fasting
Hysterical Fainting From Conversion Reaction	The symbolic expression of an unacceptable idea through body language. Skin color and vital signs may be normal; sometimes with bizarre and purposive movements; occurrence in the presence of other people.	Stressful situation

Predisposing Factors	Prodromal Manifestations	Postural Associations	Recovery
Fatigue, hunger, a hot humid environment	Restlessness, weakness, pallor, nausea, salivation, sweating, yawning	Usually occurs when standing, possibly when sitting	Prompt return of consciousness when lying down, but pallor, weakness, nausea, and slight confusion may persist for a time.
Central and peripheral neuropathies: Parkinson disease, Shy-Drager syndrome; Lewy body disease diabetes, amyloidosis; antihypertensive vasodilator drugs; prolonged bed rest	Often none	Occurs soon after the person stands up Supine hypertension is common	Prompt return to normal when lying down
Bleeding from the GI tract or trauma, potent diuretics, vomiting, diarrhea, polyuria	Light-headedness and palpitations (tachycardia) on standing up	Usually occurs soon after the person stands up	Improvement with lying down, volume repletion
Chronic bronchitis in a muscular man	Often none except for cough	May occur in any position	Prompt return to normal
Nocturia, usually in elderly or adult men	Often none	Standing to void	Prompt return to normal
Heart disease, aging decrease tolerance of abnormal rhythms.	Often none	May occur in any position	Prompt return to normal prolonged cerebral hypoperfusion cardiac arrest
Cardiac disorders	Often none. Onset is sudden.	Occurs with or after exercise	Usually a prompt return to normal
Coronary artery disease	Ischemic chest pain; often none	May occur in any position	Variable
Deep vein thrombosis, bedrest hypercoagulable states (SLE; cancer), protein S or C deficiency, antithrombin III deficiency. Estrogen therapy	Dyspnea, pleuritic chest pain	May occur in any position	Related to time to diagnosis and treatment
Anxiety	Dyspnea, palpitations, chest discomfort, numbness and tingling of the hands and around the mouth lasting for several minutes. Consciousness is often maintained.	May occur in any position	Slow improvement as hyperventilation ceases
Insulin therapy and a variety of metabolic disorders	Sweating, tremor, palpitations, hunger, headache, confusion, abnormal behavior, coma	May occur in any position	Variable, depending on severity and treatment
Hysterical personality traits	Variable	A slump to the floor, often from a standing position without injury	Variable; may be prolonged, often with fluctuating responsiveness

Table 17-4 Seizure Disorders

Seizures were reclassified in 2010 into focal and generalized to better reflect current scientific advances. Underlying causes should be identified as genetic, structural/metabolic, or unknown. The complexities of the reclassification scheme are best explored by turning to the report of the ILAE Commission on Classification and Terminology, 2005–2009, cited below, and to more detailed references. This table presents only basic concepts from this report.

Focal Seizures

Focal seizures "are conceptualized as originating within networks limited to one hemisphere. They may be discretely localized or more widely distributed. Focal seizures may originate in subcortical structures. For each seizure type, ictal onset is consistent from one seizure to another, with preferential propagation patterns that can involve the contralateral hemisphere. In some cases, however, there is more than one network, and more than one seizure type, but each individual seizure type has a consistent site of onset. Focal seizures do not fall into any recognized set of natural causes." The distinction between simple partial and partial complex is eliminated, but clinicians are urged to recognize and describe "impairment of consciousness/awareness or other dyscognitive features, localization, and progression of ictal events."

Problem	Clinical Manifestations	Postictal State
Focal Seizures Without Impairment of Consciousness or Awareness		
• With observable motor and autonomic symptoms		
Jacksonian	Tonic and then clonic movements that start unilaterally in the hand, foot, or face and spread to other body parts on the same side	Normal consciousness
Other motor	Turning of the head and eyes to one side, or tonic and clonic movements of an arm or leg without the Jacksonian spread	Normal consciousness
With autonomic symptoms	A "funny feeling" in the epigastrium, nausea, pallor, flushing, lightheadedness	Normal consciousness
• With subjective sensory or psychic phenomena	Numbness, tingling; simple visual, auditory, or olfactory hallucinations such as flashing lights, buzzing, or odors	Normal consciousness
	Anxiety or fear; feelings of familiarity (déjà vu) or unreality; dreamy states; fear or rage; flashback experiences; more complex hallucinations	Normal consciousness
Focal Seizures With Impairment of Consciousness	The seizure may or may not start with the autonomic or psychic symptoms outlined above. Consciousness is impaired, and the person appears confused. Automatisms include automatic motor behaviors such as chewing, smacking the lips, walking about, and unbuttoning clothes; also more complicated and skilled behaviors such as driving a car.	The patient may remember initial autonomic or psychic symptoms (which are then termed an *aura*), but is amnesic for the rest of the seizure. Temporary confusion and headache may occur.
Focal Seizures That Become Generalized	Partial seizures that become generalized resemble tonic–clonic seizures (see next page). Unfortunately, the patient may not recall the focal onset, and observers may overlook it.	As in a tonic–clonic seizure, described on the next page. Two attributes indicate a partial seizure that has become generalized: (1) the recollection of an *aura*, and (2) a *unilateral* neurologic deficit during the postictal period.

Source: Commission on Classification and Terminology of the International League Against Epilepsy. A proposed diagnostic scheme for people with epileptic seizures and with epilepsy: report of the ILAE Task Force on Classification and Terminology. Available at http://www.ilae-epilepsy.org/Visitors/Centre/ctf/overview.cfm#2. Accessed July 15, 2011. See also Berg AT, Berkovic SF, Brodie MJ et al. Revised terminology and concepts for organization of seizures and epilepsies: Report of the ILAE Commission on Classification and Terminology, 2005–2009. Epilepsia 2010;51:676–685.

Generalized Seizures and Pseudoseizures

Generalized seizures "are conceptualized as originating as some point within, and rapidly engaging, bilaterally distributed networks.... that include cortical and subcortical structures, but do not necessarily include the entire cortex... the location and lateralization are not consistent from one seizure to another. Generalized seizures can be asymmetric." They may begin with body movements, impaired consciousness, or both. When tonic–clonic seizures begin after age 30, suspect either a partial seizure that has become generalized or a general seizure caused by a toxic or metabolic disorder. Toxic and metabolic causes include withdrawal from alcohol or other sedative drugs, uremia, hypoglycemia, hyperglycemia, hyponatremia, and bacterial meningitis.

Problem	Clinical Manifestations	Postictal (*Postseizure*) State
Generalized Seizures		
*Tonic–Clonic (grand mal)**	The person loses consciousness suddenly, sometimes with a cry, and the body stiffens into tonic extensor rigidity. Breathing stops, and the person becomes cyanotic. A clonic phase of rhythmic muscular contraction follows. Breathing resumes and is often noisy, with excessive salivation. Injury, tongue biting, and urinary incontinence may occur.	Confusion, drowsiness, fatigue, headache, muscular aching, and sometimes the temporary persistence of bilateral neurologic deficits such as hyperactive reflexes and Babinski responses. The person has amnesia for the seizure and recalls no aura.
Absence	A sudden brief lapse of consciousness, with momentary blinking, staring, or movements of the lips and hands but no falling. Two subtypes are recognized. *Typical absences* last less than 10 second and stop abruptly. *Atypical absences* may last more than 10 second.	No aura recalled. In petit mal absences, a prompt return to normal; in atypical absences, some postictal confusion
Myoclonic	Sudden, brief, rapid jerks, involving the trunk or limbs. Associated with a variety of disorders	Variable
Myoclonic Atonic (drop attack)	Sudden loss of consciousness with falling but no movements. Injury may occur.	Either a prompt return to normal or a brief period of confusion
Pseudoseizures		
May mimic seizures but are due to a conversion reaction (a psychological disorder)	The movements may have personally symbolic significance and often do not follow a neuroanatomic pattern. Injury is uncommon.	Variable

*Febrile convulsions that resemble brief tonic–clonic seizures may occur in infants and young children. They are usually benign but occasionally may be the first manifestation of a seizure disorder.

Table
17-5
Tremors and Involuntary Movements

Tremors

Tremors are rhythmic oscillatory movements, which may be roughly subdivided into three groups: resting (or static) tremors, postural tremors, and intention tremors.

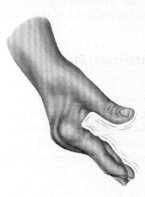 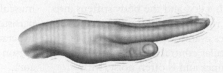 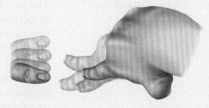

Resting (Static) Tremors

These tremors are most prominent at rest and may decrease or disappear with voluntary movement. Illustrated is the common, relatively slow, fine, pill-rolling tremor of parkinsonism, about 5 per second.

Postural Tremors

These tremors appear when the affected part is actively maintaining a posture. Examples include the fine rapid tremor of hyperthyroidism, the tremors of anxiety and fatigue, and benign essential (and sometimes familial) tremor.

Intention Tremors

Intention tremors, absent at rest, appear with movement and often get worse as the target gets closer. Causes include disorders of cerebellar pathways, as in multiple sclerosis, or any other disease of the cerebellum.

Involuntary Movements

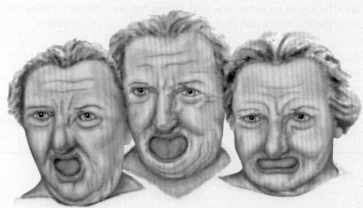

Oral–Facial Dyskinesias

Oral–facial dyskinesias are rhythmic, repetitive, bizarre movements that chiefly involve the face, mouth, jaw, and tongue: grimacing, pursing of the lips, protrusions of the tongue, opening and closing of the mouth, and deviations of the jaw. The limbs and trunk are involved less often. These movements may be a late complication of psychotropic drugs such as phenothiazines, termed *tardive* (late) dyskinesias. They also occur in long-standing psychoses, in some elderly individuals, and in some edentulous persons.

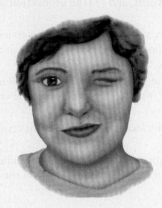

Tics

Tics are brief, repetitive, stereotyped, coordinated movements occurring at irregular intervals. Examples include repetitive winking, grimacing, and shoulder shrugging. Causes include Tourette's syndrome and drugs such as phenothiazines and amphetamines.

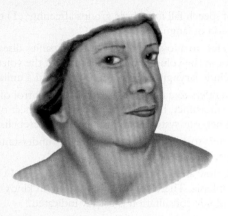

Dystonia

Dystonic movements are similar to athetoid movements, but often involve larger portions of the body, including the trunk. Grotesque, twisted postures may result. Causes include drugs such as phenothiazines, primary torsion dystonia, and as illustrated, spasmodic torticollis.

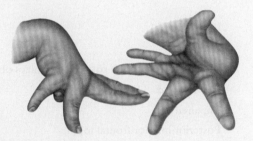

Athetosis

Athetoid movements are slower and more twisting and writhing than choreiform movements, and have a larger amplitude. They most commonly involve the face and the distal extremities. Athetosis is often associated with spasticity. Causes include cerebral palsy.

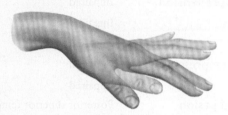

Chorea

Choreiform movements are brief, rapid, jerky, irregular, and unpredictable. They occur at rest or interrupt normal coordinated movements. Unlike tics, they seldom repeat themselves. The face, head, lower arms, and hands are often involved. Causes include Sydenham's chorea (with rheumatic fever) and Huntington's disease.

Table

17-6　**Disorders of Speech**

Disorders of speech fall into three groups affecting: (1) the voice, (2) the articulation of words, and (3) the production and comprehension of language.

- *Aphonia* refers to a loss of voice that accompanies disease affecting the larynx or its nerve supply. *Dysphonia* refers to less severe impairment in the volume, quality, or pitch of the voice. For example, a person may be hoarse or only able to speak in a whisper. Causes include laryngitis, laryngeal tumors, and a unilateral vocal cord paralysis (CN X).

- *Dysarthria* refers to a defect in the muscular control of the speech apparatus (lips, tongue, palate, or pharynx). Words may be nasal, slurred, or indistinct, but the central symbolic aspect of language remains intact. Causes include motor lesions of the central or peripheral nervous system, parkinsonism, and cerebellar disease.

- *Aphasia* refers to a disorder in producing or understanding language. It is often caused by lesions in the dominant cerebral hemisphere, usually the left.

Compared below are two common types of aphasia: (1) Wernicke's, a fluent (receptive) aphasia, and (2) Broca's, a nonfluent (or expressive) aphasia. There are other less-common kinds of aphasia, which are distinguished by differing responses on the specific tests listed. Neurologic consultation is usually indicated.

	Wernicke's Aphasia	**Broca's Aphasia**
Qualities of Spontaneous Speech	Fluent; often rapid, voluble, and effortless. Inflection and articulation are good, but sentences lack meaning and words are malformed (paraphasias) or invented (neologisms). Speech may be totally incomprehensible.	Nonfluent; slow, with few words and laborious effort. Inflection and articulation are impaired but words are meaningful, with nouns, transitive verbs, and important adjectives. Small grammatical words are often dropped.
Word Comprehension	Impaired	Fair to good
Repetition	Impaired	Impaired
Naming	Impaired	Impaired, though the patient recognizes objects
Reading Comprehension	Impaired	Fair to good
Writing	Impaired	Impaired
Location of Lesion	Posterior superior temporal lobe	Posterior inferior frontal lobe

Although it is important to recognize aphasia early in your encounter with a patient, integrate this information with your neurologic examination as you approach diagnosis.

Table

17-7 Nystagmus

Nystagmus is a rhythmic oscillation of the eyes, analogous to a tremor in other parts of the body. It has multiple causes, including impairment of vision in early life, disorders of the labyrinth and the cerebellar system, and drug toxicity. Nystagmus occurs normally when a person watches a rapidly moving object (e.g., a passing train). Study the three characteristics of nystagmus described in this table so you can correctly identify the type of nystagmus. Then refer to textbooks of neurology for differential diagnoses.

Direction of Gaze in Which Nystagmus Appears
Example: Nystagmus on Right Lateral Gaze
Nystagmus Present (Right Lateral Gaze)

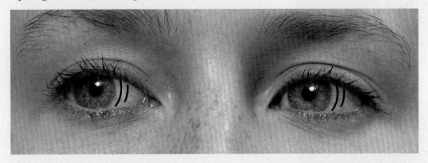

Although nystagmus may be present in all directions of gaze, it may appear or become accentuated only on deviation of the eyes (e.g., to the side or upward). On extreme lateral gaze, the normal person may show a few beats resembling nystagmus. Avoid making assessments in such extreme positions, and *observe for nystagmus only within the field of full binocular vision.*

Nystagmus Not Present (Left Lateral Gaze)

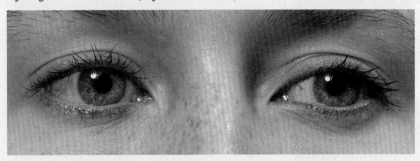

Direction of the Quick and Slow Phases
Example: Left-Beating Nystagmus—a Quick Jerk to the Left in Each Eye, Then a Slow Drift to the Right

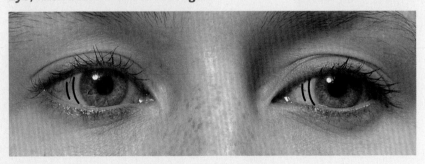

Nystagmus usually has both slow and fast movements, but *is defined by its fast phase.* For example, if the eyes jerk quickly to the patient's left and drift back slowly to the right, the patient is said to have *left-beating nystagmus.* Occasionally, nystagmus consists only of coarse oscillations without quick and slow components. It is then said to be *pendular.*

(table continues on page 756)

Table

17-7   **Nystagmus** (*continued*)

Plane of the Movements
Horizontal Nystagmus

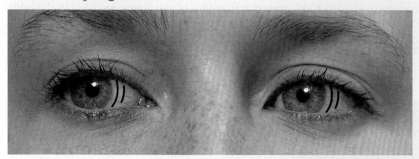

The movement of nystagmus may occur in one or more planes (i.e., horizontal, vertical, or rotary). It is the plane of the movements, not the direction of the gaze, that defines this variable.

Vertical Nystagmus

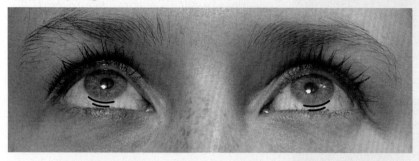

Rotary Nystagmus

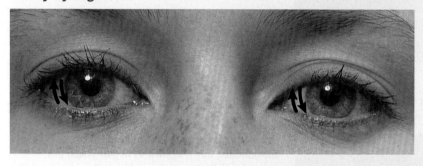

Table

17-8   **Types of Facial Paralysis**

Facial weakness or paralysis may result either from (1) a peripheral lesion of CN VII, the facial nerve, anywhere from its origin in the pons to its periphery in the face, or (2) a central lesion involving the upper motor neuron system between the cortex and the pons. A peripheral lesion of CN VII, exemplified here by a Bell's palsy, is compared with a central lesion, exemplified by a left hemispheric cerebrovascular accident. These can be distinguished by their different effects on the upper part of the face.

The lower part of the face normally is controlled by upper motor neurons located on only one side of the cortex—the opposite side. *Left hemispheric damage to these pathways, as in a stroke, paralyzes the right lower face.* The upper face, however, is controlled by pathways from both sides of the cortex. Even though the upper motor neurons on the left are destroyed, others on the right remain, and the right upper face continues to function fairly well.

CN VII—Peripheral Lesion	**CN VII—Central Lesion**

Peripheral nerve damage to CN VII paralyzes the entire right side of the face, including the forehead.

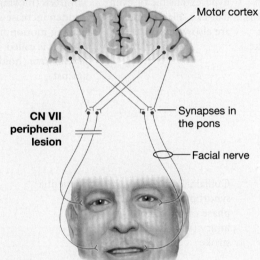

Motor cortex

CN VII peripheral lesion

Synapses in the pons

Facial nerve

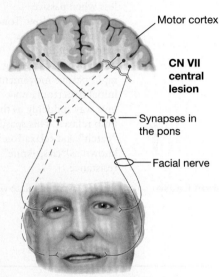

Motor cortex

CN VII central lesion

Synapses in the pons

Facial nerve

Closing Eyes

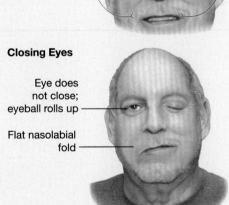

Eye does not close; eyeball rolls up

Flat nasolabial fold

Closing Eyes

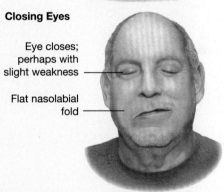

Eye closes; perhaps with slight weakness

Flat nasolabial fold

Raising Eyebrows

Forehead not wrinkled; eyebrow not raised

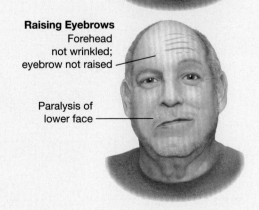

Paralysis of lower face

Raising Eyebrows

Forehead wrinkled; eyebrow raised

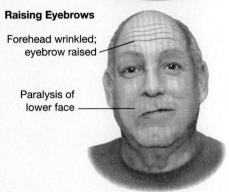

Paralysis of lower face

Table
17-9   **Disorders of Muscle Tone**

	Spasticity	Rigidity	Flaccidity	Paratonia
Location of Lesion	Upper motor neuron or corticospinal tract systems	Basal ganglia system	Lower motor neuron system at any point from the anterior horn cell to the peripheral nerves	Both hemispheres, usually in the frontal lobes
Description	Increased muscle tone (*hypertonia*) that is rate dependent. Tone is greater when passive movement is rapid, and less when passive movement is slow. Tone is also greater at the extremes of the movement arc. During rapid passive movement, initial hypertonia may give way suddenly as the limb relaxes. This spastic "catch" and relaxation is known as "clasp-knife" resistance.	Increased resistance that persists throughout the movement arc, independent of rate of movement, is called *lead-pipe rigidity*. With flexion and extension of the wrist or forearm, a superimposed rachetlike jerkiness is called *cogwheel rigidity*.	Loss of muscle tone (*hypotonia*), causing the limb to be loose or floppy. The affected limbs may be hyperextensible or even flail-like. Flaccid muscles are also weak.	Sudden changes in tone with passive range of motion. Sudden loss of tone that increases the ease of motion is called *mitgehen* (moving with). Sudden increase in tone making motion more difficult is called *gegenhalten* (holding against).
Common Cause	Stroke, especially late or chronic stage	Parkinsonism	Guillain-Barré syndrome; also initial phase of spinal cord injury (spinal shock) or stroke	Dementia

| Table 17-10 | **Abnormalities of Gait and Posture** |

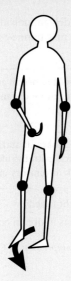

Spastic Hemiparesis

Seen in corticospinal tract lesion in stroke, causing poor control of flexor muscles during swing phase. Affected arm is flexed, immobile, and held close to the side, with elbow, wrists, and interphalangeal joints flexed. Affected leg extensors spastic; ankle plantar-flexed and inverted. Patients may drag toe, circle leg stiffly outward and forward (*circumduction*), or lean trunk to contralateral side to clear affected leg during walking.

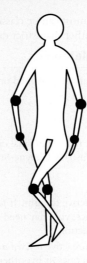

Scissors Gait

Seen in spinal cord disease, causing bilateral lower extremity spasticity, including adductor spasm, and abnormal proprioception. Gait is stiff. Patients advance each leg slowly, and the thighs tend to cross forward on each other at each step. Steps are short. Patients appear to be walking through water. Scissoring is seen in all spasticity disorders, most commonly cerebral palsy.

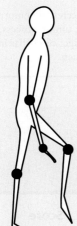

Steppage Gait

Seen in foot drop, usually secondary to peripheral motor unit disease. Patients either drag the feet or lift them high, with knees flexed, and bring them down with a slap onto the floor, thus appearing to be walking up stairs. They cannot walk on their heels. The steppage gait may involve one or both legs. Tibialis anterior and toe extensors are weak.

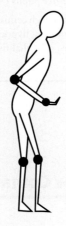

Parkinsonian Gait

Seen in the basal-ganglia defects of Parkinson disease. Posture is stooped, with flexion of head, arms, hips, and knees. Patients are slow getting started. Steps are short and shuffling, with involuntary hastening (*festination*). Arm swings are decreased, and patients turn around stiffly—"all in one piece." Postural control is poor (*retropulsion*).

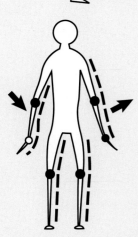

Cerebellar Ataxia

Seen in disease of the cerebellum or associated tracts. Gait is staggering, unsteady, and wide based, with exaggerated difficulty on turns. Patients cannot stand steadily with feet together, whether eyes are open or closed. Other cerebellar signs are present such as dysmetria, nystagmus, and intention tremor.

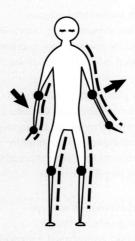

Sensory Ataxia

Seen in loss of position sense in the legs (with polyneuropathy or posterior column damage). Gait is unsteady and wide based (with feet wide apart). Patients throw their feet forward and outward and bring them down, first on the heels and then on the toes, with a double tapping sound. They watch the ground for guidance when walking. With eyes closed, they cannot stand steadily with feet together (positive Romberg sign), and the staggering gait worsens.

Although there are many causes of coma, most can be classified as either *structural* or *metabolic*. Findings vary widely in individual patients; the features listed are general guidelines rather than strict diagnostic criteria. Remember that psychiatric disorders may mimic coma.

	Toxic–Metabolic	Structural
Pathophysiology	Arousal centers poisoned or critical substrates depleted	Lesion destroys or compresses brainstem arousal areas, either directly or secondary to more distant expanding mass lesions.
Clinical Features		
• Respiratory pattern	If regular, may be normal or hyperventilation. If irregular, usually Cheyne-Stokes	Irregular, especially Cheyne-Stokes or ataxic breathing. Also with selected stereotypical patterns like "apneustic" respiration (peak inspiratory arrest) or central hyperventilation

• Pupillary size and reaction	Equal, reactive to light. If *pinpoint* from opiates or cholinergics, you may need a magnifying glass to see the reaction.
	
	May be unreactive if *fixed and dilated* from anticholinergics or hypothermia
		Unequal or unreactive to light (fixed)
		  Midposition, fixed—suggests midbrain compression
		
		  Dilated, fixed—suggests *compression* of CN III from herniation

• Level of consciousness	Changes *after* pupils change	Changes *before* pupils change
Examples of Cause	Uremia, hyperglycemia alcohol, drugs, liver failure hypothyroidism, hypoglycemia, anoxia, ischemia meningitis, encephalitis hyperthermia, hypothermia	Epidural, subdural, or intracerebral hemorrhage; cerebral infarct or embolus; tumor, abscess; brainstem infarct, tumor, or hemorrhage; cerebellar infarct, hemorrhage, tumor, or abscess

Activity		Score
Eye Opening		
None	1 = Even to supraorbital pressure	
To pain	2 = Pain from sternum/limb/supraorbital pressure	
To speech	3 = Nonspecific response, not necessarily to command	
Spontaneous	4 = Eyes open, not necessarily aware	_____
Motor Response		
None	1 = To any pain; limbs remain flaccid	
Extension	2 = Shoulder adducted and shoulder and forearm internally rotated	
Flexor response	3 = Withdrawal response or assumption of hemiplegic posture	
Withdrawal	4 = Arm withdraws to pain, shoulder abducts	
Localizes pain	5 = Arm attempts to remove supraorbital/chest pressure	
Obeys commands	6 = Follows simple commands	_____
Verbal Response		
None	1 = No verbalization of any type	
Incomprehensible	2 = Moans/groans, no speech	
Inappropriate	3 = Intelligible, no sustained sentences	
Confused	4 = Converses but confused, disoriented	
Oriented	5 = Converses and is oriented	_____
		TOTAL (3–15)*

*Interpretation: Patients with scores of 3–8 usually are considered to be in a coma.
Source: Teasdale G, Jennett B. Assessment of coma and impaired consciousness. A practical scale. Lancet 1974;304(7872):81–84.

Table
17-13 Pupils in Comatose Patients

Pupillary size, equality, and light reactions help to assess the cause of coma and to determine the region of the brain that is impaired. Remember that unrelated pupillary abnormalities, including miotic drops for glaucoma or mydriatic drops for a better view of the ocular fundi, may have preceded the coma.

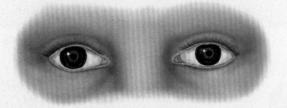

Small or Pinpoint Pupils

Bilaterally small pupils (1–2.5 mm) suggest damage to the sympathetic pathways in the hypothalamus, or metabolic encephalopathy, a diffuse failure of cerebral function that has many causes, including drugs. Light reactions are usually normal.

Pinpoint pupils (<1 mm) suggest a hemorrhage in the pons, or the effects of morphine, heroin, or other narcotics. The light reactions may be seen with a magnifying glass.

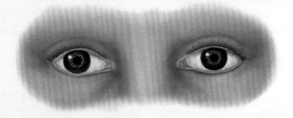

Midposition Fixed Pupils

Pupils that are in the *midposition or slightly dilated* (4–6 mm) and are *fixed to light* suggest structural damage in the midbrain.

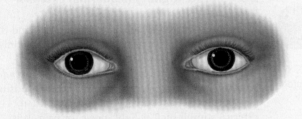

Large Pupils

Bilaterally fixed and dilated pupils may be due to severe anoxia and its sympathomimetic effects, as seen after cardiac arrest. They may also result from atropinelike agents, phenothiazines, or tricyclic antidepressants.

Bilaterally large reactive pupils may be due to cocaine, amphetamine, LSD, or other sympathetic nervous system agonists.

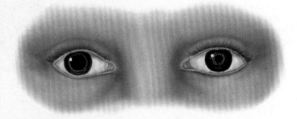

One Large Pupil

A pupil that is *fixed and dilated* warns of herniation of the temporal lobe, causing compression of the oculomotor nerve and midbrain. A single large pupil is most commonly seen in diabetic patients with infarction of CN III.

Table	
17-14	**Abnormal Postures in Comatose Patients**

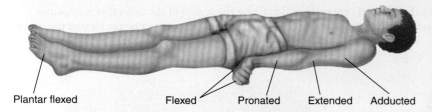

Plantar flexed   Flexed   Pronated   Extended   Adducted

Decorticate Rigidity (Abnormal Flexor Response)

In *decorticate rigidity*, the upper arms are flexed tight to the sides with elbows, wrists, and fingers flexed. The legs are extended and internally rotated. The feet are plantar flexed. This posture implies a destructive lesion of the corticospinal tracts within or very near the cerebral hemispheres. When unilateral, this is the posture of chronic spastic hemiplegia.

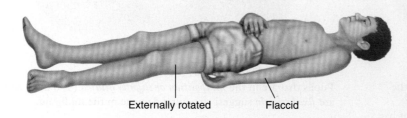

Externally rotated   Flaccid

Hemiplegia (Early)

Sudden unilateral brain damage involving the corticospinal tract may produce a *hemiplegia* (one-sided paralysis), which is flaccid early in its course. Spasticity will develop later. The paralyzed arm and leg are slack. They fall loosely and without tone when raised and dropped to the bed. Spontaneous movements or responses to noxious stimuli are limited to the opposite side. The leg may lie externally rotated. One side of the lower face may be paralyzed, and that cheek puffs out on expiration. Both eyes may be turned away from the paralyzed side.

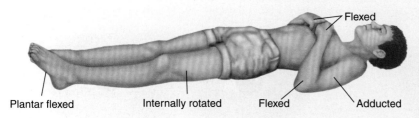

                                   Flexed

Plantar flexed   Internally rotated   Flexed   Adducted

Decerebrate Rigidity (Abnormal Extensor Response)

In *decerebrate rigidity*, the jaws are clenched and the neck is extended. The arms are adducted and stiffly extended at the elbows, with forearms pronated, wrists and fingers flexed. The legs are stiffly *extended at the knees*, with the feet plantar flexed. This posture may occur spontaneously or only in response to external stimuli such as light, noise, or pain. It is caused by a lesion in the diencephalon, midbrain, or pons, although severe metabolic disorders such as hypoxia or hypoglycemia may also produce it.

Special Populations

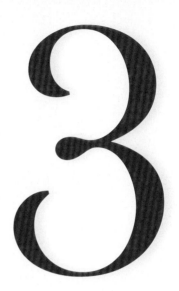

3

Special Populations

Assessing Children: Infancy Through Adolescence

Peter G. Szilagyi, MD, MPH

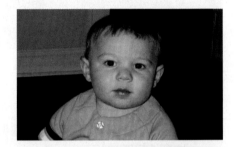

This chapter highlights clinical assessment for each pediatric age group, beginning with general principles of development and key components of health promotion. Newborns, infants, young and school-aged children, and adolescents are covered in separate sections, with relevant discussions of development, history taking, health promotion and counseling, and techniques of examination for each.

Guide to Chapter Organization

General Principles of Child Development
Health Promotion and Counseling: Key Components
Assessing the Newborn
Assessment Several Hours After Birth
Assessing the Infant
Assessing Young and School-Aged Children
Assessing Adolescents
Recording Your Findings

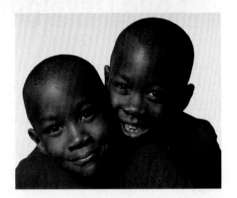

Often, neophyte and even some veteran examiners are intimidated when approaching a tiny baby or an upset child, especially under the critical eyes of anxious parents. Although it is initially challenging, you will come to enjoy almost all pediatric encounters.

Review Chapter 1, Overview: Physical Examination and History Taking, for the methods and sequence of examining adults. When examining infants and children, the sequence should vary according to the child's age and comfort level. *Perform less invasive maneuvers early and potentially distressing maneuvers near the end of the examination.* For example, palpate the head and neck and auscultate the heart and lungs early, and examine the ears and mouth and palpate the abdomen near the end. If the child reports pain in one area, examine that area last.

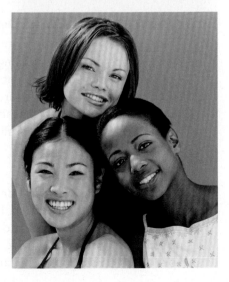

The format of the medical record is the same for both children and adults. Although the sequence of the physical examination may vary, convert your clinical findings back into the traditional written or electronic format.

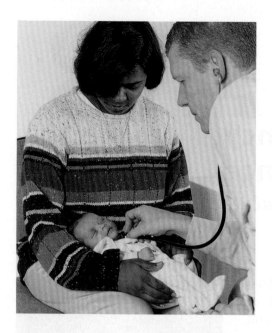

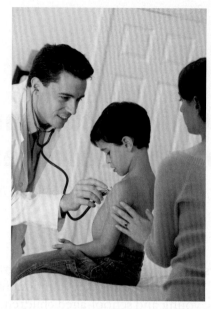

General Principles of Child Development

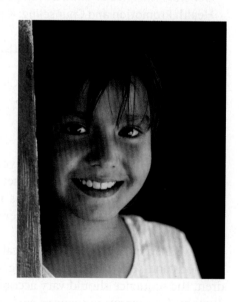

Childhood is a period of remarkable physical, cognitive, and social growth—by far the greatest in a person's lifetime. Within a few short years, children physically increase 20-fold, acquire sophisticated language and reasoning, develop complex social interactions, and become mature adults.

Understanding the normal physical, cognitive, and social development of children facilitates effective interviews and physical examinations and is the basis for distinguishing normal from abnormal findings.

Four Principles of Child Development

▶ Child development proceeds along a predictable pathway.
▶ The range of normal development is wide.
▶ Various physical, social, and environmental factors, as well as diseases, can affect child development and health.
▶ The child's developmental level affects how you conduct the history and physical examination.[1]

● The first principle of *child development* is that it *proceeds along a predictable pathway* governed by the maturing brain. You can measure age-specific milestones and use them to characterize development as normal or abnormal. Once the child reaches a milestone, he or she proceeds to the next. Because your health care visit and physical examination take place at one point in time, you need to determine where the child fits along a developmental trajectory. *Loss of milestones is cause for concern.*

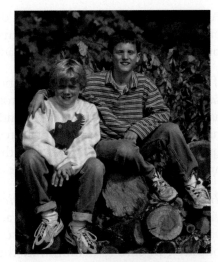

- The second principle is that the *range of normal development is wide.* Children mature at different rates. Each child's physical, cognitive, and social development should fall within a broad developmental range.

- The third principle recognizes that *various physical, social, and environmental factors, as well as diseases, can affect child development and health.* For example, chronic illnesses, child abuse, and poverty can all cause detectable physical abnormalities and alter the rate and course of development. Children with physical or cognitive disabilities may not follow the expected age-specific developmental trajectory.

- The fourth principle, specific to the pediatric examination, is that *the child's developmental level affects how you conduct the medical history and physical examination.* For example, interviewing a 5-year-old is fundamentally different from interviewing an adolescent. Both order and style differ from an adult examination. You must adapt your physical examination to the developmental level of the child while simultaneously attempting to ascertain that developmental level. An understanding of normal child development helps you achieve these tasks.

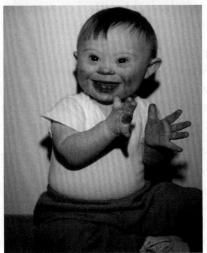

Health Promotion and Counseling: Key Components

Benjamin's Franklin's advice that "an ounce of prevention is worth a pound of cure" is particularly true for children and adolescents because prevention at a young age can result in improved health outcomes for decades. Pediatric clinicians dedicate substantial time to health supervision visits and health promotion activities.

Several national and international organizations have identified guidelines for health promotion for children.[2-5] Current concepts of health promotion include not only the detection and prevention of disease but also active promotion of the well-being of children and their families, spanning physical, cognitive, emotional, and social health.

Every interaction with a child and family is an opportunity for health promotion. From the interview to the physical examination, think of your interactions as an opportunity for two important tasks: the detection of clinical problems and the promotion of health.

Capitalize on the examination to offer age-appropriate guidance about the child's development. Provide suggestions about reading, conversing, playing music, and optimizing opportunities for gross and fine motor development.

Advise parents about upcoming developmental stages and strategies to encourage their child's development. Parents are the major agents of health promotion for children, and your advice is implemented through them.

The American Academy of Pediatrics (AAP) publishes guidelines for *health supervision visits* and the key age-appropriate components of these visits (see www.aap.org). Remember that children and adolescents who have a chronic illness or high-risk family or environmental circumstances will probably require more frequent visits and more intensive health promotion. Key health-promotion issues and strategies, tailored for specific age groups, are found throughout this chapter.

Integrate explanations of your physical findings with health promotion. Provide advice about expected maturational changes or how health behaviors can affect physical findings (e.g., exercise may reduce blood pressure and obesity). Be sure to demonstrate the relationship between healthy lifestyles and physical health. For example, give parents a copy of their child's body mass index (BMI) result along with a "prescription" for healthy living.

Childhood immunizations are a mainstay for health promotion and have been heralded as the most significant medical achievement in public health worldwide. The childhood immunization schedule changes yearly. Updates are published widely and disseminated on Web sites of the Centers for Disease Control and Prevention (CDC) (see www.cdc.gov) and the AAP.[6,7]

Screening procedures are performed at specific ages. These include growth parameters and developmental screening at all ages, blood pressure screening after age 3, and BMI screening after age 2, and vision and hearing screening at key ages. Screening procedures recommended for high-risk patients or at certain ages include tests for lead poisoning, tuberculosis exposure, anemia, dyslipidema, urinary tract infections, and sexually transmitted infections. There is variation worldwide in recommendations for screening tests; the AAP recommendations are provided at www.aap.org.[2]

Anticipatory guidance is a major component of the pediatric visit. Key areas cover a broad range of topics, from purely "medical" to developmental, social and emotional health. All these factors affect children's health.

Key Components of Pediatric Health Promotion

1. Age-appropriate developmental achievement of the child
   - Physical (maturation, growth, puberty)
   - Motor (gross and fine motor skills)
   - Cognitive (developmental milestones, language, school performance)
   - Emotional (self-efficacy, self-esteem, independence, morality)
   - Social (social competence, self-responsibility, integration with family and community)
2. Health supervision visits
   - Periodic assessment of medical and oral health
   - Children with special health care needs often require more frequent health supervision visits

(continued)

Key Components of Pediatric Health Promotion (*continued*)

3. Integration of physical examination findings with healthy lifestyles
4. Immunizations
5. Screening procedures
6. Anticipatory guidance[9]
   - Healthy habits
   - Nutrition and healthy eating
   - Safety and prevention of injury
   - Physical activity
   - Sexual development and sexuality
   - Self-responsibility and efficacy
   - Family relationships (inter-actions, strengths, supports)
   - Emotional and mental health
   - Oral health
   - Recognition of illness
   - Screen time
   - Prevention of risky behaviors
   - School and vocation
   - Peer relationships
   - Community interactions
7. Partnership between health care provider and child, adolescent, and family

Assessing the Newborn

The first year of life, infancy, is divided into the neonatal period (the first 28 days) and the postneonatal period (29 days to 1 year).

Tips for Examining Newborns

- Examine the newborn in the presence of the parents.
- Swaddle and then undress the newborn as the examination proceeds.
- Dim the lights and rock the newborn to encourage the eyes to open.
- Observe feeding if possible, particularly breast-feeding.
- Demonstrate calming maneuvers to parents (e.g., swaddling).
- Observe and teach parents about transitions as the newborn arouses.
- A typical sequence for the examination of the newborn:
  - Careful observation
  - Head, neck, heart, lungs, abdomen, genitourinary system
  - Lower extremities, back
  - Ears, mouth
  - Eyes, whenever they are spontaneously open
  - Skin, as you go along
  - Neurologic system
  - Hips

The first pediatric examination is performed immediately after delivery by obstetrical or pediatric clinicians. A comprehensive pediatric exam is generally performed within 24 hours of birth. Subsequent physical examinations occur at regular intervals or when the infant is ill. Assessment techniques for these exams are described in detail in the following sections.

If possible, do the physical examination in front of the parents so they can interact with you and ask questions. Parents may question their baby's physical appearance, so stating normal findings as you go can be reassuring. Observe parental bonding with the newborn, and watch how well the breast-feeding baby latches on and sucks. Breast-feeding is physiologically and psychologically optimal, but many mothers will need help and support at first. Early detection of difficulties and anticipatory guidance can promote and sustain breast-feeding.

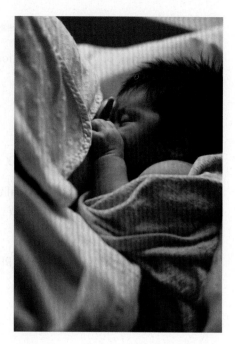

Newborns are most responsive 1 to 2 hours after a feeding, when they are neither too satiated (becoming less responsive) nor too hungry (and often agitated). Start with the newborn swaddled and comfortable. Then undress the newborn as the examination proceeds, for gradual stimulation and arousal. If the newborn becomes agitated, use a pacifier or a bottle of formula (if not breast-feeding), or allow the baby to suck on your gloved finger. Reswaddle the baby long enough to complete the parts of examination that require a quiet baby.

IMMEDIATE ASSESSMENT AT BIRTH

Examining newborns immediately after birth is important for determining general condition, developmental status, abnormalities in gestational development, and any congenital abnormalities. This examination may reveal diseases of cardiac, respiratory, or neurologic origin. Listen to the anterior thorax with your stethoscope, palpate the abdomen, and inspect the head, face, oral cavity, extremities, genitalia, and perineum. *Refer to the section "Assessing the Infant" for a complete physical examination.*

Apgar Score. The Apgar score is an assessment of the newborn immediately after birth. Its five components classify the newborn's neurologic recovery from birth and immediate adaptation to extrauterine life. Score each newborn at 1 and 5 minutes after birth according to the following table. Scoring is based on a 3-point scale (0, 1, or 2) for each component. Total scores may range from 0 to 10. Scoring may continue at 5-minute intervals until the score is >7. If the 5-minute Apgar score is 8 or more, proceed to a more complete examination.[10]

The Apgar Scoring System

Clinical Sign	Assigned Score		
	0	1	2
Heart rate	Absent	<100	>100
Respiratory effort	Absent	Slow and irregular	Good; strong
Muscle tone	Flaccid	Some flexion of the arms and legs	Active movement
Reflex irritability*	No responses	Grimace	Crying vigorously, sneeze, or cough
Color	Blue, pale	Pink body, blue extremities	Pink all over

*Reaction to suction of nares with bulb syringe

(continued)

The Apgar Scoring System (*continued*)

1-Minute Apgar Score		5-Minute Apgar Score	
8–10	Normal	8–10	Normal
5–7	Some nervous system depression	0–7	High risk for subsequent central nervous system and other organ system dysfunction
0–4	Severe depression, requiring immediate resuscitation		

Gestational Age and Birth Weight. *Classify newborns according to their gestational age of maturity and birth weight.* These classifications help predict medical problems and morbidity. Some clinical practice guidelines target infants born before a certain gestational age or below specific birth weight parameters.

Gestational age is based on specific neuromuscular signs and physical characteristics that change with gestational maturity. The *Ballard Scoring System* estimates gestational age to within 2 weeks, even in extremely premature infants. A complete Ballard Scoring System, with instructions for assessing neuromuscular and physical maturity, is included in this chapter on p. 773.[11]

Classification by Gestational Age and Birth Weight

Gestational Age

Classification	Gestational Age
▶ Preterm	▶ <34 wks
▶ Late preterm	▶ 34–36 wks
▶ Term	▶ 37–42 wks
▶ Postterm	▶ >42 wks

Birth Weight

Classification	Weight
▶ Extremely low birth weight	▶ <1,000 g
▶ Very low birth weight	▶ <1,500 g
▶ Low birth weight	▶ <2,500 g
▶ Normal birth weight	▶ ≥2,500 g

Preterm infants are at risk for both short-term complications (mainly respiratory and cardiovascular) as well as long-term sequela (e.g., neurodevelopmental).

Late preterm infants are at considerable risk for prematurity-related complications.

Postterm infants are at increased risk of perinatal mortality or morbidity such as asphyxia and meconium aspiration.

A useful classification, shown below, is derived from the gestational age and birth weight on the intrauterine growth curve.

Newborn Classifications[10]

Category	Abbreviation	Percentile
Small for gestational age	SGA	<10th
Appropriate for gestational age	AGA	10–90th
Large for gestational age	LGA	>90th

The figure on the below shows the intrauterine growth curves for the 10th and 90th percentiles and depicts the categories of maturity for newborns based on gestational age and birth weight.

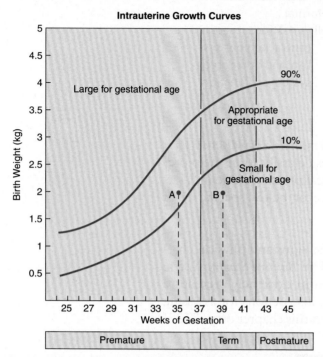

Intrauterine Growth Curves

LGA infants may experience difficulties during birth. Infants of mothers with diabetes are often LGA and may have metabolic abnormalities shortly after birth, as well as congenital anomalies.

A common complication among LGA newborns is hypoglycemia, which can result in jitteriness, irritability, cyanosis, or other health issues.

While no etiology is noted for many SGA infants, known causes include fetal, placental, and maternal factors.

Level of intrauterine growth based on gestational age and birth weight of liveborn, single, white infants. Point A represents a premature infant, while point B indicates an infant of similar birth weight who is mature but SGA; the growth curves are representative of the 10th and 90th percentiles for all of the newborns in the sampling. (Adapted from Sweet YA. Classification of the low-birth-weight infant. In Klaus MH, Fanaroff AA. Care of the high-risk neonate, 3rd ed. Philadelphia: WB Saunders, 1986. Reproduced with permission.)

The three babies shown below were all born at 32 weeks' gestational age and weighed 600 g (SGA), 1,400 g (AGA), and 2,750 g (LGA). Each of these categories has a different mortality rate, highest for preterm SGA and LGA infants, and lowest for term AGA infants.

Preterm AGA infants are more prone to respiratory distress syndrome, apnea, patent ductus arteriosus with left-to-right shunt, and infection. *Preterm SGA infants* are more likely to experience asphyxia, hypoglycemia, and hypocalcemia.

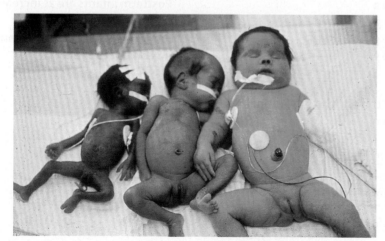

The New Ballard Score for Determining Gestational Age in Weeks

		−1	0	1	2	3	4	5
Neuromuscular Maturity	Posture							
	Square window (wrist)	>90°	90°	60°	45°	30°	0°	
	Arm recoil		180°	140°–180°	110°–140°	90°–110°	<90°	
	Popliteal angle	180°	160°	140°	120°	100°	90°	<90°
	Scarf sign							
	Heel to ear							
Physical Maturity	Skin	Sticky friable transparent	Gelatinous red, translucent	Smooth pink, visible veins	Superficial peeling and/or rash, few veins	Cracking pale areas rare veins	Parchment deep cracking no vessels	Leathery cracked wrinkled
	Lanugo	None	Sparse	Abundant	Thinning	Bald areas	Mostly bald	
	Plantar surface	heel — toe 40–50 mm: −1 <40 mm: −2	>50 mm no crease	Faint red marks	Anterior transverse crease only	Creases anterior 2/3	Creases over entire sole	
	Breast	Imperceptible	barely preceptible	flat areola no bud	Stippled areola 1–2-mm bud	Raised areola 3–4-mm bud	Full areola 5–10-mm bud	
	Eye/ear	Lids fused loosely: −1 Tightly: −2	Lids open, pinna flat stays folded	Slightly curved pinna; soft, slow recoil	Well-curved pinna; soft, but ready recoil	Formed and firm instant recoil	Thick cartilage, ear stiff	
	Genitals male	Scrotum flat, smooth	Scrotum empty, faint rugae	Testes in upper canal, rare rugae	Testes descending, few rugae	Testes down, good rugae	Testes pendulous, deep rugae	
	Genitals female	Clitoris prominent, labia flat	Prominent clitoris, small labia minora	Prominent clitoris, enlarging minora	Majora and minora equally prominent	Majora large, minora small	Majora cover clitoris and minora	

Maturity Rating

Score	Weeks
−10	20
−5	22
0	24
5	26
10	28
15	30
20	32
25	34
30	36
35	38
40	40
45	42
50	44

Asphyxiated neonates or neonates obtunded by anesthetic agents or drugs will score lower on neuromuscular maturity criteria. In such instances, scoring should be repeated at 24 to 48 hours of age. The sum of the scores for all of the neuromuscular and physical maturity items provides an estimate of gestational age in weeks, using the maturity rating scale at the lower right potion of the figure. (Redrawn from Ballard JL et al. J Pediatr 1991;119:417.)

Assessment Several Hours After Birth

During the first day of life, newborns should have a comprehensive examination. Wait until 1 or 2 hours after a feeding, when the baby is most responsive, and ask the parents to remain in the room. Follow the sequence shown on pp. 769–770. See *Techniques of Examination* (p. 780) for details on examining newborns and infants.

Observe the undressed newborn. Note the newborn's color, size, body proportions, nutritional status, and posture, as well as respirations and movements of the head and extremities. Most normal, full-term newborns lie in a symmetric position, with the limbs semiflexed and the legs partially abducted at the hip.

In *breech babies* (buttock first), the knees are flexed in utero; in a *frank breech baby*, the knees are extended in utero. In both, the hips are flexed.

Note the baby's spontaneous motor activity, with flexion and extension alternating between the arms and legs. The fingers are usually flexed in a tight fist, but may extend in slow athetoid posturing movements. You will observe brief tremors of the body and extremities during vigorous crying, and even at rest.

By 4 days after birth, tremors at rest signal central nervous system disease from various possible causes, ranging from *asphyxia* to *drug withdrawal*.

Studies by Dr. T. Berry Brazelton and others have demonstrated the wide range of abilities in newborns, which are described below. [12] Parents will be delighted by these abilities.

Asymmetric movements of the arms or legs at any time suggest *central or peripheral neurologic deficits, birth injury* (such as a fractured clavicle or brachial plexus injury), or *congenital anomalies*.

What a Newborn Can Do [12]

Core Elements

▶ Newborns use all five senses. For example, they prefer to look at human faces and turn to a parent's voice.

▶ Newborns are unique individuals. Marked differences exist in temperaments, personality, behavior, and learning.

▶ Newborns interact dynamically with caregivers—a two-way street!

Newborns who cannot perform many of these behaviors may have a neurologic condition, drug withdrawal, or a serious illness such as infection.

Examples of Complex Newborn Behavior

Habituation	Ability to selectively and progressively shut out negative stimuli (e.g., a repetitive sound)
Attachment	A reciprocal, dynamic process of interacting and bonding with the caregiver
State Regulation	Ability to modulate the level of arousal in response to different degrees of stimulation (e.g., self-consoling)
Perception	Ability to regard faces, turn to voices, quiet in presence of singing, track colorful objects, respond to touch, and recognize familiar scents

Assessing the Infant

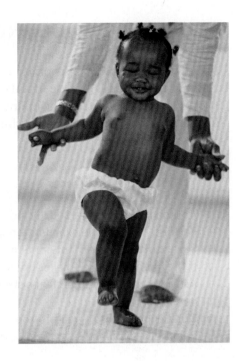

DEVELOPMENT

Physical Development. Physical growth during infancy is faster than at any other age.[13] By 1 year, the infant's birth weight should have tripled and height increased by 50%.

The figure below shows the developmental progression in infancy. Even newborns have surprising abilities, such as fixing upon and following human faces. Neurologic development progresses centrally to peripherally. Thus, newborns learn head control before trunk control and use of arms and legs before use of hands and fingers.

Activity, exploration, and environmental manipulation contribute to learning. By 3 months, normal infants lift the head and clasp the hands. By 6 months, they roll over, reach for objects, turn to voices, and possibly sit with support. With increasing peripheral coordination, infants reach for objects, transfer them from hand to hand, crawl, stand by holding on, and play with objects by banging and grabbing. A 1-year-old may be standing and putting everything in the mouth.[14]

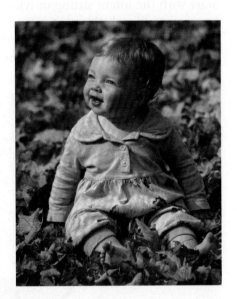

Cognitive and Language Development. Exploration fosters increased understanding of self and environment. Infants learn cause and effect (e.g., shaking a rattle produces sound), object permanence, and use of tools. By 9 months, they may recognize the examiner as a stranger deserving wary cooperation, seek comfort from parents during examinations, and actively manipulate reachable objects (e.g., equipment). Language development proceeds from cooing at 2 months, to babbling at 6 months, to saying one to three words by 1 year.[15]

Social and Emotional Development. Understanding of self and family also matures. Social tasks include bonding, attachment to caregivers, and trust that they will meet needs. Temperaments vary. Some infants are predictable, adaptable, and respond positively to new stimuli; others are less so and respond intensely or negatively. Because environment affects social development, observe the infant's interactions with caregivers.

Developmental Milestones During Infancy[13]

	Birth	1 m	2 m	3 m	4 m	5 m	6 m	7 m	8 m	9 m	10 m	11 m	12 m
Physical	Fixes/follows			Rolls over			Sits		Pulls to stand		Stands		Walks
	Head control			Grasps rattle			Thumb–finger grasp				Crawls		
Cognitive/ Language	Responds to sounds		Squeals	Imitates speech sounds			Dada/Mama specific				2 words	3 words	
Social/ Emotional	Smiles				Works for toy				Imitates activities				
	Regards face						Feeds self		Indicates wants			Uses spoon	

GENERAL GUIDELINES

Use developmentally appropriate methods such as *distraction* and *play* to examine the infant. Because infants pay attention to one thing at a time, it is relatively easy to distract the infant from the examination being performed. You can use a moving object, a flashing light, a game of peek-a-boo, tickling, or any sort of noise.

If you cannot distract the infant or make the awake infant attend to an object, your face, or a sound, consider a possible *visual* or *hearing deficit*.

Tips for Examining Infants

▶ Approach the infant gradually, using a toy or object for distraction.
▶ Perform much of the examination with the infant in the parent's lap.
▶ Speak softly to the infant or mimic the infant's sounds to attract attention.
▶ If the infant is cranky, make sure he or she is well fed before proceeding.
▶ Ask a parent about the infant's strengths to elicit useful developmental and parenting information.
▶ Don't expect to do a head-to-toe exam in a specific order. Take what the infant gives you and save the mouth and ear exam for last.

Start with the infant sitting or lying in the parent's lap. If the infant is tired, hungry, or ill, ask the parent to hold the baby against the parent's chest. Make sure appropriate toys, a blanket, or other familiar objects are nearby. A hungry infant may need to be fed first.

Many neurologic conditions can be diagnosed during this general part of the exam. For example, you can detect *hypotonia,* conditions associated with *irritability* or signs of *cerebral palsy* (see neurologic examination below).

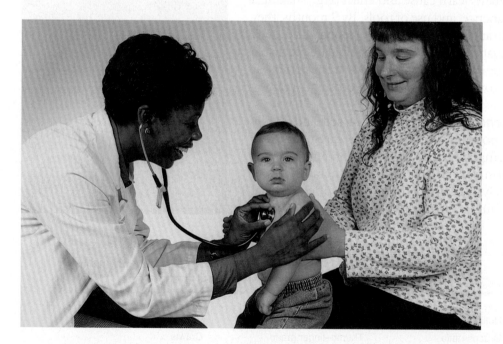

Close observation of an awake infant sitting on the parent's lap can reveal potential abnormalities such as *hypotonia* or *hypertonia*, conditions with abnormal skin color, jaundice or cyanosis, jitteriness, or respiratory problems.

Observe parent–infant interactions. Watch the parent's affect when talking about the infant. Note the parent's manner of holding, moving, dressing, and comforting the infant. Assess and comment on positive interactions, such as the obvious pride in the mother's face on the previous page.

Infants do not object to removing their clothing. To keep yourself and your surroundings dry, it is wise to leave the diaper in place throughout the examination; remove it only to examine the genitals, rectum, and hips.

Testing for Developmental Milestones

Because you want to measure the infant's best performance, check milestones at the end of the interview, just before the examination. This "fun and games" interlude also enhances cooperation during the examination. Experienced clinicians can weave the developmental examination into the other parts of the examination. The table on p. 775 shows some key physical or motor, cognitive or language, and social–emotional milestones during the first year. As an example, the infant in the photo below can sit unsupported, uses a thumb-finger grasp, and is indicating wants—an 8-month level.

The AAP recommends that health care providers use a standardized developmental screening instrument for infants as young as several months of age.[16]

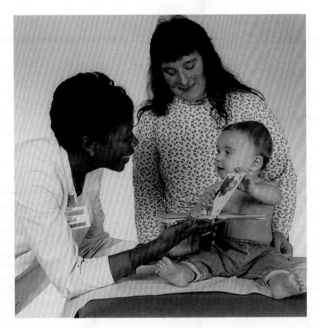

A traditional standard instrument for measuring developmental milestones throughout infancy and childhood has been the Denver Developmental Screening Test (DDST).[17] This instrument is designed to detect developmental delays in four domains of development from birth through 6 years: personal–social, fine motor–adaptive, language, and gross motor. The DDST is not a measure of intelligence, but rather a measure of developmental attainment in these four categories. It is a highly specific test (so that normal children will test as normal) but is not highly sensitive (i.e., many children with mild developmental delay score as normal).

Observation of the infant's communication with the parent can reveal abnormalities such as *developmental delay, language delay, hearing deficits,* or *inadequate parental attachment.* Likewise, such observations may identify maladaptive nurturing patterns that may stem from *maternal depression* or *inadequate social support.*

Many disorders cause delays in more than one milestone. For most children with developmental delay, the causes are unknown. Some known causes include *abnormality in embryonic development* (e.g., prenatal insult); *hereditary and genetic disorders* (e.g., inborn errors, genetic abnormalities); *environmental and social problems* (e.g., insufficient stimulation); *pregnancy or perinatal problems* (e.g., placental insufficiency, prematurity); and *childhood diseases* (e.g., infection, trauma, chronic illness).

If a cooperative infant fails items on a standardized screening instrument, developmental delay is possible, necessitating more precise testing and evaluation.

Numerous newer developmental screening instruments have been promulgated and tested on a variety of populations. Some useful ones include the Ages and Stages Questionnaire, the Early Language Milestone Scale (ELM Scale-2), the Modified Checklist for Autism in Toddlers (MCHAT), and the Parents' Evaluation of Developmental Status (PEDS). In general, these instruments have sensitivity and specificity around 70% to 80% (see Chapter 2), which is still lower than characteristics of typical clinical tests. This is due to the wide ranges of normal development, the difficulty in assessing development, and the scarcity of interventions.

Use these screening instruments as adjuncts to a comprehensive developmental examination. Suspected delays warrant further examination. For babies born prematurely, adjust expected developmental milestones for the gestational age up to 12 months.

An infant or toddler who has developmental skills that plateau or are out of sequence may have *autism* or *cerebral palsy.*

Pediatric Developmental Screening Flowchart

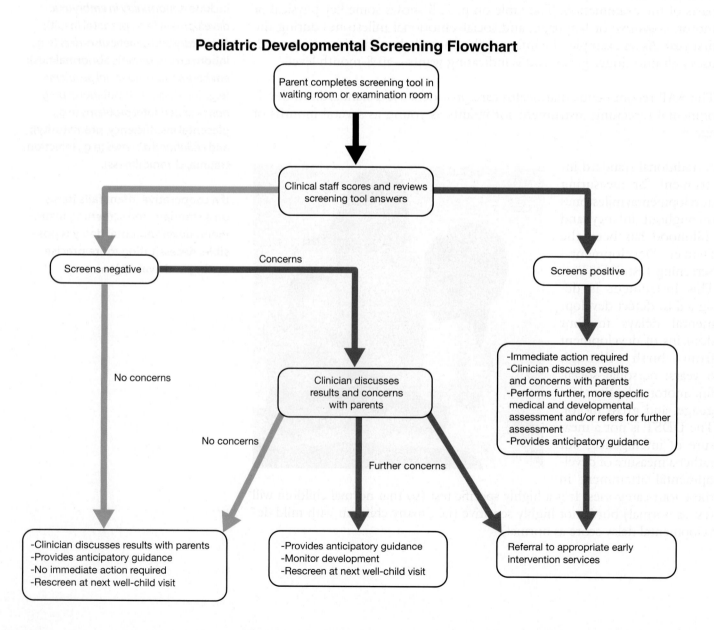

HEALTH PROMOTION AND COUNSELING: EVIDENCE AND RECOMMENDATIONS

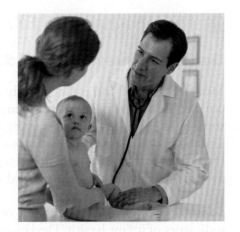

The AAP and the group Bright Futures[3] recommend health supervision visits for infants at the following ages: at birth, at 3 to 5 days, by 1 month, and at 2, 4, 6, 9, and 12 months. This is called the *Infant Periodicity Schedule*. Health supervision visits provide opportunities to answer questions for parents, assess the infant's growth and development, perform a comprehensive physical examination, and provide anticipatory guidance. Age-appropriate anticipatory guidance includes healthy habits and behaviors, social competence of caregivers, family relationships, and community interactions.

These visits provide an opportunity to plot a course for health and successful development. That infants generally are well during these visits enhances the quality of the experience. Parents usually are receptive to suggestions about health promotion, which can have major, long-term influences on the child and family. Strong interviewing skills are necessary as you discuss with families strategies to optimize the health and well-being of their infants. Review the critical components of a health supervision visit for a 6-month-old. Adjust the content to the appropriate developmental level of the infant.

Components of a Health Supervision Visit for a 6-Month-Old

Discussions With Parents
- Address parents' concerns/questions
- Provide advice
- Perform social history
- Assess development, nutrition, safety, oral health, family relationships, community

Developmental Assessment
- Use a standardized developmental instrument to measure milestones
- Assess milestones by history
- Assess milestones by examination

Physical Examination
- Perform a careful examination, including growth parameters with percentiles for age

Screening Tests
- Vision and hearing (by exam), possibly hematocrit and lead (if high risk), screen for social risk factors

Immunizations
- See schedule (AAP or CDC Web site)

Anticipatory Guidance
Healthy Habits and Behaviors
- Injury and illness prevention
    Infant seat, rolling walker, poisons, tobacco exposure
- Nutrition
    Breast-feeding or bottle, solids, limit juice, prevent choking, overfeeding
- Oral health
    No bottle in bed, fluoride, brushing teeth
Parent–Infant Interaction
- Promoting development
Family Relationships
- Time for self; babysitters
Community Interaction
- Child care, resources

TECHNIQUES OF EXAMINATION

General Survey and Vital Signs

Measurement of the infant's body size and assessment of vital signs are critical. Tables on the accompanying Web site show norms for blood pressure, height, weight, BMI (starting age 2 years), and head circumference. Compare vital signs or body proportions with age-specific norms, because they change dramatically as children grow. Some pediatric practitioners also assess pain regularly, using standardized pain scales.

Somatic Growth. Measurement of growth is one of the most important indicators of infant health. Deviations may provide an early indication of an underlying problem. Compare growth parameters with respect to normal values for age and sex, as well as prior readings on the same child, to assess trends.

Measure growth parameters carefully, using consistent technique and, optimally, the same scales to measure height and weight.

The most important tools for assessing somatic growth are the growth charts, which are published by the National Center for Health Statistics (www.cdc.gov/nchsv) and also the World Health Organization (www.who .int). All charts include height, weight, and head circumference for age, with one set for children up to 36 months and a second set for 2 to 18 years. Charts plotting weight by length as well as BMI are also available. These growth charts have percentile lines indicating the percentage of normal children above and below the child's measurement by chronologic age. Special growth charts are available for use in infants born prematurely, to correct for this result.

The AAP, NIH, and CDC now recommend that clinicians use the 2006 WHO International growth charts for children 0 to 23 months of age. CDC growth charts should be used in the United States to assess growth in children 2 to 19 years of age.

Length. For children younger than 2 years, measure body length by placing the child supine on a measuring board or in a measuring tray, as shown here. Direct measurement of the infant using a tape measure is inaccurate unless an assistant holds the child still with hips and knees extended.

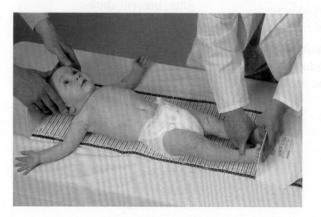

Measurement deviations beyond two standards for age, or above the 95th percentile or below the 5th percentile, are indications for more detailed evaluation. These deviations may be the first and only indicators of disease (see examples on the Web site tables). Many experts recommend using 2 standard deviations on WHO growth charts to assess abnormal growth.

A common cause of an apparent deviation in somatic growth is *measurement error*, attributed partly to the challenge of measuring a squirming infant or child. Confirm abnormalities by repeat measurement.

Although many normal infants cross percentiles on growth charts, a sudden or significant change in growth may indicate systemic disease due to various possible organ systems.

Abnormalities that can cause deviation from normal growth patterns include *Down syndrome* or *prematurity*. Growth charts are also available for children with specific conditions such as *Down syndrome* or *Turner syndrome*.

Reduced growth velocity, shown by a drop in height percentile on a growth curve, may signify a chronic condition. Comparison with normal standards is essential, because growth velocity normally is less during the second year than during the first year.

Chronic conditions causing reduced length or height include *neurologic*, *renal*, *cardiac*, and *endocrine disorders*.

Velocity growth curves are helpful in older children, especially those who are suspected of having endocrine disorders.

Weight. Weigh infants directly with an infant scale. Infants should be weighed naked or be clothed only in a diaper.

If the infant's weight is unexpectedly and significantly different than anticipated, redo the measurement to ensure accuracy.

Head Circumference. The head circumference always should be measured during the first 2 years of life, but measurement can be useful at any age to assess growth of the head. The head circumference in infants reflects the rate of growth of the cranium and the brain.

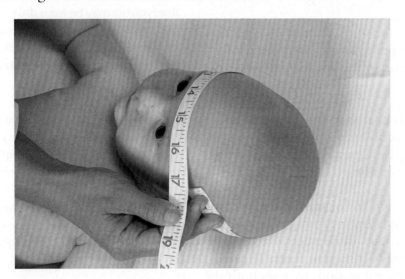

Vital Signs

Blood Pressure. Although obtaining accurate blood pressure readings in infants is challenging, this measurement is nevertheless important for some high-risk infants and should be routinely performed after age 3 years. You will need your skills in distraction or play, as shown in the accompanying photo.

The most easily used measure of systolic blood pressure in infants is the *Doppler method*, which detects arterial blood flow vibrations, converts them to systolic blood pressure levels, and transmits them to a digital read-out device.

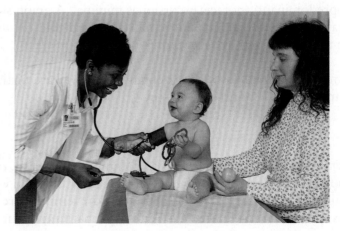

Failure to thrive is inadequate weight gain for age. Common indicators are: (a) growth <5th percentile for age; (b) drop >2 quartiles in 6 months; or (c) weight for length <5th percentile. Causes include environmental or psychosocial factors and a variety of gastrointestinal, neurologic, cardiac, endocrine, renal, and other diseases.

A small head size may result from *premature closure of the sutures* or *microcephaly*, which may be familial or due to *chromosomal abnormalities*, *congenital infections, maternal metabolic disorders*, and *neurologic insults*.

An abnormally large head size (>95th percentile or 2 standard deviations above the mean) is *macrocephaly*, which may result from *hydrocephalus, subdural hematoma*, or rare causes like *brain tumor* or *inherited syndromes*. *Familial megaloencephaly* (large head) is a benign familial condition.

Systolic blood pressure gradually increases throughout childhood. For example, normal systolic pressure in males is about 70 mm Hg at birth, 85 mm Hg at 1 month, and 90 mm Hg at 6 months (see WHO or CDC Web site).

Pulse. The heart rate of infants is more sensitive to the effects of illness, exercise, and emotion than that of adults. A graph showing normal heart rates for infants and children is available on thePoint.

Heart Rates From Birth to 1 Year

Age	Average Heart Rate	Range
Birth–1 mo	140	90–190
1–6 mo	130	80–180
6–12 mo	115	75–155

You may have trouble obtaining an accurate pulse rate in a squirming infant. Palpate the femoral arteries in the inguinal area or the brachial arteries in the antecubital fossa, or auscultate the heart.

Respiratory Rate. As with heart rate, compared with that of adults, the respiratory rate in infants has a greater range and is more responsive to illness, exercise, and emotion than that of adults. The rate of respirations per minute ranges between 30 and 60 in the newborn.

The respiratory rate may vary considerably from moment to moment in the newborn, with alternating periods of rapid and slow breathing. The sleeping respiratory rate is most reliable. Respiratory rates during active sleep compared with quiet sleep may be up to 10 breaths per minute faster. The respiratory pattern should be observed for at least 60 seconds to asses both the rate and the pattern. In infancy and early childhood, diaphragmatic breathing is predominant; thoracic excursion is minimal. A graph showing normal respiratory rates for infants and children is available on thePoint. Rates above these levels signify *tachypnea*.

Commonly accepted cutoffs for defining *tachypnea* are birth to 2 months, >60/min; 2 to 12 months, >50/min.

Temperature. Because fever is so common in children, obtain an accurate body temperature when you suspect infection, collagen vascular disease, or malignancy. Axillary and thermal-tape skin temperature recordings in infants and children are inaccurate. Auditory canal temperatures are accurate.

Causes of *sustained hypertension* in newborns include *renal artery disease* (stenosis, thrombosis), *congenital renal malformations*, and *coarctation of the aorta*.

While *sinus tachycardia* may be extremely rapid (up to 250/min), a pulse rate that is too rapid to count (usually >180/min) may indicate *paroxysmal supraventricular tachycardia*.

Bradycardia may be from drug ingestion, hypoxia, intracranial or neurologic conditions, or, rarely, cardiac arrhythmia such as heart blockage.

Extremely rapid and shallow respiratory rates are seen in newborns with *cyanotic cardiac disease* and *right-to-left shunting*, and *metabolic acidosis*.

Fever can raise respiratory rates in infants by up to 10 respirations per minute for each degree centigrade of fever.

Tachypnea and increased respiratory effort in an infant are signs of lower respiratory disease such as *bronchiolitis* or *pneumonia*.

Fever (>38.0°C or >100.4°F) in infants younger than 2 to 3 months may be a sign of *serious infection* or disease. These infants should be evaluated promptly.

The technique for obtaining a *rectal temperature* is relatively simple. One method is illustrated below. Place the infant prone, separate the buttocks with the thumb and forefinger on one hand, and with the other hand gently insert a well-lubricated rectal thermometer, to a depth of 2 to 3 cm. Keep the thermometer in place for at least 2 minutes.

Body temperature in infants and children is less constant than in adults. The average rectal temperature is higher in infancy and early childhood, usually above 99.0°F (37.2°C) until after age 3 years. Body temperature may fluctuate as much as 3°F during a single day, approaching 101°F (38.3°C) in normal children, particularly in late afternoon and after vigorous activity.

Anxiety may elevate the body temperature of children. *Excessive bundling* of infants may elevate the skin temperature but not the core temperature.

Temperature instability in a newborn may result from sepsis, metabolic abnormality, or other serious conditions. Older infants rarely manifest temperature instability.

Potentially sick febrile infants under 3 months of age may have *serious bacterial infection* and should have temperatures assessed using a rectal thermometer.

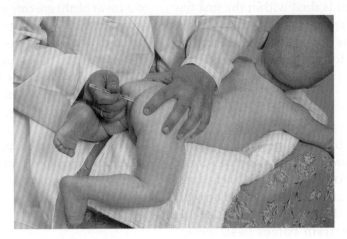

The Skin

Inspection.   Examine the skin of the newborn or infant carefully to identify both normal markings and potentially abnormal ones. The photos on pp. 786 and 787 demonstrate normal markings. The newborn's skin has a unique characteristic *texture and appearance*. The texture is soft and smooth because it is thinner than the skin of older children. Within the first 10 minutes after birth, a normal newborn progresses from generalized cyanosis to pinkness. In lighter-skinned infants, an erythematous flush, giving the skin the appearance of a "boiled lobster," is common during the first 8 to 24 hours, after which the normal pale pink coloring predominates.

Some newborns with *polycythemia* have a "ruddy" complexion. This is a reddish-purple color.

Vasomotor changes in the dermis and subcutaneous tissue—a response to cooling or chronic exposure to radiant heat—can produce a latticelike, bluish mottled appearance (*cutis marmorata*), particularly on the trunk, arms, and legs. This response to cold may last for months in normal infants. *Acrocyanosis*, a blue cast to the hands and feet when exposed to cold (see p. 786), is very common in newborns for the first few days and may recur throughout early infancy. Occasionally in newborns, a remarkable color change (*harlequin dyschromia*) appears, with transient cyanosis of one-half of the body or one extremity, presumably from temporary vascular instability.

Cutis marmorata is prominent in *premature infants* and in infants with *congenital hypothyroidism* and *Down syndrome*. If acrocyanosis does not disappear within 8 hours or with warming, *cyanotic congenital heart disease* should be considered.

The amount of melanin in the skin of newborns varies, affecting *pigmentation*. Black newborns may have a lighter skin color initially, except in the nail beds and genitalia, which are dark at birth. A dark or bluish pigmentation over the buttocks and lower lumbar regions is common in newborns of African, Asian, and Mediterranean descent. These areas, formerly called Mongolian spots, result from pigmented cells in the deep layers of the skin; they become less noticeable with age and usually disappear during childhood. Document these pigmented areas to avoid later concern about bruising.

Central cyanosis in a baby or child of any age should raise suspicion of *congenital heart disease*. The best area to look for central cyanosis is the tongue and oral mucosa, not the nail beds or the extremities.

At birth there is a fine, downy growth of hair called *lanugo* over the entire body, especially the shoulders and back. This hair is shed within the first few weeks. Lanugo is prominent in premature infants. Hair thickness on the head varies considerably among newborns and is not predictive of later hair growth. All of the original hair is shed within months, replaced with a new crop, sometimes of a different color.

Pigmented light-brown lesions (<1 to 2 cm at birth) are *café-au-lait spots*. Isolated lesions have no significance, but multiple lesions with smooth borders may suggest *neurofibromatosis* (see Table 18-2, Common Skin Rashes and Skin Findings in Newborns and Infants, p. 879).

Inspect the newborn closely for a series of common skin conditions. At birth, a cheesy white material called *vernix caseosa*, composed of sebum and desquamated epithelial cells, covers the body. Some newborns have *edema* over their hands, feet, lower legs, pubis, and sacrum; this disappears within a few days. Superficial desquamation of the skin is often noticeable 24 to 36 hours after birth, particularly in postterm babies (>40 weeks' gestation).

Skin desquamation is rarely a sign of *placental circulatory insufficiency* or *congenital ichthyosis*.

You should be able to identify four common dermatologic conditions in newborns:—*miliaria rubra, erythema toxicum, pustular melanosis*, and *milia*— which are shown on pp. 786 and 787. None of these is clinically significant.

Both erythema toxicum and pustular melanosis may appear similar to the pathologic vesiculopustular rash of *herpes simplex* or *Staphylococcus aureus skin infection*.

Note any signs of trauma from the birth process and the use of forceps or suction; these signs disappear but should prompt a careful neurologic examination.

Midline hair tufts over the lumbosacral spine region suggest a possible *spinal cord defect*.

Jaundice. Carefully examine and touch the newborn's skin to assess the level of jaundice. Normal "physiologic" jaundice, which occurs in half of all newborns, appears on the second or third day, peaks at about the fifth day, and usually disappears within a week. Jaundice can be seen best in natural

Jaundice within the first 24 hours of birth may be from *hemolytic disease of the newborn*.

daylight rather than artificial light. Newborn jaundice seems to progress from head to toe, with more intense jaundice on the upper body and less intense yellow color in the lower extremities.

To detect jaundice, apply pressure to the skin (see photos below) to press out the normal pink or brown color. A yellowish "blanching" indicates jaundice.

Another technique is to press a glass slide against the skin to empty the capillary bed and observe for color contrast.

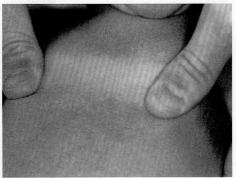

Pressing the red color from the skin allows better recognition of the yellow of jaundice. The infant on the left has no appreciable jaundice, while the infant on the right has a bilirubin level of 13 mg/dL (222 μmol/L). From Fletcher M. Physical Diagnosis in Neonatology. Philadelphia: Lippincott-Raven, 1998.

Vascular Markings. A common *vascular marking* is the "salmon patch" (also known as *nevus simplex*, "flame nevi," telangiectatic nevus, or capillary hemangioma). These flat, irregular, light pink patches (see p. 787) are most often seen on the nape of the neck ("stork bite"), upper eyelids, forehead, or upper lip ("angel kisses"). They are not true nevi, but result from distended capillaries. They often disappear by 1 year of age and are covered by the hairline.

Palpation. Palpate the newborn or infant's skin to assess the degree of hydration, or turgor. Roll a fold of loosely adherent skin on the abdominal wall between your thumb and forefinger to determine its consistency. The skin in well-hydrated infants returns to its normal position immediately upon release. Delay in return is a phenomenon called "tenting" and usually occurs in children with significant dehydration.

Late-appearing jaundice or jaundice that persists beyond 2 to 3 weeks should raise suspicions of *biliary obstruction* or *liver disease*.

A common source of jaundice during the first couple of weeks is breastfeeding jaundice which generally resolves.

A unilateral dark, purplish lesion, or "port wine stain" over the distribution of the ophthalmic branch of the trigeminal nerve may be a sign of *Sturge-Weber syndrome*, which is associated with seizures, hemiparesis, glaucoma, and mental retardation.

Significant edema of the hands and feet of a newborn girl may be suggestive of *Turner's syndrome*.

Dehydration is a common problem in infants. Usual causes are insufficient intake or excess loss of fluids from diarrhea.

Newborn Skin Findings

Finding/Description	Finding/Description

Common Nonpathologic Conditions

Acrocyanosis

This bluish discoloration usually appears in the palms and soles. *Cyanotic congenital heart disease can present with severe acrocyanosis.*

Jaundice

Physiologic jaundice occurs during days 2 to 5 of life and progresses from head to toe as it peaks. *Extreme jaundice may signify a hemolytic process or biliary or liver disease.*

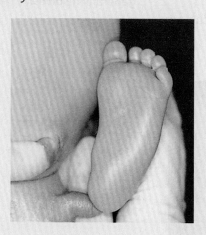

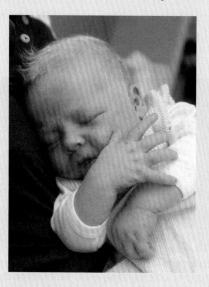

Common Benign Rashes

Miliaria rubra

Scattered vesicles on an erythematous base, usually on the face and trunk, result from obstruction of the sweat gland ducts; this condition disappears spontaneously within weeks.

Erythema toxicum

Usually appearing on days 2 to 3 of life, this rash consists of erythematous macules with central pinpoint vesicles scattered diffusely over the entire body. They appear similar to flea bites. These lesions are of unknown etiology but disappear within 1 week of birth.

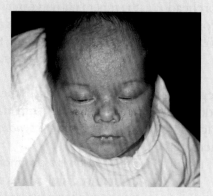

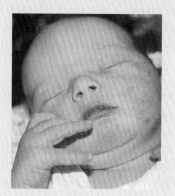

(continued)

Newborn Skin Findings (*continued*)

Finding/Description

Finding/Description

Pustular melanosis

Seen more commonly in black infants, the rash presents at birth as small vesiculopustules over a brown macular base; these can last for several months.

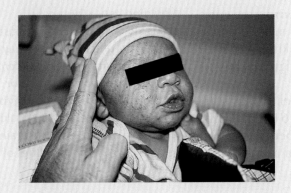

Milia

Pinhead-sized smooth white raised areas without surrounding erythema on the nose (seen here), chin, and forehead result from retention of sebum in the openings of the sebaceous glands. Although occasionally present at birth, milia usually appears within the first few weeks and disappears over several weeks.

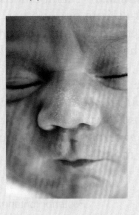

Benign Birthmarks
Eyelid patch

This birthmark fades, usually within the first year of life.

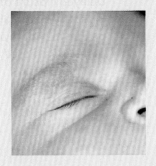

Salmon patch

Also called the "stork bite," or "angel kiss," this splotchy pink mark fades with age.

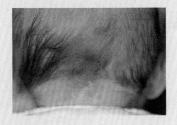

Café-au-lait spots

These light-brown pigmented lesions usually have borders and are uniform. They are noted in more than 10% of black infants. *If more than five café-au-lait spots exist, consider the diagnosis of neurofibromatosis (see Table 18-2, Common Skin Rashes and Skin Findings in Newborns and Infants, p. 879).*

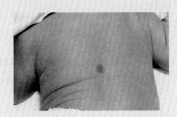

Mongolian spots

These are more common among dark-skinned babies. It is important to note them so that they are not mistaken for bruises.

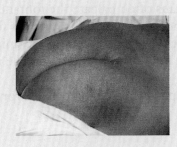

The Head

At birth, a baby's head may seem relatively large to you. A newborn's head accounts for one fourth of the body length and one third of the body weight; these proportions change, so that by adulthood, the head accounts for one eighth of the body length and about one tenth of the body weight.

Sutures and Fontanelles. Membranous tissue spaces called *sutures* separate the bones of the skull from one another. The areas where the major sutures intersect in the anterior and posterior portions of the skull are known as *fontanelles*. Examine the *sutures* and *fontanelles* carefully (see the figure below).

On palpation, the sutures feel like ridges and the fontanelles like soft concavities. The *anterior fontanelle* at birth measures 4 cm to 6 cm in diameter and usually closes between 4 and 26 months of age (90% between 7 and 19 months). The *posterior fontanelle* measures 1 cm to 2 cm at birth and usually closes by 2 months.

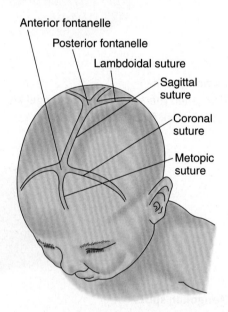

- Anterior fontanelle
- Posterior fontanelle
- Lambdoidal suture
- Sagittal suture
- Coronal suture
- Metopic suture

Carefully examine the fontanelle, because its fullness reflects *intracranial pressure*. Palpate the fontanelle while the baby is sitting quietly or being held upright. Clinicians often palpate the fontanelles at the beginning of the examination. In normal infants, the anterior fontanelle is soft and flat. A full anterior fontanelle with increased intracranial pressure is seen when a baby cries or vomits. Pulsations of the fontanelle reflect the peripheral pulse.

Inspect the scalp veins carefully to assess for dilatation.

An enlarged posterior fontanelle may be present in *congenital hypothyroidism.*

Overlap of the cranial bones at the sutures at birth, called *molding,* results from passage of the head through the birth canal; it disappears within 2 days.

A bulging, tense fontanelle is observed in infants with *increased intracranial pressure,* which may be caused by *central nervous system infections, neoplastic disease,* or *hydrocephalus* (obstruction of the circulation of cerebrospinal fluid within the ventricles of the brain; see Table 18-5, Abnormalities of the Head, p. 881).

Early closure of the fontanelles can be due to developing *microcephaly* or to *craniosynostosis* or some *metabolic abnormalities.*

Delayed closure of the fontanelles is usually a normal variant, but can be due to *hypothyroidism, megalocephaly, increased intracranial pressure* or *rickets.*

A depressed anterior fontanelle may be a sign of *dehydration.*

Dilated scalp veins are indicative of long-standing *increased intracranial pressure.*

Skull Symmetry and Head Circumference. Carefully assess *skull symmetry*. Various conditions can cause asymmetry; some are benign, while others reflect underlying pathology.

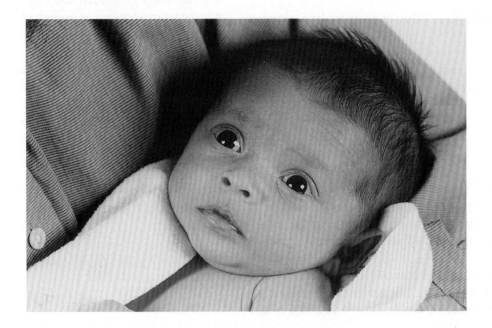

A common type of localized swelling of the scalp is a *cephalohematoma,* caused by subperiosteal hemorrhage from the trauma of birth. This swelling does not cross over suture lines and resolves within 3 weeks. As the hemorrhage resolves and calcifies, there may be a palpable bony rim with a soft center.

Look for asymmetric head swelling. A newborn's scalp may be swollen over the occipitoparietal region. This is called *caput succedaneum*, from capillary distention and extravasation of blood and fluid resulting from the vacuum effect of rupture of the amniotic sac. This swelling typically crosses suture lines and resolves in 1 to 2 days.

The premature infant's head at birth is relatively long in the occipitofrontal diameter and narrow in the bitemporal diameter (*dolichocephaly*). Usually the skull shape normalizes within 1 to 2 years. This condition can be prevented by frequent repositioning (providing "tummy time" when the infant is awake).

Pick up the infant and examine the skull shape from behind. Asymmetry of the cranial vault (*positional plagiocephaly*) occurs when an infant lies mostly on one side, resulting in a flattening of the parieto-occipital region on the dependent side and a prominence of the frontal region on the ipsilateral side. It disappears as the baby becomes more active and spends less time in one position, and symmetry is almost always restored. Interestingly, the current trend to have newborns sleep on their backs to reduce the risk for sudden infant death syndrome has resulted in more cases of positional plagiocephaly.

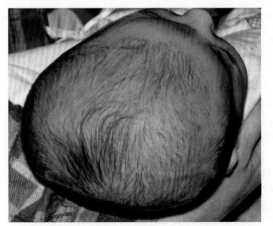

Plagiocephaly may also reflect pathology such as *torticollis* from injury to the sternocleidomastoid muscle at birth or *lack of stimulation* of the infant.

Measure the head circumference (p. 781) to detect abnormally large head size (*macrocephaly*) or small head size (*microcephaly*), both of which may signify an underlying disorder affecting the brain.

Palpate along the suture lines. A raised, bony ridge at a suture line suggests craniosynostosis.

Palpate the infant's skull with care. The cranial bones generally appear "soft" or pliable; they will normally become firmer with increasing gestational age.

Facial Symmetry. Check the *face* of infants for symmetry. In utero positioning may result in transient facial asymmetries. If the head is flexed on the sternum, a shortened chin (*micrognathia*) may result. Pressure of the shoulder on the jaw may create a temporary lateral displacement of the mandible.

Examine the face for an overall impression of the *facies;* it is helpful to compare with the face of the parents. A systematic assessment of a child with abnormal-appearing facies can identify specific syndromes.[18] The box below describes steps for evaluating facies.

Premature closure of cranial sutures causes *craniosynostosis* (p. 881), with an abnormally shaped skull. *Sagittal suture* synostosis causes a narrow head from lack of growth of the parietal bones.

In *craniotabes,* the cranial bones feel springy. Craniotabes can result from increased intracranial pressure, as with *hydrocephaly,* metabolic disturbances such as *rickets,* and infection such as *congenital syphilis.*

Micrognathia may also be part of a syndrome, such as the *Pierre Robin syndrome.*

Evaluating a Newborn or Child With Possible Abnormal Facies

Carefully review the history, especially:
- Family history
- Pregnancy
- Perinatal history

Note abnormalities on other parts of the physical examination, especially:
- Growth
- Development
- Other dysmorphic somatic features

Perform measurements (and plot percentiles), especially:
- Head circumference
- Height
- Weight

Consider the three mechanisms of facial dysmorphogenesis:
- Deformations from intrauterine constraint
- Disruptions from amniotic bands or fetal tissue
- Malformations from intrinsic abnormality in face/head or brain

Examine the parents and siblings:
- Similarity to a parent may be reassuring (e.g., large head) but may also be an indication of a familial disorder

Try to determine whether the facial features fit a recognizable syndrome, comparing with:
- References (including measurements) and pictures of syndromes
- Tables/databases of combinations of features

Most developmental and genetic syndromes with abnormal facies also have other abnormalities.

An infant with *congenital hyperthyroidism* may have coarse facial features and other abnormal facies (Table 18-6, Diagnostic Facies in Infancy and Childhood, p. 882).

A child with abnormal shape or length of palpebral fissures (see Table 18-6, Diagnositc Facies in Infancy and Childhood, p. 882):
   Upslanting (*Down syndrome*)
   Down-slanting (*Noonan's syndrome*)
   Short (*fetal alcohol effects*)

Chvostek's Sign. Percuss the cheek to check for *Chvostek's sign*, which is present in some metabolic disturbances and occasionally in normal infants. Percuss at the top of the cheek just below the zygomatic bone in front of the ear, using the tip of your index or middle finger.

The Eyes

Inspection. Newborns keep their eyes closed except during brief awake periods. If you attempt to separate their eyelids, they will tighten them even more. Bright light causes infants to blink, so use subdued lighting. Awaken the baby gently and support the baby in a sitting position; often the eyes open.

To examine the eyes of infants and young children and use some tricks to get them to cooperate. Small colorful toys are useful as fixation devices in examining the eyes.

Newborns may look at your face and follow a bright light if you catch them during an alert period. Some newborns can follow your face and turn their heads 90 degrees to each side. Examine infants for *eye movements*. Hold the baby upright, supporting the head. Rotate yourself with the baby slowly in one direction. This usually causes the baby's eyes to open, allowing you to examine the sclerae, pupils, irises, and extraocular movements. The baby's eyes gaze in the direction you are turning. When the rotation stops, the eyes look in the opposite direction, after a few nystagmoid movements.

A positive Chvostek's sign produces facial grimacing caused by repeated contractions of the facial muscles. A Chvostek's sign is noted in cases of *hypocalcemic tetany, tetanus and tetany due to hyperventilation.*

A newborn who truly cannot open an eye (even when awake and alert) may have *congenital ptosis.* Causes include birth trauma, third cranial nerve palsy, and mechanical problems.

Subconjunctival hemorrhages are common in neonates born via vaginal delivery.

Nystagmus (wandering or shaking eye movements) persisting after a few days or persisting after the maneuver described on the left may indicate *poor vision* or *central nervous system disease.*

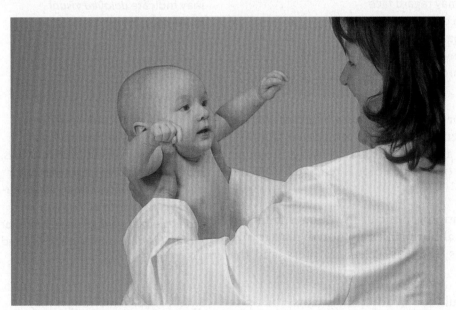

If a newborn fails to gaze at you and follow your face during alert periods, pay particular attention to the rest of the ocular examination. While this may still be a normal child, the newborn may have *visual impairment.*

During the first 10 days of life, the eyes may be fixed, staring in one direction if just the head is turned without moving the body (*doll's eye reflex*).

During the first few months of life, some infants have intermittent crossed eyes (*intermittent alternating convergent strabismus*, or *esotropia*) or laterally deviated eyes (*intermittent alternating divergent strabismus*, or *exotropia*).

Alternating convergent or divergent *strabismus* persisting beyond 3 months, or persistent strabismus of any type, may indicate *ocular motor weakness* or another abnormality in the visual system.

Look for abnormalities or congenital problems in the *sclerae* and *pupils*. Subconjunctival hemorrhages are common in newborns. The eyes of many newborns are edematous from the birth process.

Colobomas may be seen with the naked eye and represent defects in the iris.

Observe pupillary reactions by response to light or by covering each eye with your hand and then uncovering it. Although there may be initial asymmetry in the size of the pupils, over time they should be equal in size and reaction to light.

Inspect the irises carefully for abnormalities.

Brushfield's spots are a ring of white specks in the iris (see Table 18-7, Abnormalities of the Eyes, Ears, and Mouth, p. 884). Although sometimes present in normal children, these strongly suggest *Down syndrome*.

Examine the *conjunctiva* for swelling or redness. Most newborn nurseries use an antibiotic eye ointment to help prevent gonococcal eye infection.

Persistent ocular discharge and tearing since birth may be from *dacryocystitis* or *nasolacrimal duct obstruction*.

You will not be able to measure the *visual acuity* of newborns or infants. You can use visual reflexes to indirectly assess vision: direct and consensual pupillary constriction in response to light, blinking in response to bright light (*optic blink reflex*), and blinking in response to quick movement of an object toward the eyes. During the first year of life, visual acuity sharpens as the ability to focus improves. Infants achieve the following visual milestones:

Failure to progress along these visual developmental milestones may indicate *delayed visual maturation*.

Visual Milestones of Infancy[19]

Birth	Blinks, may regard face
1 month	Fixes on objects
1½–2 months	Coordinated eye movements
3 months	Eyes converge, baby reaches
12 months	Acuity around 20/50

Ophthalmoscopic Examination. For the *ophthalmoscopic examination*, with the newborn awake and eyes open, examine the red retinal (fundus) reflex by setting the ophthalmoscope at 0 diopters and viewing the pupil from about 10 inches. Normally, a red or orange color is reflected from the fundus through the pupil.

Congenital glaucoma may cause cloudiness of the cornea. A dark light reflex can result from *cataracts*, *retinopathy of prematurity*, or other disorders. A white retinal reflex (*leukokoria*) is abnormal, and *cataract*, *retinal detachment*, *chorioretinitis*, or *retinoblastoma* should be suspected.

A thorough ophthalmoscopic examination is difficult in young infants but may be needed if ocular or neurologic abnormalities are noted. The cornea can ordinarily be seen at +20 diopters, the lens at +15 diopters, and the fundus at 0 diopters.

Examine the optic disc area as you would for an adult. In infants, the optic disc is lighter in color, with less macular pigmentation. The foveal light reflection may not be visible. Look carefully for retinal hemorrhages. Papilledema is rare in infants because the fontanelles and open sutures accommodate any increased intracranial pressure, sparing the optic discs.

Small retinal hemorrhages may occur in normal newborns. Extensive hemorrhages may suggest severe *anoxia, subdural hematoma, subarachnoid hemorrhage,* or *trauma*.

The Ears

The physical examination of the ears of infants is important because many abnormalities can be detected, including structural problems, otitis media, and hearing loss.

The goals are to determine the *position*, *shape*, and *features of the ear* and to detect abnormalities. Note ear position in relation to the eyes. An imaginary line drawn across the inner and outer canthi of the eyes should cross the pinna or auricle; if the pinna is below this line, then the infant has low-set ears. Draw this imaginary line across the face of the baby on p. 789; note that it crosses the pinna.

Small, deformed, or low-set auricles may indicate associated *congenital defects*, especially renal disease.

Otoscopic examination of the newborn's ear can detect only patency of the *ear canal* because accumulated vernix caseosa obscures the tympanic membrane for the first few days of life.

A small skin tab, cleft, or pit found just forward of the tragus represents a remnant of the *first branchial cleft* and usually has no significance.

The infant's ear canal is directed downward from the outside; therefore, pull the auricle gently downward, not upward, for the best view of the eardrum. Once the tympanic membrane is visible, note that the light reflex is diffuse; it does not become cone-shaped for several months.

Otitis media (see p. 836) can occur in infants.

The *acoustic blink reflex* is a blinking of the infant's eyes in response to a sudden sharp sound. You can produce it by snapping your fingers or using a bell, beeper, or other noisemaking device approximately 1 foot from the infant's ear. Be sure you are not producing an airstream that may cause the infant to blink. This reflex may be difficult to elicit during the first 2 to 3 days of life. After it is elicited several times within a brief period, the reflex disappears, a phenomenon known as *habituation*. This crude test of hearing certainly is not diagnostic. Most newborns in the United States are given hearing screenings, which are mandatory in the majority of states.

Perinatal problems raising the risk for *hearing defects* include birth weight <1,500 g, anoxia, treatment with potentially ototoxic medications, congenital infections, severe hyperbilirubinemia, and meningitis.

Signs That an Infant Can Hear

Age	Sign
0–2 mos	Startle response and blink to a sudden noise
	Calming down with soothing voice or music
2–3 mos	Change in body movements in response to sound
	Change in facial expression to familiar sounds
3–4 mos	Turning eyes and head to sound
6–7 mos	Turning to listen to voices and conversation

In the absence of universal hearing screening, many children with *hearing deficits* are not diagnosed until as old as 2 years. Clues to hearing deficits include parental concern about hearing, delayed speech, and lack of developmental indicators of hearing.

The Nose and Sinuses

The most important component of the examination of the infant nose is to test for patency of the nasal passages. You can do this by gently occluding each nostril alternately while holding the infant's mouth closed. This normally will not cause stress because most infants are nasal breathers. Some infants are *obligate nasal breathers* and have difficulty breathing through their mouths. Do not occlude both nares simultaneously, as this will cause considerable distress.

Inspect the nose to ensure that the nasal septum is midline. You can gently insert a wide nasal speculum of the otoscope into the nose.

At birth, the maxillary and the ethmoid sinuses are present. Palpation of the sinuses of newborns is not helpful.

The nasal passages in newborns may be obstructed in *choanal atresia*. In severe cases, nasal obstruction can be assessed by attempting to pass a No. 8 feeding tube through each nostril into the posterior pharynx.

The Mouth and Pharynx

Use both inspection with a tongue blade and flashlight and palpation to inspect the mouth and pharynx. The photo below shows one method, employing the parent to hold the infant's head and arms. The newborn's mouth is edentulous, and the alveolar mucosa is smooth, with finely serrated borders. Occasionally, pearl-like retention cysts are seen along the alveolar ridges and are easily mistaken for teeth; these disappear within 1 or 2 months. Petechiae are commonly found on the soft palate after birth.

Rarely, *supernumerary teeth* are noted. These are usually dysmorphic and are shed within days but are removed to prevent aspiration.

Palpate the upper hard palate to make sure it is intact. *Epstein's pearls*, tiny white or yellow, rounded mucous retention cysts, are located along the posterior midline of the hard palate. They disappear within months.

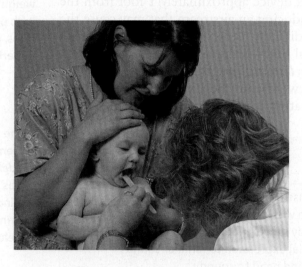

Cysts may be noted on the tongue or mouth. Thyroglossal duct cysts may open under the tongue.

Infants produce little saliva during the first 3 months. Older infants produce a lot of saliva and drool frequently.

Inspect the tongue. The frenulum varies, sometimes extending almost to the tip and other times is thick and short, limiting protrusion of the tongue (*ankyloglossia*, or *tongue tie*); these variations rarely interfere with speech or function.

You will often see a whitish covering on the tongue. If this coating is from milk, it can be easily removed by scraping or wiping it away. Use a tongue blade or your gloved finger to wipe away the coating.

The pharynx of the infant is best seen while the baby is crying. You will likely have difficulty using a tongue blade because it produces a strong gag reflex. Do not expect to be able to visualize the tonsils. Infants do not have prominent lymphoid tissue; tonsils increase in size as children grow.

Listen to the quality of the *infant's cry*. Normal infants have a lusty, strong cry. The following box lists some unusual types of infant cries.

Although unusual, a prominent, protruding tongue may signal *congenital hypothyroidism* or *Down syndrome*.

Oral candidiasis (thrush) is common in infants. The lesions are difficult to wipe away and have an erythematous raw base (see Table 18-7, Abnormalities of the Eyes, Ears, and Mouth, p. 884).

Macroglossia is associated with several systemic conditions. If associated with hypoglycemia and omphalocele, the diagnosis is likely *Beckwith-Wiedemann* syndrome.

A congenital fissure of the median line of the palate is a *cleft palate*.

Abnormal Infant Cries (If Persistent)

Type	Possible Abnormality
Shrill or high-pitched	Increased intracranial pressure. Also in newborns born to narcotic-addicted mothers.
Hoarse	Hypocalcemic tetany or congenital hypothyroidism
Continuous inspiratory and expiratory stridor	Upper airway obstruction from various lesions (e.g., a polyp or hemangioma), a relatively small larynx (*infantile laryngeal stridor*), or a delay in the development of the cartilage in the tracheal rings (*tracheomalacia*)
Absence of cry	Severe illness, vocal cord paralysis, or profound brain damage

Inspiratory stridor since birth suggests a congenital abnormality as described in this table. Stridor that appears following birth can be due to infection such as *croup, foreign body, or gastroesophageal reflux*.

There is a predictable pattern of tooth eruption and also wide variation. A rule of thumb is that a child will have one tooth for each month of age between 6 and 26 months, up to 20 primary teeth.

Natal teeth are teeth that are present at birth. They are usually simply early eruptions of normal teeth, but they can be part of syndromes.

The Neck

Palpate the *lymph nodes of the neck* and assess for any additional masses such as *congenital cysts*. Because the necks of infants are short, it is best to palpate the neck while infants are lying supine, whereas older children are best examined while sitting. Check the position of the thyroid cartilage and trachea.

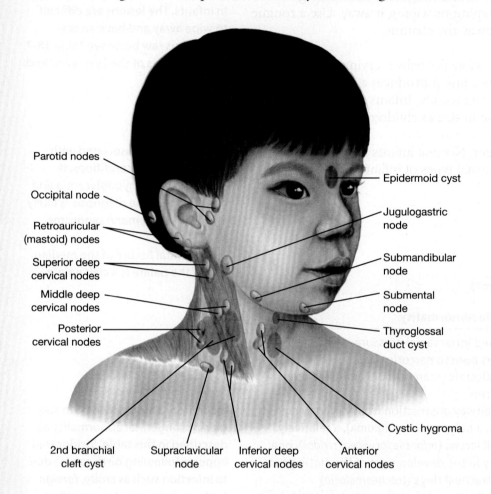

Parotid nodes

Occipital node

Retroauricular (mastoid) nodes

Superior deep cervical nodes

Middle deep cervical nodes

Posterior cervical nodes

Epidermoid cyst

Jugulogastric node

Submandibular node

Submental node

Thyroglossal duct cyst

2nd branchial cleft cyst

Supraclavicular node

Inferior deep cervical nodes

Anterior cervical nodes

Cystic hygroma

In newborns, palpate the *clavicles* and look for evidence of a fracture. If present, you may feel a break in the contour of the bone, tenderness, crepitus at the fracture site, and limited movement of the arm on the affected side.

The Thorax and Lungs

The infant's *thorax* is more rounded than that of adults. The thin chest wall has little musculature; thus, lung and heart sounds are transmitted quite clearly. The bony and cartilaginous rib cage is soft and pliant. The tip of the xiphoid process often protrudes anteriorly, immediately beneath the skin.

Branchial cleft cysts appear as small dimples or openings anterior to the midportion of the sternocleidomastoid muscle. They may be associated with a sinus tract.

Preauricular cysts and sinuses are common, pinhole-size pits, usually located anterior to the helix of the ear. They are often bilateral and may be associated with *hearing deficits*.

Thyroglossal duct cysts are located at the midline of the neck, just above the thyroid cartilage. These small, firm, mobile masses move upward with tongue protrusion or with swallowing. They are usually detected after 2 years.

Congenital torticollis, or a "wry neck," is from bleeding into the sternocleidomastoid muscle during the stretching process of birth. A firm fibrous mass is felt within the muscle 2 to 3 weeks after birth and generally disappears over months.

A *fracture of the clavicle* may occur during birth, particularly during delivery of a difficult arm or shoulder extraction.

Two types of chest wall abnormalities noted in childhood include *pectus excavatum,* or "funnel chest," and *pectus carinatum,* or "chicken breast deformity."

Inspection. Carefully *assess respirations* and *breathing patterns*. Newborns, especially those born prematurely, show periods of normal rate (30 to 40 per minute) alternating with "periodic breathing," during which respiratory rate slows markedly and may even cease for 5 to 10 seconds.

Do not rush to the stethoscope. Instead, observe the infant carefully as demonstrated on the next page. Inspection is easiest when infants are not crying; thus, work with the parents to settle the child. Observe for perhaps 1 minute, note general appearance, respiratory rate, color, nasal component of breathing, audible breath sounds, and work of breathing, as described below.

Because infants are obligate nasal breathers, observe their nose as they breathe. Look for *nasal flaring*. Observe breathing with the infant's mouth closed or during nursing or sucking on a bottle to assess for nasal patency. Listen to the sounds of breathing; note any *grunting, audible wheezing,* or *lack of breath sounds (obstruction).*

Observe two aspects of the infant's breathing: *audible breath sounds* and *work of breathing.* These are particularly relevant in assessing both upper and lower respiratory illness. Studies in countries with poor access to chest radiographs have found these signs at least as useful as auscultation.

Apnea is cessation of breathing for more than 20 seconds. It is often accompanied by bradycardia and may indicate *respiratory disease, central nervous system disease,* or, rarely, a *cardiopulmonary condition.* Apnea may be a high-risk factor for *sudden infant death syndrome (SIDS).*

In newborns and young infants, nasal flaring may be the result of *upper respiratory infections,* with subsequent obstruction of their small nares, but it may also be caused by *pneumonia* or other serious respiratory infections.

Observing Respiration—Before You Touch the Child

Type of Assessment	Specific Observable Pathology
General appearance	Inability to feed or smile
	Lack of consolability
Respiratory rate	Tachypnea (see p. 140)
Color	Pallor or cyanosis
Nasal component of breathing	Nasal flaring (enlargement of both nasal openings during inspiration)
Audible breath sounds	Grunting (repetitive, short expiratory sound)
	Wheezing (musical expiratory sound)
	Stridor (high-pitched, inspiratory noise)
	Obstruction (lack of breath sounds)
Work of breathing	Nasal flaring (excessive movement of nares)
	Grunting (expiratory noises)
	Retractions (chest indrawing):
	Supraclavicular (soft tissue above clavicles)
	Intercostal (indrawing of the skin between ribs)
	Subcostal (just below the costal margin)

Any of the abnormalities listed on the left should raise concern about underlying respiratory pathology.

Lower respiratory infections, defined as infections below the vocal cords, are common in infants and include *bronchiolitis* and *pneumonia.*

Acute stridor is a potentially serious condition; causes include *laryngotracheobronchitis (croup), epiglottitis, bacterial tracheitis, foreign body, hemangioma,* or a *vascular ring.*

In infants, abnormal work of breathing plus abnormal findings on auscultation, are the best findings for ruling in *pneumonia.* The best sign for ruling *out* pneumonia is the absence of tachypnea.

In healthy infants, the ribs do not move much during quiet breathing. Any outward movement is produced by descent of the diaphragm, which compresses the abdominal contents and in turn shifts the lower ribs outward.

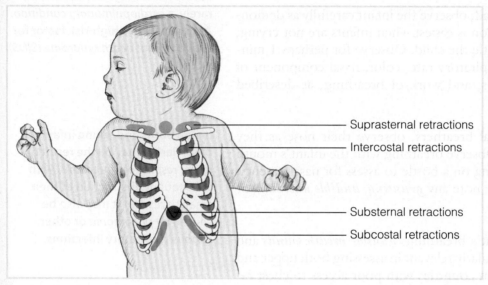

— Suprasternal retractions
— Intercostal retractions

— Substernal retractions
— Subcostal retractions

Asymmetric chest movement may indicate a space-occupying lesion. Pulmonary disease causes increased abdominal breathing and can result in *retractions (chest indrawing)*, an indicator of pulmonary disease before 2 years of age. Chest indrawing is inward movement of the skin between the ribs during inspiration. Movement of the diaphragm primarily affects breathing, with little assistance from the thoracic muscles. As mentioned in the preceding table, three types of retractions can be noted in infants: supraclavicular, intercostal, and subcostal.

Airway obstruction or lower respiratory tract disease in infants can result in the *Hoover sign*, or paradoxical (seesaw), breathing in which the abdomen moves outward while the chest moves inward during inspiration.

Thoracoabdominal paradox, inward movement of the chest and outward movement of the abdomen during inspiration (abdominal breathing), is a normal finding in newborns. It persists during active, or REM, sleep even when it is no longer seen during wakefulness or quiet sleep because of the decreased muscle tone of active sleep. As muscle strength increases and chest wall compliance decreases with age, abdominal breathing should no longer be noted. If observed, it may signify respiratory disease.

Children with *muscle weakness* may be noted to have thoracoabdominal paradox at several years of age.

Palpation. Assess tactile fremitus by *palpation*. Place your hand on the chest when the infant cries or makes noise. Place your hand or fingertips over each side of the chest and feel for symmetry in the transmitted vibrations. Percussion is not helpful in infants except in extreme instances. The infant's chest is hyperresonant throughout, and it is difficult to detect abnormalities on percussion.

Because of the excellent transmission of sounds throughout the chest, any abnormalities of tactile fremitus or on percussion suggest severe pathology, such as a large *pneumonic consolidation*.

Auscultation. After performing these maneuvers, you are ready for *auscultation*. Breath sounds are louder and harsher than those of adults because the stethoscope is closer to the origin of the sounds. It is often difficult to distinguish transmitted upper airway sounds from sounds originating in the chest. Upper airway sounds tend to be loud, transmitted symmetrically throughout the chest, and loudest as you move your stethoscope toward the neck. They are usually inspiratory, coarse sounds. Lower airway sounds are loudest over the site of pathology, are often asymmetric, and often occur during expiration.

Biphasic sounds imply severe obstruction from intrathoracic airway narrowing or severe obstruction from extrathoracic airway narrowing.

Distinguishing Upper Airway From Lower Airway Sounds in Infants

Technique	Upper Airway	Lower Airway
Compare sounds from nose/stethoscope	Same sounds	Often different sounds
Listen to harshness of sounds	Harsh and loud	Variable
Note symmetry (left/right)	Symmetric	Often asymmetric
Compare sounds at different locations (higher or lower)	Sounds louder as stethoscope is moved up chest	Often sounds louder lower in chest toward abdomen
Inspiratory vs. expiratory	Almost always inspiratory	Often has expiratory phase

Expiratory sounds usually arise from an intrathoracic source, whereas inspiratory sounds typically arise from an extrathoracic airway such as the trachea. During expiration, the diameter of the intrathoracic airways decreases because radial forces from the surrounding lung do not "tether" the airways open as occurs during inspiration. Higher flow rates during inspiration produce turbulent flow, resulting in appreciable sounds.

The characteristics of the *breath sounds*, such as vesicular and bronchovesicular, and of the adventitious lung sounds, such as crackles, wheezes, and rhonchi, are the same as those for adults, except that they may be more difficult to distinguish in infants and often occur together. Wheezes and rhonchi are common in infants. *Wheezes*, often audible without the stethoscope, occur more frequently because of the smaller size of the tracheobronchial tree. *Rhonchi* reflect obstruction of larger airways, or bronchi. *Crackles* (rales) are discontinuous sounds (see p. 314), near the end of inspiration; they are usually caused by lung disorders, are far less likely to represent cardiac failure in infants than in adults, and tend to be harsher than in adults.

The Heart

Inspection. Before examining the heart itself, observe the infant carefully for any cyanosis. Acrocyanosis in the newborn is discussed on p. 786. It is important to detect central cyanosis because it is always abnormal and because many congenital cardiac abnormalities, as well as respiratory diseases, present with cyanosis.[20]

Recognizing minimal degrees of cyanosis requires care. Look inside of the body (i.e., the inside of the mouth, the tongue, or the conjunctivae, instead of peering through the skin). A true strawberry pink is normal, whereas any hint of raspberry red suggests desaturation.

The distribution of the cyanosis should be evaluated. An oximetry reading will confirm desaturation.

Diminished breath sounds in one side of the chest of a newborn suggest unilateral lesions (e.g., *congenital diaphragmatic hernia*).

Upper respirartory infections are not serious in infants but can produce loud inspiratory sounds that are transmitted to the chest.

Wheezes in infants occur commonly from *asthma* or *bronchiolitis.*

Crackles (rales) can be heard with *pneumonia* and *bronchiolitis.*

Central cyanosis without acute respiratory symptoms suggests cardiac disease. See Table 18-9, Cyanosis in Children, p. 886 and Table 18-10, Congenital Heart Murmurs, pp. 887–888.

Cardiac Causes of Central Cyanosis in Infants and Children

Age of Onset	Potential Cardiac Cause
Immediately at birth	Transposition of the great arteries
	Pulmonary valve atresia
	Severe pulmonary valve stenosis
	Possibly Ebstein's malformation
Within a few days after birth	All of the above plus:
	Total anomalous pulmonary venous return
	Hypoplastic left heart syndrome
	Truncus arteriosus (sometimes)
	Single ventricle variants
Weeks, months, or years of life	All of the above plus:
	Pulmonary vascular disease with atrial, ventricular, or great vessel shunting

Observe the infant for *general signs of health*. The infant's nutritional status, responsiveness, happiness, and irritability are all clues that may be useful in evaluating cardiac disease. Note that noncardiac findings can be present in infants with cardiac disease.

Tachypnea, tachycardia, and hepatomegaly in infants suggest *heart failure*.

Common Noncardiac Findings in Infants With Cardiac Disease

Poor feeding	Tachypnea	Poor overall appearance
Failure to thrive	Hepatomegaly	Weakness
Irritability	Clubbing	

Observe the respiratory rate and pattern to help distinguish the degree of illness and cardiac versus pulmonary diseases. An increase in respiratory effort is expected from pulmonary diseases, whereas in cardiac disease, there may be tachypnea but not increased work of breathing until heart failure becomes significant.

A diffuse bulge outward of the left side of the chest suggests long-standing *cardiomegaly*.

Palpation. The major branches of the aorta can be assessed by evaluation of the *peripheral pulses*. All neonates should have an evaluation of all pulses at the time of their newborn examination. In neonates and infants, the brachial artery pulse in the antecubital fossa is easier to feel than the radial artery pulse at the wrist. Both temporal arteries should be felt just in front of the ear.

The absence or diminution of femoral pulses is indicative of *coarctation of the aorta*. If you cannot detect femoral pulses, measure blood pressures of the lower and upper extremities. If they are equal or lower in the legs, coarctation is likely to be present.

Feel the femoral pulses. They lie in the midline just below the inguinal crease, between the iliac crest and the symphysis pubis. Take your time to search for femoral pulses; they are difficult to detect in chubby, squirming infants. If you first flex the infant's thighs on the abdomen, this may overcome the reflex flexion that occurs when you then extend the legs.

Feel the pulses in the lower extremities using your index or middle finger. The dorsalis pedis and posterior tibial pulses (see figure) may be difficult to feel unless there is an abnormality involving aortic run-off. Normal pulses should have a sharp rise and should be firm and well localized.

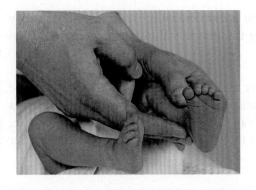

A weak or thready, difficult-to-feel pulse may reflect *myocardial dysfunction* and *heart failure*, particularly if associated with an unusual degree of tachycardia.

Although the pulses in the feet of neonates and infants are often faint, several conditions can cause full pulses, such as *patent ductus arteriosus* or *truncus arteriosus.*

As discussed on pp. 781–782, carefully measure the *blood pressure* of infants and children as part of the cardiac examination.

The *point of maximal impulse*, or *PMI*, is not always palpable in infants and is affected by respiratory patterns, a full stomach, and the infant's positioning. It is usually an interspace higher than in adults during the first few years of life because the heart lies more horizontally within the chest.

A *"rolling" heave* at the left sternal border suggests an *increase in right ventricular work*, whereas the same kind of motion closer to the apex suggests the same thing for the left ventricle.

Palpation of the chest wall will allow you to assess volume changes within the heart. For example, a hyperdynamic precordium reflects a big volume change.

Thrills are palpable when turbulence within the heart or great vessels is transmitted to the surface. Knowledge of the structures of the precordium helps pinpoint the origin of the thrill. Thrills are easiest to feel with your palm or the base of your fingers rather than your fingertips. Thrills have a somewhat rough, vibrating quality. The figure below shows locations of thrills that occur in infants and children from various cardiac abnormalities.

Patent ductus arteriosus (PDA) is associated with hyperdynamic precordium and bounding distal pulses.

Visible and palpable chest pulsations suggest a hyperdynamic state from either increased metabolic rate or inefficient pumping as a result of an underlying *cardiac defect.*

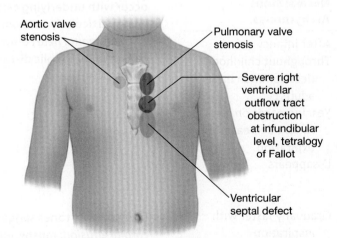

Aortic valve stenosis

Pulmonary valve stenosis

Severe right ventricular outflow tract obstruction at infundibular level, tetralogy of Fallot

Ventricular septal defect

LOCATION OF THRILLS IN INFANTS AND CHILDREN

Auscultation.   You can evaluate the *heart rhythm* more easily in infants by listening to the heart than by feeling the peripheral pulses; in older children assess the rhythm either way.

Infants and children commonly have a normal sinus dysrhythmia, with the heart rate increasing on inspiration and decreasing on expiration, sometimes quite abruptly. This normal finding can be identified by its repetitive nature, its correlation with respiration, and its involvement of several beats rather than a single beat.

Many neonates and some older children have premature atrial or ventricular beats that are often described as "skipped" beats. You can usually eradicate them by increasing their intrinsic sinus rate through exercise such as crying in an infant or jumping in an older child, although they may also be more frequent in the postexercise period. In a completely healthy child, they are usually benign and rarely persist.

Heart Sounds.   Evaluate the S_1 and S_2 heart sounds carefully. They are normally crisp. You can usually hear the second sounds (S_2) at the base separately, but they should fuse into a single sound in deep expiration. In the neonate, you should be able to detect a split S_2 if you examine the infant when the infant is completely quiet or asleep. Detecting this split eliminates many, but not all, of the more serious congenital cardiac defects.

The most common dysrhythmia in infants is *paroxysmal supraventricular tachycardia,* or *paroxysmal atrial tachycardia (PSVT, or PAT).* It can occur at any age, including in utero. It is remarkably well tolerated by some infants and children and is found on examination when the child looks perfectly healthy, may be mildly pale or has tachypnea, but has a rapid, sustained, completely regular heart rate of 240 beats per minute or more. Other children, particularly neonates, appear very ill. In older children, this dysrhythmia is more likely to be truly paroxysmal, with episodes of varying duration and frequency.

Pathologic arrhythmias in children can be from *structural cardiac lesions* but also from other causes such as *drug ingestion, metabolic abnormalities, endocrine disorders, serious infections,* and *postinfectious states,* or conduction disturbances without structural heart disease.

Characteristics of Normal Variants of Heart Rhythms in Children

Characteristics	Atrial Premature Contractions (APCs) or Ventricular Premature Contractions (VPCs)	Normal Sinus Arrhythmias
Most common age	Neonates (may occur at any time)	After infancy Throughout childhood (less common in adults)
Correlation with respiration	No	Yes: Increases on inspiration, decreases on expiration
Effect of exercise on tachycardia	Eradicated by exercise May be more frequent postexercise	Disappears
Characteristic of rhythm	Skipped or missed beat Irregularly occurring	Gradually faster with inspiration Often suddenly slower on expiration
Number of beats	Usually single abnormal beats	Several beats, usually in repetitive cycles
Severity	Usually benign	Benign (by definition)

Although VPCs generally occur in otherwise healthy infants, they can occur with underlying cardiac disease, particularly *cardiomyopathies* and *congenital heart disorders.* Electrolyte or metabolic disturbances are also causes.

Distant heart tones suggest *pericardial effusion;* mushy, less distinct heart sounds suggest *myocardial dysfunction.*

In addition to trying to detect splitting of the S_2, listen for the intensity of A_2 and P_2. The aortic, or first component of the second sound at the base, is normally louder than the pulmonic, or second component.

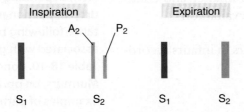

A louder-than-normal pulmonic component, particularly when louder than the aortic sound, suggests *pulmonary hypertension*.

Persistent splitting of S_2 may indicate a right ventricular volume load such as *atrial septal defect, anomalies of pulmonary venous return*, or *chronic anemia*.

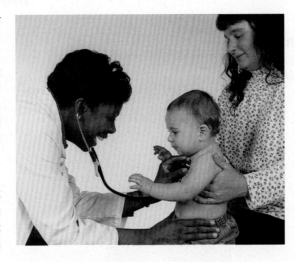

You may detect *third heart sounds*, which are low-pitched, early diastolic sounds best heard at the lower left sternal border, or apex; they reflect rapid ventricular filling. These are frequently heard in children and are normal.

The third heart sound (S_3) should be differentiated from the higher-intensity third heart sound gallop, which is a sign of underlying pathology.

Fourth heart sounds (S_4), not often heard in children, are low-frequency, late diastolic sounds, occurring just before the first heart sound.

Fourth heart sounds represent decreased ventricular compliance, suggesting *heart failure*.

You may also detect an *apparent gallop* (widely split S_2 that varies), in the presence of a normal heart rate and rhythm. This is frequently found in normal children and does not represent pathology.

A *gallop rhythm*—tachycardia plus a loud S_3, S_4, or both—is pathologic and indicates *heart failure (poor ventricular function)*.

Heart Murmurs.   One of the most challenging aspects of cardiac examination in children is the evaluation of *heart murmurs*. In addition to listening to a squirming, perhaps uncooperative child, a major challenge is to distinguish common benign murmurs from unusual or pathologic ones. Characterize heart murmurs in infants and children by noting their specific location (e.g., left upper sternal border, not just left sternal border), timing, intensity, and quality. If each murmur is delineated completely, the diagnosis is usually made, and only confirmation and amplification with laboratory tools such as ECG, chest x-ray, and echocardiography is needed.

An important rule of thumb is that, by definition, *benign murmurs in children have no associated abnormal findings*. Many (but not all) children with serious cardiac malformations have signs and symptoms other than a heart murmur obtainable on careful history or examination. Many have other noncardiac signs and symptoms, including evidence of genetic defects that may offer helpful diagnostic clues.

Any of the *noncardiac findings* that frequently accompany cardiac disease in children markedly raises the possibility that an apparently benign murmur is really pathologic.

Most children if not all will have one or more *functional, or benign, heart murmurs* before reaching adulthood.[21] It is important to identify functional murmurs by their specific qualities rather than by their intensity. You will learn to recognize the common functional murmurs of infancy and childhood, which under most circumstances do not require evaluation.

The figure below characterizes two *benign* heart murmurs in infants according to their locations and key characteristics.

Many *pathologic murmurs of congenital heart disease* are present at birth. Others are not apparent until later, depending on their severity, drop in pulmonary vascular resistance following birth, or changes associated with growth of the child. Table 18-10, Congenital Heart Murmurs, on pp. 887–888, shows examples of pathologic murmurs of childhood.

Two Common Benign Murmurs in Infants

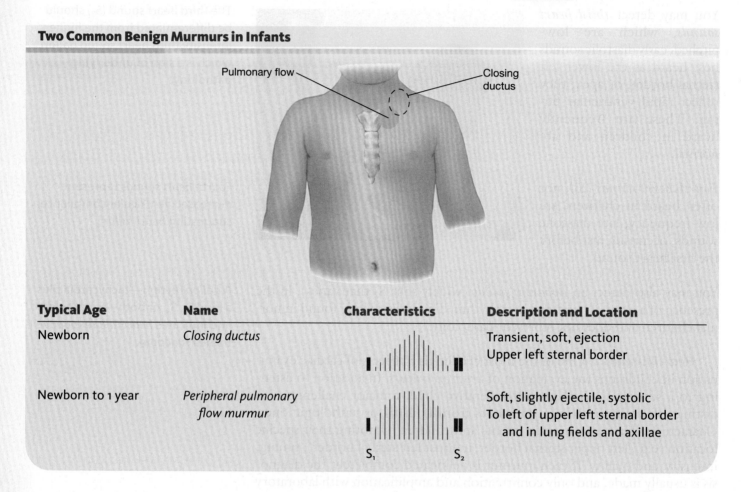

Typical Age	Name	Characteristics	Description and Location
Newborn	*Closing ductus*		Transient, soft, ejection Upper left sternal border
Newborn to 1 year	*Peripheral pulmonary flow murmur*	S_1 S_2	Soft, slightly ejectile, systolic To left of upper left sternal border and in lung fields and axillae

In some infants, you will detect a soft, somewhat ejectile murmur, not over the precordium but over the lung fields, particularly in the axillae. This represents peripheral pulmonary artery flow and is partly the result of inadequate pulmonary artery growth in utero (when there is little pulmonary blood flow) and the sharp angle at which the pulmonary artery curves backward. In the absence of any physical findings to suggest additional underlying diseases, this *peripheral pulmonary flow murmur* can be considered benign and usually disappears by 1 year.

A pulmonary flow murmur in the newborn with other signs of disease is more likely to be pathologic. Diseases may include *Williams syndrome, congenital rubella syndrome,* and *Alagille syndrome.*

Physiologic Basis for Some Pathologic Heart Murmurs

Change in Pulmonary Vascular Resistance

Heart murmurs that are dependent on a postnatal drop in pulmonary vascular resistance, allowing turbulent flow from the high-pressure systemic circuit to the lower-pressure pulmonary circuit, are not audible until such a drop has occurred. Except in premature infants, murmurs of a *ventricular septal defect* or *patent ductus arteriosus* are not expected in the first few days of life and usually become audible after a week to 10 days.

Obstructive Lesions

Obstructive lesions, such as *pulmonic and aortic stenosis,* are caused by normal blood flow through two small valves and are not dependent on a drop in pulmonary vascular resistance and are audible at birth.

Pressure Gradient Differences

Murmurs of *atrioventricular valve regurgitation* are audible at birth because of the high pressure gradient between the ventricle and its atrium.

Changes Associated With Growth of Children

Some murmurs do not follow the patterns above, but are audible due to alterations in normal blood flow and occur or change with growth. For example, even though it is an obstructive defect, *aortic stenosis* may not be audible until considerable growth has occurred and is frequently not heard until adulthood, although a congenitally abnormal valve is responsible. Similarly, the pulmonary flow murmur of an *atrial septal defect* may not be heard for a year or more because right ventricular compliance gradually increases and the shunt becomes larger, eventually producing a murmur caused by too much blood flow across a normal pulmonic valve.

A newborn with a heart murmur and central cyanosis is likely to have congenital heart disease and requires urgent cardiac evaluation.

When you detect any murmur in children, note all of the qualities as described in Chapter 9, The Cardiovascular System, to help you distinguish *pathologic murmurs* from benign murmurs. Heart murmurs that reflect underlying structural heart disease are easier to evaluate if you have a good knowledge of intrathoracic anatomy and the functional cardiac changes following birth and if you understand the physiologic basis for heart murmurs. Understanding these physiologic changes can help you to distinguish pathologic murmurs from benign heart murmurs in children.

Characteristics of specific pathologic heart murmurs in children are described in Table 18-10, Congenital Heart Murmurs, pp. 887–888.

The Breasts

The breasts of the newborn in both males and females are often enlarged from maternal estrogen effect; this may last several months. The breasts may also be engorged with a white liquid, sometimes colloquially called "witch's milk," which may last 1 or 2 weeks.

In *premature thelarche,* breast development occurs, most often between 6 months and 2 years. Other signs of puberty or hormonal abnormalities are not present.

The Abdomen

Inspection. Inspect the abdomen with the infant lying supine (and, optimally, asleep). The infant's abdomen is protuberant as a result of poorly developed abdominal musculature. You will easily notice abdominal wall blood vessels and intestinal peristalsis.

Inspect the newborn's *umbilical cord* to detect abnormalities. Normally, there are two thick-walled umbilical arteries and one larger but thin-walled umbilical vein, which is usually located at the 12-o'clock position.

A *single umbilical artery* may be associated with congenital anomalies or as an isolated anomaly.

The umbilicus in the newborn may have a long cutaneous portion (*umbilicus cutis*), which is covered with skin, or an amniotic portion (*umbilicus amnioticus*), which is covered by a firm gelatinous substance. The amniotic portion dries up and falls off within 2 weeks, whereas the cutaneous portion retracts to be flush with the abdominal wall.

An *umbilical granuloma* at the base of the navel is the development of pink granulation tissue formed during the healing process.

Inspect the area around the umbilicus for redness or swelling.

Infection of the umbilical stump (*omphalitis*) can be a serious condition.

Umbilical hernias are detectable at a few weeks of age. Most disappear by 1 year, nearly all by 5 years.

Umbilical hernias in infants are caused by a defect in the abdominal wall and can be up to 6 cm in diameter and quite protuberant with intra-abdominal pressure.

In some normal infants, you will notice a *diastasis recti*. This involves separation of the two rectus abdominis muscles, causing a midline ridge, most apparent when the infant contracts the abdominal muscles. A benign condition in most cases, it resolves during early childhood. Chronic abdominal distention may also predispose to this condition.

Auscultation. *Auscultation* of a quiet infant's abdomen is easy. You may hear an orchestra of musical tinkling bowel sounds upon placement of your stethoscope on the infant's abdomen.

An increase in pitch or frequency of bowel sounds is heard with *gastroenteritis* or, rarely, with *intestinal obstruction*.

Percussion and Palpation. You can *percuss* an infant's abdomen as you would an adult's, but may note greater tympanitic sounds because of the infant's propensity to swallow air. Percussion is useful for determining the size of organs and abdominal masses.

A silent, tympanic, distended and tender abdomen suggests *peritonitis*.

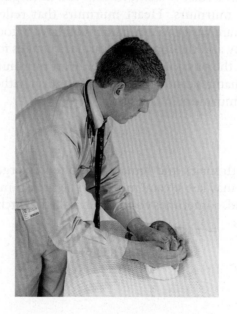

It is easy to *palpate* an infant's abdomen because infants like being touched. A useful technique to relax the infant, shown here, is to hold the legs flexed at the knees and hips with one hand and palpate the abdomen with the other. A pacifier may quiet the infant in this position.

Start gently palpating the liver low in the abdomen, moving upward with your fingers. This technique helps avoid missing an extremely enlarged liver that extends down into the pelvis. With a careful examination, you can feel the liver edge in most infants, 1 to 2 cm below the right costal margin.

An enlarged, tender liver may be due to *heart failure* or to *storage diseases*. Among newborns, causes of hepatomegaly include *hepatitis, storage diseases, vascular congestion,* and *biliary obstruction.*

One technique for assessing liver size in infants is simultaneous percussion and auscultation.[22] Percuss and simultaneously auscultate, noting a change in sound as you percuss over the liver or beyond it.

The *spleen*, like the liver, is felt easily in most infants. It is soft with a sharp edge, and it projects downward like a tongue from under the left costal margin. The spleen is moveable and rarely extends more than 1 to 2 cm below the left costal margin.

Several diseases can cause splenomegaly, including *infections, hemolytic anemias, infiltrative disorders, inflammatory* or *autoimmune diseases,* and *portal hypertension.*

Palpate the *other abdominal structures.* You will commonly note pulsations in the epigastrium caused by the aorta. This is felt on deep palpation to the left of the midline.

Abnormal abdominal masses in infants can be associated with the kidney (e.g., *hydronephrosis*), bladder (e.g., *urethral obstruction*), bowel (e.g., *Hirschsprung's disease,* or *intussusception*), and tumors.

You may be able to palpate the kidneys of infants by carefully placing the fingers of one hand in front of and those of the other behind each kidney. The descending colon is a sausagelike mass in the left lower quadrant.

Once you have identified the normal structures in the infant's abdomen, use palpation to identify abnormal masses.

In *pyloric stenosis,* deep palpation in the right upper quadrant or midline can reveal an "olive," or a 2-cm firm pyloric mass. While feeding, some infants with this condition will have visible peristaltic waves pass across their abdomen, followed by projectile vomiting.

Liver Size in Healthy Term Newborns[23]

By palpation and percussion	Mean, 5.9 ± 0.7 cm
Projection below right costal margin	Mean, 2.5 ± 1.0 cm

Male Genitalia

Inspect the male genitalia with the infant supine, noting the appearance of the penis, testes, and scrotum. The *foreskin* completely covers the *glans penis.* It is nonretractable at birth, though you may be able to retract it enough to visualize the external urethral meatus. Retraction of the foreskin in the uncircumcised male occurs months to years later. The rate of circumcision has declined recently in North America and varies worldwide, depending on cultural practices.

A *hypospadias* is present when the urethral orifice appears at some point along the ventral surface of the glans or shaft of the penis (see Table 18-12, The Male Genitourinary System, p. 890). The foreskin is incompletely formed ventrally.

Inspect the *shaft of the penis*, noting any abnormalities on the ventral surface. Make sure the penis appears straight.

A fixed, downward bowing of the penis is a *chordee;* this may accompany a hypospadias.

Inspect the *scrotum*, noting rugae, which should be present by 40 weeks' gestation. Scrotal edema may be present for several days following birth because of the effect of maternal estrogen.

Palpate the testes in the scrotal sacs, proceeding downward from the external inguinal ring to the scrotum. If you feel a testis up in the inguinal canal, gently milk it downward into the scrotum. The newborn's testes should be about 10 mm in width and 15 mm in length and should lie in the scrotal sacs most of the time.

In 3% of neonates, one or both *testes* cannot be felt in the scrotum or inguinal canal. This raises concern of *cryptorchidism*. In two-thirds of these cases, both testes are descended by 1 year of age.

In newborns with an *undescended testicle* (*cryptorchidism*), the scrotum often appears underdeveloped and tight, and palpation reveals an absence of scrotal contents (see Table 18-12, The Male Genitourinary System, p. 890).

Examine the testes for swelling within the scrotal sac and over the inguinal ring. If you detect swelling in the scrotal sac, try to differentiate it from the testis. Note whether the size changes when the infant increases abdominal pressure by crying. See if your fingers can get above the mass, trapping it in the scrotal sac. Apply gentle pressure to try to reduce the size of the mass and note any tenderness. Note whether it transilluminates.

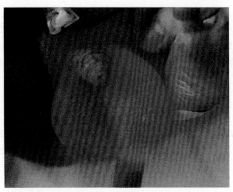

TRANSILLUMINATION OF A HYDROCELE
From Fletcher M. Physical diagnosis in neonatology. PhŠadelphia: Lippincott-Raven, 1998.

Two common scrotal masses in newborns are *hydroceles* and *inguinal hernias;* frequently both coexist, and both are more common on the right side. Hydroceles overlie the testes and the spermatic cord, are not reducible, and can be transilluminated (see photo). Most resolve by 18 months. Hernias are separate from the testes, are usually reducible, and often do not transilluminate. They do not resolve. Sometimes a thickened spermatic cord (called the *silk sign*) is noted.

Female Genitalia

Become familiar with the anatomy of an infant's female genitalia. Examine the female genitalia with the infant supine.

In the newborn female, the genitalia will be prominent due to the effects of maternal estrogen. The labia majora and minora have a dull pink color in light-skinned infants and may be hyperpigmented in dark-skinned infants. During the first few weeks of life, there is often a milky white discharge that may be blood tinged. This estrogenized appearance of the genitalia decreases during the first year of life.

Ambiguous genitalia, involving masculinization of the female external genitalia, is a rare condition caused by endocrine disorders such as *congenital adrenal hyperplasia.*

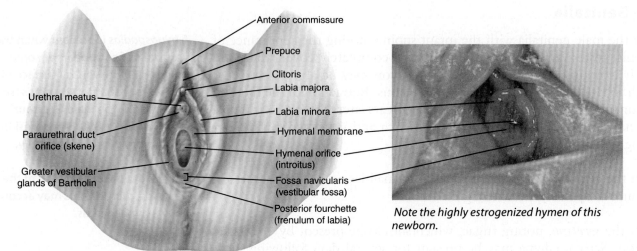

Anterior commissure
Prepuce
Clitoris
Labia majora
Urethral meatus
Labia minora
Paraurethral duct orifice (skene)
Hymenal membrane
Hymenal orifice (introitus)
Greater vestibular glands of Bartholin
Fossa navicularis (vestibular fossa)
Posterior fourchette (frenulum of labia)

Note the highly estrogenized hymen of this newborn.

This figure depicts the anatomy of a young female to best demonstrate anatomic structures.

Examine the different structures systematically, including the size of the clitoris, the color and size of the labia majora, and any rashes, bruises, or external lesions. Next, separate the labia majora at their midpoint with the thumb of each hand, or as shown in the diagrams on p. 849.

Labial adhesions occur frequently, tend to be paper thin, and often disappear without treatment.

Inspect the urethral orifice and the labia minora. Assess the hymen, which in newborns and infants is a thickened, avascular structure with a central orifice, covering the vaginal opening. You should note a vaginal opening, although the hymen will be thickened and redundant. Note any discharge.

An imperforate hymen may be noted at birth.

Rectal Examination

The rectal examination generally is not performed for infants or children unless there is question of patency of the anus or an abdominal mass. In such cases, flex the infant's hips and fold the legs to the head. Use your lubricated and gloved pinky.

A common cause of blood in the stool of infants is an *anal fissure*. These are not serious.

The Musculoskeletal System

Enormous changes in the musculoskeletal system occur during infancy. Much of the examination focuses on detection of congenital abnormalities, particularly in the hands, spine, hips, legs, and feet. Combine the musculoskeletal examination with the neurologic and developmental examination.

Careful inspection can reveal gross deformities such as dwarfism, congenital abnormalities of the extremities or digits, and annular bands that constrict an extremity.

The *newborn's hands* are clenched. Because of the palmar grasp reflex (see the discussion on the nervous system), you will need to help the infant extend the fingers. Inspect the fingers carefully, noting any defects.

Skin tags, remnants of digits, polydactyly (extra fingers), or *syndactyly* (webbed fingers) are congenital defects noted at birth.

Palpate along the *clavicle*, noting any lumps, tenderness, or crepitus; these may indicate a fracture.

A *fracture of the clavicle* can occur during a difficult birth.

Inspect the *spine* carefully. Although major defects of the spine such as *meningomyelocele* are obvious and often detected by ultrasound before birth, subtle abnormalities may include pigmented spots, hairy patches, or deep pits. These abnormalities, if present within 1 cm or so of the midline, may overlie external openings of sinus tracts that extend to the spinal canal. Do not probe sinus tracts because of the potential risk for introducing infection. Palpate the spine in the lumbosacral region, noting any deformities of the vertebrae.

Spina bifida occulta (a defect of the vertebral bodies) may be associated with defects of the spinal cord, which can cause severe neurologic dysfunction.

Examine the newborn and infant's *hips* carefully at each examination for signs of dislocation.[24] The following photos and subsequent page demonstrate the two major techniques, one to test for the presence of a posteriorly dislocated hip (*Ortolani test*) and another to test for the ability to sublux or dislocate an intact but unstable hip (*Barlow test*).[22]

A soft audible "click" heard with these maneuvers does not prove a dislocated hip, but should prompt a careful examination.

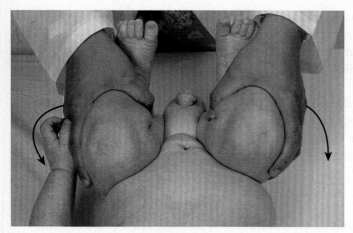

ORTOLANI TEST

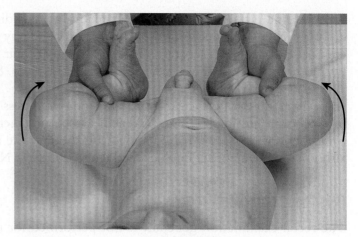

BARLOW TEST

Make sure the baby is relaxed for these techniques. For the *Ortolani test*, place the baby supine with the legs pointing toward you. Flex the legs to form right angles at the hips and knees, placing your index fingers over the greater trochanter of each femur and your thumbs over the lesser trochanters. Abduct both hips simultaneously until the lateral aspect of each knee touches the examining table.

For the *Barlow test*, place your hands in the same position as for the Ortolani test. Pull the leg forward and adduct with posterior force; that is, press in the opposite direction with your thumbs moving down toward the table and outward. Feel for any movement of the head of the femur laterally. Normally there is no movement and the hip feels "stable."

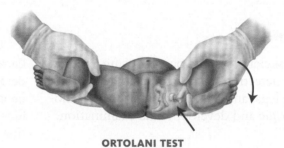

ORTOLANI TEST

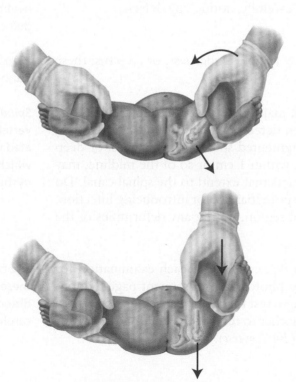

BARLOW TEST

With a developmental *dysplasia of the hip*, you feel a "clunk" as the femoral head, which lies posterior to the acetabulum, enters the acetabulum. A palpable movement of the femoral head back into place constitutes a *positive Ortolani sign*.

Developmental dysplasia of the hip is important to detect: Early treatment has excellent outcomes.

A positive Barlow sign is not diagnostic of a *dysplastic hip*, but indicates laxity and a dislocatable hip progressively, and the baby needs to be re-examined in the future. If you feel the head of the femur slipping out onto the posterior lip of the acetabulum, this constitutes a *positive Barlow sign*. If you feel this dislocation movement, abduct the hip by pressing with your index and middle fingers back inward and feel for the movement of the femoral head as it returns to the hip socket.

Children older than 3 months may have a negative Ortolani or Barlow sign and still have a *dislocated hip* due to tightening of the hip muscles and ligaments.

Test for femoral shortening using the *Galeazzi* or *Alice test*. Place the feet together and note any difference in knee heights.

Examine a newborn or infant's *legs and feet* to detect developmental abnormalities. Assess symmetry, bowing, and torsion of the legs. There should be no discrepancy in leg length. It is common for normal infants to have asymmetric thigh skin folds, but if you do detect asymmetry, make sure you perform the instability tests because dislocated hips are commonly associated with this finding.

Severe bowing of the knees can be normal, but it can also be due to *rickets* or *Blount disease*.

Most newborns are *bowlegged*, reflecting their curled-up intrauterine position.

Some normal infants exhibit twisting or *torsion of the tibia* inwardly or outwardly on its longitudinal axis. Parents may be concerned about a toeing in or toeing out of the foot and an awkward gait, all of which are usually normal. Tibial torsion corrects itself during the second year of life after months of weight bearing.

Pathologic tibial torsion occurs only in association with *deformities of the feet or hips*.

Examine the feet of newborns and infants. At birth, the feet may appear deformed from retaining their intrauterine positioning, often turned inward. You should be able to correct the feet to the neutral and even to an overcorrected position. Scratch or stroke along the outer edge to see if the foot assumes a normal position.

True *deformities of the feet* do not return to the neutral position even with manipulation.

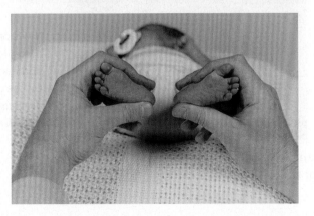

The normal newborn's foot has several benign features that may initially cause concern. The newborn's foot appears flat because of a plantar fat pad. There is often inversion of the foot, elevating the medial margin. Other babies will have adduction of the forefoot without inversion, called *metatarsus adductus*. Still others will have adduction of the entire foot. Finally, most toddlers have some pronation during early stages of weight bearing, with eversion of the foot. In all of these normal variants, the abnormal position can be easily overcorrected past midline. They all tend to resolve within 1 or 2 years.

The most common severe congenital foot deformity is talipes equinovarus or *clubfoot*.

See Table 18-13, Common Musculoskeletal Findings in Young Children, p. 890.

The Nervous System

The examination of the nervous system in infants includes techniques that are highly specific to this particular age. Unlike many neurologic abnormalities in adults that produce asymmetric localized findings, neurologic abnormalities in infants often present as developmental abnormalities such as failure to do age-appropriate tasks. Therefore, the neurologic and developmental examinations need to proceed together. A developmental abnormality should prompt you to pay particular attention to the neurologic examination.

The neurologic screening examination of all newborns should include assessment of mental status, gross and fine motor function, tone, cry, deep tendon reflexes, and primitive reflexes. More detailed examination of cranial nerve function, sensory function, and less common primitive reflexes are indicated if you suspect any abnormalities from the history or screening.[25]

The neurologic examination can reveal extensive disease but will not pinpoint specific functional deficits or minute lesions.

Mental Status.   Assess the *mental status* of newborns by observing many of the newborn activities discussed on p. 774 ("What A Newborn Can Do"). Make sure you test the newborn during alert periods. A detailed description of assessment of development is shown below.

Motor Function and Tone. Assess the *motor tone* of newborns and infants, first by carefully watching their position at rest and testing their resistance to passive movement.

Then assess *tone* as you move each major joint through its range of motion, noting any spasticity or flaccidity. Hold the baby in your hands to determine whether the tone is normal, increased, or decreased. Either increased or decreased tone may indicate intracranial disease, although such disease is usually accompanied by a number of other signs.

Sensory Function.   You can test for *sensory function* of the newborn in only a limited way. Test for pain sensation by flicking the infant's palm or sole with your finger. Observe for withdrawal, arousal, and change in facial expression. Do not use a pin to test for pain.

Cranial Nerves.   The *cranial nerves* of the newborn or infant can be tested. The following table provides useful strategies.

Signs of severe neurologic disease include *extreme irritability; persistent asymmetry of posture; persistent extension of extremities; constant turning of the head to one side; marked extension of the head, neck,* and *extremities (opisthotonus); severe flaccidity;* and *limited response to pain.*

Subtle neonatal behaviors such as fine tremors, irritability, and poor self-regulation may indicate *withdraw from nicotine* if the mother smoked during pregnancy.

Persistent irritability in the newborn may be a sign of *neurologic insult* or may reflect a variety of *metabolic, infectious,* or other *constitutional abnormalities,* or environmental conditions such as *drug withdrawal.*

Newborns with *hypotonia* often lie in a frog-leg position, with arms flexed and hands near the ears. Hypotonia can be caused by a variety of *central nervous system abnormalities* and *disorders of the motor unit.*

If changes in facial expression or cry follow a painful stimulus but no withdrawal occurs, *paralysis* may be present.

Strategies to Assess Cranial Nerves in Newborns and Infants

Cranial Nerve		Strategy
I	Olfactory	Difficult to test
II	Visual acuity	Have baby regard your face and look for facial response and tracking.
II, III	Response to light	Darken room, raise baby to sitting position to open eyes.
		Use light and test for *optic blink reflex* (blink in response to light).
		Use the otoscope (no speculum) to assess papillary responses.
III, IV, VI	Extraocular movements	Observe how well the baby tracks your smiling face.
		Use light if needed.
V	Motor	Test rooting reflex.
		Test sucking reflex (watch baby suck breast, bottle, or pacifier).
VII	Facial	Observe baby crying and smiling; note symmetry of face.
VIII	Acoustic	Test acoustic blink reflex (blinking of both eyes in response to noise).
		Observe tracking in response to sound.
IX, X	Swallow	Observe coordination during swallowing.
	Gag	Test for gag reflex.
XI	Spinal accessory	Observe symmetry of shoulders.
XII	Hypoglossal	Observe coordination of sucking, swallowing, and tongue thrusting.
		Pinch nostrils; observe reflex opening of mouth with tip of tongue to midline.

Abnormalities in the cranial nerves suggest an intracranial lesion such as *hemorrhage* or a *congenital malformation.*

Congenital facial nerve palsy can result from birth trauma or developmental deffects.

Dysphagia, or difficulty in swallowing, can occasionally be due to injury to CN IX–XII.

Deep Tendon Reflexes. The *deep tendon reflexes* are variable in newborns and infants because the corticospinal pathways are not fully developed. Their exaggerated presence or their absence has little diagnostic significance, unless this response is different from results of previous testing or extreme responses are observed.

A progressive increase in deep tendon reflexes during the first year of life may indicate central nervous system disease such as *cerebral palsy,* especially if it is coupled with increased tone.

Use the same techniques to elicit deep tendon reflexes as you would for an adult. You can substitute your index or middle finger for the neurologic hammer, as shown below.

As in adults, asymmetric reflexes suggest a lesion of the peripheral nerves or spinal segment.

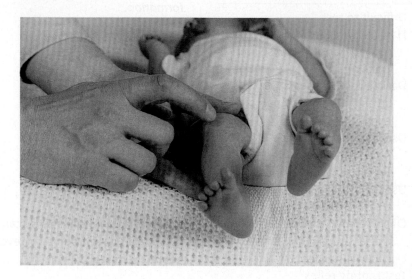

The triceps, brachioradialis, and abdominal reflexes are difficult to elicit before 6 months of age. The *anal reflex* is present at birth and important to elicit if a spinal cord lesion is suspected.

Although a normal flexion plantar response is obtained in 90% of infants, a *positive Babinski response* to plantar stimulation (dorsiflexion of big toe and fanning of other toes) can be elicited in some normal babies until 2 years of age.

Try to elicit the ankle reflex as for adults by tapping on the Achilles tendon but you often will not get a response. Another method, shown next, is to grasp the infant's malleolus with one hand and abruptly dorsiflex the ankle. You may note rapid, rhythmic plantar flexion of the newborn's foot (*ankle clonus*) in response to this maneuver. Up to 10 beats are normal in newborns and young infants; this is *unsustained ankle clonus*.

An absent anal reflex suggests loss of innervation of the external sphincter muscle caused by a spinal cord abnormality such as a congenital anomaly (e.g., *spina bifida*), *tumor*, or *injury*.

When the contractions are continuous (*sustained ankle clonus*), *central nervous system disease* should be suspected.

A newborn who is irritable, jittery and has tremors, hypertonicity, and hyperactive reflexes may have *drug withdrawal* from any of a number of drugs during pregnancy.

Neonatal abstinence syndrome results from the use of opioids by the mother while pregnant. In addition to the signs listed above, the newborn may also have autonomic signs, as well as poor feeding and seizures.

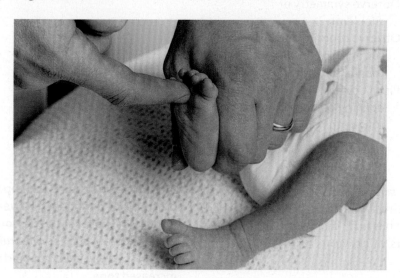

Primitive Reflexes. Evaluate the newborn and infant's developing central nervous system by assessing *infantile automatisms*, called *primitive reflexes*. These develop during gestation, are generally demonstrable at birth, and disappear at defined ages. Abnormalities in these primitive reflexes suggest neurologic disease and merit more intensive investigation.[26]

The most important primitive reflexes are illustrated below.

Development. Refer to the developmental milestones on p. 775 and to results of a standardized developmental screening instrument to learn which age-specific developmental tasks to evaluate. By observation and play with the infant, you can do both a developmental screening examination and an assessment for gross and fine motor achievement. Specifically, look for *weakness* by observing sitting, standing, and transitions. Note *station*, or the posture of sitting or standing. Assess fine motor development in a similar way, combining the neurologic and developmental examination. Key milestones include the development of the pincer grasp, ability to manipulate objects with the hands, and more precise tasks, such as building a tower of cubes or scribbling, as fine motor development progresses in a proximal to distal direction.

Assess the infant's cognitive and social–emotional development as you proceed with the comprehensive neurologic and developmental examination. Some neurologic abnormalities produce deficits or slowing in cognitive and social development. Infants who have developmental delay may have abnormalities found on the neurologic examination because much of the examination is based on age-specific norms.

A *neurologic* or *developmental abnormality* is suspected if primitive reflexes are:
- Absent at appropriate age
- Present longer than normal
- Asymmetric
- Associated with posturing or twitching

Many causes of developmental delay exist and often no cause is identified. Etiologies include *prenatal* (genetic, central nervous system, congenital hypothyroidism), *perinatal* (preterm, asphyxia, infection, trauma), and *postnatal* (trauma, infection, toxin, abuse).

Developmental delay across more than one domain (e.g., motor plus cognitive) suggests more severe disease.

Primitive Reflex

Primitive Reflex		Maneuver	Ages	
Palmar Grasp Reflex		Place your fingers into the baby's hands and press against the palmar surfaces. The baby will flex all fingers to grasp your fingers.	Birth to 3–4 months	Persistence beyond 4 months suggests pyramidal tract dysfunction. Persistence of clenched hand beyond 2 months suggests central nervous system damage, especially if fingers overlap thumb.
Plantar Grasp Reflex		Touch the sole at the base of the toes. The toes curl.	Birth to 6–8 months	Persistence beyond 8 months suggests pyramidal tract dysfunction.

(continued)

Primitive Reflex (continued)

Primitive Reflex		Maneuver	Ages	
Rooting Reflex		Stroke the perioral skin at the corners of the mouth. The mouth will open and baby will turn the head toward the stimulated side and suck.	Birth to 3–4 months	Absence of rooting indicates severe generalized or central nervous system disease.
Moro Reflex (Startle Reflex)		Hold the baby supine, supporting the head, back, and legs. Abruptly lower the entire body about 2 feet. The arms abduct and extend, hands open, and legs flex. Baby may cry.	Birth to 4 months	Persistence beyond 4 months suggests neurologic disease (e.g., cerebral palsy); persistence beyond 6 months strongly suggests it. Asymmetric response suggests fracture of clavicle or humerus or brachial plexus injury.
Asymmetric Tonic Neck Reflex		With baby supine, turn head to one side, holding jaw over shoulder. The arms/legs on side to which head is turned extend while the opposite arm/leg flex. Repeat on other side.	Birth to 2 months	Persistence beyond 2 months suggests asymmetric central nervous system development and sometimes predicts the development of cerebral palsy.
Trunk Incurvation (Galant's) Reflex		Support the baby prone with one hand, and stroke one side of the back 1 cm from midline, from shoulder to buttocks. The spine will curve toward the stimulated side.	Birth to 2 months *(continued)*	Absence suggests a transverse spinal cord lesion or injury. Persistence may indicate delayed development.

Primitive Reflex (continued)

Primitive Reflex		Maneuver	Ages	
Landau Reflex		Suspend the baby prone with one hand. The head will lift up, and the spine will straighten.	Birth to 6 months	Persistence may indicate delayed development.
Parachute Reflex		Suspend the baby prone and slowly lower the head toward a surface. The arms and legs will extend in a protective fashion.	8 months and does not disappear	Delay in appearance may predict future delays in voluntary motor development.
Positive Support Reflex		Hold the baby around the trunk and lower until the feet touch a flat surface. The hips, knees, and ankles extend, the baby stands up, partially bearing weight, sags after 20–30 seconds.	Birth or 2 months until 6 months	Lack of reflex suggests hypotonia or flaccidity. Fixed extension and adduction of legs (scissoring) suggests spasticity from neurologic disease, such as cerebral palsy.
Placing and Stepping Reflexes		Hold baby upright as in positive support reflex. Have one sole touch the tabletop. The hip and knee of that foot will flex and the other foot will step forward. Alternate stepping will occur.	Birth (best after 4 days). Variable age to disappear	Absence of placing may indicate paralysis. Babies born by breech delivery may not have placing reflex.

A normative measure of development is the developmental quotient,[27] shown here:

$$\text{Development quotient} = \frac{\text{Development age}}{\text{Chronologic age}} \times 100$$

Assess the development of an infant or child using standard scales for each type of development. Assign to a child a gross motor developmental quotient, a fine motor developmental quotient, a cognitive developmental quotient, and so forth.

Developmental Quotients

>85	Normal
70–85	Possibly delayed; follow-up needed
<70	Delayed

Case Examples of Gross and Fine Motor Development

Gross Motor Development	Fine Motor Development
A 12-month-old child who is just pulling to stand (gross motor developmental age of 9 months), cruising (10 months), and walking when both hands are held (10 mos) has a gross motor developmental age of 10 months. This child's gross motor developmental quotient is: $(\frac{10}{12} \times 100) = 83$ This child is in the gray zone, is likely to do well without intervention, but requires close follow-up.	A 12-month-old child can transfer objects from hand to hand (a fine motor developmental age of 6 months), rake objects into his palm (7 months), and pull things (7 months). He cannot hold blocks in each hand and does not have thumb and finger grasp (8–9 months). He has normal primitive reflexes (most absent), increased tone, scissoring of legs when held, spasticity, and delays on the gross motor part of the DDST. This child's fine motor developmental quotient is: $(\frac{7}{12} \times 100) = 58$ This child is delayed in fine motor development and has signs of *cerebral palsy*.

Assessing Young and School-Aged Children

DEVELOPMENT

Early Childhood: 1 to 4 Years

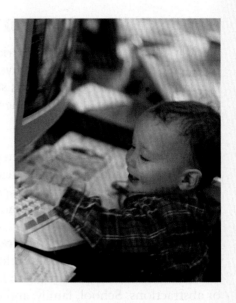

Physical Development. After infancy, the rate of physical growth slows by approximately half. After 2 years, toddlers gain about 2 to 3 kg and grow 5 cm per year. Physical changes are impressive. Chubby, clumsy toddlers transform into leaner, more muscular preschoolers.

Gross motor skills also develop quickly. Most children walk by 15 months, run well by 2 years, and pedal a tricycle and jump by 4 years. Fine motor skills develop through neurologic maturation and environmental manipulation. The 18-month-old who scribbles becomes a 2-year-old who draws lines and then a 4-year-old who makes circles.

Cognitive and Language Development. Toddlers move from sensorimotor learning (through touching and looking) to symbolic thinking, solving simple problems, remembering songs, and engaging in imitative play. Language develops with extraordinary speed. An 18-month-old with 10 to 20 words becomes a 2-year-old with three-word sentences, and a 3-year-old who converses well. By 4 years, preschoolers form complex sentences. They remain preoperational, however, without sustained logical thought processes.

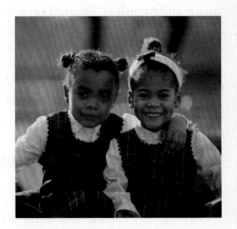

Social and Emotional Development. New intellectual pursuits are surpassed only by an emerging drive for independence. Because toddlers are impulsive and have poor self-regulation, temper tantrums are common.

Developmental Milestones During Early Childhood

	1 yr	2 yr	3 yr	4 yr	5 yr
Physical/ Motor	Walks	Throws	Jumps in place Balances on 1 foot	Hops Pedals tricycle	Skips Balances well
Cognitive/ Language	2–3 words	2–3-word phrases	Sentences	Speech all understandable	Copies figures Defines words
Social/ Emotional	Plays games (peek-a-boo)	Imitates activities	Feeds self	Imaginative Sings	Dresses self Plays games

Middle Childhood: 5 to 10 Years

Middle childhood is an active period of growth and development. Goal-directed exploration, increased physical and cognitive abilities, and achievements by trial and error mark this stage. The physical examination is more straightforward, but always consider the developmental stages and tasks that school-aged children are facing.

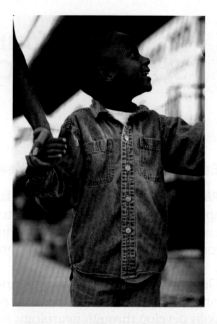

Physical Development. Children grow steadily but more slowly. Strength and coordination improve dramatically, with more participation in activities. This is also when children with physical disabilities or chronic illnesses become more aware of their limitations.

Cognitive and Language Development. Children become "concrete operational"—capable of limited logic and more complex learning. They remain rooted in the present, with little ability to understand consequences or abstractions. School, family, and environment greatly influence learning. A major developmental task is self-efficacy, or the ability to thrive in different situations. Language becomes increasingly complex.

Social and Emotional Development. Children become progressively more independent, initiating activities and enjoying accomplishments. Achievements are critical for self-esteem and developing a "fit" within major social structures—family, school, and peer activity groups. Guilt and poor self-esteem also may emerge. Family and environment contribute enormously to the child's self-image. Moral development remains simple and concrete, with a clear sense of "right and wrong."

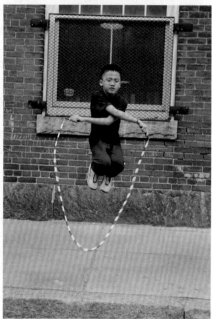

Developmental Tasks During Middle Childhood

Task	Characteristic	Health Care Needs
Physical	Enhanced strength and coordination	Screening for strengths, assessing problems
	Competence in various tasks and activities	Involving parents
		Support for disabilities
		Anticipatory guidance: safety, exercise, nutrition
Cognitive	"Concrete operational": focus on the present	Emphasis on short-term consequences
	Achievement of knowledge and skills, self-efficacy	Support; screening about skills and school performance
Social	Achieving good "fit" with family, friends, school	Assessment, support, advice about interactions
	Sustained self-esteem	Support, emphasis on strengths
	Evolving self-identity	Understanding, advice, support

THE HEALTH HISTORY

An important aspect of examining children is that parents are usually watching and taking part in the interaction, providing you the opportunity to observe the parent–child interaction. Note whether the child displays age-appropriate behaviors. Assess the "goodness of fit" between parents and child. Although some abnormal interactions may result from the unnatural setting of the examination room, others may be a consequence of interactional problems. Careful *observation* of the child's interactions with parents and the child's unstructured play in the examination room can reveal *abnormalities in physical, cognitive, and social development.*

Normal toddlers are occasionally terrified or angry at the examiner. Often, they are completely uncooperative. Most eventually warm up to you. If this behavior continues or is not developmentally appropriate, there may be an *underlying behavioral or developmental abnormality.* Older, school-aged children have more self-control and prior experience with clinicians and are generally cooperative with the examination.

Abnormalities Detected While Observing Play

Behavioral*	Social or Environmental
Poor parent–child interactions	Parental stress, depression
Sibling rivalry	Risk for abuse or neglect
Inappropriate parental discipline	
"Difficult temperament"	Neurologic
	Weakness
Developmental	Abnormal posture
Gross motor delay	Spasticity
Fine motor delay	Clumsiness
Language delay (expressive, receptive)	Attentional problems, hyperactivity
	Autistic features
Delay in social or emotional tasks	Musculoskeletal abnormalities

*Note: The child's behavior during the visit may not represent typical behavior, but your observations may serve as a springboard for discussion with parents.

Assessing Younger Children

A difficult challenge examining children in this age group is avoiding a physical struggle, a crying child, or a distraught parent. Accomplishing this successfully is one aspect of the "art of medicine" in the practice of pediatrics.

Gain the child's confidence and allay the child's fears from the start of the encounter. Your approach will vary with the circumstances of the visit. A health supervision visit allows greater rapport than a visit when the child is ill.

Let the child remain dressed during the interview to minimize the child's apprehension. It also allows you to interact more naturally and observe the child playing, interacting with the parents, and undressing and dressing.

Toddlers who are 9 to 15 months may have *stranger anxiety*, a fear of strangers that is developmentally normal. It signals the toddler's growing awareness that the stranger is new. You should not approach these toddlers quickly. Make sure they remain solidly in their parent's lap throughout much of the examination.

Some Tips for Examining Young Children (1- to 4-Year-Olds)

Useful Strategies for Examination	Useful Toys and Aids
Examine a child sitting on parent's lap. Try to be at the child's eye level.	"Blow out" the otoscope light.
First examine the child's toy or teddy bear, then the child.	"Beep" the stethoscope on your nose.
Let the child do some of the exam (e.g., move the stethoscope). Then go back and "get the places we missed."	Make tongue-depressor puppets.
	Use the child's own toys for play.
	Jingle your keys to test for hearing.
Ask the toddler who keeps pushing you away to "hold your hand." Then have the toddler "help you" with the exam.	Shine the otoscope through the tip of your finger, "lighting it up," and then examine the child's ears with it.
Some toddlers believe that if they can't see you, then you aren't there. Perform the exam while the child stands on the parent's lap, facing the parent.	Use age-appropriate books.
If 2-year-olds are holding something in each hand (such as tongue depressors), they can't fight or resist.	
Hand the child an age-appropriate book and engage the child in reading	

Engage children in age-appropriate conversation. Ask simple questions about their illness or toys. Compliment their appearance or behavior, tell a story, or play a simple game. If a child is shy, turn your attention to the parent to allow the child to warm up gradually.

With certain exceptions, physical examination does not require use of the examining table; it can be done on the floor or with the child in a parent's lap. The key is to engage the child's cooperation. For young children who resist undressing, expose only the body part being examined. When examining siblings, begin with the oldest child, who is more likely to cooperate and set a good example. Approach the child pleasantly. Explain each step as you perform it. Continue conversing with the family to provide distraction.

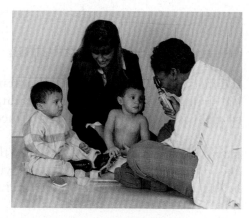

Plan the examination to start with the least distressing procedures and end with the most distressing, usually involving the throat and ears. Begin with parts that can be done with the child sitting, such as examining the eyes or palpating the neck. Lying down may make a child feel vulnerable, so change positions with care. Once a child is supine, begin with the abdomen, saving throat and ears or genitalia for last. You may need a parent's help to restrain the child for examination of the ears or throat; however, use of formal restraints is inappropriate. Patience, distraction, play, flexibility in the order of the examination, and a caring but firm and gentle approach are all key to successfully examining the young child.

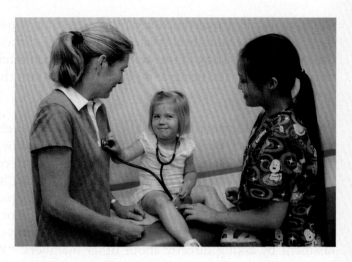

More Tips for Examining the Young Child

Use a reassuring voice throughout the examination.

Let the child see and touch the examination tools you will be using.

Avoid asking permission to examine a body part because you will do the examination anyway. Instead, ask the child which ear or which part of the body he or she would like you to examine first.

Examine the child in the parent's lap. Let the parent undress the child.

If unable to console the child, give the child a short break.

Make a game out of the examination! For example, "Let's see how big your tongue is!" or "Is Elmo in your ear? Let's see!"

Reassure parents that resistance to examination is developmentally appropriate. Some embarrassed parents scold the child, compounding the problem. Involve parents in the examination. Learn which techniques and approaches work best and are most comfortable for you.

Assessing Older Children

Examining children after they reach school age usually poses few difficulties. Although some have unpleasant memories of previous clinical encounters, most children respond well when the examiner is attuned to their developmental level.

Many children at this age are modest. Providing gowns and leaving underwear in place as long as possible are wise approaches. Suggest that children disrobe behind a curtain. Consider leaving the room while they change with parents' help. Some children may prefer opposite-sex siblings to leave, but most prefer a parent of either sex to remain in the room. Parents of children younger than 11 years should stay with them.

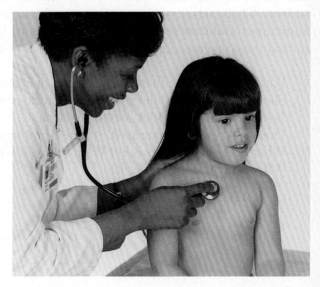

Children usually are accompanied by a parent or caregiver. Even when alone, they are often seeking health care at the request of their parent; indeed, the parent is usually sitting in the waiting room. When interviewing a child, you need to consider the needs and perspectives of both the child and the caregivers.

Establishing Rapport. Begin the interview by greeting and establishing rapport with each person present. Refer to the child by name rather than by "him" or "her." Clarify the role or relationship of all of the adults and children. "Now, are you Jimmy's grandmother?" "Please help me by telling me Jimmy's relationship to everyone here." Address the parents as "Mr. Smith" and "Ms. Smith" rather than by their first names or "Mom" or "Dad." When the family structure is not immediately clear, you may avoid embarrassment by asking directly about other members. "Who else lives in the home?" "Who is Jimmy's father?" "Do you live together?" Do not assume that just because parents are separated, only one parent is actively involved in the child's life. Same-sex parents are now relatively common.

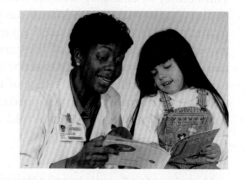

To establish rapport, meet children on their own level. Use your personal experiences with children to guide how you interact in a health care setting. Eye contact on their level, participating in playful engagement, and talking about what interests them are always good strategies. Ask children about their clothes, one of their toys, what book or TV show they like, or their adult companion in an enthusiastic but gentle style. Spending time at the beginning of the interview to calm and connect with an anxious child can put both the child and the caregiver at ease.

Working With Families. One challenge when several people are present is deciding to whom to direct your questions. While eventually you need to get information from both the child and the parent, it is useful to start with the child. Asking simple open-ended questions like "Are you sick? . . . Tell me about it," followed by more specific questions, often provides much of the clinical data. The parents can then verify the information, add details that give you the larger context, and identify other issues you need to address. Characterize symptom attributes the same way you do with adults. Sometimes children are embarrassed to begin, but once the parent has started the conversation, direct questions back to the child:

> Your mom tells me that you get stomachaches. Tell me about them.
> Show me where you get the pain. What does it feel like?
> Is it sharp like a pinprick, or does it ache?
> Does it stay in the same spot, or does it move around?
> What helps make it go away? What makes it worse?
> What do you think causes it?

The presence of family members allows you to observe how they interact with the child. A child may be able to sit still or may get restless and start fidgeting. Watch how the parents set, or fail to set, limits when needed.

Multiple Agendas. Each individual in the room, including the clinician, may have a different idea about the nature of the problem and what needs to be done about it. Discover as many of these perspectives and agendas as possible. Family members who are not present (e.g., the absent parent or grandparent) may also have concerns. Ask about those concerns, too. "If Suzie's father were here today, what questions or concerns would he have?" "Have you, Mrs. Jones, discussed this with your mother or anyone else?" "What does she think?"

For example, Mrs. Jones brings Suzie in for abdominal pain because she is worried that Suzie may have an ulcer and is also worried about Suzie's eating habits. Suzie is not worried about the belly pain, but is uneasy about the changes in her body and about getting fat. Mr. Jones thinks that Suzie's schoolwork is not getting enough attention. You, as the clinician, need to balance these concerns with what you see as a healthy 12-year-old girl in early puberty with some mild functional abdominal pain. Your goals need to include helping the family to be realistic about the range of "normal" and uncovering the concerns of each person.

The Family as a Resource. In general, family members provide most of the care and are your natural allies in promoting the child's health. Being open to a wide range of parenting behaviors helps to make this alliance. Raising a child reflects cultural, socioeconomic, and family practices. It is important to respect the tremendous variation in these practices. A good strategy is to view the parents as experts in the care of their child and yourself as their consultant. This demonstrates respect for the parents' care and minimizes their likelihood of discounting or ignoring your advice. Parents face many challenges raising children, so practitioners need to be supportive, not judgmental. Comments like, "Why didn't you bring him in sooner?" or "What did you do that for!" do not improve your rapport with the parent. Statements acknowledging the hard work of parenting and praising successes are always appreciated. "Mr. Smith, you are doing such a wonderful job with Bobby. Being a parent takes so much work and Bobby's behavior here today clearly shows your efforts." Or to the child, "Bobby you are so lucky to have such a wonderful dad."

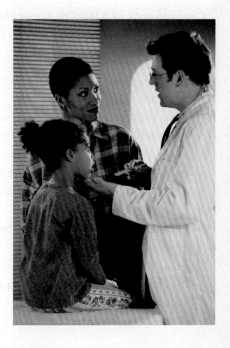

Hidden Agendas. As with adults, the chief complaint may not relate to the real reason the parent has brought the child to see you. The complaint may be a bridge to concerns that may not seem quite legitimate as a reason to go to the doctor. Try to create a trusting atmosphere that allows parents to be open about all their concerns. Ask facilitating questions like:

Do you have any other concerns about Randy?
Was there anything else that you wanted to tell/ask me today?

HEALTH PROMOTION AND COUNSELING: EVIDENCE AND RECOMMENDATIONS

Children 1 to 4 Years

The AAP and Bright Futures periodicity schedules for children include health supervision visits at 12, 15, 18, and 24 months, followed by annual visits when the child is 3 and 4 years old.[8] An additional visit at 30 months is also recommended to assess the child's development.

During these health supervision visits, clinicians address concerns and questions from parents, evaluate the child's growth and development, perform a comprehensive physical examination, and provide anticipatory guidance about healthy habits and behaviors, social competence of caregivers, family relationships, and community interactions.

This is a critical age for preventing childhood obesity: Many children begin their trajectory toward obesity between ages 3 and 4. It is also important to assess the child's development. Standardized developmental screening instruments are recommended to measure the different dimensions of a child's development (see p. 766). Similarly, it is important to differentiate normal (but potentially challenging) childhood behavior from abnormal behavioral or mental health problems.

The following box demonstrates the major components of a health supervision visit for a 3-year-old, stressing health promotion. You do not have to wait for a health supervision visit to address many of these health promotion issue; they can be addressed during other types of visits, even when the child is mildly ill.

Components of a Health Supervision Visit for a 3-Year-Old

Discussions With Parents
▶ Parental concerns
▶ Provide advice
▶ Childcare, school, social
▶ Major topic areas: development, nutrition, safety, oral health, family relationships, community

Developmental Assessment
▶ Assess milestones: gross and fine motor, social–personal, language; use a screener.

Physical Examination
▶ Careful examination, including growth parameters with percentiles for age.

Screening Tests
▶ Vision and hearing (formal testing at age 4), hematocrit and lead (if high risk or at ages 1–3), screen for social risk factors

Immunizations
▶ See AAP schedule

Anticipatory Guidance
Healthy Habits and Behaviors
▶ Injury and illness prevention
  Car seat, poisons, tobacco exposure, supervision
▶ Nutrition and Exercise
  Obesity assessment; healthy meals and snacks
▶ Oral health
  Brushing teeth; dentist
Parent–Infant Interaction
▶ Reading and fun times, limiting screen time
Family Relationships
▶ Activities, babysitters
Community Interaction
▶ Child care, resources

Children 5 to 10 Years

The AAP and Bright Futures periodicity schedules for children recommend annual health supervision visits during this period.[8] As for earlier ages, these visits present opportunities to assess the child's physical, mental, and developmental health and the parent–child relationship. Once again, health promotion should be incorporated into all interactions with children and families; take advantage of any opportunity to promote optimal health and development.

Older children enjoy talking directly with the examiner. In addition to discussing health, safety, development, and anticipatory guidance with parents, include the child in these conversations, using age-appropriate language and concepts. Discuss the child's experience and perceptions of school, and other cognitive and social activities. Focus on healthy habits such as good nutrition, exercise, reading, stimulating activities, and safety.

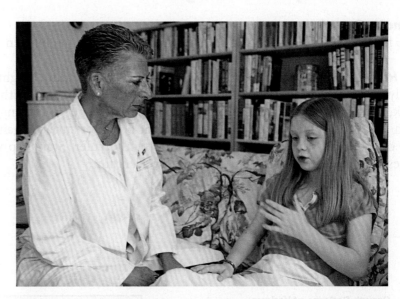

About 12% to 20% of children have some type of chronic physical, developmental, or mental condition.[28] Some behaviors that become established at this age can lead to or exacerbate chronic conditions such as obesity or eating disorders. Health promotion is critical to optimize healthy habits and minimize unhealthy ones. Helping families and children with chronic diseases deal most effectively with these disorders is a key part of health promotion.

For all children, health promotion involves assessing and promoting the family's overall health.

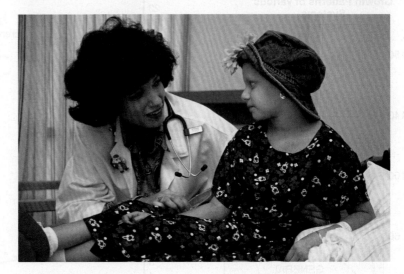

The specific components of the health supervision visit for older children are the same as the components for younger children. Emphasize school performance and experiences, as well as appropriate and safe sports and activities.

TECHNIQUES OF EXAMINATION

The order of the examination now begins to follow that used for adults. Examine painful areas last, and forewarn children about areas you are going to examine. If a child resists part of the examination, you can return to it at the end.

General Survey and Vital Signs

Somatic Growth

The figures below demonstrate somatic growth patterns in children.

Height. For children older than 2 years, measure standing height, optimally using wall-mounted stadiometers. Have the child stand with heels, back, and head against a wall or the back of the stadiometer. If using a wall with a marked ruler, make sure to place a flat board or surface against the top of the child's head and at right angles to the ruler. Stand-up weight scales with a height attachment are not very accurate.

Short stature, defined as subnormal height for age, can be a normal variant or caused by endocrine or other diseases. Normal variants include *familial short stature* and *constitutional delay.* Chronic diseases include *growth hormone deficiency,* other endocrine diseases, *gastrointestinal disease, renal* or *metabolic disease,* and *genetic syndromes.*

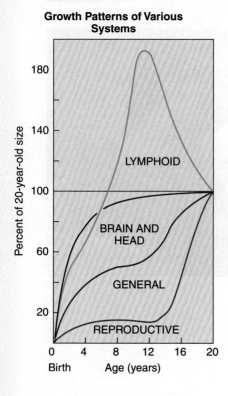

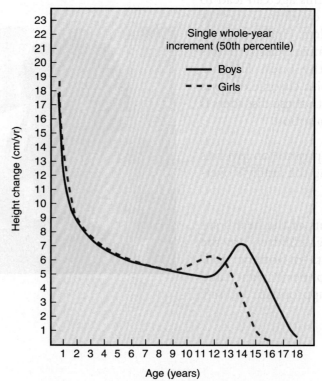

Velocity curves for length and height for boys and girls based on intervals of 1 year. (From Lowrey GH. Growth and Development of Children, 8th ed. Chicago: Mosby, 1986.)

After age 2 years, children should grow at least 5 cm per year. During puberty, growth velocity increases.

Weight. Children who can stand should be weighed in their underpants or in a gown on a stand-up scale. Use the same scales, across successive visits, to optimize comparability.

Head Circumference. In general, head circumference is measured until the child reaches 24 months. Afterward, head circumference measurement may be helpful if you suspect a genetic or a central nervous system disorder.

Body Mass Index for Age. Age- and sex-specific charts are now available to assess BMI in children. BMI in children is associated with body fat, related to subsequent health risks for obesity. BMI measurements are helpful for early detection of obesity in children older than 2 years. BMI growth charts for children take into account differences by sex and age. Obesity is now a major childhood epidemic, and it often begins before 6 to 8 years. Consequences of childhood obesity include hypertension, diabetes, metabolic syndrome, and poor self-esteem. Childhood obesity often leads to adult obesity and shortened lifespan. It is helpful to give parents their BMI results, together with information about the impact of healthy eating and physical activity.

Interpreting BMI in Children

Group	BMI-for-Age
Underweight	<5th percentile
Healthy weigh	5th–85th percentile
Overweight	85th–95th percentile
Obese	≥95th percentile

Vital Signs

Blood Pressure. Hypertension during childhood is more common than previously thought, and it is important to recognize, confirm, and appropriately manage it.

Children have elevated blood pressure during exercise, crying, and anxiety. When the procedure for measuring blood pressure is explained and demonstrated beforehand, most children are cooperative. If the blood pressure is initially elevated, you can perform blood pressure readings again at the end of the examination. Leave the cuff on the arm (deflated) and repeat the reading later. Elevated readings must always be confirmed by subsequent measurements.

Young children can have inadequate weight and height gain if caloric intake is insufficient. Etiologies of failure to thrive include *psychosocial, interactional, gastrointestinal, and endocrine disorders.*

Most children with exogenous obesity are also tall for their age. Children with endocrine causes of obesity tend to be short.

Childhood obesity is a major epidemic: 32% of U.S. children have a BMI greater than the 85th percentile, and 17% have a BMI in the 95th percentile or greater.[29] Long-term morbidity from childhood obesity spans many organ systems, including cardiovascular, endocrine, renal, musculoskeletal, gastrointestinal, and psychological. Prevention, early detection, and aggressive management are needed.

A very common cause of apparent hypertension is anxiety or "white-coat hypertension." The most frequent "cause" of an elevated blood pressure in children is probably an *improperly performed examination,* often due to an incorrect cuff size.

A proper cuff size is essential for accurate determinations of blood pressure in children. Select the blood pressure cuff as you would for adults; it should be wide enough to cover two thirds of the upper arm or leg. A narrower cuff falsely elevates the blood pressure reading, whereas a wider cuff lowers it and may interfere with proper placement of the stethoscope diaphragm over the artery.

With children, as with adults, the first Korotkoff sound indicates systolic pressure and the point at which the Korotkoff sounds disappear constitutes the diastolic pressure. At times, especially among chubby young children, the Korotkoff sounds are not easily heard. In such instances, you can use palpation to determine the systolic blood pressure, remembering that the systolic pressure is approximately 10 mm Hg lower by palpation than by auscultation.

A relatively inaccurate means is "inspection." Watch for the needle to bounce about 10 mm Hg higher than it does in auscultation. This technique is suboptimal, but sometimes is the only method for squirming children.

In children, as in adults, blood pressure readings from the thigh are approximately 10 mm Hg higher than those from the upper arm. If they are the same or lower, *coarctation of the aorta* should be suspected.

Transient hypertension in children can be caused by some common childhood medications, including those to treat asthma (e.g., prednisone) and ADHD (e.g., Ritalin).

Causes of *sustained hypertension* in childhood include primary hypertension (with no underlying etiology) and secondary hypertension (which has an underlying etiology). Causes of secondary hypertension include: renal, endocrine, and neurologic disease, vascular causes, drugs or medications and psychologic causes.

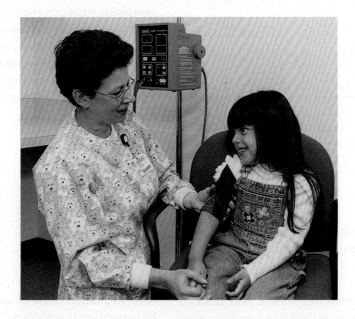

In 2004, the National Heart, Lung, and Blood Institute's National High Blood Pressure Working Group on Hypertension Control in Children and Adolescents defined normal, high-normal, and high blood pressure as follows, with measurements on at least three separate occasions[30]:

Blood Pressure

Blood Pressure Category	Average Systolic and/or Diastolic Blood Pressure for Age, Sex, and Height
Normal	<90th percentile
Prehypertensive	90th–95th percentile
Hypertensive	≥95th percentile
-stage 1	95th percentile to 5 mm Hg above 99th percentile
-stage 2	≥99th percentile plus 5 mm Hg

The epidemic of childhood obesity has also resulted in a rising prevalence of childhood hypertension.

Children who have hypertension should be evaluated extensively to determine the cause. For infants and young children, a specific cause can usually be found. An increasing proportion of older children and adolescents, however, have essential or primary hypertension. In all cases, it is important to repeat measurements to reduce the possibility that the elevation reflects anxiety. Sometimes, repeating measurements in school is a way to obtain readings in a more relaxed environment. Hypertension and obesity often coexist in children.

It is also important not to *falsely label* a child or adolescent as having hypertension, because of the stigma of labeling, potential limitations to activities, and possible side effects of treatment.

Pulse.   Average heart rates and ranges of normal are shown in the table below. Measure the heart rate over a 60-second interval.

Average Heart Rate of Children at Rest

Age	Average Rate	Range (Two Standard Deviations)
1–2 years	110	70–150
2–6 years	103	68–138
6–10 years	95	65–125

Sinus bradycardia is a heart rate <100 beats per minute in children younger than 3 years, and <60 beats per minute in children 3 to 9 years.

Respiratory Rate.   The rate of respirations per minute ranges from 20 to 40 during early childhood, and 15 to 25 during late childhood, reaching adult levels at around 15 years of age.

For young children, observe the movements of the chest wall for two 30-second intervals or over 1 minute, preferably before stimulating them. Direct auscultation of the chest or placing the stethoscope in front of the mouth is also useful for counting respirations, but the measurement may be falsely elevated if the child becomes agitated. For older children, use the same technique as that used for adults.

Children with respiratory diseases such as *bronchiolitis* or *pneumonia* have rapid respirations (up to 80 to 90/min) but *also* increased work of breathing such as grunting, nasal flaring, or use of accessory muscles.

The commonly accepted standard for tachypnea in children older than 1 year is a respiratory rate >40 breaths per minute.

The best single physical finding for ruling out pneumonia is an absence of tachypnea.

Temperature. In children, auditory canal temperature recordings are preferable because they can be obtained quickly with essentially no discomfort.

Children younger than 3 years, who appear very ill with a fever, should be evaluated for sepsis, urinary tract infection, pneumonia, or other serious infection.

The Skin

After a child's first year of life, the techniques of examination are the same as those for the adult (see Chapter 6, The Skin, Hair, and Nails.)

The Head

In examining the head and neck, tailor your examination to the child's stage of growth and development.

Even before touching the child, carefully observe the shape of the head, its symmetry, and the presence of abnormal facies. Abnormal facies may not be apparent until later in childhood; therefore, carefully examine the face as well as the head of all children.

There are diagnostic facies in childhood (Table 18-6, Diagnostic Facies in Infancy and Childhood, pp. 882–883, shows several) that reflect chromosomal abnormalities, endocrine defects, chronic illness, and other disorders.

Fetal alcohol syndrome can cause abnormal facies (p. 882) and microcephaly, as well as developmental delay.

The Eyes

The two most important components of the eye examination for young children are to determine whether the gaze is conjugate or symmetric and to test visual acuity in each eye.

Strabismus (see Table 18-7, Abnormalities of the Eyes, Ears, and Mouth, p. 884) in children requires treatment by an ophthalmologist.

Conjugate Gaze. Use the methods described in Chapter 7 for adults to assess conjugate gaze, or the position and alignment of the eyes, and the function of the extraocular muscles. The corneal light reflex test and the cover–uncover test are particularly useful in young children.

Both ocular strabismus and anisometropia (eyes with significantly different refractive errors) can result in amblyopia, or reduced vision in an otherwise normal eye. Amblyopia can lead to a "lazy eye," with permanently reduced visual acuity if not corrected early (generally by 6 years).

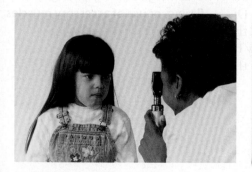
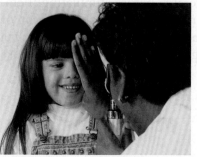

Perform the cover–uncover test as a game by having the young child watch your nose or tell you if you are smiling or not, while you cover one of the child's eyes.

The common forms of strabismus in children involve horizontal deviation: elite nasal ("eso") or temporal ("exo.") A latent strabismus ("phoria") occurs when you disrupt fixation, whereas manifest strabismus ("tropia") is present without interruption and is noted by the cover-uncover test.

Visual Acuity. It may not be possible to measure the *visual acuity* of children younger than 3 years who cannot identify pictures on an eye chart. For these children, the simplest examination is to assess for fixation preference by alternately covering one eye; the child with normal vision will not object, but a child with poor vision in one eye will object to having the good eye covered. In all tests of visual acuity, it is important that both eyes show the same result.

Reduced visual acuity is more likely among children who were born prematurely, and among those with other neurologic or developmental disorders.

Visual Acuity

Age	Acuity
3 months	Eyes converge, baby reaches
12 months	~20/200
Younger than 4 years	20/40
4 years and older	20/30

Any difference in visual acuity between the eyes (e.g., 20/20 on the left and 20/30 on the right) is abnormal.

Visual acuity in children 3 years and older can usually be formally tested using an eye chart with one of a variety of optotypes (characters or symbols).[31] A child who does not know letters or numbers reliably can be tested using pictures, symbols, or the "E" chart. Using the "E" chart, most children will cooperate by telling you in which direction the "E" is pointing.

The most common visual disorder of childhood is *myopia,* which can be easily detected using this examination technique.

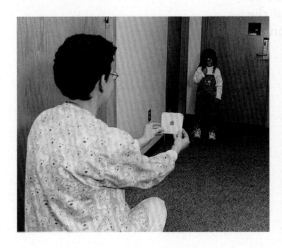
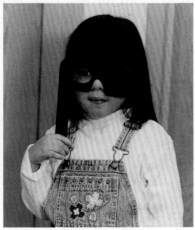

Some children develop *abnormalities in near vision,* which can lead to reading difficulties, headaches, and school problems, as well as double vision.

Visual Fields. The *visual fields* can be examined in infants and young children with the child sitting on the parent's lap. One eye should be tested at a time with the other eye covered. Hold the child's head in the midline while bringing an object such as a toy into the field of vision from behind the child. The overall method is the same as that for adults, except that you will have to make this into a game for your patient.

The Ears

Examining the *ear canal and drum* can be difficult in young children who are sensitive and fearful because they cannot observe the procedure. With a little practice, you can master this technique. Unfortunately, many young children need to be briefly restrained during this examination, which is why you may want to leave it for the end.

If the child is not too fearful, you may examine the ears with the child sitting on a parent's lap. Make a game out of the otoscopic examination, such as finding an imaginary object in the child's ear or talking playfully to allay fears. It may help to place the otoscopic speculum gently into the external auditory canal of one ear and then withdraw it so the child gets used to the procedure, before the actual examination.

Ask the parent for a preference regarding the positioning of the child for the examination. There are two common positions: the child lying down and restrained, and the child sitting in the parent's lap. If the child is held supine, have the parent hold the arms either extended (see photos on the next page) or close to the sides to limit motions. Hold the head and pull the pinna (auricle) upwards with one hand while you hold the otoscope with your other hand. If the child is on the parent's lap, the child's legs should be between the parent's legs. The parent could help by placing one arm around the child's body and using the second arm to steady the head.

Tympanic Membranes. Many students have difficulty visualizing a child's tympanic membrane. In young children, the external auditory canal is directed upward and backward from the outside, and the auricle must be pulled upward, outward, and backward to afford the best view. Hold the child's head with one hand, and with that same hand, pull up on the auricle. With your other hand, position the otoscope.

Tips for Conducting the Otoscopic Examination

Use the best angle of the otoscope.
Use the largest possible speculum.
  A larger speculum allows you to better visualize the tympanic membrane.
  A small speculum may not provide a seal for pneumatic otoscopy.
Don't apply too much pressure, which will cause the child to cry and may
  cause false-positive results on pneumatic otoscopy.
Insert the speculum ¼ to ½ inch into the canal.
First find the landmarks.
  Careful–sometimes the ear canal resembles the tympanic membrane.
Note whether the tympanic membrane is abnormal.
Remove cerumen if it is blocking your view, using
  Special plastic curettes
  A moistened microtipped cotton swab
  Flushing of ears for older children
  Special instruments that can also be purchased.

There are two ways to hold the otoscope, as illustrated by the following photos:

● The first is the method generally used in adults, with the otoscope handle pointing upward or laterally while you pull up on the auricle. Hold the lateral aspect of your hand that has the otoscope against the child's head to provide a buffer against sudden movements by the patient.

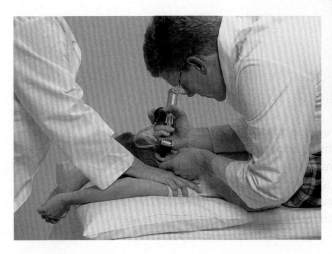
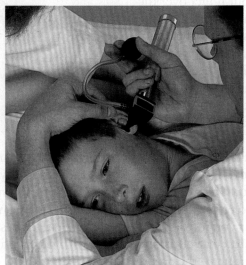

- The second is used by many pediatricians because of the different angle of the auditory canal in children. Hold the otoscope with the handle pointing down toward the child's feet, while you pull up on the auricle. Hold the head and pull up on the auricle with one hand, while you hold the otoscope with the other hand.

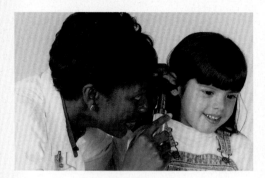
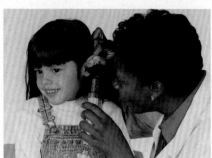

Acute otitis media is a common condition of childhood. A symptomatic child typically has a red, bulging tympanic membrane, with a dull or absent light reflex and diminished movement on pneumatic otoscopy. Purulent material may also be seen behind the tympanic membrane. See Table 18-7, Abnormalities of the Eyes, Ears, and Mouth, p. 884. The most useful symptom in making the diagnosis is ear pain, if combined with the above signs.[32,33]

You can use a *pneumatic otoscope* to improve the accuracy of diagnosis of otitis media in children. This allows you to assess the mobility of the tympanic membrane as you increase or decrease the pressure in the external auditory canal by squeezing the rubber bulb of the pneumatic otoscope.

First, check the pneumatic otoscope for leaks by placing your finger over the tip of the speculum and squeezing the bulb. Note the pressure on the bulb. Then insert the speculum, obtaining a proper seal; this is critical because failure to obtain a seal can produce a false-positive finding (lack of movement of the tympanic membrane).

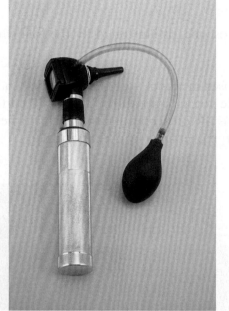

Sometimes during acute otitis media the tympanic membrane ruptures, leading to pus in the auditory canal. In these cases, you generally will not visualize the tympanic membrane.

Movement of the tympanic membrane is absent in middle ear effusion (*otitis media with effusion*).

When air is introduced into the normal ear canal, the tympanic membrane and its light reflex move inward. When air is removed, the tympanic membrane moves outward. This to-and-fro movement of the tympanic membrane has been likened to the luffing of a sail. If the tympanic membrane fails to move perceptibly as you introduce positive or negative pressure, the child is likely to have a middle ear effusion. A child with acute otitis media may flinch because of pain due to the air pressure.

Gently move and pull on the *pinna* before or during your otoscopic examination. Carefully inspect the area behind the pinna, over the mastoid bone. Many offices now use a tympanometer, which measures the compliance of the tympanic membrane and helps to diagnose a middle ear effusion.

Significant, temporary hearing loss for several months can accompany otitis media with effusion.

With *otitis externa* (but not otitis media), movement of the pinna elicits pain.

With acute *mastoiditis,* the auricle may protrude forward, and the area over the mastoid bone is red, swollen, and tender.

Formal Hearing Testing. Although formal hearing testing is necessary for accurate detection of hearing deficits in young children, you can grossly test for hearing by using the whispered voice test. Stand behind the child (so that the child cannot read your lips), cover one of the child's ear canals, and rub the tragus, using a circular motion. Whisper letters, numbers, or a word and have the child repeat it, and then test the other ear. This technique has relatively high sensitivity and specificity compared with formal testing.[34]

Younger children who fail these screening maneuvers or who have speech delay should have audiometric testing. These children may have *hearing deficits* or central auditory processing disorders.

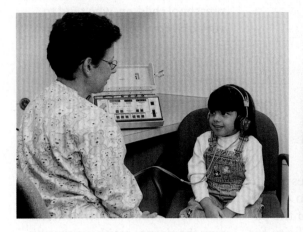
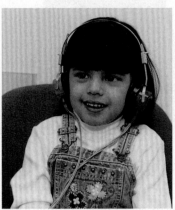

The AAP recommends that all children older than 4 years have a full-scale acoustic screening test using standardized equipment. If you do use an acoustic screening test, be sure to test the entire acoustic range, including the speaking range (500 to 6,000 Hz). The table below shows one classification of hearing ranges.

Up to 15% of school-aged children have at least mild hearing loss, emphasizing the importance of screening for hearing prior to school age.[32]

The two types of hearing loss seen in children are *conductive* and *sensorineural* hearing loss.

Causes of *conductive hearing loss* include congenital abnormalities, trauma, recurrent otitis media and tympanic membrane perforation.

Causes of *sensorineural hearing loss* include hereditary congenital infections, ototopic drugs, trauma and some infections such as meningitis.

Hearing Ranges on Formal Acoustic Screening Tests	
Normal hearing	0–20 dB
Mild hearing loss	21–40 dB
Moderate hearing loss	41–60 dB
Severe hearing loss	61–90 dB
Profound hearing loss	>90 dB

The Nose and Sinuses

Inspect the anterior portion of the nose by using a large speculum on your otoscope. Inspect the nasal mucous membranes, noting their color and condition. Look for nasal septal deviation and the presence of polyps.

Pale, boggy nasal mucous membranes are found in children with *chronic (perennial) allergic rhinitis.*

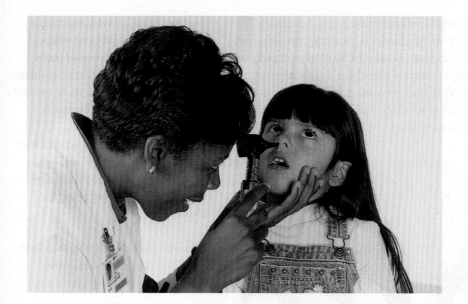

Maxillary sinuses are noted on x-rays by age 4 years, sphenoid sinuses by age 6, and frontal sinuses by age 6 to 7. The sinuses of older children can be palpated as in adults, looking for tenderness.[35] Transillumination of the paranasal sinuses of younger children has poor sensitivity and specificity for diagnosing sinusitis or fluid in the sinuses.

The Mouth and Pharynx

For anxious or young children, leave this part of the examination toward the end, because it may require parental restraint. The young, cooperative child may be more comfortable sitting in the parent's lap.

Healthy children are more likely to cooperate with this examination than sick children, especially if the sick child sees the tongue blade or has had previous experience with throat cultures.

The accompanying figure demonstrates how to get children to open their mouths. The child who can say "ahhh" will usually offer a sufficient (albeit brief) view of the posterior pharynx so that a tongue blade is unnecessary.

If you need to use the tongue blade, push down and pull slightly forward toward yourself while the child says "ahhh," being careful not to place the blade too far posteriorly, eliciting a gag reflex. Sometimes, young and anxious children will need to be restrained and will clamp their teeth and purse their lips. In these cases, carefully slip the tongue depressor between the teeth and onto the tongue. This will either allow you to push down on the tongue or elicit a gag reflex, which should permit a brief look at the posterior pharynx and tonsils. Careful planning and parental help are needed.

Examine the *teeth* for the timing and sequence of eruption, number, character, condition, and position. Abnormalities of the enamel may reflect local or general disease.

Purulent rhinitis is common in viral infections but may be part of the constellation of symptoms of *sinusitis*.

Foul-smelling, purulent, unilateral discharge from the nose may be due to a *foreign body* in the nose. This is particularly common among young preschool children, who tend to stick objects into any body orifice.

Nasal polyps are flesh-colored growths inside the nares. They are generally isolated findings but in some cases are present as part of a syndrome.

Children with purulent rhinorrhea (generally unilateral) and also headache, sore throat, and tenderness over the sinuses may have *sinusitis*.

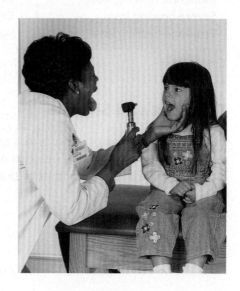

How to Get Children to Open Their Mouths (aka, "Would You Please Say 'Ahhh'?")

▶ Turn it into a game.
  ▶ "Now let's see what's in your mouth."
  ▶ "Can you stick out your *whole tongue*?"
  ▶ "I bet you can't open your mouth *really wide*!"
  ▶ "Let me see the inside of your teeth."
  ▶ "Can you pant like a dog on a hot day?"
▶ Don't show a tongue blade unless really necessary.
▶ Demonstrate first on an older sibling (or even the parent).
▶ Offer enthusiastic praise for opening their mouths a little, and encourage them to open even wider.

Dental caries are the most common health problem in children. They are particularly prevalent in impoverished populations and can cause both short-term and long-term problems.[36] Caries are highly treatable.

Carefully inspect the upper teeth, as shown in the photo. This is a common location for *nursing-bottle caries*. The technique shown in the photo, called "lift the lip," can help visualize dental caries.

Visualize the inside of the upper teeth by having the child look up at the ceiling with the mouth wide open.

The table below displays a common pattern of teeth eruption. In general, lower teeth erupt a bit earlier than upper teeth.

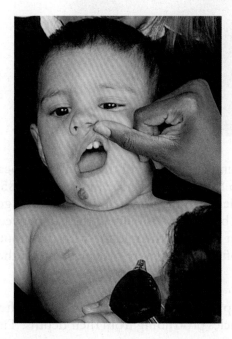

Dental caries are caused by bacterial activity. Caries are more likely among young children who have prolonged bottle-feeding ("nursing-bottle caries"). See Table 18-8, Abnormalities of the Teeth, Pharynx, and Neck, p. 885, for different stages of caries.

Staining of the teeth may be intrinsic or extrinsic. Intrinsic stains may be from tetracycline use before 8 years (yellow, gray, or brown stain). Iron preparation (black stain) and fluoride (white stain) are examples of extrinsic stains. Extrinsic stains can be polished off; intrinsic stains cannot (see Table 18-8, Abnormalities of the Teeth, Pharynx, and Neck, p. 885).

Tooth Types and Age of Eruption[37]

Tooth Type	Approximate Age of Eruption	
	Primary (mos)	Permanent (yrs)
Central incisor	5–8	6–8
Lateral incisor	5–11	7–9
Cuspids	24–30	11–12
First bicuspids	—	10–12
Second bicuspids	—	10–12
First molars	16–20	6–7
Second molars	24–30	11–13
Third molars	—	17–22

Look for abnormalities of the position of the teeth. These include malocclusion, maxillary protrusion (*overbite*), and mandibular protrusion (*underbite*). You can demonstrate the latter two by asking the child to bite down hard while either you or the child parts the lips. Observe the true bite. In normal children, the lower teeth are contained within the arch formed by the upper teeth.

Malocclusion and misalignment of teeth can be from thumb sucking, a hereditary condition, or premature loss of primary teeth.

Carefully inspect the *tongue*, including the underside. Most children will happily stick their tongue out at you, move it from side to side, and demonstrate its color (the blue tongue below is from eating candy).

Common abnormalities include *coated tongue* in viral infections, and *strawberry tongue,* found in scarlet fever.

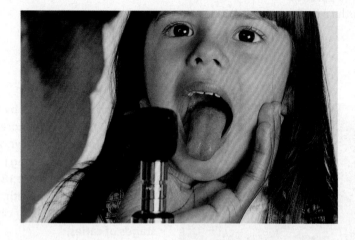

Some young children have a tight frenulum. Children who are severely "tongue-tied" might have a speech impediment. Have the child touch the tongue to the roof of the mouth to diagnose this condition, which is easily treated.

A *geographic tongue* is a benign but permanent condition in which a portion of the tongue has a rough, unusual appearance.

Note the size, position, symmetry, and appearance of the *tonsils*. The peak growth of tonsillar tissue is between 8 and 16 years (see figure on p. 885). The size of the tonsils varies considerably in children and is often categorized on a scale of 1+ to 4+, with 1+ being easy visibility of the gap between the tonsils, and 4+ being tonsils that touch in the midline with the mouth wide open. The tonsils in children often appear more obstructive than they really are.

Streptococcal pharyngitis typically produces a strawberry tongue, white or yellow exudates on the tonsils or posterior pharynx, a beefy-red uvula, and palatal petechiae.[38]

Tonsils in children usually have deep crypts on their surfaces, which often have white concretions or food particles protruding from their depths. This does not indicate disease.

A *peritonsillar abscess* is suggested by asymmetric enlargement of the tonsils and lateral displacement of the uvula.

Look for clues of a submucosal cleft palate, such as notching of the posterior margin of the hard palate or a bifid *uvula*. Because the mucosa is intact, the underlying defect is easily missed.

Acute epiglottitis is now rare in the United States because of immunization against *Haemophilus influenzae* type B. This is a contraindication to examination of the throat because of potential gagging and laryngeal obstruction.

Extremely rarely, you may encounter a child who has a sore throat and has difficulty swallowing saliva, who is sitting up stiffly in a "tripod" position (see p. 843) because of throat obstruction. Do not open this child's mouth because he may have acute epiglottitis, or obstruction from another cause.

Bacterial tracheitis can cause airway obstruction.

Note the quality of the child's voice. Certain abnormalities can change the pitch and quality of the voice.

Tonsillitis can be caused by bacteria, such as *Streptococcus,* or viruses. The "rocks in the mouth" voice is accompanied by enlarged tonsils with exudates.

Voice Changes—Clues to Underlying Abnormalities

Voice Change	Possible Abnormality
Hypernasal speech	Submucosal cleft palate
Nasal voice plus snoring	Adenoidal hypertrophy
Hoarse voice plus cough	Viral infection (croup)
"Rocks in mouth"	Tonsillitis

The epidemic of childhood obesity has resulted in many children who snore and have *sleep apnea.*

You may note an abnormal breath odor, which may help lead to a specific diagnosis.

Halitosis in a child can be caused by upper respiratory, pharyngeal, or mouth infection; foreign body in the nose; dental disease; and gastroesophageal reflux.

The Neck

Beyond infancy, the techniques for examining the neck are the same as for adults. Lymphadenopathy is unusual during infancy but very common during childhood. The child's lymphatic system reaches its zenith of growth at 12 years, and cervical or tonsillar lymph nodes reach their peak size between 8 and 16 years.

Lymphadenopathy is usually from viral or bacterial infections (see Table 18-8, Abnormalities of the Teeth, Pharynx, and Neck, p. 885).

The vast majority of enlarged lymph nodes in children are due to infections (mostly viral but frequently bacterial) and not to malignant disease, even though the latter is a concern for many parents. It is important to differentiate normal lymph nodes from abnormal ones or from congenital cysts of the neck.

Malignancy is more likely if the node is >2 cm, is hard, or is fixed to the skin or underlying tissues (i.e., not mobile), and is accompanied by serious systemic signs such as weight loss.

The figure on p. 796 demonstrates the typical anatomical locations of lymph nodes and congenital cysts of the neck.

Check for *neck mobility.* It is important to ensure that the neck of all children is supple and easily mobile in all directions. This is particularly important when the patient is holding the head in an asymmetric manner and when central nervous system disease such as meningitis is suspected.

In young children with small necks, it may be difficult to differentiate low posterior cervical lymph nodes from *supraclavicular lymph nodes* (which are always abnormal and raise suspicion for malignancy).

In children, the presence of nuchal rigidity is a more reliable indicator of meningeal irritation than *Brudzinski's sign* or *Kernig's sign*. To detect nuchal rigidity in older children, ask the child to sit with legs extended on the examining table. Normally, children should be able to sit upright and touch their chins to their chests. Younger children can be persuaded to flex their necks by having them follow a small toy or light beam. You also can test for nuchal rigidity with the child lying on the examining table, as shown here. Nearly all children with nuchal rigidity will be extremely sick, irritable, and difficult to examine. In many countries, the incidence of bacterial meningitis has plummeted because of vaccinations.

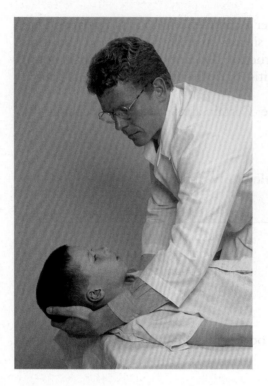

Nuchal rigidity is marked resistance to movement of the head in any direction. It suggests meningeal irritation due to *meningitis, bleeding, tumor,* or *other causes.* These children are extremely irritable and difficult to console and may have "paradoxical irritability"—increased irritability when being held.

When meningeal irritation is present, the child assumes the *tripod position* and is unable to assume a full upright position to perform the chin-to-chest maneuver.

The Thorax and Lungs

As children age, the lung examination becomes similar to that for adults. Cooperation is critical. Auscultation usually is easiest when a child barely notices (as when in a parent's lap). Let a toddler who seems fearful of the stethoscope play with it before it touches the child's chest.

With upper airway obstruction such as croup, inspiration is prolonged and accompanied by other signs such as stridor, cough, or rhonchi.

Assess the relative proportion of time spent on inspiration versus expiration. The normal ratio is about 1:1. Prolonged inspirations or expirations are a clue to disease location. Degree of prolongation and effort or "work of breathing" are related to disease severity.

With lower airway obstruction such as asthma, expiration is prolonged and often accompanied by wheezing.

Young children asked to "take deep breaths" often hold their breath, further complicating auscultation. It is easier to let preschoolers breathe normally. Demonstrate to older children how to take nice, quiet, deep breaths. Make it a game. To accomplish a forced expiratory maneuver, ask the child to blow out candles on an imaginary birthday cake or use pinwheels.

Pneumonia in young children generally is manifested by fever, tachypnea, dyspnea, and increased work of breathing.

Although *upper respiratory infections* due to viruses can cause young infants to appear quite ill, upper respiratory infections in children present with the same signs as in adults, and children generally appear well, without lower respiratory signs.

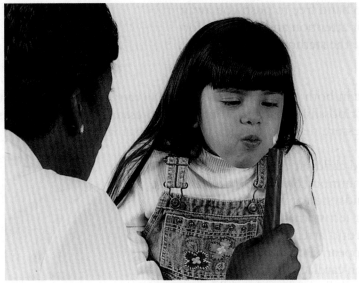

Childhood asthma is an extremely common condition throughout the world. Children with acute asthma present with varying severity and often have increased work of breathing. Expiratory wheezing and a prolonged expiratory phase, caused by reversible bronchospasm, can be heard without the stethoscope and are apparent on auscultation. Wheezes are often accompanied by inspiratory rhonchi caused by viruses that triggered the asthma.[39]

Older children will be cooperative for the respiratory examination and can even go through the maneuvers of assessing fremitus or listening to "E to A" changes (see pp. 314–315). As children grow, the evaluation by observation discussed on the previous page, such as assessing the work of breathing, nasal flaring, and grunting, becomes less helpful in assessing for respiratory pathology. Palpation, percussion, and auscultation achieve greater importance in a careful examination of the thorax and lungs.

Children in respiratory distress may assume a "tripod position" in which they lean forward to optimize airway potency. This same position can also be caused by pharyngeal obstruction (see p. 841).

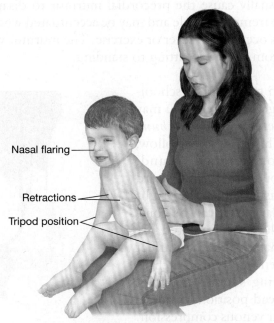

Nasal flaring

Retractions

Tripod position

A CHILD IN RESPIRATORY DISTRESS

The Heart

The examination of the heart and vascular systems in infants and children is similar to that in adults, but recognition of their fear, their inability to cooperate, and in many instances, their desire to play, will make the examination easier and more productive. Use your knowledge of the developmental stage of each child. A 2-year-old may be easiest to examine while standing or sitting on the mother's lap, facing her shoulder, or being held. Give young children something to hold in each hand. They cannot figure out

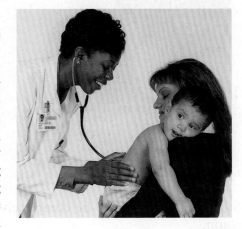

General abnormalities may suggest increased likelihood of congenital cardiac disease, as exemplified by Down syndrome or Turner's syndrome.

how to drop the object and, therefore, have no hand free to push you away. Endless chatter to small children will hold their attention and they may forget you are examining them. Let children move the stethoscope themselves, going back to listen properly.

Blood Pressure.   Measure the blood pressure in both arms and one leg at one time around age 3 to 4 years to check for possible coarctation of the aorta. Thereafter, only the right arm blood pressure needs to be measured.

In *coarctation of the aorta,* the blood pressure is lower in the legs than in the arms.

Benign Murmurs.   Preschool and school-aged children often have benign murmurs (see figure on p. 845). The most common (*Still's murmur*) is a grade I–II/VI, musical, vibratory, early and midsystolic murmur with multiple overtones, located over the mid or lower left sternal border, but also frequently heard over the carotid arteries. Carotid artery compression will usually cause the precordial murmur to disappear. This murmur may be extremely variable and may be accentuated when cardiac output is increased, as occurs with fever or exercise. The murmur will diminish as the child goes from supine to sitting to standing.

In preschool or school-aged children, you may detect a *venous hum*. This is a soft, hollow, continuous sound, louder in diastole, heard just below the right clavicle. It can be completely eliminated by maneuvers that affect venous return, such as lying supine, changing head position, or jugular venous compression. It has the same quality as breath sounds and, therefore, is frequently overlooked.

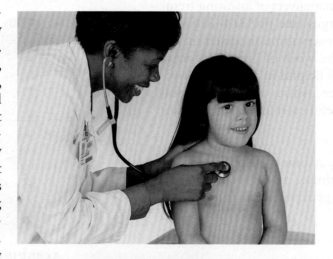

Among young children, murmurs without the recognizable features of the three common benign murmurs may signify underlying heart disease and should be evaluated thoroughly by a pediatric cardiologist.

Pathologic murmurs that signify cardiac disease can first appear after infancy and during childhood. Examples include aortic stenosis and mitral valve disease.

The murmur heard in the carotid area or just above the clavicles is known as a *carotid bruit*. It is early and midsystolic, with a slightly harsh quality. It is usually louder on the left and may be heard

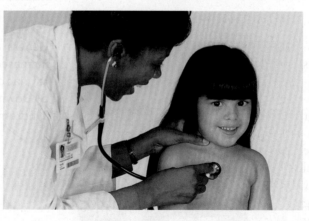

alone or in combination with the Still's murmur. It may be completely eradicated by carotid artery compression.

Location and Characteristics of Benign Heart Murmurs in Children*

Venous hum — Carotid bruit — Pulmonary flow — Still's murmur

Typical Age	Name	Characteristics	Description and Location
Preschool or early school age	*Still's murmur*		Grade I–II/VI, musical, vibratory Multiple overtones Early and midsystolic Mid/lower left sternal border Frequently also a carotid bruit
Preschool or early school age	*Venous hum*		Soft, hollow, continuous Louder in diastole Under clavicle Can be eliminated by maneuvers
Preschool and later	*Carotid bruit*		Early and midsystolic Usually louder on left Eliminated by carotid compression

*See the table on p. 863 for location and characteristics of benign heart murmurs in older children and adolescents.

The Abdomen

Toddlers and young children commonly have protuberant abdomens, most apparent when they are upright. The examination can follow the same order as for adults, except that you may need to distract the child during the examination.

Most children are ticklish when you first place your hand on their abdomens for *palpation*. This reaction tends to disappear, particularly if you distract the child with conversation and place your whole hand flush on the abdominal surface for a few moments without probing. For children who are particularly sensitive and who tighten their abdominal muscles, you can start by placing the child's hand under yours. Eventually you will be able to remove the child's hand and palpate the abdomen freely.

An exaggerated "pot-belly appearance" may indicate malabsorption from *celiac disease, cystic fibrosis,* or *constipation* or *aerophagia.*

A common condition of childhood that can occasionally cause a protuberant abdomen is *constipation.* The abdomen is often tympanitic on percussion, and stool is sometimes felt on palpation.

Try flexing the knees and hips to relax the child's abdominal wall, as shown below. Palpate lightly in all areas, then deeply, leaving the site of potential pathology to the end.

Chronic or recurrent abdominal pain is relatively common in children. Causes include both *functional disorders* and *organic disorders.*

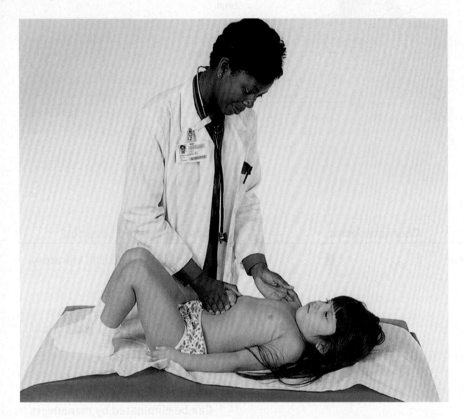

Functional disorders causing abdominal pain include *irritable bowel syndrome, functional dyspepsia,* and *childhood functional abdominal pain syndrome.*

Organic causes of chronic or recurrent abdominal pain in children include *gastritis* or *ulcer, gastroesophageal reflux, constipation,* and *inflammatory bowel disease.*

Many children present with abdominal pain from *acute gastroenteritis.* Despite pain, their physical examination is relatively normal except for increased bowel sounds on auscultation and mild tenderness on palpation.

Expected Liver Span of Children by Percussion

Age in Years	Mean Estimated Liver Span (cm)	
	Males	Females
2	3.5	3.6
3	4.0	4.0
4	4.4	4.3
5	4.8	4.5
6	5.1	4.8
8	5.6	5.1
10	6.1	5.4

The childhood obesity epidemic has resulted in many children who have extremely *obese abdomens.* While it is difficult to accurately examine these children, the steps to the examination are the same as for normal children.

One method to determine the lower border of the liver involves the *scratch test,* shown on the next page. Place the diaphragm of your stethoscope just above the right costal margin at the midclavicular line. With your fingernail, lightly scratch the skin of the abdomen along the midclavicular line, moving from below the umbilicus toward the costal margin. When your scratching finger reaches the liver's edge, you will hear a change in the scratching sound as it passes through the liver to your stethoscope.[40]

Hepatomegaly in young children is unusual. It can be caused by *cystic fibrosis, protein malabsorption,* parasites, and *tumors.*

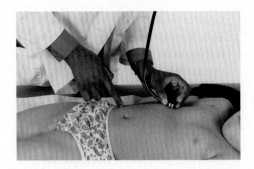 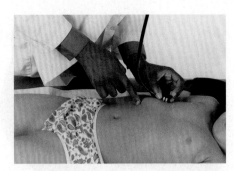

If hepatomegaly is accompanied by splenomegaly, *portal hypertension*, *storage diseases*, *chronic infections*, and *malignancy* should be considered.

The *spleen*, like the liver, is felt easily in most children. It too is soft with a sharp edge, and it projects downward like a tongue from under the left costal margin. The spleen is moveable and rarely extends more than 1 to 2 cm below the costal margin.

Various diseases can cause splenomegaly, including *infections, hematologic disorders* such as *hemolytic anemias, infiltrative disorders,* and *inflammatory* or *autoimmune diseases,* as well as congestion from *portal hypertension.*

Palpate the *other abdominal structures.* You will commonly note pulsations in the epigastrium caused by the aorta. This is felt most easily to the left of the midline, on deep palpation.

An abdominal mass felt on palpation may represent stool from constipation, or a serious condition such as a tumor.

Palpating for abdominal tenderness in an older child is the same as for the adult; however, the causes of abdominal pain are often different, encompassing a wide spectrum of acute and chronic diseases. Localization of tenderness may help you pinpoint the abdominal structures most likely to be causing the abdominal pain.

In a child with an acute abdomen, as in *acute appendicitis,* check for involuntary rigidity, rebound tenderness, a Rovsing's sign, or a positive psoas or obturator sign (see pp. 467–468).[41] *Gastroenteritis, constipation,* and *gastrointestinal obstruction* may be the causes.

Male Genitalia

Inspect the penis. The size in prepubertal children has little significance unless it is abnormally large. In obese boys, the fat pad over the symphysis pubis may obscure the penis.

There is an art to *palpation* of the young boy's scrotum and testes because many have an extremely active cremasteric reflex that may cause the testis to retract upward into the inguinal canal and thereby appear to be undescended. Examine the child when he is relaxed because anxiety stimulates the cremasteric reflex. With warm hands, palpate the lower abdomen, working your way downward toward the scrotum along the inguinal canal. This will minimize retraction of the testes into the canal.

In *precocious puberty,* the penis and testes are enlarged, with signs of pubertal changes. This is caused by a variety of conditions associated with excess androgens, including *adrenal or pituitary tumors.* Other pubertal changes also occur.

A useful technique is to have the boy sit cross-legged on the examining table, as shown here. You can also give him a balloon to inflate or an object to lift to increase intra-abdominal pressure. If you can detect the testis in the scrotum, it is descended even if it spends much time in the inguinal canal.

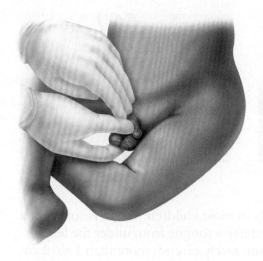

Cryptorchidism may be noted at this age. It requires surgical correction. It should be differentiated from a retractible testis.

A painful testicle requires rapid treatment; possible causes include infection such as *epididymitis* or *orchitis, torsion of the testicle,* or *torsion of the appendix testis.*

The cremasteric reflex can be tested by scratching the medial aspect of the thigh. The testis on the side being scratched will move upward.

A painless scrotal mass in a young boy is usually due to a hydrocele or a nonincarcerated inguinal hernia. Other rare causes include a varicocele or tumor.

Examine the inguinal canal as you would for adults, noting any swelling that may reflect an *inguinal hernia*. Have the boy increase abdominal pressure as described above and note whether a bulge in the inguinal canal increases.

Inguinal hernias in older boys present as they do in adult men, with swelling in the inguinal canal, particularly following a Valsalva maneuver.

Female Genitalia

The genital examination can be anxiety provoking for the older child and adolescent (especially if you are of the opposite sex), and for parents. Nevertheless, not performed, a significant finding may be missed. Depending on the child's developmental stage, explain what parts of the body you will check, and that this is part of the routine examination.

The appearance of pubic hair before 7 years should be considered *precocious puberty* and requires evaluation to determine the cause.

After infancy, the labia majora and minora flatten out, and the hymenal membrane becomes thin, translucent, and vascular, with the edges easily identified.

The genital examination is the same for all ages of children, from late infancy until adolescence. Use a calm, gentle approach, including a developmentally appropriate explanation as you do the examination. A bright light source is essential. Most children can be examined in the supine, frog-leg position.

Rashes on the external genitals can be from various causes such as physical irritation, sweating, and candidal or bacterial infections, including streptococcal infection.

If the child seems reluctant, it may be helpful to have the parent sit on the examination table with the child; alternatively, the examination may be performed while the child sits in the parent's lap. Do not use stirrups, as these may frighten the child. The following diagram demonstrates a 5-year-old girl sitting on her parent's lap with the parent holding her knees outstretched.

Vulvovaginal pruritis and *erythema* can be caused by external irritants, bubble baths, masturbatory activity, pinworms, or other infections such as *Candida* or *sexually transmitted infections*.

Examine the genitalia in an efficient and systematic manner. Inspect the external genitalia for pubic hair, the size of the clitoris, the color and size of the labia majora, and the presence of rashes, bruises, or other lesions.

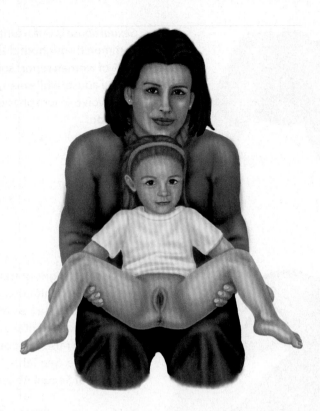

Next, visualize the structures by separating the labia with your fingers, as shown on the left below. You can also apply gentle traction by grasping the labia between your thumb and index finger of each hand, separating the labia majora laterally and posteriorly to examine the inner structures, as shown below on the right. *Labial adhesions*, or fusion of the labia minora, may be noted in prepubertal children and can obscure the vaginal and urethral orifices. They may be a normal variant.

A *vaginal discharge* in early childhood can be from *perineal irritation* (e.g., bubble baths or soaps), *foreign body, nonspecific vulvovaginitis, Candida, pinworms,* or a *sexually transmitted infection* from sexual abuse.

Vaginal bleeding is always cause for concern. Etiologies include *vaginal irritation, accidental trauma, sexual abuse, foreign body,* and *tumors. Precocious puberty* can induce menses in a young girl.

Purulent, profuse, malodorous, and blood-tinged discharge should be evaluated for the presence of *infiltration, foreign body,* or *trauma.*

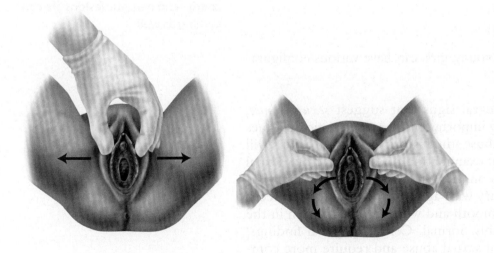

Note the condition of the labia minora, urethra, hymen, and proximal vagina. If you are unable to visualize the edges of the hymen, ask the child to take a deep breath to relax the abdominal muscles. Another useful technique is to position her in the knee–chest position, as shown on the right and below. These maneuvers will often open the hymen. You can also use saline drops to make the edges of the hymen less sticky.

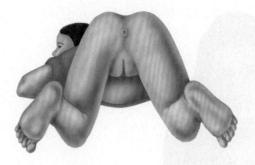

Sexual abuse is unfortunately far too common throughout the world. Up to 25% of women report some history of sexual abuse; while many of these do not involve severe physical trauma, some do.

Avoid touching the hymenal edges because the hymen is exquisitely tender without the protective effects of hormones. Examine for discharge, labial adhesions, lesions, estrogenization (indicating onset of puberty), hymenal variations (such as imperforate or septate hymen, which is rare), and hygiene. A thin, white discharge (leukorrhea) is often present. A speculum examination of the vagina and cervix is not necessary in a prepubertal child unless there is suspicion of severe trauma or foreign body.

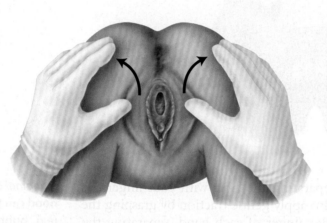

Abrasions or signs of trauma of the external genitalia can be from benign causes such as masturbation, irritants, or accidental trauma, but should also raise the possibility of *sexual abuse*. See Table 18-11, Physical Signs of Sexual Abuse, p. 889.

As demonstrated in Table 18-11, Physical Signs of Sexual Abuse, p. 889, physical signs strongly suggestive of *sexual abuse* include lacerations, ecchymoses and newly healed scars of the hymen, lack of hymenal tissue from 3 to 9 o'clock, and healed hymenal transections. Other signs such as purulent discharge and herpetic lesions are concerning as well.

The normal hymen in infants and young girls can have various configurations, as shown on the next page.

The physical examination may reveal signs that suggest *sexual abuse*, and the examination is particularly important if there are suspicious clues in the history. Even with known abuse, the majority of examinations will be unremarkable; a normal genital examination does not rule out sexual abuse. Mounds, notches, and tags on the hymen may all be normal variants. The size of the orifice can vary with age and the examination technique. If the hymenal edges are smooth and without interruption in the inferior half, the hymen is probably normal. Certain physical findings, however, suggest the possibility of sexual abuse and require more complete evaluation by an expert in the field. See Table 18-11, Physical Signs of Sexual Abuse, p. 889.

Normal Configurations of the Hymen in Prepubertal and Adolescent Females

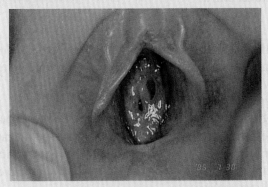

6-year-old girl with a septate hymen causing two orifices. Traction is needed to visualize the two openings.

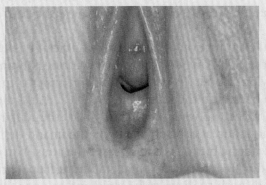

7-year-old girl with a crescent-shaped hymenal orifice

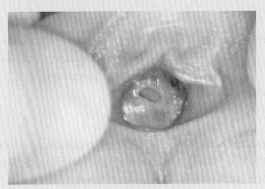

2-year-old girl with an annular orifice, located off-center, visible with labial traction

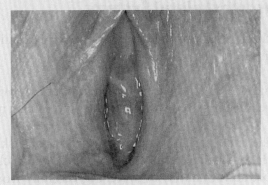

9-year-old girl with redundant labial tissue. Greater traction or a knee–chest position would reveal a normal orifice.

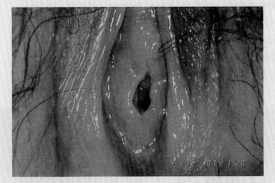

12-year-old girl with annular-shaped orifice and hormonal influence of puberty, causing thickened, pink tissue

Source of photos: Reece R, Ludwig S (eds). Child Abuse: Medical Diagnosis and Management, 2nd ed. Philadelphia: Lippincott Williams & Wilkins, 2001.

The Rectal Examination

The rectal examination is not routine but should be done whenever intra-abdominal, pelvic, or perirectal disease is suspected.

The rectal examination of the young child can be performed with the child in either the side-lying or lithotomy position. For many young children, the lithotomy position is less threatening and easier to perform. Have the child lie on the back with the knees and hips flexed and the legs abducted. Drape the child from the waist down. Provide frequent reassurance during the examination, and ask the child to breathe in and out through the mouth to relax. Spread the buttocks and observe the anus. You can use your lubricated gloved index finger, even in small children. Palpate the abdomen with your other hand, both to distract the child and to note the abdominal structures between your hands. The prostate gland is not palpable in young boys.

Anal skin tags are present in *inflammatory bowel disease* but are more often an incidental finding.

Tenderness noted on rectal examination of a child usually indicates an infectious or inflammatory cause, such as an *abscess,* or *appendicitis.*

The Musculoskeletal System

In older children, abnormalities of the upper extremities are rare in the absence of injury.

Toddlers may acquire *nursemaid's elbow* or subluxation of the radial head from a tugging injury.

The normal young child has increased lumbar concavity and decreased thoracic convexity compared with the adult, and often a protuberant abdomen.

Observe the child standing and walking barefoot. Ask the child to touch the toes, rise from sitting, run a short distance, and pick up objects. You will detect most abnormalities by watching carefully from both front and behind. To indirectly assess the child's gait pattern, note the soles of the shoes to see which side of the soles is worn down.

The cause of *acute limp* in childhood is usually trauma or injury, although infection of the bone, joint, or muscle should be considered.

During early infancy, there is a common and normal progression of increased bowlegged growth (see below left), which begins to disappear at about 18 months of age, often followed by transition toward knock-knees. The *knock-knee pattern* (as shown below right), is usually maximal by age 3 to 4 years and gradually corrects by age 9 or 10 years.

Severe bowing of the legs (genu varum) may still be physiologic bowing and will spontaneously resolve. Extreme bowing or unilateral bowing may be from pathologic causes such as *rickets* or *tibia vara (Blount's disease).*

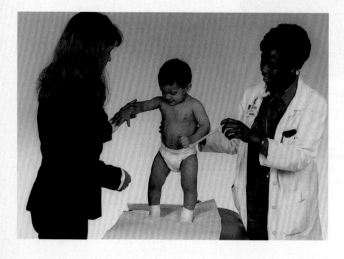
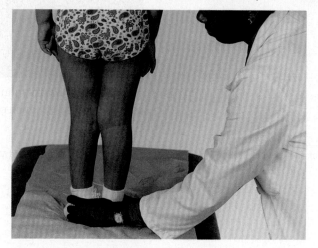

The presence of tibial torsion can be assessed in several ways[43]; one method is shown here. Have the toddler lie prone on the examination table, with the knees flexed to 90 degrees. Note the thigh–foot axis. Usually there is ±10 degrees of internal or external rotation noted by a foot pointing off in a direction. Check the position of the malleoli—they should be symmetric.

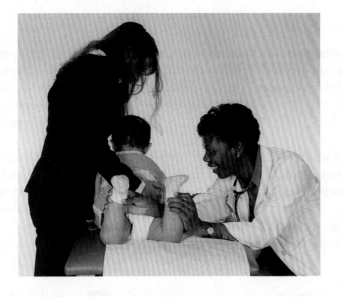

The most common lower-extremity pathology in childhood is injury from accidents. Joint injuries, fractures, sprains, strains, and serious ligament injuries such as anterior cruciate ligament tears of the knee are all too common in children.

A *chronic limp* in childhood could be caused by Blount disease, hip disorders such as *avascular necrosis of the hip*, leg length discrepancy, spinal disorder, and serious systemic disease such as leukemia.

Children may *toe in* when they begin to walk. This may increase up to 4 years of age and then gradually disappear by about 10 years of age.

Inspect any child who can stand for *scoliosis*, using techniques described under "Adolescents."

Determine any *leg shortening* that may accompany hip disease, by comparing the distance from the anterior superior spine of the ilium with the medial malleolus on each side. Straighten the child by pulling gently on the legs, and then compare the levels of the medial malleoli with each other. Put a small ink dot over the prominent malleoli and touch them together for a direct measure.

Have the child stand straight and place your hands horizontally over the iliac crests from behind. Small discrepancies can be noted. If such a discrepancy is noted and you suspect leg length discrepancy, with one iliac crest higher than the other, place a book under the shorter leg; this should eliminate the discrepancy.

Test for severe hip disease, with its associated weakness of the gluteus medius muscle. Observe from behind as the child shifts weight from one leg to the other. A pelvis that remains level when weight is borne on the unaffected side is a *negative Trendelenburg's sign*.[44] With an abnormal positive sign in *severe hip disease*, the pelvis tilts toward the unaffected hip during weight bearing on the affected side (positive Trendelenburg's sign).

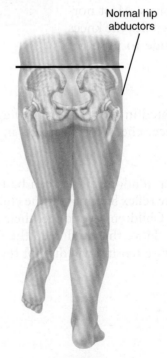
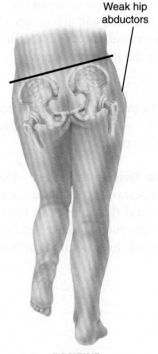

Normal hip abductors

Weak hip abductors

NEGATIVE TRENDELENBERG'S SIGN

POSITIVE TRENDELENBERG'S SIGN

The Nervous System

Beyond infancy, the neurologic examination includes the components evaluated in adults. Combine the neurologic and developmental assessment; turn this into a game with the child to assess optimal development and neurologic performance.

Children with *spastic diplegias* will often have hypotonia as infants and then excessive tone with spasticity, scissoring, and perhaps clenched fists as toddlers and young children.

Perform a structural developmental screen. Children usually enjoy this component, and you can too. Many neurologic conditions in children are accompanied by developmental abnormalities.

Problems with social interaction, verbal and nonverbal communication, restricted interests, and repetitive behaviors could be signs of *autism*.

Sensation. The sensory examination can be performed by using a cotton ball or tickling the child. This is best performed with the child's eyes closed. Do not use pin pricks.

Gait, Strength, and Coordination. Observe the child's gait while the child is walking and, optimally, running. Note any asymmetries, weakness, undue tripping, or clumsiness. Follow developmental milestones to test for appropriate maneuvers such as heel-to-toe walking (shown in the photo), hopping, and jumping. Use a toy to test for coordination and strength of the upper extremities.

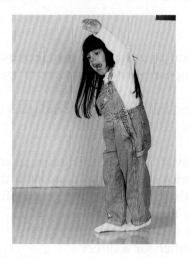

In children with uncoordinated gait, be sure to distinguish *orthopedic causes* such as positional deformities of the hip, knee, or foot from *neurologic abnormalities* such as *cerebral palsy, ataxia,* or *neuromuscular conditions*.

If you are concerned about the child's strength, have the child lie on the floor and then stand up, and closely observe the stages. Most normal children will first sit up, then flex the knees and extend the arms to the side to push off from the floor and stand up.

In certain forms of *muscular dystrophy* with weakness of the pelvic girdle muscles, children will rise to standing by rolling over prone and pushing off the floor with the arms while the legs remain extended (*Gower's sign*).

Hand preference is demonstrated in most children by age 2. If a younger child has clear hand preference, check for weakness in the nonpreferred upper extremity.

Deep Tendon Reflexes. Deep tendon reflexes can be tested as in adults. First demonstrate the use of the reflex hammer on the child's hand, assuring the child that it will not hurt. Children love to feel their legs bounce when you test their patellar reflexes. Have the child keep the eyes closed during some of this examination because tensing will disrupt the results.

Children with mild cerebral palsy may have both slightly increased tone and hyperreflexia.

Development.   You can ask children older than 3 years to draw a picture or copy objects as is done in the DDST, and then discuss their pictures to test simultaneously for fine motor coordination, cognition, and language.

Among school-aged children, the best test for development is their school performance. You can obtain school records of psychological testing results, obviating the need for the clinician to formally test an older child's development.

Distinguish between isolated delays in one aspect of development (e.g., coordination or language) and more generalized delays that occur in several components. The latter is more likely to reflect global neurologic disorders such as *mental retardation* that can be caused by many etiologies.

Cerebellar Function.   The cerebellar examination can be tested using finger-to-nose and rapid alternating movements of the hands or fingers. Children older than 5 years should be able to tell right from left, so you can assign them right–left discrimination tasks, as is done in the adult patient.

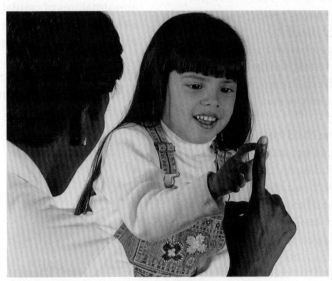

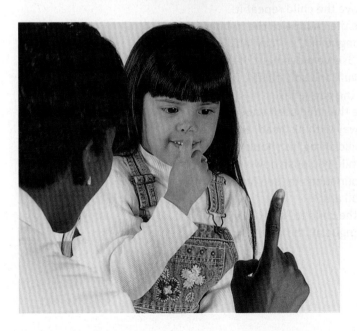

Some children with *attention deficit disorder with hyperactivity (ADHD)* will have great difficulty cooperating with your neurologic and developmental examination because of problems focusing. These children often have high energy levels, cannot stay still for extended periods, and have a history of difficulty in school or structured situations.

Delayed or disordered development in early childhood can lead to early school failure as well as social, behavioral, and emotional problems.

Cranial Nerves. The cranial nerves can be assessed quite well using developmentally appropriate strategies, as shown in the following table:

Strategies to Assess Cranial Nerves in Young Children

Cranial Nerve		Strategy
I	Olfactory	Testable in older children.
II	Visual acuity	Use Snellen chart after age 3 years.
		Test visual fields as for an adult. A parent may need to hold the child's head.
III, IV, VI	Extraocular movements	Have the child track a light or an object (a toy is preferable). A parent may need to hold the child's head.
V	Motor	Play a game with a soft cotton ball to test sensation.
		Have the child clench the teeth and chew or swallow some food.
VII	Facial	Have the child "make faces" or imitate you as you make faces (including moving your eyebrows), and observe symmetry and facial movements.
VII	Acoustic	Perform auditory testing after age 4 years.
		Whisper a word or command behind the child's back and have the child repeat it.
IX, X	Swallow and gag	Have the child stick the "whole tongue out" or "say 'ah'." Observe movement of the uvula and soft palate.
		Test the gag reflex.
XI	Spinal accessory	Have the child push your hand away with his head. Have the child shrug his shoulders while you push down with your hands to "see how strong you are."
XII	Hypoglossal	Ask the child to "stick out your tongue all the way."

Localizing neurologic signs are rare in children but can be caused by trauma, brain tumor, intracranial bleed, or infection. Children with *increased intracranial pressure* can develop cranial nerve abnormalities as well as papilledema and altered mental status.

Children with meningitis, encephalitis, or cerebral abscess can have abnormalities of cranial nerves, although they also have altered consciousness and other signs.

Although *facial nerve palsy* can be congenital, it is often caused by infection or trauma.

Assessing Adolescents

DEVELOPMENT: 11 TO 20 YEARS

Adolescence can be divided into three stages: early, middle, and late. Interview and examination techniques vary widely depending on the adolescent's physical, cognitive, and social–emotional levels of development.

Physical Development.   Adolescence is the period of transition from childhood to adulthood. The physical transformation generally occurs over a period of years, beginning at an average age of 10 in girls and 11 in boys. On average, girls end pubertal development with a growth spurt by age 14 and boys by age 16. The age of onset and duration of puberty vary widely, although the stages follow the same sequence in all adolescents. Early adolescents are preoccupied with these physical changes.

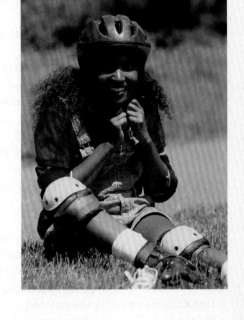

Cognitive Development.   Although less obvious, cognitive changes during adolescence are as dramatic as changes in physique. Most adolescents progress from concrete to formal operational thinking, acquiring an ability to reason logically and abstractly and to consider future implications of current actions. Although the interview and examination resemble those of adults, keep in mind the wide variability in cognitive development of adolescents and their often erratic and still limited ability to see beyond simple solutions. Moral thinking becomes sophisticated, with lots of time spent debating issues.

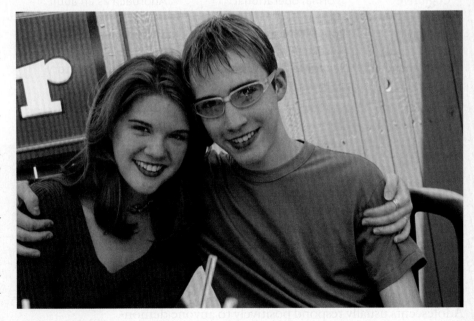

Social and Emotional Development.   Adolescence is a tumultuous time, marked by the transition from family-dominated influences to increasing autonomy and peer influence. The struggle for identity, independence, and eventually intimacy leads to stress, health-related problems, and, often, high-risk behaviors. This struggle also provides an important opportunity for health promotion.

Developmental Tasks of Adolescence

Task	Characteristic	Health Care Approaches
Early Adolescence (10- to 14-year-olds)		
Physical	Puberty (F: 10–14; M: 11–16) variable	Confidentiality; privacy
Cognitive	"Concrete operational"	Emphasis on short-term
Social		
Identity	Am I normal? Peers increasingly important	Reassurance and positive attitude
Independence	Ambivalence (family, self, peers)	Support for growing autonomy
Middle Adolescence (15- to 16-year-olds)		
Physical	Females more comfortable, males awkward	Support if patient varies from "normal"
Cognitive	Transition; many ideas	Problem solving; decision making
Social		
Identity	Who am I? Much introspection; global issues	Nonjudgmental acceptance
Independence	Limit testing; "experimental" behaviors; dating	Consistency; limit setting
Late Adolescence (17- to 20-year-olds)		
Physical	Adult appearance	Minimal unless chronic illness
Cognitive	"Formal operational"	Approach as an adult
Social		
Identity	Role with respect to others; sexuality; future	Encouragement of identity to allow growth
Independence	Separation from family; toward real independence	Support, anticipatory guidance

THE HEALTH HISTORY

The key to successfully examining adolescents is a comfortable, confidential environment. This makes the examination more relaxed and informative. Consider the teen's cognitive and social development when deciding issues of privacy, parental involvement, and confidentiality.

Adolescents usually respond positively to anyone demonstrating a genuine interest in them. Show such interest early and then sustain the connection for effective communication.

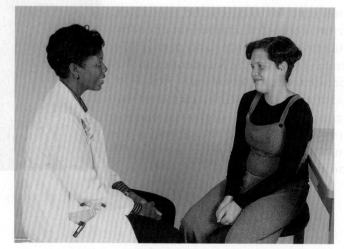

Adolescents are more likely to open up when the interview focuses on them rather than on their problems. In contrast to most other interviews, *start with specific questions* to build trust and rapport and get the conversation going. You may have to do more talking than usual, at the beginning. Chat informally about friends, school, hobbies, and family. Using silence in an attempt to get adolescents to talk or asking about feelings directly is usually not a good idea.

It is particularly important to use summarization and transitional statements and to explain what you are going to do during the physical examination. The physical examination can also be an opportunity to engage young persons. Once you have established rapport, return to more open-ended questions. At that point, make sure to ask what concerns or questions the adolescent may have. Because adolescents are often reluctant to ask their most important questions (which are sometimes about sensitive topics), ask if the adolescent has anything else to discuss. A useful phrase to use is "tell me what other questions you have."

Adolescents' behavior is related to their developmental stage, and not necessarily to chronologic age or physical maturation. Their appearance may fool you into assuming that they are functioning on a more future-oriented and realistic level. This is particularly true regarding "early bloomers," who look older than their age. The reverse can also be true, especially in teens with delayed puberty or chronic illness.

Issues of *confidentiality* are important in adolescence. Explain to both parents and adolescents that the best health care allows adolescents some degree of independence and confidentiality. It helps if the clinician starts asking the parent to leave the room for part of the interview when the child is age 10 or 11 years. This prepares both parents and teens for future visits when the patient spends time alone with the clinician.

Before the parent leaves, obtain relevant medical history from him or her, such as certain elements of past history, and clarify the parent's agenda for the visit. Adolescents need to know that you will hold in confidence what they discuss with you. However, never make confidentiality unlimited. Always state explicitly that you may need to act on information that makes you concerned about safety: "I will not tell your parents what we talk about unless you give me permission or I am concerned about your safety, for example, if you were to talk to me about killing yourself and I thought that you really were at risk to follow through, I would need to discuss it with others in order to help you."

An important goal is to help adolescents bring their concerns or questions to their parents. Encourage adolescents to discuss sensitive issues with their parents and offer to be present or help. Although young people may believe that their parents would "kill them if they only knew," you may be able to promote more open dialogue. This entails a careful assessment of the parents' perspective and the full and explicit consent of the young person.

As in middle childhood, modesty is important. The patient should remain dressed until the examination begins. Leave the room while the patient puts on a gown. Most adolescents older than 13 years prefer to be examined without a parent in the room, but this depends on the patient's developmental level, familiarity with the examiner, relationship with the parent, and culture. Ask younger adolescents and their parent their preferences. It is advisable for male clinicians to have a chaperone in the room when examining a female patient's breasts or genitalia.

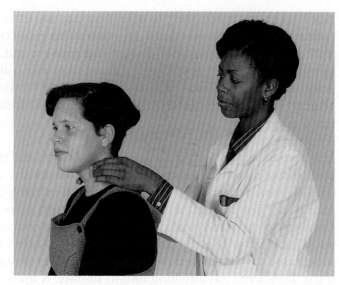

The sequence and content of the physical examination of the adolescent are similar to those in the adult. Keep in mind, however, issues unique to adolescents, such as puberty, growth, development, family and peer relationships, sexuality, decision making, and high-risk behaviors.

HEALTH PROMOTION AND COUNSELING: EVIDENCE AND RECOMMENDATIONS

The AAP recommends annual health supervision visits for adolescents.[3, 45] Be sure to include health promotion during all health encounters with youth. Adolescents with chronic problems or high-risk behaviors may require additional visits for health promotion and anticipatory guidance.

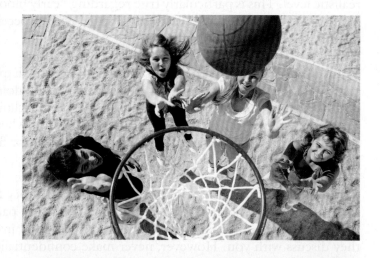

Most chronic diseases of adults have their antecedents in childhood or adolescence. For example, obesity, cardiovascular disease, addiction (to drugs, tobacco, or alcohol), and depression are all influenced by childhood and teen experiences and by behaviors established during adolescence. Most obese adults were obese as adolescents or had abnormal indicators such as elevated BMI scores. Almost all adults who are addicted to tobacco began their tobacco habits before 18 years. Therefore, a major component of health promotion for adolescents includes discussions about health behaviors or habits. Effective health promotion can help patients develop healthy habits and lifestyles and avoid several chronic health problems.

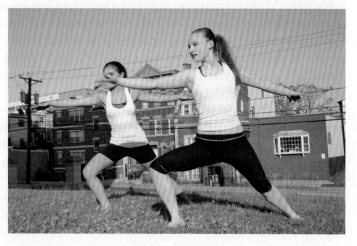

Because some health promotion topics involve confidential issues such as mental health, addiction, sexual behavior, and eating disorders, speak to adolescents (particularly older youth) privately during part of a visit that involves health supervision.

Self-completed screening questionnaires can be completed before the visit to facilitate comprehensive assessment of youth risk behaviors. This approach saves time so that you can better address the specific risk behaviors the adolescent endorses during the visit. An excellent instrument is the Guidelines for Adolescent Preventive Services (GAPS).[4, 45]

Components of a Health Supervision Visit for Adolescents 11–18 Years

Discussions With Parents
- Address parent concerns
- Provide advice
- Ask about school, activities, social interactions
- Assess youth's behaviors and habits, mental health

Discussions With Adolescent
- *Social and Emotional:* mental health, friends, family
- *Physical Development:* puberty, self-concept
- *Behaviors and Habits:* nutrition, exercise, TV or computer screen time, drug/alcohol
- *Relationships and Sexuality:* dating, sexual activity, forced sex
- *Family Functioning:* relations with parents and siblings
- *School Performance:* activities, strengths

Physical Examination
- Perform a careful examination; note growth parameters, sexual maturity ratings

Screening Tests
- Vision and hearing, blood pressure; consider hematocrit; assess emotional health and risk factors (using a validated instrument)

Immunizations
- See schedule from the AAP

Anticipatory Guidance—Teen
Promote Healthy Habits and Behaviors:
- Injury & illness prevention
  Seat belts, drunk driving, helmets, sun, weapons
- Nutrition
  Healthy meals/snacks, obesity prevention
- Oral health: dentist, brushing
- Physical activity and screen time

Sexuality:
- Confidentiality, sexual behaviors, safer sex, contraception if needed

Substance Abuse:
- Prevention strategies
- Parent–teen interaction
- Communication, rules

Social Achievement:
- Activities, school, future

Community Interaction
- Resources, involvement

Anticipatory Guidance—Parent
Positive interactions, support, safety, limit setting, family values, modeling behaviors

TECHNIQUES OF EXAMINATION

General Survey and Vital Signs

Somatic Growth.   Adolescents should wear gowns to be weighed. This is particularly important for adolescent girls being evaluated for underweight problems. Ideally, serial weights (and heights) should use the same scales.

Both obesity and eating disorders among adolescent girls are major public health problems, requiring frequent assessments of weight.

Vital Signs.   Ongoing evaluations of blood pressure are important for adolescent.[28] The average heart rate from age 10 to 14 years is 85 beats per minute, with a range of 55 to 115 beats per minute considered normal. Average heart rate for those 15 years and older is 60 to 100 beats per minute.

Causes of sustained hypertension for this age group include *primary hypertension, renal parenchymal disease,* and *drug use.*

The Skin

Examine the adolescent's skin carefully. Many adolescents will have concerns about various skin lesions, such as acne, dimples, blemishes, warts, and moles. Pay particular attention to the face and back in examining adolescents for acne.

Adolescent acne, a common skin condition, tends to resolve eventually but often benefits from proper treatment. It tends to begin during middle to late puberty.

Many adolescents spend considerable time in the sun and at tanning salons. You may detect this during a comprehensive health history or by noticing signs of tanning during the physical examination. This is a good opportunity to counsel adolescents about the dangers of excessive ultraviolet exposure, the need for sunscreen, and the risks of tanning salons.

Moles or benign nevi may appear during adolescence. Their characteristics differentiate them from atypical nevi, described on p. 880.

Counsel adolescents to begin performing a regular self-examination of the skin, as shown on pp. 179–180.

Head, Ears, Eyes, Throat, and Neck

The examination of these body parts is generally the same as for adults.

The methods used to examine the eye, including testing for visual acuity, are the same as those for adults. Refractive errors become common, and it is important to test visual acuity monocularly at regular intervals, such as during the annual health supervision visit.

An adolescent with persistent fever, tonsillar pharyngitis, and cervical lymphadenopathy may have *infectious mononucleosis.*

The ease and techniques of examining the ears and testing the hearing approach the methods used for adults. There are no ear abnormalities or variations of normal unique to this age group.

The Heart

The technique and sequence of examination are the same as those for adults. Murmurs are a continued cardiovascular issue for evaluation.

Location and Characteristics of Benign Heart Murmurs in Adolescents

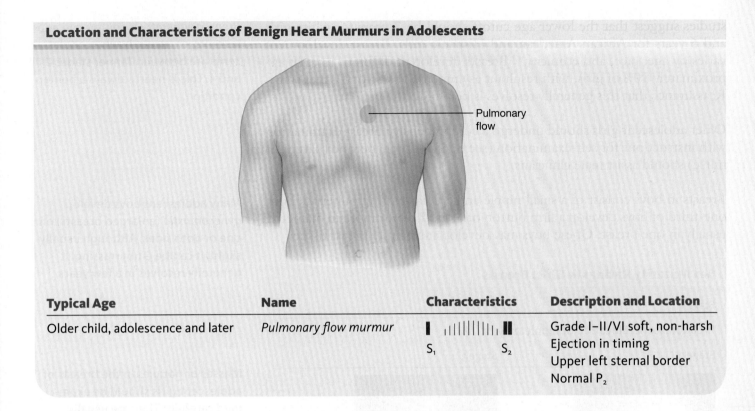

Pulmonary flow

Typical Age	Name	Characteristics	Description and Location
Older child, adolescence and later	*Pulmonary flow murmur*	S_1 S_2	Grade I–II/VI soft, non-harsh Ejection in timing Upper left sternal border Normal P_2

The benign *pulmonary flow murmur* is a grade I–II/VI soft, non-harsh murmur with the timing characteristics of an ejection murmur, beginning after the first sound and ending before the second sound but without the marked crescendo–decrescendo quality of an organic ejection murmur. If you hear this murmur, evaluate whether the pulmonary closure sound is of normal intensity and whether splitting of the second heart sound is eliminated during expiration. An adolescent with a benign pulmonary ejection murmur will have normal intensity and normally split second heart sounds.

A pulmonary flow murmur accompanied by a fixed split second heart sound suggests right-heart volume load such as an *atrial septal defect*.

This pulmonary flow murmur may also be heard in the presence of volume overload from any cause such as chronic anemia, and following exercise. It may persist into adulthood.

The Breasts

Physical changes in a girl's breasts are one of the first signs of puberty. As in most developmental changes, there is a systematic progression. Generally, over a 4-year period, the breasts progress through five stages, called Tanner stages or Tanner sex maturity rating (SMR) stages, as shown in the box on the next page. Breast buds in the preadolescent stage progress to subsequent enlargement and change in the contour of the breasts and areola. These stages are accompanied by the development of pubic hair and other secondary sexual characteristics, as shown on p. 867. Menarche usually occurs when a girl is in breast stage 3 or 4. By then, she has passed her peak growth spurt (see the figure on p. 868).

Breast buds (pea-size firm masses under the nipple) are common among both girls and boys just before puberty or early during puberty.

For years, the normal range for onset of breast development was 8 to 13 years (average, 11 years), with earlier onset considered abnormal.[46] Some studies suggest that the lower age cutoff should be 7 years for white girls and 6 years for African American and Hispanic girls. Breast development varies by age, race, and ethnicity.[47] Breasts develop at different rates in approximately 10% of girls, with resultant asymmetry of size or Tanner stage. Reassurance that this generally resolves is helpful to the patient.

Older adolescent girls should undergo a comprehensive breast examination with instructions for self-examination (see p. 427). A chaperone (parent or nurse) should assist male clinicians.

Breasts in boys consist of a small nipple and areola. During puberty, about one-third of boys develop a firm button of tissue 2 cm or more in diameter, usually in one breast. Obese boys may develop substantial breast tissue.

Breast asymmetry is common in adolescents, particularly when adolescents are between Tanner stages 2 and 4. This is nearly always a benign condition.

Many adolescent boys develop *gynecomastia* (enlarged breasts) on one or both sides. Although usually slight, it can be embarrassing. It generally resolves in a few years.

Masses or nodules in the breasts of adolescent girls should be examined carefully. They are usually *benign fibroadenomas* or *cysts;* less likely etiologies include *abscesses* or *lipomas.* Breast carcinoma is extremely rare in adolescence and nearly always occurs in families with a strong history of the disease.[48]

Sex Maturity Ratings in Girls: Breasts

Stage 1

Preadolescent. Elevation of nipple only

Stage 2

Stage 3

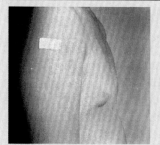

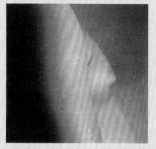

Breast bud stage. Elevation of breast and nipple as a small mound; enlargement of areolar diameter

Further enlargement of elevation of breast and areola, with no separation of their contours

Stage 4

Stage 5

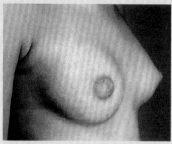

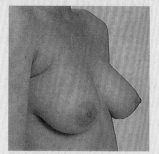

Projection of areola and nipple to form a secondary mound above the level of breast

Mature stage; projection of nipple only. Areola has receded to general contour of the breast (although in some normal individuals, the areola continues to form a secondary mound).

Photos used with permission of the American Academy of Pediatrics, *Assessment of Sexual Maturity Stages in Girls,* 1995.

The Abdomen

Techniques of abdominal examination are the same as for adults. The size of the liver approaches the adult size as the teen progresses through puberty, and is related to the adolescent's overall height. Although data are lacking about the usefulness of different techniques to assess liver size, it is likely that evidence from adult studies apply, particularly for older adolescents. Palpate the liver. If it is nonpalpable, hepatomegaly is highly unlikely. If you can palpate the lower edge, use light percussion to assess liver span.

Hepatomegaly in teens may be from *infections* such as hepatitis or infectious mononucleosis, inflammatory bowel disease, or tumors.

Male Genitalia

The genital examination of the adolescent boy proceeds like the examination of the adult male. Be aware of the embarrassment of many boys regarding this aspect of the examination.

Important anatomical changes in the male genitalia accompany puberty and help to define its progress. The first reliable sign of puberty, starting between ages 9 and 13.5 years, is an increase in the size of the testes. Next, pubic hair appears, along with progressive enlargement of the penis. The complete change from preadolescent to adult anatomy requires about 3 years, with a range of 1.8 to 5 years.

Delayed puberty is suspected in boys who have no signs of pubertal development by 14 years of age.

When examining the adolescent male, assign a sexual maturity rating. The five stages of sexual development, first described by Tanner, are outlined and illustrated on the next page. These involve changes in the penis, testes, and scrotum. In about 80% of men, pubic hair spreads farther up the abdomen in a triangular pattern pointing toward the umbilicus; this phase is not completed until the 20s.

The most common cause of delayed puberty in males is *constitutional delay,* frequently a familial condition involving delayed bone and physical maturation but normal hormonal levels.

An axiom of development is that pubertal changes follow a well-established sequence. The age range for start and completion is wide, but the sequence for each boy is the same. This progression is helpful when counseling anxious adolescents about current and future maturation and the wide range of normal for changes in puberty.

Although nocturnal or daytime ejaculation tends to begin around Sexual Maturity Rating 3, a finding on either history or physical examination of penile discharge may indicate a *sexually transmitted infection.*

In addition to constitutional delay, less common causes of *delayed puberty* in boys include primary hypogonadism or secondary hypogonadism, as well as congenital GnRH deficiency.

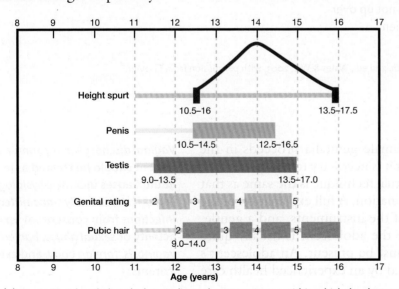

Male adolescents: Numbers below the bars indicate the ranges in age within which the changes occur.

Sex Maturity Ratings in Boys

In assigning SMRs in boys, observe each of the three characteristics separately because they may develop at different rates. Record two separate ratings: pubic hair and genital. If the penis and testes differ in their stages, average the two into a single figure for the genital rating.

		Pubic Hair	Penis	Testes and Scrotum
Stage 1		Preadolescent—no pubic hair except for the fine body hair (vellus hair) similar to that on the abdomen	Preadolescent—same size and proportions as in childhood	Preadolescent—same size and proportions as in childhood
Stage 2		Sparse growth of long, slightly pigmented, downy hair, straight or only slightly curled, chiefly at the base of the penis	Slight or no enlargement	Testes larger; scrotum larger, somewhat reddened, and altered in texture
Stage 3		Darker, coarser, curlier hair spreading sparsely over the pubic symphysis	Larger, especially in length	Further enlarged
Stage 4		Coarse and curly hair, as in the adult; area covered greater than in stage 3 but not as great as in the adult and not yet including the thighs	Further enlarged in length and breadth, with development of the glans	Further enlarged; scrotal skin darkened
Stage 5		Hair adult in quantity and quality, spread to the medial surfaces of the thighs but not up over the abdomen	Adult in size and shape	Adult in size and shape

Photos reprinted from *Pediatric Endocrinology and Growth*, 2nd ed., Wales & Wit, 2003, with permission from Elsevier.

Female Genitalia

The external examination of adolescent female genitalia proceeds in the same manner as for school-aged children. If it is necessary to complete a full pelvic examination on an adolescent, the actual technique is the same as that used for an adult, including the rectal examination. A full explanation of the steps of the examination, demonstration of the instruments, and a gentle, reassuring approach are necessary because the adolescent is usually quite anxious. A chaperone (parent or nurse) must be present. An adolescent's first pelvic examination should be performed by an experienced health care provider.

Vaginal discharge in a young adolescent should be treated as in the adult. Causes include *physiologic leukorrhea, sexually transmitted infections* from consensual sexual activity or *sexual abuse, bacterial vaginosis, foreign body,* and *external irritants.*

A girl's initial signs of puberty are hymenal changes secondary to estrogen, widening of the hips, and beginning of a height spurt, although these changes are difficult to detect. The first easily detectable sign of puberty is usually the appearance of breast buds, although pubic hair sometimes appears earlier. The average age of the appearance of pubic hair has decreased in recent years, and current consensus is that the appearance of pubic hair as early as 7 years can be normal, particularly in dark-skinned girls who develop secondary sexual characteristics at an earlier age.

Assign a sexual maturity rating to every female, irrespective of chronologic age. The assessment of sexual maturity in girls is based on both growth of pubic hair and the development of breasts.[45] The assessment (Tanner staging) of pubic hair growth is shown in the figure below. See p. 864 for breast development assessment. Counsel girls about this sequence and their current stage.

See p. 864

Pubertal development prior to the normal age ranges may signify precocious puberty, which has a variety of endocrine and central nervous system causes.

Delayed puberty (no breasts or pubic hair development by age 12) is usually caused by inadequate gonadotropin secretion from the anterior pituitary due to defective hypothalamic GnRH production. Rarer causes also exist (see p. 868).

see p. 868

Amenorrhea in adolescence can be primary (no menarche by age 16) or secondary (cessation of menses in an adolescent who had previously menstruated). While primary amenorrhea is usually due to anatomic or genetic causes, secondary amenorrhea can be due to a variety of etiologies.

Sex Maturity Ratings in Girls: Pubic Hair

Stage 1

Preadolescent—no pubic hair except for the fine body hair (vellus hair) similar to that on the abdomen

Stage 2

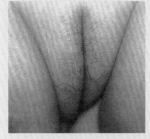

Sparse growth of long, slightly pigmented, downy hair, straight or only slightly curled, chiefly along the labia

Stage 3

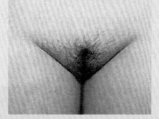

Darker, coarser, curlier hair, spreading sparsely over the pubic symphysis

Stage 4

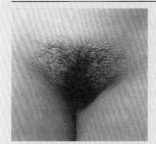

Coarse and curly hair as in adults; area covered greater than in stage 3 but not as great as in the adult and not yet including the thighs

Stage 5

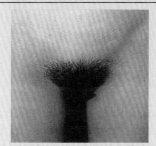

Hair adult in quantity and quality, spread on the medial surfaces of the thighs but not up over the abdomen

Photos used with permission of the American Academy of Pediatrics, *Assessment of Sexual Maturity Stages in Girls*, 1995.

Although there is a wide variation in the age of onset and completion of puberty, the stages occur in a predictable sequence, as shown below.

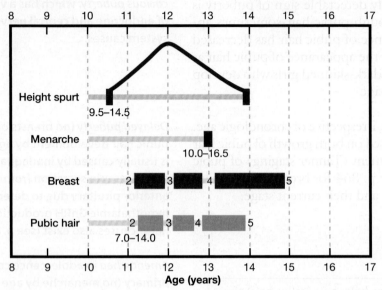

Female adolescents: Numbers below the bars indicate the ranges in age within which the changes occur.

The Musculoskeletal System

Evaluations for scoliosis and screening for participation in sports (pp. 869–871) remain common components of examination in adolescents. Other segments of the musculoskeletal examination are the same as for adults.

Assessing for Scoliosis. Make sure the child bends forward with the knees straight (Adams' bend test). Evaluate any asymmetry in positioning or gait. Scoliosis in a young child is unusual and abnormal; mild scoliosis in an older child is not uncommon.

If you detect scoliosis, use a *scoliometer* to test for the degree of scoliosis. With the patient standing, look for asymmetry of the shoulder blades or gluteal folds. Have the teen bend forward as described. Look for prominence of the posterior ribs. Place the scoliometer over the spine at a point of maximum prominence, making sure that the spine is parallel to the floor at that point, as shown above. Have the teen bend fully forward to assess lumbar scoliosis, and less so to assess thoracic scoliosis.

Delayed puberty in an adolescent female below the third percentile in height may be from Turner's syndrome or chronic disease. The two most common causes of delayed sexual development in an extremely thin adolescent girl are anorexia nervosa and chronic disease.

Obesity in females can be associated with early onset of puberty.

Several types of *scoliosis* may present during childhood. Idiopathic scoliosis (75% of cases), seen mostly in girls, is usually detected in early adolescence. As seen in the girl in this photo, the right shoulder is generally prominent. Other types include neuromuscular and congenital.

You can also use a *plumb line*, a string with a weight attached, to assess symmetry of the back. Place the top of the plumb line at C7 and have the child stand straight. The plumb line should extend to the gluteal crease (not shown here).

Scoliosis is more common among children and adolescents with neurologic or musculoskeletal abnormalities.

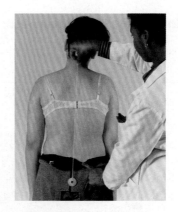

Apparent scoliosis, including an abnormal plumb line test, can be caused by a *leg-length discrepancy* (see p. 853).

The Sports Preparticipation Screening Musculoskeletal Examination. More than 25 million children and adolescents in the United States and several other countries participate in organized sports and often require "medical clearance." Start the examination with a thorough medical history, focusing on cardiovascular risk factors, prior surgeries, prior injuries, other medical problems, and a family history. The preparticipation physical examination is often the only time a healthy adolescent will see a medical professional, so it is important to include some screening questions and anticipatory guidance (see the discussion in Health Promotion and Counseling). Finally, perform a general physical, with special attention to the heart and lungs and a vision and hearing screening. Include a focused, thorough musculoskeletal examination, looking for weakness, limited range of motion, and evidence of previous injury.

A 2-minute preparticipation screening musculoskeletal examination shown below has been recommended.[49,50]

Important risk factors for sudden cardiovascular death during sports include episodes of *dizziness or palpitations, prior syncope* (particularly if associated with exercise), or family history of *sudden death* in young or middle-aged relatives.

During the preparticipation sports physical, assess carefully for *cardiac murmurs* and *wheezing* in the lungs. Also, if the adolescent has had head injuries or a concussion, perform a careful, focused neurologic examination.[49,50]

Screening Musculoskeletal Examination for Sports

Position and Instruction to Patient		Common Abnormalities From Prior Injury
Step 1: Stand straight, facing forward.	**Step 2:** Move neck in all directions.	**Step 1:** Asymmetry, swelling of joints **Step 2:** Loss of range of motion

(continued)

Screening Musculoskeletal Examination for Sports (*continued*)

Position and Instruction to Patient		Common Abnormalities From Prior Injury
Step 3: Shrug shoulders against resistance.	**Step 4:** Hold arms out to the side against resistance.	**Step 3:** Weakness of shoulder, neck, or trapezius muscles **Step 4:** Loss of strength of deltoid muscle

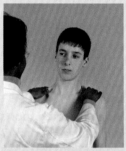 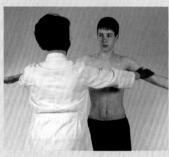

Step 5: Hold arms out to side with elbows bent 90 degrees; raise and lower arms.	**Step 6:** Hold arms out, completely bend, and straighten elbows.	**Step 5:** Loss of external rotation and injury of glenohumeral joint **Step 6:** Reduced range of motion of elbow

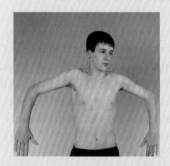 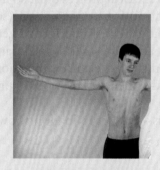

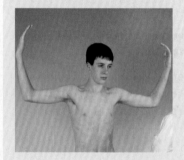 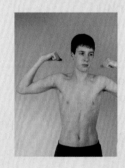

(*continued*)

Screening Musculoskeletal Examination for Sports (*continued*)

Position and Instruction to Patient		Common Abnormalities From Prior Injury

Step 7: Hold arms down, bend elbows 90 degrees, and pronate and supinate forearms.

Step 8: Make a fist, clench, and then spread fingers.

Step 7: Reduced range of motion from injury to forearm, elbow, or wrist

Step 8: Protruding knuckle, reduced range of motion of fingers from prior sprain or fracture

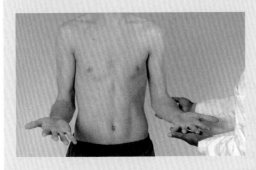

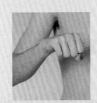

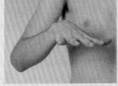

Step 9: Squat and duck-walk for four steps forward.

Step 10: Stand straight with arms at sides, facing back.

Step 9: Inability to fully flex knees and difficulty standing up from prior knee or ankle injury

Step 10: Asymmetry from scoliosis, leg-length discrepancy, or weakness from injury

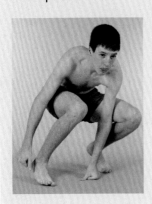

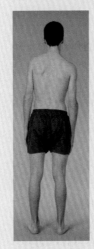

Step 11: Bend forward with knees straight and touch toes.

Step 12: Stand on heels and rise to the toes.

Step 11: Asymmetry from scoliosis and twisting of back from low back pain

Step 12: Wasting of calf muscles from ankle or Achilles tendon injury

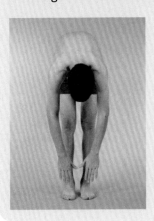

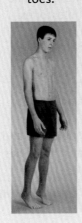

The Nervous System

The neurologic examination of the adolescent and the adult is the same. Assess the adolescent's developmental achievement according to age-specific milestones, as described on pp. 857–858.

Recording Your Findings

Initially you may use sentences to describe your findings; later you will use phrases. The style here contains phrases appropriate for most write-ups. As you read through this write-up, you note some atypical findings. Try to test yourself. See if you can interpret these findings in the context of all you have learned about the examination of children. You also will note the modifications necessary to accommodate reports from the small child's parent, rather than from the child. If you are using electronic medical records, make sure your write-up includes sufficient detail and text to adequately summarize your findings.

Recording the Examination: The Pediatric Patient

2/4/11

Brian is an active, 26-month-old boy accompanied by his mother for concern about his development and behavior.

Referral. None

Source and Reliability. Mother (Mom).

Chief Complaint: Slow development and difficult behavior.

Present Illness: Brian appears to be developing more slowly than his older sister did. He uses only single words and simple phrases, rarely combines words, and appears frustrated with not being able to communicate. People understand approximately 25% of his speech. Physical development seems normal; he can throw a ball, kick, scribble, and dress himself well. He has had no head trauma, chronic illnesses, seizures, or regression in his milestones.

   Mom also is concerned about his behavior. Brian is extremely stubborn, frequently has tantrums, gets angry easily (especially with his older sister), throws objects, bites, and physically strikes others when he doesn't get his way. His behavior seems worse around Mom, who reports that he is "fine" at his childcare center. He moves from one activity to another with an inability to sit still to read or play a game.

   Brian is an extremely picky eater who eats a large quantity of junk food and little else. He will not eat fruits or vegetables and drinks enormous quantities of juice and soda. His mother has tried everything to get him to eat healthy food, to no avail.

(continued)

The family has been under substantial stress during the past year from Brian's father being unemployed. Although Brian now has Medicaid insurance, the parents are uninsured.

Medications. One multivitamin daily.

Past History

Pregnancy. Uneventful. Mom reduced tobacco intake to a half-pack a day and drank alcohol at times. She denies use of other drugs or having infections.

Newborn Period. Born vaginally at 40 weeks; left the hospital in 2 days. Birth weight 2.5 kg (5 lbs, 8 oz). Mom does not know why Brian was small at birth.

Illnesses. Only minor illnesses; no hospitalizations.

Accidents. Required sutures last year for a facial laceration secondary to a fall on the road.

Preventive Care. Brian has had regular preventive check-ups. At the last appointment 6 months ago, his regular physician said that Brian was a bit behind on some developmental milestones and suggested a child care center that he knew was excellent, as well as increased parental attention to reading, speaking, playing, and stimulation. Immunizations are up to date. His lead level was elevated mildly last year, and Mom reports that he had "low blood." His physician recommended iron supplements and foods high in iron, but Brian really won't eat these foods.

Family History

Strong family history of diabetes (two grandparents, none with diabetes as children) and hypertension. No family history of childhood developmental, psychiatric, or chronic illnesses.

Developmental History: Sat up at 6 months, crawled at 9 months, and walked at 13 months. First words ("mama" and "car") said at approximately 1 year.

Personal and Social History: Parents are married and live with the two children in a rented apartment. Dad has not had a steady job for 1 year but has worked intermittently in construction. Mom works as a waitress part-time while Brian is in child care.

Mom had depression during Brian's first year and attended some counseling sessions, but stopped because she could not pay for them or medications. She gets support from her mother who lives 30 minutes away, and many friends, some of whom babysit occasionally.

Despite substantial family stress, Mom describes a loving and intact family. They try to eat dinner together daily, limit television, read to both children (although Brian won't sit still), and go to the nearby park regularly to play.

Environmental Exposures. Both parents smoke, although generally outside the house.

Safety. Mom reports this as a major concern: she can barely leave Brian out of her sight without him getting into something. She fears he will run under a car; the family is thinking of fencing in their small yard. Brian sits in his car seat most of the time; smoke detectors work in the home. Dad's guns are locked; medications are in a cabinet in the parents' bedroom.

(continued)

Review of Systems

General. No major illnesses.

Skin. Dry and itchy. Last year he was prescribed hydrocortisone for it.

Head, Eyes, Ears, Nose, and Throat (HEENT). *Head*: No trauma. *Eyes*: Vision fine. *Ears*: Multiple infections in the past year. Frequently ignores parents' requests; they can't tell if this is purposeful or if he can't hear well. *Nose*: Often runny; Mom wonders about allergies. *Mouth*: No dentist visit yet. Brushes teeth sometimes (a frequent source of dispute).

Neck. No lumps. Glands in neck seem large.

Respiratory. Frequent cough and whistle in chest. Mom cannot identify trigger; it tends to go away. He can run around all day without seeming to get tired.

Cardiovascular. No known heart disease. He had a murmur when younger, but it went away.

Gastrointestinal. Appetite and eating habits described above. Regular bowel movements. He is in the process of toilet training and wears pull-ups at night, but not at childcare.

Urinary. Good stream. No prior urinary tract infections.

Genital. Normal.

Musculoskeletal. He is "all boy" and never gets tired. Minor bumps and bruises occasionally.

Neurologic. Walks and runs well; seems coordinated for age. No stiffness, seizures, or fainting. Mom says his memory seems great, but his attention span is poor.

Psychiatric. Generally seems happy. Cries easily; bounces back and forth from trying to be independent to needing cuddling and comforting.

Physical Examination

Brian is an active and energetic toddler. He plays with the reflex hammer, pretending it is a truck. He appears closely bonded with his mother, looking at her occasionally for comfort. She seems concerned that Brian will break something. His clothes are clean.

Vital Signs. Ht 90 cm (90th percentile). Wt 16 kg (>95th percentile). BMI 19.8 (>95th percentile). Head circumference 50 cm (75th percentile). BP 108/58. Heart rate 90 and regular. Respiratory rate 30; varies with activity. Temperature (ear) 37.5°C. Obviously no pain.

Skin. Normal except for bruises on legs, and patchy, dry skin over external surface of elbows.

HEENT. *Head*: Normocephalic; no lesions. *Eyes*: Difficult to examine because he won't sit still. Symmetric with normal extraocular movements. Pupils 4 to 5 mm constricting. Discs difficult to visualize; no hemorrhages noted. *Ears*: Normal pinna; no external abnormalities. Normal external canals and tympanic membranes (TMs). *Nose*: Normal nares; septum midline. *Mouth*: Several darkened teeth (inside surface of upper incisors). One clear cavity on upper right incisor. Tongue normal. Cobblestoning of posterior pharynx; no exudates. Tonsils large but adequate gap (1.5 cm) between them.

(continued)

Neck. Supple, midline trachea, no thyroid palpable.

Lymph Nodes. Easily palpable (1.5 to 2 cm) tonsillar lymph nodes bilaterally. Small (0.5 cm) nodes in inguinal canal bilaterally. All lymph nodes mobile and nontender.

Lungs. Good expansion. No tachypnea or dyspnea. Congestion audible, but seems to be upper airway (louder near mouth, symmetric). No rhonchi, rales, or wheezes. Clear to auscultation.

Cardiovascular. PMI in 4th or 5th interspace and midsternal line. Normal S_1 and S_2. No murmurs or abnormal heart sounds. Normal femoral pulses; dorsalis pedis pulses palpable bilaterally.

Breasts. Normal, with some fat under both.

Abdomen. Protuberant but soft; no masses or tenderness. Liver span 2 cm below right costal margin (RCM) and not tender. Spleen and kidneys not palpable.

Genitalia. Tanner I circumcised penis; no pubic hair, lesions, or discharge. Testes descended, difficult to palpate because of active cremasteric reflex. Normal scrotum both sides.

Musculoskeletal. Normal range of motion of upper and lower extremities and all joints. Spine straight. Gait normal.

Neurologic. *Mental Status:* Happy, cooperative child. *Developmental:* Gross motor—Jumps and throws objects. Fine motor—Imitates vertical line. Language—Does not combine words; single words only, three to four noted during examination. Personal–social—Washes face, brushes teeth, and puts on shirt. Overall—Normal, except for language, which appears delayed. *Cranial Nerves:* Intact, although several difficult to elicit. *Cerebellar:* Normal gait; good balance. *Deep tendon reflexes (DTRs):* Normal and symmetric throughout with downgoing toes. *Sensory:* Deferred.

Bibliography

Citations

1. Levine MD, Carey WB, Crocker AC. Developmental–Behavioral Pediatrics, 3rd ed. Philadelphia: WB Saunders, 2002.
2. American Academy of Pediatrics. Guidelines for Health Supervision III, revised ed. Elk Grove Village, IL: Author, 2002.
3. American Academy of Pediatrics. Bright Futures. Available at http://brightfutures.aap.org/web/aboutBrightFutures.asp. Accessed February 19, 2008.
4. American Medical Association. Guidelines for Adolescent Preventive Services (GAPS). Available at http://www.ama-assn.org/ama/upload/mm/39/gapsmono.pdf. Accessed February 19, 2008.
5. United States Department of Health and Human Services. U.S. Preventive Services Task Force (USPSTF). Available at http://www.ahrq.gov/clinic/uspstfix.htm. Accessed February 19, 2008.
6. Centers for Disease Control and Prevention. Recommendations and Guidelines: 2008 Child & Adolescent Immunization Schedules. Available at http://www.cdc.gov/vaccines/recs/schedules/child-schedule.htm. Accessed February 19, 2008.

7. American Academy of Pediatrics Committee on Infectious Diseases. Recommended Immunization Schedules for Children and Adolescents—United States, 2007. Pediatrics 2007;119(1): 207–208.

8. AHRA Guide to Clinical Preventive Services. Available at http://www.ahra.gov/clinic/cps3dix.htm. Accessed July 10, 2008.

9. American Academy of Pediatrics and American College of Obstetricians and Gynecologists. Guidelines for Perinatal Care, 4th ed. Washington, DC: American Academy of Pediatrics, 1997.

10. Fuloria M, Kreiter S. The newborn examination: part 1. Emergencies and common abnormalities involving the skin, head, neck, chest, and respiratory and cardiovascular system. Am Fam Phys 2002;65(1):61–68.

11. Ballard JL, Khoury JC, Wedig K. Ballard scoring system for determining gestational age in weeks. J Pediatr 1991;119:417.

12. Brazelton TB. Working with families: opportunities for early intervention. Pediatr Clin North Am 1995;42(1):1–9.

13. Johnson CP, Blasco PA. Infant growth and development. Pediatr Rev 1997;18(7):224–242.

14. Colson ER, Dworkin PH. Toddler development. Pediatr Rev 1997;18(8):255–259.

15. Copelan J. Normal speech and development. Pediatr Rev 1995;18:91–100.

16. Identifying infants and young children with developmental disorders in the medical home: An algorithm for developmental surveillance and screening. Pediatrics 2006:118(1): 405–420.

17. Frankenburg WK, Dodds J, Archer P et al. The Denver II: A major revision and restandardization of the Denver Developmental Screening Test. Pediatrics 1992;89(1):91–97.

18. Fong CT. Clinical diagnosis of genetic diseases. Pediatr Ann 1993;22(5):277–281.

19. Hyvarinen L. Assessment of visually impaired infants. Ophthalmol Clin North Am 1994;7:219.

20. Lees MH. Cyanosis of the newborn infant: recognition and clinical evaluation. J Pediatr 1970;77:484.

21. Gessner IH. What makes a heart murmur innocent? Pediatr Ann 1997;26(2):82–91.

22. Callahan CW Jr, Alpert B. Simultaneous percussion auscultation technique for the determination of liver span. Arch Pediatr Adolesc Med 1994;148(8):873–875.

23. Reiff MI, Osborn LM. Clinical estimation of liver size in newborn infants. Pediatrics 1983;71:46–48.

24. Burger BJ, Burger JD, Bos CF et al. Neonatal screening and staggered early treatment for congenital dislocation or dysplasia of the hip. Lancet 1990;336(8730):1549–1553.

25. Zafeiriou DI. Primitive reflexes and postural reactions in the neurodevelopmental examination. Pediatr Neurol 2004; 31(1):1–8.

26. Schott JM, Rossor MN. The grasp and other primitive reflexes. J Neurol Neurosurg Psychiatry 2003;74(5):558–560.

27. Luiz DM, Foxcroft CD, Stewart R. The construct validity of the Griffiths Scales of Mental Development. Child Care Health Dev 2001;27:73–83.

28. Newacheck PW, Strickland B, Shonkoff JP et al. An epidemiologic profile of children with special health care needs. Pediatrics 1998;102:117–123.

29. Ogden CL, Carroll MD, Curtin LR et al. Prevalence of overweight and obesity in the United States, 1999–2004. JAMA 2006;295:1549–1555.

30. National High Blood Pressure Education Program Working Group on High Blood Pressure in Children and Adolescents. The Fourth Report on the Diagnosis, Evaluation, and Treatment of High Blood Pressure in Children and Adolescents. Pediatrics 2004;114:555–576.

31. Shamis DI. Collecting the "facts": vision assessment techniques: perils and pitfalls. Am Orthop J 1996;46:7.

32. Rothman R, Owens T, Simel DL. Does this child have acute otitis media? JAMA 2003;290:1633–1640.

33. Blomgren K, Pitkaranta A. Current challenges in diagnosis of acute otitis media. Intl J Ped Otorhinolaryngol 2005;69(3):295–299.

34. Pirozzo S, Papinczak T, Glasziou P. Whispered voice test for screening for hearing impairment in adults and children: systematic review. BMJ 2003;327(7421):967.

35. Wolf G, Anderhuber W, Kuhn F. Development of the paranasal sinuses in children: implications for paranasal sinus surgery. Ann Otol Rhinol Laryngol 1993;102(9):705–711.

36. Selwitz RH, Ismail AI, Pitts NB. Dental caries. Lancet 2007; 369(9555):51–59.

37. Lunt RC, Law DB. A review of the chronology of eruption of deciduous teeth. J Am Dent Assoc 1974;89:872.

38. Ebell MH, Smith MA, Barry HC et al. Does this patient have strep throat? JAMA 2000;284:2912–2918.

39. Centers for Disease Control and Prevention. National Surveillance for Asthma—United States, 1980–2004. MMWR Morb Mortal Wkly Rep 2007;56:1–60.

40. Tucker WN, Saab S, Leland SR et al. The scratch test is unreliable for determining the liver edge. J Clin Gastroenterol 1997; 25:410–414.

41. Ashcraft KW. Consultation with the specialist: acute abdominal pain. Pediatr Rev 200021:363–367.

42. Hymel KP, Jenny C. Child sexual abuse. Pediatr Rev 1996;17(7):236–249; quiz, 249–250.

43. Scherl S. Common lower extremity problems in children. Pediatr Rev 2004;25:43–75.

44. Bruce RW. Torsional and angular deformities. Pediatr Clin North Am 1996;43:867–881.

45. Elster AB, Kuznets MJ. AMA Guidelines for Adolescent Preventive Services (GAPS): Recommendations and Rationale. Baltimore, MD: Williams & Wilkins, 1993.

46. Herman-Giddens ME, Slora EJ, Wasserman RC et al. Secondary sexual characteristics and menses in young girls seen in office practice: a study from the Pediatric Research in Office Settings Network. Pediatrics 1997;99(4):505–512.

47. Biro FM, Galvez MP, Greenspan LC et al. Pubertal assessment method and baseline characteristics in a mixed longitudinal study of girls. Pediatrics [online]. August 9, 2010; doi: 10.1542/peds. 2009–3079.

48. ACOG Committee. Opinion no. 350, November 2006: Breast concerns in the adolescent. Obstet Gynecol 2006;108(5): 1329–1336.

49. Metzl JD. Preparticipation examination of the adolescent athlete: part 1. Pediatr Rev 2001;22(6):119–204.

50. Metzl JD. Preparticipation examination of the adolescent athlete: part 2. Pediatr Rev 2001;22(7):227–239.

Additional References

American Academy of Pediatrics. Bright Futures: Guidelines for Health Supervision of Infants, Children, and Adolescents, 3rd ed. Elk Grove Village, IL: American Academy of Pediatrics, 2008.

Bergen D. Human Development: Traditional and Contemporary Theories. Upper Saddle River, NJ: Pearson/Prentice Hall, 2008.

Burns CE, Dunn AM, Brady MA et al. Pediatric Primary Care: A Handbook for Nurse Practitioners, 3rd ed. St. Louis: Saunders, 2004.

Colyar MR. Well-child Assessment for Primary Care Providers. Philadelphia: FA Davis, 2003.

Dixon SD, Stein MT. Encounters with children: pediatric behavior and development, 4th ed. Philadelphia: Mosby, 2006.

Emans SJ, Laufer MR, Goldstein DP. Pediatric and Adolescent Gynecology, 5th ed. Philadelphia: Lippincott Williams & Wilkins, 2004.

Fenichel G. Clinical Pediatric Neurology: A Signs and Symptoms Approach, 5th ed. Philadelphia: Saunders, 2005.

Fuloria M, Kreiter S. The newborn examination: Part 2. Emergencies and common abnormalities involving the abdomen, pelvis, extremities, genitalia, and spine. Am Fam Phys 2002;65(2):265–270.

Grummer-Strawn LM, Reinold C, Krebs NF. Use of World Health Organization and CDC growth charts for children aged 0–59 months in the United States. MMWR 2010;59(rr09):1–15.

King TM, Tandon SD, Macias MM et al. Implementing developmental screening and referrals: Lessons learned from a national project. Pediatrics 2010;125(2):350–360.

Loughlin CE. Pulmonology. In: Robertson J, Silkofski N, eds. The Harriet Lane Handbook, 17th ed. Philadelphia: Elsevier, 2005: 613–630.

Neinstein LS. Adolescent Health Care: A Practical Guide, 4th ed. Philadelphia: Lippincott Williams & Wilkins, 2002.

Raju TNK, Higgins RD, Stark AR et al. Optimizing care and outcomes for late-preterm (near-term) infants: A summary of the workshop sponsored by the National Institute of Child Health and Human Development. Pediatrics 2006;118(3): 1207–1214.

Sass P, Hassan G. Lower extremity abnormalities in children. Am Fam Phys 2003;68:661–668.

Schonwald A, Huntington N, Chan E et al. Routine developmental screening implemented in urban primary care settings: More evidence of feasibility and effectiveness. Pediatrics 2009; 123(2):660–668.

Stellwagen L, Boies E. Care of the well newborn. Pediatr Rev 2006;27(3):89–98.

Swaiman KF, Ashwal S, Ferriero DM. Neurologic examination of the term and preterm infant. In: Pediatric Neurology: Principles & Practice, 4th ed. Philadelphia: Mosby Elsevier, 2006:47–64.

Zitelli BJ, Davis HW. Atlas of Pediatric Physical Diagnosis, 4th ed. St. Louis: Mosby, 2002.

The Bates' suite offers these additional resources to enhance learning and facilitate understanding of this chapter:

- Bates' *Pocket Guide to Physical Examination and History Taking*, 7th edition
- Bates' *Visual Guide to Physical Examination*
- thePoint online resources, for students and instructors: http://thepoint.lww.com

Table
18-1   Abnormalities in Heart Rhythm and Blood Pressure

Supraventricular Tachycardia

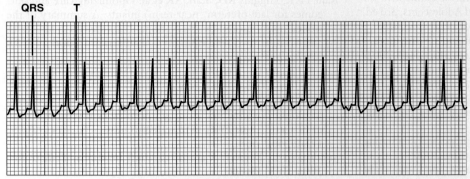

Paroxysmal supraventricular tachycardia (SVT) is the most common dysrhythmia in children. Some infants with SVT look well or may be somewhat pale with tachypnea, but have a heart rate of ≥240 beats per minute. Others are ill and in cardiovascular collapse. P waves have different morphology or are not seen.

SVT in infants is usually sustained, requiring medical therapy for conversion to a normal rate and rhythm. In older children, it is more likely to be truly paroxysmal, with episodes of varying duration and frequency.

Hypertension in Childhood—A Typical Example

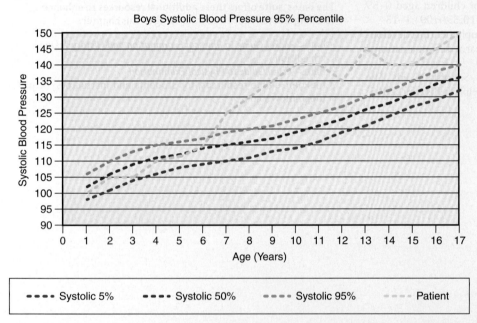

Hypertension can start in childhood.[28] Although elevated blood pressure in young children is more likely to have a renal, cardiac, or endocrine cause, older children and adolescents with hypertension are most likely to have primary or essential hypertension.

This child developed hypertension, and it "tracked" into adulthood. Children tend to remain in the same percentile for blood pressure as they grow. This tracking of blood pressure continues into adulthood, supporting the concept that adult essential hypertension often begins during childhood.

The consequences of untreated hypertension can be severe.

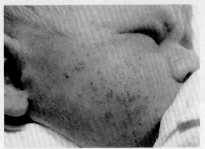

Erythema Toxicum
These common yellow or white pustules are surrounded by a red base.

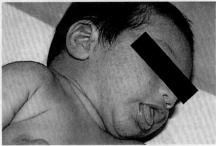

Neonatal Acne
Red pustules and papules are most prominent over the cheeks and nose of some normal newborns.

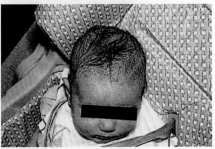

Seborrhea
The salmon red, scaly eruption often involves the face, neck, axilla, diaper area, and behind the ears.

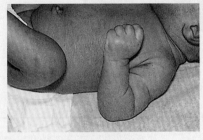

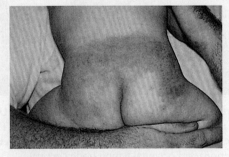

Atopic Dermatitis (Eczema)
Erythema, scaling, dry skin, and intense itching characterize this condition.

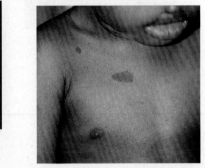

Neurofibromatosis
Characteristic features include more than 5 café-au-lait spots and axillary freckling. Later findings include neurofibromas and Lish nodules (not shown).

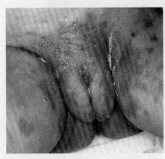

Candidal Diaper Dermatitis
This bright red rash involves the intertriginous folds, with small "satellite lesions" along the edges.

Contact Diaper Dermatitis
This irritant rash is secondary to diarrhea or irritation and is noted along contact areas (here, the area touching the diaper).

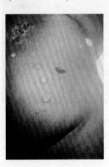

Impetigo
This infection is due to bacteria and can appear bullous or crusty and yellowed with some pus.

Table 18-3

Warts, Lesions That Resemble Warts, and Other Raised Lesions

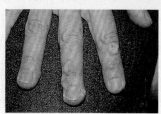

Verruca Vulgaris
Dry, rough warts on hands

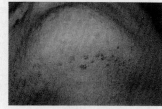

Verruca Plana
Small, flat warts

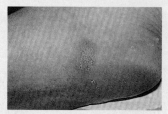

Plantar Warts
Tender warts on feet

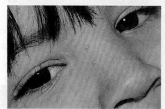

Molluscum Contagiosum
Dome-shaped, fleshy lesions

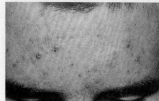

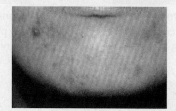

Adolescent Acne
Acne in adolescents involves open comedones (blackheads) and closed comedones (whiteheads) shown at the left, and inflamed pustules (right).

Table 18-4

Common Skin Lesions During Childhood

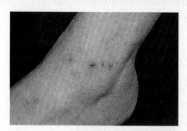

Bites
Intensely pruritic, red, distinct papules characterize these lesions.

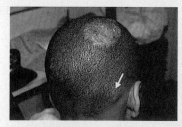

Tinea Capitis
Scaling, crusting, and hair loss are seen in the scalp, along with a painful plaque (kerion) and occipital lymph node (*arrow*).

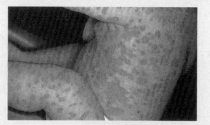

Urticaria (Hives)
This pruritic, allergic sensitivity reaction changes shape quickly.

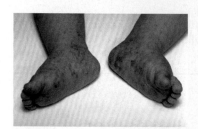

Scabies
Intensely itchy papules and vesicles, sometimes burrows, most often on extremities

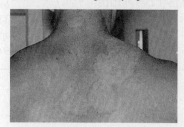

Tinea Corporis
This annular lesion has central clearing and papules along the border.

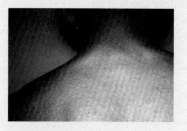

Pityriasis rosea
Oval lesions on trunk, in older children, sometimes a herald patch

Source of *Bites, Tinea Capitis, and Tinea Corporis* photos—Goodheart H. A Photoguide of Common Skin Disorders. Baltimore: Williams & Wilkins, 1999.

Table 18-5 Abnormalities of the Head

881

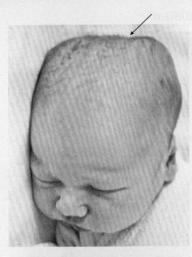

Cephalohematoma

Although not present at birth, cephalohematomas appear within the first 24 hours from subperiosteal hemorrhage involving the outer table of one of the cranial bones. The swelling, shown at the *arrow*, does not extend across a suture, though it is occasionally bilateral following a difficult birth. The swelling is initially soft, then develops a raised bony margin within a few days from calcium deposits at the edge of the periosteum. It tends to resolve within several weeks.

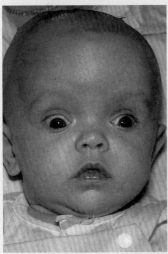

Hydrocephalus

In hydrocephaly, the anterior fontanelle is bulging, and the eyes may be deviated downward, revealing the upper scleras and creating the *setting sun* sign, as shown on the left. The setting sun sign is also seen briefly in some normal newborns. (From Zitelli BJ, Davis HW. Atlas of Pediatric Physical Diagnosis, 3rd ed. St. Louis: Mosby–Year Book, 1997. Courtesy of Dr. Albert Briglan, Children's Hospital of Pittsburgh.)

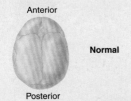

Anterior

Normal

Posterior

Craniosynostosis

Craniosynostosis is a condition of premature closure of one or more sutures of the skull. This results in an abnormal growth and shape of the skull because growth will occur across sutures that are not affected but not across sutures that are affected.

The figures demonstrate different skull shapes associated with the various types of craniosynostosis. The prematurely closed suture line is noted by the absence of a suture line in each figure. Scaphocephaly and frontal plagiocephaly are most common. The *blue shading* shows areas of maximal flattening. The *red arrows* show the direction of continued growth across the sutures, which is normal.

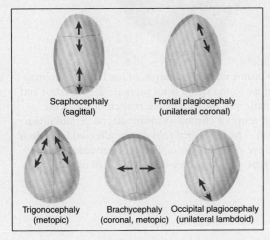

Scaphocephaly (sagittal)

Frontal plagiocephaly (unilateral coronal)

Trigonocephaly (metopic)

Brachycephaly (coronal, metopic)

Occipital plagiocephaly (unilateral lambdoid)

Table
18-6   Diagnostic Facies in Infancy and Childhood

Fetal Alcohol Syndrome

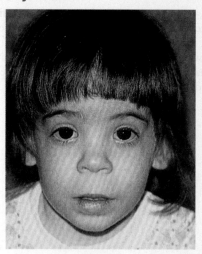

Babies born to women with chronic alcoholism are at increased risk for growth deficiency, microcephaly, and mental retardation. Facial characteristics include short palpebral fissures, a wide and flattened philtrum (the vertical groove in the midline of the upper lip), and thin lips.

Congenital Hypothyroidism

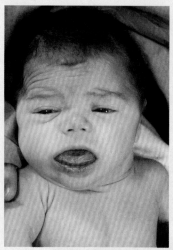

The child with congenital hypothyroidism (*cretinism*) has coarse facial features, a low-set hair line, sparse eyebrows, and an enlarged tongue. Associated features include a hoarse cry, umbilical hernia, dry and cold extremities, myxedema, mottled skin, and mental retardation. Most infants with congenital hypothyroidism have no physical stigmata; this has led to screening of all newborns in the United States and most other developed countries for congenital hypothyroidism.

Congenital Syphilis

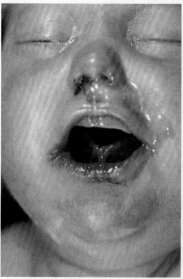

In utero infection by *Treponema pallidum* usually occurs after the 16th week of gestation and affects virtually all fetal organs. If it is not treated, 25% of infected babies die before birth and another 30% shortly thereafter. Signs of illness appear in survivors within the first month of life. Facial stigmata shown here include bulging of the frontal bones and nasal bridge depression (*saddle nose*), both from periostitis; rhinitis from weeping nasal mucosal lesions (*snuffles*); and a circumoral rash. Mucocutaneous inflammation and fissuring of the mouth and lips (*rhagades*), not shown here, may also occur as stigmata of congenital syphilis, as may craniotabes tibial periostitis (*saber shins*) and dental dysplasia (*Hutchinson's teeth*—see p. 288).

Facial Nerve Palsy

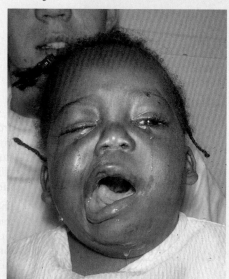

Peripheral (lower motor neuron) paralysis of the facial nerve may be from (1) an injury to the nerve from pressure during labor and birth, (2) inflammation of the middle ear branch of the nerve during episodes of acute or chronic otitis media, or (3) unknown causes (Bell's palsy). The nasolabial fold on the affected left side is flattened, and the eye does not close. This is accentuated during crying, as shown here. Full recovery occurs in ≥90% of those affected.

Down Syndrome

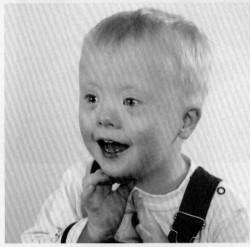

The child with Down syndrome (trisomy 21) usually has a small, rounded head, a flattened nasal bridge, oblique palpebral fissures, prominent epicanthal folds, small, low-set, shell-like ears, and a relatively large tongue. Associated features include generalized hypotonia, transverse palmar creases (*simian lines*), shortening and incurving of the fifth fingers (*clinodactyly*), Brushfield's spots (see p. 884), and mental retardation.

Battered Child Syndrome

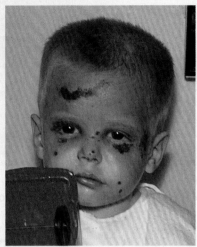

The child who has been physically abused (battered) may have old *and* fresh bruises on the head and face and may either look sad and forlorn or be actively seeking to please, sometimes even particularly involved with and attentive to the abusing parent. Other stigmata include bruises in areas (axilla and groin) not usually subject to injury rather than the bony prominences; x-ray evidence of fractures of the skull, ribs, and long bones in various stages of healing; and skin lesions that are morphologically similar to implements used to inflict trauma (hand, belt buckle, strap, rope, coat hanger, or lighted cigarette).

Perennial Allergic Rhinitis

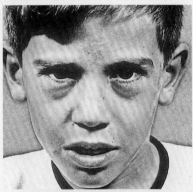

The child suffering from perennial allergic rhinitis has an open mouth (cannot breathe through the nose) and edema and discoloration of the lower orbitopalpebral grooves ("allergic shiners"). Such a child is often seen to push the nose upward and backward with a hand ("allergic salute") and to grimace (wrinkle the nose and mouth) to relieve nasal itching and obstruction.

Hyperthyroidism

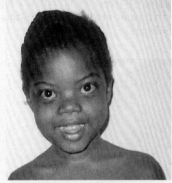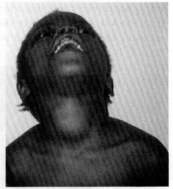

Thyrotoxicosis (*Graves' disease*) occurs in approximately 2 per 1,000 children younger than 10 years. Affected children exhibit hypermetabolism and accelerated linear growth. Facial characteristics shown in this 6-year-old girl are "staring" eyes (not true exophthalmos, which is rare in children) and an enlarged thyroid gland (*goiter*).

Table 18-7

Abnormalities of the Eyes, Ears, and Mouth

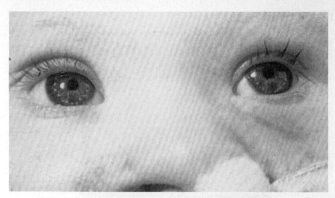

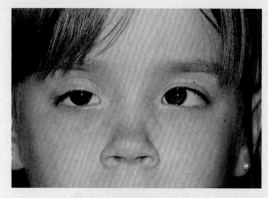

Brushfield's Spots

These abnormal speckling spots on the iris suggest Down syndrome.

Strabismus

Strabismus, or misalignment of the eyes, can lead to visual impairment. Esotropia, shown here, is an inward deviation.

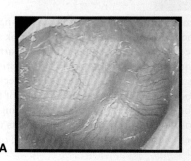 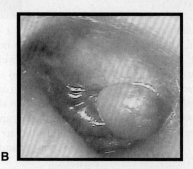 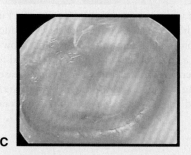

A   B   C

Otitis Media

Otitis media is one of the most common conditions in young children. The spectrum of otitis media is shown here. **(A)** Typical acute otitis media with a red, distorted, bulging tympanic membrane in a highly symptomatic child. **(B)** Acute otitis media with bullae formation and fluid visible behind the tympanic membrane. **(C)** Otitis media with effusion, showing a yellowish fluid behind a retracted and thickened tympanic membrane.

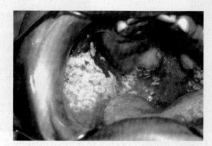

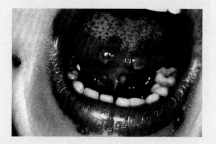

Oral Candidiasis ("Thrush")

This infection is common in infants. The white plaques do not rub off.

Herpetic Stomatitis

Tender ulcerations on the oral mucosa are surrounded by erythema.

Source of photos: *Otitis Media*—Courtesy of Alejandro Hoberman, Children's Hospital of Pittsburgh, University of Pittsburgh.

Table
18-8

Abnormalities of the Teeth, Pharynx, and Neck

Dental Caries

Dental caries is a major global health and pediatric problem. The photographs to the left show different characteristics of caries.

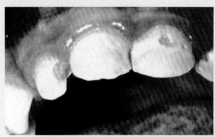

NURSING BOTTLE CARIES

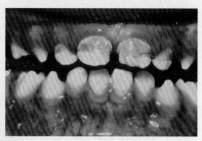

EROSION OF TEETH

Staining of the Teeth

Various causes can lead to staining of the teeth of children, including intrinsic stains such as tetracycline (*right*) or extrinsic stains such as poor oral hygiene (not shown). Extrinsic stains can be removed.

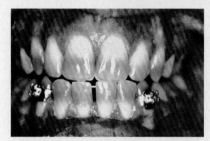

Streptococcal Pharyngitis ("Strep Throat")

This common childhood infection has a classic presentation of erythema of the posterior pharynx and palatal petechiae (*left*). A foul-smelling exudate (*right*) is also commonly noted.

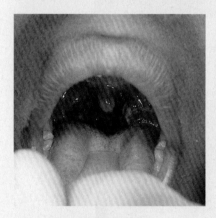

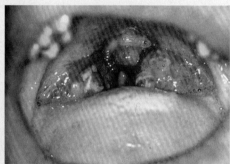

Lymphadenopathy

Enlarged and tender cervical lymph nodes are common in children. The most likely causes are viral and bacterial infections. Lymph node enlargement can be bilateral, as shown in the figure to the left.

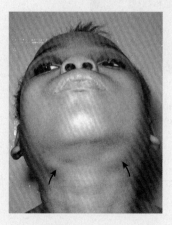

Sources of photos: *Dental Caries* and *Staining of the Teeth*—Courtesy of American Academy of Pediatrics.

Table
18-9
Cyanosis in Children

It is important to recognize cyanosis. The best location to examine is the mucous membranes. Cyanosis is a "raspberry" color, whereas normal mucous membranes should have a "strawberry" color. Try to identify the cyanosis in these photographs before reading the captions.

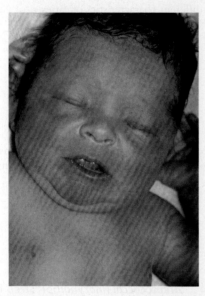

Generalized Cyanosis

This baby has total anomalous pulmonary venous return and an oxygen saturation level of 80%.

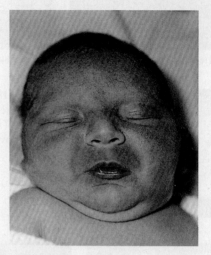

Perioral Cyanosis

This baby has mild cyanosis above the lips, but the mucous membranes remain pink.

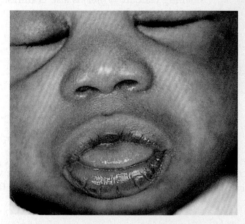

Bluish Lips, Giving Appearance of Cyanosis

Normal pigment deposition in the vermilion border of the lips gives them a bluish hue, but the mucous membranes are pink.

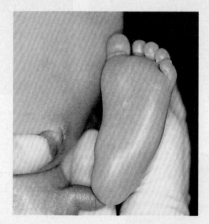

Acrocyanosis

This commonly appears on the feet and hands of babies shortly after birth. This infant is a 32-week-old newborn.

Source of photos (except *Generalized Cyanosis*): Fletcher M. Physical Diagnosis in Neonatology. Philadelphia: Lippincott-Raven, 1998.

Table 18-10 **Congenital Heart Murmurs**

Some heart murmurs reflect underlying heart disease. If you understand their physiologic causes, you will more readily be able to identify and distinguish them from innocent heart murmurs. Obstructive lesions result when blood flows through valves that are too small. Because this problem does not depend on the drop in pulmonary vascular resistance following birth, these murmurs are audible at birth. Defects with left-to-right shunts, on the other hand, depend on the drop in pulmonary vascular resistance. High-pressured shunts such as ventricular septal defect, patent ductus arteriosus, and persistent truncus arteriosus are not heard until 1 week or more after birth. Low-pressured left-to-right shunts, such as in atrial septal defects, may not be heard for considerably longer, usually first being noted at 1 year or more. Many children with congenital cardiac defects have combinations of defects or variations of abnormalities, so findings on cardiac examination may not follow these classic patterns. This table shows a limited selection of the more common defects.

Congenital Defect and Mechanism	Characteristics of the Murmur	Associated Findings
Pulmonary Valve Stenosis Usually a normal valve anulus with fusion of some or most of the valve leaflets, restricting flow across the valve *Mild* 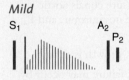 *Severe* 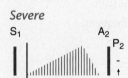	*Location.* Upper left sternal border *Radiation.* In mild degrees of stenosis, the murmur may be heard over the course of the pulmonary arteries in the lung fields. *Intensity.* Increases in intensity and duration as the degree of obstruction increases *Quality.* Ejection, peaking later in systole as the obstruction increases	Usually a prominent ejection click in early systole Pulmonary component of the second sounds at the base (P_2) becomes delayed and softer, disappearing as obstruction increases. Inspiration may increase murmur; expiration may increase click. Growth is usually normal. Newborns with severe stenosis may be cyanotic from right-to-left atrial shunting and rapidly develop heart failure.
Aortic Valve Stenosis Usually a bicuspid valve with progressive obstruction, but there may be a dysplastic valve or damage from rheumatic fever or degenerative disease 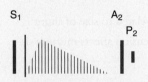	*Location.* Midsternum, upper right sternal border *Radiation.* To the carotid arteries and suprasternal notch; may also be a thrill *Intensity.* Varies, louder with increasingly severe obstruction *Quality.* An ejection, often harsh, systolic murmur	May be an associated ejection click The aortic closure sound may be increased in intensity. There may be a diastolic murmur of aortic valve regurgitation. Newborns with severe stenosis may have weak or absent pulses and severe heart failure. May not be audible until adulthood even though the valve is congenitally abnormal
Tetralogy of Fallot Complex defect with ventricular septal defect, infundibular and usually valvular right ventricular outflow obstruction, malrotation of the aorta, and right-to-left shunting at ventricular septal level *With Pulmonic Stenosis*  *With Pulmonic Atresia* 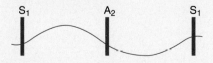	*General.* Variable cyanosis, increasing with activity *Location.* Mid-to-upper left sternal border. If pulmonary atresia, there is no systolic murmur but the continuous murmur of ductus arteriosus flow at upper left sternal border or in the back. *Radiation.* Little, to upper left sternal border, occasionally to lung fields *Intensity.* Usually grade III–IV *Quality.* Midpeaking, systolic ejection murmur	Normal pulses The pulmonary closure sound is usually not heard. May have abrupt hypercyanotic spells with sudden increase in cyanosis, air hunger, altered level of awareness Failure to gain weight with persistent and increasingly severe cyanosis Long-term persistence of cyanosis accompanied by clubbing of fingers and toes Persistent hypoxemia leads to polycythemia, which will accentuate the cyanosis.

(table continues on page 888)

Table
18-10 Congenital Heart Murmurs *(continued)*

Transposition of the Great Arteries

A severe defect with failure of rotation of the great vessels, leaving the aorta to arise from the right ventricle and the pulmonary artery from the left ventricle

General. Intense generalized cyanosis

Location. No characteristic murmur. If present, it may reflect an associated defect such as VSD.

Radiation and Quality. Depends on associated abnormalities

Single loud second sound of the anterior aortic valve

Frequent rapid development of heart failure

Frequent associated defects, as described at the left

Ventricular Septal Defect

Blood going from a high-pressured left ventricle through a defect in the septum to the lower-pressured right ventricle creates turbulence, usually throughout systole.

Small to Moderate

Location. Lower left sternal border

Radiation. Little

Intensity. Variable, only partially determined by the size of the shunt. Small shunts with a high pressure gradient may have very loud murmurs. Large defects with elevated pulmonary vascular resistance may have no murmur. Grade II–IV/VI with a thrill if grade IV/VI or higher.

Quality. Pansystolic, usually harsh, may obscure S_1 and S_2 if loud enough

With large shunts, there may be a low-pitched middiastolic murmur of relative mitral stenosis at the apex.

As pulmonary artery pressure increases, the pulmonic component of the second sounds at the base increases in intensity. When pulmonary artery pressure equals aortic pressure, there may be no murmur, and P_2 will be very loud.

In low-volume shunts, growth is normal.

In larger shunts, heart failure may occur by 6–8 weeks; poor weight gain.

Associated defects are frequent.

Patent Ductus Arteriosus

Continuous flow from aorta to pulmonary artery throughout the cardiac cycle when ductus arteriosus does not close after birth

Small to Moderate

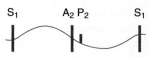

Location. Upper left sternal border and to left

Radiation. Sometimes to the back

Intensity. Varies depending on size of the shunt, usually grade II–III/VI.

Quality. A rather hollow, sometimes machinery-like murmur that is continuous throughout the cardiac cycle, although occasionally almost inaudible in late diastole, uninterrupted by the heart sounds, louder in systole

Full to bounding pulses

Noticed at birth in the premature infant who may have bounding pulses, a hyperdynamic precordium, and an atypical murmur

Noticed later in the full-term infant as pulmonary vascular resistance falls

May develop heart failure at 4–6 weeks if large shunt

Poor weight gain related to size of shunt

Pulmonary hypertension affects murmur as above.

Atrial Septal Defect

Left-to-right shunt through an opening in the atrial septum, possible at various levels

Location. Upper left sternal border

Radiation. To the back

Intensity. Variable, usually grade II–III/VI

Quality. Ejection but without the harsh quality

Widely split second sounds throughout all phases of respiration, normal intensity

Usually not heard until after age of 1 year

Gradual decrease in weight gain as shunt increases

Decreased exercise tolerance, subtle, not dramatic

Heart failure is rare.

Table
18-11 Physical Signs of Sexual Abuse

Possible Indications

1. Marked and immediate dilatation of the anus in knee–chest position, with no constipation, stool in the vault, or neurologic disorders
2. Hymenal notch or cleft that extends >50% of the inferior hymenal rim (confirmed in knee–chest position)
3. Condyloma acuminata in a child older than 3 years
4. Bruising, abrasions, lacerations, or bite marks of labia or perihymenal tissue
5. Herpes of the anogenital area beyond the neonatal period
6. Purulent or malodorous vaginal discharge in a young girl (culture and view all discharges under a microscope for evidence of a sexually transmitted infection)

Strong Indications

1. Lacerations, ecchymoses, and newly healed scars of the hymen or the posterior fourchette
2. No hymenal tissue from 3 to 9 o'clock (confirmed in various positions)
3. Healed hymenal transections, especially between 3 and 9 o'clock (complete cleft)
4. Perianal lacerations extending to external sphincter

A child with concerning physical signs must be evaluated by a sexual abuse expert for a complete history and sexual abuse examination.

Any physical sign must be evaluated in light of the entire history, other parts of the physical examination, and laboratory data.

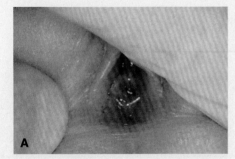

A

Acute hemorrhage and ecchymoses of tissues (10-month-old)

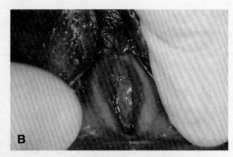

B

Erythema and superficial abrasions to the labia minora (5-year-old)

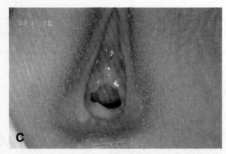

C

Healed interruption of hymenal membrane at 9 o'clock (4-year-old)

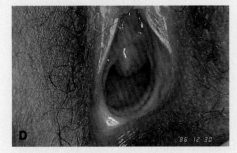

D

Narrowed posterior ring continuous with floor of vagina (12-year-old)

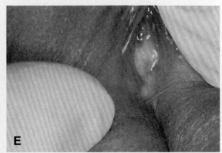

E

Copious vaginal discharge and erythema (9-year-old)

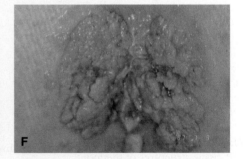

F

Extensive condylomata around the anus (2-year-old)

Source: Reece R, Ludwig S, eds. Child Abuse Medical Diagnosis and Management, 2nd ed. Philadelphia: Lippincott Williams & Wilkins, 2001.

Table
18-12

The Male Genitourinary System

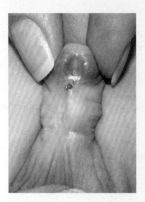

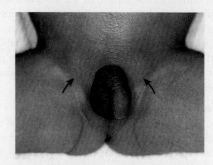

Hypospadias

Hypospadias is the most common congenital penile abnormality. The urethral meatus opens abnormally on the ventral surface of the penis. One form is shown above; more severe forms involve openings on the lower shaft or scrotum.

Undescended Testicle

You should distinguish between undescended testes, shown above (with testes in the inguinal canals—see *arrows*), from highly retractile testes from an active cremasteric reflex.

Sources of photos: *Hypospadias*—Courtesy of Warren Snodgrass, MD, UT–Southwestern Medical Center at Dallas; *Undescended Testicle*—Fletcher M. Physical Diagnosis in Neonatology. Philadelphia: Lippincott-Raven, 1998.

Table
18-13

Common Musculoskeletal Findings in Young Children

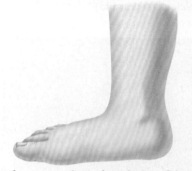

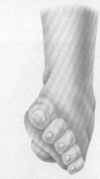

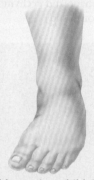

Flat feet or *pes planus* from laxity of the soft-tissue structures of the foot

Inversion of the foot (*varus*)

Metatarsus adductus in a child. The forefoot is adducted and not inverted.

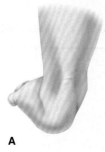
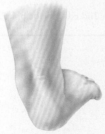

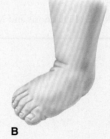
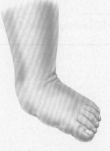

A

B

Pronation in a toddler. (**A**) When viewed from behind, the hindfoot is everted. (**B**) When viewed from the front, the forefoot is everted and abducted.

Table
18-14 **The Power of Prevention: Vaccine-Preventable Diseases**

This table shows photographs of children with vaccine-preventable diseases. Childhood vaccines have been named the single most important medical intervention in the world in terms of influence on public health. Because of vaccinations, we hope you will never see many of these conditions, but you should be able to identify them. Try to identify the diseases before reading the captions.

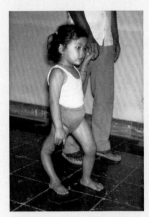

Polio
The deformed leg of this child is from polio.

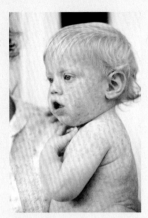

Measles
Characteristic rash of measles

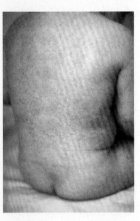

Rubella
Rubella rash on a child's back

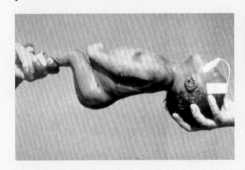

Tetanus
Rigid newborn with neonatal tetanus

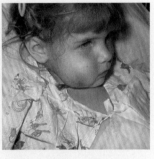

Haemophilus influenzae
Type b
Periorbital cellulitis from this invasive bacterial disease

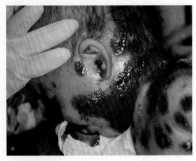

Varicella
An infant with a severe form of varicella

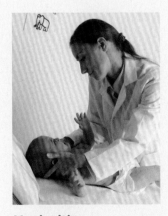

Meningitis

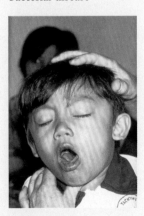

Pertussis

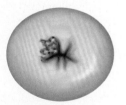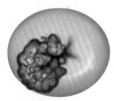

Cervical Cancer
Largely prevented through vaccination by human papillomavirus vaccine.

Sources of photos: *Polio*—Courtesy of World Health Organization; *Haemophilus influenzae*—Courtesy of American Academy of Pediatrics; *Varicella*—Courtesy of Barbara Watson, MD, Albert Einstein Medical Center and Division of Disease Control, Philadelphia Department of Health; *Tetanus*—Courtesy of Centers for Disease Control and Prevention. *Pertussis*—Courtesy of the Immunization Action Coalition.

The Pregnant Woman

This chapter focuses on the history and physical examination of the healthy pregnant woman. The techniques of examination are similar to those of the nonpregnant woman; however, the clinician must distinguish normal variations arising from pregnancy from abnormal findings. This chapter emphasizes common anatomic and physiologic changes that evolve throughout pregnancy, elements of the health history specific to the pregnant woman, recommendations for health promotion during pregnancy, and physical examination techniques specific to the prenatal period.

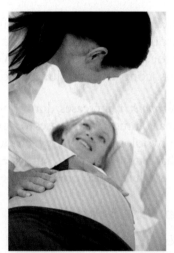

Anatomy and Physiology

Physiologic Hormonal Changes

During pregnancy, hormonal alterations lead to extensive variations in many of the major body systems. Because these normal physiologic changes produce the visible changes in anatomy, hormonal and physiologic changes are presented first in this chapter. These complex changes are summarized briefly here.

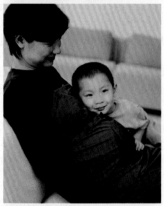

- *Estrogen* promotes endometrial growth that supports the early embryo.[1] This hormone appears to stimulate prolactin output in the anterior lobe of the pituitary gland, which readies breast tissue for lactation.[1] Estrogen also contributes to the hypercoagulable state that puts pregnant women at higher risk for thromboembolic events.[2]

- *Progesterone* also affects numerous body systems. Rising progesterone leads to increased tidal volume and alveolar minute ventilation, though respiratory rate remains constant; respiratory alkalosis and subjective shortness of breath result from these changes.[3] Lower esophageal sphincter tone results from rising levels of estradiol and progesterone, contributing to gastroesophageal reflux. Progesterone relaxes tone in the ureters and bladder, causing hydronephrosis and an increased risk of bacteriuria.[4]

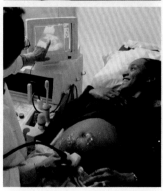

- *Human chorionic gonadotropin (HCG).* HCG is produced by the placenta and supports progesterone synthesis in the corpus luteum, effectively preventing the early embryo from being lost to menstruation. Serum and urine pregnancy assays test for this hormone, which is only present at clinically significant levels during pregnancy and selected pathologic states (such as gestational trophoblastic disease).[1]

- *Human placental lactogen* and other hormones have been implicated in the insulin resistance and hyperglycemia associated with gestational diabetes (GDM).[5] Half of all women who have GDM during a pregnancy will go on to develop type 2 diabetes during their lifetime.[6]

- *Thyroid hormone* (T3 and free T4) and *thyroid stimulating hormone* (TSH) levels fluctuate, usually within the normal range, due to HCG's stimulation of the TSH receptor.[7]

- *Relaxin* is secreted by the corpus luteum and placenta, promoting ligamentous laxity in the sacroiliac joints and pubic symphysis in preparation for passage of the baby.[8] Weight gain, especially around the gravid uterus, contributes to lumbar lordosis and other musculoskeletal strain.

- *Erythropoietin* increases during pregnancy, which raises erythrocyte mass.[9] Plasma volume also increases to a greater extent, causing relative hemodilution and physiologic anemia, which can protect against blood loss during birth. Cardiac output increases but systemic vascular resistance decreases, resulting in a net fall in blood pressure, especially during the second trimester.[10]

Anatomic Changes

Changes in the breasts, urogenital tract, and abdomen are the most visible signs of pregnancy. To refresh your understanding of the anatomy and physiology of these body systems, review Chapter 9, Abdomen; Chapter 10, Breasts and Axillae; and Chapter 14, Female Genitalia.

Breasts. The breasts enlarge moderately due to hormonal stimulation causing increased vascularity and glandular hyperplasia. By the third gestational month, breasts become more nodular. The nipples become larger and more erectile, with darker areolae and more pronounced Montgomery glands. The venous pattern over the breasts visibly increases as pregnancy progresses. In the second and third trimesters, some women secrete colostrum, a thick, yellowish, nutrient-rich precursor to milk. Breast tenderness may make them more sensitive during examination.

Uterus. Muscle cell hypertrophy, increases in fibrous and elastic tissue, and development of blood vessels and lymphatics all contribute to the growth of the uterus. In the first trimester, the uterus is confined to the pelvis and shaped like an inverted pear; it may retain its prior anteverted (forward-leaning), retroverted (backward-leaning), or

36 wks
32 wks
28 wks
24 wks
20 wks
16 wks
12–14 wks

GROWTH PATTERNS OF THE UTERINE FUNDUS BY WEEKS OF PREGNANCY

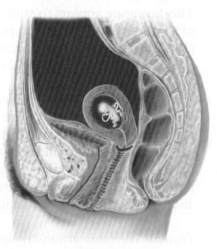

FIRST TRIMESTER

retroflexed (backward-bent) position. By 12 to 14 weeks, the gravid uterus becomes externally palpable as it expands into a globular shape beyond the pelvic brim.

Beginning in the second trimester, the enlarging fetus pushes the uterus into an anteverted position that encroaches on the space usually occupied by the bladder, triggering frequent voiding. Intestines are displaced laterally and superiorly. The uterus stretches its own supporting ligaments, causing "round ligament pain" in the lower quadrants. Often, slight dextrorotation to accommodate the rectosigmoid structures on the left side of the pelvis leads to greater discomfort on the right side.[10] Growth patterns of the gravid uterus are shown above. Sagittal diagrams of the gravid abdomen in each trimester appear on the right.[11]

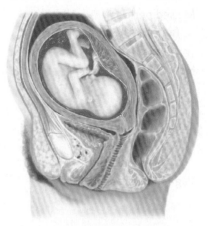

SECOND TRIMESTER

Vagina. Increased vascularity throughout the pelvis during pregnancy gives the vagina a bluish color, known as *Chadwick's sign*. Vaginal walls appear deeply rugated due to thicker mucosa, loosening of connective tissue, and hypertrophy of smooth muscle cells. Normal vaginal secretions may become thick, white, and more profuse. Increased glycogen stores in the vaginal epithelium give rise to a proliferation of *Lactobacillus acidophilus,* which lowers the pH in the vagina. This acidification protects against some vaginal infections, but at the same time, increased glycogen may contribute to higher rates of vaginal candidiasis.[12]

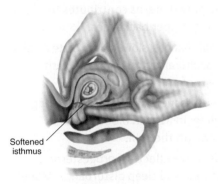

Softened isthmus

HEGAR'S SIGN

Cervix. *Chadwick's sign* is also apparent as cyanosis of the cervix. *Hegar's sign* is the palpable softening of the cervical isthmus, the portion of the uterus that narrows into the cervix, illustrated at the left. The cervical canal fills with a tenacious mucous plug that protects the uterine environment from outside pathogens.

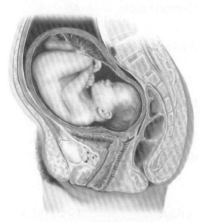

THIRD TRIMESTER

Adnexae. Early in pregnancy the corpus luteum, the ovarian follicle that has discharged its ovum, may be prominent enough to be felt on the affected ovary as a small nodule; this disappears by midpregnancy.

External Abdomen. As the skin over the abdomen stretches to accommodate the fetus, purplish *striae gravidarum* ("stretch marks") may appear. A *linea nigra*, a brownish black pigmented vertical stripe along the midline skin, may develop. As tension on the abdominal wall increases with advancing pregnancy, the rectus abdominis muscles may separate at the midline; this is termed *diastasis recti.* If diastasis is severe, especially in multiparous women, only a layer of skin, fascia, and peritoneum may cover the anterior uterine wall, and fetal parts may be palpable through this muscular gap.[13]

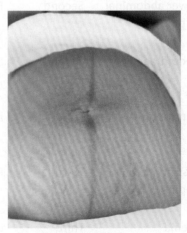

STRIAE AND LINEA NIGRA

Common Concerns During Pregnancy and Their Explanations

Common Concerns	Trimester	Explanation
Missed periods (amenorrhea)	All	High levels of estrogen, progesterone, and HCG build up the endometrium and prevent menses, causing missed periods which are often the first noticeable sign of pregnancy.
Heartburn	All	Progesterone relaxes the lower esophageal sphincter, allowing gastric contents to reflux into the esophagus. The gravid uterus also exerts physical pressure against the stomach, contributing to reflux symptoms.[14]
Urinary frequency	All	Increases in blood volume and filtration rate through the kidneys result in increased urine production, while pressure from the gravid uterus reduces potential space for the bladder. Dysuria or suprapubic pain should be investigated for urinary tract infection.
Vaginal discharge	All	Asymptomatic milky white discharge, *leukorrhea*, results from increased secretions from vaginal and cervical epithelium due to vasocongestion and hormonal changes. Any foul-smelling or pruritic discharge should be investigated.
Constipation	All	Constipation results from slowed gastrointestinal transit due to hormonal changes, dehydration from nausea and vomiting, and iron supplementation in prenatal vitamins.[14]
Hemorrhoids	All	Hemorrhoids may be caused by constipation, decreased venous return from increasing pressure in the pelvis, and changes in activity level during pregnancy.[14]
Backache	All	Hormonally induced relaxation of joints and ligaments contribute to musculoskeletal aches. Lordosis required to balance the gravid uterus contributes to lower back strain. Breast growth may contribute to upper backaches.
Nausea and/or vomiting	First	This is poorly understood but may arise from hormonal changes, slowed gastrointestinal peristalsis, alterations in smell and taste, and sociocultural factors. In *hyperemesis gravidarum* there is vomiting with weight loss in >5% of prepregnancy weight.
Breast tenderness/ tingling	First	Pregnancy hormones stimulate the growth of breast tissue, which causes swelling that may result in aching, tenderness, and tingling. Increased blood flow may also result in delicate veins becoming visible beneath the skin.
Fatigue	First/Third	Related to rapid change in energy requirements, sedative effects of progesterone, changes in body mechanics due to the gravid uterus, and sleep disturbance. Many women report increased energy and well-being during the second trimester.
Lower abdominal pain	Second	Rapid growth in the second trimester causes tension and stretching of round ligaments that support the uterus, causing sharp or cramping pain with movement or positional change.
Abdominal striae	Second or third	Stretching of the skin and tearing of the collagen in the dermis contribute to thin, usually pink, bands, or *striae gravidarum* (stretch marks). These may persist or fade over time after the pregnancy ends.
Contractions	Third	Irregular and unpredictable uterine contractions (*Braxton Hicks contractions*) are rarely associated with labor. Contractions that become regular or painful should be evaluated for onset of labor.
Loss of mucous plug	Third	Passage of the mucous plus often occurs during labor but may happen prior to the onset of contractions. As long as there are no regular contractions, bleeding, or loss of fluid, loss of the mucous plug is unlikely to herald the onset of labor.
Edema	Third	Decreased venous return, obstruction of lymphatic flow, and reduced plasma colloid oncotic pressure commonly cause lower extremity edema. However, hand and face edema may signal preeclampsia.

The Health History

Common Concerns

> ▶ Initial prenatal history
>> ▶ Confirmation of pregnancy
>> ▶ Symptoms of pregnancy
>> ▶ Concerns and attitudes toward the pregnancy
>> ▶ Current health and past medical history
>> ▶ Past obstetric history
>> ▶ Risk factors for maternal and fetal health
>> ▶ Family history
>> ▶ Plans for breast-feeding
> ▶ Determining gestational age and expected date of delivery

Prenatal care focuses on optimizing health and minimizing risk for the mother and fetus. The goals of the initial prenatal visit are to confirm the pregnancy, assess the health of the mother and risks of complications, and counsel the mother about expectations for the pregnancy. Subsequent visits review specific exam findings in the mother and fetus, employ timely preventive screenings, and assess any interim changes to health status.

Initial Prenatal History. Initial prenatal visits should occur early in pregnancy but may not happen until later stages of gestation; tailor your history to the timing of this visit within the gestational cycle.

Ask about *confirmation of pregnancy*: Has the patient had a confirmatory urine pregnancy test, and when? When was her last menstrual period (LMP)? Has she had an ultrasound to establish dates? Explain that serum pregnancy tests are rarely required to confirm pregnancy.

Ask about *symptoms of pregnancy*: Does she have missed periods, breast tenderness, nausea or vomiting, fatigue, or urinary frequency?

See the table on "Common Concerns during Pregnancy and Their Explanations" for a list of normal as well as concerning symptoms, p. 896.

Ask about *concerns and attitudes toward the pregnancy*: How does the patient feel about the pregnancy? Is she excited, concerned, or scared? Was the pregnancy planned and desired? If not desired, does she plan to keep the pregnancy to term, terminate, or consider adoption? Is a partner, father of the baby, or other family support network involved? Elicit this information in an open-ended fashion, without conveying judgment. Be open to diverse family structures, such as extended families supporting young single mothers and pregnancies conceived by sperm donation. Be prepared to counsel patients when challenging answers arise, such as an admission that a pregnancy resulted from a coerced sexual act, or a reply that a pregnancy is not desired.

Ask about *current health and past medical history*. Does she have any acute or chronic medical concerns, past or present? Pay particular attention to issues that affect pregnancy, such as abdominal surgeries, hypertension, diabetes, cardiac conditions including any that were surgically corrected in childhood, asthma, hypercoagulability states involving lupus or anticardiolipin antibodies, mental health disorders including postpartum depression, HIV, sexually transmitted infections (STIs), abnormal Pap smears, and exposure to diethylstilbestrol (DES) in utero.

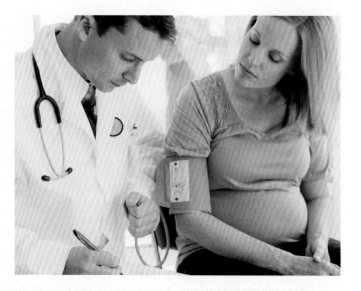

Ask about the patient's *past obstetric history*. How many prior pregnancies has she had? How many were term deliveries, preterm deliveries, spontaneous or therapeutic abortions, and how many resulted in living children? Were there any pregnancy complications such as diabetes, hypertension, preeclampsia, intrauterine growth restriction, or preterm labor? Were there any labor and delivery complications such as large babies (fetal macrosomia), fetal distress, or emergency interventions? Were deliveries by normal vaginal delivery, assisted delivery (vacuum or forceps), or cesarean section?

Ask about the patient's *risk factors* for maternal and fetal health: Does she use tobacco, alcohol, or illicit drugs? Does she take any medications, over-the-counter drugs, or herbal preparations? Does she have any toxic exposures at work, home, or otherwise? Is her nutritional intake adequate, or is she at risk from problems stemming from obesity? Does she have an adequate social support network and income source? Are there unusual sources of stress at home or work? Is there any history of physical abuse or domestic violence?

Ask about *family history*. Are there any genetically transmitted diseases in the family such as sickle cell anemia, cystic fibrosis, or muscular dystrophy, among others? Have babies in the family had any congenital problems?

Ask about *plans for breast-feeding*. Breast-feeding in infancy offers protection to the baby against a variety of infectious and noninfectious conditions, and some evidence suggests a protective effect on the mother against breast cancer and other conditions as well.[15] Educational interventions during pregnancy, as well as clinician encouragement, increase subsequent rates of breast-feeding initiation and duration, though it is unclear precisely which interventions are most effective.[16]

Determining Gestational Age and Expected Date of Delivery. Accurate dating is best done early and contributes to appropriate management of the pregnancy. Dating establishes the timeframe for reassuring the patient about normal progress, establishing paternity, timing screening tests, tracking fetal growth, and effectively triaging preterm and postdates labor.

- *Gestational age.* To establish gestational age, count the number of weeks and days from the first day of the LMP. Counting this *menstrual age* from the LMP, although biologically distinct from date of conception, is the standard means of calculating fetal age, yielding an average pregnancy length of 40 weeks. Rarely, the actual date of conception is known (as with in vitro fertilization), and in these cases a *conception age* may be employed, which is 2 weeks less than the menstrual age. However, this number should never be used to make clinical judgments that rely on the menstrual age for standards of care.

- *Expected date of delivery (EDD).* The expected date of delivery is 40 weeks from the first date of the LMP. Using *Naegele's rule*, the EDD can be estimated by taking the LMP, adding 7 days, subtracting 3 months, and adding 1 year.

- *Tools for calculations.* Pregnancy wheels and online calculators are commonly used to expedite these calculations. However, pregnancy wheels vary widely in quality and accuracy, and are often produced as marketing tools by pharmaceutical companies. Simple online calculators may be less variable, but should be checked for accuracy before routine use.

- *Limitations on pregnancy dating.* Patients' recall of the LMP is highly variable. Even when recalled accurately, LMP can be biased by hormonal contraceptives or menstrual irregularities such as lengthy cycles. LMP dating should be checked against physical exam markers such as fundal height, and any wide discrepancies should be clarified by ultrasound evaluation. It has almost become the standard of care to obtain dating ultrasounds for every pregnancy regardless of the certainty of the LMP.

Concluding the Initial Visit. Once your examination is complete and your patient has dressed, reaffirm your commitment to her health and her concerns during pregnancy. Review your findings and ask if she has any further questions. If further pregnancy confirmation, dating, or screening tests are required, discuss the next steps. Reinforce the importance of regular prenatal care and review the sequence of future visits. Record your findings in the prenatal record.

Subsequent Prenatal Visits. Though little evidence exists regarding the optimal number of prenatal appointments, obstetric visits traditionally follow a set schedule: monthly until 30 gestational weeks, then biweekly until 36 weeks, then weekly until delivery.[10] Update and document the history at every visit, especially fetal movement felt by the patient, contractions, leakage of fluids, and vaginal bleeding. The physical examination findings at every visit should include vital signs (especially blood pressure and weight), fundal height, verification of fetal heart rate (FHR), and determination of fetal position and activity, as described in Techniques of Examination to follow.

Health Promotion and Counseling: Evidence and Recommendations

Important Topics for Health Promotion and Counseling

▶ Nutrition
▶ Weight gain
▶ Exercise
▶ Substance abuse
▶ Domestic violence
▶ Prenatal laboratory screening
▶ Immunizations

Nutrition. Evaluate the nutritional status of the mother during the first prenatal visit, paying particular attention to issues of inadequate nutrition as well as obesity.

● *Take a diet history.* What does the patient typically eat for each meal? How often does she eat? Is she experiencing severe nausea that prevents adequate intake? Does she have any prior issues that affect her diet such as diabetes, eating disorders, or history of bariatric surgery?

● *Review examination and laboratory findings.* Measure the height and weight, then calculate the body mass index (BMI); note that later in pregnancy, BMI is biased by the gravid uterus. Hematocrit is used to screen for anemia, which may reflect nutritional deficiency, underlying medical issues, or a normal state relative to pregnancy.

● *Recommend a multivitamin.* Prenatal vitamins should include 0.4 to 0.8 mg of folic acid, 30 mg of iron, and a variety of other routine vitamins.[17] No particular brand has been shown to be clinically superior.

● *Caution the patient about foods to avoid.* Pregnant patients should avoid unpasteurized dairy products, soft cheeses, raw eggs, and delicatessen meats due to the risk of *Listeria, Salmonella,* and toxoplasmosis.[18] Large amounts of soluble vitamins, especially vitamin A, can become toxic. Ingestion of large sea-going fish including shark, swordfish, mackerel, and tuna, should be minimized due to their concentration of mercury and possible effects on the neurologic development in the fetus; this recommendation is controversial because some nutrients from seafoods also contribute to healthy development of the fetal brain.[17,19]

● *Make a nutritional plan.* In general, the pregnant woman will need to increase her oral intake by only 300 calories per day.[18] Review weight and exercise goals tailored to her BMI (see below). Small frequent meals may help with mild nausea. A team-based approach involving dieticians or behavioral health specialists may be most effective in complex cases such as gestational diabetes or disordered eating behaviors.

Weight Gain. Weight gain should be closely monitored during pregnancy, as both excessive and inadequate weight gain are associated with poor birth outcomes. Ideally, patients should begin pregnancy with a BMI as close to the normal range as possible. The patient should be weighed at each visit with results plotted on a graph for the patient and provider to review and discuss. Weight gain recommendations from the Institute of Medicine were updated recently to accommodate changing demographics, including higher rates of obesity, greater propensity for chronic disease when entering pregnancy, older age at conception, and other issues. These newer guidelines consider the health of both the mother and the developing fetus.[20]

Recommendations for Total and Rate of Weight Gain During Pregnancy, by Prepregnancy BMI, 2009

Prepregnancy BMI	BMI*	Total Weight Gain (lbs)	Rates of Weight Gain† 2nd and 3rd Trimester (lbs/wk)
Underweight	<18.5	28–40	1 (1–1.3)
Normal weight	18.5–24.9	25–35	1 (0.8–1)
Overweight	25–29.9	15–25	0.6 (0.5–0.7)
Obese (includes all classes)	≥30	11–20	0.5 (0.4–0.6)

*To calculate BMI go to www.nhlbisupport.com/bmi/

†Calculations assume a 0.5–2 kg (1.1–4.4 lbs) weight gain in the first trimester

Source: Rasmussen KM, Yaktine AL (eds) and Institute of Medicine. Committee to Re-examine IOM Pregnancy Weight Guidelines. Weight gain during pregnancy: re-examining the guidelines. Washington, DC: National Academies Press, 2009. Available at http://www.iom.edu/ Reports/2009/Weight-Gain-During-Pregnancy-Reexamining-the-Guidelines.aspx. Accessed February 26, 2011.

Exercise. Pregnant women should engage in 30 minutes of moderate exercise or more on most days of the week unless there are contraindications.[21] Women initiating exercise during pregnancy should be cautious and consider programs developed specifically for pregnant women. Water-based exercises can temporarily help alleviate musculoskeletal aches, but immersion in hot water should be avoided. After the first trimester, women should avoid exercise in the supine position, which compresses the inferior vena cava, resulting in dizziness and decreased placental blood flow. Because the center of gravity shifts in the third trimester, advise against exercises that may cause loss of balance. Contact sports or activities that risk abdominal trauma are unwise in all trimesters. Pregnant women should avoid overheating, dehydration, and any exertion that causes notable fatigue or discomfort.[10]

Substances of Abuse. Abstinence from substances of abuse is the immediate goal during pregnancy. As with other difficult topics, an open-ended non-judgmental approach often leads to better outcomes between the clinician and patient than judgmental or directive approaches to care. Universal screening can uncover subtle issues and help you address these topics in a neutral manner.

- *Tobacco.* Tobacco use accounts for a third of all low-birth-weight babies and many other poor pregnancy outcomes, including placental abruption and preterm labor.[10] Cessation is the goal, but any decrease in usage is favorable.[22]

- *Alcohol.* Fetal alcohol syndrome, the neurodevelopmental sequela of alcohol exposure during fetal development, is the leading cause of preventable mental retardation in the United States. No safe dose of alcohol is known during fetal development, thus several professional organizations recommend that women abstain throughout pregnancy.[10] Support for abstinence may come from counseling, inpatient treatment, Alcoholics Anonymous, or a variety of other programs.

- *Illicit drugs.* Illegal drugs have a variety of effects on fetal development; if issues of addiction arise, women should be referred for treatment immediately. Women using illicit drugs are often at risk for infectious diseases such as HIV and hepatitis C, and should be counseled and screened accordingly.

- *Abuse of prescription drugs.* Ask about unusual use of narcotics, stimulants, benzodiazepines, and other commonly abused prescription drugs.

Domestic Violence. Pregnancy is a time when risk of intimate partner violence increases. Pre-existing patterns of abuse may intensify from verbal to physical abuse or from mild to severe physical abuse. Up to one in five women experiences some form of abuse during pregnancy, which has been associated with delayed prenatal care, low infant birth weight, or even murder of the mother and fetus.[23,24]

The American College of Obstetrics and Gynecology recommends universal screening of all women for domestic violence without regard to socioeconomic status.[25] Again, a direct, nonjudgmental approach will help you gain comfort with this difficult topic. One question may be, "Since you've been pregnant, have you been hit, slapped, or otherwise hurt by anyone?"[10] Nonverbal clues include frequent last-minute changes to appointments, unusual behavior during visits, partners who refuse to leave the patient alone, and bruises or other injuries. Admission of abuse may arise only after several visits because of fear about safety and reprisal.

When abuse becomes apparent, ask the patient how you can best help her. Respect the limits she places on sharing information, and presume that she knows best how to handle her own situation (with the caveat that, if minor children are involved, you may be forced to report certain behaviors to authorities). Maintain an updated list of shelters, counseling centers, hotline numbers, and other trusted local referrals. Plan future appointments at accelerated intervals. Finally, complete a thorough physical exam as much as she permits, and document all injuries on a body diagram.

National Domestic Violence Hotline

▶ Web site: www.thehotline.org
▶ 1-800-799-SAFE (7233)
▶ TTY for hearing impaired: 1-800-787-3224

Prenatal Laboratory Screenings. An initial standard prenatal screening panel includes blood type and Rh, antibody screen, complete blood count—especially hematocrit and platelet count, rubella titer, syphilis test, hepatitis B surface antigen, HIV test, STI screen for gonorrhea and chlamydia, and urinalysis with culture. Timed screenings include an oral glucose tolerance test for gestational diabetes around 24 weeks, and a vaginal swab for group B *streptococcus* between 35 to 37 weeks' gestation. Pursue additional tests related to the mother's risk factors, such as screening for aneuploidy, screening for Tay-Sachs or other genetic diseases, amniocentesis, or checking for infectious diseases such as hepatitis C.[26]

Immunizations. Pregnant women should be up to date on tetanus vaccination.[27] Influenza vaccination is indicated if the patient is in the second or third trimester during the influenza season. The following vaccines are safe during pregnancy: pneumococcal, meningococcal, and hepatitis B. The following vaccines are NOT safe during pregnancy: measles/mumps/rubella, polio, varicella; however, all women should have rubella titers drawn during pregnancy and be immunized after birth if found to be nonimmune.[28] Rho (D) immunoglobulin, or RhoGAM, should be given to all Rh-negative women at 28 weeks' gestation and again within 3 days of delivery to prevent sensitization to an Rh-positive infant.[26]

Techniques of Examination

As you begin the examination, show respect for your patient's comfort and privacy, as well as her individual and cultural sensitivities. If this is a first visit, complete the history while she is clothed. If partners or children are present, ask the patient if she prefers that they stay or leave the room during the physical examination. Ask if she has ever had a pelvic examination; if not, take time to explain the process and seek her cooperation with each component. Cultural constraints regarding modesty should be balanced against the need to complete the examination. Note that if your patient has a history of sexual assault, she may resist examination of the pelvis; however, this may also reflect reasonable personal or cultural boundaries. To ease examination of the breasts and abdomen, ask the patient to gown with the opening in front.

Positioning. In early pregnancy, there are no special concerns regarding positioning the patient. In later trimesters, the semisitting position with the knees bent, as shown below, affords greater comfort by reducing the weight of the gravid uterus on the abdominal vessels. By contrast, the supine position causes the uterus to overlie the vertebral column and compress the descending aorta and inferior vena cava. For this reason, avoid asking the pregnant woman to spend long periods lying on her back. Most portions of the exam (except the pelvic exam) should be done in the sitting or left-side-lying position.

Compression interferes with venous return from the lower extremities and pelvic vessels, causing the patient to feel dizzy and faint, the *supine hypotensive syndrome*.

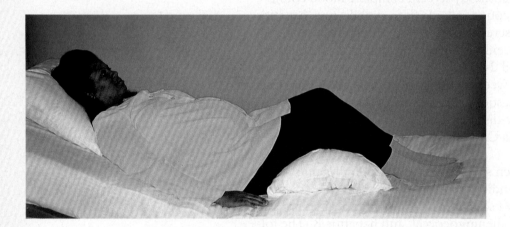

Between portions of the examination, allow the patient to sit upright again, taking care that she feels acclimated before she stands. Offer her time to empty her bladder, especially prior to the pelvic examination, which you should complete relatively quickly.

Examining Technique and Equipment. Your touch and the motions of your hands are especially important as you examine the pregnant woman. Warm your hands and recall that the palmar surfaces of your fingertips are the most sensitive. Use them to apply firm yet gentle palpation with smooth continuous contact with the skin rather than abrupt pressure or kneading. Whenever possible the fingers should be held together and flat against the abdominal or pelvic surface to minimize discomfort.

Before beginning the examination, gather the equipment listed below.

Equipment for Examining the Pregnant Woman

▶ *Gynecologic speculum and lubrication*: Because of vaginal wall relaxation during pregnancy, a larger than usual speculum may be needed.

▶ *Sampling materials*: Because of the increased vascularity of vaginal and cervical structures, the cervical brush may cause bleeding that interferes with Pap smear samples, so the Ayre wooden spatula or "broom" sampling device is preferred during pregnancy. Additional swabs may be needed to screen for sexually transmitted infections, group B strep, and wet mount preparations.

▶ *Tape measure*: A plastic or paper tape measure is used to assess the size of the uterus after 20 gestational weeks.

▶ *Doppler FHR monitor and gel*: A "Doppler" or "Doptone" is a handheld device used to assess FHR after 10 weeks of gestation when applied externally to the gravid belly. A fetoscope (an elongated bell on a stethoscopelike device) was used historically, but is no longer in common practice.

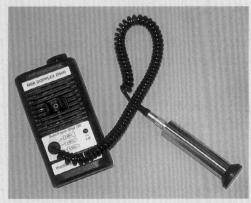

GENERAL INSPECTION

Observe the general health, emotional state, nutritional status, and neuro-muscular coordination of the woman as she walks into the room and climbs onto the exam table.

HEIGHT, WEIGHT, AND VITAL SIGNS

Measure the height and weight. Calculate the BMI with standard tables, using 19 to 25 as normal for the prepregnant state.

Tolerance of first-trimester weight loss due to nausea and vomiting depends on prepregnancy BMI, but losses in excess of 5% of pre-pregnancy weight are considered excessive, representing *hyperemesis gravidarum,* and may lead to adverse pregnancy outcomes.[29]

Take the blood pressure at every visit. A baseline prepregnancy reading helps determine a patient's usual range. In the second trimester, blood pressure normally drops below the nonpregnant state. All elevations in blood pressure must be characterized and closely monitored, as hypertension can be both an independent diagnosis and a marker of preeclampsia.

Chronic hypertension is systolic BP >140 or diastolic BP >90 documented before pregnancy, before 20 weeks, and after 12 weeks postpartum.

Gestational hypertension is SBP >140 or DBP >90 first documented after 20 weeks without proteinuria.

Preeclampsia is SBP >140 or DBP >90 after 20 weeks with proteinuria.[30]

HEAD AND NECK

Face the seated patient and observe the head and neck, paying particular attention to the following features:

- *Face.* Irregular brownish patches around the forehead, cheeks, nose, and jaw are known as *chloasma* or *melasma*, the "mask of pregnancy," a normal skin finding during pregnancy.

  Facial edema after 20 gestational weeks may reflect *preeclampsia* and should be investigated.

- *Hair.* Hair may become dry, oily, or sparse during pregnancy; mild hirsutism on the face, abdomen, and extremities is also common.

  Localized patches of hair loss should not be attributed to pregnancy (though postpartum hair loss is common).

- *Eyes.* Assess the conjunctivae and sclera for signs of pallor and jaundice.

  Anemia may cause conjunctival pallor.

- *Nose.* Inspect the mucous membranes and septum. Nasal congestion and nose bleeds are more common during pregnancy.[31]

  Erosions and perforations of the nasal septum are seen in use of intranasal cocaine.

- *Mouth.* Examine the teeth and gums. Gingival enlargement with bleeding is common during pregnancy.

  Dental problems are associated with poor pregnancy outcomes, so dental referrals should be made liberally for tooth and gum pain or infections.[10]

- *Thyroid gland.* Modest symmetric enlargement is normal on inspection and palpation.[1]

  Significant thyroid enlargement, goiters, and nodules are abnormal and require investigation.

THORAX AND LUNGS

Count the respiratory rate, which should remain normal throughout pregnancy.

Inspect the thorax for contours and breathing patterns.

Percuss to observe diaphragmatic elevation that may be seen as early as the first trimester.

Auscultate for clear breath sounds without wheezes, rales, or rhonchi.

Dyspnea accompanied by increased respiratory rate, cough, rales, or respiratory distress raises concerns of possible infection, asthma, pulmonary embolus, or peripartum cardiomyopathy.

HEART

Palpate the apical impulse, which may be rotated upward and leftward toward the fourth intercostal space by the enlarging uterus.

Auscultate the heart. Listen for a *venous hum* or continuous *mammary souffle* (pronounced *soo*-fl) often found during pregnancy due to increased blood flow through normal vessels.[32] The mammary souffle is commonly heard during late pregnancy or lactation, is strongest in the second or third intercostal space at the sternal border, and is typically both systolic and diastolic, though only the systolic component may be audible.

See also Chapter 9, Cardiovascular System, pp. 333–403.

Assess dyspnea and signs of heart failure for possible *peripartum cardiomyopathy*, particularly in the late stages of pregnancy.

Listen for murmurs.

Murmurs may signal anemia. Investigate any diastolic murmur.

BREASTS

The breast examination is similar to that of a nonpregnant woman but with some notable differences.

See also Chapter 10, Breasts and Axillae, pp. 405–431.

Inspect the breasts and nipples for symmetry and color. Normal changes include a marked venous pattern, darkened nipples and areolae, and prominent Montgomery's glands.

Inverted nipples need attention at the time of birth if breast-feeding is planned.

Palpate for masses and axillary lymph nodes. Normal breasts may be tender and nodular during pregnancy.

Pathologic masses may be difficult to isolate but should receive immediate attention. Severe focal tenderness with erythema in *mastitis* requires immediate treatment.

Compress each nipple between your thumb and index finger; colostrum may express from the nipples during later trimesters.

Bloody or purulent discharge should not be attributed to pregnancy.

ABDOMEN

To prepare for this portion of the exam, help the patient move into a semi-sitting position with knees flexed, as shown on p. 904.

Inspect the abdomen for striae, scars, size, shape, and contour. Purplish *striae* and *linea nigra* are normal in pregnancy.

Scars can confirm prior surgery, but external cesarean scars may not match the orientation of the scar on the uterus, which is critical in evaluating appropriateness for vaginal births after cesarean section.

Palpate the abdomen for:

- *Organs and masses.* The mass of the gravid uterus is expected.

- *Fetal movement.* The examiner can usually feel movements externally after 24 gestational weeks; the mother can usually feel these by 18 to 24 weeks.[10] Maternal sensation of fetal movement is traditionally known as "quickening."

If fetal movement cannot be felt after 24 weeks, consider error in calculating gestational age, fetal death or severe morbidity, or false pregnancy. Confirm fetal health and gestational age with a formal ultrasound.

- *Uterine contractility.* Irregular uterine contractions occur as early as 12 weeks and may be triggered by external palpation during the third trimester. During contractions, the abdomen feels tense or firm to the examiner, obscuring the palpation of fetal parts; after the contraction, the palpating fingers sense the relaxation of the uterine muscle.

Before 37 weeks, regular uterine contractions with or without pain and bleeding are abnormal, suggesting preterm labor.

- *Measure the fundal height* if gestational age is >20 weeks. With a plastic or paper tape measure, locate the pubic symphysis and place the "zero" end of the tape measure where you can firmly feel that bone. Then extend the tape measure to the very top of uterine fundus and note the number of centimeters measured. Though subject to error between 16 and 36 weeks, measurement in centimeters should roughly equal the number of weeks' gestation.[33,34] At 20 weeks, the fundus should reach the umbilicus.

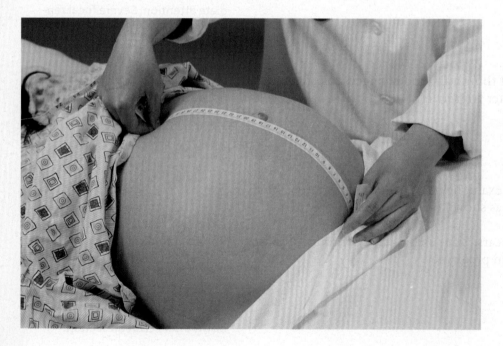

If fundal height is *4 cm larger* than expected, consider multiple gestation, a large fetus, extra amniotic fluid, or uterine leiomyoma. If fundal height is *4 cm smaller than expected*, consider low level of amniotic fluid, missed abortion, intrauterine growth retardation, or fetal anomaly. Both of these conditions should be investigated by formal ultrasound.

Auscultate the fetal heart tones. The Doppler fetal rate monitor ("Doppler" or "Doptone") is the standard instrument used for this measurement, and can detect the fetal rate (FHR) as early as 10 weeks' gestation.

Lack of audible fetal heart tones may indicate fewer weeks' gestation than expected, fetal demise, false pregnancy, or observer error; inability to locate the FHR should always be investigated with formal ultrasound.

- *Location.* From 10 to 18 weeks' gestation, the FHR is located along the midline of the lower abdomen. After that time, the FHR is best heard over the back or chest and depends on fetal position; the Leopold maneuvers can help identify the position. (See pp. 912–914.)

After 24 weeks, auscultation of more than one FHR in different locations with varying rates suggests multiple gestation.

- *Rate.* The FHR ranges between 120 and 160 beats per minute (BPM). A heart rate of 60 to 90 BPM is usually maternal but an adequate FHR should be confirmed.

Sustained dips in FHR, or "decelerations," have a wide differential diagnosis but always warrant investigation, at least by formal FHR monitoring.

- *Rhythm.* FHR should vary 10 to 15 BPM from second to second, especially later in the pregnancy. After 32 to 34 weeks, the FHR should become more variable and increased with fetal activity. This subtlety can difficult to assess with a Doppler but can be traced with a formal FHR monitor if any questions arise.

Lack of beat-to-beat variability is difficult to discern with a handheld Doppler, but this finding warrants investigation with a formal FHR monitor.

GENITALIA

For this portion of the exam, the patient will need to be supine with feet placed in stirrups. Be prepared with needed equipment, and minimize the time she will need to be in this position to avert dizziness and hypotension from uterine compression of the major abdominal vessels.

External Genitalia. Inspect the external genitalia. Relaxation of the vaginal introitus and enlargement of the labia and clitoris are normal changes of pregnancy. In multiparous women, scars from perineal lacerations or episiotomy incisions may be present.

Inspect for labial varicosities, cystoceles, and rectoceles.

Labial varicosities may arise during pregnancy and become tortuous and painful. Cystoceles and rectoceles may be pronounced from the muscle relaxation of pregnancy.

Palpate the Bartholin's and Skene's glands for tenderness and cysts.

See also Chapter 14, Female Genitalia, pp. 539–575.

Internal Genitalia. Prepare for both a speculum and bimanual examination.

Speculum Examination. Relaxation of perineal and vulvar structures during pregnancy may minimize, but not eliminate, discomfort from the speculum exam. Because increased vascularity of vaginal and cervical structures promotes friability, insert and open the speculum gently to prevent tissue trauma and bleeding.

- *Inspect the cervix for color, shape, and closure.* A parous cervix may look irregular because of healed lacerations from prior births.

A pink cervix suggests a non-pregnant state. Cervical erosion, erythema, discharge, or irritation suggests cervicitis and warrants investigation for STIs.

- *Perform a Pap smear if indicated,* and collect other vaginal specimens such as STI cultures, wet mount samples, or group B strep swabs as appropriate.

- *Inspect the vaginal walls* as you withdraw the speculum. Check for color, relaxation, rugae, and discharge. Normal findings include bluish color, deep rugae, and increased milky white discharge, or *leukorrhea.*

Investigate abnormal vaginal discharges for possible *candida* or for bacterial vaginosis, which can affect pregnancy outcome.

Bimanual Examination. The bimanual examination is often easier during pregnancy, due to pelvic floor relaxation. Avoiding sensitive urethral structures, insert two lubricated fingers into the introitus, palmar side down, with slight pressure downward on the perineum. Maintaining downward pressure on the perineum, gently turn the fingers palmar side up.

- *Cervix.* Because of softening during pregnancy, or Hegar's sign, the cervix may be difficult to distinguish at first. Estimate the cervical length by palpating the lateral surface of the cervical tip to the lateral fornix. Prior to 34 to 36 weeks' gestation, the cervix should retain its initial length of 3 cm or greater. Locate the cervical os. The *external os* may be open to admit a fingertip in multiparous women. The *internal os,* the narrow passage between the endocervical canal and the uterine cavity, should be closed until late pregnancy, regardless of parity. The surface of a multiparous cervix may feel irregular because of healed lacerations from prior births.

Cervical opening or shortening (effacement) prior to 37 weeks may indicate preterm labor.

- *Uterus.* With your internal fingers placed at either side of the cervix and the external hand on the patient's abdomen, use the internal fingers to gently lift the uterus upward toward the abdominal hand. Capture the fundal portion of the uterus between your two hands and assess the uterine size, keeping in mind the contours of the gravid uterus at various gestational intervals, as noted on p. 894. Palpate for shape, consistency, and position.

An irregularly shaped uterus suggests uterine *leiomyomata,* or fibroids, or a *bicornuate uterus,* one with two distinct cavities separated by a septum.

- *Adnexa*. Palpate the right and left adnexa. The corpus luteum may be palpable as a small nodule on the affected ovary during the first weeks after conception. After the first trimester, adnexal masses become difficult to feel.

- *Pelvic floor*. Evaluate pelvic floor strength as you withdraw the examining fingers.

Adnexal tenderness or masses early in gestation require ultrasonic evaluation to rule out ectopic pregnancy. Acute pelvic inflammatory disease is rare in pregnancy, especially after the first trimester, because the adnexae are sealed by the gravid uterus and mucous plug.

ANUS AND RECTUM

Anus. Inspect for external hemorrhoids. If present, note their size, location, and any evidence of thrombosis.

Hemorrhoids often engorge during late pregnancy; they may be painful, bleed, or thrombose.

Rectum and Rectovaginal Septum. Rectal examination is not standard in prenatal care unless symptoms warrant investigation, such as rectal bleeding or masses. Rectovaginal examination is limited to conditions compromising the integrity of the rectovaginal septum. This examination may assist in determining the size of a retroverted or retroflexed uterus, but transvaginal ultrasound provides superior information, if available.

EXTREMITIES

Ask the woman to resume sitting or to lie on her left side. *Inspect* the legs for varicose veins.

Varicose veins may begin or worsen during pregnancy.

Palpate the extremities for edema in the pretibial, ankle, and pedal distributions, which are rated on a 0 to 4+ scale. Physiologic edema is common in advanced pregnancy, during hot weather, and in women who stand for long periods of time; this is due to decreased venous return from the lower extremities.

See Chapter 12, Peripheral Vascular System, for grades of edema, pp. 505–506. Unilateral severe edema with calf tenderness warrants evaluation for *deep vein thrombosis*. Hand or facial edema after 20 gestational weeks should be investigated for the possibility of *preeclampsia*.

Elicit the knee and ankle deep tendon reflexes.

Hyperreflexia may signal preeclampsia; however, this must be compared to recorded baseline reflexes because individual variation is great.[35]

SPECIAL TECHNIQUES

Leopold Maneuvers

Leopold maneuvers are used to determine the fetal position within the maternal abdomen beginning in the second trimester; accuracy is greatest after 36 weeks' gestation.[17] These exam findings can help ascertain the adequacy of fetal growth and the readiness for vaginal birth by assessing:

- The upper and lower fetal pole, namely. the proximal and distal fetal parts

- The maternal side where the fetal back is located

- The descent of the presenting part into the maternal pelvis

- The extent of flexion of the fetal head

- The estimated size/weight of the fetus (an advanced skill that will not be addressed further here)

Common deviations include *breech presentation* (when parts other than the head, such as buttocks or foot, present at the maternal pelvis), and lack of engagement of the presenting part in the maternal pelvis at term. If discovered prior to term, breech presentations may sometimes be corrected by rotational maneuvers.

First Maneuver (Upper Fetal Pole). Stand at the woman's side, facing her head. Palpate the uppermost part of gravid uterus gently, with the fingertips together, to determine what fetal part is located at the fundus (the "upper fetal pole").

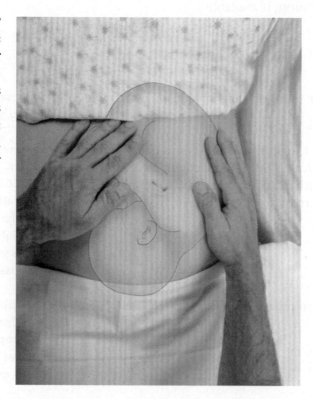

The fetal buttocks are usually at the upper fetal pole; they feel firm but irregular, and less globular than the head. The fetal head feels firm, round, and smooth. Occasionally, neither part is easily palpated at the fundus, as when the fetus is in a transverse lie.

Second Maneuver (Sides of the Maternal Abdomen). Place one hand on each side of the woman's abdomen, capturing the fetal body between them. Steady the uterus with one hand and palpate the fetus with the other, looking for the back on one side and extremities on the other.

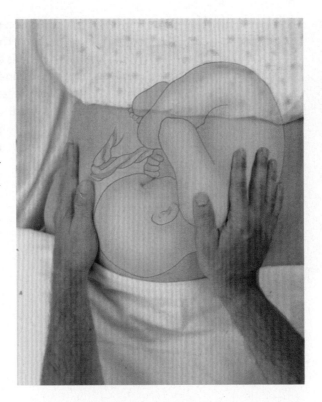

By 32 weeks' gestation, the examiner's hand on the fetal back feels a smooth, firm surface as long or longer than the hand itself. The examiner's hand on the fetal arms and legs feels irregular bumps, and may sense kicking if the fetus is awake and active.

Third Maneuver (Lower Fetal Pole and Descent Into Pelvis). Face the woman's feet. Place the flat palmar surfaces of the fingertips on the fetal pole just above the pubic symphysis. Palpate the presenting fetal part for texture and firmness to distinguish head from buttock. Judge the descent (or engagement) of the presenting part into the maternal pelvis. Alternatively, Pawlik's grip may be employed by using the thumb and fingers of one hand to grasp the lower fetal pole and assess the presenting part and descent into pelvis; however, this tends to be uncomfortable to the gravid patient.

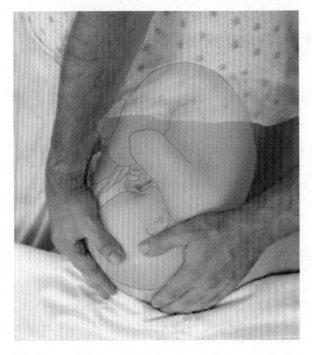

Again, the fetal head feels very firm and globular; the buttocks feel firm but irregular, and less globular than the head. When the fetal head is the presenting part, this is referred to as a *vertex* or *cephalic* presentation. If the most distal part of the lower fetal pole cannot be palpated due to interference from the bony pelvis, it is usually engaged in the pelvis. If you can depress the tissues over the maternal bladder without touching the fetus, the presenting part is proximal to your fingers.

Fourth Maneuver (Flexion of the Fetal Head). This maneuver assesses the flexion or extension of the fetal head, presuming that the fetal head is the presenting part in the pelvis. Still facing the woman's feet, with your hands positioned on either side of the gravid uterus, identify the fetal front and back sides. Using one hand at a time, slide your fingers down each side of the fetal body until you reach the "cephalic prominence," that is, where the fetal brow or occiput juts out.

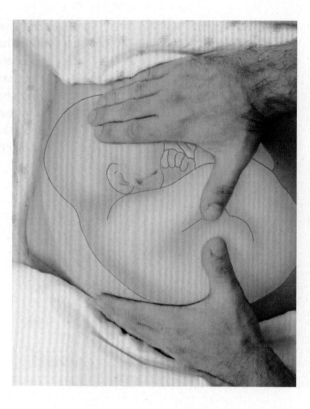

If the cephalic prominence juts out along the line of the fetal back, the head is extended. If the cephalic prominence juts out along the line of the fetal anterior side, the head is flexed.

Recording Your Findings

Like many specialties, obstetrics utilizes a very specific vocabulary, not all of which can be covered in this text.

- Pregnant women are described in terms of number of pregnancies (gravida) and labors (para) they have experienced. Parity is further broken down into *term deliveries, preterm deliveries, abortions* (spontaneous + therapeutic), and *living children,* which, listed in that order yields the mnemonic "TPAL."

- This is expressed in "Gs and Ps"; for example, a woman who has had two prior children and is pregnant with her third (with no other pregnancies) would be referred to simply as a "G2P2." A woman with two early-term losses, 3 living children who delivered at term, and a current pregnancy, would be referred to as a "G6,P3023." This shorthand allows obstetricians to track large amounts of data succinctly.

Typically, the presentation of a pregnant patient follows a standardized pattern: age, Gs and Ps, weeks of gestation, means of determining gestational age (ultrasound versus LMP), followed by chief complaint, then important historical and exam findings. Two sample presentations are given on the next page.

Recording the Physical Examination—
The Pregnant Woman

"32-year-old G3,P1102 at 18 weeks' gestation as determined by LMP presents to establish prenatal care. Patient endorses fetal movement; denies contractions, vaginal bleeding, and leakage of fluids. On external exam, low transverse cesarean scar is evident; fundus is palpable just below umbilicus. On internal exam, cervix is open to fingertip at the external os but closed at the internal os; cervix is 3 cm long; uterus enlarged to size consistent with 18-week gestation. Speculum exam shows leucorrhea with positive Chadwick's sign. FHT by Doppler are between 140 and 145 BPM."

OR

"21-year-old G1,P1000 at 33 weeks' gestation as determined by 19-week ultrasound presents with chief complaint of decreased fetal movement. Patient endorses minimal fetal movement over the last 24 hours; denies contractions, vaginal bleeding, and leakage of fluids. On external exam, nontender gravid abdomen with no scars is noted; fundus is measured at 32 cm; fetus is vertex but not engaged in pelvis by Leopold maneuvers. On internal exam, cervix is closed, thick, and high; speculum exam shows thin grey discharge with clue cells on wet mount. FHT by Doppler are between 155 and 160 BPM."

Describes examination of healthy pregnant woman at 18 weeks' gestation.

Describes examination of somewhat complex presentation of a pregnant woman at 33 weeks' gestation.

Bibliography

Citations

1. Cunningham FG, Leveno KL, Bloom SL et al (eds). Williams Obstetrics, 22nd ed. New York: McGraw Hill, Medical Publishers Division, 2005.
2. Moore L, Bilello KL, Murin S. Sex and gender issues and venous thromboembolism. Clin Chest Med 2004;25:281–297.
3. McCormack MC, Wise RA. Respiratory physiology in pregnancy. Respir Med 2009;1:1–8.
4. Swift SE, Ostergard DR. Effects of progesterone on the urinary tract. Int Urogynecol J 1993;4:232–236.
5. Kuhl C. Etiology and pathogenesis of gestational diabetes. Diabetes Care 1998;21(Suppl 2):B19–26.
6. Kim C, Newton KM, Knopp RH. Gestational diabetes and the incidence of type II diabetes: a systematic review. Diabetes Care 2002;25:1862–1868.
7. Glinoer D, de Nayer PD, Bourdoux P et al. Regulation of maternal thyroid during pregnancy. J Clin Endocrinol Metab 1990;71:276–287.
8. Becker I, Woodley SJ, Stringer MD. The adult human pubic symphysis: a systematic review. J Anat 2010;217:475–487.
9. Milman N, Graudal N, Nielsen OJ et al. Serum erythropoietin during normal pregnancy: relationship to hemoglobin and iron status markers and impact of iron supplementation in a longitudinal, placebo-controlled study on 118 women. Int J Hematol 1997;66(2):159–168.
10. Ratcliffe SD, Baxley EG, Cline MK et al (eds). Family Medicine Obstetrics. Philadelphia: Mosby Elsevier, 2008.
11. Andersen HF, Johnson TR, Barclay ML et al. Gestational age assessment. I. Analysis of individual clinical observations. Am J Ostet Gynecol 1981;139:173–177.
12. Creasy R, Resnik R, Iams J. Maternal Fetal Medicine: Principles and Practice, 5th ed. Philadelphia: Saunders, 2004.
13. Boisonnault JS, Blaschak MJ. Incidence of diastasis rectus abdominis during the childbearing year. Phys Ther 1988;68: 1082–1086.
14. Greenberger NJ, Blumberg RS, Burakoff R. Current Diagnosis and Treatment: Gastroenterology, Hepatology, & Endoscopy. New York: McGraw Hill Companies, 2009.
15. Freund C, Mirabel L, Annane K et al. Breastfeeding and breast cancer. Gynecol Obstet Fertil 2005;33:739–744.
16. U.S. Preventive Services Task Force. Primary care interventions to promote breastfeeding: U.S. Preventive Services Task Force recommendation statement. Ann Intern Med 2008; 149:560–564.
17. Kirkham C, Harris S, Grzybowski S. Evidence-based prenatal care: part I. general prenatal care and counseling issues. Am Fam Physician 2005;71:1307–1316.
18. Kaiser L, Allen LH, American Dietetic Association. Position of American Dietetic Association: nutrition and life style for a healthy pregnancy outcome. J Am Diet Assoc 2008;108:553–561.
19. Hibbeln JR, Davis JM, Steer C et al. Maternal seafood consumption during pregnancy and neurodevelopmental outcomes in childhood (ALSPAC study): an observational cohort study. Lancet 2007;369(9561):578–585.
20. Rasmussen KM, Yaktine AL (eds) and Institute of Medicine. Committee to Reexamine IOM Pregnancy Weight Guidelines. Weight Gain During Pregnancy: Re-examining the Guidelines. Washington, DC: National Academies Press, 2009. Available

BIBLIOGRAPHY

at http://www.iom.edu/Reports/2009/Weight-Gain-During-Pregnancy-Reexamining-the-Guidelines.aspx. Accessed February 26, 2011.

21. American College of Obstetricians and Gynecologists (ACOG). Exercise during pregnancy and the postpartum period. ACOG Committee Opinion, No 267. Obstet Gynecol 2002;99:171–173.

22. U.S. Preventive Services Task Force. Counseling and interventions to prevent tobacco use and tobacco-caused disease in adults and pregnant women: U.S. Preventive Services Task Force reaffirmation recommendation statement. Ann Intern Med 2009;150:551–555.

23. Gazmararian JA, Lazorick, S, Spitz AM et al. Prevalence of violence against pregnant women. JAMA 1996;275:1915–1920.

24. Boy A, Salihu HM. Intimate partner violence and birth outcomes: a systematic review. Int J Fertil Womens Med 2004;49:159–164.

25. American College of Obstetrics and Gynecology (ACOG). Psychosocial risk factors: perinatal screening and intervention. ACOG Committee Opinion, No 343. Obstet Gynecol 2006; 108:469–477.

26. Kirkham C, Harris S, Grzybowski S. Evidence-based prenatal care: part I. general prenatal care and counseling issues. Am Fam Physician 2005;71:1307–1316.

27. Murphy TV, Slade BA Broder KR et al. Prevention of pertussis, tetanus, and diphtheria among pregnant and postpartum women and their infants recommendations of the Advisory Committee on Immunization Practices (ACIP). MMWR 2008;57(26):723.

28. Centers for Disease Control and Prevention. Measles, mumps, and rubella—vaccine use and strategies for elimination of measles, rubella, and congenital rubella syndrome and control of mumps: recommendations of the Advisory Committee on Immunization Practices (ACIP). MMWR 1998;47 (RR-8): 18, 32–33.

29. Quinlan JD, Hill DA. Nausea and vomiting of pregnancy. Am Fam Physician 2003;68:121–128.

30. Leeman L, Fontaine P. Hypertensive disorders of pregnancy. Am Fam Physician 2008;78:93–100.

31. Ellegård EK. Clinical and pathogenetic characteristics of pregnancy rhinitis. Clin Rev Allergy Immunol 2004;26:149–159.

32. Elkayam U, Gleicher N. Cardiac Problems in Pregnancy: Diagnosis and Management of Maternal and Fetal Heart Disease, 3rd ed. New York: John Wiley & Sons, 1998.

33. Belizan JM, Villar J, Nardin JC et al. Diagnosis of intrauterine growth retardation by a simple clinical method: measurement of uterine height. Am J Obstet Gynecol 1987;131:643–646.

34. Persson B, Strangenberf M, Lunnell NL et al. Prediction of size of infants at birth by measurement of symphysis fundus height. Br J Obstet Gynaecol 1986;93:206–211.

35. Karumanchi SA, Lindheimer MD. Advances in the understanding of eclampsia. Curr Hypertens Rep 2008;10:305–312.

Additional References

American College of Obstetricians and Gynecologists, Committee on Health Care for Underserved Women. ACOG Committee Opinion No. 361. Breastfeeding: maternal and infant aspects. Obstet Gynecol 2007;109(2 Pt 1):479–480.

Balsells M, García-Patterson A, Gich I et al. Maternal and fetal outcome in women with type 2 versus type 1 diabetes mellitus: a systematic review and metaanalysis. J Clin Endocrinol Metab 2009;94:4284–4291.

Bell R, Bailey K, Cresswell T et al, Northern Diabetic Pregnancy Survey Steering Group. Trends in prevalence and outcomes of pregnancy in women with pre-existing type I and type II diabetes. BJOG 2008;115:445–452.

Blenning CE, Paladine H. An approach to the postpartum office visit. Am Fam Physician 2005;72:2491–2496.

Cunningham FG, Williams JW. Williams Obstetrics, 23rd ed. New York: McGraw-Hill Medical, 2010.

Fraser DC, Cooper MS, Myles MF. Myles Textbook for Midwives, 15th ed. New York: Churchill Livingstone Elsevier, 2009.

Grote NK, Bridge JA, Gavin AR et al. A meta-analysis of depression during pregnancy and the risk of preterm birth, low birth weight, and intrauterine growth restriction. Arch Gen Psychiatry 2010;67:1012–1024.

Mahmud M, Mazza D. Preconception care of women with diabetes: a review of current guideline recommendations. BMC Womens Health 2010;10:5.

Musters C, McDonald E, Jones I. Management of postnatal depression. BMJ 2008;337:a736.

Nicholson W, Bolen S, Witkop CT et al. Benefits and risks of oral diabetes agents compared with insulin in women with gestational diabetes: a systematic review. Obstet Gynecol 2009; 113:193–205.

U. S. Preventive Services Task Force. Screening for family and intimate partner violence: recommendation statement. Ann Intern Med 2004;140:382–386.

U.S. Preventive Services Task Force. Screening for gestational diabetes mellitus: U.S. Preventive Services Task Force Recommendation Statement. Ann Intern Med 2008;148:759–765.

The Bates' suite offers these additional resources to enhance learning and facilitate understanding of this chapter:

- Bates' *Pocket Guide to Physical Examination and History Taking*, 7th edition
- Bates' *Visual Guide to Physical Examination*
- thePoint online resources, for students and instructors: http://thepoint.lww.com

The Older Adult

Older Americans now number more than 39 million and are expected to reach 88 million by 2050.[1,2] Americans are living longer than previous generations: Life span at birth is currently 84 years for women and 82 years for men. The percentage of those older than 85 years is projected to double by 2050 to over 4% of the U.S. population. Hence, the *"demographic imperative"* to societies worldwide is to maximize not only life span but also the "health span" so that older adults maintain full function as long as possible, enjoying rich and active lives in their homes and communities.

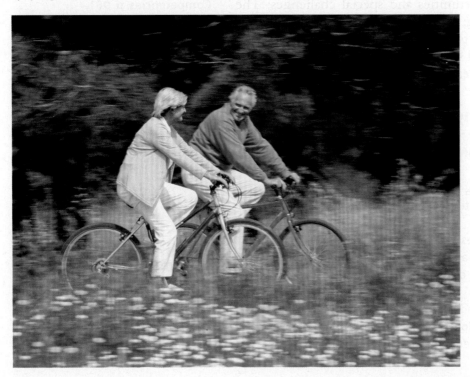

Although statistics fall into groupings by decades, aging is hardly chronologic, bound by time in years, but encompasses a wealth of wisdom and lived experience in addition to the diverse spectrum of health and illness. The aging population is highly heterogeneous—in disposition, social networks, level of physical activity, and biology. Frailty is one of society's common myths about aging; more than 95% of Americans older than 65 years live in the community, and only 4% reside in institutional facilities.[1] Functional status supersedes disability as a measure of healthy aging. Over the past 20 years, adults over 65 have reported fewer functional limitations. Those reporting at least one functional limitation have declined from 49% to 42%, even though over 80% report at least one chronic condition.[3] However, recent trends suggest that obesity may increase future levels of disability, especially in African American and Hispanic adults ages 60 to 69.[4,5] Studies show that successful aging is not strictly medical, but rests on variables such as positive outlook, outdoor exercise, and social contacts.[6] Even terminology about aging is in flux. This chapter uses the term "older adult" and at times "senior." Because evidence is slender about preferred designations, take the time to find out which terms your patients prefer.

Promoting healthy aging calls for new goals in clinical care—"an informed activated patient interacting with a prepared proactive team, resulting in high quality satisfying encounters and improved outcomes" and a distinct set of clinical attitudes and skills.[7,8] New paradigms highlight the importance of shifting assessment to *geriatric conditions* that fall outside traditional disease models but are strongly linked to activities of daily living, present in almost 50% of older adults.[9] Managing these conditions—cognitive impairment, falls, incontinence, low body mass index, dizziness, impaired vision and hearing—presents special opportunities and special challenges: The focus on healthy or "successful" aging; the need to understand and mobilize family, social, and community supports; the importance of skills directed to functional assessment, "the sixth vital sign"; and the opportunities for promoting the older adult's long-term health and safety.

See discussion of geriatric conditions and syndromes on p. 928.

See Table 20-1, Minimum Geriatrics Competencies, p. 961.

Chapter Overview: The Aging Adult

▶ Anatomy and Physiology: Changes of Aging
▶ The Health History
  ▶ Approach to the Patient: adjusting the office environment; shaping the content and pace of the visit; eliciting symptoms; responsiveness to the cultural dimensions of aging
  ▶ Special Areas of Concern: activities of daily living; instrumental activities of daily living; medications; acute and persistent pain; smoking and alcohol; nutrition; frailty; advance directives and palliative care
▶ Health Promotion and Counseling
  ▶ Includes when to screen, vision and hearing, exercise, immunizations, household safety and fall prevention, cancer screening, depression, dementia, mild cognitive impairment and cognitive decline, and elder mistreatment and abuse
▶ Techniques of Examination
  ▶ Functional Assessment, including The 10-Minute Geriatric Screener and assessing risk for falls
  ▶ Physical Examination of the Older Adult
▶ Recording your findings

Anatomy and Physiology

Primary aging reflects changes in physiologic reserves over time that are independent of and not induced by any disease. These changes are especially apt to appear during periods of stress, such as exposure to fluctuating temperatures, dehydration, or even shock. Decreased cutaneous vasoconstriction and sweat production can impair responses to heat; declines in thirst may delay recovery from dehydration; and the physiologic drops in maximum cardiac output, left ventricular filling, and maximum heart rate seen with aging may impair the response to shock.

At the same time, the aging population displays marked heterogeneity. Investigators have identified vast differences in how people age and have distinguished "usual" aging, with its complex of diseases and impairments, from "optimal" aging. Optimal aging occurs in those people who escape debilitating disease entirely and maintain healthy lives late into their 80s and 90s. Studies of centenarians show that genes account for approximately 20% of the probability of living to 100, with healthy lifestyles accounting for approximately 20% to 30%.[10,11] These findings provide compelling evidence for promoting optimal nutrition, strength training and exercise, and daily function for older adults to delay unnecessary depletion of physiologic reserves.

Vital Signs

Blood Pressure.   In Western societies, systolic blood pressure tends to rise from childhood through old age. The aorta and large arteries stiffen and become atherosclerotic. As the aorta becomes less distensible, a given stroke volume causes a greater rise in systolic blood pressure; *systolic hypertension* with a *widened pulse pressure* often ensues. Diastolic blood pressure stops rising at approximately the sixth decade. At the other extreme, some elderly people develop a tendency toward *postural (orthostatic) hypotension*—a sudden drop in blood pressure when they rise to standing.

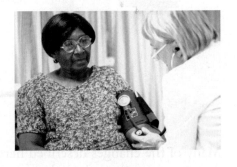

Heart Rate and Rhythm.   In older adults, resting heart rate remains unchanged, but pacemaker cells decline in the sinoatrial node, as does maximal heart rate, affecting response to physiologic stress.[12] Older adults are more likely to have abnormal heart rhythms such as atrial or ventricular ectopy. Asymptomatic rhythm changes are generally benign. However, some rhythm changes cause *syncope*, or temporary loss of consciousness.

Respiratory Rate and Temperature.   Respiratory rate is unchanged, but changes in temperature regulation lead to susceptibility to *hypothermia*.

Skin, Nails, and Hair.   With age, the skin wrinkles, becomes lax, and loses turgor. The vascularity of the dermis decreases, causing lighter skin to look paler and more opaque. Skin on the backs of the hands and forearms appears thin, fragile, loose, and transparent. There may be purple patches or macules, termed *actinic purpura,* that fade over time. These spots and patches come from blood that has leaked through poorly supported capillaries and spread within the dermis.

Nails lose luster with age and may yellow and thicken, especially on the toes.

Hair undergoes a series of changes. Scalp hair loses its pigment, producing graying. Hair loss on the scalp is genetically determined. As early as 20 years, a man's hairline may start to recede at the temples; hair loss at the vertex follows. In women, hair loss follows a similar but less severe pattern. In both sexes, the number of scalp hairs decreases in a generalized pattern, and the diameter of each hair gets smaller. Less familiar, but probably more important clinically, is normal hair loss elsewhere on the body— the trunk, pubic areas, axillae, and limbs. As women reach age 55 years, coarse facial hairs appear on the chin and upper lip but do not increase further thereafter.

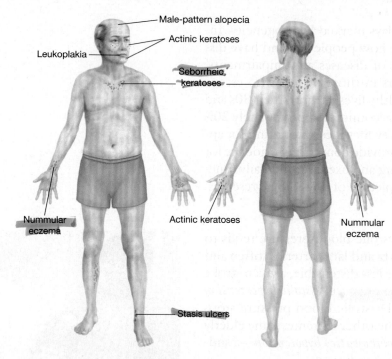

Many of the changes described here pertain to lighter-skinned people and do not necessarily apply to those with darker skin tones. For example, Native American men have relatively little facial and body hair compared with lighter-skinned men and should be evaluated according to their own norms.

Head and Neck

Eyes and Visual Acuity.   The eyes, ears, and mouth bear the brunt of old age. The fat that surrounds and cushions the eye within the bony orbit may atrophy, so the eyeball appears to recede. The skin of the eyelids becomes wrinkled, occasionally hanging in loose folds. Fat may push the fascia of the eyelids forward, creating soft bulges, especially in the lower lids and the inner third of the upper lids. Because of fewer lacrimal secretions, older patients may complain of dry eyes. The corneas lose some of their luster.

The pupils become smaller, making it more difficult to examine the ocular fundi. The pupils may also become slightly irregular but should continue to respond to light and near effort.

Visual acuity remains fairly constant between 20 and 50 years. It diminishes gradually until approximately 70 years and then more rapidly. Nevertheless, most elderly people retain good to adequate vision (20/20 to 20/70 as measured by standard charts). Near vision, however, begins to blur noticeably for virtually everyone. From childhood on, the lens gradually loses its elasticity, and the eye grows progressively less able to accommodate and focus on nearby objects. Ensuing *presbyopia* usually becomes noticeable during the fifth decade.

Aging affects the lenses and increases risk for *cataracts, glaucoma*, and *macular degeneration*. Thickening and yellowing of the lenses impair the passage of light to the retinas, requiring more light for reading and doing fine work. Cataracts affect 1 in 10 people in their 60s and 1 in 3 people in their 80s. Because the lens continues to grow over the years, it may push the iris forward, narrowing the angle between iris and cornea and increasing the risk of *narrow-angle glaucoma*.

See Chapter 7, Head and Neck, pp. 205–291.

Hearing.   Acuity of hearing, like that of vision, usually diminishes with age. Early losses, which start in young adulthood, involve primarily the high-pitched sounds beyond the range of human speech and have relatively little functional significance. Gradually, loss extends to sounds in the middle and lower ranges. When a person fails to catch the upper tones of words while hearing the lower ones, words sound distorted and are difficult to understand, especially in noisy environments. Hearing loss associated with aging, known as *presbycusis*, becomes increasingly evident, usually after 50 years.

Mouth, Teeth, and Lymph Nodes.   There are diminished salivary secretions and a decreased sense of taste; medications or various diseases can contribute considerably to such changes. Decreased olfaction and increased sensitivity to bitterness and saltiness also affect taste. Teeth may wear down, become abraded, or be lost to dental caries or periodontal disease. If a person has no teeth, the lower portion of the face looks small and sunken, with accentuated "purse-string" wrinkles radiating from the mouth. Overclosure of the mouth may lead to maceration of the skin at the corners, or *angular cheilitis*. The bony ridges of the jaws that once surrounded the tooth sockets are gradually resorbed, especially in the lower jaw.

See Chapter 7, The Head and Neck, pp. 205–291.

The frequency of palpable cervical nodes gradually diminishes with age and, according to one study, falls below 50% between 50 and 60 years. In contrast to the lymph nodes, the submandibular glands become easier to feel.

Thorax and Lungs.   As people age, their capacity for exercise decreases. The chest wall becomes stiffer and harder to move, respiratory muscles may weaken, and the lungs lose some of their elastic recoil. Lung mass declines, and residual volume increases. An increase in closing volumes of small airways cells predisposes to atelectasis and risk of pneumonia. The speed of breathing out with maximal effort gradually diminishes, and cough becomes less effective.

Skeletal changes associated with aging may accentuate the dorsal curve of the thoracic spine, producing kyphosis from osteoporotic vertebral collapse and increasing the anteroposterior diameter of the chest. The resulting "barrel chest," however, has little effect on function.

Cardiovascular System.

A number of changes occur in the neck vessels, cardiac output, heart sounds, and murmurs.

Review the effects of aging on blood pressure and heart rate described on p. 344.

Neck Vessels. Lengthening and tortuosity of the aorta and its branches occasionally result in kinking or buckling of the carotid artery low in the neck, especially on the right. The resulting pulsatile mass, occurring chiefly in women with hypertension, may be mistaken for a carotid aneurysm—a true dilatation of the artery. A tortuous aorta occasionally raises the pressure in the jugular veins on the left side of the neck by impairing their drainage within the thorax.

In older adults, systolic bruits heard in the middle or upper portions of the carotid arteries suggest, but do not prove, partial arterial obstruction from atherosclerosis. In contrast, cervical bruits in younger people are usually innocent.

Cardiac Output. Myocardial contraction is less responsive to stimulation from β-adrenergic catecholamines. Heart rate drops but stroke volume increases, so cardiac output is maintained. Diastolic dysfunction arises from decreased early diastolic filling and greater dependence on atrial contraction.

Risk of heart failure increases with loss of atrial contraction and onset of atrial fibrillation.

Extra Heart Sounds—S_3 and S_4. A physiologic *third heart sound*, commonly heard in children and young adults, may persist as late as age 40 years, especially in women. After age 40, however, an S_3 strongly suggests heart failure from volume overload of the left ventricle, as in coronary artery disease or valvular heart disease (e.g., mitral regurgitation). In contrast, a *fourth heart sound* is seldom heard in young adults other than well-conditioned athletes. An S_4 can be heard in otherwise healthy older people, but often suggests decreased ventricular compliance and impaired ventricular filling.

See Table 9-8, Extra Heart Sounds in Diastole, p. 398.

Cardiac Murmurs. Middle-aged and older adults commonly have a *systolic aortic murmur*. This murmur is detected in approximately one-third of people close to 60 years, and in more than half of those reaching 85 years. Aging thickens the bases of the aortic cusps with fibrous tissue. Calcification follows, resulting in audible vibrations. Turbulence produced by blood flow into a dilated aorta may further augment this murmur. In most people, the process of fibrosis and calcification, known as *aortic sclerosis*, does not impede blood flow. In some, the aortic valve leaflets become calcified and immobile, resulting in *aortic stenosis* and outflow obstruction. A brisk carotid upstroke may help distinguish aortic sclerosis from aortic stenosis with its delayed upstroke, but clinical differentiation between aortic sclerosis and aortic stenosis may be difficult. Both carry increased risk for cardiovascular morbidity and mortality.

Similar changes alter the mitral valve, usually approximately one decade later than aortic sclerosis. Calcification of the mitral valve annulus, or valve ring, impedes normal valve closure during systole, causing the systolic murmur of *mitral regurgitation.* This murmur may become pathologic as volume overload increases in the left ventricle.

Peripheral Vascular System.   Aging itself confers relatively few clinically important changes for the peripheral vascular system. Although arterial and venous disorders, especially atherosclerosis, affect older adults more frequently, they probably cannot be considered part of normal aging. Peripheral arteries tend to lengthen, become tortuous, and feel harder and less resilient. These changes do not necessarily indicate atherosclerosis, however, or pathologic changes in the coronary or cerebral vessels.

The common changes in skin, nails, and hair discussed earlier do not arise from arterial disease, though they may accompany it. Loss of arterial pulsations is not typical, however, and demands careful evaluation. An important concern is possible aneurysm in the abdominal aorta in older adults with abdominal or back pain, especially those who are male, smoke, and have coronary disease. Rarely, the temporal arteries in those older than 50 years may become subject to *giant cell,* or *temporal arteritis,* leading to loss of vision in 15% of those affected, and to complaints of headache and jaw claudication. Mean age of onset is 72 years. An important concern is possible aneurysm in the abdominal aorta in older adults with abdominal or back pain, especially those who are male, smoke, and have coronary disease.

Breasts and Axillae.   The normal adult breast may be soft, but also granular, nodular, or lumpy. This uneven texture represents physiologic nodularity. It may be bilateral and palpable throughout or only in parts of the breast. With aging, the female breasts tend to diminish as glandular tissue atrophies and is replaced by fat. The breasts often become flaccid and more pendulous. The ducts surrounding the nipple may become more easily palpable as firm, stringy strands. Axillary hair diminishes.

Abdomen.   During the middle and later years, fat tends to accumulate in the lower abdomen and near the hips, even when total body weight is stable. This accumulation, together with weakening of the abdominal muscles, often produces a soft, more protruding abdomen. Occasionally, patients interpret this change as fluid or evidence of disease.

Aging may blunt the manifestations of acute abdominal disease. Pain may be less severe, fever is often less pronounced, and signs of peritoneal inflammation, such as muscular guarding and rebound tenderness, may be diminished or even absent.

See Chapter 11, The Abdomen, pp. 433–487.

Male and Female Genitalia; Prostate.   As men age, sexual interest appears to remain intact, although frequency of intercourse declines. Several physiologic changes accompany decreasing testosterone levels. Erections become more dependent on tactile stimulation and less responsive to erotic cues. The penis decreases in size, and the testicles drop lower in the scrotum. Protracted illnesses, more than aging, lead to decreased testicular size. Pubic hair may decrease and become gray. Erectile dysfunction, or the inability to have an erection, affects approximately 50% of older men. Vascular causes are the most common, both atherosclerotic arterial occlusive disease and corpora cavernosa venous leak.[13] Chronic diseases such as diabetes, hypertension, dyslipidemia, and smoking, as well as medication side effects, all contribute to prevalence of erectile dysfunction.

In women, ovarian function usually starts to diminish during the fifth decade; on average, menstrual periods cease between 45 and 52 years. As estrogen stimulation falls, many women experience hot flashes, sometimes for up to 5 years. Symptoms range from flushing, sweating, and palpitations to chills and anxiety. Sleep disruption and mood changes are common. Women may report vaginal dryness, urge incontinence, or dyspareunia. Several vulvovaginal changes occur: pubic hair becomes sparse as well as gray; the labia and clitoris become smaller. The vagina narrows and shortens, and the vaginal mucosa becomes thin, pale, and dry, with loss of lubrication. The uterus and ovaries diminish in size. Within 10 years after menopause, the ovaries are usually no longer palpable. The suspensory ligaments of the adnexa, uterus, and bladder may also relax. Sexuality and sexual interest are often unchanged, particularly when women are untroubled by partner issues, partner loss, or unusual work or life stress.[14]

In men, proliferation of prostate epithelial and stromal tissue, termed *benign prostatic hyperplasia (BPH)*, begins in the third decade, yet prostate enlargement results in only about 50%, and symptoms occur in only about half of men with enlargement.[15] Symptoms of urinary hesitancy, dribbling, and incomplete emptying can often be traced to causes other than BPH, such as coexisting disease, use of medication, and lower tract abnormalities. Hyperplasia continues to increase prostate volume until the seventh decade, then appears to plateau. These changes are androgen dependent.

Musculoskeletal System. Musculoskeletal changes continue throughout the adult years. Soon after maturity, subtle losses in height begin; significant shortening is obvious by old age. Most loss of height occurs in the trunk as intervertebral discs become thinner and the vertebral bodies shorten or even collapse from osteoporosis. Flexion at the knees and hips may also contribute to shortened stature. Alterations in the discs and vertebrae also contribute to the kyphosis of aging and increase the anteroposterior diameter of the chest, especially in women. For these reasons, the limbs of an elderly person tend to look long in proportion to the trunk.

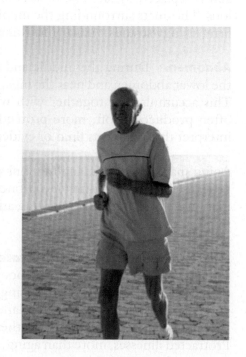

With aging, skeletal muscles decrease in bulk and power, and ligaments lose some of their tensile strength. Range of motion diminishes, partly because of osteoarthritis. Sarcopenia is the loss of lean body mass and strength with aging.[16] The mechanism responsible for muscle loss is not fully understood. Nonetheless, there is a substantial body of evidence that strength training in older adults can slow or reverse this process.

Nervous System. Aging may affect all aspects of the nervous system, from mental status to motor and sensory function and reflexes. Age-related losses can exact a heavy toll. Older adults experience the death of loved ones and friends, retirement from valued employment, diminution in income, decreased physical capacities including impairments in vision and hearing, and often growing social isolation. Moreover, the aging brain experiences biologic changes. Brain volume and the number of cortical brain cells decrease, and both microanatomical and biochemical changes have been identified. Nevertheless, most adults adapt well to growing older. They maintain self-esteem, adapt to their changing capacities and circumstances, and eventually prepare themselves for death.

Most older adults do well on mental status examinations, but selected impairments may become evident, especially at advanced ages. Many older people complain about their memories. "Benign forgetfulness" is the usual explanation and may occur at any age. This term refers to difficulty recalling the names of people or objects or certain details of specific events. Identifying this common phenomenon, when appropriate, may assuage worries about Alzheimer's disease. In addition to this circumscribed forgetfulness, elderly people retrieve and process data more slowly and take more time to learn new material. Their motor responses may slow, and their ability to perform complex tasks may diminish.

Frequently, the clinician must try to distinguish these age-related changes in the nervous system from manifestations of specific mental disorders more prevalent with aging, such as *depression* and *dementia*. Sorting out these ailments may be difficult, because both mood disturbances and cognitive changes can alter the patient's ability to recognize or report symptoms. Older patients are also more susceptible to *delirium*, a temporary state of confusion that may be the first clue to infection or problems with medications. The clinician must learn to recognize these conditions promptly and to protect the patient from harm. Some findings that would be abnormal in younger people, however, occur so often in the elderly that they can be attributed to aging alone, such as the changes in hearing, vision, extraocular movements, and pupillary size, shape, and reactivity described earlier.

Review Chapter 5, Behavior and Mental Status, The Mental Status Examination, pp. 151–160, and Table 20-4, Delirium and Dementia, p. 964.

Changes in the motor system are common. Older adults move and react with less speed and agility than younger ones, and skeletal muscles decrease in bulk. The hands of an aged person often look thin and bony as a result of atrophy of the interosseous muscles, causing muscle wasting in the backs of the hands that leaves concavities or grooves. As illustrated on pp. 708–709, this change may first appear between the thumb and the hand (first and second metacarpals) but may also be seen between the other metacarpals. Small muscle wasting may also flatten the thenar and hypothenar eminences of the palms. Arm and leg muscles can also show signs of atrophy, exaggerating the apparent size of adjacent joints. Muscle strength, though diminished, is relatively well maintained.

Occasionally, an older person develops a benign essential tremor in the head, jaw, lips, or hands that may be confused with parkinsonism. Unlike parkinsonian tremors, however, benign tremors are slightly faster and disappear at rest, and there is no associated muscle rigidity.

See Chapter 17, The Nervous System, Table 17-5, Tremors and Involuntary Movement, pp. 752–753.

Aging may also affect vibratory sense and reflexes. Older adults frequently lose some or all vibration sense in the feet and ankles (but not in the fingers or over the shins). Less commonly, position sense may diminish or disappear. The gag reflex may be diminished or absent. Abdominal reflexes may diminish or disappear. Ankle reflexes may be symmetrically decreased or absent, even when reinforced. Less commonly, knee reflexes are similarly affected. Partly because of musculoskeletal changes in the feet, the plantar responses become less obvious and more difficult to interpret. If other neurologic abnormalities accompany these changes, or if atrophy and reflex changes are asymmetric, you should search for an explanation other than age alone.

The Health History

APPROACH TO THE PATIENT

As you talk with older adults, begin to refine your usual techniques for obtaining the Health History. Your demeanor should convey respect, patience, and cultural awareness. Be sure to address patients by an appropriate title and their last name.

Approach to the Older Adult Patient

▶ Adjusting the office environment
▶ Shaping the content and pace of the visit
▶ Eliciting symptoms
▶ Addressing the cultural dimensions of aging

Adjusting the Office Environment. First, take the time to adapt the environment of the office, hospital, or nursing home to put your patient at ease. Recall the physiologic changes in temperature regulation, and make sure the office is neither too cool nor too warm. Brighter lighting helps compensate for changes in lens proteins; a well-lit room allows the older adult to see your facial expressions and gestures. Face the patient directly, sitting at eye level.

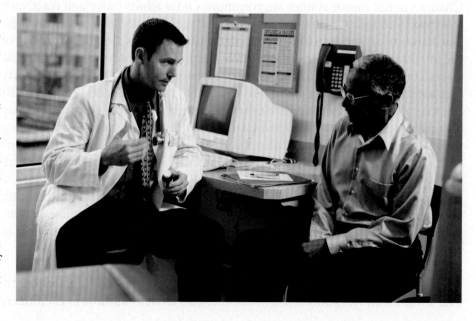

More than 50% of older adults have hearing deficits, especially loss of high-tone discrimination, so a quiet room, free of distractions or noise, is most conducive to good communication. In the hospital setting, turn off the radio or television before starting your discussions. If appropriate, consider using a "pocket talker," a microphone that amplifies your voice and connects to an earpiece inserted by the patient. Adopt low speaking tones, and make sure the patient is using glasses, hearing aids, and dentures when needed to assist with communication. Patients with quadriceps weakness benefit from chairs with higher seating and a wide stool with a handrail leading up to the examining table.[17]

Shaping the Content and Pace of the Visit. With older adults, plan to alter the traditional format of the initial or follow-up visit. From middle age on, people begin to measure their lives in terms of years left rather than years lived. Older people often reminisce about the past and reflect on previous experiences. Listening to this process of life review provides important insights and helps you support patients as they work through painful feelings or recapture joys and accomplishments.

At the same time, it is important to balance the need to assess complex problems with the patient's endurance and possible fatigue. To provide enough time to fully listen to the patient but prevent exhaustion, make ample use of brief and well-validated screening tools,[18] information from home visits and the medical record, and reports from family members, caregivers, and allied health disciplines. Consider dividing the initial assessment into two visits. Two or more shorter visits may be less fatiguing and more productive because older patients frequently need more time to respond to questions, and their explanations may be slow and lengthy.

See "10-Minute Geriatric Screener," p. 942.

Eliciting Symptoms in the Older Adult. Eliciting the history from older adults calls for an astute clinician: Patients may accidentally or purposefully underreport symptoms; the presentation of acute illnesses may be different; common symptoms may mask a geriatric syndrome; patients may have cognitive impairment.

Underreporting. Older patients tend to overestimate their health when affected by increasing disease and disability.[17] It is best to start the visit with open-ended questions like "How can I help you today?" Older patients may be reluctant to report their symptoms. Some are afraid or embarrassed; others try to avoid medical expenses or the discomforts of diagnosis and treatment. Still others overlook their symptoms, thinking they are merely part of aging, or they may simply forget about them. To reduce the risk for late recognition and delayed intervention, adopt more directed questions or health screening tools, and consult with family members and caregivers.

Atypical Presentations of Illness. Acute illnesses present differently in older adults. Older patients with infections are less likely to have fever. In those with myocardial infarction, reports of chest pain fall with increasing age, and complaints of shortness of breath, syncope, stroke, and acute confusion become more common.[19] Older patients with hyperthyroidism and hypothyroidism present with fewer symptoms and signs. In hyperthyroidism, fatigue, weight loss, and tachycardia comprise the most common symptom triad in patients age 50 or older.[20] Older patients are more likely to have anorexia and atrial fibrillation; heat intolerance, increased sweating, and hyperreflexia are considerably rarer. In hypothyroidism, fatigue and weakness are common but notably nonspecific; the usual chilliness, paresthesias, weight gain, and cramps found in younger patients are uncommon.

Geriatric Conditions and Syndromes. Managing an increasing number of interrelated conditions calls for recognizing the symptom clusters typical of different *geriatric syndromes.* These are understood to have the following features: multifactorial origin; typically in older, often frail adults; often precipitated by an acute event; episodic; and often followed by functional decline. Because consensus on the definition is still in flux, some prefer the term *geriatric conditions,* or "a collection of symptoms and signs common in older adults not necessarily related to a specific disease."[9] Examples of geriatric syndromes or conditions include delirium, cognitive impairment, falls, dizziness, depression, urinary incontinence, and functional impairment.[21] Student clinicians need to learn about these syndromes because one symptom may relate to several others in a pattern unfamiliar to the patient. Searching for the usual "unifying diagnosis" may pertain to fewer than 50% of older adults.[22]

Cognitive Impairment. Finally, the student must be knowledgeable about how cognitive impairment affects the patient's history. Evidence suggests that when older patients do report symptoms, their reports are reliable and contain more symptoms than reports from family or collateral sources.[23–25] When compared with unimpaired counterparts, even elders with mild cognitive impairment provide sufficient history to reveal concurrent disorders. Use simple sentences with prompts about necessary information. For patients with more severe impairments, confirm key symptoms with family members or caregivers in the patient's presence and with his or her consent.

Learn to recognize and avoid stereotypes that distort your appreciation of each patient as unique, with a treasure of life experiences. Discover how older patients see themselves and their situations. Listen for their priorities, goals, and coping skills. Such knowledge strengthens your alliance with older patients as you plan for their care and treatment.

Tips for Communicating Effectively With Older Adults

▶ Provide a well-lit, moderately warm setting with minimal background noise and safe chairs and access to the examining table.

▶ Face the patient and speak in low tones; make sure the patient is using glasses, hearing devices, and dentures, if needed.

▶ Adjust the pace and content of the interview to the stamina of the patient; consider two visits for initial evaluations when indicated.

▶ Allow time for open-ended questions and reminiscing; include family and caregivers when needed, especially if the patient has cognitive impairment.

▶ Make use of brief screening instruments, the medical record, and reports from allied disciplines.

▶ Carefully assess symptoms, especially fatigue, loss of appetite, dizziness, weight loss, and pain, for clues to underlying disorders.

▶ Make sure written instructions are in large print and easy to read.

Addressing Cultural Dimensions of Aging. Clinicians must acquire new knowledge, awareness, and skills to improve health and health care delivery for the rapidly growing number of older adults of diverse ethnic backgrounds.[3] In fact, the demographic imperative for older adults is primarily an *ethnogeriatric imperative,* "because by mid-century more than one in three older Americans is projected to be from one of the four populations designated as 'minority,'" as seen in the adjacent graph.[26]

- *Hispanic Americans* over age 65 will jump from 2.7 million in 2008, or 6.8% of older adults, to 17.5 million in 2050, or 19.8% of the older population.[2]

- *African American* older adults will increase from 3.3 million, or 8.5%, to 10.5 million in 2050, or 11.9%.

- *Asian Americans* and other ethnic groups, although smaller in number, will increase from 1.7 million to 10 million, or from 4.6% to 11.2%.

- *Non-Hispanic whites* will almost double in number from 31.2 million to 51.8 million, but will drop from 80.4% to 58.5% of the older adult population by 2050.

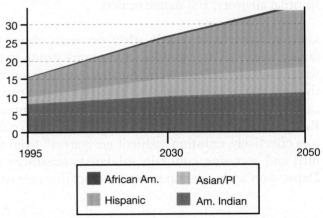

Projected Percentage of Minority Age Groups 65 and Older

Legend: African Am., Asian/PI, Hispanic, Am. Indian

Source: Yeo, F. How will the U.S. healthcare system meet the challenge of the ethnogeriatric imperative? J Am Geriatr Soc 2009;57:1278–1235.

These broad categories in federal reporting hardly capture how older adults of different cultures experience suffering, illness, and decisions about care. Cultural differences affect the epidemiology of illness and mental health, the process of acculturation in families, individual concerns about aging, choices about healers and when to pursue symptoms, the potential for misdiagnosis, and disparities in health outcomes.[27–29] Culture shapes beliefs about the entire spectrum of aging: work and retirement, perceptions of health and illness, the utility of medications, use of health care proxies, and preferences about dying, to name just a few. Health disparities vary markedly in different populations; some are more prevalent and some are less so.[26] Learning about these variations can help tailor interventions for better protection of all. Despite advances in *ethnogeriatrics,*[30] information on racial and ethnic disparities in later life regarding chronic disease, activities of daily living, and self-rated health status remains "limited and inconsistent," and guidelines for providing individualized culturally appropriate care are sparse.[31]

The ***ETHIC(S)*** mnemonic helps clinicians escape the pitfalls of group-labeling by expanding individual history taking to include *Explanation, Treatment, Healers, Negotiate, Intervention, Collaborate, and Spirituality.*[32] However, this model may miss important information about cultural identity, social supports, and views about health care.[33] Experts recommend letting patients establish their cultural identity by probing four key areas during the patient interview: the individual's cultural identity; cultural explanations of the individual's illness; cultural factors related to the psychosocial environment and levels of function; and cultural elements in the clinician–patient relationship. Take the time to visit the Stanford Geriatrics Education Center Web site to test your "ethnogeriatric IQ"[34] and explore

See Table 20-2, Disparities in Health Status of U.S. Older Adults, p. 962.

See Table 20-3, Interviewing Older Adults: Enhancing Culturally Appropriate Care, p. 963.

the Stanford curriculum in ethnogeriatrics.[35] Review the components of self-awareness needed for cultural competency, and learn culturally specific ways to convey respect to older adults and reflect appropriate nonverbal communication. Direct eye contact or handshaking, for example, may not be culturally appropriate. Among the immigrant and refugee groups with particular heath care needs are Vietnamese, Laotians, Haitians, Somalis, Russians and Eastern Europeans, Afghans, and Bosnians. Identify critical life experiences that affect the patient's outlook and psyche arising from the country of origin or migration history. Ask about family decision making, spiritual advisors, and native healers.

Cultural values particularly affect decisions about the end of life. Elders, family, and even an extended community group may make these decisions with or for the older patient. Such group decision making is in contrast to the patient autonomy and informed consent that many contemporary health care providers value, expect, and automatically assume to be desired by all.[36] Being sensitive to the stresses of migration and acculturation, using translators effectively, enlisting "patient navigators" from the family and community, and accessing culturally validated assessment tools like the Geriatric Depression Scale are important for empathic care of older adults.[37]

See Chapter 3, Demonstrating Cultural Humility—A Changing Paradigm, pp. 73–77.

See Chapter 3, Interviewing and the Health History, on working with translators, pp. 81–82.

SPECIAL AREAS OF CONCERN WHEN ASSESSING COMMON OR CONCERNING SYMPTOMS

Common Concerns

▸ Activities of daily living
▸ Instrumental activities of daily living
▸ Medications
▸ Acute and persistent pain
▸ Smoking and alcohol
▸ Nutrition
▸ Frailty
▸ Advance directives and palliative care

Symptoms in the older adult can have many meanings and interconnections, as we have seen previously in geriatric conditions and syndromes (p. 928). Explore the meaning of these symptoms as you would with all patients, and review the Common or Concerning Symptoms sections in previous chapters. For older adults, be sure to place these symptoms in the context of your overall functional assessment. Several areas warrant special attention as you gather the health history. Approach the following areas with extra thoroughness and sensitivity, always focusing on helping the older adult to maintain optimal level of function and well-being.

Activities of Daily Living.   Learning how older adults, especially those with chronic illness, function in terms of daily activities is essential and provides an important baseline for future evaluations. First, ask about the capacity to perform the *activities of daily living (ADLs);* these consist of basic self-care abilities. Then move on to inquiries about capacity for higher level functions, the *instrumental activities of daily living (IADLs).* Can the patient perform these activities independently, does he or she need some help, or is the patient entirely dependent on others?

You may wish to start with an open-ended request like "Tell me about your typical day" or "Tell me about your day yesterday." Then move to a greater level of detail . . . "You got up at 8 AM? How is it getting out of bed? . . . What did you do next?" Ask how things have changed, who is available for help, and what helpers actually do. Remember that assessing the patient's safety is one of your priorities.

Activities of Daily Living and Instrumental Activities of Daily Living

Physical Activities of Daily Living (ADLs)	Instrumental Activities of Daily Living (IADLs)
Bathing	Using the telephone
Dressing	Shopping
Toileting	Preparing food
Transferring	Housekeeping
Continence	Laundry
Feeding	Transportation
	Taking medicine
	Managing money

Medications. Prescription drug statistics expose the rationale for obtaining a complete drug history.[7] Those older than 65 years receive approximately 30% of all prescriptions. Approximately 80% of older adults have at least one chronic disease and take at least one prescription drug each day. Roughly 30% of 65-and-over adults take more than eight prescribed drugs each day. Older adults have more than 50% of all reported adverse drug reactions causing hospital admission, reflecting pharmacodynamic changes in the distribution, metabolism, and elimination of drugs that place them at increased risk.

Take a thorough *medication history,* including name, dose, frequency, and indication for each drug. Be sure to explore all components of polypharmacy, including suboptimal prescribing, concurrent use of multiple drugs, underuse, inappropriate use, and nonadherence. Ask about use of over-the-counter medications, vitamin and nutritional supplements, and mood-altering drugs such as narcotics, benzodiazepines, and recreational substances. Assess medications for drug interactions. Be particularly careful when treating *insomnia,* estimated to occur in 40% of older adults. A *sleep history* provides information essential for diagnosis; a *sleep diary* may be especially helpful in uncovering the origins of a poor sleep pattern.[38] Increased exercise may be the best remedy. Types of sleep disorders and recommended management are described in the 2009 guidelines.[39]

Recall that medications are the most common modifiable risk factor associated with falls. Review strategies for avoiding polypharmacy. It is wise to keep the number of drugs prescribed to a minimum and to "start low, go slow" with respect to dosing. Learn about drug–drug interactions and the *Beers criteria* listing drugs contraindicated in older adults.[40,41] Although it is derived from an inpatient study, review the GeroNet Adverse Drug Reaction (ADR) Risk Score to help prevent unnecessary illness and hospital admissions.[42] Patients with scores >3 to 4 are at high risk for ADRs.

GeroNet Risk Score for ADRs

Variable	OR (95% CI)	Points
>4 Comorbid conditions	1.31 (1.04–1.64)	
Heart Failure	1.79 (1.39–2.30)	1
Liver disease	1.36 (1.06–1.74)	1
No. of drugs		1
≤5	1 [Reference]	0
5–7	1.90 (1.35–2.68)	1
≥8	4.07 (2.93–5.65)	4
Previous ADR	2.41 (1.79–3.23)	2
Renal failure (GFR <60 mL/min)	1.21 (0.96–1.51)	1

Source: Onder G, Petrovic M, Balamurugan T et al. Less is more. Development and validation of a score to assess risk of adverse drug reactions among the in-hospital patients 65 years or older. Arch Intern Med 2010;170:1142–1148.

Acute and Persistent Pain. Pain and associated complaints account for 80% of clinician visits. Prevalence of pain may reach 25% to 50% in community-dwelling adults and 40% to 80% in nursing home residents. Pain usually arises from musculoskeletal complaints such as back and joint pain.[43] Headache, neuralgias from diabetes and herpes zoster, nighttime leg pain, and cancer pain are also common. Older patients are less likely to report pain, leading to undue suffering, depression, social isolation, physical disability, and loss of function. The American Geriatrics Society favors the term *persistent pain,* because "chronic pain" is associated with negative stereotypes.[44]

Pain is subjective, so some view pain as a spectrum disorder rather than "the fifth vital sign." See discussion, pp. 127–130.

Characteristics of Acute and Persistent Pain

Acute Pain	Persistent Pain
Distinct onset	Lasts more than 3 months
Obvious pathology	Often associated with psychological or functional impairment
Short duration	Can fluctuate in character and intensity over time
Common causes: postsurgical, trauma, headache	Common causes: arthritis, cancer, claudication, leg cramps, neuropathy, radiculopathy

Source: Reuben DB, Herr KA, Pacala JT, et al. Geriatrics at Your Fingertips: 2004, 6th ed., p. 119. Malden, MA: Blackwell Publishing, Inc., for the American Geriatrics Society, 2004.

Accurate assessment is the basis of effective treatment. Inquire about pain *each time* you meet with an older patient. Assessing pain in older adults is challenging. Patients may not want to report symptoms because of fears of additional testing, costs, or progression of disease.[45] There may be cognitive or verbal impairments, or barriers of trust, language, or cultural understanding. The patient may report multiple conditions that complicate assessment. Nonetheless, evidence shows that pain reporting by patients with even mild to moderate cognitive impairment is reliable. Ask specifically, "Are you having any pain right now? How about during the past week?" Be alert for signs of untreated pain, such as use of the terms "burning," "discomfort," or "soreness," depressed affect, and nonverbal change in posture or gait. Many multidimensional and unidimensional pain scales are available. Unidimensional scales such as the Visual Analog Scale, graphic pictures, and the Verbal 0–10 Scale have all been validated and are easiest to use.[43,46] Recruit caregivers or family members for relevant history in patients with severe cognitive deficits.

Learn to distinguish acute pain from persistent pain, and thoroughly investigate its cause. In older adults, confusion, restlessness, fatigue, or irritability may all arise from conditions causing pain. Assessing pain includes comprehensive evaluation of its effects on quality of life, social interactions, and functional level. Multidisciplinary assessment is warranted if the cause cannot be identified and risks of disability and comorbidity are high. Study the many modalities of pain relief, ranging from analgesics to the full range of nonpharmacologic therapies, especially those that engage patients directly and actively in their treatment plan and build self-reliance. Patient education alone has been shown effective.[44] Relaxation techniques, tai chi, acupuncture, massage, and biofeedback can avert adding more medications.

See the *10-Minute Geriatric Screener* for functional assessment on p. 942.

Smoking and Alcohol. *Smoking* is harmful at all ages. At each visit, advise smokers, approximately 13% of older adults, to quit.[47] The commitment to stop smoking may take time, but quitting is a crucial step to reducing risk for heart disease, pulmonary disease, malignancy, and loss of daily function.

At-risk drinking guidelines are lower for adults over 65, due to physiologic changes that amplify harm from *alcohol*, as well as frequent comorbid illness and risk of drug interactions. No more than three drinks on any occasion or seven drinks a week are recommended.[48] The estimated prevalence of alcohol-related problems in older adults ranges from 2% to 22%, hovering around 10% in recent studies.[49–51] Lifelong prevalence of alcohol dependency and abuse ranges from 4% to 8%.[52] Rates of alcoholism in older patients in the hospital, emergency room, and clinic settings has been reported at 21%, 24%, and 36%, respectively. Alcohol accounts for roughly 1% of hospital admissions in this age group. Harmful and hazardous drinking may encompass a much broader group depending on functional status, medications, and comorbidities, including anxiety and depression.[53]

Despite the prevalence of alcohol-related problems, rates of detection and treatment are low. Screening all older adults is especially important, because many medications have adverse interactions with alcohol, and up to 30% of older adult drinkers exacerbate co-morbid ailments like cirrhosis, gastrointestinal bleeding or reflux disease, gout, hypertension, diabetes, insomnia, gait disorders, and depression.[54] Look for the clues shown in the box below, especially in elders with recent bereavement or losses, pain, disability or depression, or a family history of alcohol disorders.

Detecting Alcohol-Use Disorders in Older Adults: Clinical Clues

▶ Memory loss, cognitive impairment
▶ Depression, anxiety
▶ Neglect of hygiene, appearance
▶ Poor appetite, nutritional deficits
▶ Sleep disruption
▶ Hypertension refractory to therapy
▶ Blood sugar control problems
▶ Seizures refractory to therapy
▶ Impaired balance and gait, falls
▶ Recurrent gastritis and esophagitis
▶ Difficulty managing warfarin dosing

Source: American Geriatrics Society. Screening recommendation: clinical guidelines for alcohol use disorders in older adults. Available at http://www.annalsoflongtermcare.com/article/5143. Accessed February 15, 2011.

Use the CAGE questions to uncover problem drinking. Although symptoms and signs are subtler in older adults, making early detection more difficult, the four CAGE questions remain sensitive and specific in this age group, using the conventional cutoff score of 2 or more.[53,54]

See Chapter 3, Interviewing and the Health History, Alcohol and Illicit Drugs, pp. 88–89.

Nutrition. Taking a diet history and using the Rapid Screen for Dietary Intake and the Nutrition Screening Checklist are especially important in older adults. Prevalence of undernutrition increases with age, affecting 5% to 10% of elderly outpatients and 30% to 50% of hospitalized elders.[55] Those with chronic disease are particularly at risk, especially those with poor dentition, oral or gastrointestinal disorders, depression or other psychiatric illness, and drug regimens that affect appetite and oral secretions. For underweight elders, the serum albumin is an independent risk factor for all-cause mortality.[56]

Frailty. *Frailty* is a multifactorial geriatric condition or syndrome characterized by an age-related lack of adaptive physiological capacity that can occur even in the absence of identifiable illness. Depending on scoring criteria and the population studied, prevalence ranges from 4% to 22%.[57] Frailty is characterized by loss of muscle mass, decreased energy and exercise intolerance, and decreased physiological reserve, with increasing vulnerability to physiological stressors.[58] Screen your patients for the presence of three of the five central components identified in the Cardiovascular Health Study and pursue related interventions: unintentional weight loss, slow walking speed, self-reported exhaustion, low energy expenditure, and weakness.[59]

Advance Directives and Palliative Care. Many older patients are interested in expressing their wishes about end-of-life decisions and would like providers to initiate these discussions before any serious illness develops.[60] More than a quarter of older adults may require surrogate decision making at the end of life.[61] Advance care planning involves several tasks: providing information, invoking the patient's preferences, identifying proxy decision makers, and discussion by relating these decisions to a current illness or experiences with relatives or friends. Ask about preferences relating to written "Do Not Resuscitate" orders specifying life support measures "if the heart or lungs were to stop or give out." Second, encourage the patient to establish in writing a health care proxy or durable power of attorney for health care, "someone who can make decisions reflecting your wishes in case of confusion or emergency." These conversations, although difficult at first, convey your respect and concern for patients and help them and their families prepare openly and in advance for a peaceful death.[62] Encourage these discussions in an office setting rather than in the uncertain and stressful environment of emergency or acute care.

For patients with advanced or terminal illnesses, include the review of advance directives in an overall plan for palliative care.[63] The goal of palliative care is "to relieve suffering and improve the quality of life for patients with advanced illnesses and their families through specific knowledge and skills, including communication with patients and family members; management of pain and other symptoms; psychosocial, spiritual, and bereavement support; and coordination of an array of medical and social services."[64] To ease patient and family distress, focus on your communication skills: Make good eye contact; ask open-ended questions; respond to anxiety, depression, or changes in the patient's affect; show empathy; and be sure to consult caregivers.

See also Chapter 3, The Patient With Altered Capacity, pp. 78–79, and Death and the Dying Patient, pp. 90–92.

Health Promotion and Counseling: Evidence and Recommendations

Important Topics for Health Promotion and Counseling in the Older Adult

- When to screen
- Vision and hearing
- Exercise
- Immunizations
- Household safety and fall prevention
- Cancer screening
- Depression
- Dementia, mild cognitive impairment, and cognitive decline
- Elder mistreatment and abuse

When to Screen. As the life span for older adults extends into the 80s, new issues for screening emerge. Given the heterogeneity of the aging population, guiding principles for deciding who might benefit from screening and when screening might be stopped are helpful, especially because evidence for making screening decisions is not always available. In general, base screening decisions on each older person's particular circumstances, rather than age alone. Three factors should be considered: life expectancy, time interval until benefit from screening accrues, and patient preference.[65] The American Geriatrics Society recommends that if life expectancy is short, give priority to treatment that will benefit the patient in the time that remains. Consider deferring screening if it places added burdens on the older adult with multiple medical problems, a shortened life expectancy, or dementia. Tests that help with prognosis and planning, however, are still warranted even if the patient would not pursue treatment.[66]

Vision and Hearing. Screening for age-related changes in *vision* and *hearing* is important to help older adults maintain optimal function, and is included in the 10-Minute Geriatric Screener. Test *vision* objectively using an eye chart. Asking the patient about any *hearing* loss may be adequate, followed by the whisper test and more formal testing if indicated. Among adults over 65 years, 17% have trouble seeing and 35% have trouble hearing.[3]

See 10-Minute Geriatric Screener, p. 942.

See Chapter 7, The Head and Neck, techniques for assessing hearing, pp. 235–238.

Exercise. Recommend regular aerobic exercise to improve strength and aerobic capacity, increase physiologic reserve, improve energy for doing ADLs, and slow onset of disability. Recent studies show that exercise improves psychological well-being, including anxiety and depression, and reduces risk of cognitive decline and dementia.[67]

In its updated 2009 recommendations, the American College of Sports Medicine advocates a physically active lifestyle with moderate intensity exercise for at least 10 to 30 minutes a day or up to 150 minutes a week.[67] Those limited by chronic conditions "should be as physically active as their abilities and conditions allow." The ideal exercise program should include aerobic exercise for endurance, muscle strengthening exercises against resistance, and flexibility exercises. Those with risk of falling or impaired mobility should also do balance exercises. For older adults who are deconditioned or functionally limited, "the intensity and duration of physical activity should be low at the outset"; for those with chronic conditions "the progression of activities should be individual and tailored to tolerance and preference." In the very frail, strength and balance exercise may need to precede aerobic activity. The College notes that "although no amount of physical activity can stop the biological aging process, there is evidence that regular exercise can minimize the physiological effects of an otherwise sedentary lifestyle and increase active life expectancy by limiting the development and progression of chronic disease and disabling conditions."

Immunizations. Offer your patients vaccines for influenza, pneumonia, zoster (shingles), and tetanus/diphtheria (Td). Vaccination rates still lag for targeted groups, especially Hispanics and African Americans.

See also Chapter 8, The Thorax and Lungs, Immunizations, pp. 304–305.

Older Adult Immunizations 2010–2011

Influenza vaccine.[68] The following groups should receive the influenza vaccine each year:

- *All adults ≥50 years*
- Adults with chronic pulmonary and cardiovascular disorders including asthma (but excluding hypertension), and renal, hepatic, neurologic, hematologic or metabolic disorders including diabetes
- Adults who are immunosuppressed from medication or HIV
- Residents of nursing homes and other chronic care facilities; adults with morbid obesity (BMI ≥40)
- Household contacts and caregivers of children under 5 years and adults ≥50 years, especially those with medical conditions placing them at risk for severe complications from influenza

Pneumococcal vaccine[69]

- *All adults ≥65 years;* for those with their first vaccination at age 65, only one vaccination is needed. Those vaccinated before age 65 should be revaccinated at age 65 years or later if at least 5 years have passed since their previous dose.
- *Adults ages 19–64 years* should also be vaccinated if they fall in the following groups: chronic conditions from heart disease (except hypertension), lung disease including asthma, diabetes, cochlear implants, alcoholism, liver disease, smoking, and cerebrospinal fluid leaks; functional or anatomic asplenia; and immunocompromise from HIV, malignancy, medications, transplants, and renal failure and nephritic syndrome

Zoster vaccine[70]

- *All adults ≥60 years*, regardless of whether they have already had either chicken pox or shingles. Vaccination reduces herpes zoster infection by over 50% and postherpetic neuralgia by over 65%.
- The vaccine should not be given to adults with a history of a primary or acquired immunodeficiency state, including leukemia, lymphoma, or other malignant neoplasm affecting the bone marrow or lymphatic system, or with HIV/AIDs or to those receiving immunosuppressive therapy, including high-dose corticosteroids.

Tetanus/diphtheria (Td) vaccine[71,72]

- *Adults* with an uncertain or incomplete history of primary vaccination, should receive three doses of Td or Tdap (Td plus acellular pertussis), then a Td booster every 10 years.
- Adults ≤65 years should get Tdap if they have never received Tdap previously and/or have contact with infants ≤12 months of age to protect against pertussis.

Household Safety and Fall Prevention. Emergency room visits for household injuries are increasing at a rapid rate, particularly for adults older than 75 years. In a 2002 special report, the U.S. Consumer Product Safety Commission estimated that almost 1.5 million adults older than 65 years were treated for injuries related to household products, including more than 60% with falls. Emergency room visits and deaths were most likely to involve yard

See also Assessing and Preventing Falls, pp. 943–944.

and garden equipment, ladders and stepstools, personal use items like hair dryers and flammable clothing, and bathroom and sports injuries. Encourage older adults to adopt corrective measures for poor lighting, chairs at awkward heights, slippery or irregular surfaces, and environmental hazards.

Home Safety Tips for Older Adults

▶ Handrails on both sides of any stairway
▶ Well-lit stairways, paths, and walkways
▶ Rugs secured by nonslip backing or adhesive tape
▶ Grab bars and nonslip mat or safety strips in the bath or shower
▶ Smoke alarms and plan for escaping fire

Cancer Screening. Cancer screening recommendations for older adults remain controversial, primarily due to limited evidence, especially for adults over ages 70 to 75.[54,65] Geriatricians currently advise *individualized decision making* based on: (1) estimated life expectancy, usually beyond 5 years; (2) the potential benefits and harms from screening, including risk of dying from the disease being screened; and (3) the potential benefits and harms according to the individual's values and preferences. Current recommendations of the U.S. Preventive Services Task Force (USPSTF) are summarized below.[73] Detailed discussions of screening guidelines are available through the American Geriatrics Society.[74]

See also discussions about screening for breast cancer, pp. 415–417, prostate cancer, pp. 580–583 , cervical cancer, pp. 548–550, and colorectal cancer, p. 585.

Screening Recommendations for Older Adults: U.S. Preventive Services Task Force

▶ **Breast cancer (2009):** Recommends mammography every 2 years for women ages 50 to 74; cites insufficient evidence for women ≥75 years.
▶ **Cervical cancer (2003):** Recommends against routine screening for women older than age 65 if they have had adequate recent screening with normal Pap smears and are not otherwise at high risk for cervical cancer, based on fair evidence
▶ **Colorectal cancer (2008):** Recommends screening with colonoscopy every 10 years, sigmoidoscopy every 5 years with high-sensitivity fecal occult blood tests (FOBTs) every 3 years, or FOBTs every year beginning age 50 years through age 75 years. Recommends against routine screening for adults ages 76 to 85 years, due to moderate certainty that the net benefit is small.
▶ **Prostate cancer (2008):** States that evidence is insufficient to balance the benefits and harms of screening for men <75 years; recommends against screening men ≥75 years.
▶ **Skin cancer (2009), lung cancer (2004):** States that evidence is insufficient to balance the benefits and harms of whole-body skin examinations or screening for lung cancer.

Depression. *Depression* affects approximately 10% of older men and 18% of older women, but is both underdiagnosed and undertreated.[3,75] In older adults, only two screening questions are needed, reaching a sensitivity of 100% and specificity of 77%.[76–78]

See Chapter 5, Behavior and Mental Status, Depression, pp. 149–150.

- "Over the past 2 week have you felt down, depressed, hopeless?" (screens for depressed mood)

- "Over the past 2 weeks have you felt little interest or pleasure in doing things?" (screens for anhedonia)

Positive responses should prompt further investigation with scales such as the Geriatric Depression Scale.[79] Depressed men over age 65 years are at increased risk for suicide and require particularly careful evaluation.

Dementia, Mild Cognitive Impairment, and Cognitive Decline. *Dementia* is "an acquired syndrome of decline in memory and at least one other cognitive domain such as language, visuospatial, or executive function sufficient to interfere with social or occupational functioning in an alert person."[80] Alzheimer's disease (AD), the predominant form of dementia, affects 13% of Americans over age 65, or roughly 5.1 million people.[81,82] As the aging population increases, by 2050 prevalence will exceed 13 million cases.[83] Risk factors include advancing age, family history, and the gene mutation apolipoprotein (APOE) ε4. Risk of AD more than doubles in first-degree relatives. Risk doubles in the presence of one APOE ε4 allele and increases fivefold or more in the presence of two alleles.[84]

Diagnosis of AD is challenging: the mechanisms of disease are still under intense investigation; the absence of a consistent and uniformly applied definition of disease continues to hamper investigation of risk factors; between 60% and 90% of Alzheimer patients have coexisting ischemic disease; and distinguishing *age-related cognitive decline* from *mild cognitive impairment* and AD remains problematic.[81,83,85] Presence of delirium and depression can further complicate diagnosis.[86] Some distinguishing clues have emerged from the current literature.

See Table 20-4, Delirium and Dementia, p. 964, and Table 20-5, Screening for Dementia: The Mini-Cog, p. 965.

- ***Age-related cognitive decline:*** suggested by mild forgetfulness, difficulty remembering names, mildly reduced concentration. Such symptoms are sporadic and do affect function.

- ***Mild cognitive impairment (MCI):*** evidence of memory impairment without cognitive deficits or functional decline. AD develops at a higher frequency in MCI patients, progressing to AD at a rate of approximately 12% to 15% per year.[87–89]

- ***Alzheimer's disease:*** normal alertness but progressive global deterioration of cognition in multiple domains, including short-term memory, but with sparing of memory for remote events; subtle language errors; visuospatial perceptual difficulties; and changes in executive function, or the ability to perform sequential tasks such as IADLs. Memory difficulties may take the form of repeating questions, losing objects, or confusion when performing tasks such as shopping. Later stages include impaired judgment and disorientation progressing to aphasia, apraxia, left–right confusion, and ultimately dependence of IADLs. Psychosis and agitation may also occur.

Screening with the *Mini Mental State Examination* or the *Mini-Cog* is recommended, although it may not be definitive. It is important to obtain collateral information from family members and caretakers. Formal neuropsychological testing may also be necessary. For a current summary and screening tools, download the overview from the American Geriatrics Society, *A Guide to Dementia Diagnosis and Treatment*.[90]

See Table 20-5, Screenings for Dementia: The Mini-Cog, p. 965.

Once you identify cognitive changes, investigate contributing factors such as medications, metabolic abnormalities, depression, delirium, and other medical and psychiatric conditions, including vascular risks such as diabetes and hypertension. Counsel families about the challenges for caregivers and review household safety. The NIHSeniorHealth Web site is especially helpful.[91] Learn the laws about reporting *drivers with dementia* in your state. Consult the American Academy of Neurology Evidence-Based Practice Parameter for drivers with dementia, updated in 2010, and the National Highway Traffic Safety Administration for simulations and other resources for assessing impaired drivers.[92–94] Foster patient and family discussion of arranging for health proxies, power of attorney, and advance directives while the patient can still contribute to active decision making.

See Chapter 3, The Patient with Altered Capacity, pp. 78–79.

Elder Mistreatment and Abuse. Finally, screen vulnerable older adults for possible *elder mistreatment*, which includes abuse, neglect, exploitation, and abandonment. Prevalence ranges from 1% to 10%, depending on the population studied, and is even higher among older adults with depression and dementia.[95,96] Most studies rely on self-report, so many more cases remain undetected.[97] Self-neglect is a growing national concern and represents more the 505 of adult protective service referrals. Several screening instruments are available, but no single instrument has emerged for rapid yet accurate assessment of these important problems.[97,98]

Techniques of Examination

As you have seen, assessment of the older adult does not follow the traditional format of the history and physical examination. It calls for enhanced interviewing techniques, special emphasis on daily function and key topics related to older adult health, and a focus on functional assessment during the physical examination. Because of its importance to the health of older adults and the order of your assessment, this section begins with Assessing

Functional Status: the "Sixth Vital Sign." This segment includes how to evaluate risk for falls, one of the greatest threats to health and well-being in older adults. Next, are elements of the traditional "head-to-toe" examination tailored to the older adult.

ASSESSING FUNCTIONAL STATUS: THE "SIXTH VITAL SIGN"

During assessment of older adults, place a special premium on maintaining the patient's health and well-being. In a sense, all visits are opportunities to promote the patient's independence and optimal level of function. Although the specific goals of care may vary, preserving the patient's functional status, the "sixth vital sign," is of primary importance. Functional status specifically means the ability to perform tasks and fulfill social roles associated with daily living across a wide range of complexity.[99] Your assessment of functional status begins as the patient enters the room. Several validated and time-efficient assessment tools can facilitate this approach.

Assessing *functional status* provides a baseline for establishing interventions to optimize the health of your older patients and for identifying *geriatrics conditions and syndromes* that can be modified or prevented, such as cognitive impairment, falls, incontinence, low body mass index, dizziness, impaired vision and hearing. Deficits in function are now recognized as better predictors of patient outcome and mortality after hospitalization than the admitting diagnoses. The USPSTF in 2010 outlined new prevention recommendations for older adults that better recognize the multifactorial nature of geriatric syndromes and bundles recommendations on related topics, such as osteoporosis, vitamin D supplementation, and prevention of falls, so that they are "more consistent, interlinked, and comprehensive" and directed at interventions that are effective.[100]

One useful performance-based assessment tool is the *10-Minute Geriatric Screener*, which is brief, has high interrater agreement, and can be easily used by office staff.[101] It covers three important areas of geriatric assessment: cognitive, psychosocial, and physical function. It includes vision, hearing, and questions about urinary incontinence, an often hidden source of social isolation and distress in up to 30% of older women and 15% to 28% of men.[102] For elucidating causes of incontinence, two mnemonics may be helpful: DIAPERS, (Delirium, Infection, Atrophic urethritis/vaginitis, Pharmaceuticals, Excess urine output from conditions like hyperglycemia or heart failure, Restricted mobility, and Stool impaction) and DDRRIIPP (Delirium, Drug side effects, Retention of feces, Restricted mobility, Infection of urine, Inflammation, Polyuria, and Psychogenic).

10-Minute Geriatric Screener

Problem	Screening Measure	Positive Screen

Vision	Two parts:
	  Ask: "Do you have difficulty driving, or watching television, or reading, or doing any of your daily activities because of your eyesight?"
	If yes, then:
	  Test each eye with Snellen chart while patient wears corrective lenses (if applicable).
		Yes to question and inability to read >20/40 on Snellen chart

Hearing	Use audioscope set at 40 dB. Test hearing using 1,000 and 2,000 Hz.	Inability to hear 1,000 or 2,000 Hz in both ears or either of these frequencies in one ear
Leg mobility	Time the patient after asking: "Rise from the chair. Walk 20 feet briskly, turn, walk back to the chair, and sit down."	Unable to complete task in 15 seconds

Urinary incontinence	Two parts:
	  Ask: "In the last year, have you ever lost your urine and gotten wet?"
	If yes, then ask:
	  "Have you lost urine on at least 6 separate dates?"
		Yes to both questions

Nutrition/weight loss	Two parts: Ask: "Have you lost 10 lbs over the past 6 months without trying to do so?" Weigh the patient.	Yes to the question or weight <100 lbs
Memory	Three-item recall	Unable to remember all three items after 1 minute
Depression	Ask: "Do you often feel sad or depressed?"	Yes to the question

Physical disability	Six questions: "Are you able to . . . :
	  "Do strenuous activities like fast walking or bicycling?"
	  "Do heavy work around the house like washing windows, walls, or floors?"
	  "Go shopping for groceries or clothes?"
	  "Get to places out of walking distance?"
	  "Bathe, either a sponge bath, tub bath, or shower?"
	  "Dress, like putting on a shirt, buttoning and zipping, or putting on shoes?"
		No to any of the questions

Source: Moore AA, Siu AL. Screening for common problems in ambulatory elderly: clinical confirmation of a screening instrument. Am J Med 1996;100:438–440.

Further Assessment for Preventing Falls.   A preponderance of evidence links falls, a multifactorial geriatric syndrome, to fatal and nonfatal injuries, mortality, and burgeoning medical costs that exceed $20 billion annually.[103] Falls are also linked to declines in function and early admission to long-term care facilities. At least one-third of adults aged 65 years or older fall at least once a year, and falls are the leading cause of fatal and nonfatal injuries in this age group. Investigators point out that falls "are not purely random events but can be predicted by assessing a number of risk factors."[104] Several recent reviews and meta-analyses have identified risk factors and effective interventions more precisely. In 2010, the American Geriatrics Society and British Geriatrics Society updated their algorithm for preventing falls in older adults (see p. 944).[105] Study the algorithm and note the key features you should incorporate into your practice:

- Screen fall risk for all community-dwelling older adults

- Identify *high-risk older adults*, namely those with a single fall in the past 12 months with abnormal gait and balance and those with two or more falls in the prior 12 months, an acute fall, and/or difficulties with gait and balance

- Assess older adults at high risk by conducting:

  - A detailed fall history, medication review, and history of relevant risk factors such as acute and chronic medical problems

  - A detailed assessment of gait, balance, mobility, and lower extremity joint function; neurologic function, lower extremity muscle strength; cardiovascular status; visual acuity, and examination of the feet and footwear

  - Functional assessment

  - Environmental assessment

- Implement multifactorial/multicomponent interventions to address identified risks and prevent falls

Although study methodologies for fall interventions vary greatly, evidence is strongest for the following: gait, balance, and strength training, particularly over an extended period, reported to reduce falls by about 13%; vitamin D supplementation of 700 IU to 1,000 IU daily, which reduces falls by 17%; and minimization or withdrawal of psychoactive and other medications.[104,106–109] Multifactorial interventions appear to be more effective than interventions targeted to specific risk factors, reducing falls by 6%, increasing to 11% when there is fall risk management. Additional prevention strategies that have been evaluated include reducing home hazards, vision correction, and improved management of chronic conditions such as change in postural blood pressure, and numerous types and combinations of exercise. Gait velocity and hand grip are also emerging as possible predictors of falls.[110,111]

Prevention of Falls in Older Persons Living in the Community

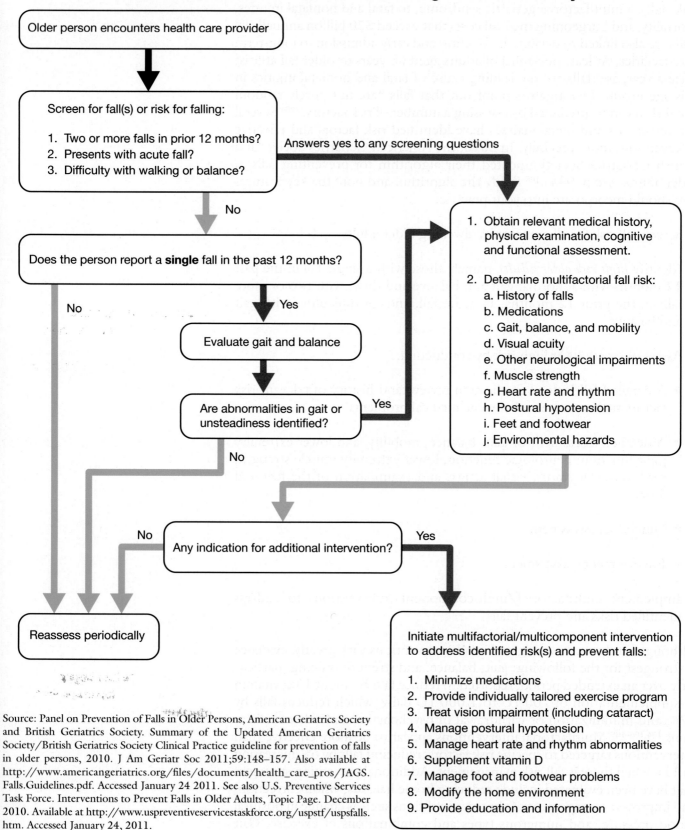

Source: Panel on Prevention of Falls in Older Persons, American Geriatrics Society and British Geriatrics Society. Summary of the Updated American Geriatrics Society/British Geriatrics Society Clinical Practice guideline for prevention of falls in older persons, 2010. J Am Geriatr Soc 2011;59:148–157. Also available at http://www.americangeriatrics.org/files/documents/health_care_pros/JAGS. Falls.Guidelines.pdf. Accessed January 24 2011. See also U.S. Preventive Services Task Force. Interventions to Prevent Falls in Older Adults, Topic Page. December 2010. Available at http://www.uspreventiveservicestaskforce.org/uspstf/uspsfalls. htm. Accessed January 24, 2011.

PHYSICAL EXAMINATION OF THE OLDER ADULT

General Survey.   Deepen the observations about the patient that you have been compiling since the visit began. What is the patient's apparent state of health and degree of vitality? What about mood and affect? Is screening for cognitive changes needed? Note the patient's hygiene and how the patient is dressed. How does the patient walk into the room? Move onto the examining table? Are there changes in posture or involuntary movements?

Flat or impoverished affect occurs in *depression, Parkinson's disease,* or *Alzheimer's disease.*

See Table 20-5, Screening for Dementia: The Mini-Cog, p. 965, for a brief and validated screening tool for dementia.[112,113]

Undernutrition, slowed motor performance, loss of muscle mass, or weakness suggests frailty. Kyphosis or abnormal gait can impair balance and increase risk of falls.

Vital Signs.   Measure blood pressure using recommended techniques (see pp. 119–124), checking for increased systolic blood pressure (SBP) and widened pulse pressure (PP), defined as SBP minus diastolic blood pressure (DBP). With aging, SBP and peripheral vascular resistance increase, whereas DBP decreases. In the "oldest old," those 80 years of age and older, blood pressure targets of 140 to 150/70 to 80 appear optimal.[114–118]

Isolated systolic hypertension (SBP ≥140) after age 50 triples the risk for coronary heart disease in men and increases risk of stroke; PP ≥60 is a risk factor for cardiovascular and renal disease and stroke.[119,120]

Assess the patient for orthostatic hypotension, defined as a drop in SBP of ≥20 mm Hg or DBP of ≥10 mm Hg within 3 minutes of standing. Measure blood pressure and heart rate in two positions: supine after the patient rests for up to 10 minutes; then within 3 minutes.

Review the JNC 7 categories of prehypertension to help you with early detection and treatment of hypertension (p. 124).

Orthostatic hypotension occurs in 20% of older adults and in up to 50% of frail nursing home residents, especially when they first arise in the morning. Symptoms include lightheadedness, weakness, unsteadiness, visual blurring, and, in 20% to 30% of patients, syncope. Causes include medications, autonomic disorders, diabetes, prolonged bed rest, volume depletion, amyloidosis, and cardiovascular disorders.[121–125]

Measure heart rate, respiratory rate, and temperature. The apical heart rate may yield more information about arrhythmias in older patients. Use thermometers accurate for lower temperatures. Obtain oxygen saturation using a pulse oximeter.

Respiratory rate ≥25 breaths per minute indicates lower respiratory infection; also heart failure and chronic obstructive pulmonary disease exacerbation.

Hypothermia is more common in older patients.

Weight and height are especially important in the elderly and are needed for calculation of the body mass index. Weight should be measured at every visit.

Skin.   Note physiologic changes of aging, such as thinning, loss of elastic tissue and turgor, and wrinkling. Skin may be dry, flaky, rough, and often itchy *(asteatosis)*, with a latticework of shallow fissures that creates a mosaic of small polygons, especially on the legs.

Observe any patchy changes in color. Check the extensor surface of the hands and forearms for white depigmented patches, or *pseudoscars*, and for well-demarcated vividly purple macules or patches, *actinic purpura*, that may fade after several weeks.

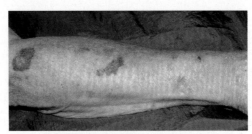

ACTINIC PURPURA—FOREARM

Look for changes from sun exposure. Areas of skin may appear weather beaten, thickened, yellowed, and deeply furrowed; there may be *actinic lentigines*, or "liver spots," and *actinic keratoses*, superficial flattened papules covered by a dry scale.

Inspect for the benign lesions of aging, namely *comedones*, or blackheads, on the cheeks or around the eyes; *cherry angiomas*, which often appear early in adulthood; and *seborrheic keratoses*, raised yellowish lesions that feel greasy and velvety or warty.

Distinguish such lesions from a *basal cell carcinoma*, initially a translucent nodule that spreads and leaves a depressed center with a firm elevated border, and from a *squamous cell carcinoma*, a firm reddish-appearing lesion often emerging in a sun-exposed area. A dark raised asymmetric lesion with irregular borders may be a *melanoma*. See Table 6-9, Skin Tumors, p. 194, and Table 6-10, Benign and Malignant Nevi, p. 195.

Watch for any painful vesicular lesions in a dermatomal distribution.

Suspect *herpes zoster* from reactivation of latent varicella-zoster virus in the dorsal root ganglia. Risk increases with age and impaired cell-mediated immunity.[126]

In older bed-bound patients, especially those emaciated or neurologically impaired, inspect the skin thoroughly for damage or ulceration.

Pressure sores may develop from obliteration of arteriolar and capillary blood flow to the skin or from shear forces during movement across sheets or when lifted upright incorrectly. See Table 6-13, Pressure Ulcers, p. 200.

Head and Neck. Conduct a careful and thorough evaluation of the head and neck.

See Chapter 7, The Head and Neck, pp. 205–291.

Inspect the eyelids, the bony orbit, and the eye. The eye may appear recessed from atrophy of fat in the surrounding tissues. Observe any *senile ptosis* arising from weakening of the levator palpebrae, relaxation of the skin, and increased weight of the upper eyelid. Check the lower lids for ectropion or *entropion*. Note yellowing of the sclera, and *arcus senilis*, a benign whitish ring around the limbus.

See Table 7-7, Variations and Abnormalities of the Eyelids, p. 266, and Table 7-9, Opacities of the Cornea and Lens, p. 268.

Test visual acuity, using a pocket Snellen chart or wall-mounted chart. Note any *presbyopia*, the loss of near vision arising from decreased elasticity of the lens related to aging.

More than 40 million Americans have refractive errors.

The pupils should respond to light and near effort. Except for possible impairment in upward gaze, extraocular movements should remain intact.

Using your ophthalmoscope, carefully examine the lenses and fundi.

Cataracts, glaucoma, and macular degeneration all increase with aging.[127]

Inspect each lens carefully for any opacities. Do not depend on the flashlight alone because the lens may look clear superficially.

Cataracts are the world's leading cause of blindness. Risk factors include cigarette smoking, exposure to UV-B light, high alcohol intake, diabetes, medications (including steroids), and trauma. See Table 7-9, Opacities of the Cornea and Lens, p. 268.

In older adults, the fundi lose their youthful shine and light reflections, and the arteries look narrowed, paler, straighter, and less brilliant. Assess the cup-to-disc ratio, usually 1:2 or less.

Retinal microvascular disease is linked to cerebral microvascular changes and cognitive impairment.[128]

An increased cup-to-disc ratio suggests open angle *glaucoma,* caused by irreversible optic neuropathy and leading to loss of peripheral and central vision and blindness. Prevalence is three to four times higher in African Americans than in the general population.[129]

Inspect the fundi for colloid bodies causing alterations in pigmentation, called *drusen*.

Macular degeneration causes poor central vision and blindness.[130] Types include *dry atrophic* (more common but less severe) and *wet exudative*, or neovascular. Drusen may be hard and sharply defined, or soft and confluent with altered pigmentation, shown below and on p. 232.

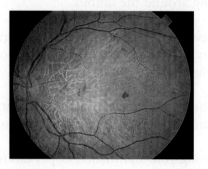

Test hearing by occluding one ear and using the techniques for whispered voice or an audioscope. Be sure to inspect the ear canals for cerumen, because removal can quickly improve hearing.

See techniques for testing hearing, pp. 235–238. Asking if hearing loss is present is an effective screening method. Patients who report hearing loss have an LR of 2.2 for impairment, with an LR of 0.13 if they report no hearing loss. Proceed to audiometry for those saying yes; check acuity to whispered voice for saying no (LR 6 if no acuity; LR 0.03 if acuity intact).[131,132]

Examine the oral cavity for odor, appearance of the gingival mucosa, any caries, mobility of the teeth, and quantity of saliva. Inspect closely for lesions on any of the mucosal surfaces. Ask the patient to remove dentures so you can check the gums for denture sores.

Malodor is present in poor oral hygiene, periodontitis, and caries. *Gingivitis* may arise from periodontal disease. Dental plaque and cavitation may cause caries. Increased tooth mobility from abscesses or advanced caries warrants removal to prevent aspiration. Decreased salivation may develop from medications, radiation, Sjögren's syndrome, or dehydration. Lesions may arise from *oral tumors,* usually on the lateral borders of the tongue and floor of the mouth.[133]

Continue with your usual examination of the thyroid gland and lymph nodes.

Thorax and Lungs. Complete the usual examination, making note of subtle signs of changes in pulmonary function.

Increased anteroposterior diameter, purse-lipped breathing, and dyspnea with talking or minimal exertion suggest *chronic obstructive pulmonary disease.*

Cardiovascular System. Review your findings from measurement of the blood pressure and heart rate.

Isolated systolic hypertension and a widened pulse pressure are cardiac risk factors, prompting a search for *left ventricular hypertrophy (LVH).*

As with younger adults, begin by inspecting the jugular venous pressure, palpating the carotid upstrokes, and listening for any overlying carotid bruits.

A *tortuous atherosclerotic aorta* can raise pressure in the left jugular veins by impairing drainage into the right atrium. It may also cause kinking of the carotid artery low in the neck on the right, chiefly in women with hypertension; this can be mistaken for a *carotid aneurysm.*

Carotid bruits can be heard in *aortic stenosis* in and *carotid stenosis* (increases risk of ipsilateral stroke).

Assess the point of maximal impulse (PMI), then auscultate S_1 and S_2. Listen also for the extra sounds of S_3 and S_4.

Sustained PMI is present in LVH; diffuse PMI in heart failure (see pp. 372–374)

In older adults an S_3 suggests dilatation of the left ventricle from heart failure or cardiomyopathy; an S_4 often accompanies hypertension.

Beginning in the second right interspace, listen for cardiac murmurs in all areas of auscultation (see pp. 379–382). Describe the timing, shape, location of maximal intensity, radiation, intensity, pitch, and quality of each murmur you detect.

A systolic crescendo–decrescendo murmur in the second right interspace suggests *aortic sclerosis* or *aortic stenosis,* seen respectively in approximately 30% and 2% of community-dwelling older adults. Both carry increased risk for cardiovascular disease and death.[134]

For systolic murmurs over the clavicle, check for delay between the brachial and radial pulses.

Delay present during simultaneous palpation (but not compression) of the brachial and radial pulses denotes *aortic stenosis.*[135]

A harsh holosystolic murmur at the apex suggests *mitral regurgitation,* common in older adults.

Breasts and Axillae.   Palpate the breasts carefully for lumps or masses. Include palpation of the tail of Spence that extends into the axilla. Examine the axillae for lymphadenopathy. Note any scaly, vesicular ulcerated lesions on or near the nipple.

Lumps or masses in older women, and, more rarely, in older men, mandate further investigation for possible breast cancer.

Paget's disease is less common, but peaks between the ages of 50 and 60 years.[136]

Abdomen.   Continue your usual examination of the abdomen. Check for any bruits over the aorta, renal arteries, and femoral arteries. Inspect the upper abdomen; palpate to the left of the midline for any aortic pulsations. Try to assess the width of the aorta by pressing more deeply with one hand on each of its lateral margins (see p. 465).

Bruits are present in atherosclerotic vascular disease.

Widened aorta and pulsatile mass occur in *abdominal aortic aneurysm.*

Peripheral Vascular System.   Auscultate the abdomen for bruits, as above, and assess the width of the abdominal aorta in the epigastric area; examine for a pulsatic mass.

Consider *abdominal aortic aneurysm* if aortic width is ≥3 cm or with a pulsatile mass, especially in older male smokers with coronary disease.

Palpate pulses carefully.

Diminished or absent pulses may indicate *arterial occlusion.* Consider confirmation with an office ankle–brachial index (see Table 12-3, Using the Ankle-Brachial Index, p. 516). Note that ≤33% of patients with peripheral vascular disease have symptoms of claudication.[137]

Female Genitalia and Pelvic Examination.[138]   Take special care to explain the steps of the examination and allow time for careful positioning. Ask an assistant to help the older woman move onto the examining table, then into the lithotomy position. Raising the head of the table may make her more comfortable. For the woman with arthritis or spinal deformities who cannot flex her hips or knees, an assistant can gently raise and support the legs, or help the woman into the left lateral position.

Inspect the vulva for changes related to menopause such as thinning of the skin, loss of pubic hair, and decreased distensibility of the introitus. Identify any labial masses. Note that bluish swellings may be varicosities. Bulging of the anterior vaginal wall below the urethra may indicate a urethrocele or urethral diverticulum.

Benign masses include condylomata, fibromas, leiomyomas, and sebaceous cysts. See Table 14-3, Bulges and Swellings of the Vulva, Vagina, and Urethra, p. 570.

Look for any vulvar erythema.

Look for erythema with satellite lesions results in infection with *Candida;* erythema with ulceration or necrotic center in vulvar *carcinoma.* Multifocal reddened lesions with white scaling plaques are seen in extramammary *Paget's disease,* an intraepithelial adenocarcinoma.

Inspect the urethra for *caruncles*, or prolapse of fleshy erythematous mucosal tissue at the urethral meatus. Note any enlargement of the clitoris.

Clitoral enlargement may accompany *androgen-producing tumors* or use of androgen creams.

Spread the labia, press downward on the introitus to relax the levator muscles, and gently insert the speculum after moistening it with warm water or a water-soluble lubricant. If you find severe vaginal atrophy, a gaping introitus, or an introital stricture from estrogen loss, you will need to vary the size of the speculum.

Inspect the vaginal walls, which may be atrophic, and the cervix. Note any thin cervical mucus or vaginal or cervical discharge.

Estrogen-stimulated cervical mucus with ferning is seen with use of hormone replacement therapy, in *endometrial hyperplasia*, and *estrogen-producing tumors*.

Discharge may accompany vaginitis or cervicitis. See Table 14-2, Vaginal Discharge, p. 569.

Use an endocervical brush (or less commonly, a wooden spatula) to obtain endocervical cells for the Pap smear. Consider using a blind swab if the atrophic vagina is too small.

See Table 14-7, Positions of the Uterus, p. 573, and Table 14-8, Abnormalities of the Uterus, p. 574.

After removing the speculum, ask the patient to bear down to detect uterine prolapse, cystocele, urethrocele, or rectocele.

Perform the bimanual examination. Check for motion of the cervix and for any uterine or adnexal masses.

Mobility of the cervix is restricted with inflammation, malignancy, or surgical adhesion. Look for enlarging uterine fibroids, or leiomyomas, in *malignant leiomyosarcoma*; palpable ovaries in *ovarian cancer*

Perform the rectovaginal examination if indicated. Assess for uterine and adnexal irregularities through the anterior rectal wall, and check for rectal masses. Change gloves if blood from the bimanual examination is on the vaginal examining glove to obtain an accurate stool sample.

A uterus that is enlarged, fixed, or irregular may indicate adhesions or possible malignancy. Rectal masses are found in *colon cancer*.

Male Genitalia and Prostate. Examine the penis, retracting the foreskin if present. Examine the scrotum, testes, and epididymis.

Findings include smegma, penile cancer, and scrotal hydroceles.

Proceed with the rectal examination, paying special attention to any rectal masses and any nodularity or masses of the prostate. Note that the anterior and median lobes of the prostate are inaccessible to rectal palpation, limiting the utility of the digital rectal examination for detecting prostate enlargement or possible malignancy.

Rectal masses suggest *colon cancer*, *prostate hyperplasia* and in prostate enlargement; *prostate cancer* is possible if nodules or masses are present.

Musculoskeletal System. Begin your evaluation with the *10-Minute Geri-atric Screener* on p. 942. Be sure to include the test for leg mobility, also known as the *timed "get up and go" test* for gait and balance, an excellent screen for risk of falling. Ask the patient to get up from a chair, walk 10 feet, turn, and return to the chair. Most older adults can complete this test in 10 seconds.

If the patient has joint deformities, deficits in mobility, pain with movement, or a delayed "get up and go," conduct a more thorough examination. Apply the techniques for examining individual joints and pursue a more compre-hensive neurological examination.

Look for degenerative joint changes in *osteoarthritis;* joint inflammation in *rheumatoid* or *gouty arthritis.*

See Chapter 16, The Musculoskele-tal System; see Tables 16-1 to 16-10, pp. 668–679.

Timed Get Up and Go Test

Performed with patient wearing regular footwear, using usual walking aid if needed, and sitting back in a chair with armrest.

On the word, "Go," the patient is asked to do the following:

1. Stand up from the arm chair
2. Walk 3 m (in a line)
3. Turn
4. Walk back to chair
5. Sit down

Time the second effort.
Observe patient for postural stability, steppage, stride length, and sway.

Scoring:
▶ **Normal:** completes task in <10 seconds
▶ **Abnormal:** completes task in >20 seconds

Low scores correlate with good functional independence; high scores cor-relate with poor functional independence and higher risk of falls.

Reproduced from: Get-up and Go Test. In: Mathias S, Nayak USL, Isaacs B. "Balance in elderly patient" The "Get Up and Go" Test. Arch Phys Med Rehabil 1986;67:387–389; Podsiadlo D, Richardson S. The Timed "Up and Go": A test of basic functional mobility for frail elderly persons. J Am Geriatr Soc 1991;39:142–148.

Nervous System. As with the musculoskeletal examination, begin your evaluation with the *10-Minute Geriatric Screener* (p. 942).

Pursue further examination if you note any deficits. Focus especially on memory and affect.

Learn to distinguish delirium from depression and dementia (see Table 20-4). Search carefully for underly-ing causes.[139,140] See Table 20-5, Screening for Dementia: The Mini-Cog, p. 965.

Pay close attention to gait and balance, particularly standing balance; timed 8-foot walk; stride characteristics like width, pace, and length of stride; and careful turning.

Abnormalities of gait and balance, especially widening of base, slowing and lengthening of stride, and difficulty turning, are correlated with risk for falls.[107,110]

Note that standard neuromuscular tests have not been shown to predict impairments in mobility.[141] Although neurologic abnormalities are common in the older population, their prevalence without identifiable disease increases with age, ranging from 30% to 50%.[142] Examples of age-related abnormalities include unequal pupil size, decreased arm swing and spontaneous movements, increased leg rigidity and abnormal gait, presence of the snout and grasp reflexes, and decreased toe vibratory sense.

Search for evidence of flexed posture, tremor, rigidity, bradykinesia, micrographia, shuffling gait, and difficulty rising from a chair.

These findings are seen in *Parkinson's disease,* found in 1% of adults 65 years or older and 2% of those 85 years or older.[143,144] Tremor is slow frequency, occurs at rest, has a "pill-rolling" quality, and is aggravated by stress and inhibited during sleep or movement. *Essential tremor* if bilateral and symmetric, positive family history, and diminished by alcohol.

Persistent blinking after glabellar tap and difficulty walking heel-to-toe are also common in *Parkinson's disease.*

Recording Your Findings

Note that initially you may use sentences to describe your findings; later you will use phrases. The style below contains phrases appropriate for most write-ups. As you read through this physical examination, you will notice some atypical findings. Try to test yourself. See if you can interpret these findings in the context of all you have learned about the examination of the older adult.

See Table 20-6, Managing Older Adults: The Siebens Domain Management Model, p. 966, for an alternative way to organize the record and patient care.

Recording the Physical Examination—The Older Adult

Mr. J is an older adult who appears healthy but overweight, with good muscle bulk. He is alert and interactive, with good recall of his life history. He is accompanied by his son.

Vital Signs: Ht (without shoes) 5′ 10″. Wt (dressed) 195 lbs. BMI 28. BP 145/88 right arm, supine; 154/94 left arm, supine. Heart rate (HR) 98 and regular. Respiratory rate (RR) 18. Temperature (oral) 98.6°F.

10-Minute Geriatric Screener (see p. 942)
Vision: Patient reports difficulty reading. Visual acuity 20/60 on Snellen chart.

Needs further evaluation for glasses and possibly hearing aid.

Hearing: Cannot hear whispered voice in either ear. Cannot hear 1,000 or 2,000 Hz with audioscope in either ear.

Leg Mobility: Can walk 20 feet briskly, turn, walk back to chair, and sit down in 14 seconds.

Urinary Incontinence: Has lost urine and gotten wet on 20 separate days.

Needs further evaluation for incontinence, including "DIAPERS" assessment (see p. 941), prostate examination, and postvoid residual, which is normally ≤50 mL (requires bladder catheterization).

Nutrition: Has lost 15 lbs over the past 6 months without trying.

Needs nutritional screen, p. 934.

Memory: Can remember three items after 1 minute.

Depression: Does not often feel sad or depressed.

Physical Disability: Can walk fast but cannot ride a bicycle. Can do moderate but not heavy work around the house. Can go shopping for groceries or clothes. Can get to places out of walking distance. Can bathe each day without difficulty. Can dress, including buttoning and zipping, and can put on shoes.

Consider exercise regimen with strength training.

Physical Examination
Skin. Warm and moist. Nails without clubbing or cyanosis. Hair thinning at crown.

Head, Eyes, Ears, Nose, Throat (HEENT). Scalp without lesions. Skull NC/AT. Conjunctiva pink, sclera muddy. Pupils 2 mm constricting to 1 mm, round, regular, equally reactive to light and accommodation. Extraocular movements intact. Disc margins sharp, without hemorrhages or exudates. Mild arteriolar narrowing. TMs with good cone of light. Weber midline. AC ≥ BC. Nasal mucosa pink. No sinus tenderness. Oral mucosa pink. Dentition fair. Caries present. Tongue midline, slight beefy redness. Pharynx without exudates.

Neck. Supple. Trachea midline. Thyroid lobes slightly enlarged, no nodules.

Lymph Nodes. No cervical, axillary, epitrochlear, or inguinal lymph nodes.

Thorax and Lungs. Thorax symmetric. Kyphosis noted. Lungs resonant with good excursion. Breath sounds vesicular. Diaphragms descend 4 cm bilaterally.

(continued)

Cardiovascular. JVP 6 cm above the left atrium. Carotid upstrokes brisk, without bruits. PMI tapping, in the 5th ICS, 9 cm lateral to the midsternal line. II/VI harsh holosystolic murmur at the apex, radiating to the axilla. No S_3, S_4, or other murmurs.

Abdomen. Scaphoid, with active bowel sounds. Soft, nontender. No masses or hepatosplenomegaly. Liver span 7 cm in right midclavicular line; edge smooth and palpable at the RCM. No CVAT.

Genitourinary. Circumcised male. No penile lesions. Testes descended bilaterally, smooth.

Rectal. Rectal vault without masses. Stool brown, negative for occult blood.

Extremities. Warm and without edema. Calves supple.

Peripheral Vascular. Pulses 2+ and symmetric.

Musculoskeletal. Mild degenerative changes at the knees, with quadriceps wasting. Good range of motion in all joints.

Neurological. Oriented to person, place, and time. Mini-Mental State: score 29. Cranial nerves II–XII intact. Motor: Decreased quadriceps bulk. Tone intact. Strength 4/5 throughout. RAMs, finger-to-nose intact. Gait with widened base. Sensation intact to pinprick, light touch, position, and vibration. Romberg negative. Reflexes 2+ and symmetric, with plantar response downgoing.

Bibliography

Citations

1. Administration on Aging. Census data and population estimates, 2009. Available at http://www.aoa.gov/AoARoot/Aging_Statistics/Census_Population/Index.aspx. Accessed January 8, 2011.
2. Administration on Aging. A Profile of Older Americans: 2009. Available at http://www.aoa.gov/AoARoot/Aging_Statistics/Profile/2009/docs/2009profile_508.pdf. Accessed January 8, 2011.
3. Federal Interagency Forum on Aging Related Statistics. Older Americans 2010: Key Indicators of Well-Being. Available at http://www.agingstats.gov/agingstatsdotnet/Main_Site/Data/2010_Documents/Docs/OA_2010.pdf. Accessed January 9, 2011.
4. Seeman TE, Merkin SS, Crimmins EM et al. Disability trends among older Americans: National Health and Nutrition Examination Surveys, 1988–1994 and 1999–2004. Am J Public Health 2010;100:100–107.
5. Alley DE, Chang VW. The changing relationship of obesity and disability, 1988-2004. JAMA 2007;298:2020–2027.
6. Strawbridge WJ, Cohen RD, Shema SJ et al. Successful aging: predictors and associated activities. Am J Epidemiol 1996;144:135–41.
7. Bodenheimer T, Wagner EH, Brumbach, K. Improving primary care for patients with chronic illness. JAMA 2002;288:1775–1779.
8. Geriatrics Interdisciplinary Advisory Group, American Geriatrics Society. Interdisciplinary care for older adults with complex needs: American Geriatrics Society Position Statement. J Am geriatric soc 2006;54:849–852.
9. Cigolle CT, Langad KM, Kabeto MU et al. Geriatric conditions and disability: the health and retirement study. Ann Intern Med 2007;147:156–164.
10. Perls TT. Understanding the determinants of exceptional longevity. Ann Intern Med 2003;139(5):445–449.
11. Rowe JW, Kahn RL. Human aging: usual and successful. Science 1987;237:143–149.
12. Taffet GE. Physiology of aging. In: Cassel CK, Leipzig RM, Cohen HJ, et al., eds. Geriatric Medicine, 4th ed. New York: Springer, 2003:27–36.
13. Tenover JL. Sexuality, sexual function, androgen therapy, and the aging male. In Halter JB, Ouslander JG, Tinetti ME et al (eds). Hazzard's Geriatric Medicine and Gerontology, 6th ed. New York: McGraw-Hill, 2009.
14. Kaiser FE. Sexual function and the older woman. In Cassel CK, Leipzig RM, Cohen HJ et al (eds). Geriatric Medicine, 4th ed. New York: Springer, 2003.
15. DeBeau CE. Benign prostatic hyperplasia. In Cassel CK, Leipzig RM, Cohen HJ et al (eds). Geriatric Medicine, 4th ed. New York: Springer, 2003.
16. Evans WJ. Skeletal muscle loss: cachexia, sarcopenia, and inactivity. Am J Clin Nutr 2010;91:1123S–1127S.
17. Tangarorong GL, Kerins GJ, Besdine RW. Clinical approach to the older patient: an overview. In Cassel CK, Leipzig RM, Cohen HJ et al (eds). Geriatric Medicine, 4th ed. New York: Springer, 2003.

18. Iowa Geriatric Education Center, University of Iowa. Geriatric Assessment Tools. Available at http://www.healthcare.uiowa.edu/igec/tools. Accessed January 7, 2011.

19. Bayer AJ, Chadna JS, Farag RR et al. Changing presentation of myocardial infarction with increasing old age. J Am Geriatr Soc 1986;34:263–266.

20. Trivalle C, Dulcet J, Chasssagrie P et al. Differences in the signs and symptoms of hyperthyroidism in older and younger patients. J Am Geriatrr Soc 1996;44:50–53.

21. Tinetti ME, Williams CS, Gill TM. Dizziness among older adults: a possible geriatric syndrome. Ann Intern Med 2000; 132:337–344.

22. Fried LP, Sotrer DJ, King DE et al. Diagnosis of illness presentation in the elderly. J Am Geriatr Soc 1991;39:117–123.

23. Davis PB, Robins LBN. History-taking in the elderly with and without cognitive impairment. J Am Geriatr Soc 1989; 37:249–255.

24. Ferraro KF, Su YP. Physician-evaluated and self-reported morbidity for predicting disability. Am J Public Health 2000; 90:103–108.

25. Kuczmarski MF, Kuczmarski RJ, Najjar M. Effects of age on validity of self-reported height, weight and body mass index: findings from the third National Health and Nutrition Examination Survey, 1988-1994. J Am Diet Assoc 2001; 101:28–34.

26. Yeo, F. How will the U.S. healthcare system meet the challenge of the ethnogeriatric imperative? J Am Geriatr Soc 2009; 57:1278–1235.

27. Goldstein MZ, Griswold K. Practical geriatrics: cultural sensitivity and aging. Psychiatric Serv 1998;49:769–771.

28. Lee SJ, Moody-Ayers SY, Landfeld CS et al. The relationship between self-rated health and mortality in older black and white Americans. J Am Geriatr Soc 2007;55:1624–1629.

29. Sudore RL, Mehta KM, Simonsick EM et al. Limited literacy in older people and disparities in health and healthcare access. J Am Geritr Soc 2006;54:770–776.

30. Severence JS, Yeo G. Ethnogeriatric education: a collaborative project of Geriatric Education Centers. Gernontol Geriatric Educ 2006;26:33–38.

31. August KJ, Sorkin DH. Racial and ethnic disparities in indicators of physical health status: do they still exist throughout late life? J Am Geriatr Soc 2010;58:2009–2015.

32. Kobylarz FA, Heath JM, Lide RC. The ETHNIC(S) mnemonic: a clinical tool for ethnogeriatric education. J Am Geriatr Soc 2002;50:1852–1859.

33. Aggarwal NK. Reassessing cultural evaluations in geriatrics: insights from cultural psychiatry. J Am Geriatr Soc 2010; 58:2191–2196.

34. Stanford Geriatrics Education Center. "Test your Ethnogeriatric IQ." Available at http://sgec.stanford.edu/training/iq.html. Accessed January 14, 2011.

35. Stanford Geriatric Education Center. Curriculum in Ethno-Geriatrics. Available at http://sgec.stanford.edu/training/ethno.html. Accessed January 14, 2011.

36. Nunez GR. Culture, demographics, and critical care issues: an overview. Crit Care Clin 2003;19:619–639.

37. Xakellis G, Brangman SA, Ladson H et al. Curricular framework: core competencies in multicultural geriatric care. J Am Geriatr Soc 2004;52:137–142.

38. Spielman AJ, Yang C, Glovinsky PB. Assessment techniques for insomnia. In Kryger M, Roth T, Dement WC (eds). Principles and Practice of Sleep Medicine, 4th ed. Philadelphia: Saunders, 2005.

39. Bloom HG, Ahmed I, Alessi CA et al. Evidence-based recommendations for the assessment and management of sleep disorders in older persons. J Am Geriatr Soc 2009;57:761–789.

40. Fick DM, Cooper JW, Wade WE et al. Updating the Beers criteria for potentially inappropriate medication use in older adults: results of a U.S. consensus panel of experts. Arch Intern Med 2003;163:2716–2724.

41. Reuben DB, Herr KA, Pacala JT et al. Geriatrics at your fingertips, 6th ed. Malden MA: Blackwell Science Inc., for the American Geriatrics Society, 2004.

42. Onder G, Petrovic M, Balamurugan T et al. Less is more. Development and validation of a score to assess risk of adverse drug reactions among the in-hospital patients 65 years or older. Arch Intern Med 2010;170:1142–1148.

43. Ferrell BA. Acute and chronic pain. In Cassel CK, Leipzig RM, Cohen HJ et al (eds). Geriatric Medicine, 4th ed. New York: Springer, 2003.

44. American Geriatrics Society Panel on the Pharmacologic Management of Persistent Pain in Older Persons. Pharmacologic management of persistent pain in older persons. J Am Geriatr Soc 2009;57:1331–1346.

45. Charlton JE, ed. Core curriculum for Professional Education in Pain, 3rd ed. Seattle: Internaional Association for the Study of Pain, 2005. Available at http://www.iasp-pain.org/AM/Template.cfm?Section=Publications&Template=/CM/HTMLDisplay.cfm&ContentID=2307#TOC. Accessed January 16, 2011.

46. American Medical Association. Pain Management Module 5: Assessing and Treating Pain in Older Adults. Available at http://www.ama-cmeonline.com/pain_mgmt/module05/index.htm. Accessed January 16, 2011.

47. Moore AA, Karno MP, Grella CE et al. Alcohol, tobacco, and nonmedical drug use in older U.S. adults: data from the 2001/02 National Epidemiologic Survey of Alcohol and Related Conditions. J Am Geriatr Soc 2009;57:2275–2281.

48. National Institute on Aging. Age Page: Alcohol Use in Older People. Available at http://www.nia.nih.gov/HealthInformation/Publications/alcohol.htm. Accessed January 16, 2011.

49. Jones TV, Lindsey BA, Yount P et al. Alcoholism screening questionnaires: are they valid in elderly medical outpatients? J Gen Intern Med 1993;8:674–678.

50. Fink A, Morton SC, Beck JC et al. The alcohol-related problems survey: identifying hazardous and harmful drinking in older primary care patients. J Am Geriatr Soc 2002;50:1717–1722.

51. Moore AA, Giuli L, Gould R et al. Alcohol use, comorbidity, and mortality. J Am Geriatr Soc 2006;54:757–762.

52. Callahan CM, Tierney WM. Health services use and morality among older primary care patients with alcoholism. J Am Geriatr Soc 1995;43:1378–1383.

53. Kirchner JE, Zubritsky C, Cody M et al. Alcohol consumption among older adults in primary care. J Gen Intern Med 2007;22:92–97.

54. American Geriatrics Society. Screening recommendation: clinical guidelines for alcohol use disorders in older adults. Available at http://www.annalsoflongtermcare.com/article/5143. Accessed January 15, 2011.

55. Takahashi PY, Okhravi HR, Lim LS et al. Preventive health care in the elderly population: a guide for practicing physicians. May Clinic Proc 2004;79:416–4127.

56. Corti MC, Guralnik JM, Salive ME et al. Serum albumin level and physical disability as predictors of mortality in older persons. JAMA 1994;272:1036–1042.

57. Song X, Mitnitski A, Rockwood K. Prevalence and 10-year outcomes of frailty in older adults in relation to deficit accumulation. J Am Geriatr Soc 2010;58:681–687.

58. Espinoza SE, Fried LP. Risk factors for frailty in the older adult. Clin Geratr 2007;15:37–44.

59. Fried LP, Tangen CM. Watson J et al. Cardiovascular Health Study Collaborative Research Group. Frailty in older adults: evidence for a phenotype. J Gerontol A Biol Sci Med Sci 2001;56:M146–M156.

60. Tulsky JA. Doctor-patient communication issues. In Cassel CK, Leipzig RM, Cohen HJ et al (eds). Geriatric Medicine, 4th ed. New York: Springer, 2003.

61. Silviera MJ, Kim SYH, Langa KM. Advance directives and outcomes of surrogate decision making before death. N Engl J Med 2010;363:1211–1218.

62. Callahan D. The value of achieving a peaceful death. In: Cassel CK, Leipzig RM, Cohen HJ et al (eds). Geriatric Medicine, 4th ed. New York: Springer, 2003:351–360.

63. Qaseem A, Snow V, Shekelle P et al. Clinical Guidelines: Evidence-based interventions to improve the palliative care of pain, dyspnea, and depression at the end of life: a clinical practice guideline from the American College of Physicians. Ann Intern Med 2008;148:141–146.

64. Morrison RS, Meier DE. Clinical practice: palliative care. N Engl J Med 2004;350:2582–2590.

65. Walter LC, Covinsky KE. Cancer screening in elderly patients. A framework for individualized decision-making. JAMA 2001;285:2750–2756.

66. American Geriatrics Society Ethics Committee, American Geriatrics Society. Health screening decisions for older adults: AGS position paper. J Am Geriatr Soc 2003;51:270–271.

67. American College of Sports Medicine, Chodzko-Zajko W, Proctor DN, Flatarone Singh MAF et al. American College of Sports Medicine position stand. Exercise and physical activity for older adults. Med Sci Sports Exerc 2009;41:1510–1530.

68. Centers for Disease Control and Prevention. 2010-2011 Influenza prevention and control recommendations. Available at http://www.cdc.gov/flu/professionals/acip/flu_vax1011.htm. Accessed January 16, 2011.

69. Morbidity and Mortality Weekly Report. Updated recommendations for prevention of invasive pneumococcal disease among adults using the 23-valent pneumococcal polysaccharide vaccine (PPV23). MMWR 2010;59:1102–1105, September 3, 2010. Also available at http://www.cdc.gov/mmwr/preview/mmwrhtml/mm5934a3.htm#tab. Accessed January 16, 2010.

70. Centers for Disease Control and Prevention. Vaccines and Preventable Diseases: Herpes Zoster vaccination for health professionals. Updated January 2011. Available at http://www.cdc.gov/vaccines/vpd-vac/shingles/hcp-vaccination.htm#recommendations. Accessed January 16, 2011.

71. Centers for Disease Control and Prevention. Preventing tetanus, diphtheria, and pertussis among adults: use of tetanus toxoid, reduced diphtheria toxoid and acellular pertussis vaccine. Recommendations of the Advisory Committee on Immunization Practices (ACIP) and recommendation of ACIP, supported by the Healthcare Infection Control Practices Advisory Committee (HICPAC), for use of Tdap among health-care personnel. MMWR 2006;55:1–33, December 15, 2006.

72. Centers for Disease Control and Prevention. Updated Recommendations for Use of Tetanus Toxoid, Reduced Diphtheria Toxoid and Acellular Pertussis (Tdap) Vaccine from the Advisory Committee on Immunization Practices, 2010. MMWR 2011;60:13–15, January 16 2011. Available at http://www.cdc.gov/mmwr/preview/mmwrhtml/mm6001a4.htm. Accessed January 16, 2011.

73. U.S. Preventive Services Task Force. Recommendations for adults. Available at http://www.uspreventiveservicestaskforce.org/adultrec.htm. Accessed January 16, 2011.

74. American Geriatrics Society. Cancer screening in older adults: guidelines and controversies. Annual scientific meeting—May 2010. Available at http://www.americangeriatrics.org/annual_meeting/2010_meeting_handouts/saturday/cancer_screening. Accessed January 16, 2011.

75. Unutzer J. Late-life depression. N Engl J Med 2007;357:2269–2276.

76. Fancher TL, Kravitz R. In the clinic: depression. Ann Intern Med 2010;152:ITC5-1–18.

77. Whooley MA, Avins AL, Miranda J et al. Case-finding instruments for depression. Two questions are as good as many. J Gen Intern Med 1997;12:439–445.

78. Chunyu LMM, Friedman B, Conwell Y et al. Validity of the Patient Health Questionnaire 2 (PHQ-2) in identifying major depression in older people. J Am Geriatr Soc 2007;55:596–602.

79. Brink TL, Yesavage JA. Geriatric Depression Rating Scale. Available at http://www.stanford.edu/~yesavage/Testing.htm. Accessed January 22, 2010.

80. U.S. Preventive Services Task Force. Screening for dementia: recommendations and rationale. June 2003. Available at http://www.uspreventiveservicestaskforce.org/3rduspstf/dementia/dementrr.htm. Accessed January 22, 2011.

81. Daviglus ML, Bell CC, Berrettini W et al. National Institutes of Health State-of-the Science Conference Statement: preventing Alzheimer disease and cognitive decline. Ann Intern Med 2010;153:176–181.

82. Alzheimer's Association. 2010 Alzheimer's disease: facts and figures. Available at http://www.alz.org/documents_custom/report_alzfactsfigures2010.pdf. Accessed January 7, 2010.

83. Querforth HW, LaFerla FM. Mechanisms of disease. Alzheimer's disease. New Engl J Med 2010;362:329–344.

84. Mayeux R. Early Alzheimer's disease. N Engl J Med 2010;362:2194–2201.

85. Blass DM, Rabins PV. In the clinic: dementia. Ann Intern Med 2008;148:ITC4-1–ITC4-16.

86. Wong CL, Holrroyd-Leduc J, Simel DL et al. Does this patient have delirium? Value of bedside instruments. JAMA 2010;304:779–786.

87. Farias ST, Mungas D, Reed BR et al. Progression of mild cognitive impairment to dementia in clinic- vs community-based cohorts. Arch Neurol 2009;66:1151–1157.

88. Tschanz JT, Weklsg-Bohmer KA, Leketsos CG et al. Conversion to dementia from mild cognitive disorder: the Cache County Study. Neurology 2006;67:229–234.

89. Busse A, Hensel A, Guhne U et al. Mild cognitive impairment: long-term course of four clinical subtypes. Neurology 2006;67:2176–2185.

90. American Geriatrics Society. A guide to dementia diagnosis and treatment, 2010. Available at http://dementia.americangeriatrics.org/documents/AGS_PC_Dementia_Sheet_2010v2.pdf. Accessed January 7, 2010.

91. National Institutes of Health. NIHSeniorHealth. Caring for someone with Alzheimer's. Updated April 18, 2008. Available at http://nihseniorhealth.gov/alzheimerscare/toc.html. Accessed January 23, 2011.

92. Iverson DJ, Gronseth GS, Reger MA et al. Practice Parameter update: evaluation and management of driving risk in dementia. Report of the Quality Standards Subcommittee of the American Academy of Neurology. Neurology 2010;74:1316–1324.

93. National Highway Traffic safety administration. Impaired driving. Available at http://www.nhtsa.gov/Impaired. Accessed January 22, 2010.

94. Dyer CB, Pickens S, Burnett J. Vulnerable drivers: when it is no longer safe to drive. JAMA 2007;298:1448–1450.

95. Acierno R, Hernandez MA, Amstadter AB et al. Prevalence and correlates of emotional, physical, sexual, and financial abuse and potential neglect in the United States: the National Elder Mistreatment Study. Am J Public Health 2010;100:292–297.

96. Dong X, Simon MA, Wilson RS et al. Decline in cognitive function and risk of elder self-neglect: finding from the Chicago Health Aging Project. J Am Geriatr Soc 2010;58:2292–2299.

97. Cohen M, Levin SH, Gagin R et al. Elder abuse: disparities between older people's disclosure of abuse, evident signs of abuse, and high risk of abuse. J Am Geriatr Soc 2007;55:1224–1230.

98. Fulmer T. Screening for mistreatment of older adults. Am J Nurs 2008;108:52–59.

99. Koretz B, Reuben DB. Instruments to assess functional status. Also see Reuben DB. Comprehensive geriatric assessment and systems approaches to geriatric care. In: Cassel CK, Leipzig RM, Cohen HJ et al (eds). Geriatric Medicine, 4th ed. New York: Springer, 2003:185–204.

100. Leipzig RM, Whitlock EP, Wolff TA et al. Reconsidering the approach to prevention recommendations for older adults. Ann Intern med 2010;153:809–814.

101. Moore AA, Siu AL. Screening for common problems in ambulatory elderly: clinical confirmation of a screening instrument. Am J Med 1996;100:438–440.

102. Fung CH, Spencer B, Eslami M et al. Quality indicators for the screening and care of urinary incontinence in vulnerable elders. J Am Geriatr Soc 2007;55:S443–S449.

103. Michael YL, Whitlock WP, Lin JS et al. Primary care—relevant interventions to prevent falling in older adults: a systematic evidence review for the U.S. Preventive Services Task Force. Ann Intern Med 2010;153:815–825.

104. Sherrington C, Whitney JC, Lord SR et al. Effective exercise for the prevention of falls: a systematic review and meta-analysis. J Am Geriatr Soc 2008;56:2234–243.

105. Panel on Prevention of Falls in Older Persons, American Geriatrics Society and British Geriatrics Society. Summary of the Updated American Geriatrics Society/British Geriatrics Society Clinical Practice guideline for prevention of falls in older persons, 2010. J Am Geriatr Soc 2011;59:148–157. Also available at http://www.americangeriatrics.org/files/documents/

health_care_pros/JAGS.Falls.Guidelines.pdf. Accessed January 24, 2011. See also U.S. Preventive Services Task Force. Interventions to Prevent Falls in Older Adults, Topic Page. December 2010. Available at http://www.uspreventiveservicestaskforce.org/uspstf/uspsfalls.htm. Accessed January 24, 2011.

106. Tinetti ME, Kumar C. The patient who falls: "It's always a trade-off." JAMA 2010;303:258–266.

107. Cooper R, Kuh D, Hardy R. Objectively measured physical capability levels and mortality: systematic review and meta-analysis. BMJ 2010;341:4427–4439.

108. Bischoff-Ferrari HA, Dawson-Hughes B, Staehelin HB et al. Fall prevention with supplemental and active forms of vitamin d: a meta-analysis of randomized controlled trials. BMJ 2009;339:3692–3703.

109. Gillespie LD, Robertson MC, Gillespie WJ et al. Interventions for preventing falls in older people living in the community. Cochrane Database Syst Rev 2009; Apr 15:CD007146.

110. Montero-Odasso M, Schapira M, Soriano ER et al. Simple gait velocity assessment predicts adverse events in healthy seniors aged 75 years and older. J Gerontol A Biol Sci Med Sci 2005;60:1304–1309.

111. Sirkisian CA, Bruenwald TL, Boscardin WJ et al. Preliminary evidence for subdimensions of geriatric frailty: the MacArthur study of successful aging. J Am Geriatr Soc 2008;56:2292–2297.

112. Borson S, Scanlan JM, Brush M et al. The Mini-Cog: a cognitive "vital signs" measure for dementia screening in multilingual elderly. Int J Geriatric Psychiatry 2000;15:1021–1027.

113. Borson S, Scanlan JM, Chen P et al. The Mini-Cog as a screen for dementia: validation in a population-based sample. J Am Geriatr Soc 2003;51:1451–1454.

114. Beckett NS, Peters R, Fletcher AE et al. Treatment of hypertension in patients 80 years of age or older. N Engl J Med 2008;358:1887–1898.

115. Denardo SJ, Gong Y, Nichols WW et al. Blood pressure and outcomes in very old hypertensive coronary artery disease patients: an INVEST study. Am J Med 2010;123:719–726.

116. Oates DJ, Berlowitz DR, Glickman ME et al. Blood pressure and survival in the oldest old. J Am Geriatr Soc 2007;55:383–388.

117. Chaudry SI, Krumholz HM, Foody JM. Systolic hypertension in older persons. JAMA 2004;292:1974–1080.

118. Lloyd-Jones DM, Evans JC, Levy D. Hypertension in adults across the age spectrum: current outcomes and control in the community. JAMA 2005;294:466–472.

119. Papademetriou V. Comparative prognostic value of systolic, diastolic, and pulse pressure. Am J Cardiol 2003;91:433–435.

120. Vaccarino V, Berger AK et al. Pulse pressure and risk of cardiovascular events in the systolic hypertension in the elderly program. Am J Cardiol 2001;88:980–986.

121. Gupta V. Orthostatic hypotension in the elderly: diagnosis and treatment. Am J Med 2007;120:841–847.

122. Carlson JE. Assessment of orthostatic blood pressure: measurement technique and clinical applications. South Med J 1999;92:167–173.

123. Consensus Committee of the American Autonomic Society and the American Academy of Neurology. Consensus statement on the definition of orthostatic hypotension, pure autonomic failure, and multiple system atrophy. Neurology 1996;46:1470.

124. McGee S, Abernathy WB, Simel DL. Is this patient hypovolemic? JAMA 1999;281:1022–1029.

125. Ooi WL, Barrett S, Hossain M et al. Patterns of orthostatic blood pressure change and their clinical correlates in a frail elderly population. JAMA 1997;227:1299–1304.

126. Kimberlin DW, Whitley RJ. Varicella-zoster vaccine for the prevention of herpes zoster. N Engl J Med 2007;356:1338–1343.

127. Rowe S, Maclean CH. Quality indicators for the care of vision impairment in vulnerable elders. J Am Geriatr Soc 2007; 55:S450–S456.

128. Liew G, Mitchell P, Wong TY et al. Retinal microvascular signs and cognitive impairment. J Am Geriatric Soc 2009;57: 1892–1896.

129. Friedman DS, Jampel HD, Munoz B et al. The prevalence of open-angle glaucoma among blacks and whites 73 years and older: the Salisbury Eye Evaluation Glaucoma Study. Arch Ophthalmic 2006;124:1625–1630.

130. Bourla DH, Young TA. Age-related macular degeneration: a practical approach to a challenging disease. J Am Geriatr Soc 2006;54:1130–1135.

131. Ragia A, Thavendiranathan P, Detsky AS. Does this patient have hearing impairment? JAMA 2006;295:416–428.

132. Swan IRC, Browning GG. The whispered voice as a screening test for hearing impairment. J Royal Col Gen Pract 1985;35:197.

133. Gonsalves WC, Wrightson AS, Henry RG. Common oral conditions in older persons. Am Fam Physician 2008;78: 845–852.

134. Otto CM, Lind BK, Kitzman DW et al. Association of aortic-valve sclerosis with cardiovascular mortality and morbidity in the elderly. JAMA 1999;341:142–147.

135. Leach RM, McBrien DJ. Brachioradial delay: a new clinical indicator of the severity of aortic stenosis. Lancet 1990;335: 1199–1201.

136. Caliskan M, Gatti G, Sosnovskikh et al. Paget's disease of the breast: the experience of the European Institute of Oncology and review of the literature. Breast Cancer Res Treat 2008;112:513–521.

137. McDermott MM, Greenland P, Liu K et al. The ankle brachial index is associated with leg function and physical activity: the walking and leg circulation study. Ann Intern Med 2002;136:873–883.

138. Dumesic DA. Pelvic examination: what to focus on in menopausal women. Consultant 1996;36:39–46.

139. Holsinger T, Deveau J, Boustani M et al. Does this patient have dementia? JAMA. 2007;297:2391–404.

140. Wong CL, Holroyd-Leduc J, Simel DL et al. Does this patient have delirium? Value of bedside instruments. JAMA 2010;304:779–786.

141. Tinetti ME, Glinter SF. Identifying mobility dysfunction in elderly patients. JAMA 1988;259:1190–1193.

142. Odenheimer G, Funkenstein HH, Beckett L et al. Comparison of neurologic changes in "successful aging" persons vs the total aging population. Arch Neurol 1994;51: 573–580.

143. Rao G, Fisch L, Srinivasan S et al. Does this patient have Parkinson disease? JAMA 2003;289:347–353.

144. Jankovic J. Parkinson's disease: clinical features and diagnosis. J Neurol Neurosurg Psychiatry 2008;78:368–376.

Additional References

Administration on Aging. U.S. Department of Health and Human Services. Available at http://www.aoa.gov/AoARoot/Index.aspx. Accessed January 8, 2011.

Ahmed A. Clinical manifestations, diagnostic assessment, and etiology of heart failure in older adults. Clin Geriatr Med 2007;23:11–30.

American Geriatrics Society. Available at http://www.americangeriatrics.org. Accessed June 22, 2008.

American Geriatrics Society. A pocket guide to common immunizations for the older adult (≥65 years). Available at http://www.americangeriatrics.org/files/documents/AGS_PocketGuide.pdf. Accessed January 7, 2010.

American Geriatrics Society. Ethnogeriatrics Steering Committee. Doorway Thoughts: Cross-cultural Health Care for Older Adults. Sudbury, MA: Jones and Bartlett, 2004.

American Medical Association. Pain Management Module 5: Assessing and Treating Pain in Older Adults. Available at http://www.ama-cmeonline.com/pain_mgmt/printversion/ama_painmgmt_m5.pdf. Accessed January 16, 2011.

Beckett NS, Peters R, Fletcher AE et al, for the HYVET Study Group. Treatment of hypertension in patients 80 years of age or older. N Engl J Med 2008;78:1887–1898.

Bhattacharya J, Choudhry K, Lakdawalla DN. Chronic disease and trends in severe disability in working age populations. Med Care 2008;46:92–100.

Blazer DG, Steffens DC (eds). American Psychiatric Publishing Textbook of Geriatric Psychiatry, 4th ed. Arlington, VA: American Psychiatric Publishing Inc., 2009.

Bloom HG, Ahmed I, Alessi CA et al. Evidence-based recommendations for the assessment and management of sleep disorders in older persons. J Am Geriatr Soc 2009;57:761–789.

Bobrie G, Genes N, Vaur L et al. Is "isolated home" hypertension as opposed to "isolated office" hypertension a sign of greater cardiovascular risk? Arch Intern Med 2001;161:2295–2211.

Carolan Doerflinger DM. How to try this: the mini-cog. Am J Nurs 2007;107:62–71.

Chobanion AV. Isolated systolic hypertension in the elderly. N Engl J Med 2007;357:789–796.

Cooper-DeHoff RM, Gong Y, Handberg EM et al. Tight blood pressure control and cardiovascular outcomes among hypertensive patients with diabetes and coronary artery disease. JAMA 2010;304:61–68.

Delancey JO, Asthont-Miller JA. Pathophysiology of adult urinary incontinence. Gastroenterology 2004;126(Suppl 1):S23–S32.

Donowitz GR, Cox HL. Bacterial community-acquired pneumonia in older patients. Clin Geriatr Med 2007;23:515–534.

Duthie EH, Katz PR, Malone ML (eds). Practice of Geriatrics, 4th ed. Philadelphia: Saunders, 2007.

Ene-Stroescu D, Gorbien MJ. Gouty arthritis. A primer on late-onset gout. Geriatrics 2005;60(7):24–31.

Gavi S, Hensley J. Diagnosis and management of type 2 diabetes in adults: a review of the ICSI guideline. Geriatrics 2009;64: 12–17, 29.

Goldbdrg LR. In the clinic. Heart failure. Ann Intern Med 2010;152:ITC6-1–ITC6-16.

Hazzard WR, Halter JB. Hazzard's Geriatric Medicine and Gerontology, 6th ed. New York: McGraw-Hill, 2009.

Hyde Z, Flicker L, Hankey GJ et al. Prevalence of sexual activity and associated factors in men aged 75 to 95 years. Ann Intern Med 2010;153:693–702.

Inouye SK. Delirium in older persons. New Engl J Med 2006;354:1157–1165.

Inouye SK, van Dyck CH, Alessi CA et al. Clarifying confusion: the confusion assessment method. A new method for detection of delirium. Ann Intern Med 1990;113:941–94. See also Inouye SK. The Confusion Assessment Method (CAM) Training Manual and Coding guide, Developed February 25, 1991; last updated September 10, 2009. Available at http://www.hospitalelderlifeprogram.org/pdf/The%20Confusion%20Assessment%20Method.pdf. Accessed January 29, 2011.

Kales HC, Mellow AM. Race and depression: does race affect the diagnosis and treatment of late-life depression? Geriatrics 2006;61:18–21.

Kobylarz FA, Pomidor A, Heath JM. SPEAK. A mnemonic tool for addressing health literacy concerns in geriatric clinical encounters. Geriatrics 2006;61:20–26.

Lorenz KA, Lynn J, Dy SM et al. Clinical guidelines: evidence for improving palliative care at the end of life: a systematic review. Ann Intern Med 2008;148:147–159.

Nakasato YR, Carnes BA. Health promotion in older adults. Promoting successful aging in primary care settings. Geriatrics 2006;61:27–31.

National Institutes of Health. NIHSeniorHealth. Available at http://nihseniorhealth.gov/index.html. Accessed January 8, 2011.

Norton P, Brubaker L. Urinary incontinence in women. Lancet 2006;367(9504):57–67.

Nusbaum MR, Lenahan P, Sadovsky R. Sexual health in aging men and women: addressing the physiologic and psychological sexual changes that occur with age. Geriatrics 2005;60:18–23.

Nutt JG, Wooten GF. Diagnosis and initial management of Parkinson's disease. N Engl J Med 2005;353:1021–1027.

Reuben D. Medical care for the final years of life: "when you're 83, it's not going to be 20 years." JAMA 2009;302:2686–2694.

Romero-Ortuno R, Cogan L, Foran T et al. Continuous noninvasive orthostatic blood pressure measurements and their relationship with orthostatic intolerance, falls, and frailty in older people. J Am Geriatr Soc 2011;59:655–665.

Scalf LA, Shenefelt PD. Contact dermatitis: diagnosing and treating skin conditions in the elderly. Geriatrics 2007;62:14–19.

Sessums LL, Zembrzuska H, Jackson JL. Does the patient have medical decision-making capacity? JAMA 2011;306:420–427.

Staats DO. Preventing injury in older adults. Geriatrics 2008;63:12–17.

Studenski S, Perera S, Patel K. Gait speed and survival in older adults. JAMA 2011;305:50–58.

Swindell WR, Ensrud KE, Cawthon PM et al. Indicators of "healthy aging" in older women (65–69 years of age). A data-mining approach based on prediction of long-term survival. BMC Geriatr 2010;10:55.

Tseng HF, Smith N, Harpaz R et al. Herpes zoster vaccine in older adults and the risk of subsequent herpes zoster disease. JAMA 2011;305:160–166.

Velickovic M, Gracies JM. Movement disorders. Keys to identifying and treating tremor. Geriatrics 2002;57:32–36.

Vistamehr S, Shelsta HN, Pammisano PC et al. Glaucoma screening in a high-risk population. J Glaucoma 2006;15:534–540.

Walter LC, Covinsky KE. Cancer screening in elderly patients—a framework for individualized decision making. JAMA 2011;285:2750–2756.

Walter LC, Lewis CL, Barton MB. Screening for colorectal, breast, and cervical cancer in the elderly: a review of the evidence. Am J Med 2005;118:1078–1086.

Weiner DK. Office management of chronic pain in the elderly. Am J Med 2007;120:306–315.

The Bates' suite offers these additional resources to enhance learning and facilitate understanding of this chapter:

- Bates' *Pocket Guide to Physical Examination and History Taking*, 7th edition
- Bates' *Visual Guide to Physical Examination*
- thePoint online resources, for students and instructors: http://thepoint.lww.com

| Table |
| 20-1 | **Minimum Geriatric Competencies*** |

Medication Management

1 Explain impact of age-related changes on drug selection and dose, based on knowledge of age-related changes in renal and hepatic function, body composition, and central nervous system sensitivity.
2 Identify medications, including anticholinergic, psychoactive, anticoagulant, analgesic, hypoglycemic, and cardiovascular drugs that should be avoided or used with caution in older adults and explain the potential problems associated with each.
3 Document a patient's complete medication list, including prescribed, herbal and over-the-counter medications, and for each medication provide the dose, frequency, indication, benefit, side effects, and an assessment of adherence.

Cognitive and Behavioral Disorders

4 Define and distinguish among the clinical presentations of delirium, dementia, and depression.
5 Formulate a differential diagnosis and implement initial evaluation in a patient who exhibits cognitive impairment.
6 Urgently initiate a diagnostic workup to determine the root cause (etiology) of delirium in an older patient.
7 Perform and interpret a cognitive assessment in older patients for whom there are concerns regarding memory or function.
8 Develop an evaluation and nonpharmacologic management plan for agitated, demented, or delirious patients.

Self-Care Capacity

9 Assess and describe baseline and current functional abilities (instrumental activities of daily living, activities of daily living, and special senses) in an older patient by collecting historical data from multiple sources and performing a confirmatory physical examination.
10 Develop a preliminary management plan for patients presenting with functional deficits, including adaptive interventions and involvement of interdisciplinary team members from appropriate disciplines, such as social work, nursing, rehabilitation, nutrition, and pharmacy.
11 Identify and assess safety risks in the home environment, and make recommendations to mitigate these.

Falls, Balance, Gait Disorders

12 Ask all patients >65 years, or their caregivers, about falls in the last year, watch the patient rise from a chair and walk (or transfer), then record and interpret the findings.
13 For a patient who has fallen, construct a differential diagnosis and evaluation plan that addresses the multiple etiologies identified by history, physical examination, and functional assessment.

Health Care Planning and Promotion

14 Define and differentiate among types of code status, health care proxies, and advanced directives in the site where one is training.
15 Accurately identify clinical situations where life expectancy, functional status, patient preference, or goals of care should override standard recommendations for screening tests in older adults.
16 Accurately identify clinical situations where life expectancy, functional status, patient preference, or goals of care should override standard recommendations for treatment in older adults.

Atypical Presentation of Disease

17 Identify at least three physiologic changes of aging for each organ system and their impact on the patient, including their contribution to homeostenosis (the age-related narrowing or homeostatic reserve mechanisms).
18 Generate a differential diagnosis based on recognition of the unique presentations of common conditions in older adults, including acute coronary syndrome, dehydration, urinary tract infection, acute abdomen, and pneumonia.

Palliative Care

19 Assess and provide initial management of pain and key nonpain symptoms based on patient's goals of care.
20 Identify the psychological, social, and spiritual needs of patients with advanced illness and their family members, and link these identified needs with the appropriate interdisciplinary team members.
21 Present palliative care (including hospice) as a positive, active treatment option for a patient with advanced disease.

Hospital Care for Elders

22 Identify potential hazards of hospitalization for all older adult patients (including immobility, delirium, medication side effects, malnutrition, pressure ulcers, procedures, peri- and postoperative periods, and hospital-acquired infections) and identify potential prevention strategies.
23 Explain the risks, indications, alternatives, and contraindications for indwelling (Foley) catheter use in the older adult patient.
24 Explain the risks, indications, alternatives, and contraindications for physical and pharmacologic restraint use.
25 Communicate the key components of a safe discharge plan (e.g., accurate medication list, plan for follow-up), including comparing/contrasting potential sites for discharge.
26 Conduct a surveillance examination of areas of the skin at high risk for pressure ulcers and describe existing ulcers.

*These pertain primarily to medical students but are generalizable to the health care team.

Source: Association of American Medical Colleges/John A. Hartford Foundation, Inc. A Consensus Conference on Competencies in Geriatrics Education, October 5, 2007.

Table 20-2 — Disparities in Health Status of U.S. Older Adults Compared to Non-Hispanic Whites

Populations	More Prevalent	Less Prevalent	Populations	More Prevalent	Less Prevalent
African American	Heart disease Hypertension Cerebrovascular disease Diabetes mellitus Most cancers (especially prostate) Glaucoma Vascular dementia Fair or poor SRH Activity limitation Untreated dental caries	Osteoporosis Respiratory disease	Filipino (cont'd)	Liver cancer Lung cancer (m) Thyroid cancer (f)	
			Hmong	Diabetes mellitus Hepatitis B Posttraumatic stress disorder	
American Indian or Alaska Native*	Diabetes Fair or poor SRH Activity limitation Accidents (m) Alcoholism Cervical cancer (f) Kidney disease Liver disease Tuberculosis Rheumatoid arthritis Hearing problems Vision problems	Cancer Cerebrovascular disease	Japanese	Depression Suicide Diabetes mellitus Hemorrhagic stroke Vascular dementia Esophageal cancer Stomach cancer Colorectal cancer Liver cancer Osteoporosis (f)	
Southwestern and Oklahoma Tribes	Gallbladder cancer		Korean	Fair or poor SRH Liver cancer (m) Diabetes mellitus	
Alaska Natives	Esophageal cancer Liver cancer		Vietnamese	Depression Cervical cancer (f) Hepatitis B Liver cancer Thyroid cancer (f)	
Asian American (undifferentiated)	Tuberculosis	Heart disease Hypertension Cerebrovascular disease Cancer (most kinds) Respiratory disease Hip fracture	Native Hawaiian and Pacific Islander	Heart disease Hypertension Diabetes mellitus	
			Guamanian	Parkinson's disease	
			Hispanic or Latin American (undifferentiated)	Fair or poor SRH Activity or functional limitations	Heart disease Cancer (most types) Cerebrovascular disease Respiratory disease Accidents
Asian Indian	Depression Insulin resistance				
Cambodian	Severe headache and dizziness Posttraumatic stress disorder		Dominican	Dementia Arthritis Hypertension	
Chinese	Diabetes mellitus (f) Depression Suicide (f) Vascular dementia Esophageal cancer Nasopharyngeal cancer (m) Liver cancer Pancreatic cancer (f) Colorectal cancer Hepatitis B	Breast cancer (f) Ovarian cancer (f) Prostate cancer (m) Colon cancer (f)	Mexican	Diabetes mellitus Depression (f) Cervical cancer (f) Liver cancer Lung cancer (m) Untreated dental caries	Hip fracture or osteoporosis Hypertension Arthritis
			Puerto Rican	Diabetes mellitus Liver cancer Heart disease (f) Dementia Arthritis Cataracts Depression Hypertension	
Filipino	Diabetes mellitus Hypertension Gout	Breast cancer (f)			

SRH = self-rated health; (f) = female; (m) = male

Source: Yeo, F. How will the U.S. healthcare system meet the challenge of the ethnogeriatric imperative? J Am Geriatr Soc 2009;57:1278–1235.

Cultural Dimension	Interview
Cultural Identity of the Individual	Where are you and your family from? What is your ancestry? Are there cultural differences between you and your parents or you and your significant other? Do you feel a strong connection to any groups of people? If so, whom? What foods do you eat? What holidays do you celebrate? What languages do you speak? With whom do you speak these languages? What languages would you like to speak with me? What types of activities do you enjoy? What are your sources for news and entertainment? Has this changed over time?
Cultural Explanations of the Individual's Illness	Do you or anyone else have a name for the problem you're having now? Why do you think it's happening to you? What will make it better or worse? When did it start and when do you think you'll get better? Has anyone else you know had this problem? What activities has this problem stopped you from doing that you, your family, or your friends expect? Who else have you seen for help with this problem? Should I talk to anyone else you trust to help you with this problem?
Cultural Factors Related to Psychological Environment and Levels of Functioning	Who lives at home with you? Can they help with this problem? Who else can help you? Is anything going on to make this problem better or worse? How has this problem affected your life? Is it preventing you from working? Moving, grooming, feeding, or sleeping? Do people close to you understand how you feel?
Cultural Elements of the Clinician–Patient Relationship	Do you think your friends or family would be upset if you spoke to me about the problem? What can I do to make you feel more comfortable? How often can you see me? Do you have any wishes for or concerns about treatment? What are your thoughts about medications? Can I share your answers with anyone else you trust?

Source: Aggarwal NK. Reassessing cultural evaluations in geriatrics: insights from cultural psychiatry. J Am Geriatr Soc 2010;58:2191–2196.

Table 20-4 — Delirium and Dementia

Delirium and dementia are common and important disorders that affect multiple aspects of mental status. Both have many possible causes. Some clinical features of these two conditions and their effects on mental status are compared below. A delirium may be superimposed on dementia.

	Delirium	Dementia
Clinical Features		
Onset	Acute	Insidious
Course	Fluctuating, with lucid intervals; worse at night	Slowly progressive
Duration	Hours to weeks	Months to years
Sleep/Wake Cycle	Always disrupted	Sleep fragmented
General Medical Illness or Drug Toxicity	Either or both present	Often absent, especially in Alzheimer's disease
Mental Status		
Level of Consciousness	Disturbed. Person less alert to clearly aware of the environment and less able to focus, sustain, or shift attention	Usually normal until late in the course of the illness
Behavior	Activity often abnormally decreased (somnolence) or increased (agitation, hypervigilance)	Normal to slow; may become inappropriate
Speech	May be hesitant, slow or rapid, incoherent	Difficulty in finding words, aphasia
Mood	Fluctuating, labile, from fearful or irritable to normal or depressed	Often flat, depressed
Thought Processes	Disorganized, may be incoherent	Impoverished. Speech gives little information
Thought Content	Delusions common, often transient	Delusions may occur
Perceptions	Illusions, hallucinations, most often visual	Hallucinations may occur
Judgment	Impaired, often to a varying degree	Increasingly impaired over the course of the illness
Orientation	Usually disoriented, especially for time. A known place may seem unfamiliar.	Fairly well maintained, but becomes impaired in the later stages of illness
Attention	Fluctuates, with inattention. Person easily distracted, unable to concentrate on selected tasks	Usually unaffected until late in the illness
Memory	Immediate and recent memory impaired	Recent memory and new learning especially impaired
Examples of Cause	Delirium tremens (due to withdrawal from alcohol)	*Reversible:* Vitamin B_{12} deficiency, thyroid disorders
	Uremia	*Irreversible:* Alzheimer's disease, vascular dementia (from multiple infarcts), dementia due to head trauma
	Acute hepatic failure	
	Acute cerebral vasculitis	
	Atropine poisoning	

Table
20-5

Screening for Dementia: The Mini-Cog

Administration

The test is administered as follows:

1. Instruct the patient to listen carefully to and remember 3 unrelated words and then to repeat the words.

2. Instruct the patient to draw the face of a clock, either on a blank sheet of paper or on a sheet with the clock circle already drawn on the page. After the patient puts the numbers on the clock face, ask him or her to draw the hands of the clock to read a specific time.

3. Ask the patient to repeat the 3 previously stated words.

Scoring

Give 1 point for each recalled word after the clock drawing test (CDT) distractor.
Patients recalling none of the three words are classified as demented (Score = 0).
Patients recalling all three words are classified as nondemented (Score = 3).
Patients with intermediate word recall of 1–2 words are classified based on the CDT (Abnormal = demented; Normal = nondemented).

Note: The CDT is considered normal if all numbers are present in the correct sequence and position, and the hands readably display the requested time.

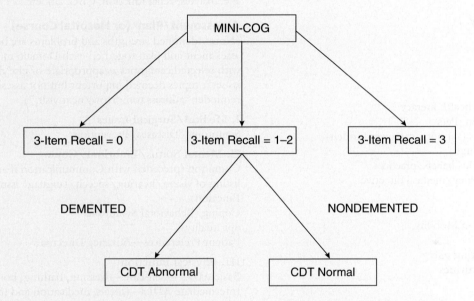

Source: From Borson S, Scanlan J, Brush M et al. The Mini-Cog: a cognitive 'vital signs' measure for dementia screening in multi-lingual elderly. Int J Geriatr Psychiatry 2000;15(11):1021–1027. Copyright John Wiley & Sons Limited. Reproduced with permission.

| Table 20-6 | **Managing Older Adults: The Siebens Domain Management Model** |

One framework to guide care of older adults is the Siebens Domain Management Model.[a,b] With practicality as a goal, the model organizes a patient's health-related problems and strengths into four domains: I. Medical/Surgical Issues; II. Mental Status/Emotions/Coping; III. Physical Function; and IV. Living Environment. Using these domain headings helps make care planning and documentation efficient and comprehensive and promotes interdisciplinary teamwork.

Format for Provider History & Physical Reports
(Modify as needed for Follow-Up Visits)
Revised with Siebens Domain Management Model (SDMM)[a]

Subjective[b]

Chief Concern or Reason for Visit (follow-up)

History of Present Illness
Symptoms/Workups to date/Patient's Perspective/Worries

Medications

Allergies

Past Medical History
Health maintenance

Family History

Social History
Education/functional health literacy
Marital status, Children, Pets
Nature of relationships (support/caregiver burden)
Alcohol/Tobacco/Drugs
Spirituality and Religious beliefs, practices
Health Power of Attorney/medical directive

Functional History
Prior level of function in Mobility,
Self-care
Medication mgmt, paying bills
Work/Leisure/Fun activities

Review of Systems
Inclusive of sexuality

Objective[b]

Pertinent Physical Exam
Vital Signs and pertinent organ systems

Cognition, Affect
Mobility—moving in bed, getting out of bed or a chair, walking, etc.

Pertinent Labs
Electrolytes, renal function, CBC, alb, etc.

Assessment/Plan[b] (or Hospital Course)
(Note: Identified strengths and problems are best listed with assessment and plan together; each Domain must, ideally, be listed with selected categories as appropriate or else described as "no issues"; topics deemed important but not assessed can be listed with reminder "address tomorrow/next visit.")

I. Medical/Surgical Issues
Symptoms/Diseases/Prevention

II. Mental Status/Emotions/Coping
Cognition (preceded with Communication if any issues including a listing of vision/hearing/speech/language issues)
Emotions
Coping/Behavioral Symptoms
Spirituality
Patient Preferences—Advance Directives

III. Physical Function
Basic ADLs—(self-care—dressing, bathing, home mobility, etc.)
Intermediate ADLs—(meals, medication and money management, etc.)
Advanced ADLs—(sexuality, work, parenting, leisure/fun, driving, general physical activity/exercise, etc.)

IV. Living Environment
A. Physical (home, adaptations, community)
B. Social (family supports/coping, social interactions, etc.)
C. Financial (health insurance, personal income, etc.) & Community Resources

---

[a]Siebens H. Applying the Domain Management Model in Treating Patients with Chronic Diseases Jt. Comm J Qual Improvement 2001;27:302–314.
[b]Note that information is also organized in the familiar SOAP format–Subjective, Objective, Assessment, Plan.
© Hilary C. Siebens, MD, 2005
Also available at: www.siebenspcc.com.

Index

Page numbers followed by b indicate in-chapter boxed material; those followed by t indicate end-of-chapter tables.

A

ABCD method, for melanoma screening, 175, 175b, 179, 180b, 195t
Abdomen. *See also specific organs*
  anatomy of, 433–435
  examination techniques for, 452–469
    for abdominal wall mass, 469
    in adolescents, 865
    for aorta, 465
    for appendicitis, 467–468
    for ascites, 466–467
    auscultation, 454–455
    for bladder, 465
    in children, 845–847
    for cholecystitis, 468
    in infants, 806–807
    inspection, 452–454
    for kidneys, 463–464
    for liver, 457–461
    in older adults, 950
    palpation, 455–456
    percussion, 455
    during pregnancy, 907–909
    recording findings, 469, 469b
    for spleen, 461–463
    for ventral hernias, 468
  in health history, 436–447
    gastrointestinal tract and, 438–445
    urinary tract and, 445–446
  health promotion and counseling and, 447–451
  in older adults, 923
  in physical examination, 21
  during pregnancy, 895
  protuberant, 483t
  quadrants of, 434–435
  sounds in, 484t
  tender, 485t–486t
Abdominal aorta, anatomic considerations, 434
Abdominal aortic aneurysm, 465, 950
  in older adults, 465
  risk factors for, 465
  screening for, 498
Abdominal fullness, 441
Abdominal masses
  assessment of, 469, 483t
  categories of, 456
Abdominal pain, 472t–473t
  in children, 847
  following meals, 496
  gastrointestinal symptoms in, 440–441
  lower acute, 440
  lower chronic, 440
  during pregnancy, 896b
  rebound tenderness, 457
  types of, 436–437
  upper acute, 438
  upper chronic, 438–439
Abdominal reflexes, 730
Abdominal wall
  assessment of mass, 469, 483t
  localized bulges in, 482t
  tenderness of, 485t
Abducens nerve, 684, 685b
  of children, 856b
  examination of, 704
  of infant, 813b
  paralysis of, 270t
Abduction
  of fingers, 635
  of hip, 647b, 648
  of shoulder, 621b
  of thumb, 635
  of wrist, 632b
Abduction stress test, 657b
Abductor group, of hip muscles, 644
ABI (ankle–brachial index), 496–497, 516t
Absence seizure, 751t
Abstract thinking, 159–160
Abuse
  child, 90, 883t
    battered child syndrome, 883t
    sexual, 850, 889t
  domestic violence, during pregnancy, 902–903, 903b
  elder, 940
  family violence, 89–92, 90b
Acetabulum, 643
Achalasia, 474t
Achilles tendinitis, 656
Achilles tendon, 656, 659, 660
  ruptured, 656
Acholic stools, 444
Acid reflux, 439
Acne, 189t
  in adolescents, 862, 880t
  neonatal, 879t
  primary, 192t
  secondary, 192t
Acoustic blink reflex, 793
Acoustic nerve, 684, 685b
  of children, 856b
  examination of, 706
  of infant, 813b
Acoustic neuroma, 263t
Acquired immunodeficiency syndrome (AIDS), skin conditions due to, 197t–198t
Acrocyanosis, in infants, 783, 786b0, 886t
Acromegaly, facies in, 264t
Acromioclavicular arthritis, 673t
Acromioclavicular joint, 615–616
  examination technique for, 623b

Acromion, 615–616, 618
Actinic keratosis, 194t, 946
Actinic lentigines, 196t, 946
Actinic purpura, 919, 946
Active listening, in interviewing, 58
Activities of daily living (ADLs), older adults and, 930–931, 931b
Acute abdomen, 457
Acute coronary syndrome, 346
Acute necrotizing ulcerative gingivitis, 287t
Acute stress disorder, 168t
Adam's bend test, 868
Addiction, defined, 88b
Addison's disease, skin conditions due to, 198t
Adduction
  of fingers, 635
  of hip, 647b, 649
  of shoulder, 621b
  of thumb, 635
  of wrist, 632b
Adduction stress test, 657b
Adductor group, of hip muscles, 644
Adductor tubercle, 650, 653
Adhesive capsulitis, 673t
Adie's pupil, 269t
Adipose tissue, 171
  of breast, 406
ADLs (activities of daily living), older adults and, 930–931, 931b
Adnexa, during pregnancy, 911
Adnexal masses, 562, 575t
Adolescents, 857–871
  acne in, 862, 880t
  contraception methods in, 552–553
  development of, 857, 858b
  examination techniques for, 862–871
    abdomen, 865
    breasts, 863–864, 864b
    female genitalia, 866–868, 867b
    general survey, 862
    head, ears, eyes, neck, and throat, 862
    heart, 862–863, 863b
    male genitalia, 865, 866b
    musculoskeletal system, 868–869, 869b–871b
    nervous system, 872
    recording findings, 872–875
    skin, 862
    vital signs, 862
  health history in, 858–860
  health promotion and counseling and, 860–861, 861b
  sexual maturity assessment in, 542
    females, 863–864, 864b, 867–868, 867b
    males, 865, 866b
  sports preparticipation screening, 869, 869b–871b

Adult illness, in health history, 9
Advanced directives, 935
Adventitia, of artery, 489–490
Adventitious breath sounds, 313, 314b, 318, 330t–331t
Affect, in mental status examination, 148b, 153
Afferent fibers, 684, 688–689
African Americans
  aging of, 929
  breast cancer in women, 411
  cardiovascular disease in, 696
  cardiovascular disease screening for, 351–352, 352b
  health status disparities in older adults, 962t
Afterload, 342
Aging. *See also* Older adults
  optimal, 918–919
Agoraphobia, 168t
Air conduction, 234, 238, 706
Airway obstruction, in children
  lower, 842
  upper, 842
Alcohol use
  asking questions about, 88–89
  CAGE questionnaire for, 88–89, 145b, 448
  in health history, 9
  in older adults, 933–934, 934b
  during pregnancy, 902
  screening for, 145b, 150, 447–448, 448b
  stroke and, 698b
Alertness, 735b
Alice test, 811
Allen test, 507
Allergic rhinitis, perennial, 837, 883t
Allergies
  in health history, 9
  rhinorrhea and, 210
Alopecia areata, 201t
Alternative health practices, in health history, 10
Alveolar mucosa, 242
Alveoli, 299
Alzheimer's disease, 925, 939–940
Ambiguous genitalia, 808
Amblyopia, 832
Amenorrhea, 543b, 544
  in adolescents, 867
  during pregnancy, 896b
Amnestic disorders, 159
Anabolic agents, osteoporosis and, 609
Anal canal, 577–578
Anal fissure, 594t
Analgesia, defined, 721
Anal lesions, 475t
Anal reflex, 731, 814
Anal sphincter, 577–578
Anatomical snuffbox, 630
Anesthesia, defined, 721
Aneurysm
  abdominal aortic, 465, 496, 950
    in older adults, 465
    risk factors for, 465
    screening for, 498
  dissecting aortic, chest pain in, 322t–323t
Angina pectoris, 300, 322t–323t
  coronary heart disease and, 345–346
Angioedema, of lip, 282t
Angioma
  cherry, 193t, 946
  spider, 193t
Angry patient, interviewing, 80–81
Angular cheilitis, 921
Anhedonia, 149
Anisocoria, 225, 269t, 703

Ankle
  anatomy of, 658–660
  assessment of reflexes in, 728–730
    of infant, 814
  dorsiflexion at, testing, 715
  examination techniques for, 660–662
  movements of, 661b
  plantar flexion at, testing, 715
Ankle–brachial index, 496–497, 516t
Ankle clonus, 729–730, 814
Ankylosing spondylitis, 638, 641
Ankylosis, 611
Annulus fibrosis, 637
Anorectal fistula, 594t
Anorectal junction, 577–578
Anorexia, 441
Anorexia nervosa, clinical features of, 136t
Anserine bursa, 652–653, 655
Anserine bursitis, 652, 655
Anterior cruciate ligament, tear of, 609
Anterior cruciate ligament (ACL), 650, 652, 658b
Anterior drawer sign, 658b
Anterior naris, 238
Anterior talofibular ligament, 660
Anterior triangle, of neck, 247
Anteroposterior (AP) diameter, 306
Anticipatory guidance
  with adolescents, 861b
  with young children, 826b
Antihelix, 232
Antiresorptive agents, osteoporosis and, 609
Antisocial personality disorder, 146b
Anus
  abnormalities of, 593t–594t
  anatomy and physiology of, 577–578
  examination techniques for
    female, 592
    male, 586–588
    during pregnancy, 911
    recording findings, 592, 592b
Anxieties, 156b
Anxiety
  chest pain and, 301
  hyperventilation and, 301, 324t–325t
  in mental status examination, 148–149
  screening questions for, 144b
  stranger, 822
Anxiety disorders, 148, 168t
Aorta, 334–335
  coarctation of the, 125, 800
  examination techniques for, 465
  tortuosity of, 922, 949
Aortic aneurysm
  abdominal, 465, 496
    in older adults, 465
    risk factors for, 465
    screening for, 498
  dissecting, chest pain in, 322t–323t
Aortic regurgitation, 339, 402t
Aortic sclerosis, 922, 949
Aortic stenosis, 339, 401t
  in older adults, 922, 949
  syncope in, 748t–749t
Aortic valve, 335
Aortic valve stenosis, 887t
Apgar score, 770, 770b–771b
Aphasia, 153, 154b, 754t
  Broca's, 754t
  Wernicke's, 754t
Aphonia, 754t
Aphthous ulcer, 245, 290t
Apical impulse, 344
  examination techniques for, 372–374

Apley scratch test, 624b
Apnea
  in infants, 797
  sleep, in children, 841
Apocrine glands, 172
Apparent gallop, 803
Appendicitis
  acute, 472t–473t, 486t
  assessment techniques for, 467–468
  in children, 847
Appendix, anatomic considerations, 435
Apprehension sign, 673t
Appropriate for gestational age (AGA), 771b, 772
Aqueous humor body, 217
Arcus senilis, 947
Areola, 405, 407
Argyll Robertson pupils, 269t
Arm(s)
  arteries of, 490
  in coordination assessment, 716
  lymph nodes of, 493
  peripheral vascular system, examination techniques, 499–501
Arrhythmias, 125
  electrocardiogram patterns of, 391t, 392t
  in infants, 878t
  syncope in, 748t–749t
Arterial insufficiency
  chronic, 517t, 518t
  examination techniques for, 508–509
Arterial ischemia, symptoms of, 496
Arterial occlusion, 514t–515t
Arterial pulses. *See also* Pulse
  abnormalities of, 393t
  of arm, 490
  defined, 343
  feeling for difficult, 504b
  in infants, 800–801
  influences on, 343b
  of leg, 491
  physiology of, 343–344
  recommended grading of, 500
Arteries
  anatomy and physiology of, 489–491
  of arm, 490
  of leg, 491
Arteriovenous crossing, 273t
Arteritis, giant cell, headache due to, 260t–261t
Arthralgia, 603
Arthritis
  acromioclavicular, 673t
  acute septic, 603
  in ankle and feet, 660–662
  of elbow, 674t
  gonococcal, 603
  gouty
    of feet, 678t
    joint pain in, 670t–671t
  in hands, 675t
  of hip, 648–649
  of knee, 653
  in older adults, 952
  osteoarthritis, 670t–671t
    of hand, 630–631, 675t
  posttraumatic, 631
  psoriatic, 631
  rheumatoid, 603, 611
    acute, 675t
    chronic, 675t
    in feet, 660
    hand deformities in, 630–631, 675t
    joint pain in, 670t–671t

signs of, 611b
of spine, 638
Articular capsule, of shoulder, 617
Articular cartilage, 599
Articular facets, 636, 636b
Articular processes, 636
Articular structures, 598
Ascites, assessment of, 466–467, 483t
Asian Americans
  aging of, 929
  health status disparities in older adults, 962t
Assessment. *See also* Health history; Physical
    examination
  clinical data and, 30–40
    clustering data into single *vs.* multiple
        problems, 38–39
    displaying, 45–49
    integrating, 49–51
    prevalence and predictive value of, 46,
        46b–48b, 48–49
    problem list, 37–38, 38b
    quality of, 39–40, 40b
    recording, 40–43
    sifting through, 39
  clinical reasoning and, 27–30
    integrating, 49–51
    steps in, 27–30, 27b
    types of, 27
  determining scope of, 4–6
  objective data *vs.* subjective data in, 6, 6b
  plan for care and, 25–26, 30
    example, 35b–37b
    overview, 25–26
Asteatosis, 946
Astereognosis, 722
Asterixis, 733
Asthma
  in children, 843
  dyspnea in, 324t–325t
  hemoptysis in, 326t
  physical findings in, 331t
Asymmetric tonic neck reflex, 816b
Asymmetric weakness, 692
Ataxia, 691–692, 717
  cerebellar, 759t
  sensory, 759t
Ataxic breathing, 140t
Atelectasis, physical findings in, 330t
Atheroma, 490
  complex, 490
Atherosclerosis, 495, 503, 514t–515t
Atherosclerotic peripheral arterial disease, 495,
    503, 514t–515t
Athetosis, 753t
Atonic seizure, 751t
Atrial fibrillation, 125, 391t, 392t
  stroke and, 698b
Atrial flutter, 391t, 392t
Atrial premature contractions, 392t, 802b
Atrial septal defect, 888t
Atrioventricular node, 341
Atrioventricular valves, 335
Atrophy, muscular, 708
Attachment, in newborn, 774b
Attention, in mental status examination, 147b,
    148, 158
Attention deficit/hyperactivity disorder
    (ADHD), 855
Auditory acuity, examination techniques for,
    236, 237b
Auditory nerve, 234
Auricle, 232, 235
Auricular lymph node, posterior, 250

Auscultation
  of abdomen, 454–455
    in infants, 806
  defined, 18b
  of heart, 376–382
    chest wall relations, 340
    in children, 844–845
    heart murmurs, 379–382, 380b
    heart sounds, 376–382
    in infants, 801–805
  of lungs
    in children, 842–843
    in infants, 798–799, 799b
  of thorax
    anterior, 318
    posterior, 311–314, 312b, 314b
Auscultatory gap, 122
Autonomic nervous system (ANS), 220, 683
Autonomy, in patient care, 92b
AV block, 391t
Avoidant personality disorder, 146b
Axillae
  examination techniques for, in older adults, 950
  of older adults, 923
  in physical examination, 20
Axillary lymph nodes, 405
Axillary temperature, 126
Axillary vein, 405
Axiohumeral muscle group, 617
Axioscapular muscle group, 617
Axons, 682

B

Babinski reflex, in infant, 814
Babinski response, 730–731
  in infants, 813b
Back
  movements of, 641b–642b
  in physical examination, 20
Back pain
  low, 668t
    in health history, 601–602
    incidence, 605–606
    lumbosacral radiculopathy and, 732–733
    during pregnancy, 896b
Bacterial pneumonia, hemoptysis in, 326t
Bacterial vaginosis, 569t
Baker's cyst, 655
Balance
  "get up and go" test for, 952b
  in older adults, 952
  risk of fall and, 961t
Balanitis, 527
Ball-and-socket joints, 600, 600b
Ballard scoring system, for gestational age, 773
Balloon sign, 655
Ballotting of the patella, 656
Barlow test, 809–810
Barrel chest, 327t
Bartholin glands
  anatomic considerations, 539–540
  examination of, 556
Basal cell carcinoma, of skin, 173–174,
    194t
  of ear, 278t
  in older adults, 946
Basal ganglia, 682
  lesions of, 745t
Basal ganglia system, 687b
  damage to, 688
Battered child syndrome, 883t
Beau's lines, 203t

Beers criteria, 932
Behavior
  in mental status examination, 152–153
  motor, 152
Behavioral change, motivational interviewing
    for, 72, 72b, 101t
Bell, of stethoscope, 377
Bell's palsy, 706
Bending, lateral
  of neck, 641b
  of spine, 642b
Beneficence, in patient care, 92b
Benign prostatic hyperplasia (BPH), 580, 592t,
    595t, 924
Bethesda system, for Pap smear classification,
    550b
Biceps reflex, assessment of, 726
Biceps tendon, palpation of, 619
Bicipital groove, of humerus, 615–616
Bicipital tendinitis, 673t
Biliary colic, 472t–473t
Bilirubin, in jaundice, 443–444, 444b
Bimanual examination, of female genitalia, 561
  in older adults, 951
  during pregnancy, 910–911
Biot's breathing, 140t
Bipolar disorders, 167t
Birth weight, assessment of, 771, 771b
Bladder
  anatomic considerations, 434–435
  examination techniques for, 465
  intraurethral pressure, 435
  neuroregulatory control of, 435
Bladder distention, 465
Bleeding
  abnormal uterine, 543b, 544, 544b
  postmenopausal, 543b, 545
  vaginal, in children, 849
Blind, legally, 222
Bloating, 439
Blocking, 155b
Blood
  coughing up, 302, 326t
  in urine, 446
  vomiting, 441
Blood pressure
  assessment of, 119–123, 121b, 360
    ambulatory, 119–120
    in anxious patients, 125
    automated devices, 119–120
    in children, 844
    cuff for, 120, 121b
    Doppler method for, 781
    of infants, 781–782
    in obese or thin patient, 125
    in older adults, 919, 945
    during pregnancy, 906
    unequal in arms and legs, 125
  in children, 829–831, 831b, 844
  classification of, 124, 124b
  diastolic, 123
  diet and, 112–113, 139t
  high. *See* Hypertension
  in infants, 781–782
  Korotkoff sounds, 122, 124–125, 830
  low, 124
  normal range for, 124b
  orthostatic hypotension, 124, 748t–749t,
    919
  physiology of, 343–344
  systolic, 123
Blount disease, 853
Body dysmorphic disorder, 165t

skin, 173–177
  basal cell carcinoma, 173–174, 946
  melanoma, 174b, 946
  mole inspection and, 175, 175b
  in older adults, 946
  prevention of, 175
  skin self-examination for, 175, 175b
  squamous cell carcinoma, 173–174, 946
  total-body skin examination for, 175, 175b
  squamous cell carcinoma, 173–174, 194t, 196t, 946
  of stomach, 472t–473t
  of testis, 528, 536t
  of tongue, 246
  of vulva, 568t
Candidal diaper dermatitis, 879t
Candidal vaginitis, 569t
Candidiasis, oral, 285t, 289t, 795, 884t
Canker sore, 290t
Capacity
  altered, interviewing and, 78–79
  defined, 79
Capillaries, anatomy of, 491
Capillary beds, 494–495
Caput succedaneum, 789
Carcinoma
  basal cell, 173–174, 194t, 278t, 946
  of cervix, 572t
  on floor of mouth, 290t
  of lip, 283t
  pancreatic, skin conditions due to, 198t
  of penis, 535t
  squamous cell, 173–174, 194t, 196t, 946
  of tongue, 246
  of vulva, 568t
Cardiac apex, anatomic considerations, 334
Cardiac chambers
  anatomic considerations, 333–335
  pressure gradients in, 336–338
Cardiac conduction system, 341–342
Cardiac cycle, 336–338
Cardiac examination, 369–385
  in adolescents, 862–863, 863b
  auscultation, 376–382
    heart murmurs, 379–382, 380b
    heart sounds, 376–382
  in infants, 799–805
  inspection and palpation in, 370–375
    aortic area, 375
    left ventricular area, 372–374
    pulmonic area, 375
    right ventricular area, 371, 374–375
  integrating, 383
  in older adults, 949
  percussion, 375
  during pregnancy, 907
  sequence for, 369b
  special techniques in, 383–385
    recording findings, 385, 385b
    systolic murmur identification, 383, 488b
Cardiac output, 342–343
Cardinal directions of gaze, 221
Cardinal techniques, for physical examination, 17, 18b
Cardiomegaly, in infants, 800
Cardiomyopathy, hypertrophic, 384, 384b, 401t, 748t–749t
Cardiovascular disease
  coronary heart disease (CHD), chest pain and, 345–346
  ideal cardiovascular health and, 348–349
  incidence, 347–348

screening for
  African Americans, 351–352, 352b
  challenges of, 348
  lifetime risk factors, 353–354
  major risk factors, 352b–353b
  risk factor reduction goals, 348–349
  women, 350–351, 351b
  stroke and, 696
Cardiovascular system. See also under Heart entries
  age-related changes, 344
  anatomy and physiology of, 333–345
    cardiac cycle of, 336–338
    cardiac output of, 342–343
    conduction system of, 341–342
  examination techniques for, 360–385
    blood pressure, 360
    brachial pulse, 369
    carotid pulse, 367–369
    heart, 369–385
    heart rate, 360
    integration of, 383
    jugular venous pressure, 361–365, 364b
    jugular venous pulsations, 365–366
    in older adults, 949
    special techniques, 383–385
  in health history, 345–347
  health promotion and counseling and, 347–360, 347b
  in older adults, 922–923
  in physical examination, 21
  during pregnancy, 894
  in review of systems, 11
  special techniques, systolic murmur identification, 384, 384b
Carotene, 172
Carotenemia, 184t
Carotid artery
  anatomic considerations, 248, 362
  examination techniques for, 253–254
  vs. jugular vein pulsation, 364b
Carotid artery disease, stroke and, 698b
Carotid bruit, 368
  in children, 844, 845b
  in older adults, 949
Carotid pulse
  bruits, 368
  examination techniques for, 367–369
  thrills, 368
Carpal tunnel, 629
Carpal tunnel syndrome, 630
  examination techniques for, 632–634, 712–713
Cartilage, articular, 599
Cartilaginous joints, 599
Caruncle, urethral, 570t
Cataracts, 212
  nuclear, 268t
  in older adults, 921, 947
  peripheral, 268t
Cauda equina, 683–684
Cauda equina compression, 640
Cauda equina syndrome, 602
Cellulitis, acute, 514t–515t
Central cyanosis, 172, 177, 799, 800b
Central lymph nodes, 407–408
Central nervous system, 681–682
  brain, 681–682
  disorders of, 744t–745t
  spinal cord, 683
Central sensitization pain, 130b
Cephalohematoma, 789, 881t
Cerebellar ataxia, 718, 759t
Cerebellar lesions, 745t

Cerebellar system, 687b
  assessment of, in children, 855
  disorders of, 688, 715–718
Cerebellum, 681, 683
Cerebral cortex, lesions of, 744t
Cerebrum, 681–682
Cervical broom, 559b, 951
Cervical cancer, 891t
Cervical lymph nodes
  anterior superficial, 251
  deep cervical chain, 250–251
  posterior, 250
  superficial, 250
Cervical myelopathy, 669t
Cervical polyp, 571t
Cervical radiculopathy, 669t, 712
Cervical scrape, 560b
Cervical vertebrae, anatomy of, 636b
Cervicitis, mucopurulent, 572t
Cervix
  abnormalities of, 572t
  anatomy of, 540–541
  cancer of, 572t
    human papilloma virus and, 548
    risk factors for, 548
    screening for, 549–550, 549b, 550b, 938b
  inspection of, 558–559
  of older adults, 951
  os of, 540–541, 572t
  during pregnancy, 895, 910
  variations in surface of, 571t
Chadwick's sign, 895
Chalazion, 267t
Chancroid, 534t
Chart review, prior to interviewing, 64
Cheilitis
  actinic, 282t
  angular, 282t, 921
Chemicals, irritating, hemoptysis in, 326t
Chemoprevention
  in breast cancer, 418
  in prostate cancer, 583
Cherry angioma, 193t, 946
Chest. See also Heart; Lung(s); Thorax
  anatomical terms for locations on, 298
  deformities of, 327t
Chest expansion, assessment of, 307
Chest indrawing, in infants, 798
Chest pain, 300–301
  angina pectoris, 300, 322t–323t
  anxiety and, 301, 322t–323t
  in health history, 345–346
  sources of, 300b
  in various disorders, 322t–323t
Chest wall
  abnormalities of, in infants, 796
  anatomy of, 293–295
  cardiac auscultatory findings on, 340
  locating findings on, 294–295
Cheyne-Stokes breathing, 140t
Chicken pox, 196t, 199t
Chief complaint, in health history, 7b, 8
Child abuse, 90, 883t
  battered child syndrome, 883t
  sexual, 889t
Child development
  in adolescents, 857, 858b
  assessment of, 815, 818
  in early childhood (1 to 4 years), 819
  in infants, 775, 777–778, 815, 818
  in middle childhood (5 to 10 years), 820
  principles of, 766–767, 766b

Childhood illness, in health history, 9
Children. *See also* Infants
  assessment of
    older, 823–825
    at play, 821b
    younger, 821–823, 822b–823b
  cardiovascular system of, 344
  development of, 819–820
  diagnostic facies in, 882t–883t
  ears of, abnormalities of, 884t
  epilepsy in, 694
  examination techniques for, 828–856
    abdomen, 845–847
    ears, 834–837, 835b
    eyes, 832–834
    female genitalia, 848–851
    general survey, 828–832
    head, 832
    heart, 843–845
    male genitalia, 847–848
    mouth and pharynx, 838–841
    musculoskeletal system, 852–853
    neck, 841–842
    nervous system, 854–856
    nose and sinuses, 837–838
    recording findings, 872–875
    rectum, 852
    skin, 831
    thorax and lungs, 842–843
    vital signs, 829–832
  eyes of, abnormalities of, 884t
  health history in, 821–825, 822b–823b
  health promotion and counseling and,
      767–769, 826–827
    anticipatory guidance, 768
    health supervision visits, 768
    immunizations, 768
    key components of, 768b–769b
  hymen configurations in, 889t
  male genitalia of, 890t
  mouth of, abnormalities of, 884t
  musculoskeletal system of, abnormalities in,
      890t
  skin lesions in, 880t
  teeth of, abnormalities of, 885t
Chill, shaking, 106
Chilliness, 106
Chills, 106
Chlamydia, 551–552, 559
Chloasma, 906
Cholecystitis
  acute, 472t–473t, 486t
  assessment techniques for, 468
Cholesterol, high. *See* Dyslipidemia
Chondrodermatitis helicis, 278t
Chondromalacia, 654
Chorea, 753t
Chorioretinitis, healed, 277t
Chronic obstructive pulmonary disease (COPD)
  anteroposterior (AP) diameter in, 306
  dyspnea in, 324t–325t
  forced expiratory time in, 319
  in older adults, 949
  physical findings in, 331t
Chronic pain, defined, 128
Chvostek's sign, 791
Ciliary body, 217
Circumlocutions, 153
Circumstantiality, 155b
Clanging, 155b
Clarifying, during interview, 59–61
Claudication, intermittent, 495, 514t–515t

Claus Model, 413
Clavicle, 615–616
  fracture of, at birth, 796, 809
Clinical breast examination (CBE), 416
Clinical data, 30–40
  challenges of, 38–40
  clustering data into single *vs.* multiple
      problems, 38–39
  displaying, 45–49
  integrating with clinical reasoning, 49–51
  prevalence and predictive value of, 46, 46b–
      48b, 48–49
  problem list, 37–38, 38b
  quality of, 39–40, 40b
  recording, 40–43
  sifting through, 39
Clinical reasoning, 27–30
  clinical data integrating with, 49–51
  hypothesis in, 28–29, 28b–29b
  steps in, 27–30, 27b
  types of, 27
Clinical record
  checklist for, 40–43
  problem list, 37–38, 38b
  progress notes for, 53t
Clitoris, 539, 951
Clubbing of fingers, 202t
Clubfoot, 811
Cluster headache, 207, 259t
Coarctation of the aorta, 125, 800, 830, 844
Cognitive development
  of adolescents, 857, 858b
  of children, 819–820
  of infants, 775, 815, 818
Cognitive function
  higher, 148b, 159–160
  in mental status examination, 148b, 157–159
Cognitive impairment
  age-associated mild cognitive impairment,
      939–940
  mild cognitive impairment, 939
  in older adults, 928, 939–940
Cold sore, 282t
Colitis, ulcerative
  diarrhea due to, 476t–477t
  skin conditions due to, 199t
Collaborative partnerships, cultural humility
      and, 76b, 77
Colles' fracture, 630
Colloid oncotic pressure, 494–495
Colobomas, 792
Colon
  anatomic considerations, 434–435
  cancer of. *See* Colorectal cancer
Colonoscopy, 450b, 451, 585
  in older adults, 938b
Colorectal cancer
  constipation and, 475t
  diarrhea in, 476t–477t
  in older adults, 951
  risk factors for, 451
  screening for, 450–451, 450b, 585, 938b
Colostrum, 894
Columnar epithelium, 540–541, 571t
Coma, 735b
  Glasgow Coma Scale, 760t
  structural, 760t
  toxic-metabolic, 760t
Comatose patient
  examination techniques for, 734–738
    airway, breathing, and circulation, 734–735
    cardinal don'ts, 734b

  level of consciousness, 735
    neurologic examination in, 736–738
  postures in, 762t
  pupils in, 761t
Comedones, 946
Communication
  cultural humility and, 76–77, 76b
  nonverbal, in interviewing, 61
  with older adults, 926–928, 928b
Communitarianism, 92
Compartment syndrome, 514t–515t
Comprehensive assessment, 4–5, 5b
  health history, adult, 6–13, 7b
  physical examination, adult, 13–23
Comprehensive health history, 56
Compulsions, 156b
Conception age, 899
Conduction system, cardiac, 341–342
Conductive hearing loss, 209, 234, 237–238,
      281t, 706
Condylar joints, 600, 600b
Condyle, of mandible, 613
Condyloma acuminatum, 568t
Condyloma latum, 568t
Condylomata acuminata, 534t
Cone of light, 233
Confabulation, 155b
Confidentiality
  adolescents and, 859
  in patient care, 92b
Confusing patients, interviewing, 78
Congenital heart murmurs, 887t–888t
  aortic valve stenosis, 887t
  atrial septal defect, 888t
  patent ductus arteriosus, 888t
  pulmonary valve stenosis, 887t
  tetralogy of Fallot, 887t
  transposition of the great arteries, 888t
  ventricular septal defect, 888t
Congenital hypothyroidism, 788, 882t
Congenital ptosis, 791
Congenital syphilis, 882t
Congenital torticollis, 796
Congestive heart failure, 384
  in infants, 800–801, 803
Conjunctiva
  anatomic considerations, 215–216
  examination techniques for, 224, 254–255
Conjunctivitis, 262t
Consciousness
  level of
    in comatose patient, 735
    in general survey, 114
    in mental status examination, 152
  loss of, in health history, 693
Consensual reaction to light, 219, 225–226
Consent, informed, 93
Consolidation, 328t
  physical findings in, 330t
Constipation, 443, 475t
  in children, 845
  during pregnancy, 896b
Constructional ability, 160
Contraception methods, health promotion and
      counseling, 552–553
Contractions, during pregnancy, 896b, 908
Convergence, 228
Conversion disorder, 165t
Coordination
  assessment of, in children, 854
  motor assessment of, 715–719
Coracoid process, 615–616, 618

Depersonalization, 156b
Depression, 167t
  constipation related to, 475t
  delirium and dementia in, 700
  low back pain and, 606
  major depressive episode, 167t
  in older adults, 925, 939, 961t
  screening for, 144b, 149–150
de Quervain's tenosynovitis, 630–631, 633, 712
Derailment, 155b
Dermatitis
  atopic, 197t
  in infants
    atopic, 879t
    candidal, 879t
    contact diaper, 879t
Dermatofibroma, 188t
Dermatomes, 689
  assessment of, 723–724
  defined, 723
Dermatomyositis, 198t, 692
Dermis, 171
Dermoscopy, 176
Detrusor muscle, 435
Developmental disorders, dysconjugate patterns in, 270t
Developmental milestones
  of adolescence, 858b
  for children
    early childhood, 819
    middle childhood, 820b
  for infants, 775, 777–778
    visual, 792, 792b
Developmental quotient, 818
DEXA scanning, 607
Dextrocardia, 371
Diabetes
  cardiovascular disease and, 352b, 353b, 355–356
  peripheral neuropathies and, 699
  screening and diagnosis, 356b
  skin conditions due to, 198t
  in stroke, 697b
Diabetic neuropathies, 699
Diabetic retinopathy, 786
Diagnosis, working, 29–30
Diagnostic hypothesis, 71. *See also* Hypothesis
Diaphragm, 299
  of stethoscope, 377
Diarrhea, 476t–477t
  acute, 442, 476t–477t
  chronic, 442, 476t–477t
  osmotic, 476t–477t
  secretory, 476t–477t
  voluminous, 476t–477t
Diarrheal syndrome, 476t–477t
Diastasis recti, 482t, 806, 895
Diastole
  defined, 336
  extra sounds in, 379b, 398t
Diastolic blood pressure, 123, 360
Diastolic heart murmurs, 382, 402t
Diencephalon, 681–682, 684
Diet. *See also* Nutrition
  assessing intake, 110
  blood pressure and, 112–113, 139t
  food sources of nutrients, 139t
  in health history, 10
  health promotion and counseling and, 108–113, 109b

healthy fats *vs.* unhealthy fats, 359b
  nutrition screening, 137t
  recommendations for weight loss, 111–112, 112b
  resources for, 110, 111b, 112
Diethylstilbestrol (DES), cervical abnormalities due to, 572t
Differential diagnosis, 8, 71
Digital rectal examination (DRE), 581–582, 586–592
Diphtheria, 285t
Diplopia, 209, 692, 704
Direct reaction to light, 219, 225
Disc, herniated, assessment for, 732–733
Discomfort
  defined, 438–439
  lower abdomen, 440
  upper abdomen, 438–439
Discriminative sensations, assessment of, 722–723
Disease, *vs.* illness, 68
Disease/illness distinction model, 68
Disequilibrium, 263t, 691–692
Dislocation
  anterior of humerus, 673t
  anterior of shoulder, 618
  of hip, in infants, 809–810
  posterior of elbow, 627
Dissecting aortic aneurysm, chest pain in, 322t–323t
Disseminated intravascular coagulation (DIC), skin conditions due to, 198t
Dissociative disorder, 165t
Distal interphalangeal joints
  of fingers, 628, 631
  of toes, 659
Distal radioulnar joint, 628
Distal weakness, 692
Distraction, during pediatric examination, 776
Distress, signs of, 114
Diverticulitis, 475t
  acute, 472t–473t, 486t
Dizziness, 209–210, 263t, 691
DNR (do-not-resuscitate order), 91
Dolichocephaly, 789
Doll's eye reflex, 791
Doll's eyes movements, 736–737
Domestic violence, 89–90, 90b
  during pregnancy, 902–903, 903b
Do-not-resuscitate orders (DNR), 91
Dopone, for fetal heart rate, 905b
Doppler method, for blood pressure assessment, 781
Dorsalis pedis artery, pulse assessment at, 504
  in infants, 801
Dorsiflexion, 661b
Dorsiflexor muscles, 659, 659 0
Down syndrome, 843
  facies in, 883t
Dress
  in general survey, 115
  in mental status examination, 152–153
Drop arm sign, 625b
Drop attack, 751t
Dropped-arm test, 623
Drug–drug interactions, 932
Drug use
  constipation due to, 475t
  diarrhea due to, 475t
  in health history, 9

illicit
  asking questions about, 89
  during pregnancy, 902
  older adults and, 931–932, 932b, 961t
  urinary incontinence due to, 480t–481t
  vertigo due to, 263t
Drusen, 232, 277t, 948
Dry atrophic macular degeneration, 232
Dual diagnosis, 141
Duchenne muscular dystrophy, 708
Dullness
  in abdomen, 455
  percussion note, 317
Dull percussion note, 310, 310b
Duodenum, anatomic considerations, 434
Dupuytren's contracture, 611, 630, 676t
Durable power of attorney for health care, 79
Dynamic stabilizers, of shoulder, 615
Dysarthria, 153, 692, 707, 754t
Dysdiadochokinesis, 716
Dysesthesias, 693
Dyskinesias, oral–facial, 752t
Dyslipidemia
  ATP III guidelines, 357b
  cardiovascular disease and, 352b, 353b, 356–357, 357b
  skin conditions due to, 198t
  in stroke, 697b
Dysmenorrhea, 543b, 544
Dysmetria, 717
Dyspareunia, 546
Dyspepsia, 438–439, 472t–473t
Dysphagia, 439, 441–442, 474t
  esophageal, 474t
  oropharyngeal, 474t
Dysphonia, 754t
Dyspnea, 301, 346–347
  paroxysmal nocturnal, 347
  in various disorders, 324t–325t
Dysthymic disorder, 167t
Dystonia, 753t
Dysuria, 445

E

Ear canal, 232–233
  examination techniques for, 235–236
Eardrum
  abnormalities of, 279t–280t
  anatomic considerations, 233–234
  examination techniques for, 235–236
  normal, 279t
Ear(s)
  abnormalities of, in children, 884t
  anatomy of, 232–234
  equilibrium and, 234
  examination techniques for, 235–238
    for adolescents, 862
    for children, 834–837, 835b
    for infants, 793
  external, 232
  in health history, 209–210
  hearing pathways and, 234
  inner, 234
  lumps on or near, 278t
  middle, 233–234
  in physical examination, 20
  in review of systems, 11
Eating disorders
  anorexia nervosa, 136t
  bulimia nervosa, 136t
Ecchymosis, 193t

Eccrine glands, 172
ECG (electrocardiogram)
  heart rhythm patterns, 391t
  normal findings, 341–342
  overview, 341
Echoing, during interview, 61
Echolalia, 155b
Ectocervix, 540
Ectropion, 266t, 540, 947
Eczema
  atopic, 185t
  in infants, 879t
Edema
  dependent, 347
  of foot and leg, 505–506
  in health history, 347
  peripheral causes of, 513t
  pitting, 505, 513t
  during pregnancy, 896b, 906, 911
  scrotal, 535t
Efferent fibers, 684
Effusion
  pleural, 331t
  serous, 280t
Egophony, 314
Ejaculation, 523
  in adolescents, 865
  premature, 523
Ejaculatory duct, 519–520
Elastic laminae, 490
Elbow
  anatomic considerations, 626
  examination techniques for, 626–627
  extension at, testing, 710–711
  flexion at, testing, 710–711
  movements of, 627b
  swollen or tender, 674t
Elder abuse, 940
Elders. See Older adults
Electrocardiogram (ECG)
  heart rhythm patterns, 391t
  normal findings, 341–342
  overview, 341
Emotional cues, in interview, 69–70
Emotional development
  of adolescents, 857, 858b
  of children, 819–820
  of infants, 775, 815, 818
Empathetic response, 58
Empowerment, patient, during interview,
    62–63, 63b
Encouragement, during interview, 60
Endocarditis, infectious, skin conditions
    due to, 198t
Endocervical brush, 560b
Endocrine system, in review of systems, 13
End-of-life decisions, 935
Endometriosis, 547
Entropion, 266t, 947
Environment
  adapting for older adults, 926–927
  for interview, 65
  for physical examination, 14
Epicondylitis
  lateral, 627, 674t
  medial, 627, 674t
Epidermis, 171
Epidermoid cyst, 528, 568t
Epididymis
  abnormalities of, 537t
  anatomy of, 519–520
  palpation of, 528

Epididymitis, 537t
  tuberculous, 537t
Epigastric hernia, 482t
Epigastric pain, 437–438
Epiglottitis, acute, 840
Epilepsy, 694
Episcleritis, 267t
Epistaxis, 211
Epitrochlear lymph nodes, 20, 493, 501
Epstein's pearls, 794
Epulis, 287t
Erectile dysfunction, 523
Erection, 520
Erythema, 184t
  vulvar, 950
Erythema infectiosum, 199t
Erythema multiforme, 196t
Erythema nodosum, 514t–515t
Erythema toxicum, 786b0, 879t
Erythropoietin, during pregnancy, 894
Esophageal cancer, 474t
Esophageal dysphagia, 474t
Esophageal spasm, diffuse, 474t
  chest pain in, 322t–323t
Esophageal stricture, 474t
Esophagitis, reflux, chest pain in, 322t–323t
Esotropia, 270t, 791
Essential tremor, in older adults, 953
Estrogen, during pregnancy, 893
Estrogen replacement therapy, in
    menopause, 553
Ethics, 92–95
  defined, 92
  feminist, 92
  informed consent and, 93
  medical, 92
  Tavistock principles, 94, 94b
ETHIC(S) mnemonic, cultural
    considerations, 929
Ethmoid sinus, 239
Ethnicity. See Cultural considerations
Ethnogeriatric imperative, 929
Eustachian tube, 233
Eversion, of ankle, 661b
Evidence-based decision-making, 28
Exercise
  counseling about, 359–360
  in health history, 10
  health promotion and counseling for, 113,
    113b, 605, 605b
  moderate and vigorous activity, 113b
  in older adults, 936
  during pregnancy, 901
  stroke and, 697b
Exophthalmos, 254, 266t
Exostoses, 235
Exotropia, 270t, 791
Expiration, 299
Extension
  of ankle, 661b
  of elbow, 627b
  of fingers, 634
  of hip, 647b, 648
  of knee, 656b
  of neck, 641b
  of shoulder, 621b
  of spine, 642b
  of thumb, 635
  of wrist, 632b
Extensor group, of hip muscles, 644
External acoustic meatus, 613
External ear, 232

External rotation
  of hip, 647b, 649
  of knee, 656b
  of shoulder, 622b, 624b
Extra-articular structures, 598–599
Extraocular movements
  examination techniques for, 226–228, 704
  in infants, 791
  overview, 221
Extraocular muscles
  examination techniques for, 226–228
  movements of, 226–227
Extremities. See also Arm(s); Leg(s)
  examination techniques for, during
    pregnancy, 911
  lower, in physical examination, 21–22
Eyebrows, 223
Eyelid patch, 787b
Eyelids
  abnormalities of, 266t
  anatomic considerations, 215
  examination techniques for, 223–224, 254–255
  of older adults, 920, 947
Eyes
  abnormalities of, in children, 884t
  anatomy of, 215–220
  autonomic nerve supply to, 220
  dysconjugate gaze, 270t
  examination techniques for, 221–232
    in adolescents, 862
    in children, 832–834
    in infants, 791–792
  extraocular movements, 221
  fundi of
    diabetic retinopathy, 276t
    hypertensive, 275t
    light-colored spots in, 277t
    normal, 275t
    red spots and streaks in, 274t
  headache due to disorder of, 260t–261t
  in health history, 207–208
  lumps and swelling around, 267t
  muscles of, 221, 226–228
  of older adults, 920, 947
  optic disc of
    abnormalities of, 272t
    natural variations of, 271t
  in physical examination, 20
  position and alignment of, 223
  pupillary abnormalities of, 269t
  pupillary reactions and, 219–220
  red reflex, 229
  in review of systems, 11
  visual fields and, 218
  visual pathways and, 218–219

F

Face
  abnormalities of, 264t
  examination techniques for, 215
  during pregnancy, 906
Faces Pain Scale, for pain, 128
Facial expression
  in general survey, 115
  in mental status examination, 153
Facial nerve, 684, 685b
  of children, 856b
  examination of, 706
  of infant, 813b
  lesion of, 757t
  palsy of, 882t

Hemiparesis
  defined, 710
  spastic, 759t
Hemiplegia, 710
  posture in, 762t
Hemochromatosis, skin conditions due to, 198t
Hemoglobin, in skin color, 172
Hemoptysis, 302, 326t
Hemorrhage
  subarachnoid
    assessment for, 731–732
    headache due to, 260t–261t
  subconjunctival, 262t
Hemorrhagic stroke, 697
Hemorrhoids
  external, 593t
  internal, 593t
  during pregnancy, 896, 911
Hepatitis
  A, 448–449
  B, 449
  C, 449–450
  risk factors for, 444b, 448–450
Hepatitis B immunization, 449, 449b
Hepatomegaly, 487t
  in adolescents, 865
  in children, 846–847
Hernia
  epigastric, 482t
  examination techniques for, 529–530
  femoral, 521, 538t
  incisional, 482t
  inguinal, 521, 529, 538t, 646
    in children, 848
    in females, 563
    in infants, 808
  scrotal, 530, 535t
  umbilical, 482t, 806
  ventral, assessment techniques for, 468
Herniated disc, 640, 732–733
Herpes simplex, 186t, 188t
  genital, 534t, 568t
  on lip, 282t
Herpes zoster, 188t, 199t, 946
Herpetic stomatitis, 884t
Hinge joints, 600, 600b
Hip dysplasia, in infants, 809–810
Hip(s)
  anatomy of, 643–644
  examination techniques for, 645–649
    in infants, 809–810
  flexion deformity of, 648
  motor assessment of
    abduction, 713
    adduction, 713
    extension, 714
    flexion, 713
  movements of, 647b, 649
Hispanic Americans
  aging of, 929
  health status disparities in older adults, 962t
Histrionic personality disorder, 146b
Hives, 188t, 197t, 880t
HIV infection
  in females, 552
  health promotion and counseling for,
    524–526, 552
  incidence, 525, 552
  in males, 524–526
  screening guidelines, 552
Hoarseness, 211
Holosystolic heart murmur, 380, 399t

Hoover sign, 798
Hormone replacement therapy (HRT)
  in breast cancer, 411
  in menopause, 553
Hormones
  changes during pregnancy, 893–894
  of ovaries, 541
  placental, 894
Horner's syndrome, 269t, 703–704
Household safety, in older adults, 938b
Houston, valves of, 577–578
HSV 6, 199t
Human chorionic gonadotropin (hCG), during
    pregnancy, 893–894
Human immunodeficiency virus (HIV)
  in females, 552
  health promotion and counseling for,
    524–526, 552
  incidence, 525, 552
  in males, 524–526
  screening guidelines, 552
Human papilloma virus (HPV)
  cervical cancer and, 548
  vaccine for, 550
Human placental lactogen, during pregnancy, 894
Humeroulnar joint, 626
Humerus, 615
  anterior dislocation of, 673t
  in elbow joint, 626
  in shoulder anatomy, 615–616
Hutchinson's teeth, 288t
Hydration, in infants, 785
Hydrocele, 528–529, 535t, 808
Hydrocephalus, 881t
Hydrostatic pressure, 494
Hymen, 539
  imperforate, 557
  normal configurations, 850, 851b
Hyoid bone, 248
Hyperalgesia, defined, 721
Hyperemesis gravidarum, 896b, 905
Hyperesthesia, defined, 721
Hyperkinetic ventricular impulse, 394t
Hyperopia, 208, 230
Hyperpnea, 140t
Hyperpyrexia, defined, 126
Hyperreflexia, 725
Hyperresonance, percussion note, 310,
    310b, 317
Hypertension
  in adolescents, 862
  assessment of. See Blood pressure, assessment of
  cardiovascular disease and, 352b, 353b,
    354–355
  in children, 830–831
  chronic, during pregnancy, 906
  classification of, 124b, 354b
  gestational, 906
  in infants, 782, 878t
  isolated systolic, 124, 945
  lifestyle modifications for, 358, 358b
  masked, 119
  ocular, 213
  in older adults, 919, 945, 949
  in retinal artery, 273t
  in stroke, 697b
  white coat, 119, 125
Hypertensive retinopathy, 275t
Hyperthyroidism, 212, 291t
  in children, 883t
  effects on eye, 226–228
  skin conditions due to, 198t

Hypertrophic cardiomyopathy, syncope in,
    748t–749t
Hypertrophy, muscular, 708
Hyperventilation, 140t
  anxiety and, 301, 324t–325t
  hypocapnia due to, 748t–749t
Hypervolemia, 364
Hypesthesia, defined, 721
Hypocapnia, 748t–749t
Hypochondriasis, 165t
Hypogastric pain, 437
Hypoglossal nerve, 246, 684, 685b
  of children, 856b
  examination of, 707–708
  of infant, 813b
Hypoglycemia, syncope in, 748t–749t
Hypomanic episode, 167t
Hyporeflexia, 725
Hypospadias, 527, 535t, 807, 890t
Hypotension, 124
  orthostatic, 124
    defined, 945
    in older adults, 919, 945
    syncope in, 748t–749t
Hypothalamus, 682
Hypothenar atrophy, 630, 676t, 708
Hypothermia, 126
  causes of, 127
  defined, 126
  in older adults, 919, 945
Hypothesis
  in clinical reasoning, 28–29, 28b–29b
  diagnostic, 71
  interviewing and, 71
Hypothyroidism, 212, 291t, 728
  congenital, 788, 882t
  skin conditions due to, 198t
Hypotonia, 709
  in newborn, 812
Hypovolemia, 363

I

IADLs (instrumental activities of daily living),
    older adults and, 931, 931b
Ichthyosis vulgaris, 190t
Icterus, 443–444
Idiopathic pain, 130b
Iliac crest, 433, 637, 643, 646
Iliac spine, 433
  anterior superior, 643, 646
  posterior superior, 643, 646
Iliac tubercle, 643, 646
Iliopectineal bursa, 644
Iliopsoas bursa, 644
Ilium, 643
  wing of, 643
Illness, *vs.* disease, 68
Illusions, 157
Immunizations, 768
  adult
    influenza, 304, 304b
    pneumococcal disease, 304, 305b
  childhood, 891t
  in health history, 9
  in older adults, 936, 937b
  during pregnancy, 903
Impetigo, 190t
  in infants, 879t
Impingement syndrome, 672t
Incisional hernia, 482t

Incoherence, 155b
Incontinence. *See* Urinary incontinence
Incus, 233
Indigestion, 440
Infantile automatisms, 815, 815b–817b
Infants (first year)
    cry of, 795, 795b
    cyanosis in, 886t
    developmental milestones for, 775, 777–778
    development of, 775, 815, 818
    ears of, abnormalities of, 884t
    examination techniques for
        abdomen, 806–807
        breasts, 805
        ears, 793
        eyes, 791–792
        female genitalia, 808–809
        general survey, 780–783
        head, 788–791
        heart, 799–805
        hips, 809–810
        male genitalia, 807–808
        mouth and pharynx, 794–795
        musculoskeletal system, 809–811
        neck, 796
        nervous system, 812–818, 818b
        nose and sinuses, 794
        rectal examination, 809
        skin, 783–787
        thorax and lungs, 796–799
        vital signs, 781–783
    eyes of, abnormalities of, 884t
    head of, abnormalities of, 881t
    health promotion and counseling and, 778, 778b
    health supervision visits for, 778, 778b
    heart murmurs in
        normal variants of, 801, 802b, 803–804, 804b
        pathologic, 802, 804–805, 805b
    heart rhythm abnormalities in, 878t
    hypertension in, 782, 878t
    male genitalia, abnormalities of, 890t
    mouth of, abnormalities of, 884t
    newborns. *See* Newborn(s)
    preterm, 771–772, 789
    skin of, abnormalities of, 879t
    vital signs, 781–783
Infection. *See also specific infections*
    constipation due to, 475t
    diarrhea due to, 476t–477t
    umbilical hernia in, 482t
Infectious endocarditis, 198t
Inferior vena cava, 335, 491
Inflammation
    in joint pain, 603
    meningeal, 731–732, 842
Inflammatory bowel disease (IBD), diarrhea due to, 476t–477t
Inflammatory diarrhea, 476t–477t
Influenza immunizations
    in adults, 304, 304b
    in older adults, 936, 937b
Informed consent, 93
Infraspinatus muscle, 616
    examination technique for, 625b
Inguinal canal, 521
Inguinal hernia, 521, 529–530, 538t
    in children, 848
    in females, 563
    in infants, 808
Inguinal ligament, 646

Inguinal lymph nodes, 493–494, 502, 521
Inguinal ring, 521
Inguinal structures, 646
Initial survey, thorax, 306
Inner ear, 234
Insect bites, 189t, 880t
Insight, in mental status examination, 148, 148b, 157
Insomnia, in older adults, 931
Inspection
    of abdomen, 452–454
        in infants, 806
    of axillae, 425
    of breast, female, 420–421
    in cardiac examination, 370–375
    defined, 18b
    of elbow, 626
    of eyes, infants, 791–792
    female genitalia
        cervix, 558–559
        external, 556
        vagina, 560
    of hip, 645–646
    of inguinal hernia, 529
    of knee, 652–653
    of lungs, in infants, 797–798
    of male genitalia, 527
    of penis, 527
    of scrotum, 528
    of shoulder, 618
    of skin, 177–178
        for infants, 783–785
    of spine, 637–638, 639b
    of thorax
        anterior, 315
        posterior, 306
    of wrist and hand, 629–630
Inspiration, 299
Instrumental activities of daily living (IADLs), older adults and, 931, 931b
Intelligence, limited, interviewing and, 84
Intention tremors, 752t
Intercarpal joints, 628
Interdental papillae, 242
Intermittent claudication, 495, 514t–515t
Internal capsule, 682–683
Internal rotation
    of hip, 647b, 650
    of knee, 656b
    of shoulder, 622b, 624b
Interphalangeal joints
    distal, 659
    proximal, 659
Interpreter, working with, 81–82, 82b
Intervertebral discs, 637
    herniated, 640
Intervertebral foramen, 636, 636b
Interviewing, 55–95
    adapting for special situations, 77–92
        across language barriers, 81–82, 82b
        with angry patient, 80–81
        with challenging patients, 77
        with confusing patients, 78
        with crying patient, 80
        patients with altered capacity, 78–79
        patients with impaired hearing, 83–84
        patients with impaired vision, 84
        patients with limited intelligence, 84
        patients with low literacy, 82–83
        patients with personal problems, 84
        seductive patients, 84
        with silent patients, 77–78

        talkative patient, 79–80
        with talkative patients, 79–80
    Brief Action Planning, 102t
    chart review prior to, 64
    clinical behavior and appearance, 65
    cultural considerations in, 73–77
    environment and, 65
    ethics and, 92–95
    goals for, 64
    health history format for, 56
    motivational, 72, 72b, 101t
    note taking and, 67
    patient-centered, 55
    preparation, 64–65
    self-reflection and, 73
    sensitive topics in, 85–92, 85b
        alcohol and drugs, 88–89, 88b
        death and dying patient, 90–91
        family violence, 89–90, 90b
        guidelines for, 85, 85b–86b
        mental health history, 87–88
        sexual history, 86–87, 87b
    sequence of, 63b, 65–73
        clarifying patient's story, 59–61, 70–71
        closing, 72–73
        diagnostic hypothesis, 71
        establishing agenda, 67–68
        establishing rapport, 65–67
        inviting patient's story, 68
        patient's perspective, 68–69, 69b–70b
        responding to emotional cues, 69–70
    techniques for, 58–64, 58b
        active listening, 58
        empathetic response, 58
        empowering patient, 62–63, 63b
        nonverbal communication, 61
        partnering, 62
        questioning, 59–61, 59b
        reassurance, 61
        summarization, 62
        transition, 62
        validation, 61
Intestinal obstruction
    acute mechanical, 472t–473t
    constipation and, 475t
Intima of artery, 489–490
Intracranial pressure, increased, in infants, 788
Intraurethral pressure, 435
Introitus, 539
Intussusception, 475t
Inversion, of ankle, 661b
Involuntary movements
    in health history, 694
    motor assessment of, 708
    types of, 752t–753t
Iris, 215
    examination techniques for, 225
Iritis, acute, 262t
Iron, food sources of, 139t
Irritability, in newborn, 812
Irritable bowel syndrome, 475t, 476t–477t
Ischemia, mesenteric, 472t–473t
Ischemic stroke. *See also* Stroke
    defined, 695
Ischial (ischiogluteal) bursa, 644, 647
Ischial (ischiogluteal) bursitis, 647
Ischial tuberosity, 640, 644
Ischiogluteal bursa, 644
Ischium, 643
Isometric handgrip, 385
Isthmus, of uterus, 540

Palpebral fissure, 215
Palpitations, 346
Pancreas
  anatomic considerations, 434
  cancer of, 198t, 472t–473t
Pancreatitis
  acute, 472t–473t, 486t
  chronic, 472t–473t
  skin conditions due to, 198t
Panic disorder, 148, 168t
Pannus, 483t
Pansystolic (holosystolic) heart murmur,
    380, 399t
Papanicolaou (Pap) smear
  in cervical cancer screening, 549–550,
    549b, 550b
  classification of, 550b
  guidelines for, 549–550, 549b
  during pregnancy, 910
  specimen collection, 559, 559b–560b
Papilledema, 272t
  detection of, 230b–231b
Papilloma, 426
Papules, 188t, 196t
Parachute reflex, 817b
Paradoxical breathing, 798
Paradoxical pulse, 368, 393t
Paralysis
  defined, 710
  facial, 757t
  flaccid, 737
Paranasal sinuses, 239. See also Sinuses
Paranoid schizoid personality disorder, 145b
Paraphasias, 153
Paraphimosis, 527
Paraplegia, defined, 710
Parasternal muscles, 299
Parasympathetic nervous system, 683
Paratonia, 758t
Paraurethral glands
  anatomic considerations, 539
  examination of, 564
Paravertebral muscles, 640
Paresis, defined, 710
Parietal bone, 214
Parietal lobe, 681–682
Parietal pain, 437
Parietal pleura, 298
Parkinsonian gait, 759t
Parkinson's disease
  abnormal facies in, 264t
  tremors in, 953
Paronychia, 202t
Parotid duct, 214, 244
Parotid gland, 214
  enlargement of, 264t
Paroxysmal atrial tachycardia, 802
Paroxysmal nocturnal dyspnea, 347
Paroxysmal supraventricular tachycardia, 782, 802
Pars flaccida, 233, 236
Pars tensa, 233, 236
Partnering, in interviewing, 62
Past history, in health history, 7b, 9
Patella, ballotting of the, 656
Patellar tendon, 650, 653–654
Patellofemoral compartment, 654
Patellofemoral grinding test, 654
Patellofemoral joint, 650
Patellofemoral syndrome, 654
Patent ductus arteriosus, 403t, 801, 888t
Pathologic process, in clinical reasoning, 28
Pathophysiologic problems, 28

Patient assessment. See Assessment
Patient-centered interviewing, 55
Patient comfort, during physical examination,
    15–16
Patient record, 26
Patient's perspective, 68–69, 69b–70b
Pectoralis major muscle, 405
Pectoral lymph nodes, 407–408, 425
Pectus carinatum, 796
Pectus excavatum, 796
Pediatrics. See Adolescents; Children; Infants
Pedicle, 636b
Pediculosis pubis, 556
Pelvic examination, 553–564, 554b
  in adolescents, 866–868, 867b
  approach to, 553–554
  bimanual examination, 561
  cervix, 558–559
  equipment for, 555
  external genitalia, 556
  indications for, 554
  lubricant use in, 563b
  in older adults, 950–951
  ovaries, 561–562
  Pap smear specimen collection, 559,
    559b–560b
  patient positioning, 556
  pelvic muscles, 562
  in rape victims, 555
  rectovaginal examination, 563
  speculum use in, 557–559
  tips for successful, 554b
  uterus, 561
  vagina, 560
Pelvic floor
  examination of, 562
  during pregnancy, 911
Pelvic inflammatory disease (PID), 575t
Pelvic muscles, examination of, 562
Pelvic pain
  acute, 548
  chronic, 548
Pelvic tilt, 639b
Penile discharge, 523
Penis
  abnormalities of, 535t
  anatomy and physiology of, 519–520
  cancer of, 535t
  of children, 847
  development of, Tanner stages for, 865, 866b
  examination techniques for, 527
  of infants, 807–808
  lesions of, 523
  of older adults, 923–924
Peptic ulcer, 472t–473t
Perception(s)
  in mental status examination, 147b, 157
  in newborn, 774b
Percussion
  of abdomen, 455
    in infants, 806–807
  in cardiac examination, 375
  defined, 18b
  of kidneys, 464
  of liver, 457–458
  of spleen, 461–462
  of thorax
    anterior, 317–318
    posterior, 308–311, 310b
Percussion notes, 309–311, 310b
  in various disorders, 330t–331t
Perforating veins, 492

Pericardial friction rub, 403t
Pericarditis, chest pain in, 322t–323t
Perimenopause, 544
Perineum, 539
Periodicity schedule, infant, 778, 778b
Periodic physical examination, 5–6
Peripheral arterial disease, 495–496, 496b
  atherosclerotic, 495, 503, 514t–515t
  risk factor for lower extremity, 497b
Peripheral cataracts, 268t
Peripheral cyanosis, 172
Peripheral nerves, 684, 686
Peripheral nervous system, 683–686, 685b, 686
  anatomic considerations, 745t
  cranial nerves in, 684, 685b
  disorders of, 745t
  peripheral nerves, 684, 686
Peripheral neuropathies, 721
  diabetes and, 699
  mononeuropathy, 745t
  polyneuropathy, 745t
Peripheral vascular disease
  arterial, 489, 495–496, 496b
    painful, 514t–515t
    risk factors for, 497b
    screening for, 496–498, 497b
    skin conditions due to, 199t
  venous, 489, 514t–515t
Peripheral vascular system
  anatomy and physiology of, 489–495
    arteries, 489–491
    veins, 491–492
  examination techniques for, 498–510, 498b,
    499b
    arms, 499–501
    arterial insufficiency, 508–509
    arterial supply to hand, 507–508
    in infants, 800–801
    legs, 501–507
    mapping varicose veins, 509
    in older adults, 950
    recording findings, 510, 510b
    venous valve competency, 509–510
  in health history, 495–496
  health promotion and counseling and,
    496–498, 497b
  of older adults, 923
  in physical examination, 21–22
  in review of systems, 12
Peritoneal inflammation, 486t
Peritonitis, assessment for, 457
Periumbilical pain, 437
Perpendicular lighting, 14
Perseveration, 155b
Personal history, in health history, 7b, 10
Personal hygiene
  in general survey, 115
  in mental status examination, 152–153
Personality disorders, 145, 145b–146b
Pertussis, 891t
Pes planus, 890t
Petechiae, oral, 286t
Petechia purpura, 193t
Petersen speculum, 555
Peutz-Jeghers syndrome, 283t
Peyronie's disease, 535t
Phalen's sign, 634
Pharyngitis, 211, 284t
  streptococcus, 840, 885t
Pharynx
  abnormalities of, 284t–286t
  anatomic considerations, 244

hyperactive, 725
hypoactive, 725
in older adults, 926
optic blink, 792
in physical examination, 22
primitive, in newborn, 815, 815b–817b
recording findings for, 739
spinal, 689–690
Reflex esophagitis, chest pain in, 322t–323t
Reflex hammer, 725
Refractive error, 230
Regurgitation, 439, 441
Reinforcement, in deep tendon reflexes
    assessment, 726
Reiter's syndrome, skin conditions due
    to, 199t
Relaxin, during pregnancy, 894
Reliability, of a test, 43b
Remote memory, 158
Renal artery disease, screening for, 497–498
Reproductive system. See Female genitalia; Male
    genitalia
Respirations. See also Breathing; Respiratory rate
    assessment of, in comatose patient, 736
Respiratory infection, upper, in children, 842
Respiratory rate
    abnormal, 140t
    assessment of, 126
    in children, 831–832
    in infants, 782, 797
    normal, 126, 140t
    in older adults, 919, 945
Respiratory system. See also Lung(s)
    in review of systems, 11
Resting tremors, 752t
Restless leg syndrome, 694
Rest pain, 514t–515t
Retching, 440
Retention cyst, 571t
Reticular activating (arousal) system, 683
Retina, inspection of, 229–231, 231b–232b
Retinal artery
    hypertensive, 273t
    normal, 273t
Retinal hemorrhage, 274t
Retinopathy
    diabetic, 276t
    hypertensive, 275t
Retraction signs, in breast cancer, 431t
Retroflexion, of uterus, 573t
Retrograde filling test, 509–510
Retroversion, of uterus, 573t
Review of systems, in health history, 7b,
    10–13
Rheumatic fever, 603, 611
Rheumatoid arthritis, 603, 611
    acute, 675t
    chronic, 675t
    in feet, 660
    hand deformities in, 630–631, 675t
    joint pain in, 670t–671t
    skin conditions due to, 199t
Rheumatoid nodules
    on ear, 278t
    of elbow, 674t
Rhinitis, 240
    perennial allergic, 837, 883t
    purulent, 838
Rhinorrhea, 210
RhoGAM immunization, 903
Rhonchi, 314, 314b, 329t
    in infants, 799

Ribs
    anatomic considerations, 293–295
    fractured, 319
Riedel's lobe, 487t
Right atrium, 334–335
Right ventricle, 333–335
Right ventricular impulses, abnormalities
    of, 394t
Rigidity, 457, 709, 758t
Rinne test, 238, 281t, 706
Ritualistic behavior, 148
Rocky Mountain Spotted fever, skin conditions
    due to, 199t
Romberg test, 718
Rooting reflex, 816b
Roseola infantum, 199t
Rotation
    external
        of hip, 647b, 649
        of knee, 657b
        of shoulder, 622b, 624b
    internal
        of hip, 647b, 649
        of knee, 657b
        of shoulder, 622b, 624b
    of neck, 641b
    of spine, 642b
Rotator cuff
    compression, 623
    examination techniques for, 624b–625b
    tear, 618, 620, 623, 672t
    tendinitis, 672t
Routine clinical check-up, 5–6
Rovsing's sign, 468, 847
Rubella, 199t, 891t
Rubeola, 199t
Rubor, 509
R wave, 341

S

Sacroiliac joint, 640, 643, 646
Sacroiliac notch, 640
Sacrum, 643
Safety, in older adults, 937–938, 938b
Saliva, decreased, in older adults, 948
Salmon patch, 785, 787b
Salpingitis, acute, 485t
Saphenous vein
    great, 492
    small, 492
Sarcoidosis, dyspnea in, 324t–325t
Scabies, 189t
Scale, skin lesion, 190t
Scalene muscles, 299
Scalp, examination techniques for, 215
Scaphoid fracture, 630
Scapula, 615
    winging of, 733–734
Scapulohumeral muscle group, 616
Scapulothoracic articulation, 615
Scars, 190t
Schizoaffective disorder, 169t
Schizoid personality disorder, 145b
Schizophrenia, 155b, 169t
Schizophreniform disorder, 169t
Schizotypal personality disorder, 145b
Sciatica, 602, 668t
    assessment for, 732–733
Sciatic nerve, examination techniques for, 640
Scissors gait, 759t

Sclera, examination techniques for, 224
Scleroderma, 474t
    skin conditions due to, 199t
Sclerosis, tuberous, skin conditions due to, 199t
Scoliosis, 618, 639, 662
    in adolescents, 868–869
    in children, 853
Scotomas, 208
Screening tests, in health history, 9
Scrotal edema, 535t
Scrotal hernia, 530, 535t
Scrotum
    abnormalities of, 535t
    anatomy of, 519–520
    in boys, 847–848
    development of, Tanner stages for, 865, 866b
    examination techniques for, 528–529
    in infants, 807
    lesions of, 523–524
        in infants, 808
    swelling of, 529
Sebaceous glands, 172
Seborrhea, in infants, 879t
Seborrheic keratosis, 194t, 946
Secondary prevention, 347
Secretory diarrhea, 476t–477t
Seizures, 750t–751t
    acute symptomatic, 694
    focal, 750t
    generalized, 751t
        focal that become, 750t
    in health history, 694
    pseudoseizures, 751t
Self-awareness, cultural humility and, 76, 76b
Self-care capacity, in older adults, 961t
Self-reflection, interviewing and, 73
Semilunar valves, 335
Semimembranosus bursa, 652
Seminal vesicles, 519–520, 577
Sensation, loss of, in health history, 693
Sensitivity, of a test, 44b, 46b
Sensorineural hearing loss, 209, 234, 237–238,
    281t, 706
Sensory ataxia, 759t
Sensory cortex, lesions of, 722–723
Sensory (afferent) fibers, 684, 688–689
Sensory pathways, 688–689
    damage to, 689
Sensory system
    assessment of, 719–724
        in children, 854
        dermatomes, 723–724
        discriminative sensations, 722–723
        light touch, 721
        in newborn, 812
        pain, 721
        proprioception, 721–722
        recording findings, 739
        temperature, 721
        testing patterns, 720
        vibration, 721
    in physical examination, 22
Septic arthritis, 603
Serous effusion, 280t
Serratus anterior muscle, 405
Sexual abuse, child, 850, 889t
Sexual dysfunction
    female, 546
    male, 523
Sexual history, taking, 86–87, 87b
    female, 546
    male, 522–524, 522b

Sexually transmitted infections (STI)
  in females, 547, 551–552, 568t
    health promotion and counseling, 524–526, 551–552, 585
    incidence, 524–525, 551
  in males, 523–526, 534t
Sexual maturity, Tanner stages for, 542
  in females, 555, 863–864, 864b, 867–868, 867b
  in males, 865, 866b
Sexual orientation, 522–523, 546
Sexual response
  female, 546
  male, 523
S₁ heart sound, 371, 376, 379b, 395t
  in infants, 802–803
S₂ heart sound, 371, 376, 379b, 396t
  apparent gallop, 803
  in infants, 802–803
  split, 802
S₃ heart sound, 374–375
  in infants, 803
  in older adults, 922, 949
S₄ heart sound, 374–375
  in infants, 803
  in older adults, 922, 949
Shortness of breath, 346–347
Short process of malleus, 233, 236
Short stature, 116, 828
Shoulder girdle, 615
Shoulder(s)
  anatomy of, 615–618
    bony structures, 615–616
    bursae of, 617–618
    joints of, 616
    muscle groups of, 616–617
  examination techniques for, 618–625
    inspection, 618
    maneuvers, 623, 623b–625b
    palpation, 618–620
    range of motion, 620, 620b–622b
  frozen, 673t
  movements of, 620b–622b
  painful, 672t–673t
Sickle cell anemia, skin conditions due to, 199t
Siebens Domain Management Model, for older adults, 966t
Sigmoidoscopy, 450b, 451
Silent patients, interviewing, 77–78
Sinus arrhythmia, 392t
Sinuses
  anatomy of, 239
  examination techniques for
    in children, 837–838
    infants, 794
  in health history, 210
  palpation of, 241
  paranasal, 239
  in physical examination, 20
  in review of systems, 11
  transillumination of, 255–256
Sinusitis, 241
  in children, 838
  headache due to, 260t–261t
Sinus node, 341
Situs inversus, 371
Skene's glands, 539
Skin
  anatomy of, 171–172
  cancer of, 173–177
    basal cell carcinoma, 173–174, 946
    melanoma, 174b, 946

mole inspection and, 175, 175b
  in older adults, 946
  prevention of, 175
  skin self-examination for, 175, 175b
  squamous cell carcinoma, 173–174, 946
  total-body skin examination for, 175
changes in pigmentation, 183t–184t
color of, 115, 171–172, 177, 183t–184t
conditions and joint pain, 604b
diseases related to, 198t–199t
examination techniques for, 177–180
  in adolescents, 862
  infants, 783–787
  in older adults, 946
in health history, 173
health promotion and counseling and, 173–177
in infants, 879t
lesions of
  acne, 192t
  anatomic location and distribution, 185t
  benign and malignant nevi, 195t
  during childhood, 880t
  examination techniques for, 178–179
  examples, 196t–197t
  patterns and shapes, 186t
  primary, 187t–189t
  purpuric, 193t
  secondary, 190t–191t
  self-examination, 175, 175b, 179, 180b
  vascular, 193t
in newborn(s), 783–787
in older adults, 919–920, 946
in physical examination, 20
pressure ulcers, 178–179, 200t
recording findings, 181, 181b
in review of systems, 11
Skin self-examination, for skin cancer, 175, 175b, 179, 180b
Skull, examination techniques for, 215
Skull symmetry, of infants, 789–790
Sleep apnea, in children, 841
Sleep diary, 931
Sleep history, 931
Small for gestational age (SGA), 771b, 772
Small pox, 189t
Smoking
  cardiovascular disease and, 352b, 353b
  cessation of, 302–304, 303b
  effects of, 303b
  health counseling about, 359, 359b
  in older adults, 933
  during pregnancy, 902
  in stroke, 697b
Snellen chart, 221
Social development
  of adolescents, 857, 858b
  of children, 819–820
  of infants, 775, 815
Social history, in health history, 7b, 10
Social phobia, 149, 168t
Sodium, food sources of, 139t
Sodium intake, blood pressure and, 112–113
Soft palate, 239, 244
  assessment of, 707
Soleus muscle, 656
Somatic growth
  of adolescents, 862
  of children, 828–829
  of infants, 780–781
Somatic nervous system, 683
Somatic pain, 129b
Somatization disorder, 165t

Somatoform disorders, 142, 165t
Somatoform symptom, 142
Spastic diplegia, 854
Spastic hemiparesis, 759t
Spasticity, 709, 758t
Specificity, of a test, 44b, 46b
Specula, for pelvic examination
  during pregnancy, 905b, 910
  procedure for, 557–559
  types of, 555
Speech
  disorders of, 754t
  in mental status examination, 148, 153, 154b
Spermatic cord
  abnormalities of, 537t
  anatomy of, 519–520
  palpation of, 528
  torsion of, 537t
  varicocele of, 537t
Spermatocele, 537t
Sphenoid sinus, 239
Spheroidal joints, 600, 600b
Sphygmomanometer, selection of, 120, 121b
Spider angioma, 193t
Spider vein, 193t
Spina bifida, 639
Spina bifida occulta, 809
Spinal accessory nerve, 684, 685b
  of children, 856b
  examination of, 707
  of infant, 813b
Spinal cord
  anatomy of, 683
  lesions of, 744t
  segments of, 683
Spinal cord syndromes, 719
Spinal nerves, 684, 686
Spinal reflexes, 689–690
  cutaneous stimulation reflexes, 690b, 730–731
    abdominal, 730
    anal, 731
    plantar, 730–731
  deep tendon reflexes, 689–690, 690b
    ankle, 728–730
    assessment of, 725–730
    biceps, 726
    brachioradialis, 727
    in children, 854
    knee, 728
    in newborn, 813–814
    supinator, 727
    triceps, 727
Spinal roots, lesions of, 745t
Spinal stenosis, 495
Spine
  anatomy of, 635–637, 636b
  examination techniques for, 637–642
  movements of, 641b–642b
Spinothalamic tract, 688
Spinous process, 295, 636, 636b, 637, 640, 643
Spleen
  anatomic considerations, 434
  examination techniques for, 461–463
    in children, 847
    in infants, 807
    palpation, 462–463
    percussion, 461–462
Splenic percussion sign, 461–462
Splenius capitis muscle, 637
Splenomegaly, 461, 463
  in infants, 807

Vestibular neuronitis, 263t
Vestibule, 238, 539
Vibration sense
  assessment of, 721
  in older adults, 925–926
Violence, family, 89–90, 90b
  during pregnancy, 902–903, 903b
Viral exanthems, skin conditions due to, 199t
Visceral pain, abdominal, 436–437
Visceral pleura, 298
Visceral tenderness, abdominal, 485t
Vision changes, in health history, 212–213
Visual acuity
  examination techniques for, 221–222
    in children, 832–834, 833, 833b
    in infants, 792
  in older adults, 920–921, 947
Visual Analog Scale, for pain, 128
Visual fields, 218
  defects in, 222, 265t, 703
  examination techniques for, 222–223
    in children, 834
  optic nerve and, 703
Visual impairment
  in infants, 791
  interviewing and, 84
  in older adults, 936
Visual pathways, 218–219
Vital signs, 105, 119–127. *See also* Blood
    pressure; Heart rate; Heart rhythms;
    Respiratory rate; Temperature, body
  in adolescents, 862
  blood pressure, 119–125
  in children, 829–832
  documentation, 131
  examination techniques for, infants (first year),
    780–783
  heart rate, 126
  heart rhythm, 126
  in infants, 781–783
  in older adults, 919, 945–946
  pain as fifth, 105, 127–130
  in physical examination, 20
  during pregnancy, 905–906
  respiratory rate, 126
  temperature, 126–127
Vitamin D
  food sources of, 139t
  osteoporosis and, 608
  recommended dietary intake for, 608b
Vitiligo, 183t, 187t
Vitreous body, 217

Vitreous floaters, 232
Voice
  assessment of, 707
    in children, 841, 841b
  hoarseness, 211
Voice sounds, transmitted, 314
  normal, 328t
  in pneumonia, 328t
  in various disorders, 330t–331t
Volume overload, 343, 394t
Voluminous diarrhea, 476t–477t
Vomiting, 440–441
  hematemesis, 441
  during pregnancy, 896b, 905
von Recklinghausen's syndrome, 198t
Vulva, 539
  bulges and swelling of, 570t
  carcinoma of, 568t
  lesions of, 568t
  of older adults, 950
  vulvovaginal symptoms, 545
Vulvar erythema, 950
Vulvovaginal symptoms, 545

W

Waist circumference, 117
Warmth, in joint examination, 611b
Warts
  in children, 880t
  genital, 534t, 568t
  plantar, 679t, 880t
Weakness
  asymmetric, 692
  distal, 692
  in health history, 106, 692
  proximal, 692
  symmetric, 692
Weber test, 237, 281t, 706
Weight
  at birth, 771
  body mass index (BMI) and
    calculation of, 117, 117b, 118t
    in children, 829, 829b
    classification by, 110, 110b
    obesity and, 110, 110b
  of children, 829
  counseling about, 359, 359b
  in general survey, 116–117
  in health history, 107–108
  health promotion and counseling and,
    108–113, 109b

of infants, 781
of older adults, 946
physical activity and, 605, 605b
steps to maintain optimal, 109b, 110
Weight gain
  drugs associated with, 107
  in health history, 107
  during pregnancy, 901, 901b
Weight loss
  causes of, 107, 117
  counseling about, 359, 359b
  in health history, 17–18
  in older adults, 946
  during pregnancy, 896b, 905
  recommendations for, 111–112, 112b
Wernicke's aphasia, 754t
Wet exudative macular degeneration, 232
Wharton's ducts, 244
Wheal, 188t, 197t
Wheezes, 301, 314, 329t
Wheezing, in infants, 799
Whiplash, 669t
Whispered pectoriloquy, 315
Whisper voice test, 236, 237b
White coat hypertension, 119, 125
Whiteley Index, 145b
White matter
  of brain, 682
  of spinal cord, 686
Winging of scapula, 733–734
Women, cardiovascular disease screening
    for, 350–351, 351b
Wong-Baker Faces Pain Scale, for pain,
    128
Working diagnosis, 29–30
Work of breathing, in infants, 797
Wrist
  anatomy of, 628–629
  examination techniques, 629–634
  extension at, testing, 711
  movements of, 632

X

Xanthelasma, 267t
Xiphoid process, 293, 433–434

Z

Zoster vaccine, 936, 937b
Zygomatic arch, 613
Zygomatic bone, 214